MW01257670

Non-Neoplastic Kidney Diseases

ATLAS OF NONTUMOR PATHOLOGY

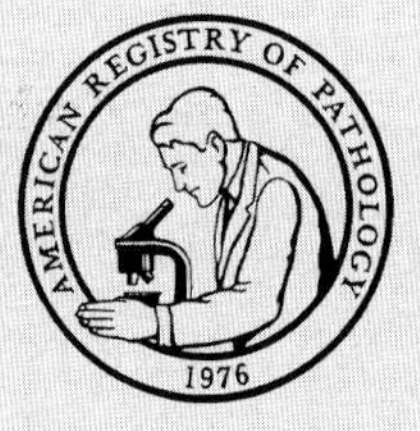

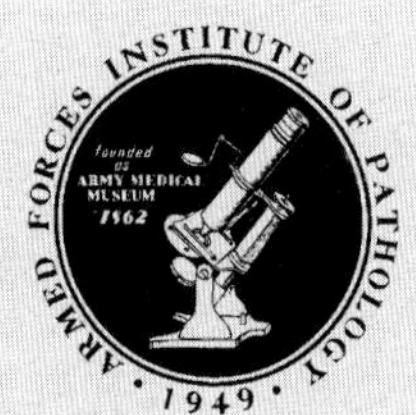

ARP PRESS

Silver Spring, Maryland

Editorial Director: Kelley A. Squazzo
Production Editor: Dian S. Thomas
Editorial/Scanning Assistant: Mirlinda Q. Caton
Copyeditor: Audrey Kahn
Scanning Technician: Kenneth Stringfellow

ATLAS OF NONTUMOR PATHOLOGY

First Series
Fascicle 4

Non-Neoplastic Kidney Diseases

Vivette D. D'Agati, MD

J. Charles Jennette, MD

Fred G. Silva, MD

Published by the
American Registry of Pathology
Washington, DC
in collaboration with the
Armed Forces Institute of Pathology
Washington, DC

2005

ATLAS OF NONTUMOR PATHOLOGY

Manuscript Reviewed by:
Jay Bernstein, MD
Mark Haas, MD, PhD
Michael Kashgarian, MD

Available from the American Registry of Pathology
Armed Forces Institute of Pathology
Washington, DC 20306-6000
www.afip.org
ISBN: 1-881041-96-4

INTRODUCTION TO SERIES

This is the fourth Fascicle of the Atlas of Nontumor Pathology, a complementary series to the Armed Forces Institute of Pathology (AFIP) Atlas of Tumor Pathology, first published in 1949.

For several years, various individuals in the pathology community have suggested the formation of a new series of monographs concentrating on this particular area. In 1998, an Editorial Board was appointed and outstanding authors chosen shortly thereafter.

The purpose of the atlas is to provide surgical pathologists with ready expert reference material most helpful in their daily practice. The lesions described relate principally to medical non-neoplastic conditions. Many of these lesions represent complex entities and, when appropriate, we have included contributions from internists, radiologists, and surgeons. This has led to some increase in the size of the monographs but the emphasis remains on diagnosis by the surgical pathologist.

Previously, the Fascicles have been available on CD-ROM format as well as in print. In order to provide the widest possible advantages of both modalities, we have formatted the print Fascicle on the World Wide Web. Use of the Internet allows cross-indexing within the Fascicles as well as linkage to PubMed.

Our goal is to continue to provide expert information at the lowest possible cost. Therefore, marked reductions in pricing are available to residents and fellows as well as to pathology faculty and other staff members purchasing the Fascicles on a subscription basis.

We believe that the Atlas of Nontumor Pathology will serve as an outstanding reference for surgical pathologists as well as an important contribution to the literature of other medical specialties.

Donald West King, MD
Leslie H. Sobin, MD
J. Thomas Stocker, MD
Bernard Wagner, MD

PREFACE

Since its introduction in the late 1950s, percutaneous renal biopsy has become the gold standard for the diagnosis of medical diseases of the kidney. The advent of percutaneous needle biopsy and its increasing use over the last half century forged the transition from autopsy-based studies of the kidney to modern biopsy-based pathologic interpretation. The diagnosis of medical diseases of the kidney is one of the few areas in pathology where the standard work-up requires the systematic integration of light microscopy, immunofluorescence microscopy, and transmission electron microscopy, which in turn must be correlated with presenting clinical, serologic, and radiographic findings. This reliance on multiple diagnostic modalities makes our specialty uniquely challenging and rewarding.

Many of the renal conditions we recognize today as distinct disease entities were identified through the close collaboration between renal pathologists and nephrologists in order to define the cardinal pathologic features, presentation, optimal therapy, and outcome. Over the last 50 years, the art of renal biopsy interpretation has been refined through the routine application of multiple, thin (2 to 3 micron), serial paraffin sections stained with a battery of histologic stains (including hematoxylin and eosin, periodic acid–Schiff, Masson trichrome, and Jones methenamine silver), cryostat serial sections stained by direct immunofluorescence for detection of immune reactants (including IgG, IgM, IgA, kappa and lambda light chains, C3, C1q, and fibrin), semithin plastic sections, and transmission electron microscopy—all of which have become standard technologies in the renal pathologist's armamentarium. This multidisciplinary approach to renal biopsy interpretation, as well as the use of repeat biopsy in selected cases to gauge the efficacy of treatment, has helped to elucidate pathogenetic mechanisms and define the natural history of disease. It is not surprising that approximately half of the chapters in any of the major textbooks of nephrology have headings that incorporate pathology-based terms and diseases—a testament to the central role that renal pathology has played in the evolution of the specialty.

This one-volume Atlas of Renal Pathology covers the major diagnostic disease categories in twenty-six chapters. Although specialized, renal pathology need not be difficult if the subject is approached in a systematic fashion. To this end, we have organized the chapters around standardized disease entities or patterns of disease, including congenital and hereditary diseases, acquired diseases of the native kidney (primarily affecting glomerular, tubulointerstitial, and vascular compartments), and diseases of the renal allograft. The terminology we have used is that preferred by most practicing North American pathologists. Wherever possible, we have tried to remain consistent with the widely recognized International Nomenclature of Disease, a joint project of the Council for International Organizations of Medical Sciences and the World Health Organization. Although the Atlas provides comprehensive coverage of the major common disease entities and their variants, it also includes many rare, but no less important, conditions. The extensive collection of images is the focal point, balanced by an informative, pithy text and the selective use of illustrative tables. If a "picture is worth a thousand words," this volume is actually 5000 pages long with over 1.5 million "words" (in virtual terms, seven times its present size)!

We are happy for this opportunity to leave to posterity the best of our renal pathology slide collections, which we have worked so hard to amass over the years. It is gratifying to know that they will be put to good use in the training of succeeding generations of young pathologists. Most of the images and case studies were collected from the following institutions: 1) the Renal Pathology Laboratory, Department of Pathology, Columbia University, College of Physicians & Surgeons in New York City, founded in 1973 by Dr. Conrad L. Pirani, and under the direction of Dr. Vivette D'Agati since 1985; 2) the Renal Pathology Laboratory at the University of North Carolina under the direction of Dr. J. Charles Jennette; 3) the Renal Pathology Laboratory at the University of Oklahoma, initially under the direction of Dr. Fred G. Silva, now under the able direction of Dr. Zoltan Laszik; and 4) the Southwest Pediatric Nephrology Study Group under the direction of Dr. Ron Hogg, Dallas. We are also grateful for the many outstanding images contributed by our friends and colleagues in the renal community throughout the world.

This anthology of renal disease would not have been possible without the contributions of the many patients afflicted with kidney disease and the many dedicated physicians who care for them. We are also indebted to the members of the Renal Pathology Society for their support, collegiality, and stimulating discussions over the past 20 years.

Finally, we remember with respect and affection the seminal influence of Dr. Conrad L. Pirani, one of the founding fathers of our discipline, who died on May 28, 2005 at the age of 90. With deepest gratitude, we dedicate this Atlas in his memory.

Vivette D. D'Agati, MD
Renal Pathology Laboratory
Columbia University, College of Physicians & Surgeons

J. Charles Jennette, MD
Department of Pathology and Laboratory Medicine
University of North Carolina

Fred G. Silva, MD
Department of Pathology
Emory University and The Medical College of Georgia

ACKNOWLEDGMENTS

I acknowledge above all my husband, Edward G. Imperatore. Without his steadfast support and encouragement, my career in academic medicine would not have been possible. I thank my children, Edward A. and Paul V., who have given me so much love and were never jealous of the weekends taken from them. I thank my mentor, Dr. Conrad L. Pirani, who inspired me and provided the scholarly foundation on which to build my own experience. Thanks to my former Chairman, Dr. Donald West King, for supporting my early career at Columbia, and my current Chairman, Dr. Michael Shelanski, for fostering the rich intellectual environment in which my laboratory has flourished. I thank my associate, Dr. Glen Markowitz, for his friendship and generous support throughout this project. I thank my dear colleagues and co-authors, Dr. Fred G. Silva and Dr. J. Charles Jennette, for sharing so freely the wisdom of their vast experience in the years before and during this endeavor. I cannot forget to acknowledge the many patients whose biopsies illuminate the pages of this book and the dedicated technical staff of the Columbia Renal Pathology Laboratory that labored over them. Finally, I acknowledge my parents, Vivette P. and Dr. Vincent C. D'Agati, for teaching me by example that many of life's most rewarding activities combine love of learning and hard work.

Vivette D. D'Agati, MD

I acknowledge the continuous support of my loving wife, Yvonne, throughout my career. She may not know much renal pathology but she knows a lot of renal pathologists. I acknowledge the seminal role on my career of Dr. Fred Dalldorf who was responsible for initiating my interest in renal pathology. I have learned a great deal while teaching others and thus I thank all the renal pathology fellows who have come to Chapel Hill over the past three decades, especially my first fellow and good friend, Dr. Samy Iskandar. I thank my longstanding nephrologist colleague, Dr. Ronald Falk, who has prodded me to integrate clinical relevance into my approach to renal pathology. I thank the other renal pathologists who now are at UNC and have afforded me the time to work on this text, Drs. Sharan Singh, David Thomas, and Volker Nickeleit. I thank my wonderful daughters, Jennifer and Caroline, and my granddaughters, Olivia and Augusta, for their understanding and tolerance of my long hours devoted to my fascination with renal pathology.

J. Charles Jennette, MD

I would like to acknowledge the unending support of my wife, Jean Dixon Silva, for this and all my academic ventures over the last three decades. I thank all the outstanding teachers/mentors that I have had throughout the years and the University of Oklahoma which supported me in the early years. In addition, many thanks to the following individuals who have provided encouragement, wisdom, and mentorship over the years: Dr. Conrad L. Pirani, Master Renal Pathologist and my Academic Mentor in Renal Pathology; Dr. Donald West King, my former Chair of the Department of Pathology, Columbia University College of Physicians & Surgeons and my other Academic Father; and Drs. Vernie Stembridge and John Childers, my Texas Rangers, Mentors, Advisors, and Friends at the University of Texas/Southwestern Medical School/Dallas. Finally to my mother and father, Valerie and Fred Silva, who taught me so much, and my daughter, Lindsay Kathleen Silva, who has brought so much joy to my life.

Fred G. Silva, MD

Permission to use copyrighted illustrations has been granted by:

American Society of Nephrology

J Am Soc Nephrol 1997;8:1930–4. For table 26-4.

J Am Soc Nephrol 2004;15:501–3. For table 13-3.

Elsevier Science, Inc.

Am J Kidney Dis 1994;24:130–41. For table 15-3.

Atlas of Renal Pathology 1999:136–57. For table 21-1.

Med Clin North Am 1997;81:653–77. For figures 8-1 and 8-3.

Robbins Pathologic Basis of Disease (the Kidney), 6th ed., 1999. For table 23-1.

Uropathology 1989. For table 24-1.

John Wiley & Sons

Arthritis Rheum 1994;37:187–92. For table 15-2.

Lippincott Williams and Wilkins

Atlas of Genitourinary Tract Disorders, 1988. For figure 2-35.

Heptinstall's Pathology of the Kidney, 5th ed., 1998. For table 14-4.

Medicine 1985;64:219–27. For table 14-1.

Renal Disease: Classification and Atlas, Parts I and II, 1987. For figures 2-2, 2-12, 2-15, 15-54, 16-44, 16-45, 16-46, and 16-47.

Massachusetts Medical Society

New Engl J Med 1997;337:1512–23. For table 15-5.

Oxford University Press

Nephrol Dial Transplant 1998;13(Suppl. 1):16–20. For figure 15-38.

Publishers of the Netter Collection

CIBA Collection of Medical Illustrations, 1973. For figures 1-1, 1-5, 1-6 and 1-7.

UroCor, Inc.

Metabolic Management System, Oklahoma, 2001. For figures 23-4, 23-7, 23-10, 23-11, 23-13, and 23-14.

CONTENTS

1 NORMAL RENAL ANATOMY, HISTOLOGY, AND DEVELOPMENT

EMBRYOLOGY OF THE KIDNEY

The kidneys develop from bilateral masses of intermediate mesoderm called the nephrogenic cords, which are located between the dorsal somites and the mesoderm of the lateral plate, behind the embryonic coelom (1,2). In each elongated nephrogenic cord, three successive excretory systems are formed during the third to fourth weeks of gestation (fig. 1-1): first, the transient pronephros, the most cranial; second, the mesonephros, the middle segment; and third, the metanephros, the caudal segment and the direct precursor of the adult kidney.

The metanephros has two parts: the metanephric mesenchyme (metanephric blastema) and the ureteric bud epithelium. The ureteric bud arises from the caudal end of the mesonephric duct where it curves medially to join the cloaca. The proximal end of the ureteric bud proceeds cranially and dorsally toward the metanephric blastema, while its distal end extends caudally as the embryo grows and elongates. The cranial tip of the ureteric bud swells slightly, creating an ampulla (figs. 1-2, 1-3A). As the ampulla contacts the metanephric blastema, the ampulla undergoes rapid branching. There is mutual induction of differentiation by the metanephric blastema and the ureteric bud. The branches of the ureteric bud ultimately cause nephron development by inducing the metanephric blastemal mesenchyme to form glomeruli and tubules. The ureteric bud gives rise to the collecting ducts, calyces, renal pelvis, and ureter, and the metanephric blastema gives rise to the remainder of the kidney.

The ampullary tips induce condensations of metanephric blastema to become nephrons composed of glomeruli, proximal tubules, loops of Henle, distal tubules, interstitium, and vessels. Some of the blastemal cells in each condensation form a hollow nephrogenic vesicle. Other blastemal nests form separate solid caps for the next divisions of the ampulla. Each of

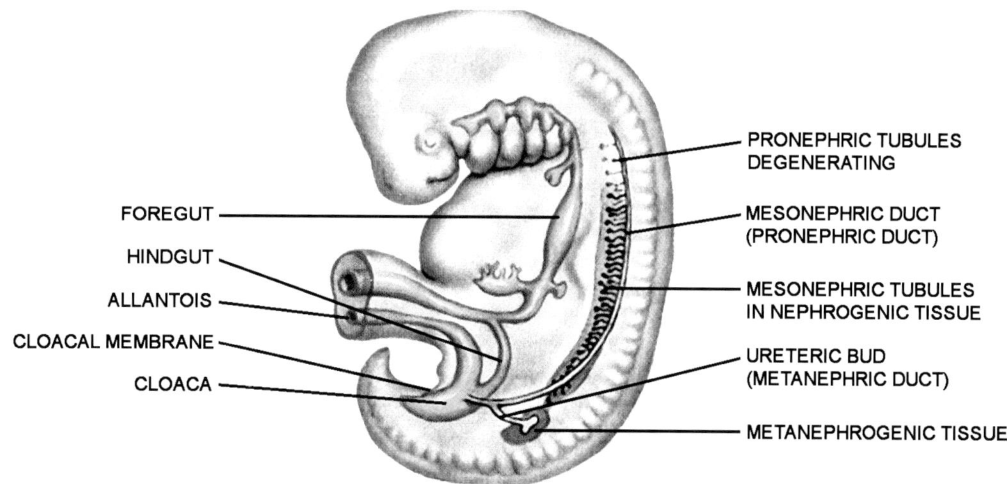

Figure 1-1

DIAGRAM OF PRONEPHROS, MESONEPHROS, AND METANEPHROGENIC TISSUE

The ureteric bud arises from the mesonephric duct and branches into the metanephrogenic tissue (metanephric blastema). (Plate 28 from Netter HN. Kidneys, ureters, and urinary bladder. The CIBA collection of medical illustrations, Vol. 6. Summit, NJ: CIBA Pharmaceutical Co; 1973:30.)

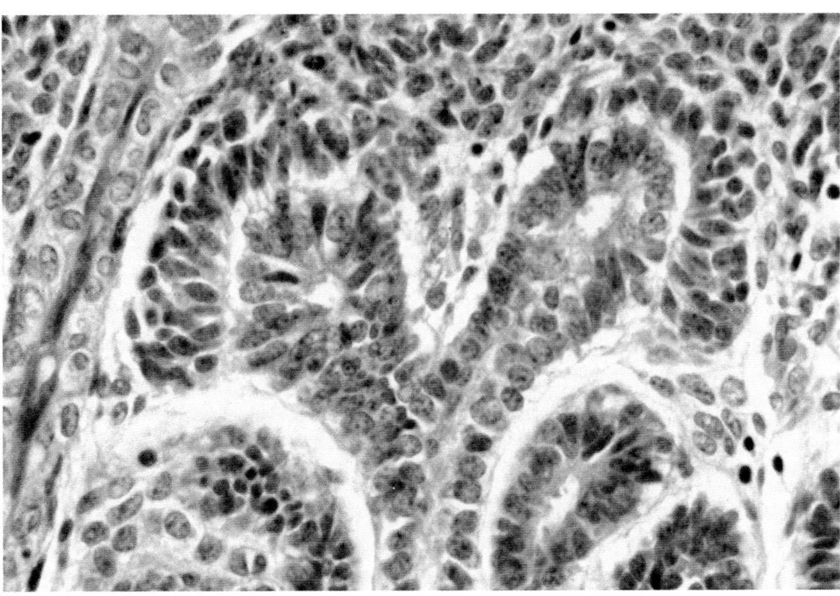

Figure 1-2

URETERIC BUD AMPULLA AND METANEPHRIC BLASTEMA

Two ampullae have formed at the terminus of a branch of a ureteric bud in the outer renal cortex of this 19-week fetus. The overlying metanephric blastema is being induced to condense into the anlage of a nephron (hematoxylin and eosin [H&E] stain).

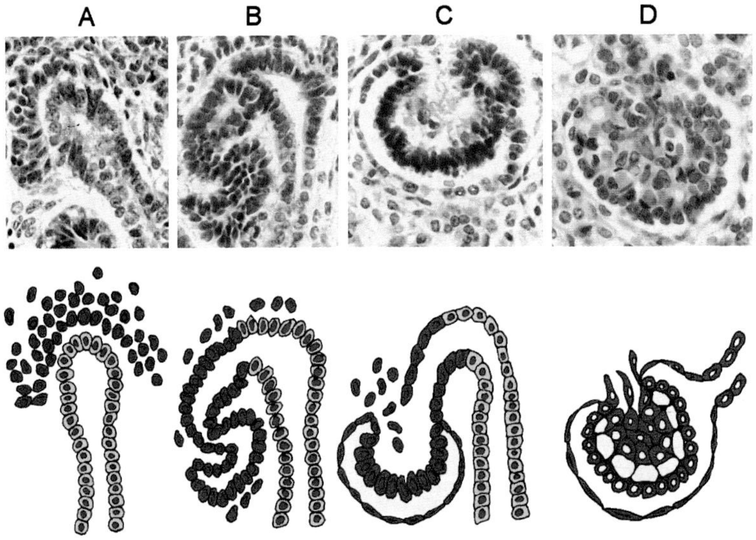

A B C D

Figure 1-3

STAGES OF NEPHROGENESIS

The stages of nephrogenesis in the photomicrographs above are depicted in the diagrams below. Cells in green are derived from the ureteric bud and those in red from the metanephric blastema. A ureteric bud ampulla induces metanephric blastema to condense (A) and then form a nephrogenic vesicle that elongates into an S-shaped structure (B). A communication forms between the upper end of the vesicle and the ureteric ampulla. An invagination forms in the lower end of the vesicle (C). Capillaries grow into this invagination to become the glomerular capillary tuft (D). The cells in the near wall of the invagination remain columnar and become the epithelial cells that overlie glomerular capillaries (podocytes), while the cells in the far wall flatten and become the epithelial cells that line Bowman's capsule (C,D).

the hollow nephrogenic vesicles elongates and folds back on itself to generate an S-shaped structure (fig. 1-3). The proximal portion of the upper limb of the S-shaped body becomes continuous, joining with the ampullary lumen of the adjacent ureteric bud (fig. 1-3B). The upper and middle portions of the nephrogenic vesicle elongate and differentiate to form the proximal and distal convoluted tubules, and the loop of Henle. The lower portion of the nephrogenic vesicle develops an invagination that receives the developing capillaries that become the glomerular tuft (fig. 1-3C). The layer of cells on the opposite wall of the vesicle flattens and forms the parietal layer of Bowman's capsule. The layer of cells in contact with the ingrowing capillaries remains columnar (fig. 1-3C) and is stretched over the developing glomerular tuft capillaries to form the glomerular visceral epithelium (podocytes) (fig. 1-3D).

The next step in nephrogenesis is the formation of the nephron arcades. Each ampulla is capable of inducing the formation of further nephrons. With the induction of additional nephrons, the attachment of the tubule of the older nephron shifts away from the ampulla as it progresses on toward the capsule, inducing the formation of more nephrons along the way. Thus, the nephrons that are induced by the same ampulla are joined together in an arcade of 4 to 7 nephrons aligned along a collecting duct. During the course of the next 14 weeks, although no further ampullary ureteric bud divisions occur, the already-formed ampullae advance to the peripheral renal cortex. From 36 weeks to term, no further nephrons are produced although they continue to mature. The nephrons in the outer cortex are the last to mature because this is the zone that is reached last by the ureteric bud ampullae. During the final weeks of gestation, the loops of Henle continue to increase in length. The proximal and distal tubules become longer and more tortuous.

The development of the differentiated nephrons proceeds from the corticomedullary junction to the cortical surface. Therefore, the subcapsular cortical zone of the developing kidney contains the most immature glomeruli (fig. 1-4). These subcapsular immature glomeruli often persist into infancy.

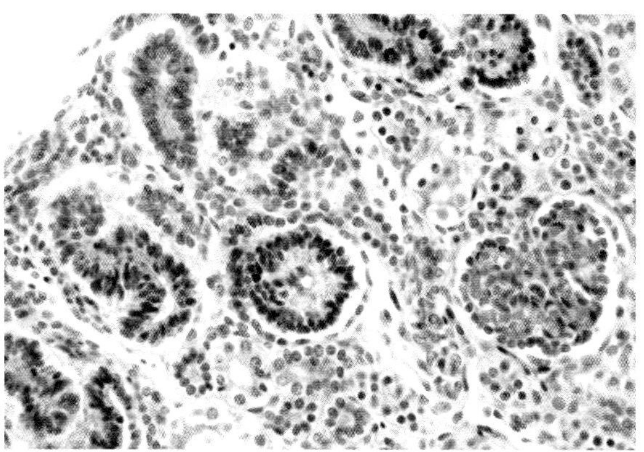

Figure 1-4

FETAL KIDNEY

The capsular surface of this kidney from a 19-week fetus is to the left and the deeper cortex to the right. The subcapsular zone contains developing nephrons, including an S-shaped nephrogenic vesicle. To the far right is a relatively mature glomerulus. This figure illustrates the gradient of maturation that occurs during renal development (H&E stain).

GROSS ANATOMY OF THE KIDNEY

The kidneys are paired, bean-shaped organs in the retroperitoneum, anterior to the transversalis fascia (3,5,6). They extend from approximately the 12th thoracic to the 3rd lumbar vertebrae, with the left kidney slightly more craniad than the right. The positions vary slightly with changes in posture and with respiration. Normally, the left kidney is nearer the midline than the right. The renal hilum does not face exactly midline, but is oriented slightly anteriorly.

A thin fibrous capsule envelops the kidneys and provides a smooth covering. The renal capsule is easily stripped off, although numerous fine processes of connective tissue and a few small blood vessels are disrupted during this procedure. An adherent capsule suggests parenchymal disease that has caused fibrosis between the capsule and the kidney. The renal capsule attaches to the renal hilum at the renal pelvis. After the capsule is stripped, the normal renal surface is smooth, glistening, and deep red-brown. A pale or granular surface indicates disease. In infants, grooves that are the remnants of the lobular configuration of the fetal kidney often are present on the renal surface. Minor vestiges of fetal lobulation may persist in adult kidneys.

The kidneys each weigh approximately 120 to 180 g in the normal adult man, and are approximately 11 x 6 x 3 cm. The left kidney is slightly larger than the right. In women, the kidneys are a little smaller. The total renal mass of the kidney correlates with body surface area and weight.

The medial surface of the kidney (renal hilum) has a concavity with an elongated opening, called the renal sinus; this contains adipose tissue, connective tissue, nerves, blood and lymphatic vessels, and the renal pelvis and calyces (fig. 1-5) (3,6). The calyces are funnel-like and collect the urine from the medullary papillae and transmit it to the renal pelvis. The muscular renal pelvis also is funnel-like and empties into the ureter.

Renal Parenchyma

The sectioned, normal renal parenchyma has a dark red-brown outer cortex, and a lighter-colored inner medulla that forms conical structures

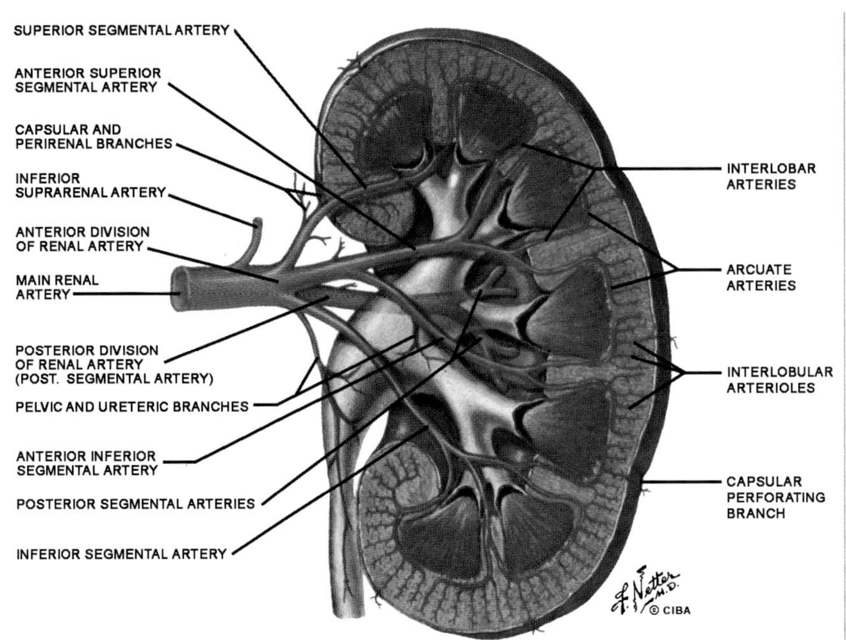

Figure 1-5

KIDNEY ANATOMY

This drawing depicts a kidney cut open to reveal the distribution of the renal arteries and the configuration of the urinary collecting system within the renal sinus. The papillary tips of the medullary pyramids are projecting into the calyces, which attach to the renal pelvis. Note the distribution of the interlobar, arcuate, and interlobular arteries. (Plate 14 from Netter HN. Kidneys, ureters, and urinary bladder. The CIBA collection of medical illustrations, Vol. 6. Summit, NJ: CIBA Pharmaceutical Co; 1973:6.)

called pyramids. The papillae are the pyramidal tips that protrude into the calyces (fig. 1-5). Normally, each kidney contains approximately 7 to 15 papillae. Six or fewer papillae indicate hypoplasia. Adjacent pyramids may be fused to form compound papillae, especially at the upper and lower poles of the kidneys.

For gross pathologic examination of an entire kidney, it is very important to cut the kidney so that all renal papillae can be inspected. This can be accomplished by cutting slightly into the convex outer surface of the kidney with a large blade, stopping when the renal collecting system is entered. Then, instead of continuing the bisection with the same large blade, it is better to continue opening or bisecting the kidney using scissors, cutting along the renal pelvic collecting system and opening the renal pelvis in this way. With this technique, one is ensured of seeing all renal papillae and having an unobstructed view of the renal pelvis and major calyces.

The renal parenchyma is composed of lobes. Each lobe is centered on a medullary pyramid, which is partially enveloped by a cap of renal cortex and by extensions of cortex, the columns of Bertin, that surround the outer medulla. The renal cortex is approximately 1-cm thick.

A smaller functional unit of the kidney is the lobule. The most widely used definition of lobule is the cortical parenchyma between two interlobular arteries with a central medullary ray. The term also has been used for the renal cortex between two medullary rays containing nephrons that receive blood from one central interlobular artery.

Renal Blood Vessels and Lymphatics

There is a very large blood flow to the kidney, amounting to approximately one fourth to one fifth of the cardiac output. It is one of the most vascular organs, gram for gram, in the human body. The main renal artery arises from the aorta and divides into the anterior and posterior segmental branches at the renal hilus (fig. 1-5). The segmental arteries divide into the interlobar arteries, which course between the renal lobes in the renal sinus. The interlobar arteries penetrate the renal parenchyma at the corticomedullary junction, where they become the arcuate arteries that arch over the convex outer surface of the medulla at the junction with the cortex. The arcuate arteries give rise to the interlobular arteries, which ascend into the renal cortex. Afferent arterioles branch off the interlobular arteries and terminate in the glomerular tuft capillaries. These arteries and arterioles are end vessels, which means that if they are occluded, the tissues they supply

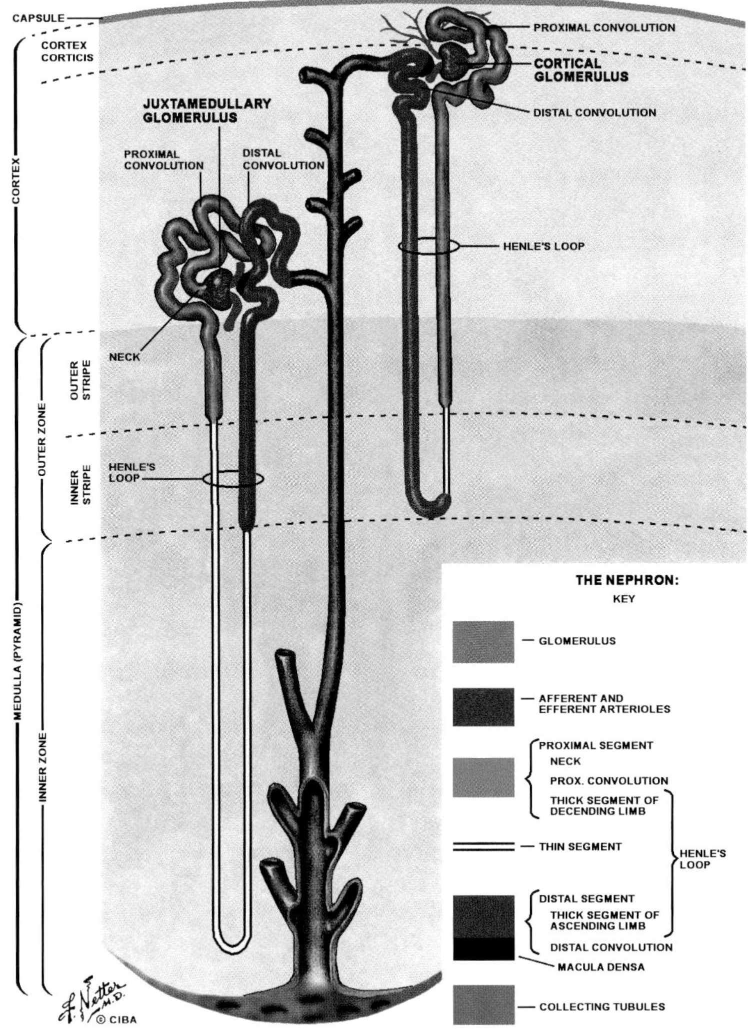

Figure 1-6

NEPHRONS

The tubule of the outer cortical glomerulus has a short loop that turns back at the border between the inner and outer medulla, whereas the juxtamedullary glomerulus has a long loop that extends far into the inner medulla. The outer stripe of the outer medulla contains no thin limbs, the inner stripe has thin and thick limbs, and the inner medulla has only thin limbs of the loop of Henle. These differences in the distribution of thick and thin limbs are the most useful marker for identifying these zones microscopically. (Plate 5 from Netter HN. Kidneys, ureters, and urinary bladder. The CIBA collection of medical illustrations, Vol. 6. Summit, NJ: CIBA Pharmaceutical Co; 1973:6.)

downstream become ischemic, possibly resulting in injury or necrosis.

Blood leaves the glomerular capillaries through the efferent arterioles, which then branch to form the extensive peritubular capillary network of the renal cortex. The efferent arterioles leading from the juxtamedullary glomeruli descend into the outer renal medulla where they give rise to the rich vascular bundles containing the vasa recta that supply blood to the medullary regions. Blood from these capillaries drains into the interlobular/arcuate/interlobar veins, which run parallel with the arteries and merge to leave the kidney as the renal vein.

Networks of lymphatic vessels accompany the arteries in the cortex and the vasa recta in the medulla (4). They merge into multiple larger lymphatic channels that exit the kidney at the hilum and connect to periaortic lymph nodes.

HISTOLOGY OF THE KIDNEY

The functional unit of the kidney, the nephron, consists of a glomerulus and the associated tubules (fig. 1-6) (11,23,25,29). Each human kidney contains between 0.7 and 1.2 million nephrons. Only the renal cortex contains glomeruli. The renal tubule consists of the three major divisions: the proximal tubule, the loop of Henle, and the distal tubule. The distal tubule continues into a collecting duct (also called a collecting tubule). As discussed earlier, the collecting ducts are derived embryologically from the ureteric

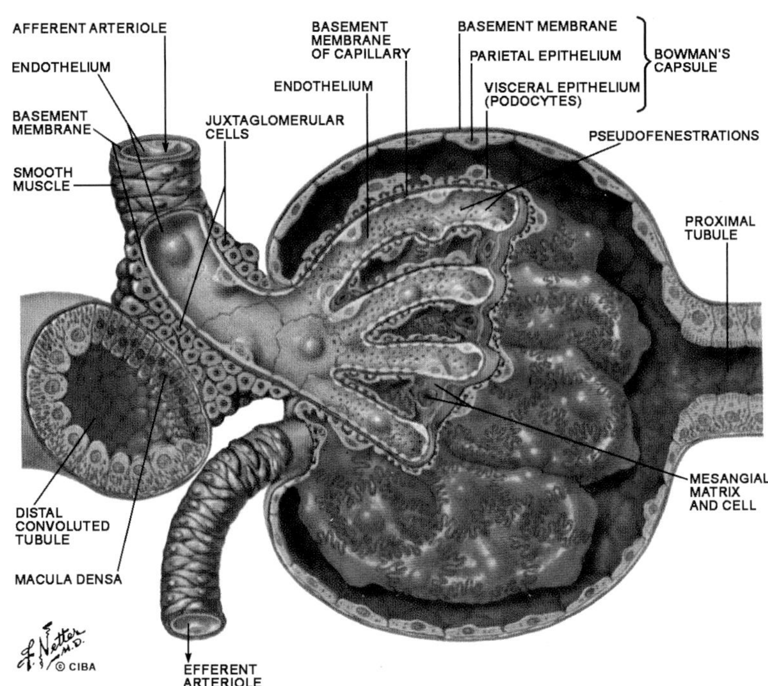

Figure 1-7

GLOMERULUS

This three-dimensional drawing has a cut away showing the lumen of the afferent arteriole and several capillary branches. Note the endothelial fenestrations. In the three-dimensional surface of the podocytes, the foot processes of adjacent podocytes interdigitate. (Plate 6 from Netter HN. Kidneys, ureters, and urinary bladder. The CIBA collection of medical illustrations, Vol. 6. Summit, NJ: CIBA Pharmaceutical Co; 1973:7.)

bud, whereas the remainder of the upstream nephron is derived from the metanephric blastema. The loop of Henle is defined as including the proximal straight portion of the proximal tubule (also called the pars recta of the proximal tubule), the thin limb of Henle, and the thick ascending limb of the distal tubule (pars recta of the distal tubule).

The nephrons originating from outer and middle cortical glomeruli have short loops of Henle. These short loops turn back in the inner stripe of the outer medulla (fig. 1-6). The juxtamedullary nephrons arise from the glomeruli located near the corticomedullary junction and have long loops of Henle, which course deep into the inner medulla before turning back. The complex microscopic architecture of the nephron reflects its complicated and diverse functions.

Glomeruli

A glomerulus is an intricate structure composed of capillaries, mesangial cells, endothelial cells, visceral epithelial cells (podocytes), parietal epithelial cells, and various components of basement membrane and matrix (fig. 1-7). The parietal epithelial cells and their basement membrane form Bowman's capsule, which is continuous with the visceral epithelium at the hilum of the glomerulus and with the proximal tubular epithelium at the origin of the proximal tubule. Bowman's space contains the ultrafiltrate of plasma that will be processed further by the nephron to become urine. At the glomerular hilum, the afferent arterioles enter and branch into the glomerular capillaries. The capillaries eventually coalesce into the efferent arterioles, which exit at the hilum. The lumens of the glomerular capillaries are lined by specialized fenestrated endothelium which sits partly on the capillary wall glomerular basement membrane and partly on the capillary face of the mesangium (figs. 1-8, 1-9).

The mesangium, which is composed of mesangial cells (specialized smooth muscle cells) and surrounding collagenous matrix, forms the structural core of the glomerulus and is continuous at the hilum with the extraglomerular cells of the juxtaglomerular apparatus and the muscularis of the hilar arterioles (8,9,15,20). The capillary face of the mesangium is covered by the capillary endothelium and the sides of the mesangium are covered by the paramesangial basement membrane (figs. 1-9, 1-10). Thus, the glomerular basement membrane does not completely surround glomerular capillary lumens

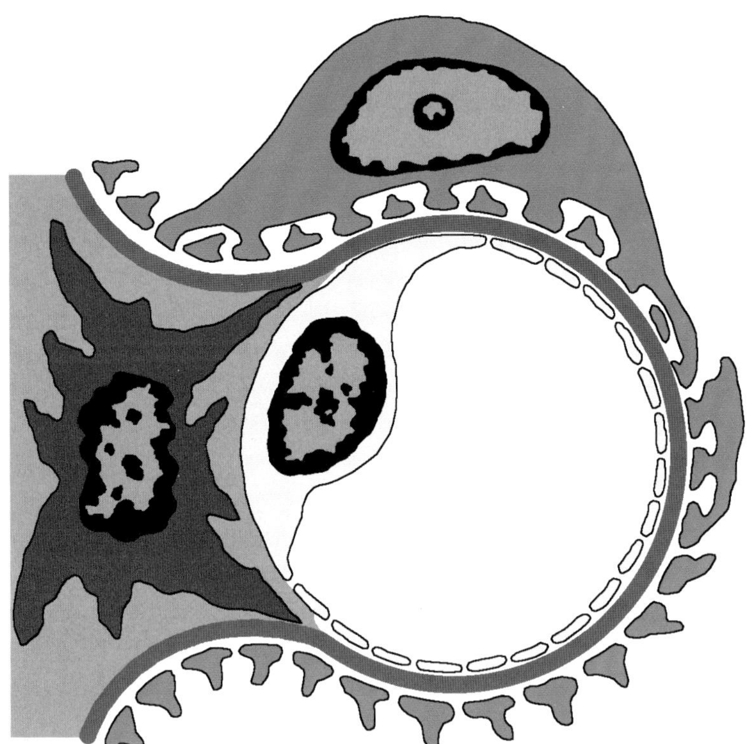

Figure 1-8

GLOMERULAR CAPILLARY

Diagram depicting a fenestrated endothelial cell (yellow) with its nucleus located over the mesangium. The glomerular basement membrane surrounds the outer capillary wall but then splays out over the mesangium as the paramesangial basement membrane.

Figure 1-9

GLOMERULAR CAPILLARY

This transmission electron micrograph shows the same structures diagramed in figure 1-8. Beginning in the midline on the right and moving to the left, there is the urinary space, podocyte with foot processes, glomerular basement membrane, fenestrated peripheral endothelial cytoplasm, capillary lumen, endothelial cell body with nucleus over the face of the mesangium, and (at the far left) the mesangial cell with paramesangial basement membrane above and below.

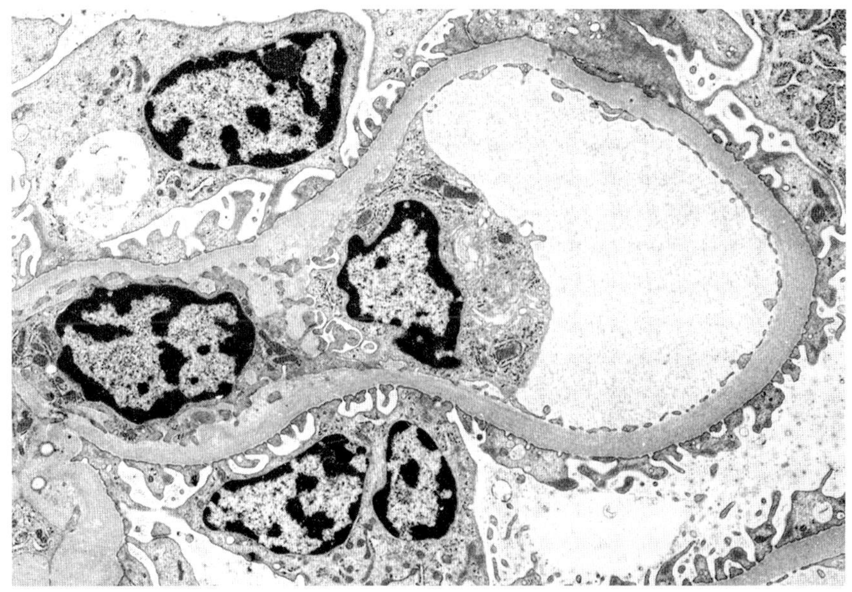

but rather splays out over the mesangium to form the paramesangial basement membrane. This provides a direct route of access between the circulation and the mesangium, and vice versa. In fact, small projections of mesangial cytoplasm may extend between endothelial cells to come in direct contact with the capillary lumens (30). Fluid and macromolecules can traffic from the capillary lumens through the mesangium to the hilum (20). Cell membrane dense bodies (attachment plaques), which are a feature of smooth muscle cells in general, are useful ultrastructural markers of mesangial cells in diagnostic material (fig. 1-10). These dense

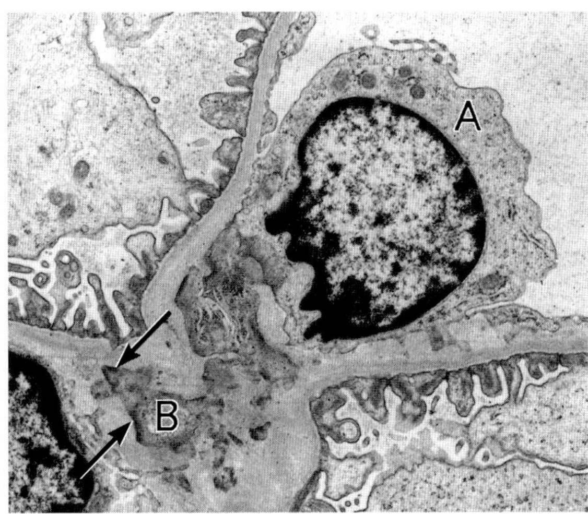

Figure 1-10

MESANGIUM

This transmission electron micrograph shows an endothelial cell body (A) overlying the luminal side of the mesangium. The dense bodies of the cell membrane (arrows) help identify islands of mesangial cytoplasm (B) that are surrounded by matrix. Intact foot processes are external to the paramesangial and the capillary wall basement membranes.

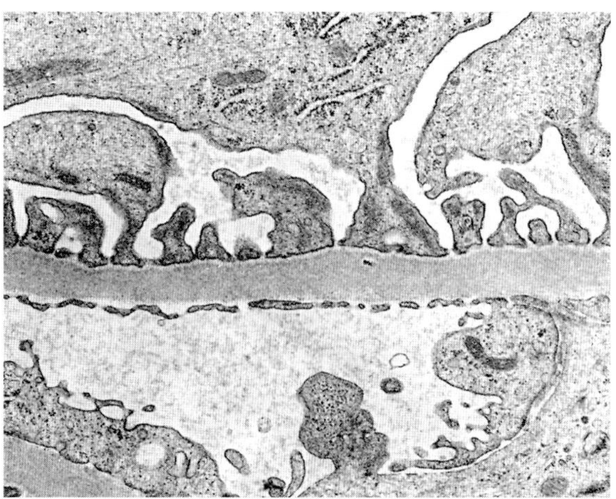

Figure 1-11

GLOMERULAR CAPILLARY WALL

At the top of this transmission electron micrograph is a podocyte cell body and foot processes with intervening urinary space. The soles of the foot processes rest on the thin lamina rara externa, which is less electron dense than the much thicker lamina densa just below. A more irregular lamina lucida interna lies between the bottom of the lamina densa and the fenestrated endothelium.

bodies are the sites of attachment of mesangial cytoskeletal elements to the inside of the cell membrane, and of matrix or glomerular basement membrane molecules to the outside of the cell membrane (cell surface). This allows mesangial contraction to influence glomerular function. Mesangial cells send out processes that attach to the matrix and to the glomerular basement membrane, especially at the juncture of the basement membrane of the capillary wall and paramesangium (16,26). These processes allow the mesangial cell to control capillary diameter.

Glomerular capillary endothelial cells are usually oriented with the nucleus overlying the mesangium (figs. 1-9, 1-10). A thin layer of endothelial cytoplasm, which has numerous fenestrations approximately 75 to 100 nm in diameter, covers most of the surface of the capillary lumen. In the capillary walls away from the mesangium, the endothelium sits on the inner aspect of the glomerular basement membrane (fig. 1-9).

The major constituent of the glomerular basement membrane is type IV collagen (7); other important components are entactin, fibronectin, laminin, and sulfated proteoglycans (21). The glomerular basement membrane is 250- to 350-nm thick in adults, increased from approximately 150 nm at birth. Electron microscopy demonstrates three layers: the lamina lucida (lamina rara) interna, the lamina densa, and the lamina lucida (lamina rara) externa (fig. 1-11). Both the endothelial cells and podocytes contribute to the synthesis of the glomerular basement membrane.

The visceral epithelial cells or podocytes are highly specialized cells that cover the external surface of the glomerular basement membrane and thus line the glomerular surface of Bowman's space (the urinary space of the glomerulus) (22). The opposite wall of Bowman's space is lined by less specialized, flat epithelial cells forming the parietal epithelium. Podocytes (visceral glomerular epithelial cells) have three components: the cell body containing the nucleus; the major processes that radiate out from the cell body; and the foot processes (pods) that interdigitate with foot processes from adjacent podocytes and sit on the surface of the glomerular basement membrane (11,25). Interdigitation of the foot process is seen best in three dimensions (fig. 1-7). In cross section, the foot processes appear as a row of pods (feet)

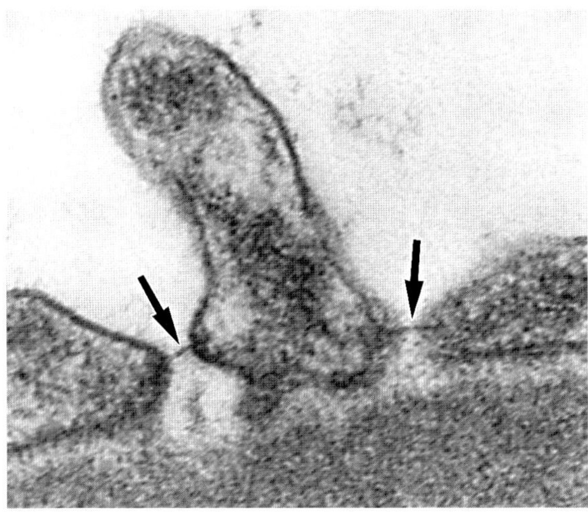

Figure 1-12

PODOCYTE FOOT PROCESS AND SLIT DIAPHRAGMS

High-magnification transmission electron micrograph shows two slit diaphragms, which are modified adherens junctions that link adjacent foot processes. The lamina lucida externa is between the soles of the foot processes and the lamina densa of the glomerular basement membrane.

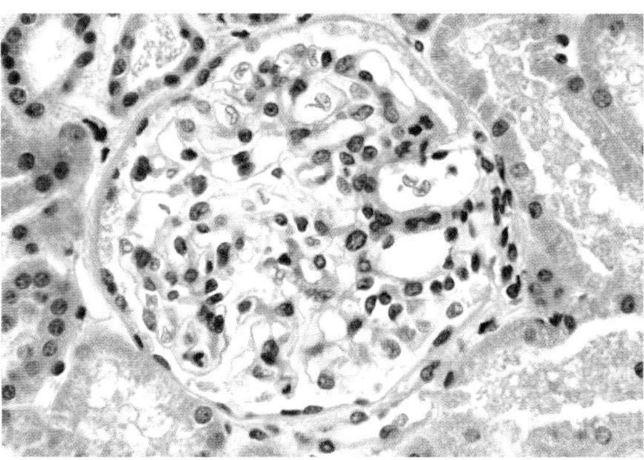

Figure 1-13

NORMAL GLOMERULUS

H&E stain allows an assessment of the general cellularity and architectural features of glomeruli and other elements of the renal parenchyma. In this normal glomerulus, note the parietal epithelial cells lining Bowman's capsule, the podocytes lining the outer surface of the glomerular tuft, the thin capillary walls, the patent capillary lumens, the small amount of mesangial matrix, and the attachment of the hilum (on the right).

with their soles sitting on top of the lamina lucida externa (figs. 1-8–1-12). At high magnification, a slit diaphragm can be seen stretching between adjacent foot processes (fig. 1-12). This is a modified adherens junction (20). Much is known about the molecular composition of podocytes, and this is relevant to a variety of diseases that are discussed later, such as congenital nephrotic syndrome and focal segmental glomerulosclerosis (10,22). Important podocyte constituents include nephrin, podocin, podocalyxin, synaptopodin, CD2-associated protein, P-cadherin, and alpha-actinin-4 (10,27,28). A detailed discussion of the function of these molecules is beyond the scope of this text.

The various components of the glomeruli can be evaluated by light microscopy, especially when special stains are used. Stains that often are used for pathologic evaluation of renal tissue include hematoxylin and eosin (H&E) (fig. 1-13), periodic acid–Schiff (PAS) (fig. 1-14), Masson trichrome (fig. 1-15), and Jones methenamine silver (JMS) (fig. 1-16). Each glomerular component should be examined systematically: Bowman's capsule, parietal epithelial cells, podocytes, glomerular basement membrane, endothelium, capillary lumen, and mesangium.

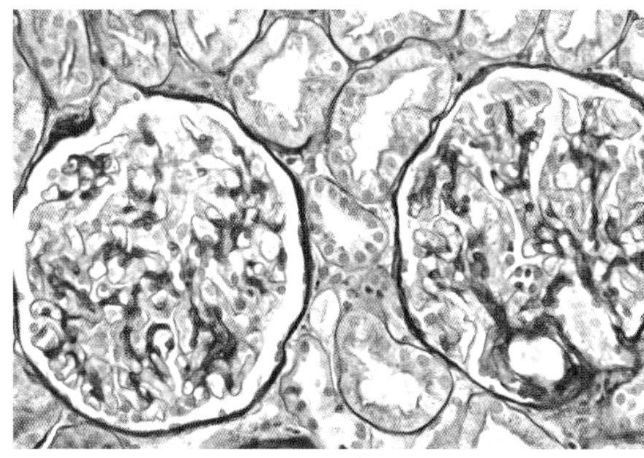

Figure 1-14

NORMAL GLOMERULUS

Periodic acid–Schiff (PAS) stain allows a more accurate assessment of the glomerular basement membranes, mesangial matrix, and tubular basement membranes. The glomerulus on the right is sectioned to show an intraglomerular portion of the efferent arteriole. The PAS stain also helps identify normal proximal tubules because their epithelial cells have prominent apical PAS-positive brush borders. Most of the tubules in this field are proximal tubules with brush borders. There is a distal tubule in the center of the photomicrograph, which has a smaller diameter and epithelial cells without a prominent brush border. Note the scant interstitial tissue of the normal cortex.

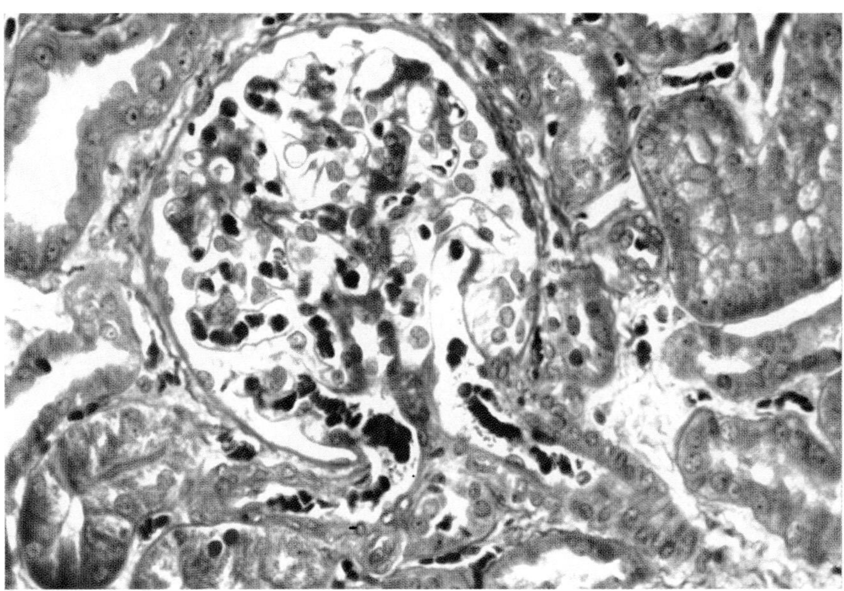

Figure 1-15

NORMAL GLOMERULUS

Masson trichrome staining does not add much to the evaluation of normal glomeruli, but is helpful in the examination of diseased renal tissue because it can help identify scarring, hyalinosis, immune deposits, and fibrinoid necrosis. This midcortical glomerulus is sectioned through the hilum to show both the afferent arteriole on the right and the efferent arteriole on the left. The efferent arteriole is slightly smaller and branches soon after exiting the tuft.

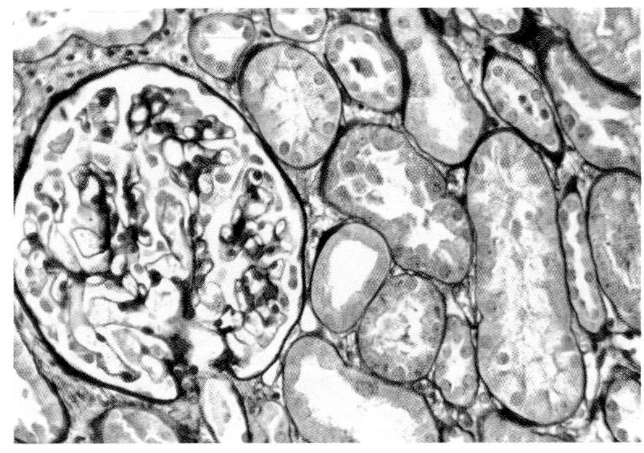

Figure 1-16

NORMAL GLOMERULUS

The Jones methenamine silver (JMS) stain accentuates basement membranes even better than the PAS stain. Note the small amount of mesangial matrix in this normal glomerulus. The tubulointerstitial compartment demonstrates the normal back-to-back arrangement of tubules in the renal cortex, with very little intervening interstitium.

Vasculature

The vasculature of the kidney is structurally and functionally very complex (11,13,16,25,28). All arteries and arterioles have an intima, muscularis, and adventitia. In normal kidneys of young individuals, there is little or no separation of endothelial cells from the underlying elastica or muscularis (fig. 1-17). With aging and in many pathologic conditions, there is a thickening of the intima by the deposition of connective tissue.

The main renal artery, interlobar arteries, and arcuate arteries have an internal and external elastic lamina on either side of a well-developed muscularis. The interlobular arteries have an internal elastic lamina but no well-defined external elastic lamina (fig. 1-17). Interlobular arteries have 3 to 5 layers of smooth muscle cells in the media. Terminal afferent arterioles and efferent arterioles have no identifiable internal or external elastic lamina, and have 1 to 4 layers of smooth muscle cells in the media (fig. 1-15).

The afferent arteriole breaks up into capillaries immediately after entering the glomerulus. The efferent arteriole has an intraglomerular segment that forms before it exits at the hilum (8). This can be seen by light microscopy as a profile of vessel wall with muscularis in the glomerular tuft (fig. 1-14). The efferent arterioles that exit from glomeruli in the middle and outer cortex have 1 or 2 layers of myocytes and are of smaller diameter than the afferent arterioles to the same glomeruli. However, the efferent arterioles that exit from juxtamedullary glomeruli are larger in diameter than the afferent arterioles to the same glomeruli and have 3 to 4 layers of myocytes. Efferent arterioles from outer glomeruli arborize after a short distance and become the cortical peritubular capillaries. Efferent ar-

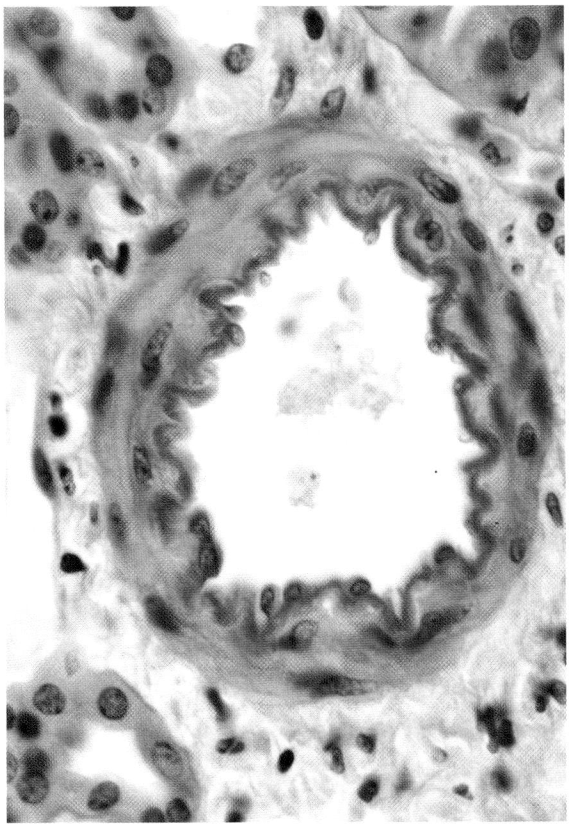

Figure 1-17

INTERLOBULAR ARTERY

This PAS-stained section shows an interlobular artery that has a muscularis composed of 2 to 3 layers of myocytes, a well-defined internal elastic lamina, and no discernable intimal space between the endothelium and elastica.

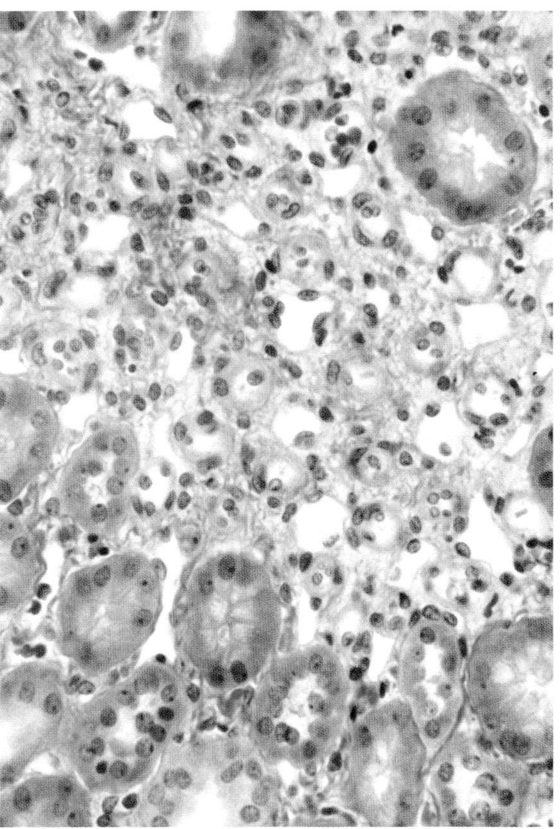

Figure 1-18

VASCULAR BUNDLE

This cross section of a vascular bundle (center of field) in the outer medulla shows thick-walled descending vasa recta and thin-walled ascending vasa recta. At the periphery of the bundle are thick limbs of the loop of Henle (Masson trichrome stain).

terioles from deeper glomeruli, especially from juxtamedullary glomeruli, give rise to multiple vasa recta, which loop down into the medulla to form a plexus around tubules. Descending and ascending vasa recta are grouped into vascular bundles. Cross sections of vascular bundles show thick-walled descending vasa recta and thin-walled ascending vasa recta (fig. 1-18). Peritubular capillaries have focal fenestrations and a very thin basement membrane (fig. 1-19).

Tubules and Interstitium

The renal tubules comprise 80 to 90 percent of the volume of the normal renal cortex. In most of the normal renal cortex, the tubules are back-to-back, with most of the intervening space occupied by thin-walled vessels lying in little, if any, interstitium (figs. 1-14, 1-16). There is substantially more interstitium in the medulla surrounding the medullary collecting ducts, thin loops of Henle, and associated straight portions of the proximal and distal tubules (figs. 1-20–1-22) (17,20). The most conspicuous interstitium in the cortex is the adventitia around the larger vascular bundles that contain the arteries, veins, and lymphatics. The peritubular interstitium contains only sparse fibroblasts and a few trafficking leukocytes. In the medulla, there is a gradual increase in the amount of interstitial tissue from the outer medulla to the papillary tip. Although few interstitial cells are noted in the cortex, they are readily identified in the medulla. Interstitial cells in the inner medulla often have conspicuous cytoplasmic lipid and

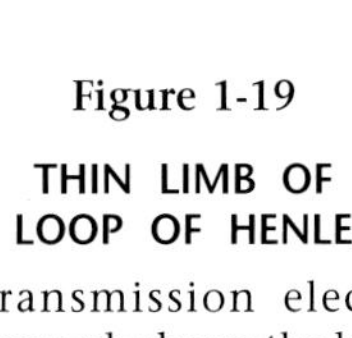

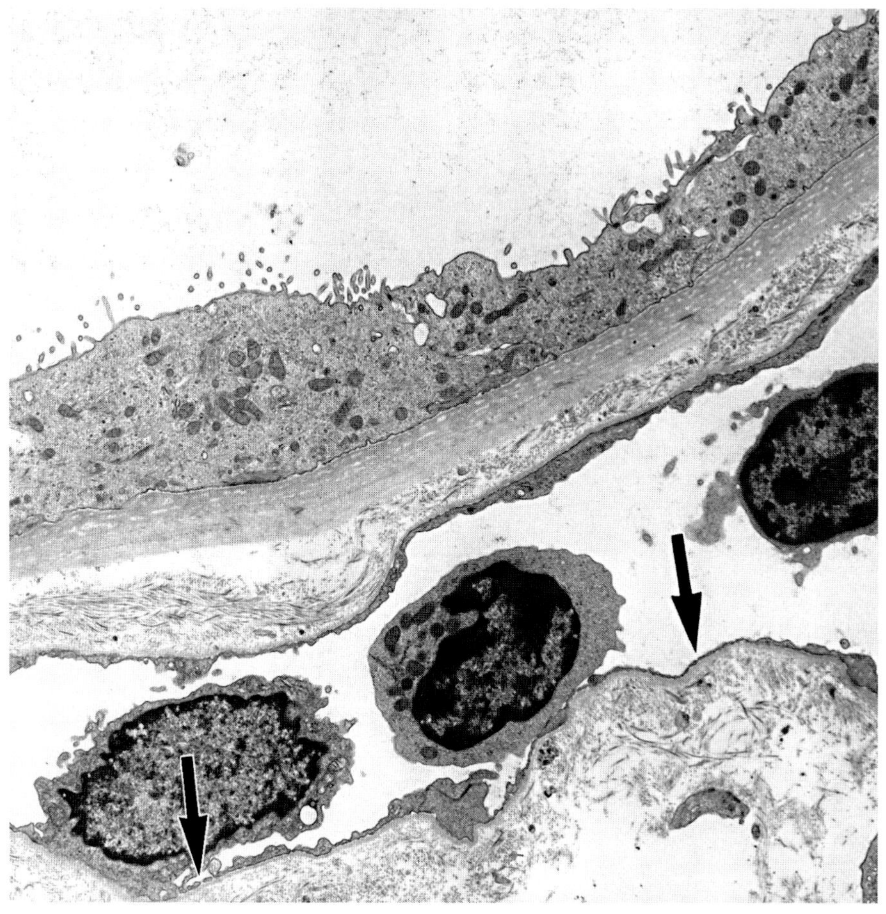

Figure 1-19

THIN LIMB OF LOOP OF HENLE

Transmission electron micrograph shows the lumen of a thin limb of the loop of Henle at the top lined by a flat epithelial cell. Adjacent to the tubule is a peritubular capillary with focal fenestrations (arrows).

Figure 1-20

INNER STRIPE OF OUTER MEDULLA

The presence of a collecting duct (center), thin limbs of the loop of Henle (on left with hyaline casts), and thick limbs of the loop of Henle (on right) indicate that this is the inner stripe of the outer medulla (refer to figure 1-6 for orientation). The collecting duct has a tall epithelium with pale cytoplasm and distinct cell boundaries. The thin limbs have a very flat epithelium and might be mistaken for small vessels if not for the casts. The thick limbs have low acidophilic cytoplasm (H&E stain).

usually are oriented at right angles to the vessels and tubules (18). A pathologic increase in the cortical interstitium is readily detected by routine light microscopy, but an abnormal increase in the medullary interstitium is more difficult to detect.

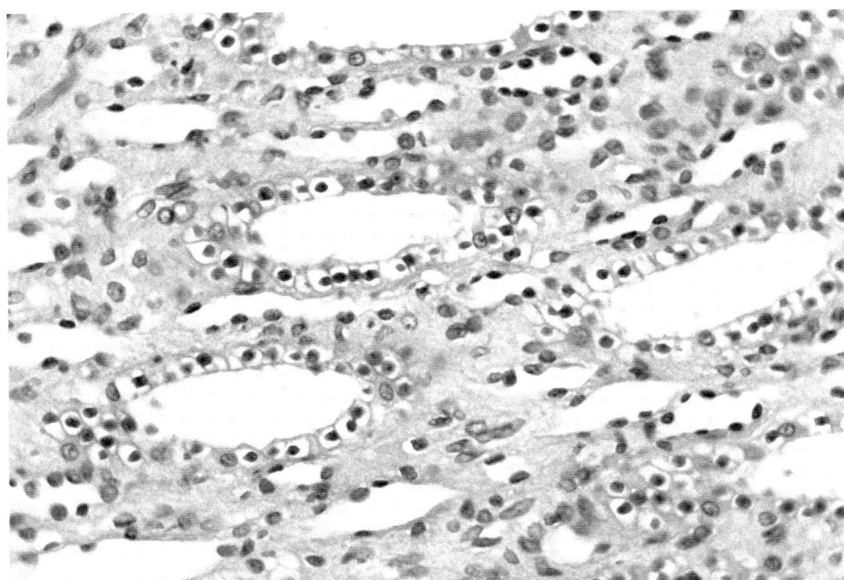

Figure 1-21

INNER MEDULLA

This oblique section through the inner medulla shows numerous collecting ducts lined by cuboidal epithelial cells with clear cytoplasm. The cell borders are distinct because of the lack of lateral interdigitations. The smaller tubules with a very flat epithelium are thin limbs of the loop of Henle. There are no thick limbs in the inner medulla (see figure 1-6) (H&E stain).

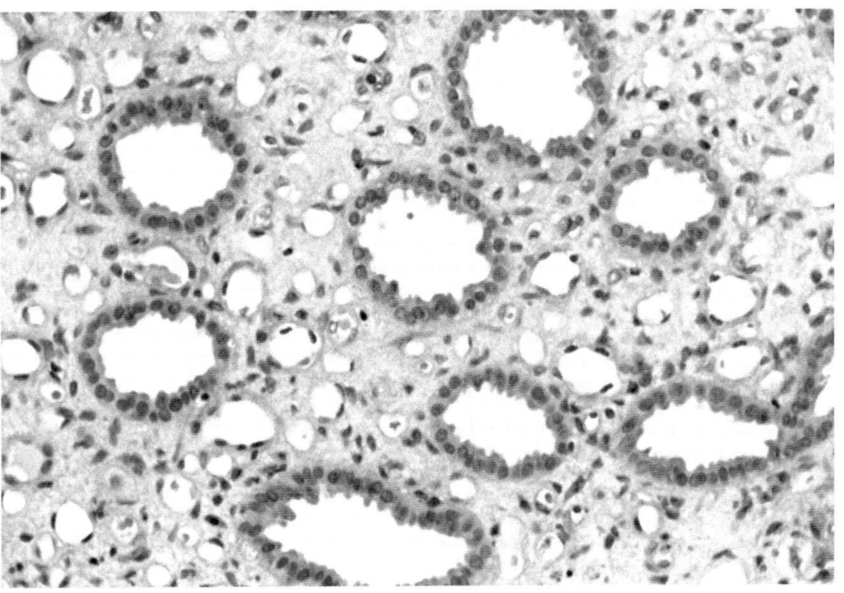

Figure 1-22

PAPILLARY TIP

A cross section through a papillary tip shows terminal collecting ducts (ducts of Bellini). Most of the thin-walled structures are thin limbs of the loop of Henle, but some are small peritubular capillaries (H&E stain).

Although the normal tubular system of each nephron can be divided morphologically and functionally into more than 15 structurally and functionally different segments (11,14,19,29), the major divisions are into proximal and distal tubules and loop of Henle (see fig. 1-6). The proximal convoluted tubules and distal tubules in the cortex of the normal kidney can be distinguished with reasonable accuracy. The epithelium of the proximal convoluted tubules has abundant eosinophilic cytoplasm and a prominent apical microvillous brush border. The brush border is seen best with special stains, such as PAS (see fig. 1-14). By electron microscopy, the cells of the cortical proximal tubule have tall brush borders, numerous large elongated mitochondria, and extensive basolateral infoldings of the cell membrane that interdigitate with adjacent cells (fig. 1-23). The proximal tubule is divided into the initial pars convoluta (proximal convoluted tubule in the cortex) and the pars recta (straight portion, which is located in the medulla) (see fig. 1-6). Tight junctions (zonula occludens) separate the intercellular space from the tubular lumen.

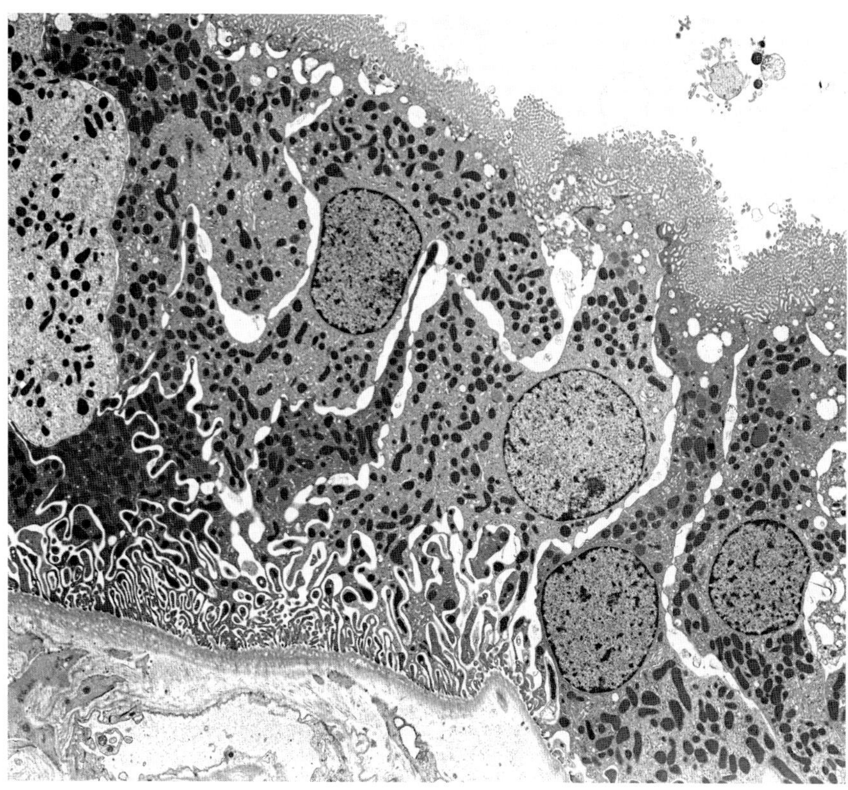

Figure 1-23

PROXIMAL CONVOLUTED TUBULE EPITHELIUM

Transmission electron micrograph shows a prominent brush border with clear endocytic vesicles just below. The cytoplasm has numerous elongated mitochondria. Fixation has caused slight contraction of the cells, which facilitates identification of the basolateral interdigitations.

A rich endocytic-lysosomal system is beneath the apical border (fig. 1-23). The prominence of the basolateral interdigitations and the number and size of mitochondria diminish in the distal pars recta of the proximal tubule. Here, interdigitations are sparse and the mitochondria are smaller and rounder (fig. 1-24).

The thin limb of the loop of Henle extends from the end of the straight portion (pars recta) of the proximal tubule to the beginning of the thick ascending limb of the distal tubule. It has a very thin epithelium and a delicate basement membrane (figs. 1-19–1-22) (23,29). Short-loop nephrons arising in the outer and middle cortex have a short, descending thin-limb segment that does not extend below the inner strip of the outer medulla while long-loop nephrons arising in the juxtamedullary cortex have long, descending thin limbs that extend into the papillary tip before looping back toward the cortex (see fig. 1-6). The transition of the proximal tubule to the descending thin limb demarcates the border between the outer and inner stripe of the outer medulla. The border between the outer medulla and the inner medulla is the point where the short loops turn back toward the cortex and the ascending thin limbs from long-loop nephrons turn into the thick ascending limbs. The epithelium of the thin limb of the loop of Henle is flat and nondescript by light microscopy (figs. 1-20–1-22). Electron microscopy reveals varying degrees of basolateral interdigitations, varying numbers of organelles, and different intercellular junctions at different sites along the loop. In most locations, interdigitations, organelles, and microvilli are sparse (fig. 1-19).

The distal tubule consists of the thick ascending limb (medullary and cortical), the macula densa, and the distal convoluted tubule (11,14, 29). The ascending thin limb abruptly becomes the thick ascending limb of the distal tubule at the border between the inner and outer medulla (see fig. 1-6). Electron microscopy reveals numerous basolateral interdigitations associated with many elongated mitochondria. This is similar to the finding in proximal tubules, however, the thick ascending limb cells can be distinguished from proximal tubule epithelium by their lack of apical brush borders of microvilli, smaller size, and more cubical shape.

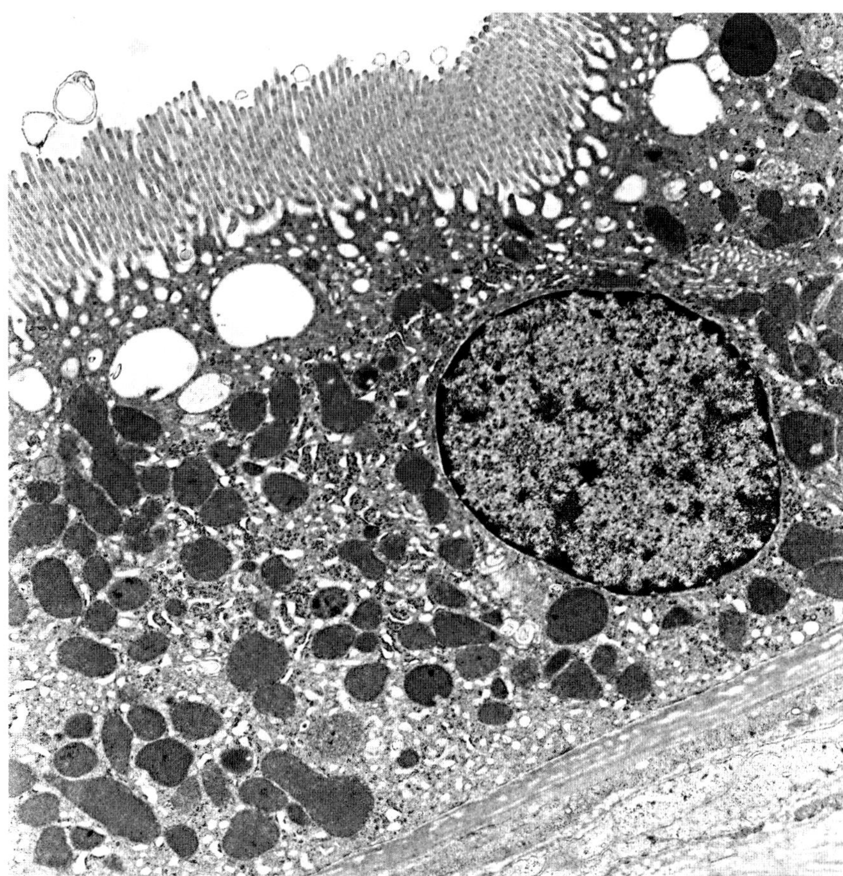

Figure 1-24

PARS RECTA PROXIMAL TUBULE EPITHELIUM

Compared to the cells in figure 1-23, there are fewer basolateral interdigitations and rounder mitochondria. The prominent brush border identifies the cell as part of the proximal tubule.

Immunohistochemistry demonstrates the production of Tamm-Horsfall protein by the thick ascending limb. Tamm-Horsfall protein is a major constituent of most tubular casts. The thick ascending limb terminates with the macula densa, which is described later as a component of the juxtaglomerular apparatus. The distal convoluted tubule arises after the macula densa and ends in an indistinct junction with a collecting duct. An intervening connecting tubule usually cannot be clearly delineated histologically in humans. Distal tubular epithelial cells are smaller than proximal tubular epithelial cells, have less eosinophilic cytoplasm, have more centrally placed nuclei, and lack a PAS-positive apical brush border (see fig. 1-14). Often it is histologically difficult, if not impossible, to accurately separate the distal tubules from cortical segments of collecting ducts. The distal convoluted tubule has cells with an ultrastructure similar to that of the thick ascending limb, but the former are larger (fig. 1-25).

The cells of the collecting duct are cuboidal in the cortex, and increase in height as they descend toward the papilla (figs. 1-20–1-22). Electron microscopy identifies two distinct cell types in the collecting ducts: principal cells (collecting duct cells) and intercalated cells (dark cells). Principal cells have relatively pale cytoplasm because of a paucity of organelles. Ultrastructurally, there are numerous infoldings of the basal cell membrane but unlike many cells elsewhere in the nephron, there are minimal or no lateral interdigitations. Thus, by light microscopy, a more distinct boundary often can be seen between cells in the collecting duct compared to the proximal and distal tubules where there are extensive lateral interdigitations (figs. 1-20–1-22). Intercalated cells have more cytoplasmic organelles (e.g., numerous vesicles, mitochondria, and ribosomes) and thus have more electron-dense cytoplasm than principal cells. As the collecting tubules course through the medulla toward the papillary tip,

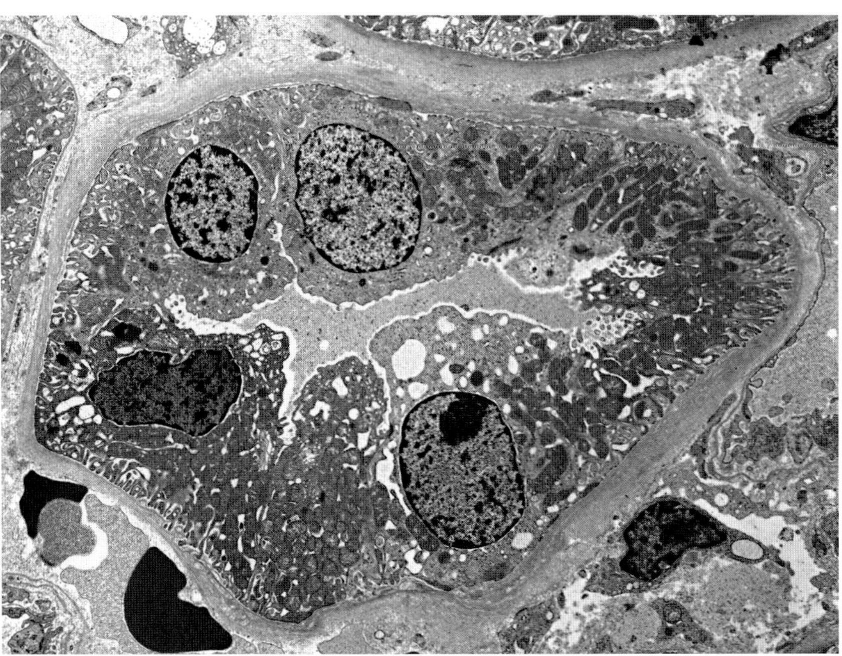

Figure 1-25

DISTAL CONVOLUTED TUBULE EPITHELIUM

The epithelial cells have numerous basolateral interdigitations, abundant mitochondria, and sparse microvilli.

intercalated cells become less frequent and the epithelium becomes taller, with paler cytoplasm. Near the papillary tip, the collecting ducts (tubules) coalesce into larger collecting ducts (the ducts of Bellini) that have taller epithelium (fig. 1-22). These ducts open onto the papillary surfaces where the epithelium merges with the transitional epithelium of the extrarenal urinary tract. The calyces and renal pelvis are lined by transitional epithelium (urothelium).

A variety of lectins and antibodies can precisely separate different segments of normal and diseased tubules. These, however, are not used for routine diagnostic evaluation.

Juxtaglomerular Apparatus

The juxtaglomerular apparatus is located at the vascular pole of the glomerulus (8,11,14,29). The vascular components are the terminal portion of the afferent arteriole and the initial portion of the efferent arteriole. The extraglomerular mesangial cells (lacis cells, or Goormaghtigh cells) are modified smooth muscle cells that are part of the juxtaglomerular apparatus (see fig. 1-16). They are in continuity with the intraglomerular mesangial cells (also of smooth muscle cell lineage) and the smooth muscle cells of the hilar arterioles (8,9). The tubular component of the juxtaglomerular apparatus is the adjacent specialized portion of the distal tubule called the macula densa (figs. 1-7, 1-26). The macula densa is the only part of the tubular system of the nephron with "reversed polarity," that is, the nuclei are apical, with the Golgi apparatus and endocytic apparatus concentrated in the basal cytoplasm. This indicates that the bulk of synthesized molecules are directed toward the glomerulus rather than the tubular lumen (molecules involved in tubuloglomerular feedback). The cells of the macula densa are taller than those of the surrounding epithelium and the nuclei appear closely packed. The macula densa contacts the hilum of the same glomerulus that gave rise to the tubule that it is a part of. The broadest contact is with the extraglomerular mesangial cells (fig. 1-26).

Sympathetic nerves are the neural component of the juxtaglomerular apparatus and course along the arterioles but do not enter the glomeruli. Renin granules are in the cytoplasm of clusters of cells in the muscularis of the afferent arteriole in the juxtaglomerular apparatus and occasionally in the extraglomerular mesangial cells and efferent arterioles. These cytoplasmic granules can be identified by light microscopy using a Bowie stain, by immunohistochemistry using antibodies to renin, or by electron microscopy as membrane-bound electron-dense granules.

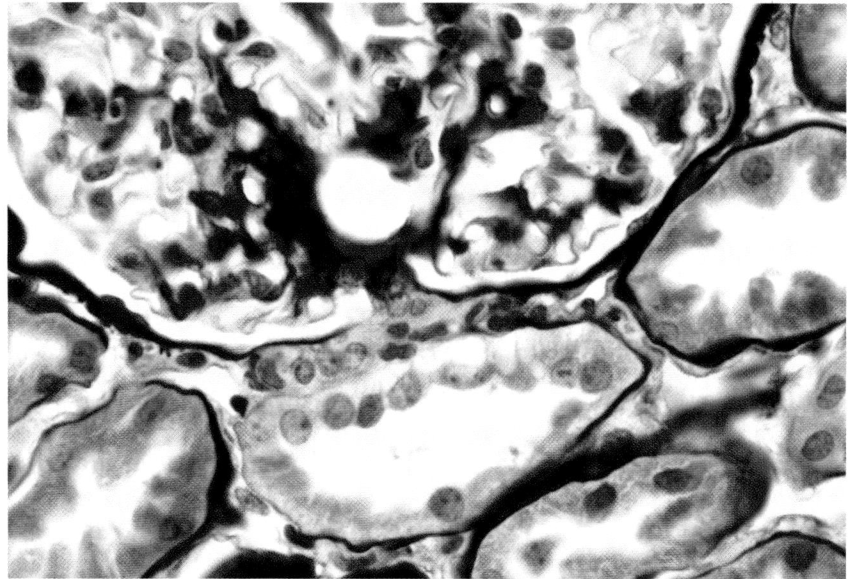

Figure 1-26

JUXTAGLOMERULAR APPARATUS

This JMS stain with an H&E counterstain shows the macula densa separated from the glomerular hilum by extraglomerular mesangial cells. The arteriolar component of the juxtaglomerular apparatus is not in the plane of section. Note the "reversed polarity" of the epithelial cells in the macula densa, with the nuclei in an apical position and cytoplasmic clearing in the basal area caused by the Golgi apparatus.

REFERENCES

Embryology

1. Netter FH. Kidneys, ureters, and urinary bladder. The CIBA collection of medical illustrations, Vol. 6. Summit, NJ: CIBA Pharmaceutical Products; 1973.
2. Risdon RA, Woolf AS. Development of the kidney. In: Jennette JC, Olson JL, Schwartz MM, Silva FG, eds. Hepinstall's pathology of the kidney. Philadelphia: Lippincott-Raven; 1998:67–84.

Gross Anatomy

3. A handbook of kidney nomenclature and nosology: criteria for diagnosis, including laboratory procedures. International Committee for Nomenclature and Nosology of Renal Disease. Boston: Little, Brown; 1975:1–37.
4. Kriz W, Bankir L. A standard nomenclature for structure of the kidney. The Renal Commission of the International Union of Physiological Sciences (IUPS). Kidney Int 1988;33:1–7.
5. Netter FH. Kidneys, ureters, and urinary bladder. The CIBA collection of medical illustrations, Vol. 6. Summit, NJ: CIBA Pharmaceutical Products; 1973.
6. Risdon RA, Woolf AS. Anatomy. In: Jennette JC, Olson JL, Schwartz MM, Silva FG, eds. Hepinstall's pathology of the kidney, 5th ed. Philadelphia: Lippincott-Raven; 1998:3–66.

Histology of the Kidney

7. Boutaud A, Borza DB, Bondar O, et al. Type IV collagen of the glomerular basement membrane. Evidence that the chain specificity of network assembly is encoded by the noncollagenous NC1 domains. J Biol Chem 2000;275:30716–24.
8. Elger M, Sakai T, Kriz W. The vascular pole of the renal glomerulus of rat. Adv Anat Embryol Cell Biol 1998;139:1–98.
9. Elger M, Sakai T, Winkler D, Kriz W. Structure of the outflow segment of the efferent arteriole in rat superficial glomeruli. Contrib Nephrol 1991; 95:22–33.
10. Endlich K, Kriz W, Witzgall R. Update in podocyte biology. Curr Opin Nephrol Hypertension 2001;10:331–40.
11. A handbook of kidney nomenclature and nosology: criteria for diagnosis, including laboratory procedures. International Committee for Nomenclature and Nosology of Renal Disease. Boston: Little, Brown; 1975:1–37.
12. Kriz W. Structural organization of renal medullary circulation. Nephron 1982;31:290–5.
13. Kriz W, Bachmann S. Pre- and postglomerular arterioles of the kidney. J Cardiovasc Pharmacol 1985;7(Suppl 3):S24–30.
14. Kriz W, Bankir L. A standard nomenclature for structure of the kidney. The Renal Commission of the International Union of Physiological Sciences (IUPS). Kidney Int 1988;33:1–7.

15. Kriz W, Elger M, Lemley KV, Sakai T. Mesangial cell-glomerular basement membrane connections counteract glomerular capillary and mesangium expansion. Am J Nephrol 1990;10(Suppl 1):4–13.
16. Kriz W, Elger M, Lemley K, Sakai T. Structure of the glomerular mesangium: a biomechanical interpretation. Kidney Int Suppl 1990;30:S2–9.
17. Kriz W, Napiwotzky P. Structural and functional aspects of the renal interstitium. Contrib Nephrol 1979;16:104–8.
18. Lemley KV, Kriz W. Anatomy of the renal interstitium. Kidney Int 1991;39:370–81.
19. Madsen KM, Brenner BM. Structure and function of the renal tubule and interstitium. In: Tisher CC, Brenner BM, eds. Renal pathology with clinical and functional correlations, 2nd ed. Philadelphia: Lippincott; 1994:661–98.
20. Makino H, Hironaka K, Shikata K, et al. Mesangial matrices act as mesangial channels to the juxtaglomerular zone. Tracer and high-resolution scanning electron-microscopic study. Nephron 1994;66:181–8.
21. Miner JH. Renal basement membrane components. Kidney Int 1999;56:2016–24.
22. Mundel P, Shankland S. Podocyte biology and response to injury. J Am Soc Nephrol 2002;13:3005–15.
23. Netter FH. Kidneys, ureters, and urinary bladder. The CIBA collection of medical illustrations, Vol. 6. Summit, NJ: CIBA Pharmaceutical Products; 1973.
24. Reiser J, Kriz W, Kretzler M, Mundel P. The glomerular slit diaphragm is a modified adherens junction. J Am Soc Nephrol 2000;11:1–8.
25. Risdon RA, Woolf AS. Anatomy. In: Jennette JC, Olson JL, Schwartz MM, Silva FG, eds. Hepinstall's pathology of the kidney, 5th ed. Philadelphia: Lippincott-Raven; 1998:3–66.
26. Sakai T, Kriz W. The structural relationship between mesangial cells and basement membrane of the renal glomerulus. Anat Embryol 1987;176:373–86.
27. Schwarz K, Simons M, Reiser J, et al. Podocin, a raft-associated component of the glomerular slit diaphragm, interacts with CD2AP and nephrin. J Clin Invest 2001;108:1621–9.
28. Simons M, Schwarz K, Kriz W, et al. Involvement of lipid rafts in nephrin phosphorylation and organization of the glomerular slit diaphragm. Am J Pathol 2001;159:1069–77.
29. Tisher CC. Functional anatomy of the kidney. Hosp Pract 1978;13:53–65.
30. Vodenicharov A. Peculiarities of the connection between mesangial and glomerular endothelial cells in the domestic-swine kidney. Anat Histol Embryol 1995;24:227–31.

2 CONGENITAL ABNORMALITIES INCLUDING CYSTIC DISEASES

INTRODUCTION

Congenital renal diseases are present with birth (con genesis). They may be pathologically apparent at birth (e.g., multicystic renal dysplasia) or have delayed phenotypic expression (e.g., adult-onset autosomal dominant polycystic kidney disease). They are caused by inherited genetic abnormalities, genetic mutations that occur during embryogenesis, or somatic developmental abnormalities that are acquired during embryogenesis or fetal development, including mistimed or misplaced gene expression (2–5). Congenital anomalies of the kidney and urinary tract account for more than 50 percent of abdominal masses in neonates, are the most common cause of end-stage renal disease (ESRD) in infants, and are identified in approximately 0.5 percent of pregnancies (3,5).

POTTER'S SEQUENCE

Potter's sequence (formerly *Potter's syndrome*, also known as *oligohydramnios sequence*) is a combination of gross abnormalities caused by any disease that results in severe intrauterine impairment of urine production or by other causes of oligohydramnios (1). Potter's sequence can be caused by bilateral urinary tract obstruction, bilateral renal agenesis, bilateral renal aplasia, severe bilateral renal dysplasia, autosomal recessive polycystic kidney disease, or leakage of amniotic fluid.

Patients have a beak-like nose, receding chin, low-set ears, pulmonary hypoplasia, abnormally bent lower extremities (talipes, equinovarus), and joint contractures (arthrogryposis) (fig. 2-1). The external abnormalities are caused by the absence of the cushioning effect of the amniotic fluid, which allows the fetus to be compressed by the walls of the uterus. The pulmonary hypoplasia is caused by the lack of normal maturational stimuli from the amniotic fluid as well as compression of the chest wall by the uterus. Enlarged cystic or dysplastic kidneys can add to the pulmonary compression by elevating the diaphragm.

RENAL AGENESIS

Definition. Renal agenesis is the complete absence of renal tissue, and may be unilateral or bilateral.

Clinical Features. The incidence of renal agenesis is 1 in 500 to 3,200 births (14). Bilateral renal agenesis is not compatible with unassisted extrauterine life. Most infants with this anomaly are stillborn. Unilateral renal agenesis causes no immediate renal functional impairment because the remaining single kidney undergoes sufficient hypertrophy to maintain normal renal function. Later in life, hypertension, proteinuria, and progressive renal failure may develop because of the induction of secondary focal segmental glomerulosclerosis (14, 17). Most patients with unilateral renal agenesis, however, never develop clinically significant renal abnormalities and the agenesis is identified only as an incidental finding, for example, during postmortem examination.

Gross Findings. By definition, renal agenesis is characterized by complete absence of one or both kidneys (fig. 2-2). In most patients, the ureter and bladder trigone also are completely absent (17). Less than a quarter of patients have a vestigial distal ureter. With unilateral renal agenesis, the remaining kidney undergoes hypertrophy. Unilateral and bilateral renal agenesis often are accompanied by other congenital anomalies, such as internal and external genital tact malformations, imperforate anus, rectal atresia, rectourethral fistula, and a variety of cardiovascular and neural tube defects. Bilateral renal agenesis may be accompanied by atresia or absence of the bladder and urethra. More severe caudal regression manifests as absence of the distal gut, external genitalia, and sacrum, and fusion of vestigial lower extremities (sirenomelia).

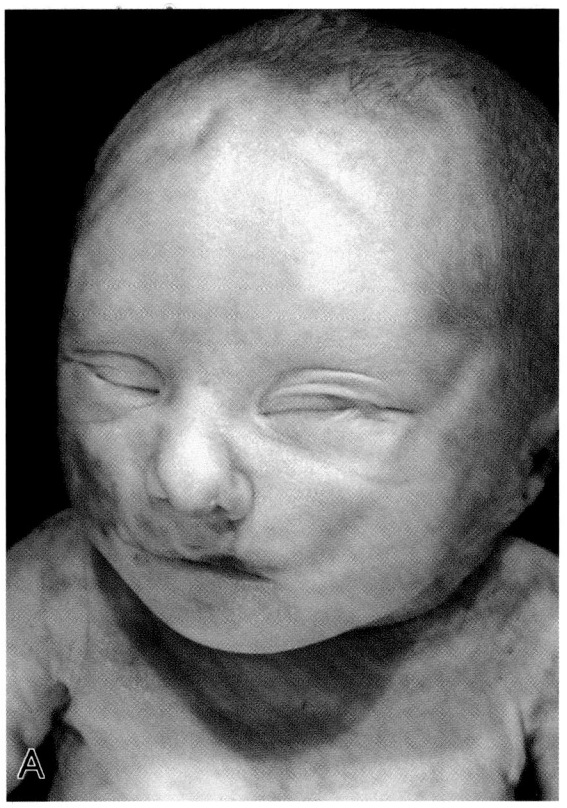

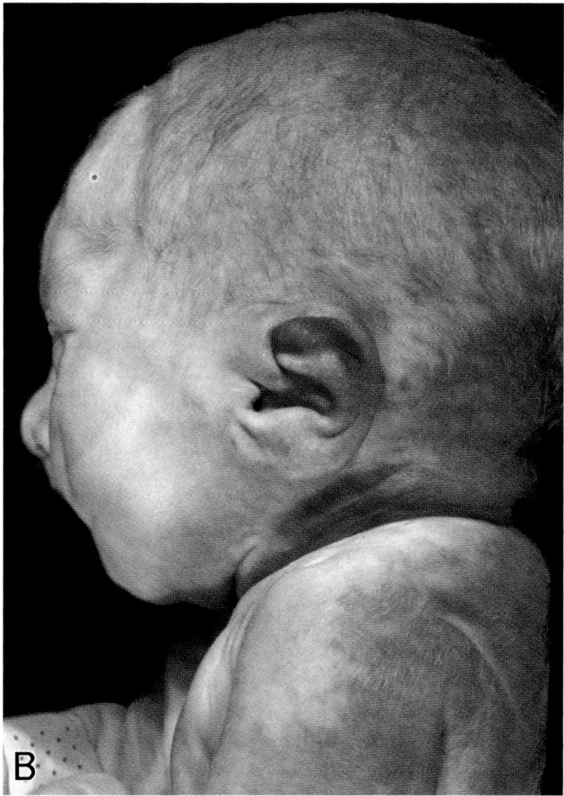

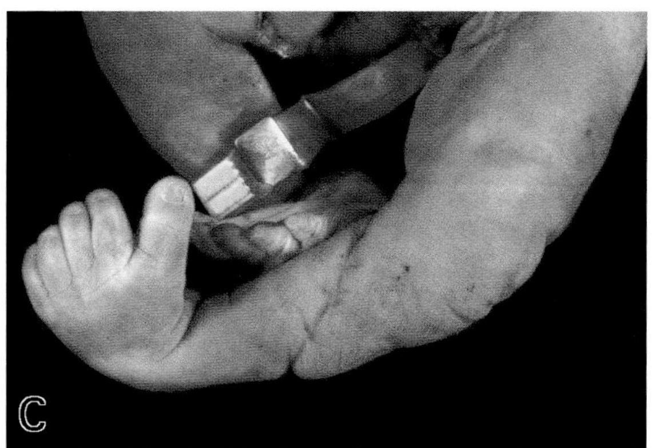

Figure 2-1

POTTER'S SEQUENCE (OLIGOHYDRAMNIOS SEQUENCE)

Manifestations include a beak-like nose (A,B), receding chin (B), low-set ears (B), and abnormally bent lower extremities (C).

As noted earlier, bilateral renal agenesis causes Potter's sequence.

Light Microscopic Findings. If there is renal tissue to examine microscopically, even if it is very aberrant, the diagnosis is not renal agenesis. With unilateral renal agenesis, the remaining contralateral kidney undergoes compensatory hypertrophy, with enlargement of glomeruli and tubules. Patients with unilateral renal agenesis are at increased risk for developing secondary focal segmental glomerulosclerosis in the single remaining kidney as a result of the overwork (14). When this happens, histologic evaluation of this kidney reveals the microscopic findings of focal segmental glomerular sclerosis (often with preferential perihilar involvement and hyalinosis) and glomerular enlargement (glomerulomegaly).

Differential Diagnosis. The major differential diagnostic consideration is renal aplastic dysplasia. Unilateral or bilateral aplastic dysplasia may result in a very small amount of malformed

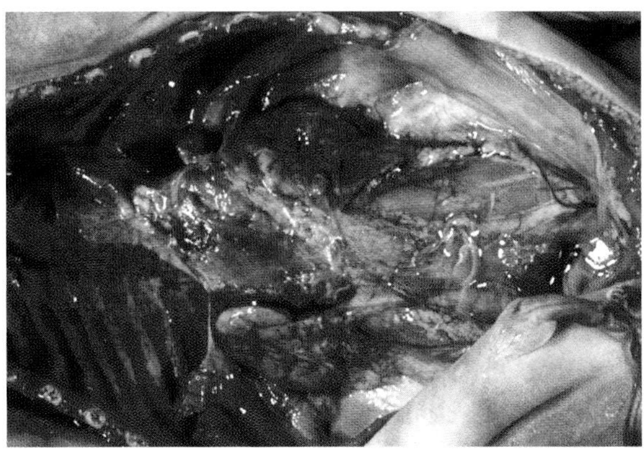

Figure 2-2

BILATERAL RENAL AGENESIS

In the absence of molding by the kidneys, the adrenal glands are disk shaped. (Fig. 11-2 from Churg J, Bernstein J, Risdon RA, Sobin LH. Renal disease: classification and atlas. Part II. New York: Igaku-Shoin; 1987:139.)

renal tissue that is difficult or impossible to identify by gross inspection. The dysplastic tissue may only be found by histologic examination of tissue at the site where the kidney should be. This is aided by the presence of an intact ureter because this points to the appropriate site for histologic examination; however, the ureter usually is absent when there is aplastic dysplasia. Imaging studies, such as ultrasound, can help differentiate renal agenesis from aplasia (8).

Etiology and Pathogenesis. The most likely cause of renal agenesis is failure of the ureteric bud to develop from the mesonephric duct (15). Without the inductive influence of the ureteric bud, the metanephric blastema does not differentiate into renal parenchyma. Renal agenesis can be caused by genetic or environmental factors or by the interaction of the two. Genes that can be mutated to cause renal agenesis include *PAX2* on chromosome 10 and *WT1* on chromosome 11 (17). Maternal risk factors for the development of renal agenesis in a child are diabetes, alcohol ingestion, and age less than 18 years.

Treatment and Prognosis. Bilateral renal agenesis results in stillbirth in approximately 40 percent of affected infants. Most who are born alive are premature and die shortly after birth because of respiratory insufficiency secondary to pulmonary hypoplasia (16). Unilateral renal agenesis is asymptomatic unless secondary focal segmental glomerulosclerosis develops.

RENAL HYPOPLASIA AND OLIGOMEGANEPHRONIC HYPOPLASIA

Definition. Renal hypoplasia is a reduction in renal mass caused by too little genesis of normal renal tissue, i.e., genesis of too few nephrons. Simple hypoplasia has no histologic abnormalities. Oligomeganephronic hypoplasia (oligomeganephronia) is characterized by marked compensatory hypertrophy caused by overwork as a result of the reduced number of nephrons (7). Most patients with hypoplasia who have reduced glomerular filtration rates develop oligomeganephronic hypoplasia (13). Simple renal hypoplasia is rare compared to oligomeganephronic hypoplasia, probably because the reduced renal function leads to compensatory nephron hypertrophy.

Clinical Features. Hypoplasia often results in a reduced glomerular filtration rate because of the reduced number of nephrons. Renal function often is stable throughout early childhood but may decline in late childhood or adulthood if secondary focal segmental glomerulosclerosis develops (11). Proteinuria also accompanies the development of focal segmental glomerulosclerosis. Especially with oligomeganephronic hypoplasia, polyuria, polydipsia, and salt wasting may develop. Renal hypoplasia occurs as an isolated abnormality or as a component of a maldevelopment syndrome, such as the renal-coloboma syndrome with renal hypoplasia and optic nerve colobomas (13).

Gross Findings. Hypoplastic kidneys are by definition small (usually less than 50 percent expected weight for gestational or postnatal age). Renal hypoplasia may be unilateral or bilateral. Oligomeganephronic hypoplasia usually is bilateral whereas simple hypoplasia usually is unilateral. Hypoplastic kidneys may be reniform or rounder than normal. The cut surface reveals six or fewer renal lobes, which is best determined by counting the number of medullary papillary tips. There may be only one lobe (a unipapillary or unireniculate kidney). The distinction between cortex and medulla is well preserved.

Light Microscopic Findings. The renal histology shows normal differentiation with varying degrees of nephron hypertrophy, dependent upon the extent and duration of the hypoplasia. There are no discernible histologic abnormalities or only minor glomerular enlargement

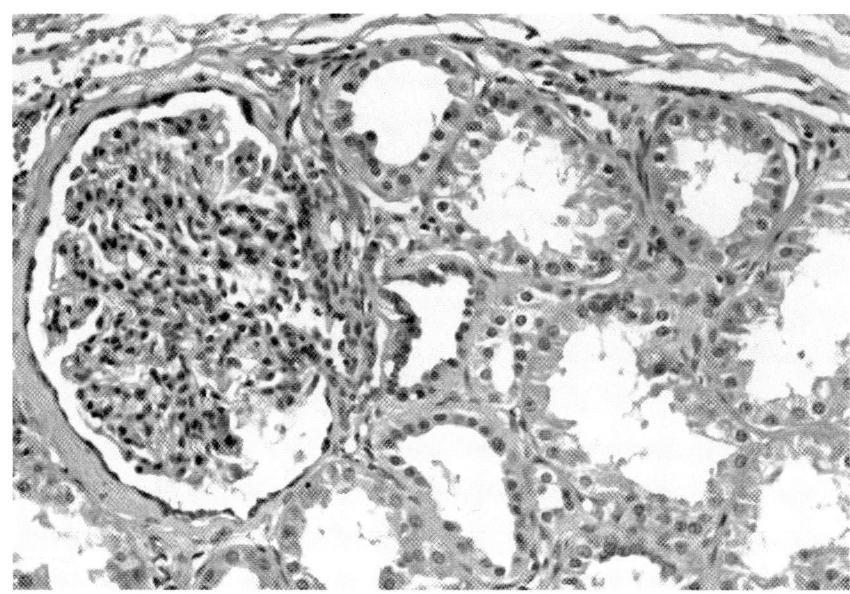

Figure 2-3

OLIGOMEGANEPHRONIC HYPOPLASIA

Nephronomegaly in a 17-g kidney removed for diagnosis from a 6-year-old child with bilateral small kidneys. A renal transplant was required because of severe renal insufficiency. The glomerulus is at least three times normal size for this age and has an increase in all cellular elements. The surrounding tubules also are enlarged (hematoxylin and eosin [H&E] stain).

with unilateral simple hypoplasia. Bilateral hypoplasia is likely to manifest changes of oligomeganephronic hypoplasia. Histologically, oligomeganephronic hyperplasia is characterized by not only glomerular enlargement but also by tubular enlargement (fig. 2-3) (7,12). There is no well-established criterion for the extent of glomerular enlargement required to separate oligomeganephronic hypoplasia from simple renal hypoplasia. A reasonable criterion is a glomerular diameter three times greater than expected for age-matched healthy controls. The enlarged glomeruli often are called hypertrophied although they in fact have hyperplasia of all elements. There are more capillaries and more mesangial segments than in normal glomeruli, which of course is accompanied by an increase in all glomerular cell types.

Oligomeganephronic hypoplasia predisposes to the development of secondary focal segmental glomerulosclerosis (11). Thus, histologic examination may reveal the features of focal segmental glomerular sclerosis and hyalinosis that are typical for other forms of secondary focal segmental glomerulosclerosis caused by glomerular overwork. Focal interstitial fibrosis and tubular atrophy usually accompany the glomerular sclerosis.

Differential Diagnosis. Renal hypoplasia must be differentiated from reduced renal size caused by other congenital or acquired pathologic processes. In the fetus or neonate, the major differential consideration is aplastic dysplasia, which can be readily distinguished histologically. Atrophy and scarring are the major causes of reduced renal size after the neonatal period. A diagnosis of hypoplasia should be made only when a small kidney has normal renal histology other than compensatory nephron hypertrophy.

Etiology and Pathogenesis. There are multiple genetic and environmental factors that can contribute to the development of renal hypoplasia. One mechanism involves genetic mutations in the *PAX2* gene on chromosome 10 (13). Patients with a mutation in this gene may have renal coloboma syndrome or isolated renal hypoplasia. The *PAX2* gene product plays a critical role in the development of the urogenital tract, eyes, and central nervous system. Experimental studies suggest that gene mutations induce renal hypoplasia by causing reduced branching of the ureteric bud and increased apoptosis in the metanephric blastema (13).

Another pathogenic mechanism of renal hypoplasia is abnormal positioning of the site of contact between the ureteric bud and the metanephric blastema (15). If this site is proximal or distal to the usual site, the blastema that is reached by the inductive stimuli from the ureteric bud contains fewer cells and thus gives rise to fewer nephrons.

Treatment and Prognosis. Bilateral renal hypoplasia is an important cause of ESRD in children (13). Severe bilateral hypoplasia causes renal

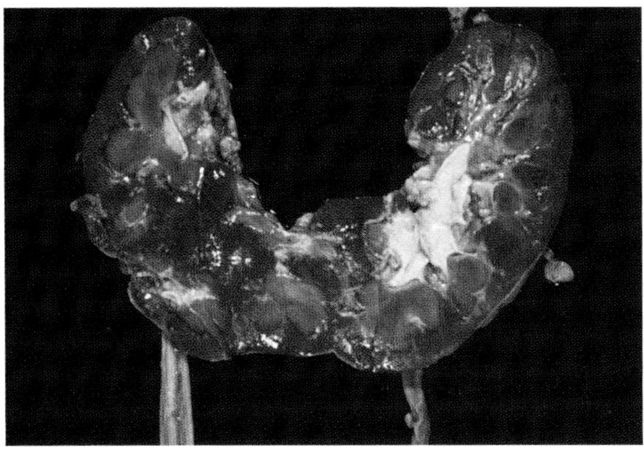

Figure 2-4

HORSESHOE KIDNEY

This horseshoe kidney was fused at the lower pole. It caused no symptoms and was an incidental finding at the time of postmortem examination.

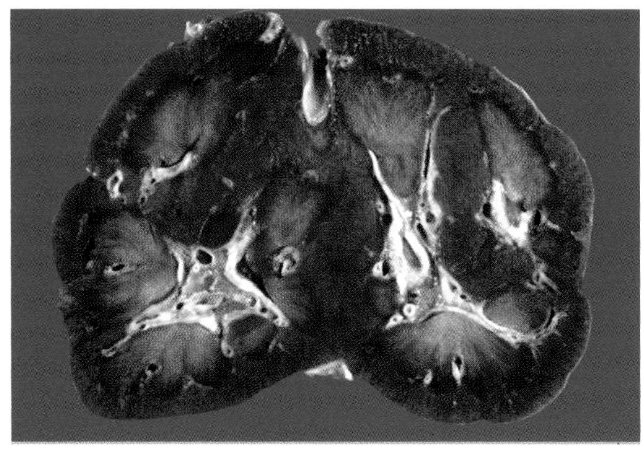

Figure 2-5

FUSED KIDNEY

This fused kidney was found in the pelvis and had two separate collecting systems. (Courtesy of Dr. S. S. Iskandar, Winston Salem, NC.)

insufficiency from birth. Delayed-onset renal failure may be caused by the development of secondary focal segmental glomerulosclerosis. Clinically, this manifests as proteinuria and progressive renal failure. Angiotensin converting enzyme inhibitors may have a beneficial effect on the outcome of the secondary focal segmental glomerulosclerosis. If the renal insufficiency is severe, renal replacement therapy may be required. Babies can be dialyzed from birth and children as young as 1 year of age can receive renal transplants.

ECTOPIC, FUSED, AND SUPERNUMERARY KIDNEYS

Definition. Ectopic kidneys are sited in abnormal locations, usually in the pelvis (9,10). Renal ectopia may involve only one kidney, or it may be bilateral. The ureter drains into the appropriate side of the bladder in simple ectopia, whereas the ureter crosses the midline and drains into the opposite side of the bladder in crossed ectopia. Fused kidneys often are ectopic, for example, nearer the midline or in the pelvis. Supernumerary kidneys, which of necessity are ectopic, are extremely rare.

Clinical Features. Ectopic, fused, and supernumerary kidneys often are asymptomatic. They may come to attention as palpable masses. Because of their abnormal location, the routes of the blood vessels and urinary tracts that lead to them are abnormal, which may predispose to obstruction, infection, stone formation, and trauma (9). Concurrent urinary tract abnormalities, which often accompany malpositioned kidneys, also add to the risk of infection. Congenital abnormalities in other organs may be present (10).

Gross Findings. Ectopic kidneys that are not fused typically have a reniform shape. They often are abnormally rotated, for example, rotated ventrally so that the pelvis and ureter are positioned more to the front than the medial side of the kidney. Of necessity, blood vessels must follow unusual routes to reach ectopic kidneys. Some ectopic kidneys are hypoplastic, which in some instances may be caused by inadequate blood supply but more likely results from aberrant induction of metanephric blastemal differentiation. The ureters of ectopic kidneys may be more tortuous than normal, especially the proximal portion, which may have to drape over a malrotated or fused kidney, causing obstruction and hydronephrosis.

Fused kidneys have varying shapes. Horseshoe kidneys are fused at one pole (usually the lower) (fig. 2-4); complete fusion of the kidneys most often produces a formless mass in the pelvis (pancake kidney) that gives rise to two or more ureters (fig. 2-5).

Supernumerary kidneys are rare and usually occur below the lower pole of a normally positioned kidney. The ureter from a supernumerary kidney enters the bladder independently or joins the ureter from the ipsilateral kidney before it enters the bladder.

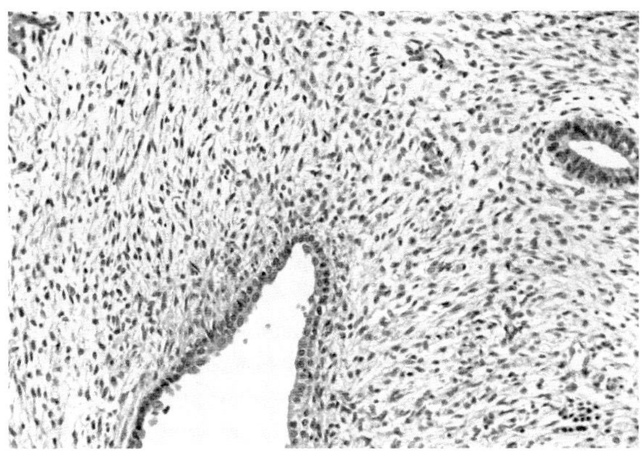

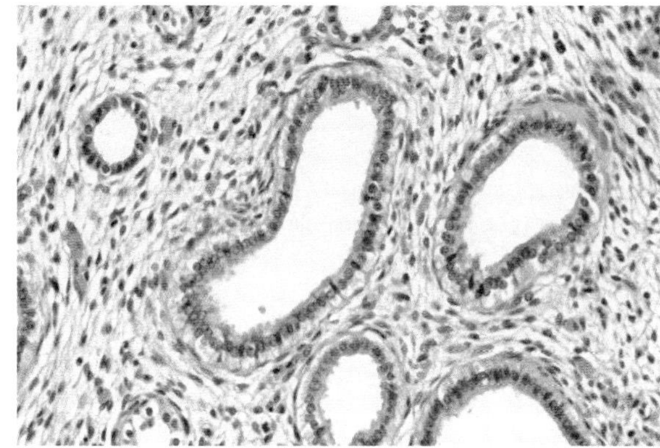

Figure 2-6

RENAL DYSPLASIA

The presence of primitive ducts surrounded by whorls of poorly differentiated mesenchyme is the hallmark of renal dysplasia. The ducts are lined by cuboidal and columnar epithelium.

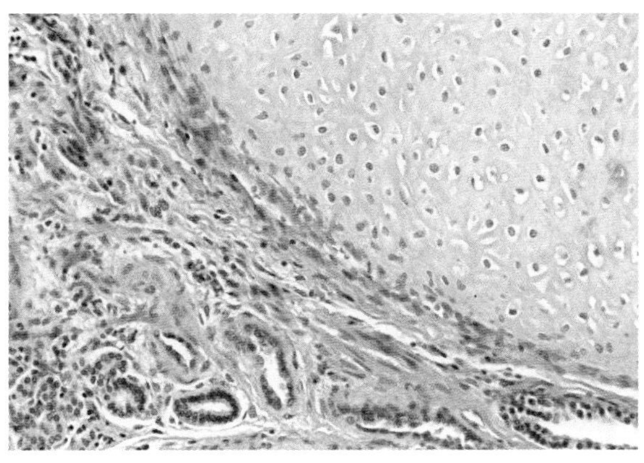

Figure 2-7

RENAL DYSPLASIA WITH CARTILAGE

The island of heterotopic cartilage is adjacent to mesenchymal stroma and primitive tubules.

Light Microscopic Findings. The histology of ectopic and fused kidneys is normal other than some gross architectural disarray at sites of fusion. Pathologic changes secondary to acquired diseases that are more frequent in ectopic and especially fused kidneys, for example, those of chronic pyelonephritis, obstructive nephropathy, or nephrolithiasis, may be observed.

Differential Diagnosis. The major differential diagnostic considerations are clinical rather than pathologic. An ectopic or fused kidney may be palpated during physical examination or seen by imaging studies and misinterpreted as a neoplasm. This has resulted in unnecessary and sometimes very damaging surgery. For example, removal of fused pelvic kidneys has resulted in total ablation of renal tissue. With modern imaging techniques, such a misdiagnosis should be exceedingly rare.

Etiology and Pathogenesis. Renal ectopia probably results from an aberrant site of interaction between the ureteric bud and the metanephric blastema (15), or from abnormal migration of the kidney during organogenesis (10). Fused kidneys result when the two ureteric buds are so close together that the metanephric mesenchyme that they induce overlaps and thus forms a fused mass of renal tissue (6).

Treatment and Prognosis. In the absence of secondary complications such as infection or obstruction, no treatment is necessary.

RENAL DYSPLASIA

Definition. Renal dysplasia is aberrant differentiation of renal parenchyma that does not proceed beyond the production of undifferentiated tubular structures surrounded by primitive mesenchyme (fig. 2-6), sometimes with accompanying divergent differentiation that results in heterotopic tissue such as cartilage (fig. 2-7). The abnormal tubules/ducts may develop into cysts of varying size, however, cyst development is not required for a pathologic diagnosis of renal dysplasia. Although cysts often are a conspicuous feature of renal dysplasia, this category of disease is usually not included as a nosologic variant of polycystic kidney disease.

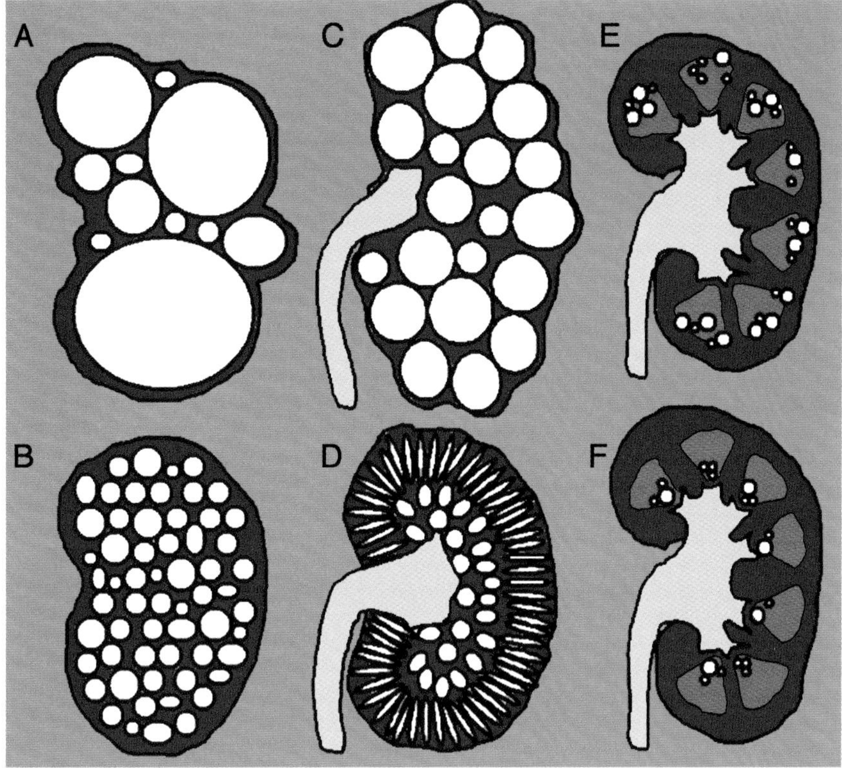

Figure 2-8

PATTERNS OF CYST FORMATION IN DYSPLASIA AND POLYCYSTIC DISEASES

A: A kidney with multicystic dysplasia is not reniform and has multiple cysts of markedly varying sizes.

B: A kidney with diffuse cystic dysplasia is reniform and studded with numerous round cysts of somewhat similar diameter.

C: A kidney with autosomal dominant polycystic kidney disease is distorted by numerous round, variably sized cysts, often greater than 1 cm in diameter.

D: A kidney with autosomal recessive polycystic kidney disease has elongated cysts in the cortex that are perpendicular to the capsule, and rounder cysts in the medulla.

E: A kidney with nephronophthisis-medullary cystic disease complex has variably sized cysts predominantly at the corticomedullary junction.

F: A medullary sponge kidney has cysts primarily confined to the medullary papillary tips.

There are several distinct patterns of dysplasia, including *multicystic dysplasia, aplastic dysplasia, hypoplastic dysplasia, obstructive dysplasia,* and *diffuse dysplasia* (Table 2-1; fig. 2-8). An archaic term for multicystic dysplasia is *Potter's type II cystic disease* and for obstructive dysplasia, *Potter's type IV cystic disease* (27).

Clinical Features. Dysplastic kidneys may be large or small. Kidneys with multicystic dysplasia typically are large. In patients with a multicystic dysplastic kidney, the most common clinical manifestation is a unilateral palpable flank mass detected soon after birth. Small multicystic kidneys may not become apparent until many years later or during postmortem examination. Unilateral renal multicystic dysplasia is the most common cause of an abdominal mass lesion in neonates and occurs in approximately 1 in 5,000 live births and 0.5 percent of autopsies (18,19).

Whereas multicystic dysplasia is rarely bilateral and usually not associated with multisystem syndromic anomalies, diffuse dysplasia usually is bilateral and often occurs as a component of a syndrome of congenital anomalies (Table 2-2). Most of these syndromes have an autosomal recessive inheritance or are a result of trisomies.

Obstructive dysplasia and sometimes hypoplastic dysplasia may manifest in neonates as urinary retention with large, hypertrophied

Table 2-1

CONGENITAL RENAL DISEASES

Congenital Renal Diseases That Arise Early During Organogenesis
Renal agenesis
Renal hypoplasia
Simple hypoplasia
Oligomeganephronic hypoplasia
Renal ectopia and fusion
Renal dysplasia (also see Table 2-2)
Aplastic dysplasia
Multicystic dysplasia
Diffuse cystic and noncystic dysplasia
Obstructive dysplasia
Segmental dysplasia with ectopic ureter
Hypoplastic dysplasia
Congenital Renal Diseases That Arise Late During Organogenesis After Nephron Formation
Polycystic kidney disease
Autosomal dominant polycystic kidney disease (*PKD*)[a]
Autosomal recessive polycystic kidney disease (*PKHD*)
Glomerulocystic disease
Isolated glomerulocystic disease
Combined with other congenital renal diseases
Renal disease with predominately medullary cysts
Nephronophthisis-medullary cystic disease complex (*NPHP, MCKD*)
Medullary sponge kidney
Multisystem syndromes with renal cysts (also see Table 2-2)
Tuberous sclerosis (*TSC*)
Von Hippel-Lindau syndrome (*VHL*)

[a]Responsible genes in parentheses.

Table 2-2

PARTIAL LISTING OF SYNDROMES THAT MAY HAVE RENAL DYSPLASIA AS A COMPONENT[a]

Syndrome	Inheritance
Acrocephaloysyndactyly (Apert's) syndrome	AD[b]
Asphyxiating thoracic dystrophy syndrome	AR
Bardet-Biedl syndrome	AR
Beckwith-Wiedemann syndrome	AD
Branchio-oto-renal syndrome	AD
Camptomelic dysplasia	AR
Cerebro-hepato-renal (Passarge's) syndrome	AR
Fryns' syndrome	AR
Goemine's syndrome	XL
Goldstone's syndrome	AR
Hall-Pallister syndrome	NF
Ivemark's syndrome	AR
Marden-Walker syndrome	AR
Meckel-Gruber syndrome	AR
Dandy-Walker syndrome	AR
Miranda-Feingold variant	AR
Orofacial digital syndrome	XL
Senior-Loken syndrome	AR
Short rib polydactyly syndrome	AR
Trisomy 16-18 (Edwards') syndrome	
Trisomy 13-15 (Patau's) syndrome	
Trisomy 21 (Down's) syndrome	
Zellweger's cerebrohepatorenal syndrome	AR

[a]From references 18, 25, and 26.

[b]AD = autosomal dominant; AR = autosomal recessive; XL = X-linked; NF = nonfamilial.

bladders. Hydronephrosis and pyelonephritis are frequent complications.

Gross Findings. Renal dysplasia can be unilateral or bilateral, and the involved kidney can be abnormally large or very small. The cut surface of a dysplastic kidney typically reveals a loss of lobular architecture, with absent or markedly distorted calyces and medullary pyramids (fig. 2-9). The urinary tracts in approximately 90 percent of patients with dysplastic kidneys have gross abnormalities, such as ureteral agenesis, ureteral atresia, ureteropelvic junction obstruction, ureterovesical stenosis, or posterior urethral valves. This is always the case with obstructive dysplasia and least often the case with bilateral diffuse cystic dysplasia. When ureters are present, the upper portion often is thin and atretic.

Aplastic renal dysplasia results in tiny rudimentary dysplastic kidneys. These often appear as small irregular islands of nondescript tissue in the retroperitoneal fat, sometimes containing small cysts (fig. 2-10, top). Histology is required to confirm that this is aplastic dysplastic renal tissue (fig. 2-10, bottom). Unilateral multicystic dysplasia may undergo involution over time and thus a distinction between involuted multicystic dysplasia and aplastic dysplasia may not be possible in adults without knowledge of the size of the involved kidney during infancy.

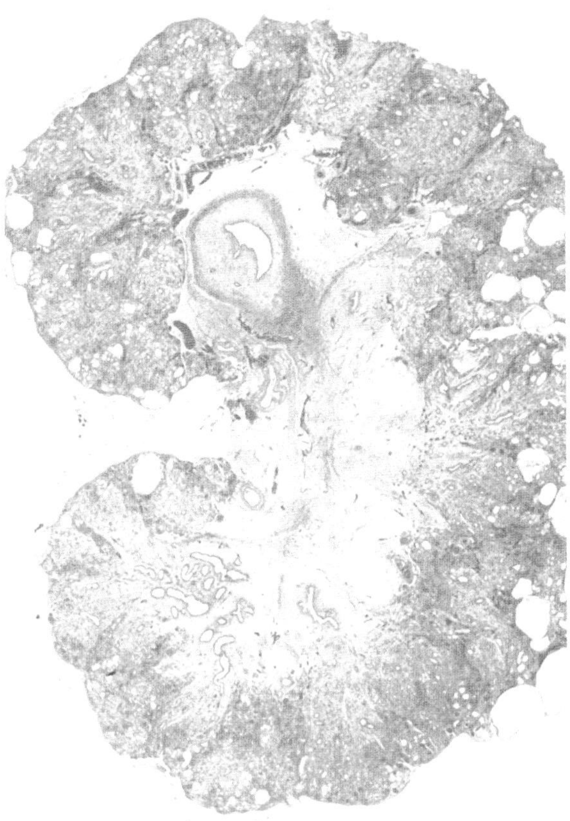

Figure 2-9

DIFFUSE RENAL DYSPLASIA

Low-power magnification shows diffuse renal dysplasia with relatively few cysts. There is no pelvis or calyces. Most of the tissue is pale blue undifferentiated mesenchyme with scattered primitive ducts and tubules (periodic acid–Schiff [PAS] stain).

Multicystic renal dysplasia, which is usually unilateral, is characterized by a kidney enlarged by multiple cysts ranging from microscopic to several centimeters in diameter (figs. 2-8, 2-11). The kidney does not have the usual bean-like (reniform) shape but rather resembles an irregular mass of multiple, variably sized cysts.

Diffuse renal dysplasia is characterized by bilateral, symmetric involvement with preservation the reniform shape (figs. 2-12, 2-13). The dysplasia usually is cystic, with relatively uniformly sized cysts evenly distributed throughout both kidneys. In a minority of patients, the cysts are inconspicuous or absent (fig. 2-9). The term *diffuse noncystic dysplasia* is used when cysts are absent and *diffuse cystic dysplasia* when cysts

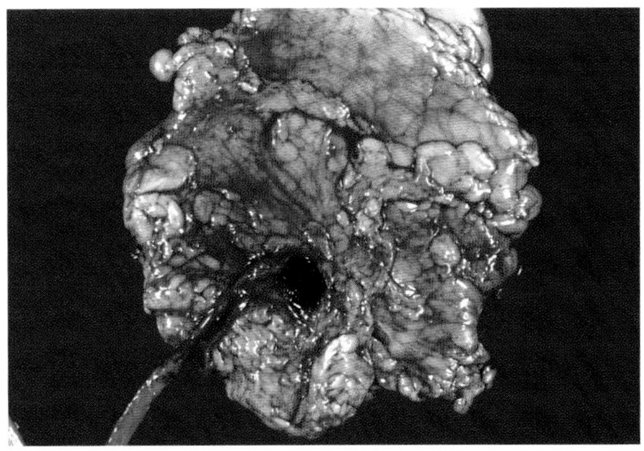

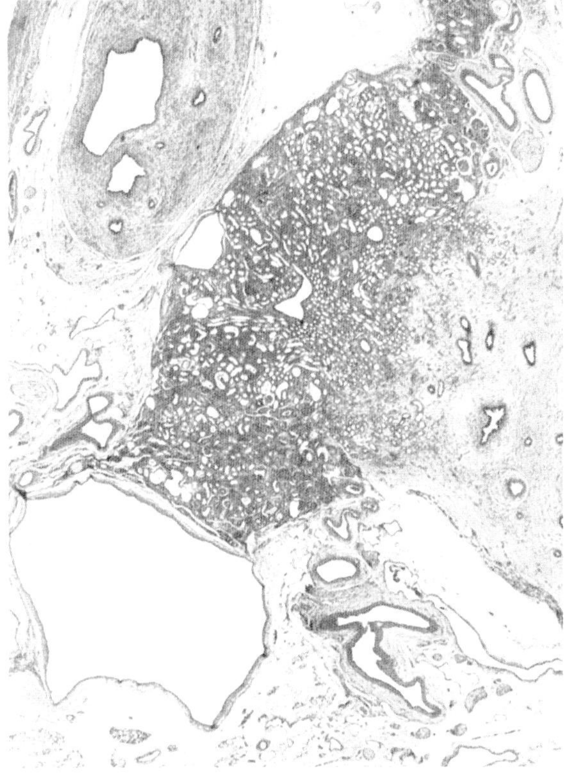

Figure 2-10

APLASTIC RENAL DYSPLASIA

The adult patient had no renal dysfunction but was found to have no identifiable kidney on the right side. The left kidney was enlarged. The patient died of an unrelated cause and at autopsy a right ureter was found but it appeared to end blindly in the retroperitoneal adipose tissue at a small focus of dark discoloration (top). Histologic examination of this area revealed a small amount of dysplastic renal tissue that was 2 cm x 3 cm in cross section (bottom). In the photomicrograph of this tissue, which shows over half of the total cross section, there is a central zone of well-differentiated nephrons surrounded by dysplastic tissue with several cysts. The left kidney was histologically unremarkable except for compensatory hypertrophy.

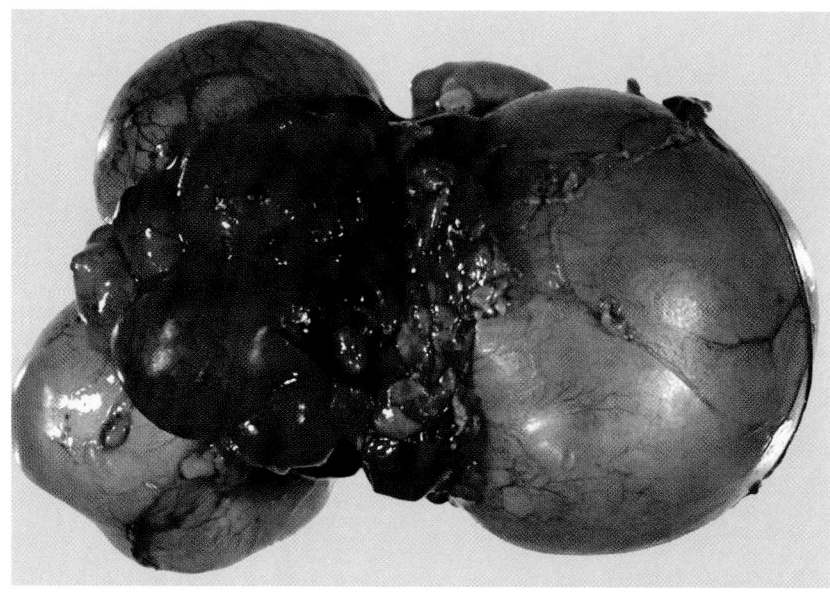

Figure 2-11

MULTICYSTIC RENAL DYSPLASIA

This mass of variably sized cysts does not have a reniform shape.

are present (25). Diffuse renal dysplasia often occurs as a component of a malformation syndrome (Table 2-2).

By definition, obstructive dysplasia is associated with, and may be caused by, congenital urinary tract obstruction. Associated urinary tract abnormalities include posterior urethral valves, urethral atresia, megaureter syndromes, and prune belly syndrome (19). The gross features of hydronephrosis and bladder hypertrophy often accompany obstructive dysplasia (fig. 2-14). The changes associated with acute and chronic pyelonephritis also may develop.

Duplex ectopic ureters are associated with dysplasia of the segment of renal parenchyma that they drain, probably through the mechanism of obstructive dysplasia. This usually affects the upper pole of the kidney but may involve the lower pole (fig. 2-15). The ectopic ureter typically ends with a cystic dilation called a ureterocele.

Hypoplastic dysplasia results in a small misshapen kidney with features that overlap with those of multicystic dysplasia or, more frequently, obstructive dysplasia. Such kidneys may have multiple conspicuous cysts like multicystic dysplasia, however, they are small rather than large. Usually, there is evidence of hydronephrosis, ureteral obstruction, or vesicoureteral reflux, which suggests that this is a variant of obstructive dysplasia.

Light Microscopic Findings. The histologic hallmark of renal dysplasia is primitive tubules and ducts lined by cuboidal or columnar epithelium and surrounded by poorly differentiated mesenchymal tissue (see figs. 2-6, 2-7, 2-9) (18,22,27). There may be scattered foci of heterotopic tissue, most often cartilage (see fig. 2-7), adipose tissue, or smooth muscle, however, this is not a prerequisite. Cartilage is found most often in the subcapsular area (19). Foci of hematopoiesis may be present (fig. 2-16). Small nodular foci of undifferentiated metanephric blastema are identified rarely (17). The tubules and ducts can have varying degrees of dilation, including overt cyst formation (fig. 2-13). Cysts typically have thin fibrous walls lined by flattened epithelium. Malformed, vestigial glomeruli may be seen within the dysplastic tissue. Glomerular cysts may occur, especially with obstructive dysplasia. In dysplastic medullary tissue, there are many fewer tubules (ducts) than normal, usually with no identifiable loops of Henle. This results in a higher ratio of interstitium to tubules/ducts.

Extensive parenchymal injury to fetal and neonatal kidney tissue may secondarily cause focal glomerular sclerosis, parietal epithelial hyperplasia, or both. The epithelial hyperplasia, which resembles the crescent formation caused by glomerulonephritis, is most frequently observed with obstructive dysplasia (fig. 2-17). This

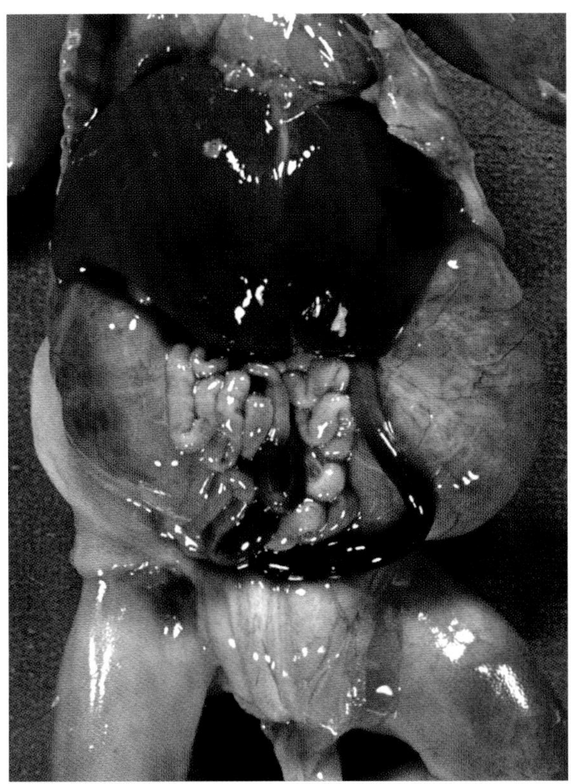

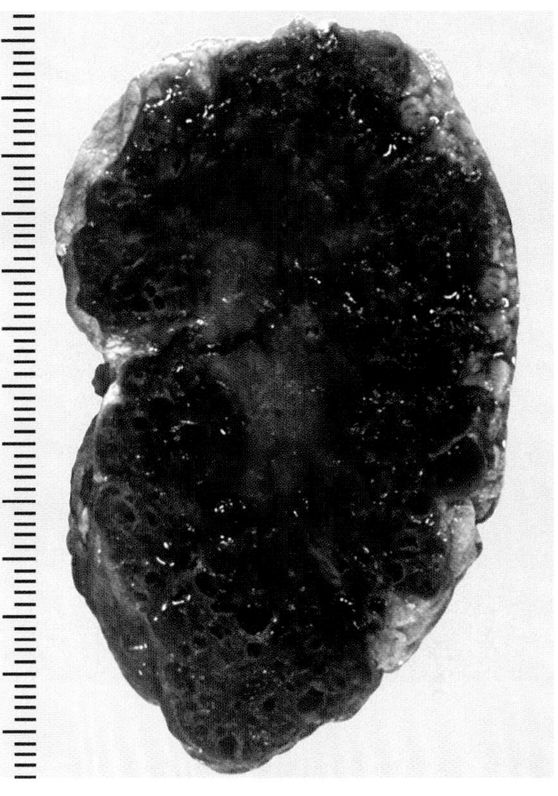

Figure 2-12

DIFFUSE CYSTIC RENAL DYSPLASIA

Left: This term fetus with Meckel-Gruber syndrome has markedly enlarged kidneys that bulge from the abdomen. The kidneys have a reniform shape.

Right: The cut surface reveals numerous cysts that do not vary as much in size as the cysts of multicystic dysplasia. (Figs. 12-16, 12-18 from Churg J, Bernstein J, Risdon RA, Sobin LH. Renal disease: classification and atlas. Part II. New York: Igaku-Shoin; 1987:157, 159.)

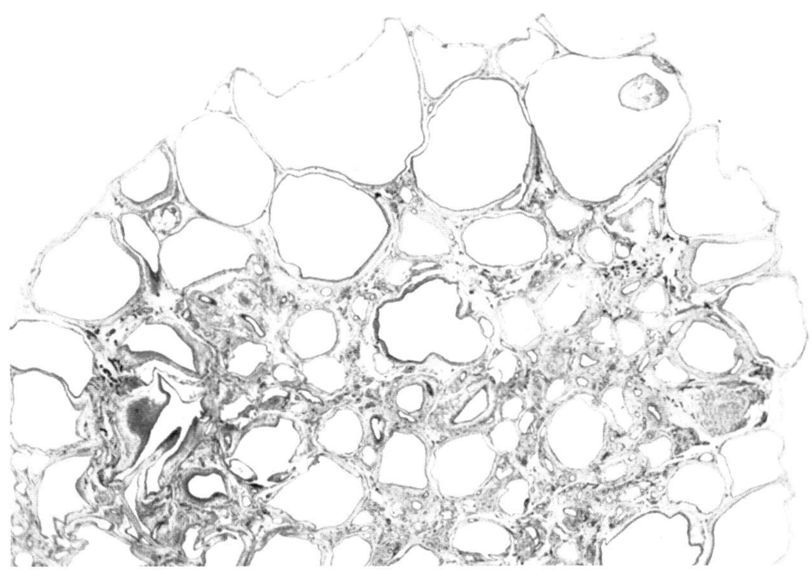

Figure 2-13

DIFFUSE CYSTIC RENAL DYSPLASIA

Low-power magnification shows numerous, relatively round cysts with a small amount of intervening dysplastic renal tissue. There are no differentiated nephrons (Jones methenamine silver [JMS] stain).

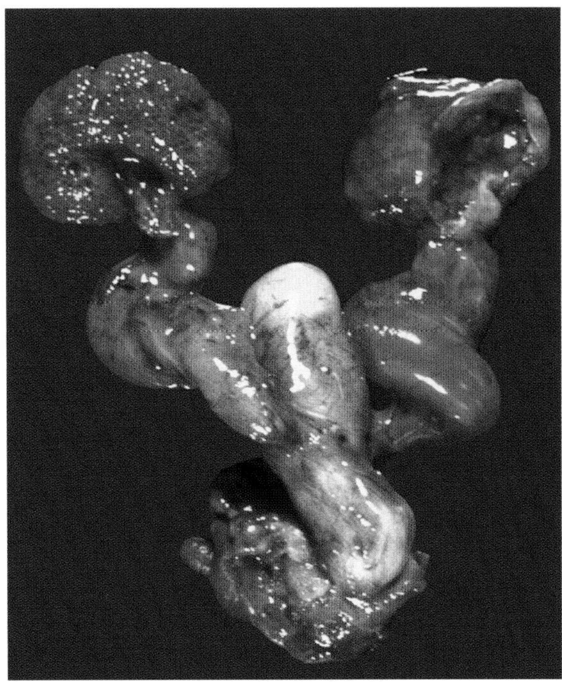

Figure 2-14

OBSTRUCTIVE RENAL DYSPLASIA

These cystic kidneys and dilated ureters are from a 19-week fetus that was stillborn after a pregnancy complicated by oligohydramnios. The fetus had bladder outlet obstruction caused by aplasia of the prostatic urethra. (Courtesy of Dr. H. Liapis, St. Louis, MO.)

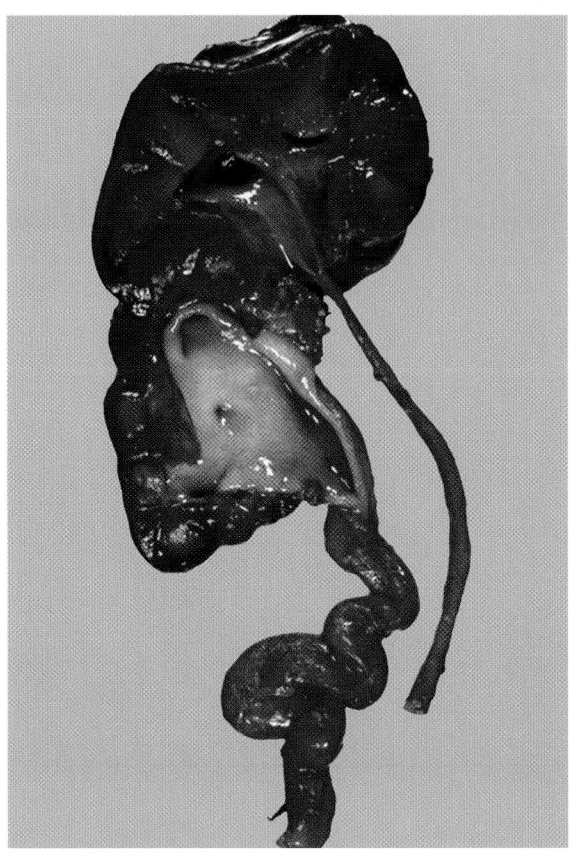

Figure 2-15

SEGMENTAL RENAL DYSPLASIA WITH ECTOPIC URETER

The dilation of the duplicate ureter at the lower portion of the kidney is indicative of obstruction. The renal tissue drained by this ureter is dysplastic. (Fig. 10-5 from Churg J, Bernstein J, Risdon RA, Sobin LH. Renal disease: classification and atlas. Part II. New York: Igaku-Shoin; 1987:127.)

reactive change should not be confused with true glomerulonephritis with crescent formation.

Differential Diagnosis. The clinical differential diagnosis for a large, unilateral, multicystic dysplastic kidney is an abdominal neoplasm, especially Wilms' tumor or neuroblastoma. This usually can be resolved by imaging studies. Aplastic dysplasia must be differentiated from agenesis. The former is diagnosed when a small focus of dysplastic renal parenchyma is identified and the latter when it is not. Diffuse cystic dysplasia must be distinguished from autosomal recessive or early-onset autosomal dominant polycystic kidney disease. The identification of primitive mesenchyme and undifferentiated tubules between the cysts indicates dysplasia. In addition, by gross inspection, autosomal recessive polycystic kidney disease has radially oriented cysts whereas diffuse cystic dysplasia has randomly oriented, more rounded cysts.

Congenital hydronephrosis caused by obstruction of the ureteropelvic junction is distinct from obstructive dysplasia. This condition usually is caused by congenital abnormalities in the smooth muscle in the wall of the ureter at the junction with the pelvis, and results in varying degrees of hydronephrosis with parenchymal atrophy. The most extreme expression results in a large cystic-appearing mass (giant hydronephrosis) with essentially total atrophy of the renal parenchyma caused by pressure and obstruction by the cystically dilated calyces (figs. 2-18, 2-19).

Congenital mesoblastic nephroma has a prominence of stroma tissue with spindle-shaped cells. This stroma may surround entrapped tubular structures. The possibility of segmental

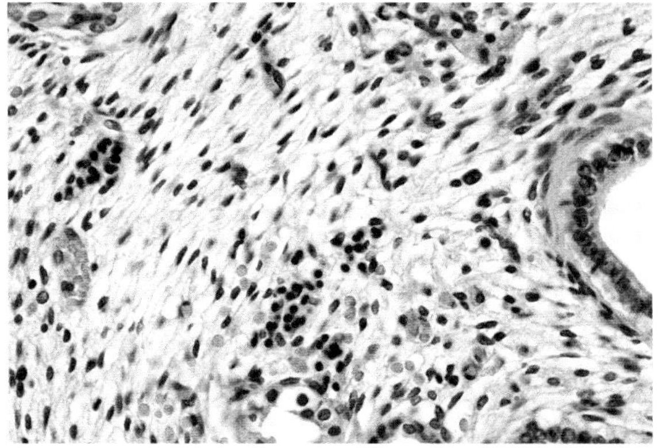

Figure 2-16

RENAL DYSPLASIA WITH HEMATOPOIESIS

Islands of normoblasts with dense round nuclei are scattered in the poorly differentiated mesenchyme of a dysplastic kidney.

dysplasia may be raised by this appearance, however, the overall histologic pattern is quite distinct from dysplasia because the stroma is dense rather than loose like mesenchyme, and the tubules have differentiated features.

Etiology and Pathogenesis. Dysplasia results from abnormal metanephric differentiation. The genetic basis for dysplasia is variable. Multicystic dysplasia is rarely familial and thus is probably not caused by a genetic abnormality in most patients. Aplastic renal dysplasia and diffuse dysplasia are more often hereditary, especially if they are accompanied by congenital anomalies in other organs. There are many syndromes of congenital abnormalities in multiple organs that are associated with dysplasia (Table 2-2); this is probably because many of the genes that are important for renal development, such as hepatocyte growth factor and *PAX2*, are also important for development in other tissues (20).

The importance of ureteric development in the induction of dysplasia is reflected in the frequency of gross and microscopic abnormalities in the ureter and bladder in patients with renal dysplasia (21). Many genetic and nongenetic processes cause abnormalities in the development of the ureteric bud and ureter. Intrinsic abnormalities, such as failure of the ureteric bud to elongate or canalize, and extrinsic abnormalities that secondarily impinge on ureter development or patency, such as extrinsic compression by overlying blood vessels (21), occur. Abnormalities in the ureteric bud, ureters, or distal urinary tract rather than primary defects in the metanephric blastema probably cause most cases of multicystic dysplasia and obstructive dysplasia.

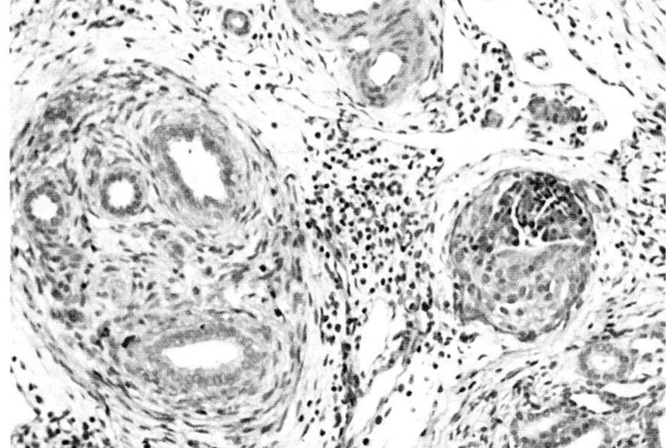

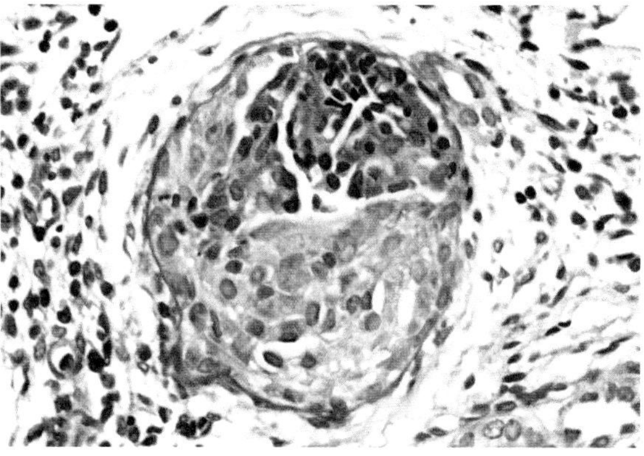

Figure 2-17

GLOMERULAR EPITHELIAL HYPERPLASIA WITH OBSTRUCTIVE DYSPLASIA

Top: The low magnification shows a background of typical renal dysplasia and a glomerulus with epithelial hyperplasia.

Bottom: The higher magnification reveals histologic features that resemble crescent formation in glomerulonephritis, however, in the setting of obstructive dysplasia, a diagnosis of glomerulonephritis should not be made on the basis of this finding alone.

In many instances, the phenotype of the congenital renal anomaly is influenced by a combination of genetic and environmental factors (21,23). This is illustrated by hereditary renal adysplasia. In affected family members, who all share the same genetic defect, the renal anomaly may be unilateral or bilateral renal agenesis, aplastic dysplasia, or multicystic dysplasia (23).

Experimental observations indicate that for the metanephric blastema to differentiate into

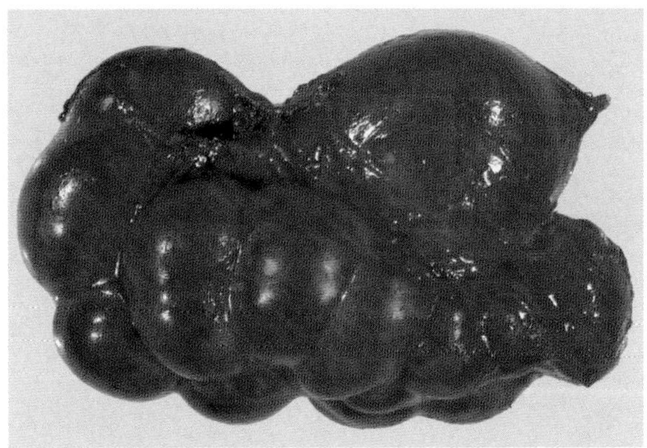

Figure 2-18

GIANT HYDRONEPHROSIS

Giant hydronephrosis is caused by congenital ureteropelvic junction stenosis. The external appearance resembles multicystic dysplasia or autosomal dominant polycystic kidney disease.

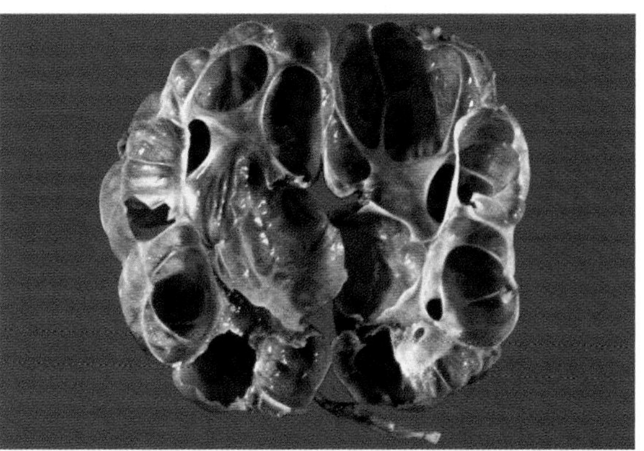

Figure 2-19

GIANT HYDRONEPHROSIS

The cut surfaces of a kidney with giant hydronephrosis reveal a dilated interconnecting pelvis and calyces, with extensive, if not total, atrophy of the renal parenchyma. The ureters are of normal diameter distal to the ureteropelvic stenosis.

normal nephrons rather than evolving into dysplasia, at least two inductive events must occur (21). First, molecular signals must be received by the blastema that prevent the mesenchyme from undergoing excessive apoptosis. Second, diffusion-limited molecules must trigger mesenchymal differentiation into the epithelial components of the nephron. Too little of both processes causes renal agenesis or aplastic dysplasia. Inhibition of apoptosis in the absence of the differentiation signal causes diffuse cystic dysplasia. There also are later signals that induce apoptosis of the residual undifferentiated mesenchyme that is left over after nephrogenesis; for example, angiotensin and its receptors have a role in this process (21). Mutations in these genes could result in residual primitive mesenchyme, which is a major feature of renal dysplasia.

Treatment and Prognosis. Severe bilateral renal dysplasia causes Potter's sequence and is often lethal because of the pulmonary hypoplasia. Unilateral renal dysplasia may cause no signs or symptoms during life and only be detected during postmortem examination. Bilateral obstructive or hypoplastic dysplasia frequently causes substantial renal insufficiency on the basis of the renal and urinary tract anomalies alone, and this may progress because of secondary hydronephrosis and pyelonephritis. A large, unilateral, multicystic dysplastic kidney, which may cause discomfort because of hemorrhage, infarction, or inflammation, is adequately treated by removal. The prognosis for patients with diffuse cystic dysplasia often is influenced as much or more by concomitant abnormalities in other organs in addition to the kidneys (Table 2-2).

AUTOSOMAL DOMINANT POLYCYSTIC KIDNEY DISEASE

Definition. Polycystic kidney disease encompasses a clinically and pathologically heterogeneous group of congenital renal diseases that are characterized by numerous cysts within the renal parenchyma (see Table-2-1; fig. 2-8). By convention, dysplasia with multiple cysts is not considered a form of polycystic kidney disease (35). The two major categories of polycystic kidney disease are autosomal dominant polycystic kidney disease and autosomal recessive polycystic kidney disease. Medullary cystic disease and medullary sponge kidney also are often grouped with these two diseases but have very different clinical and pathologic characteristics.

Autosomal dominant polycystic kidney disease was once called *adult polycystic kidney disease* because it most often manifests during adulthood. The latter term is inappropriate because autosomal dominant polycystic kidney disease manifests at any age. Another archaic term for this category of disease is *Potter's type III cystic disease* (49).

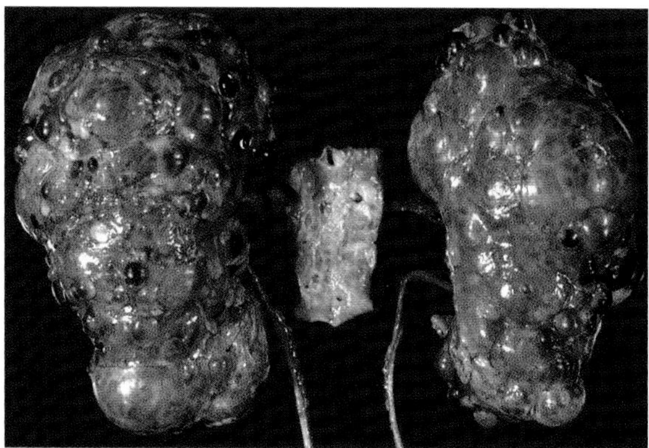

Figure 2-20

AUTOSOMAL DOMINANT POLYCYSTIC KIDNEY DISEASE

Both kidneys are massively enlarged (more than 3 kg each) and have numerous bulging cysts. The ureters are unremarkable.

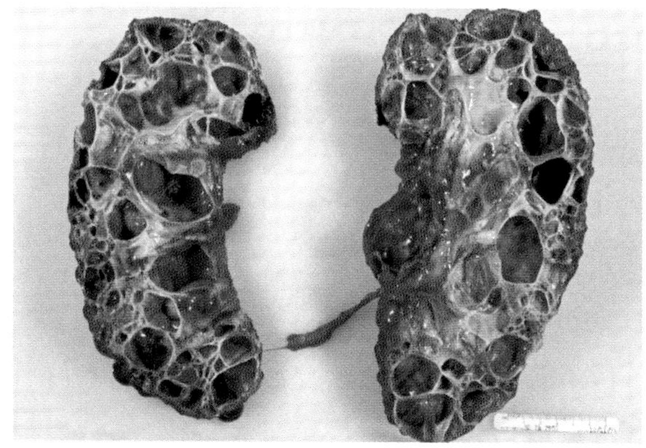

Figure 2-21

AUTOSOMAL DOMINANT POLYCYSTIC KIDNEY DISEASE

The cut surfaces reveal no identifiable residual renal parenchyma. An unremarkable ureter and a somewhat tubular pelvis can be seen entering the kidney on the right.

Clinical Features. The prevalence of autosomal dominant polycystic kidney disease is 1 in 200 to 1,000 population (33,34). It causes approximately 10 percent of ESRD in the United States and is the third leading cause of ESRD, following diabetes and hypertension (33,37). Patients usually develop symptoms during the third to fifth decades of life. However, autosomal dominant polycystic kidney disease may cause clinical manifestations at any age or may remain clinically silent throughout life. A few patients develop clinically significant disease as infants or children (41,43), and there are rare examples manifesting in utero with massive enlargement of cystic kidneys (45). Autosomal dominant polycystic kidney disease with intrauterine expression can cause Potter's sequence (35). If overt disease develops during the first year of life, it often progresses to ESRD during childhood (41,43). Autosomal dominant polycystic kidney disease that develops later in childhood may asymmetrically involve the kidneys, and result in fewer extrarenal manifestations than disease that first becomes clinically apparent in adults.

Once renal cysts become large, manifestations include a sense of heaviness in the loins, bilateral flank and abdominal masses, hematuria (including blood clots in the urine), and progressive renal failure usually beginning during the fourth decade of life. Approximately 50 percent of patients with autosomal dominant polycystic kidney disease have ESRD by 60 years of age. During the course of the disease, most patients develop hypertension; about half, hematuria; and about a quarter, nephrolithiasis.

Extrarenal expressions of autosomal dominant polycystic kidney disease include cystic manifestations in liver, pancreas, meninges, and seminal vesicles, and noncystic manifestations in blood vessels and heart (46). About 20 percent of patients have a prevalence of liver cysts during the third decade of life and 75 percent after the sixth decade. Cystic liver disease is more severe in women and appears to be influenced by estrogen (46). Liver cysts usually are asymptomatic and do not cause liver failure. When symptoms are present, they are due to enlargement and compression of adjacent structures.

Approximately 10 percent of patients have identifiable intracranial aneurysms, which are more frequent in individuals from families with a history of aneurysms. About 20 percent of patients have mitral valve prolapse. Aortic abnormalities include dilation of the aortic root and dissection of the thoracic aorta (46).

Gross Findings. Once cysts are fully developed, the kidneys become markedly enlarged bilaterally, averaging approximately 2.5 kg in severely affected adults and usually ranging from 2.0 to 4.0 kg (figs. 2-20, 2-21) (34,44). Both kidneys are similar in size in most patients, but

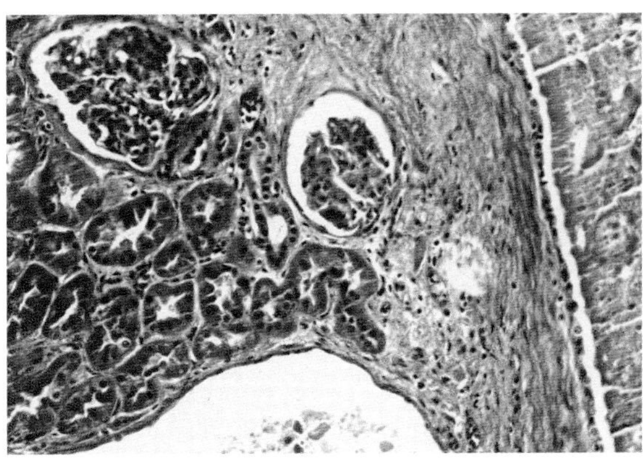

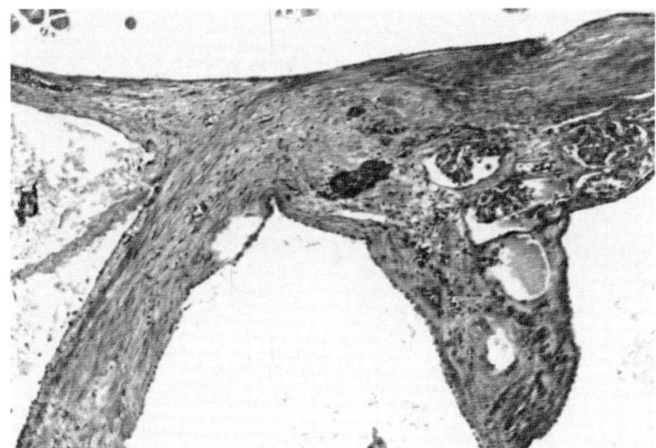

Figure 2-22

AUTOSOMAL DOMINANT POLYCYSTIC KIDNEY DISEASE

There may be relatively intact renal parenchyma between the cysts (left), however, with advanced disease, the intervening renal tissue has marked atrophy and fibrosis (right). The cysts are lined by cuboidal to flat epithelium.

about a quarter of patients have a greater than 30 percent difference between the two kidneys. Asymmetric involvement is seen more often in children than adults.

The external contour of the kidney is cobbled by numerous spherical cysts, most of which range from 0.5 to 5.0 cm in diameter. The cysts typically are filled with clear to yellow fluid, unless there has been hemorrhage (34). The cyst contents sometimes seem to be under pressure because they spurt out when the cyst is cut. With hemorrhage, cysts may contain fluid or clotted blood. Cysts occur in both the cortex and medulla. The distinction between the cortex and medulla is obscured by advanced cystic transformation but persists at earlier stages. The calyces often are markedly distorted by the cysts. The pelvis may be normal or more tubular than usual. The ureters are unaffected.

Additional gross pathologic findings are hepatic cysts in 33 percent of patients, splenic cysts in 10 percent, pancreatic cysts in 5 percent, colonic diverticula in 80 percent, and cerebral arterial aneurysms in 20 percent. Dissection of the thoracic aorta and cervicocephalic arteries also occurs but is uncommon (47). There is an increased risk for renal cell carcinoma in patients with autosomal dominant polycystic kidney disease (30).

Light Microscopic Findings. The cysts usually are lined by a single layer of cuboidal to columnar to flat epithelium (fig. 2-22) (34,44). There often are scattered foci of multilayered proliferations of epithelial cells that may even form polypoid projections into the cyst lumen. Renal cell carcinoma may arise from these foci of hyperplasia (fig. 2-23) (30). The cysts usually appear empty or filled with pale acidophilic material in standard sections. Fresh or degenerated blood may be seen in the cysts as a result of hemorrhage. Cysts arise anywhere along the nephron. Initially, they have patent connections to the nephron lumens, but eventually, the cysts are completely isolated from the nephrons from which they arise (44). As cysts increase in number and size, they compress and eventually replace the normal renal parenchyma. Usually, however, residual distorted renal parenchyma can be identified between the cysts. In the cortex, this includes well-differentiated glomeruli.

Cystic dilation of Bowman's space around glomeruli may occur. Glomerular cysts are most conspicuous in autosomal dominant polycystic kidney disease that occurs in infancy and childhood (fig. 2-24) (44). This raises the pathologic differential diagnostic consideration of glomerulocystic disease, which is discussed later in this chapter.

As the disease advances, the residual parenchyma progressively disappears through cystic transformation and atrophy. Varying degrees of chronic inflammation, fibrosis, and hemosiderin pigmentation are seen in the interstitial tissue. Coagulative necrosis from infarction is rare. Evidence of acute and chronic pyelonephritis may complicate the histologic features.

Hepatic cysts usually are only a few millimeters in diameter, but cysts several centimeters in diameter may occur (39,44). The cysts seem to arise in portal tracts and are lined by a single layer of epithelium that resembles biliary epithelium. Unlike cystic hepatic disease, the cysts of autosomal recessive polycystic kidney disease usually are not associated with substantial adjacent fibrosis. Pancreatic cysts are associated with ductal proliferation and, usually, mild fibrosis.

Differential Diagnosis. Multiple, simple renal cysts may be so numerous that they raise the possibility of polycystic renal disease (34). Simple renal cysts are common acquired lesions that occur in about half of the population over 50 years of age. They usually occur in the outer cortex, bulging the capsule. They typically are lined by nondescript flat epithelium. Simple cysts may occur in kidneys that have no evidence of other parenchymal diseases but are more frequent in kidneys with advanced chronic disease of any type. The extreme expression of this is the acquired cystic disease that occurs in patients with ESRD who are maintained on chronic dialysis. This is discussed later in the chapter.

Early-onset autosomal dominant polycystic kidney disease must be distinguished from autosomal recessive polycystic kidney disease (41,42) and diffuse cystic dysplasia. The latter is readily distinguished histologically by the presence of typical dysplastic mesenchyme and

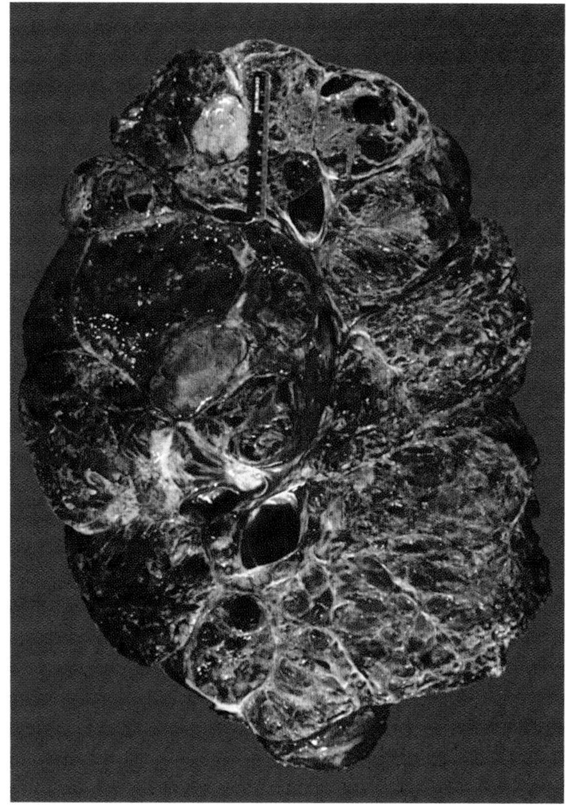

Figure 2-23

AUTOSOMAL DOMINANT POLYCYSTIC KIDNEY DISEASE WITH RENAL CELL CARCINOMA

Several cysts contain tan fleshy tissue that histologically proved to be renal cell carcinoma.

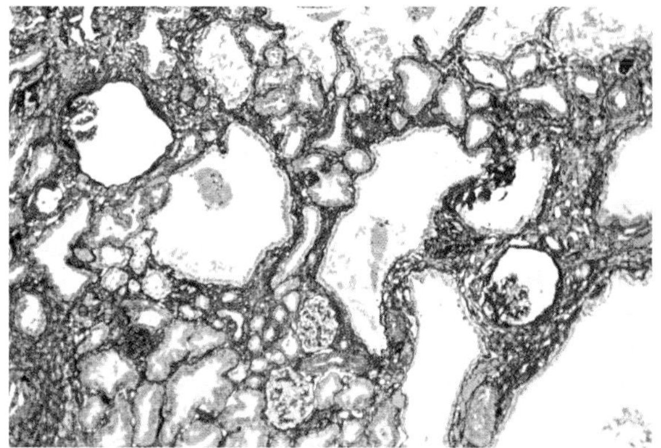

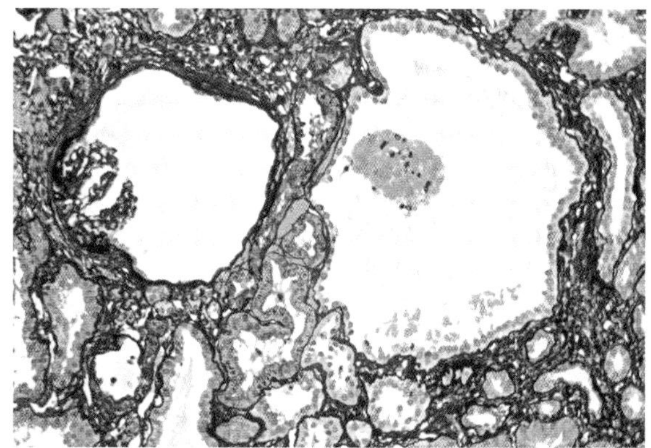

Figure 2-24

CHILDHOOD AUTOSOMAL DOMINANT POLYCYSTIC KIDNEY DISEASE

The cysts in this young child with autosomal dominant polycystic kidney disease involved many different segments of the nephrons, including glomeruli. Two glomerular cysts are seen at low-power magnification (left) and one is seen better at higher magnification (right). The glomerular cyst is lined by flat epithelium that resembles the parietal epithelium of Bowman's capsule, whereas other cysts have cuboidal epithelium (JMS stain).

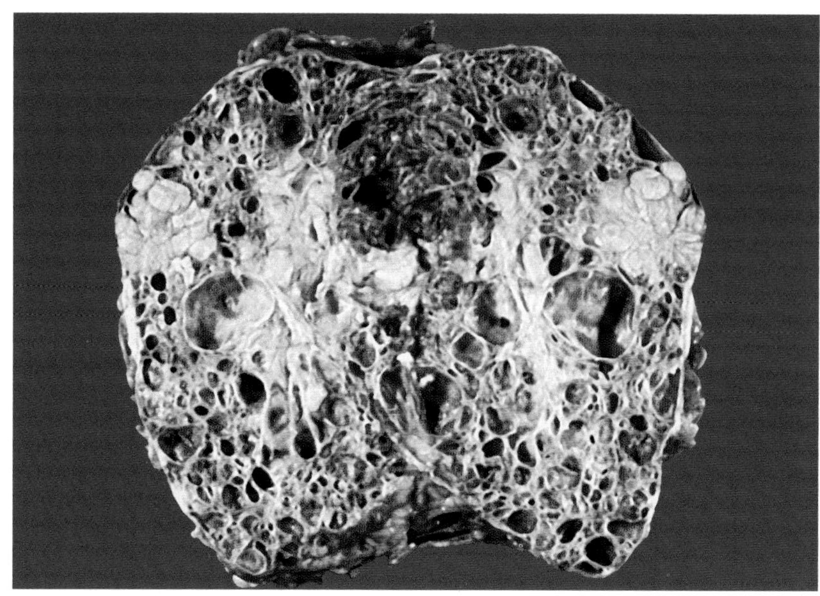

Figure 2-25

ACQUIRED RENAL CYSTIC DISEASE WITH RENAL CELL CARCINOMA

This bivalved kidney has diffuse cystic changes that were acquired during many years of hemodialysis for ESRD. Superimposed on the cystic disease is a multifocal clear cell renal cell carcinoma that can be seen as multiple foci of solid yellow tissue filling or displacing cysts.

primitive tubules and ducts. Early-onset autosomal dominant polycystic kidney disease often has glomerular cysts (fig. 2-24), whereas these essentially never occur with autosomal recessive polycystic kidney disease. In addition, cysts arise in all different segments of the nephron in the former (fig. 2-24), and only from collecting ducts in the latter.

The differential diagnosis for a kidney with numerous cysts affecting multiple sites along the nephron includes tuberous sclerosis and von Hippel-Lindau syndrome. The distinctive features of these hereditary diseases are discussed later in this chapter.

Acquired renal cystic disease may resemble autosomal dominant polycystic kidney disease pathologically (fig. 2-25), but the clinical context and histologic findings of the underlying ESRD usually clearly distinguish this acquired condition. Acquired renal cystic disease occurs in most patients who have been dialyzed for 5 or more years and also occurs in the end-stage kidneys that remain in patients who have received renal transplants (32,34). The kidneys usually weigh less than 200 g and thus are much smaller than kidneys with autosomal dominant polycystic kidney disease. The cysts are embedded in a background of scarred parenchyma and are lined by flat to cuboidal to columnar epithelium. Foci of epithelial hyperplasia are common. Acquired renal cystic disease predisposes to the formation of renal cell carcinoma, possibly from the foci of epithelial hyperplasia within the cysts (fig. 2-25) (32).

Etiology and Pathogenesis. Autosomal dominant polycystic kidney disease usually is inherited as an autosomal dominant trait, however, it may arise as a spontaneous mutation. The genetic abnormality responsible for approximately 85 percent of cases is in the polycystic kidney disease 1 gene (*PKD1*) on chromosome 16, which codes for polycystin-1 (37). *PKD2* on chromosome 4 and *PKD3*, which code for polycystin-2 and polycystin-3, account for 15 percent and less than 1 percent of cases, respectively.

The mechanism of cyst formation is not completely understood, but appears to involve abnormalities in tubular epithelial cell differentiation, proliferation, and secretion, which in turn may be influenced by abnormalities in cell-cell interaction and ion channel function (29,31,37). Cysts arise from many segments of the nephron, and eventually separate from the nephrons to form isolated cysts that continue to enlarge through epithelial proliferation in the cyst walls and fluid secretion into the cyst lumens (31). The proliferation may be monoclonal in some cysts. The delayed onset of cyst formation may be because of a requirement for acquired disruption of a second allele before the germline mutation can cause the formation of the cyst in the kidneys or liver (36,46).

Polycystin-1 and polycystin-2 are expressed in vascular smooth muscle cells in arteries (40,47) and in hepatocytes (37). This is the likely basis for the vascular and hepatic abnormalities that occur in patients with autosomal dominant polycystic kidney disease.

Treatment and Prognosis. Once renal function begins to deteriorate, the rate of deterioration accelerates with time. There is a progressive increase in renal cyst volume and overall renal size, with a concomitant reduction in renal parenchyma and glomerular filtration rate (33). In a study of 324 patients with autosomal dominant polycystic kidney disease in 80 families, the mean age when ESRD was attained was 54 years (45). There was no difference between men and women. Differences in outcome among and within families appear to be multifactorial, but the nature of the genetic mutation has a significant influence (45). Patients with onset of overt disease in infancy have a worse prognosis.

Management of hypertension is an important consideration in most patients. Bacterial infection (pyelonephritis) also is a frequent problem and requires more aggressive antibiotic therapy than typical pyelonephritis because the cysts provide a somewhat protected environment for the infection (35). The most important extrarenal manifestation is the increased risk of intracranial arterial aneurysms. Patients with autosomal dominant polycystic kidney disease have a five-fold increased risk of rupture of an intracranial aneurysm (40). Once rupture occurs, the mortality rate is greater than 35 percent from that episode, and subsequent ruptures may occur. Prospective identification of large cysts and intervention may be beneficial (40).

AUTOSOMAL RECESSIVE POLYCYSTIC KIDNEY DISEASE

Definition. Autosomal recessive polycystic kidney disease is a genetic disease that causes cystic dilation of renal collecting ducts predominantly, with variable involvement of the liver by cystic and fibrotic changes (35). This disease once was called *infantile polycystic kidney disease* because it typically causes markedly enlarged and cystic kidneys in utero that are apparent at birth. This is no longer an acceptable term because autosomal recessive polycystic kidney disease may not become clinically apparent until later in childhood, and other cystic diseases, including autosomal dominant polycystic kidney disease, may be present in infancy. Another archaic term for this category of disease is *Potter's type I cystic disease* (49).

Clinical Features. Autosomal recessive polycystic kidney disease is much less frequent than the autosomal dominant variant. It occurs in 1 in 10,000 to 50,000 live births (35,44). Most infants are stillborn or die in the perinatal period, usually because of respiratory insufficiency caused by pulmonary hypoplasia that results from oligohydramnios and thoracic compression by the enlarged kidneys. Infants who survive into the neonatal period are at risk for developing uremia after varying intervals of time, depending on the severity of the cyst formation. Patients with adequate renal function usually have urine concentrating defects and mild proteinuria. Prolonged survival may be complicated by renal failure with systemic hypertension, hepatic fibrosis with portal hypertension, or both (35,49). Children with prolonged survival are at risk for having chronic lung disease, probably as a result of some degree of pulmonary maldevelopment in utero.

Gross Findings. The kidneys typically are markedly enlarged relative to the expected size for gestational age (35,44,49). They may be so large that they interfere with the delivery of the infant. The enlargement is bilateral and symmetric. Although grossly enlarged, the kidneys are reniform and have a relatively smooth external surface. Close inspection of the external surface reveals numerous, relatively round cysts up to several millimeters in diameter lying beneath the opaque capsule (fig. 2-26). Close inspection of the cut surfaces reveals elongated, fusiform cysts in the cortex that are arranged perpendicular to the capsule, thus producing a radial pattern (figs. 2-8, 2-27). The medulla also has cysts, which are more rounded than those in the cortex (figs. 2-8, 2-28). The calyces are distorted but the renal pelvis and ureter are unremarkable.

Light Microscopic Findings. The most distinctive feature is numerous elongated cortical cysts with their long axis perpendicular to the renal capsule (figs. 2-28, 2-29). The cysts arise predominantly from collecting ducts, but a few cysts may be located in ascending limbs of the

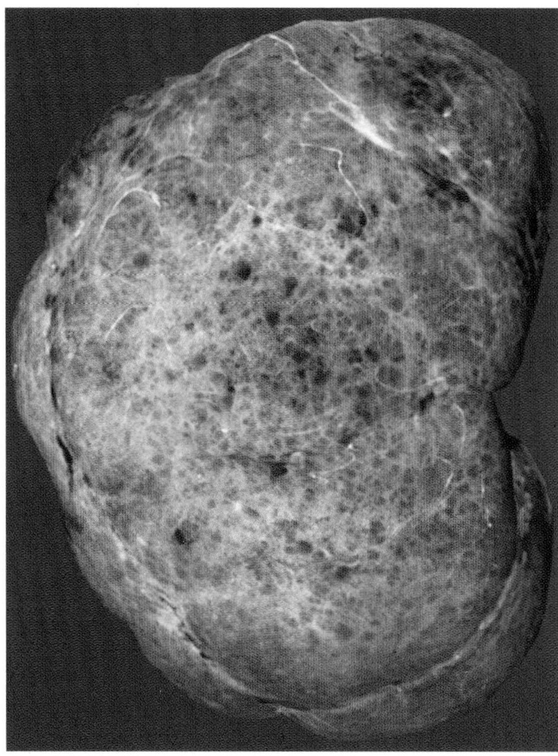

Figure 2-26

AUTOSOMAL RECESSIVE POLYCYSTIC KIDNEY DISEASE

The external surface of a kidney from a 2-month-old girl with autosomal recessive polycystic kidney disease. Myriad cysts that are relatively round from this perspective can be seen through the capsule. (Courtesy of Dr. D. A. Hill, Memphis, TN.)

loop of Henle and proximal tubules (44). Branching may be seen in the cysts, which supports their origin from collecting ducts. Medullary cysts usually are round or oval rather than elongated (fig. 2-28). During gestational weeks 14 to 26, there is a transient phase with more conspicuous cystic change in the proximal tubules, although even during this phase, most cysts arise from collecting ducts (36). Most cysts are lined by a single layer of cuboidal epithelium (fig. 2-29) (49). Typically, these cysts account for the majority of the cortex. Other parenchymal elements are compressed between the cysts. Dysplastic renal tissue is not a feature of autosomal recessive polycystic kidney disease. Interstitial fibrosis usually is minimal, however, this increases in children who survive to an older age.

The cysts become rounder with time if the patient survives beyond the perinatal period, and thus pathologic differentiation between autosomal recessive polycystic kidney disease and childhood autosomal dominant polycystic kidney disease becomes more challenging. Patients who survive past the perinatal period may have a predominance of cysts in the papillary and medullary collecting ducts, which can prompt confusion with medullary sponge kidney. The concurrence of biliary dysgenesis distinguishes atypical, predominantly medullary expression of autosomal recessive polycystic kidney disease from medullary sponge kidney.

Virtually all patients with autosomal recessive polycystic kidney disease have some degree of hepatic biliary dysgenesis (44). The hepatic lesion is characterized by bile duct dysgenesis and dilation (fig. 2-30), surrounded by fibrosis (fig. 2-31) (44,49). In two dimensions, the abnormal bile ducts have a distinctive angulated branching. Three-dimensional reconstruction shows that the abnormal bile ducts form interconnecting sacs and cisterns in the expanded portal zones (44). This configuration is similar to the embryonic stage in bile duct formation and thus appears to be a form of developmental arrest, which is the basis for the term biliary dysgenesis.

There is a reciprocal relationship between the severity of renal cystic disease and the severity of hepatic fibrosis, as well as a reciprocal relationship between the severity of cyst formation and patient survival (28,49). Patients who do not survive beyond the perinatal period typically have renal cysts in approximately 90 percent of collecting ducts but have only minimal hepatic fibrosis. Patients who survive for several months typically have cysts in about half of their collecting ducts and have mild hepatic fibrosis. The minority of patients who survive for longer than a few years have cysts in less than 25 percent of collecting ducts but develop moderate to severe hepatic fibrosis.

Differential Diagnosis. Autosomal recessive polycystic kidney disease must be distinguished from early-onset autosomal dominant polycystic kidney disease (41,42) and diffuse cystic dysplasia. The latter is readily distinguished histologically by the presence of typical dysplastic mesenchyme and primitive tubules and ducts. Early-onset autosomal dominant polycystic kidney disease often has glomerular cysts (fig. 2-24), whereas these essentially never occur with

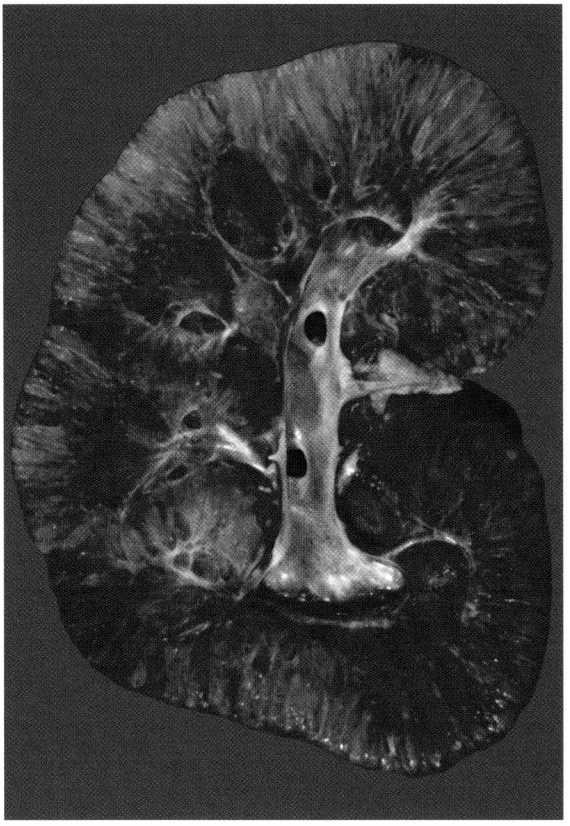

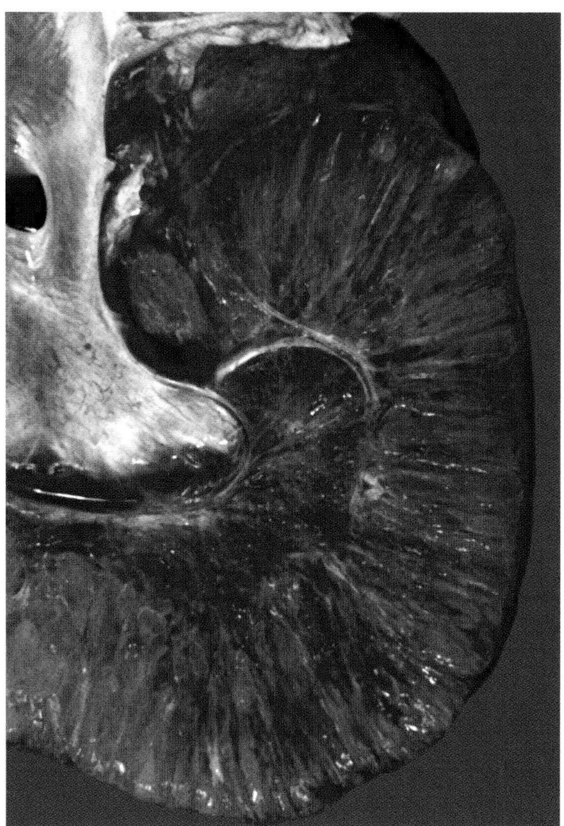

Figure 2-27

AUTOSOMAL RECESSIVE POLYCYSTIC KIDNEY DISEASE

The cut surface of the kidney seen in figure 2-26 shows the ablation of normal architecture by the cysts (left) and the radial arrangement of elongated cysts (right). The pelvis and calyces are present. (Courtesy of Dr. D. A. Hill, Memphis, TN.)

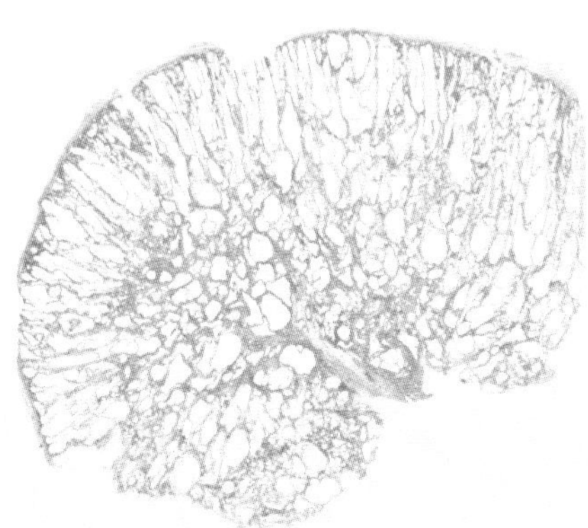

Figure 2-28

AUTOSOMAL RECESSIVE POLYCYSTIC KIDNEY DISEASE

Low-power magnification shows the extensive displacement of parenchyma by mostly elongated cysts oriented predominantly at right angles to the capsule.

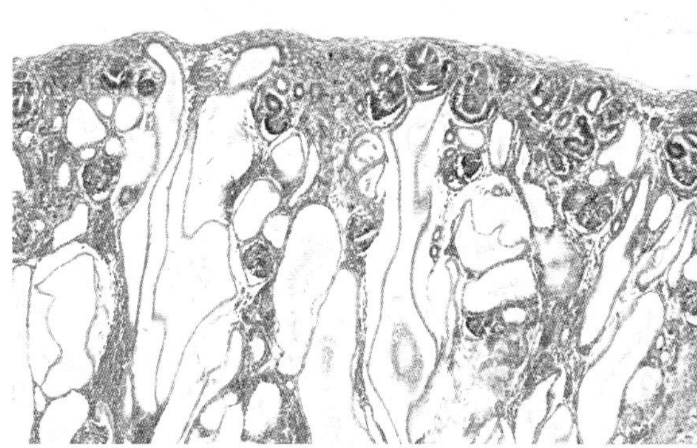

Figure 2-29

AUTOSOMAL RECESSIVE POLYCYSTIC KIDNEY DISEASE

In the subcapsular zone, there are immature glomeruli, and in the deeper cortex, there are a few mature glomeruli between the elongated cysts. The cysts are lined by a single layer of cuboidal epithelium.

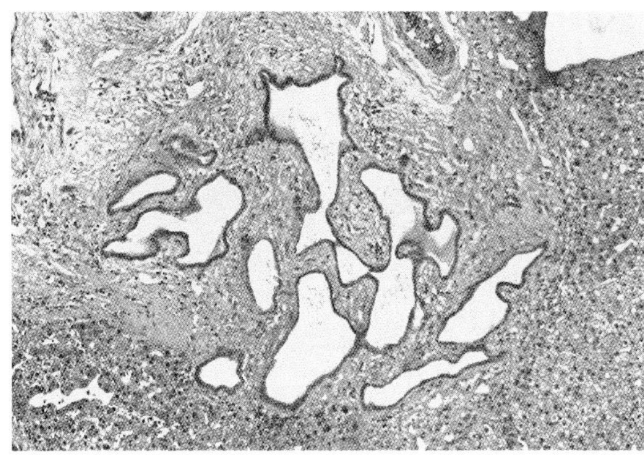

Figure 2-30

HEPATIC BILIARY DYSGENESIS WITH AUTOSOMAL RECESSIVE POLYCYSTIC KIDNEY DISEASE

This expanded portal area has dilated, interconnecting biliary radicals that are surrounded by fibrous tissue. (Courtesy Dr. J. Woosley, Chapel Hill, NC.)

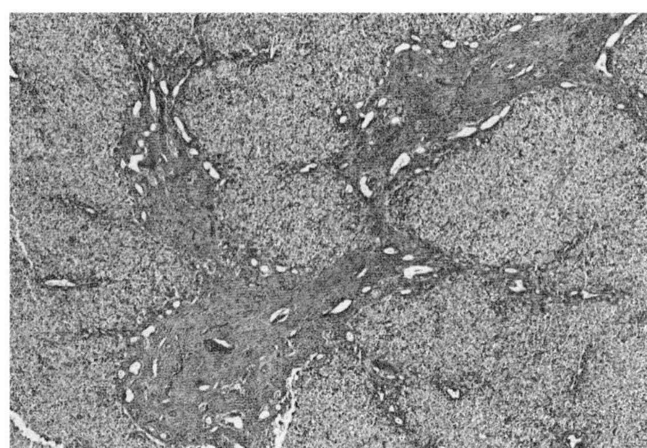

Figure 2-31

HEPATIC FIBROSIS WITH AUTOSOMAL RECESSIVE POLYCYSTIC KIDNEY DISEASE

This low-power photomicrograph shows bands of fibrous tissue associated with the abnormal bile duct proliferation.

autosomal recessive disease. In addition, the former has cysts arising in all different segments of the nephron whereas autosomal recessive disease has cysts arising predominantly from collecting ducts.

Etiology and Pathogenesis. The gene that is mutated in autosomal recessive polycystic kidney disease is the *PKHD1* gene on chromosome 6 (38,48). The gene product, fibrocystin, is a member of a class of proteins that is involved in the regulation of cell proliferation and cell adhesion. The gene is expressed in adult and fetal kidney, liver, and pancreas. Mutations in the *PKHD1* gene apparently disturb the differentiation of renal collecting ducts and hepatic biliary ducts, which results in polycystic kidney disease and biliary dysgenesis.

Treatment and Prognosis. If patients survive past the perinatal period, they are at risk for developing progressive renal failure, systemic hypertension, chronic lung disease, and portal hypertension. Artificial ventilation, bilateral nephrectomy, venovenous hemofiltration, and peritoneal dialysis can be used to support neonates who appear to have a reasonable likelihood of eventually having adequate pulmonary function for survival (35). For those who survive past the perinatal period, management includes control of hypertension and urine concentrating defects. If renal insufficiency is present, management of osteodystrophy and anemia (e.g., with erythropoietin) is important. Dialysis or transplantation are indicated if the patient develops ESRD.

GLOMERULOCYSTIC DISEASE

Definition. Glomerulocystic disease is defined by cystic ectasia of Bowman's capsule in a substantial number of glomeruli (50). This is a histologic phenotype of injury that occurs both as an isolated finding, and, most often, as a component of other congenital or acquired renal diseases, for example, glomerular cysts may be conspicuous in autosomal dominant polycystic kidney disease (especially with childhood onset), nephronophthisis-medullary cystic disease, tuberous sclerosis, obstruction, and dysplasia, especially syndromic diffuse cystic dysplasia (52,54).

Clinical Features. Patients with primary glomerulocystic disease usually have some degree of renal insufficiency, hypertension, and hematuria (54). Ultrasound typically demonstrates large, hyperechoic kidneys. Patients with glomerular cysts as a component of another congenital renal disease have the clinical manifestations of that disease.

Gross Findings. Kidneys with glomerulocystic disease as the only or major pathologic abnormality usually are enlarged, but may be of normal or small size (50,52,54). When small, medullary papillae may be abnormal or absent (54). Glomerular cysts can be seen at the renal surface as spherical structures up to 8 mm in

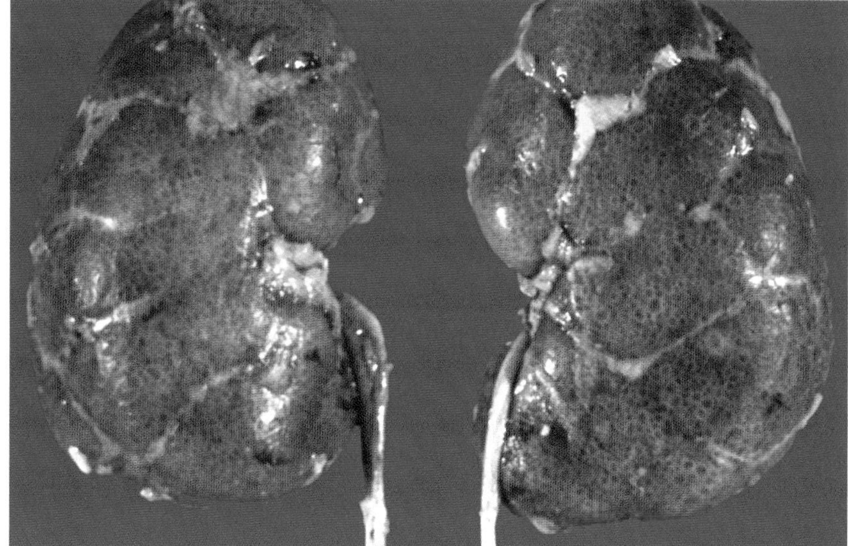

Figure 2-32

GLOMERULOCYSTIC DISEASE

Numerous round cysts are seen through the capsule. (Courtesy of Dr. S. S. Iskandar, Winston Salem, NC.)

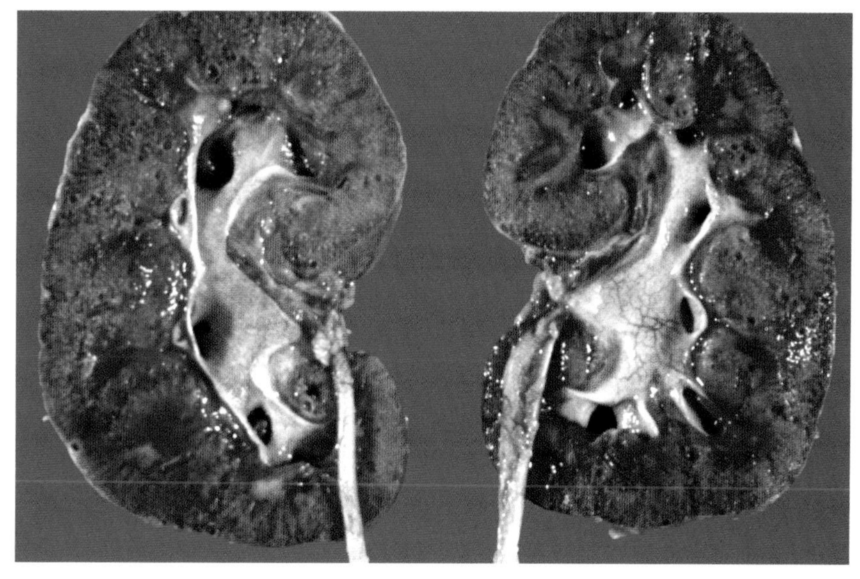

Figure 2-33

GLOMERULOCYSTIC DISEASE

The cut surfaces of the kidneys shown in figure 2-32 show numerous small round cysts scattered throughout the cortex and columns of Bertin. The medullary pyramids lack cysts, distinguishing this from autosomal dominant polycystic kidney disease and autosomal recessive polycystic kidney disease. (Courtesy of Dr. S. S. Iskandar, Winston Salem, NC.)

diameter (fig. 2-32) (53). When glomerular cysts are numerous, the external appearance of the kidney may resemble autosomal recessive polycystic kidney disease, however, the cut surface reveals predominantly round rather than radially arranged elongated cysts and the medulla is spared (fig. 2-33). When glomerular cysts accompany other renal diseases, such as polycystic kidney disease, tuberous sclerosis, or renal dysplasia, these processes usually determine the dominant gross findings.

Light Microscopic Findings. Glomerular cysts are lined by flat to cuboidal epithelium and usually contain a glomerular tuft (fig. 2-34) (50,52). The lining epithelium is rarely multilayered. The glomerular tuft within a cyst may appear normal or may have an atrophic, immature or even vestigial appearance. At a single plane of section, glomerular cysts may appear devoid of glomerular structures, but step sections usually reveal a tuft in most cysts. Glomerular cysts may have a patent communication with proximal tubules (53). Varying degrees of interstitial fibrosis, tubular atrophy, and interstitial infiltration by chronic inflammatory cells usually are present.

Figure 2-34

GLOMERULOCYSTIC DISEASE

Progressively higher-powered magnifications (A–C) show glomerular cysts with marked dilation of Bowman's space, residual immature glomerular tufts, and a single layer of flat epithelium that resembles the normal parietal epithelial cells of Bowman's capsule. At the lowest magnification (A), there is no dysplasia and no cystic changes in other portions of the nephrons.

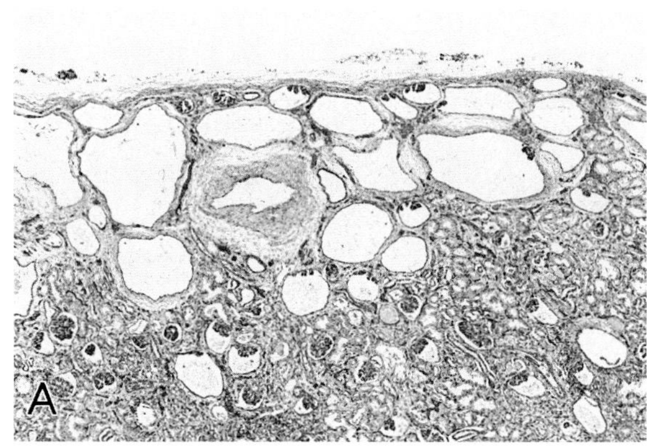

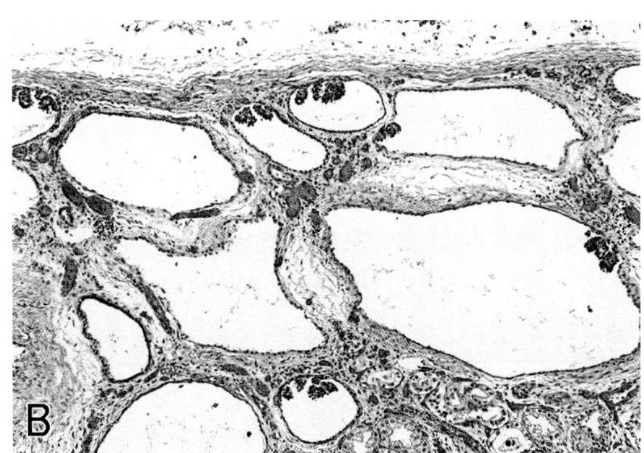

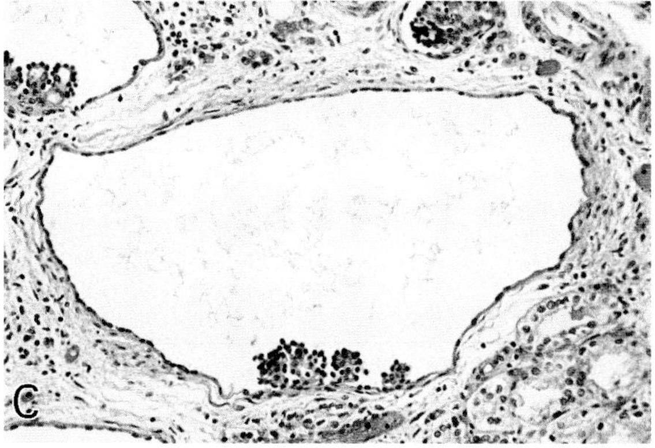

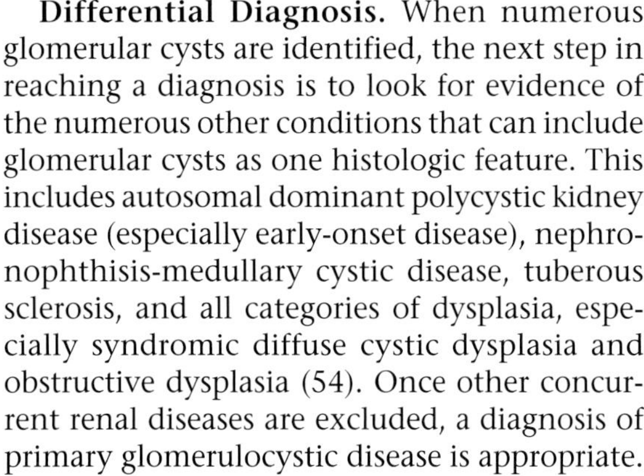

Differential Diagnosis. When numerous glomerular cysts are identified, the next step in reaching a diagnosis is to look for evidence of the numerous other conditions that can include glomerular cysts as one histologic feature. This includes autosomal dominant polycystic kidney disease (especially early-onset disease), nephronophthisis-medullary cystic disease, tuberous sclerosis, and all categories of dysplasia, especially syndromic diffuse cystic dysplasia and obstructive dysplasia (54). Once other concurrent renal diseases are excluded, a diagnosis of primary glomerulocystic disease is appropriate.

Etiology and Pathogenesis. Because of the many different settings in which glomerulocystic changes are found, multiple etiologies are possible. For example, in autosomal dominant polycystic kidney disease, the genetic mutation that causes cystic dilation in all other segments of the nephron appears capable of causing cystic dilation of Bowman's capsule. Glomerulocystic disease with no other renal abnormality (i.e., primary glomerulocystic disease) can be sporadic or familial (51,54). Familial forms usually have an autosomal dominant inheritance. A specific example is a familial form of glomerulocystic disease that is caused by a mutation in the gene for hepatocyte nuclear factor (HNF)-1-beta (51). At least in some forms of primary glomerulocystic disease, the cyst formation is not a result of obstruction or stenosis of the outflow into the proximal tubule (53).

Treatment and Prognosis. The clinical course is extremely variable and often is dependent more on the course of an associated disorder, such as polycystic kidney disease or renal dysplasia. Isolated glomerulocystic disease may progress to ESRD.

NEPHRONOPHTHISIS-MEDULLARY CYSTIC DISEASE COMPLEX

Definition. Nephronophthisis-medullary cystic disease complex is a group of familial chronic tubulointerstitial renal diseases that often have cysts located predominantly at the corticomedullary junction. Nephronophthisis is an autosomal recessive disease that usually progresses to early-onset renal failure whereas medullary cystic disease is an autosomal dominant disease usually with late-onset renal failure (57,58). The diseases are grouped into the nephronophthisis-medullary cystic disease complex because of overlapping pathologic and clinical features.

Clinical Features. Nephronophthisis-medullary cystic disease complex has an incidence of 1 in 50,000 to 100,000, and accounts for 10 to 25 percent of ESRD in children (57,58). All expressions of nephronophthisis-medullary cystic disease complex share the clinical features of polyuria, polydipsia, anemia, and insidious onset of renal failure (57,58). Virtually all patients with autosomal recessive nephronophthisis progress to ESRD by 25 years of age. Because of the absence of edema and hypertension, the renal disease often is not recognized until there is advanced renal failure. Patients with autosomal dominant medullary cystic disease usually do not develop ESRD until the third decade of life. Nephronophthisis, but not medullary cystic disease, is associated with a variety of extrarenal abnormalities, including retinitis pigmentosa (Senior-Loken syndrome), hepatic fibrosis, skeletal defects, and cerebellar vermis aplasia.

Gross Findings. Kidney size is normal or slightly decreased (55,57,58,62). Depending on the extent of chronic tubulointerstitial injury, the external surface is variably granular. With advanced disease, the kidneys are shrunken and fibrotic. In approximately two thirds to three quarters of patients, the cut surfaces of the kidneys reveal multiple 1- to 15-mm cysts, predominantly at the corticomedullary junction (fig. 2-35). The cysts may also be found in the deeper medulla. These grossly discernible cysts are larger and more frequent late in the course of disease. Not all patients have identifiable cysts, thus cysts are not required for a pathologic diagnosis of nephronophthisis-medullary cystic disease complex.

Light Microscopic Findings. The most ubiquitous but somewhat nonspecific histologic finding is marked focal thickening and replication of basement membranes in nonatrophic tubules (figs. 2-36, 2-37) (55,57,58,62). This basement membrane thickening often affects half or more tubules. The thickened basement membranes may have a very frilly or loose woven appearance, sometimes resembling a puff pastry in cross section (fig. 2-36, right). The remaining tubules have normal or thinned basement membranes. Longitudinal sections

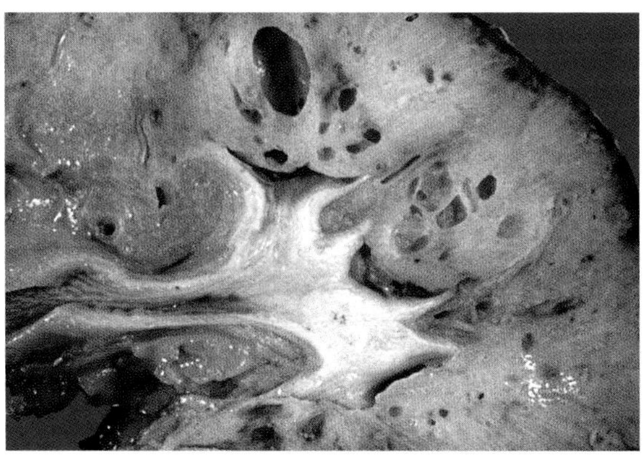

Figure 2-35

NEPHRONOPHTHISIS-MEDULLARY CYSTIC DISEASE COMPLEX

There are numerous cysts in the medulla but the cortex is relatively spared. The cortex is thinned because of chronic tubulointerstitial disease. (Fig. 1-29 from Weiss MA, Mills SE. Atlas of genitourinary tract disorders. Philadelphia: J.B. Lippincott; 1988:1-13.)

through tubules may show alternating foci of thickened and thinned basement membrane. With progressive chronic disease, interstitial fibrosis, tubular atrophy, and chronic inflammation increase. All atrophic tubules have thickened basement membranes, which thus is a nonspecific feature. Islands of Tamm-Horsfall protein may be found in the interstitium (55). Dilated and tortuous tubules are seen most often at the corticomedullary junction. Cyst formation is most frequent in distal tubules. Cysts are lined by a single layer of cuboidal to flat epithelium. With advanced disease, there are varying numbers of glomeruli with segmental or global sclerosis, and periglomerular fibrosis (fig. 2-37).

Electron Microscopic Findings. The tubular basement membrane abnormalities are apparent by electron microscopy (fig. 2-38) (55). There is marked focal thickening and lamination of some tubular basement membranes and thinning of others. Abrupt transitions between thick and thin segments may be observed. These changes are qualitatively similar to ones seen in other chronic renal diseases, but are more extensive.

Differential Diagnosis. The pathologic changes alone, especially in renal biopsy specimens, often are relatively nonspecific. Similar

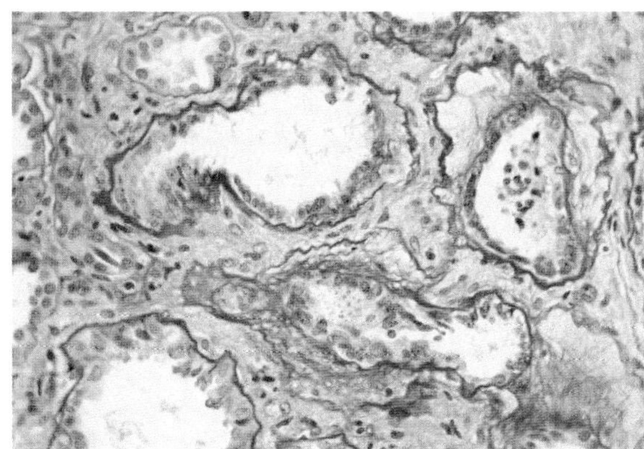

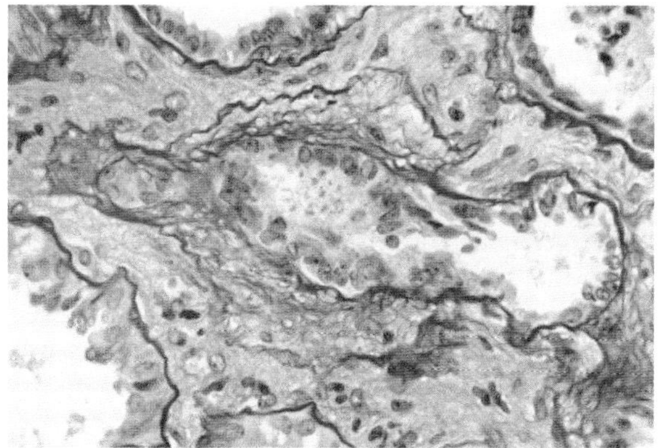

Figure 2-36

NEPHRONOPHTHISIS-MEDULLARY CYSTIC DISEASE COMPLEX

Lower- (left) and higher-powered (right) magnifications show extensive, focally variable thickening and lamination of tubular basement membranes.

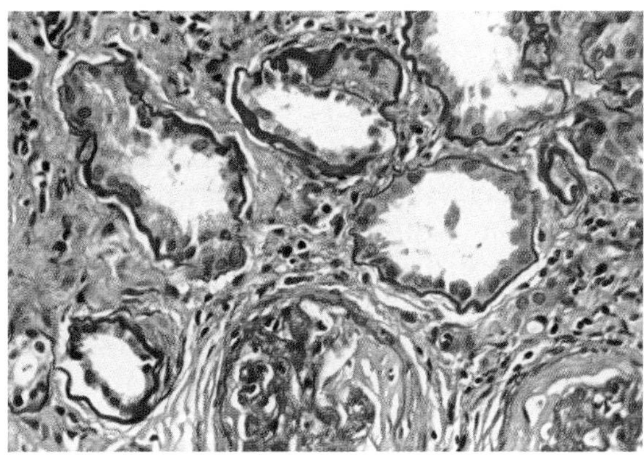

Figure 2-37

NEPHRONOPHTHISIS-MEDULLARY CYSTIC DISEASE COMPLEX

There is extensive thickening and focal lamination of the tubular basement membranes, interstitial fibrosis and chronic inflammation, and glomerular scarring.

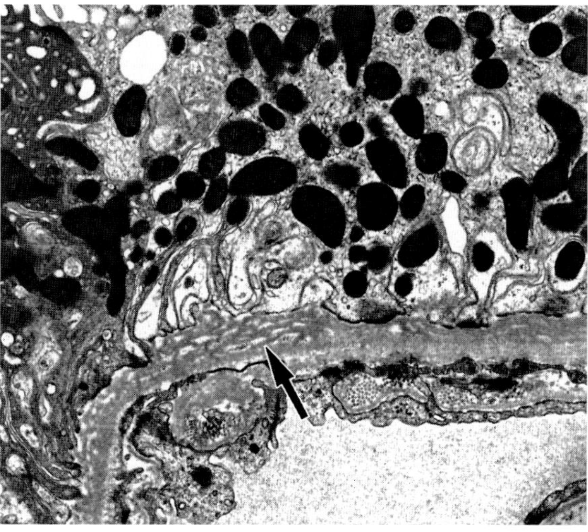

Figure 2-38

NEPHRONOPHTHISIS-MEDULLARY CYSTIC DISEASE COMPLEX

Transmission electron micrograph demonstrates thickening and lamination of the proximal tubular basement membranes (arrow). (Courtesy of Dr. A. Cohen, Los Angeles, CA.)

changes occur with many forms of chronic parenchymal disease, particularly chronic tubulointerstitial nephritis. Focal irregular thickening of basement membranes in tubules that are not atrophic should raise the possibility of nephronophthisis-medullary cystic disease complex. A conclusive diagnosis, however, requires integration of pathologic, clinical, and family history data.

When medullary cysts are prominent, the gross pathologic differential includes medullary sponge kidney. The cysts in medullary sponge kidney essentially always involve the papillary tips whereas the cysts are predominantly at the corticomedullary junction in nephronophthisis-medullary cystic disease complex (see fig. 2-8). In addition, calcification is common in the cysts of medullary sponge kidney but not nephronophthisis-medullary cystic disease complex.

Etiology and Pathogenesis. Structural and functional abnormalities in the tubules, especially in the distal nephron, appear to be the common final pathway of injury caused by the different genetic defects that produce the nephronophthisis-medullary cystic disease complex. Defects in multiple genes can result in autosomal recessive nephronophthisis (e.g., *NPHP1* on chromosome 2, *NPHP2* on chromosome 9, *NPHP3* on chromosome 3, *NPHP4* on chromosome 1) or autosomal dominant medullary cystic disease (*MCKD1*, *MCKD2*). The specific gene involved can influence the clinical phenotype. For example, mutations in *NPHP2* causes early onset of disease in infancy, *NPHP1* and *NPHP4* cause disease with onset in childhood, and *NPHP3* causes disease with onset in adolescence (median, 19 years of age) (60). There is evidence that the genetic abnormalities may cause a defect in the interaction of tubular epithelial cells with basement membrane matrix that results in progressive degenerative changes (57).

Treatment and Prognosis. There is no treatment for the primary abnormality. Therapy is thus directed at managing the consequences of the injury, including correction of abnormalities in electrolytes, acid-base balance, and water balance (57). Osteodystrophy, secondary hyperparathyroidism, and anemia also must be managed in patients with renal failure. All patients eventually require renal replacement therapy. The disease does not recur in renal transplants.

MEDULLARY SPONGE KIDNEY

Definition. Medullary sponge kidney is defined by congenital cystic dilation of the terminal collecting ducts (ducts of Bellini) in the medullary pyramids (56,61).

Clinical Features. Patients are asymptomatic unless the disease is complicated by nephrolithiasis, infection, or hematuria (61,63). Thus the true prevalence is unknown, however, estimates range from 1 in 5,000 to 20,000 (62,63). There is no sex predilection. The disease is diagnosed clinically by imaging techniques. In the absence of complications, medullary sponge kidney causes only mild concentrating and acidification defects. Five to 20 percent of patients who have nephrolithiasis have medullary sponge kidney (63). Patients, especially females, are at increased risk for pyelonephritis irrespective of the presence of nephrolithiasis. Medullary sponge kidney may be associated with a variety of congenital abnormalities in one or more other organs, including Ehler-Danlos syndrome, Beckwith-Wiedemann syndrome, hemihypertrophy, pyloric stenosis, and cardiac malformations.

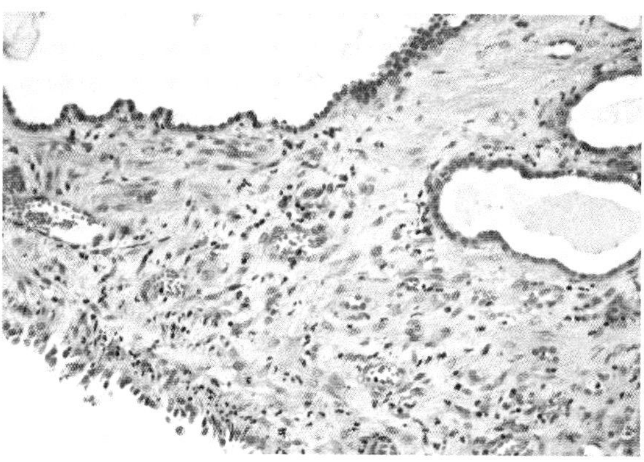

Figure 2-39

MEDULLARY SPONGE KIDNEY

This section through the papillary tip shows the urothelial surface at the lower left. There is slight infiltration by neutrophils, consistent with bacterial infection. Within the papillary tip are portions of three cysts lined by cuboidal epithelium.

Gross Findings. Kidneys usually are of normal size, but about a third of patients have slight renal enlargement (62). The cut surfaces reveal 1- to 8-mm cysts in medullary pyramids, most numerous at the papillary tips (see fig. 2-8). The disease can be unilateral or bilateral, and often is asymmetric among pyramids in one kidney and between kidneys (56,62). Some patients have involvement of only a few pyramids while others have involvement of most pyramids. Cysts may contain irregular calculi, clotted blood, or both. Ulceration of the cyst wall may accompany stones (61). Chronic inflammatory and erosive changes caused by acute and chronic pyelonephritis may be present.

Light Microscopic Findings. Cysts appear to be arising from distal collecting ducts, including the ducts of Bellini (fig. 2-39). They usually are lined by columnar to cuboidal epithelium, which may be multilayered focally (61,62). Occasionally, cysts are lined by transitional or metaplastic squamous epithelium (62). Some ducts are dilated but not overtly cystic. Cyst lumens may contain mineralized material, clotted blood, or leukocytes. Histologic features of acute or chronic infection may be identified (fig. 2-39). The interstitium around cysts that do not have

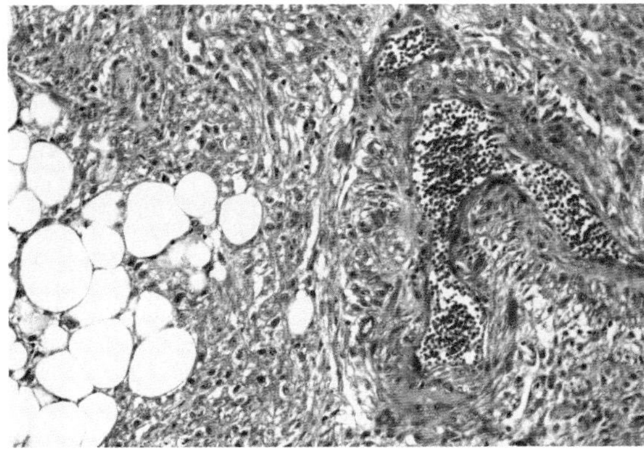

Figure 2-40

RENAL ANGIOMYOLIPOMA IN TUBEROUS SCLEROSIS

The angiomyolipoma has a zone of adipose tissue that merges with a zone of smooth muscle cells, which contains a blood vessel. Some of the smooth muscle cells in the muscularis of the vessel seem to be streaming out into the surrounding sheet of smooth muscle cells.

evidence of infection or nephrolithiasis has increased cellularity but no leukocytic infiltration. Cysts with stones may have ulceration of the epithelial lining and adjacent interstitial inflammation.

Differential Diagnosis. Medullary sponge kidney must be distinguished from nephronophthisis-medullary cystic disease complex. The former essentially always involves the papillary tips whereas papillary tip involvement is rare with nephronophthisis-medullary cystic disease complex, which has a predilection for the corticomedullary junction. In addition, calcification is common in the cysts of medullary sponge kidney but does not occur in the cysts of nephronophthisis-medullary cystic disease complex.

Etiology and Pathogenesis. Most cases of medullary sponge kidney are sporadic, however, familial examples occur. In one kindred with an autosomal dominant inheritance of renal abnormalities, medullary sponge kidney was one of a variety of expressions of ureteral developmental abnormalities (59). This supports the concept that an abnormality in ureteric bud development may be the basis for medullary sponge kidney.

Treatment and Prognosis. The cystic malformations themselves cause no clinically significant renal dysfunction. Management is directed at preventing or controlling secondary nephrolithiasis and infection (63). In the absence of infection or lithiasis, hemorrhage may occur but resolves spontaneously.

TUBEROUS SCLEROSIS

Definition. Tuberous sclerosis is an autosomal dominant disorder characterized by hamartomas in one or more organs, especially the kidney, skin, brain, eye, liver, lung, and bone (68). The most common renal lesions are angiomyolipomas and cysts. A subset of patients has concurrent tuberous sclerosis and early-onset autosomal dominant polycystic kidney disease (64).

Clinical Features. Tuberous sclerosis has a prevalence of approximately 1 in 10,000. The clinical features are extremely variable because of involvement of different organs in different patients. Frequent features include cutaneous angiofibromas, ungual fibromas, retinal astrocytomas, and seizures and mental retardation. More than half of patients have renal involvement with angiomyolipomas, cysts, or both. The renal involvement often is asymptomatic. Angiomyolipomas may cause abdominal pain and a palpable abdominal mass. Large bilateral angiomyolipomas can cause renal insufficiency. Large angiomyolipomas are at risk of rupture with exsanguinating hemorrhage. Concurrent tuberous sclerosis and autosomal dominant polycystic kidney disease often causes ESRD during childhood.

Gross Findings. Approximately 50 percent of patients have renal angiomyolipomas; 5 percent, cysts without hamartomas; and 10 percent, both (69). Renal angiomyolipomas are multinodular or lobulated, firm to fleshy lesions measuring up to 20 cm or more in diameter. They may be single or multiple in one or both kidneys, and are usually clearly demarcated from the adjacent renal parenchyma. The cut surfaces typically are variegated yellow to pink to tan, and may have evidence of recent or remote hemorrhage. Small foci of necrosis may be present. Cysts are occasionally seen within a hamartoma.

Cysts usually are scattered in the renal cortex and medulla. They vary in size from a few millimeters to several centimeters. Concurrent tuberous sclerosis and autosomal dominant polycystic kidney disease results in cystic changes similar to those of autosomal dominant polycystic kidney disease alone.

Light Microscopic Findings. The angiomyolipomas are composed of admixed well-differentiated adipose tissue, smooth muscle cells, and blood vessels (fig. 2-40). Most of the adipocytes appear mature, but there may be a few foci of lipoblasts with central nuclei. In addition to the unremarkable normal vasculature of the lesion, the characteristic vascular components are large, tortuous, thick-walled vessels. There may be asymmetric fibrous intimal thickening. The muscularis is very cellular, and, at the periphery, often seems to stream off into adjacent islands and interconnecting bands of smooth muscle cells (fig. 2-40). The smooth muscle cells may have slight pleomorphism and scattered mitotic figures. Microhamartomas may occur in glomerular segments (68). These appear as solid nodular lesions composed of polygonal to round cells that probably are proliferating mesangial (smooth muscle) cells and endothelial cells.

The cysts appear to arise from any component of the nephron and thus occur in the cortex and medulla. Glomerular cysts may be conspicuous. The cysts often are lined by multilayered epithelium that may have a papillary configuration.

Differential Diagnosis. A major differential diagnostic consideration if cysts are very prominent is autosomal dominant polycystic kidney disease. The identification of small angiomyolipomas between the cysts excludes the latter, although concurrent tuberous sclerosis and polycystic kidney disease is also a possibility (67). Tuberous sclerosis should be considered in the differential diagnosis whenever cysts arise from multiple sites in the nephron. For example, if there are conspicuous glomerular cysts as well as cysts arising from tubules, the possibility of tuberous sclerosis should be considered. Such a diagnosis requires clinical information about the presence or absence of features of tuberous sclerosis. Strong suspicion obviously is raised by a nephrectomy specimen with an angiomyolipoma and cysts. However, a renal biopsy specimen with scattered glomerular and tubular cysts should at least raise this possibility.

Etiology and Pathogenesis. Tuberous sclerosis is caused by mutations in multiple different genes (64). Mutations in the *TSC1* gene on chromosome 9, which codes for hamartin, or in the *TSC2* gene on chromosome 16, which codes for tuberin, cause indistinguishable disease. The *TSC2* gene and the *PKD1* gene are adjacent to each other on chromosome 16. Large mutations that disrupt both genes cause concurrent tuberous sclerosis and severe early-onset autosomal dominant polycystic kidney disease (64).

Treatment and Prognosis. Large bilateral hamartomas or severe cystic disease can cause renal failure; however, most patients with tuberous sclerosis do not require nephrologic management.

VON HIPPEL-LINDAU SYNDROME

Definition. Von Hippel-Lindau syndrome is an autosomal dominant disease characterized by retinal angiomatosis or hemangioblastoma of the central nervous system accompanied by renal cell carcinoma, renal cysts, pancreatic cysts, or pheochromocytoma (66,68).

Clinical Features. The incidence of von Hippel-Lindau syndrome is 1 in 30,000 to 50,000. Lesions develop and progress over time, with most patients becoming symptomatic during the second to fourth decades of life.

More than half of patients with von Hippel-Lindau syndrome have renal cysts that can be identified by renal imaging studies. These cysts rarely cause symptoms, but there is occasional abdominal discomfort or pain. Approximately a quarter of patients have renal cell carcinoma. The signs and symptoms are the same as those for primary renal cell carcinoma.

Gross Findings. The renal cysts usually are bilateral. They typically are scattered throughout both kidneys and are up to 5 cm or more in diameter. Most cyst walls are very thin; however, they may have focal excrescences caused by epithelial hyperplasia or intracystic renal cell carcinoma (68). Compared to primary renal cell carcinoma, renal cell carcinoma in von Hippel-Lindau syndrome is more often bilateral and more often has a cystic component.

Light Microscopic Findings. The cyst lining has varying proportions of flat epithelium interspersed with foci of hyperplasia that may form papillary projections into the cyst lumen (fig. 2-41). Small renal cell carcinomas may be identified arising from cyst walls.

Differential Diagnosis. The differential diagnosis for a kidney with numerous cysts affecting multiple sites along the nephron includes autosomal dominant polycystic kidney disease,

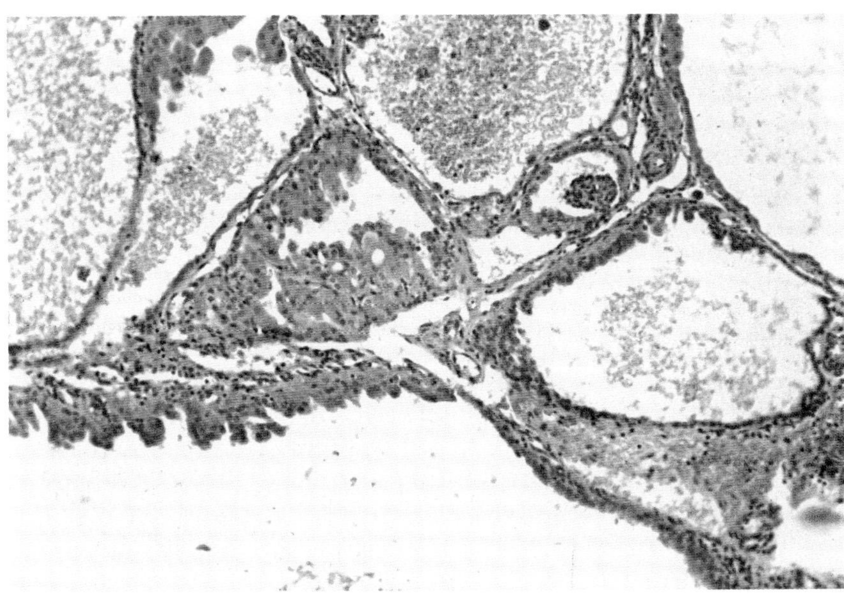

Figure 2-41

RENAL CYSTS IN VON HIPPEL-LINDAU SYNDROME

The cysts are lined by multilayered epithelium with papillary projections. (Courtesy of Dr. S. Seshan, New York, NY.)

tuberous sclerosis, and von Hippel-Lindau syndrome. Of course, the concurrence of renal cell carcinoma and renal cysts always points to von Hippel-Lindau syndrome. A careful family history, ophthalmologic examination, blood pressure determination, and imaging studies of the abdomen and brain are necessary.

Acquired renal cystic disease in patients who are on dialysis and those who have received renal transplants is another setting in which multiple cysts and multiple renal cell carcinomas occur (65). The clinical context allows recognition of this process.

Etiology and Pathogenesis. Von Hippel-Lindau syndrome is caused by a mutation in the *VHL* gene, which is a tumor suppressor gene on chromosome 3 (66). In the kidney, this appears to set the stage for aberrant proliferation of the epithelium that can be expressed as a benign or malignant proliferation, resulting in epithelial cysts or renal cell carcinomas, respectively.

Treatment and Prognosis. Renal cell carcinoma accounts for about half the deaths caused by von Hippel-Lindau syndrome. The control of hypertension is important in patients with pheochromocytomas. Surgical resection may be warranted for renal cell carcinomas or pheochromocytomas.

REFERENCES

Introduction

1. Limwongse C, Clarren SK, Cassidy SB. Syndromes and malformations of the urinary tract. In: Barratt TM, Avner ED, Harmon WE, eds. Pediatric nephrology. Baltimore: Lippincott, Williams, & Wilkins; 1999:427–52.
2. Pohl M, Bhatnagar V, Mendoza SA, Nigam SK. Toward an etiological classification of developmental disorders of the kidney and upper urinary tract. Kidney Int 2002;61:10–9.
3. Pope JC 4th, Brock JW 3rd, Adams MC, Stephens FD, Ichikawa I. How they begin and how they end: classic and new theories for the development and deterioration of congenital anomalies of the kidney and urinary tract, CAKUT. J Am Soc Nephrol 1999;10:2018–28.
4. Risdon RA, Woolf AS. Developmental defects and cystic diseases of the kidney. In: Jennette JC, Olson JL, Schwartz MM, Silva FG, eds. Heptinstall's pathology of the kidney. Philadelphia: Lippincott-Raven; 1998:1149–205.
5. Woolf AS. A molecular and genetic view of human renal and urinary tract malformations. Kidney Int 2000;58:500–12.

Abnormal Amount and Location

6. Bard J. The molecular basis of nephrogenesis and congenital kidney disease. Arch Dis Child 1992;67:983–4.
7. Fetterman GH, Habib R. Congenital bilateral oligonephronic renal hypoplasia with hypertrophy of nephrons (oligoméganéphronie): studies by microdissection. Am J Clin Pathol 1969;52:199.
8. Hiraoka M, Tsukahara H, Ohshima Y, Kasuga K, Ishihara Y, Mayumi M. Renal aplasia is the predominant cause of congenital solitary kidneys. Kidney Int 2002;61:1840–4.
9. Kazanis I, Daskalopoulos G, Dolapsakis G, Vlazakis S, Dimitrakopoulos C. Solitary crossed renal ectopia. Arch Ital Urol Androl 1999;71:197–8.
10. Limwongse C, Clarren SK, Cassidy SB. Syndromes and malformations of the urinary tract. In: Barratt TM, Avner ED, Harmon WE, eds. Pediatric nephrology. Baltimore: Lippincott, Williams, & Wilkins; 1999:427–52.
11. McGraw M, Poucell S, Sweet J, Baumal R. The significance of focal segmental glomerulosclerosis in oligomeganephronia. Int J Pediatr Nephrol 1984;5:67–72.
12. Ng WL, Cheung MF, Chan CW, Yu CL. Oligomeganephronic renal hypoplasia. Pathology 1980;12:639–45.
13. Nishimoto K, Iijima K, Shirakawa T, et al. PAX2 gene mutation in a family with isolated renal hypoplasia. J Am Soc Nephrol 2001;12:1769–72.
14. Parikh CR, McCall D, Englelman C, Schrier RW. Congential renal agenesis: case-control analysis of birth characteristics. Am J Kidney Dis 2002;39:689–94.
15. Pope JC 4th, Brock JW 3rd, Adams MC, Stephens FD, Ichikawa I. How they begin and how they end: classic and new theories for the development and deterioration of congenital anomalies of the kidney and urinary tract, CAKUT. J Am Soc Nephrol 1999;10:2018–28.
16. Risdon RA, Woolf AS. Developmental defects and cystic diseases of the kidney. In: Jennette JC, Olson JL, Schwartz MM, Silva FG, eds. Heptinstall's pathology of the kidney. Philadelphia: Lippincott-Raven; 1998:1149–205.
17. Woolf AS. A molecular and genetic view of human renal and urinary tract malformations. Kidney Int 2000;58:500–12.

Dysplasia

18. Kissane JM. Renal cysts in pediatric patients. A classification and overview. Pediatr Nephrol 1990;4:69–77.
19. Limwongse C, Clarren SK, Cassidy SB. Syndromes and malformations of the urinary tract. In: Barratt TM, Avner ED, Harmon WE, eds. Pediatric nephrology. Baltimore: Lippincott, Williams, & Wilkins; 1999:427–52.
20. Matsell DG. Renal dysplasia: new approaches to an old problem. Am J Kidney Dis 1998;32:535–43.
21. Pope JC 4th, Brock JW 3rd, Adams MC, Stephens FD, Ichikawa I. How they begin and how they end: classic and new theories for the development and deterioration of congenital anomalies of the kidney and urinary tract, CAKUT. J Am Soc Nephrol 1999;10:2018–28.
22. Risdon RA, Woolf AS. Developmental defects and cystic diseases of the kidney. In: Jennette JC, Olson JL, Schwartz MM, Silva FG, eds. Heptinstall's pathology of the kidney. Philadelphia: Lippincott-Raven; 1998:1149–205.
23. Squiers EC, Morden RS, Bernstein J. Renal multicystic dysplasia: an occasional manifestation of the hereditary renal adysplasia syndrome. Am J Med Genet Suppl 1987;3:279–84.
24. Vogler CA, Sotelo-Avila C, Ramon-Garcia G, Salinas-Madrigal L. Nodular renal blastema and metanephric hamartomas in children with urinary tract malformations: a morphologic spectrum of abnormal metanephric differentiation. Semin Diagn Pathol 1988;5:122–31.
25. Watkins SL, McDonald RA, Avner ED. Renal dysplasia, hypoplasia, and miscellaneous cystic disorders. In: Barratt TM, Avner ED, Harmon WE, eds. Pediatric nephrology, 4th ed. Baltimore: Lippincott Williams & Wilkins; 1999:415–25.
26. Woolf AS. A molecular and genetic view of human renal and urinary tract malformations. Kidney Int 2000;58:500–12.
27. Zerres K, Volpel MC, Weiss H. Cystic kidneys. Genetics, pathologic anatomy, clinical picture, and prenatal diagnosis. Hum Genet 1984;68:104–35.

Polycystic Kidney Disease

28. Blyth H, Ockenden BG. Polycystic disease of kidney and liver presenting in childhood. J Med Genet 1971;8:257–84.
29. Grande JP. Polycystin: from structure to function. Kidney Int 2000;57:1770–1.
30. Gregoire JR, Torres VE, Holley KE, Farrow GM. Renal epithelial hyperplastic and neoplastic proliferation in autosomal dominant polycystic kidney disease. Am J Kidney Dis 1987;9:27–38.
31. Hanaoka K, Guggino WB. cAMP regulates cell proliferation and cyst formation in autosomal polycystic kidney disease cells. J Am Soc Nephrol 2000;11:1179–87.
32. Hoshida Y, Nakanishi H, Shin M, Satoh T, Hanai J, Aozasa K. Renal neoplasias in patients receiving dialysis and renal transplantation: clinicopathological features and p53 gene mutations. Transplantation 1999;68:385–90.

33. King BF, Reed JE, Bergstralh EJ, Sheedy PF 2nd, Torres VE. Quantification and longitudinal trends of kidney, renal cyst, and renal parenchyma volumes in autosomal dominant polycystic kidney disease. J Am Soc Nephrol 2000;11:1505–11.
34. Kissane JM. Renal cysts in pediatric patients. A classification and overview. Pediatr Nephrol 1990;4:69–77.
35. McDonald RA, Watkins SL, Avner ED. Polycystic kidney disease. In: Barratt TM, Avner ED, Harmon WE, eds. Pediatric nephrology, 4th ed. Baltimore: Lippincott Williams & Wilkins; 1999:459–74.
36. Nakanishi K, Sweeney WE Jr, Zerres K, Guay-Woodford LM, Avner ED. Proximal tubular cysts in fetal human autosomal recessive polycystic kidney disease. J Am Soc Nephrol 2000;11:760–3.
37. Ong AC, Harris PC, Davies DR, et al. Polycystin-1 expression in PKD1, early-onset PKD1, and TSC2/PKD1 cystic tissue. Kidney Int 1999;56:1324–33.
38. Onuchic LF, Furu L, Nagasawa Y, et al. PKHD1, the polycystic kidney and hepatic disease 1 gene, encodes a novel large protein containing multiple immunoglobulin-like plexin-transcription-factor domains and parallel beta-helix 1 repeats. Am J Hum Genet 2002;70:1305–17.
39. Patterson M, Gonzalez-Vitale JC, Fagan CJ. Polycystic liver disease: a study of cyst fluid constituents. Hepatology 1982;2:475–8.
40. Pirson Y, Chauveau D, Torres V. Management of cerebral aneurysms in autosomal dominant polycystic kidney disease. J Am Soc Nephrol 2002;13:269–76.
41. Proesmans W, Van Damme B, Casaer P, Marchal G. Autosomal dominant polycystic kidney disease in the neonatal period: association with a cerebral arteriovenous malformation. Pediatrics 1982;70:971–5.
42. Pyrah LN. Medullary sponge kidney. J Urol 1966;95:274–83.
43. Rapola J, Kaariainen H. Polycystic kidney disease. Morphological diagnosis of recessive and dominant polycystic kidney disease in infancy and childhood. APMIS 1988;96:68–76.
44. Risdon RA, Woolf AS. Developmental defects and cystic diseases of the kidney. In: Jennette JC, Olson JL, Schwartz MM, Silva FG, eds. Heptinstall's pathology of the kidney. Philadelphia: Lippincott-Raven; 1998:1149–205.
45. Rossetti S, Burton S, Strmecki L, et al. The position of the polycystic kidney disease 1 (PKD1) gene mutation correlates with the severity of renal disease. J Am Soc Nephrol 2002;13:1230–37.
46. Torres VE. Extrarenal manifestations of autosomal dominant polycystic kidney disease. Am J Kidney Dis 1999;34:xlv–xlviii.
47. Torres VE, Cai Y, Chen X, et al. Vascular expression of polycystin-2. J Am Soc Nephrol 2001;12:1–9.
48. Ward CJ, Hogan MC, Rossetti S, et al. The gene mutated in autosomal recessive polycystic kidney disease encodes a large, receptor-like protein. Nat Genet 2002;30:259–69.
49. Zerres K, Volpel MC, Weiss H. Cystic kidneys. Genetics, pathologic anatomy, clinical picture, and prenatal diagnosis. Hum Genet 1984;68:104–35.

Glomerulocystic Disease

50. Bernstein J, Landing BH. Glomerulocystic kidney diseases. Prog Clin Biol Res 1989;305:27–43.
51. Bingham C, Bulman MP, Ellard S, et al. Mutations in the hepatocyte nuclear factor-1beta gene are associated with familial hypoplastic glomerulocystic kidney disease. Am J Hum Genet 2001;68:219–24.
52. Joshi VV, Kasznica J. Clinicopathologic spectrum of glomerulocystic kidneys: report of two cases and a brief review of literature. Pediatr Pathol 1984;2:171–86.
53. Liu JS, Ishikawa I, Saito Y, Nakazawa T, Tomosugi N, Ishikawa Y. Digital glomerular reconstruction in a patient with a sporadic adult form of glomerulocystic kidney disease. Am J Kidney Dis 2000;35:216–20.
54. McDonald RA, Watkins SL, Avner ED. Polycystic kidney disease. In: Barratt TM, Avner ED, Harmon WE, eds. Pediatric nephrology, 4th ed. Baltimore: Lippincott Williams & Wilkins; 1999:459–74.

Medullary Cystic Disease

55. Cohen AH, Hoyer JR. Nephronophthisis. A primary tubular basement membrane defect. Lab Invest 1986;55:564–72.
56. Higashihara E, Nutahara K, Tago K, Ueno A, Niijima T. Unilateral and segmental medullary sponge kidney: renal function and calcium excretion. J Urol 1984;132:743–5.
57. Hildebrandt F. Nephronophthisis. In: Barratt TM, Avner ED, Harmon WE, eds. Pediatric nephrology, 4th ed. Baltimore: Lippincott Williams & Wilkins; 1999:453–8.
58. Hildebrandt F, Waldherr R, Kutt R, Brandis M. The nephronophthisis complex: clinical and genetic aspects. Clin Invest 1992;70:802–8.
59. Klemme L, Fish AJ, Rich S, Greenberg B, Senske B, Segall M. Familial ureteral abnormalities syndrome: genomic mapping, clinical findings. Pediatr Nephrol 1998;12:349–56.

60. Omran H, Sasmaz G, Haffner K, et al. Identification of a gene locus for Senior-Loken syndrome in the region of the nephronophthisis type 3 gene. J Am Soc Nephrol 2002;13:75–9.
61. Pyrah LN. Medullary sponge kidney. J Urol 1966;95:274–83.
62. Risdon RA, Woolf AS. Developmental defects and cystic diseases of the kidney. In: Jennette JC, Olson JL, Schwartz MM, Silva FG, eds. Heptinstall's pathology of the kidney. Philadelphia: Lippincott-Raven; 1998:1149–205.
63. Watkins SL, McDonald RA, Avner ED. Renal dysplasia, hypoplasia, and miscellaneous cystic disorders. In: Barratt TM, Avner ED, Harmon WE, eds. Pediatric nephrology, 4th ed. Baltimore: Lippincott Williams & Wilkins; 1999:415–25.

Tuberous Sclerosis and von Hipple-Lindau Disease

64. Brook-Carter PT, Peral B, Ward CJ, et al. Deletion of the TSC2 and PKD1 genes associated with severe infantile polycystic kidney disease—a contiguous gene syndrome. Nat Genet 1994;8:328–32.
65. Hoshida Y, Nakanishi H, Shin M, Satoh T, Hanai J, Aozasa K. Renal neoplasias in patients receiving dialysis and renal transplantation: clinicopathological features and p53 gene mutations. Transplantation 1999;68:385–90.
66. Latif F, Tory K, Gnarra J, et al. Identification of the von Hippel-Lindau disease tumor suppressor gene. Science 1993;260:1317–20.
67. Mitnick JS, Bosniak MA, Hilton S, Raghavendra BN, Subramanyam BR, Genieser NB. Cystic renal disease in tuberous sclerosis. Radiology 1983;147:85–7.
68. Risdon RA, Woolf AS. Developmental defects and cystic diseases of the kidney. In: Jennette JC, Olson JL, Schwartz MM, Silva FG, eds. Heptinstall's pathology of the kidney. Philadelphia: Lippincott-Raven; 1998:1149–205.
69. Stillwell TJ, Gomez MR, Kelalis PP. Renal lesions in tuberous sclerosis. J Urol 1987;138:477–81.

3 CONGENITAL NEPHROTIC SYNDROME

Congenital nephrotic syndrome is a term applied to the development of nephrotic syndrome at birth or within the first 3 months of life (9,10, 37). Some cases are even detectable before birth. By contrast, *infantile nephrotic syndrome* refers to the occurrence of nephrotic syndrome in infants between 3 and 12 months of age (10). The manifestations of nephrotic syndrome in the first months of life include heavy proteinuria, edema, hypoalbuminemia, and hyperlipidemia.

With the application of renal biopsy, genetic analysis, and serologic measurement of antibodies to infectious agents, it has become clear that congenital and infantile nephrotic syndromes are caused by a variety of distinct clinical-pathologic conditions (Tables 3-1–3-3). Some conditions are unique to this young age group (Finnish-type congenital nephrotic syndrome, diffuse mesangial sclerosis, congenital syphilis, and congenital toxoplasmosis); other glomerular diseases occur as well in older children and adults (such as minimal change disease, focal segmental glomerulosclerosis, diffuse mesangial hypercellularity, membranous glomerulopathy, lupus nephritis, mercury intoxication, alpha-1-antitrypsin deficiency, and hemolytic uremic syndrome). In most cases, renal biopsy is essential to differentiate between these entities. This chapter focuses primarily on congenital nephrotic syndrome of the Finnish type and diffuse mesangial sclerosis.

CONGENITAL NEPHROTIC SYNDROME OF THE FINNISH TYPE

Definition. Congenital nephrotic syndrome of the Finnish type (CNF) is an inherited disorder of autosomal recessive transmission that manifests as severe, unremitting nephrotic syndrome within the first 3 months of life.

Table 3-1

MAJOR CAUSES OF CONGENITAL NEPHROTIC SYNDROME (ONSET AT BIRTH OR WITHIN FIRST 3 MONTHS OF LIFE)

Genetic
- Congenital nephrotic syndrome of the Finnish type (CNF)
- Diffuse mesangial sclerosis (DMS)
  - Isolated DMS
  - Associated with Denys-Drash syndrome
- Epidermolysis bullosa (focal segmental glomerulosclerosis)

Infectious
- Congenital syphilis (membranous glomerulopathy)
- Congenital toxoplasmosis (mesangial proliferative glomerulonephritis)

Idiopathic
- Minimal change disease
- Diffuse mesangial hypercellularity
- Focal segmental glomerulosclerosis
- Membranous glomerulopathy

Other
- Hemolytic uremic syndrome
- Lupus nephritis

Table 3-2

MAJOR CAUSES OF INFANTILE NEPHROTIC SYNDROME (ONSET 3 TO 12 MONTHS OF AGE)

Genetic
- Diffuse mesangial sclerosis (DMS)
  - Isolated
  - Associated with Denys-Drash syndrome
- Steroid-resistant nephrotic syndrome (SRNS)

Infectious
- Congenital human immunodeficiency virus (HIV) infection (focal sclerosis or minimal change disease)
- Congenital syphilis (membranous glomerulopathy)
- Cytomegalovirus (proliferative glomerulonephritis)

Idiopathic
- Minimal change disease
- Diffuse mesangial hypercellularity
- Focal segmental glomerulosclerosis
- Membranous glomerulopathy

Other
- Hemolytic uremic syndrome (thrombotic microangiopathy)
- Alpha-1-antitrypsin deficiency (membranoproliferative glomerulonephritis)
- Lupus nephritis (any World Health Organization [WHO] class)
- Mercury poisoning (membranous glomerulopathy)

Table 3-3

MAJOR GENETIC FORMS OF CONGENITAL AND INFANTILE NEPHROTIC SYNDROME

Disease	Gene	Locus	Product	Inheritance	Onset
CNF[a]	*NPHS1*	19q12-13	nephrin	autosomal recessive	<0-3 mos
DMS[b]	*WT1*	11p13	WT1	autos recessive/sporadic	0-9 mos
SRNS	*NPHS2*	1q25-31	podocin	autosomal recessive	3 mos-5 yrs

[a]CNF = congenital nephrotic syndrome of the Finnish type; DMS = diffuse mesangial sclerosis; SRNS = steroid-resistant nephrotic syndrome.

[b]Includes cases of Denys-Drash syndrome.

Clinical Features. Over half the cases have occurred in Finland, with an incidence of 1.2 in 10,000 live births (15). The frequency of genetic carriers has been estimated at 1 in 200 in Finland. However, the disease also occurs, at a lower incidence, in many countries throughout Europe and North America, and in diverse ethnic groups. The incidence in North America has been estimated at 1 in 50,000.

A prenatal diagnosis of CNF is suspected as early as 16 to 18 weeks of gestation if elevated alpha-fetoprotein levels are detected in the maternal serum or the amniotic fluid, reflecting fetal proteinuria (35). Affected fetuses are often born prematurely with postural deformities, such as contractures of the knees and elbows (28). There is an increased incidence of breech birth and other malpresentations. These abnormalities are likely due to constriction of the fetus by an abnormally large placenta. In fact, a high placental/fetal weight ratio (over 0.25) is a heralding feature of this disease.

The infant is typically small for gestational age, with widened cranial fontanelles and a small low-bridged nose. One quarter of infants have edema at birth; the remainder develop nephrotic syndrome within the first 3 months of life. Ascites often produces breathing difficulties due to compression of the lungs by a markedly distended abdomen.

The level of proteinuria is extremely high, ranging from 1 to 6 g/day (massive levels for an infant). Initially, the proteinuria is highly selective, resembling that seen in minimal change disease. As the disease progresses, the proteinuria becomes increasingly poorly selective. Serum albumin levels are extremely low, averaging less than 0.5 g/dL. Other features include microhematuria and signs of tubular dysfunction, including aminoaciduria and glycosuria. Although renal function is usually normal at birth, there is a progressive decline in the glomerular filtration rate over the first 3 to 4 years of life.

Few infants survive to an age when end-stage renal failure would develop (about age 4 to 8 years of age). Many die within the first year of life from complications of unremitting nephrotic syndrome, particularly from infections and sepsis; the latter are caused by a marked reduction in plasma immunoglobulin (Ig)G, approaching agammaglobulinemic levels (13). Other complications include growth retardation, delayed motor and mental development, hypercoagulability leading to thrombotic events, hypothyroidism due to urinary loss of thyroid-binding globulin, vitamin D deficiency due to loss of vitamin D–binding protein, and iron deficiency.

Gross Findings. At autopsy, the kidneys are enlarged and pale, with smooth, swollen cortices (2). The ratio of kidney to body weight at birth is generally increased, exceeding twice normal. The cause of the large swollen kidney likely relates to tubular dilatation and interstitial edema. In addition, there is quantitative evidence of an increased number of nephrons (40). Minute cortical cysts may be identified with a hand-magnifying lens.

Light Microscopic Findings. The histologic findings vary with the stage of the disease (27). The earliest manifestation is focal cystic dilatation of the proximal tubules (figs. 3-1, 3-2). This change is usually first observed in the inner cortex and the corticomedullary junction. Over time, cysts spread to involve the outer cortex, with relative sparing of the inner medulla (figs. 3-3, 3-4). Lectin studies have revealed the majority of cysts to be proximal in origin, although

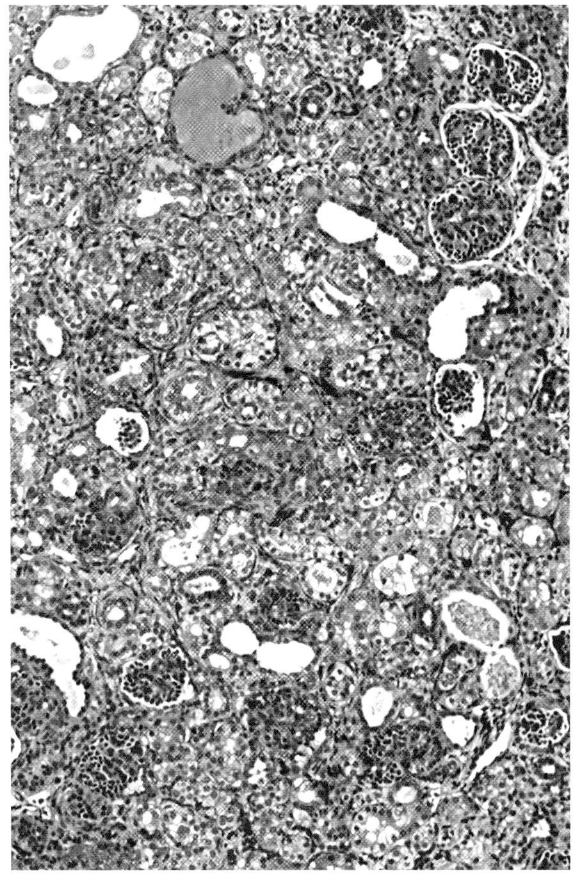

Figure 3-1

CONGENITAL NEPHROTIC SYNDROME OF THE FINNISH TYPE

Early disease shows focal tubular cysts, some of which contain proteinaceous casts (hematoxylin and eosin [H&E] stain).

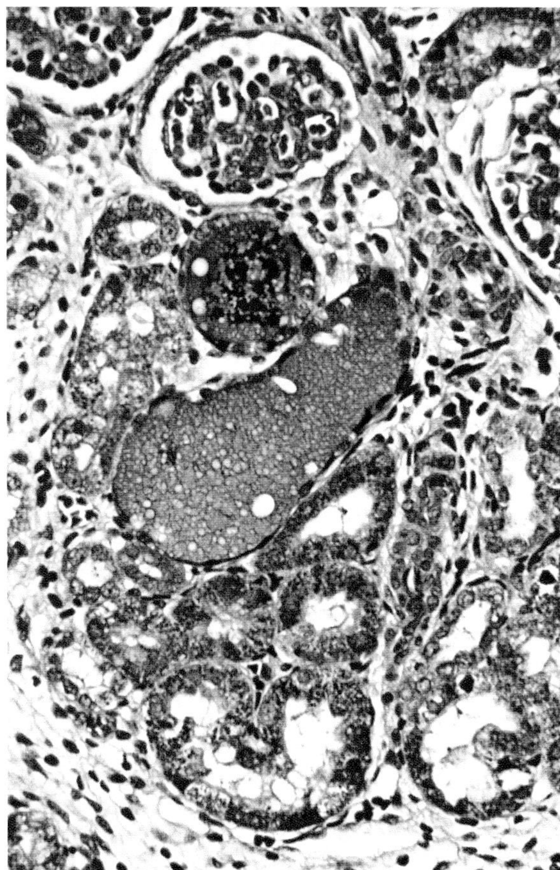

Figure 3-2

CONGENITAL NEPHROTIC SYNDROME OF THE FINNISH TYPE

An example from a 20-week fetal abortus shows a focal tubular cyst and normal-appearing glomeruli (Masson trichrome stain).

the distal tubules may be involved as the disease evolves. Cysts increase in number and size with age, reaching a maximum diameter of 100 to 400 µm. Some cysts contain proteinaceous eosinophilic casts, whereas others appear empty (fig. 3-5). The epithelium of the proximal tubule often contains intracytoplasmic protein resorption droplets, that are periodic acid–Schiff (PAS) positive and trichrome red (fig. 3-6). Clear lipid resorption droplets may also be seen in the proximal tubular cells (fig. 3-7). The epithelium lining the cyst may become flattened and atrophic. Although cysts are highly characteristic of the disease, not all cases of CNF manifest cysts (fig. 3-8): the incidence of tubular cysts varies from 67 to 75 percent in reported series.

Although glomerular changes are generally inconspicuous by light microscopy in the early stages of disease, they become more obvious as the disease progresses. There are no pathognomonic glomerular findings. Some patients have normal-appearing glomeruli (fig. 3-9). The number of infantile glomeruli is usually consistent with gestational age, although a few investigators have reported increased or reduced numbers of microglomeruli compared to normal age-matched controls. In some cases, the earliest manifestation is an increase in mesangial cellularity and matrix, producing slight glomerular enlargement (figs. 3-10, 3-11). These mesangial alterations are usually confined to the mature glomeruli and spare the fetal glomeruli.

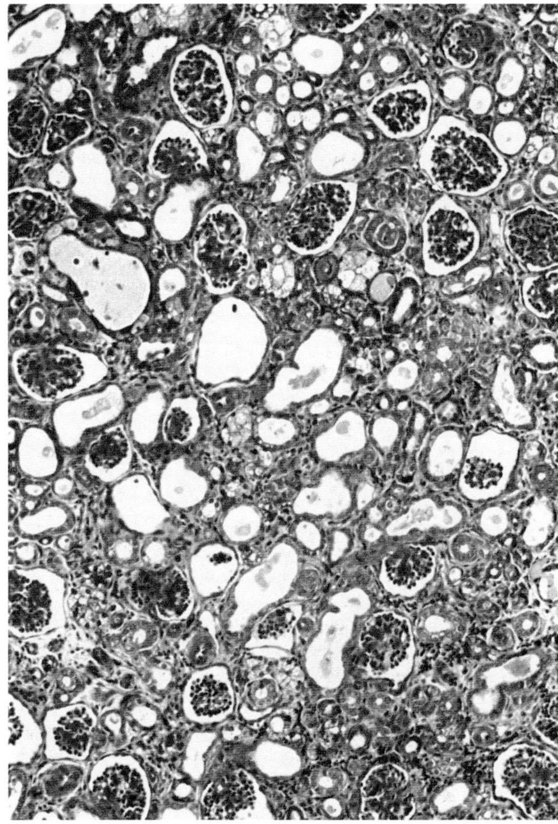

Figure 3-3

CONGENITAL NEPHROTIC SYNDROME OF THE FINNISH TYPE

Biopsy from a 2-month-old infant shows extensive tubular cysts and focal immature glomeruli (Masson trichrome stain).

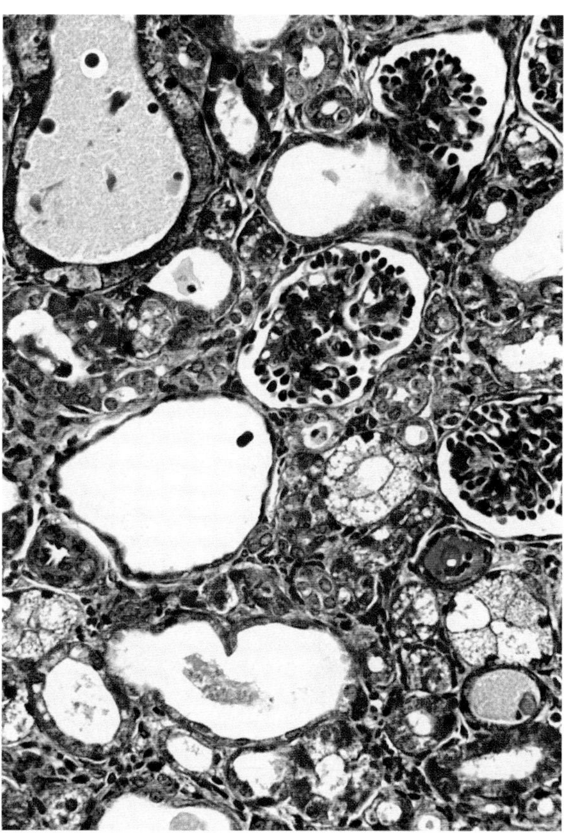

Figure 3-4

CONGENITAL NEPHROTIC SYNDROME OF THE FINNISH TYPE

High-power view shows numerous tubular cysts lacking casts. Some of the tubular cysts are lined by flattened epithelium (Masson trichrome stain).

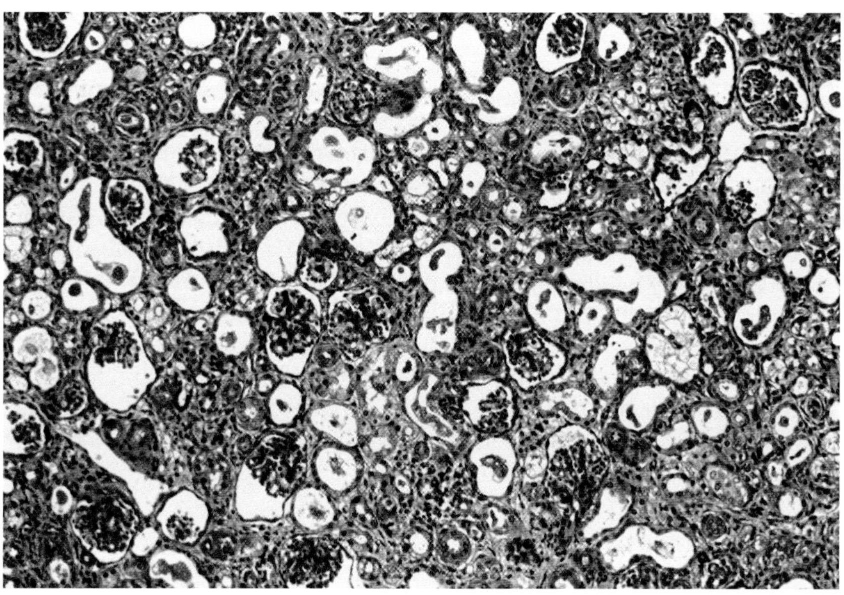

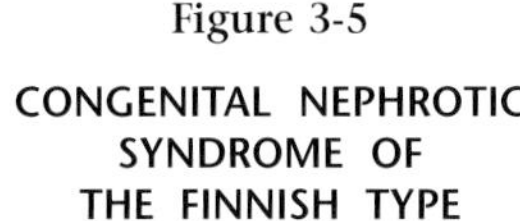

Figure 3-5

CONGENITAL NEPHROTIC SYNDROME OF THE FINNISH TYPE

There are numerous tubular cysts, most of which contain small hyaline casts (periodic acid–Schiff [PAS] stain).

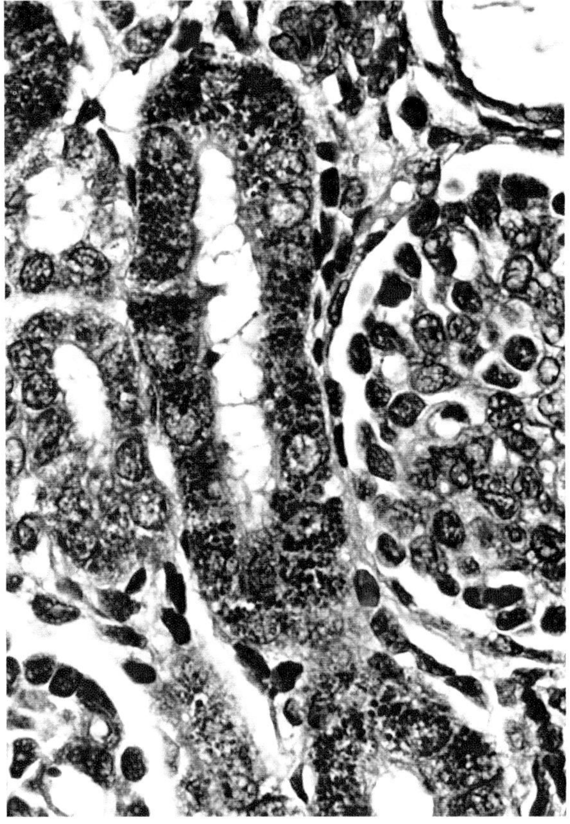

Figure 3-6

CONGENITAL NEPHROTIC SYNDROME OF THE FINNISH TYPE

Proximal tubular epithelial cells contain numerous protein resorption droplets that stain red (fuchsinophilic) with the trichrome stain.

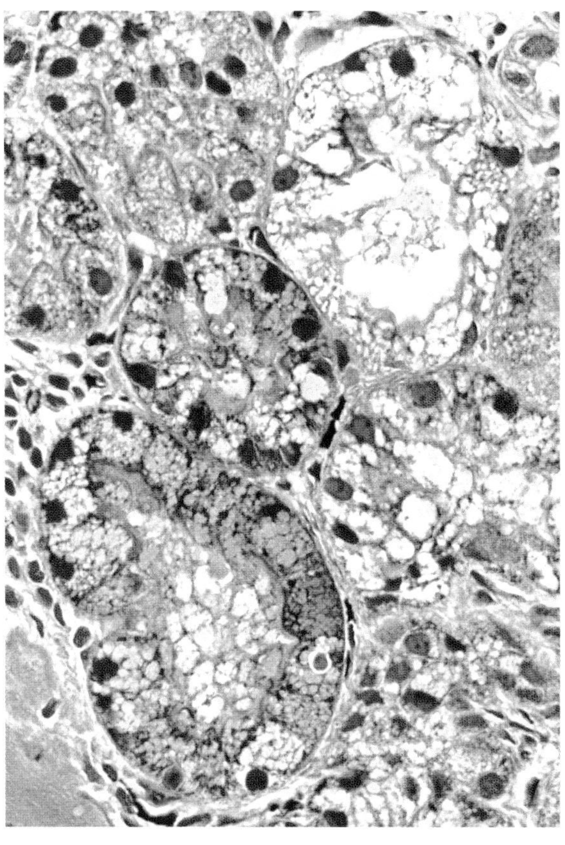

Figure 3-7

CONGENITAL NEPHROTIC SYNDROME OF THE FINNISH TYPE

The proximal tubular epithelium contains abundant clear lipid resorption droplets (Masson trichrome stain).

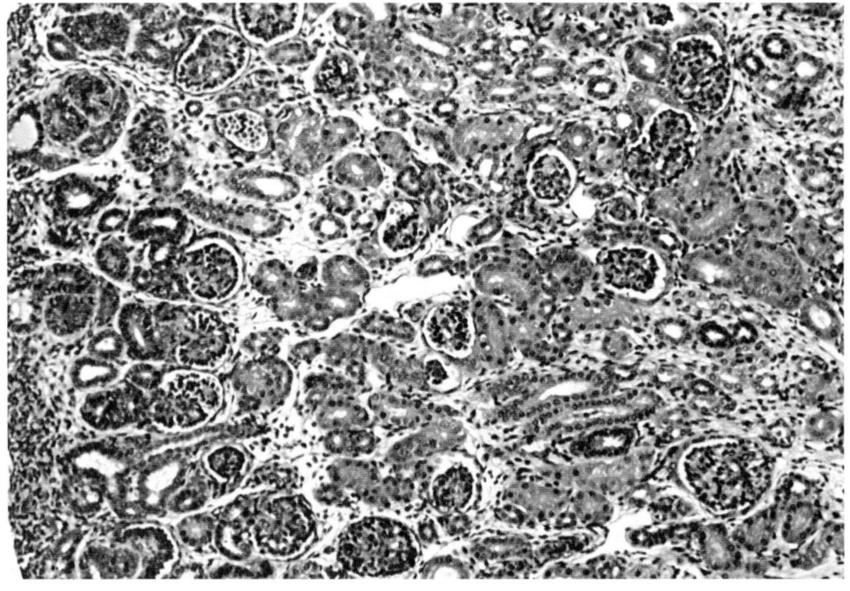

Figure 3-8

CONGENITAL NEPHROTIC SYNDROME OF THE FINNISH TYPE

Low-power view of the kidney of a 20-week fetal abortus shows no obvious abnormalities. The normal nephrogenic zone is visible to the left. The fetus was aborted following detection of elevated alpha-fetoprotein levels in maternal amniotic fluid, indicating fetal proteinuria (H&E stain).

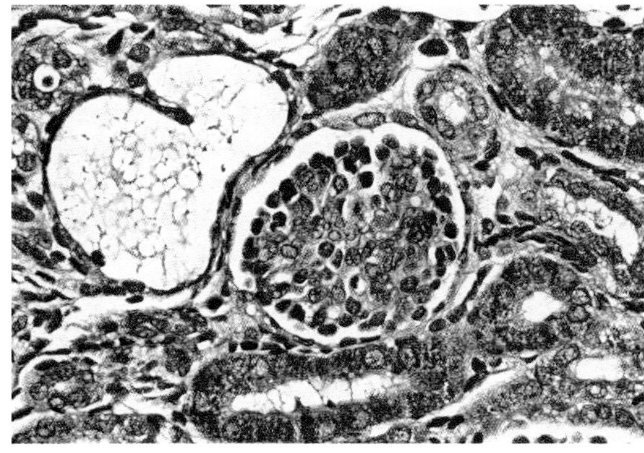

Figure 3-9

CONGENITAL NEPHROTIC SYNDROME OF THE FINNISH TYPE

Glomeruli from this 20-week fetal abortus appear normal by light microscopy. There is a rare tubular cyst with an attenuated epithelial lining (Masson trichrome stain).

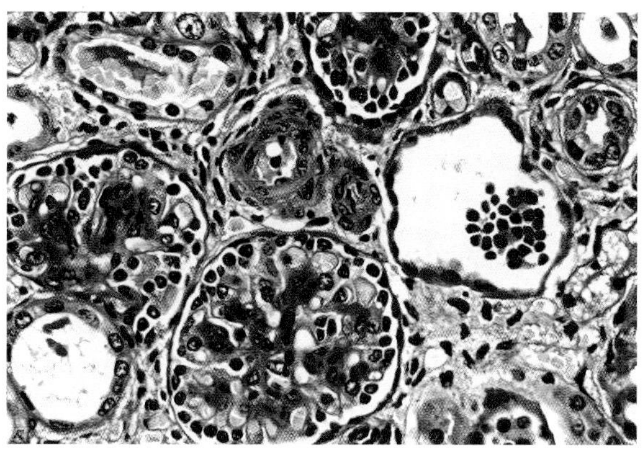

Figure 3-10

CONGENITAL NEPHROTIC SYNDROME OF THE FINNISH TYPE

Glomeruli with mild global mesangial hypercellularity alternate with immature fetal glomeruli (PAS stain).

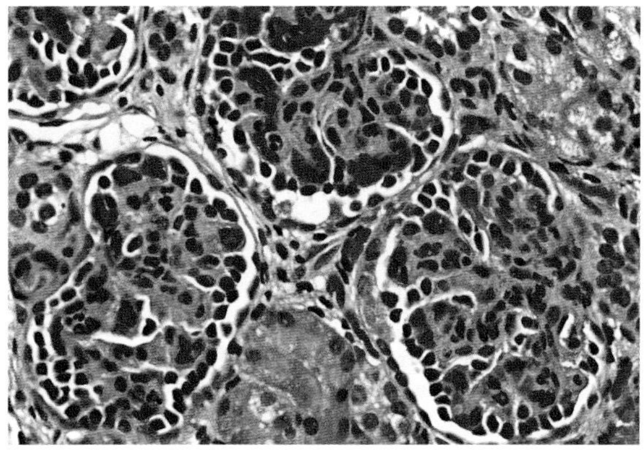

Figure 3-11

CONGENITAL NEPHROTIC SYNDROME OF THE FINNISH TYPE

Example from a 1-month-old infant. Prominent diffuse and global mesangial hypercellularity has caused accentuated glomerular lobularity (H&E stain).

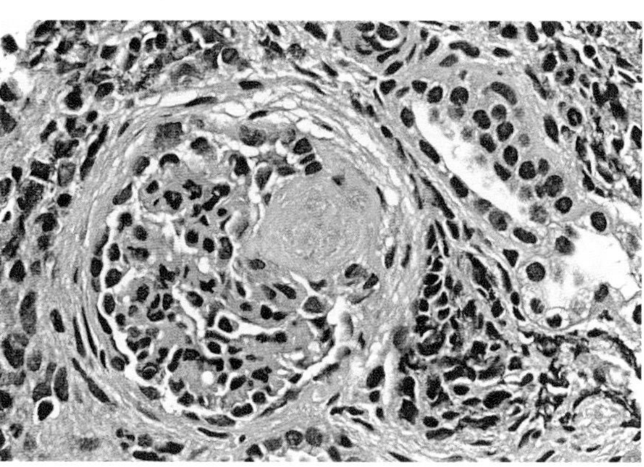

Figure 3-12

CONGENITAL NEPHROTIC SYNDROME OF THE FINNISH TYPE

Evolution to focal segmental glomerulosclerosis and hyalinosis may be found in some glomeruli (H&E stain).

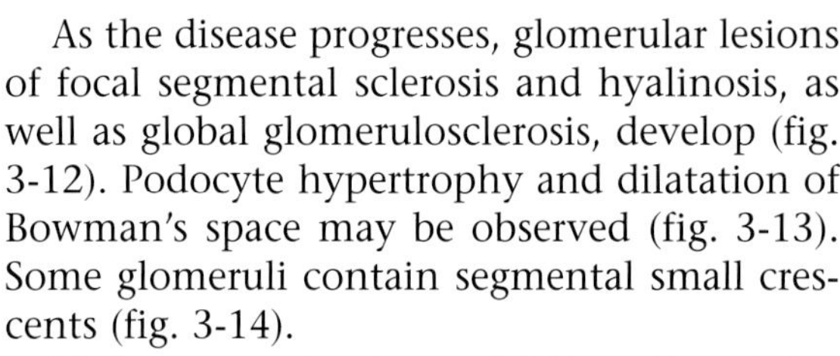

As the disease progresses, glomerular lesions of focal segmental sclerosis and hyalinosis, as well as global glomerulosclerosis, develop (fig. 3-12). Podocyte hypertrophy and dilatation of Bowman's space may be observed (fig. 3-13). Some glomeruli contain segmental small crescents (fig. 3-14).

With progression to renal failure, there is increasing global glomerulosclerosis, tubular atrophy, and interstitial fibrosis. The fibrotic interstitium may contain a sparse lymphoid infiltrate. Vascular lesions are inconspicuous; however, in infants who develop accelerated hypertension, arteriolar fibrinoid necrosis may be observed.

Immunofluorescence Findings. By immunofluorescence, there are usually no immune reactants detectable in the glomeruli. As the disease progresses, however, IgM and complement (C)3 can be found in the lesions of segmental and global glomerulosclerosis. Most impressive is the tu-

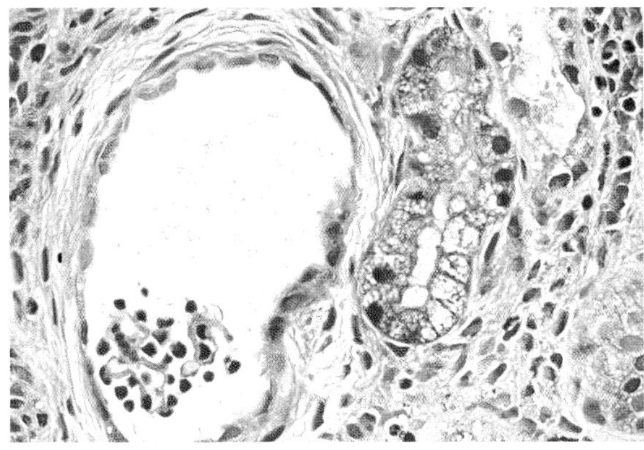

Figure 3-13

CONGENITAL NEPHROTIC SYNDROME OF THE FINNISH TYPE

An infantile glomerulus with dilatation of Bowman's space forms a glomerular microcyst (Masson trichrome stain).

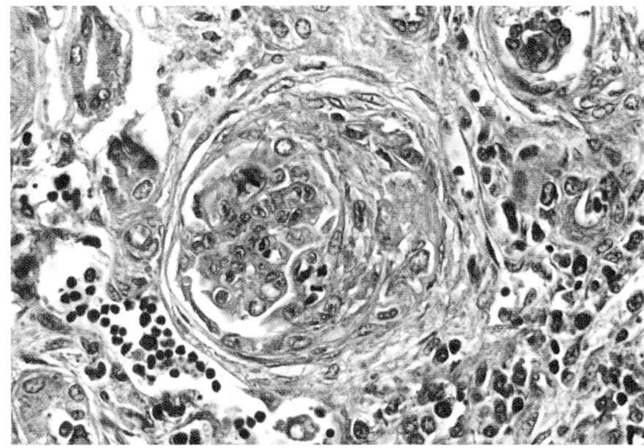

Figure 3-14

CONGENITAL NEPHROTIC SYNDROME OF THE FINNISH TYPE

A glomerulus with segmental epithelial hyperplasia forms a small crescent (Masson trichrome stain).

bular staining for albumin and immunoglobulins, corresponding to intracytoplasmic protein resorption droplets (fig. 3-15).

Electron Microscopic Findings. The electron microscopic findings are variable and nonspecific (1). The nonsclerotic glomeruli display extensive, often complete effacement of the foot processes, resembling that seen in minimal change disease (fig. 3-16). The podocytes are often enlarged, with swollen cytoplasm, intracytoplasmic transport vesicles, and microvillous cytoplasmic transformation.

In some patients, lamellation of the lamina densa, resembling that seen in hereditary nephritis, occurs. Sometimes, there is widening of the lamina rara interna. In glomeruli with lesions of focal segmental glomerulosclerosis, the findings are similar to those observed in idiopathic focal segmental glomerulosclerosis: detachment of podocytes, intervening layering of loosely woven basement membrane material, inframembranous hyalinosis, and marked effacement of the processes with podocyte hypertrophy and microvillous projections.

In specimens examined from therapeutic abortions in the second trimester, it is important to remember that the degree of foot process fusion is best assessed by evaluation of the most mature, inner cortical glomeruli (fig. 3-17). This is because developing nephrons do not develop discrete foot processes until the termi-

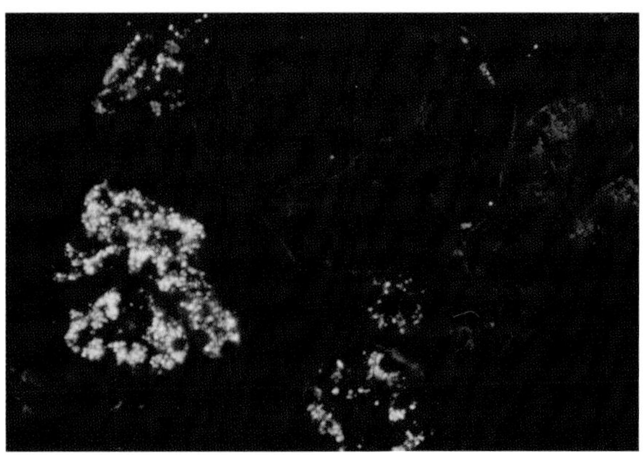

Figure 3-15

CONGENITAL NEPHROTIC SYNDROME OF THE FINNISH TYPE

By immunofluorescence, there are abundant protein resorption droplets within the proximal tubular cells that stain with antisera to albumin (immunofluorescence micrograph).

nal stages of glomerulogenesis and podocyte maturation. Thus, in the outer nephrons, the normal cytoarchitecture of immature podocytes should not be mistaken for the acquired lesions of foot process effacement.

Differential Diagnosis. The clinical-pathologic distinction between CNF and diffuse mesangial sclerosis (DMS) may be difficult because of the widely overlapping morphologic features and absence of pathognomonic findings.

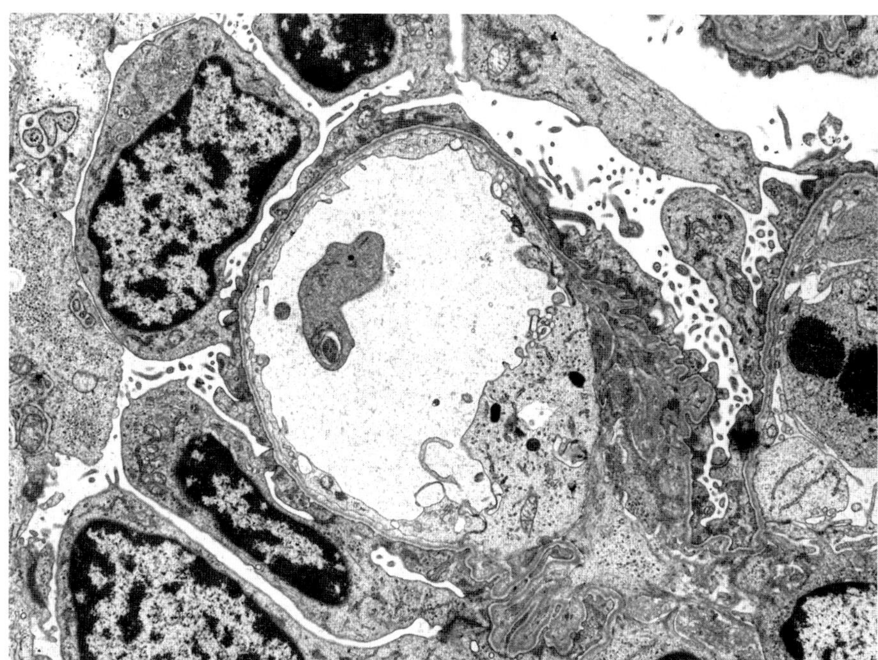

Figure 3-16

CONGENITAL NEPHROTIC SYNDROME OF THE FINNISH TYPE

There is complete effacement of the foot process, with podocyte hypertrophy. The glomerular basement membranes are thin, appropriate for the age of 1 week (electron micrograph).

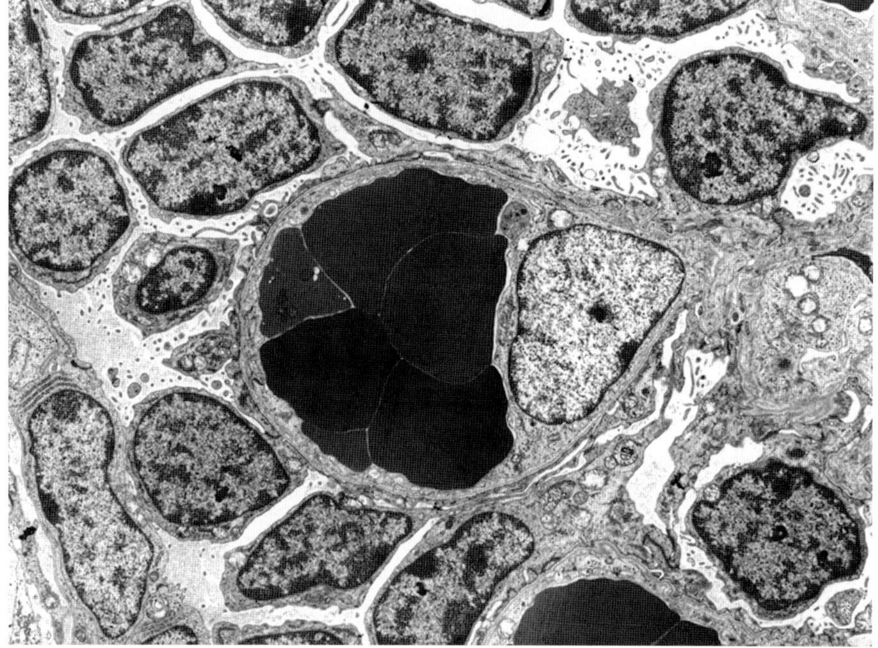

Figure 3-17

CONGENITAL NEPHROTIC SYNDROME OF THE FINNISH TYPE

An immature glomerulus from a 20-week fetal abortus shows crowning of the podocytes, with no identifiable foot process architecture and focal microvillous transformation of the podocyte cytoplasm (electron micrograph).

Although cysts are most characteristic of CNF, they may also occur as a nonspecific finding in DMS. Moreover, not all cases CNF manifest tubular cysts on biopsy. Mesangial widening may occur in both conditions. Mesangial hypercellularity is more likely to be a feature of CNF, but mesangial sclerosis is more characteristic of DMS. Both conditions may develop focal segmental and global glomerulosclerosis and both have similar ultrastructural findings.

Most helpful in differentiating the two are the timing of the onset of the disease, the rapidity of the course to renal failure, the prominence of hypertension as a clinical feature, and the perinatal history. CNF has an earlier onset (usually in utero or at birth) compared to the delayed onset of DMS (several weeks to 12 months of age). Because of its onset in utero, CNF is much more likely to be associated with a large placenta, malpresentation, and low birth weight. Severe hypertension and rapid progression to renal failure are more typical of DMS. At the present time, information on the potential diagnostic utility of the immunohistochemical study of the distribution of the gene products, nephrin and *WT1* (the Wilms' tumor gene), in renal biopsies is lacking. Genetic analysis for the major mutations of CNF is performed in specialized laboratories in Europe and the United States, and will hopefully become more widely available in the future.

The differential diagnosis also includes the entities listed in Table 3-1 (see section on differential diagnosis of diffuse mesangial sclerosis).

Etiology and Pathogenesis. Early investigations by Vernier et al. (43) demonstrated reduced staining of the glomerular basement membrane by the cationic dye polyethyleneimine, suggesting a reduction in anionic sites. This observation led to the hypothesis that the disease was caused by defective incorporation of heparan sulfate proteoglycan moieties into the glomerular basement membrane (25,38,42). However, this has not been confirmed by subsequent studies in which the normal expression of glomerular basement membrane type IV collagen, laminin, and heparan sulfate proteoglycan was observed (34).

In 1998, the genetic basis of the disease was uncovered with the identification and cloning of the responsible gene (*NPHS1*) in Finnish patients (20). The gene has been localized to chromosome 19q13.1. It spans 26 kb and contains 29 exons. The gene product, known as nephrin, is renal limited and podocyte specific. It consists of a 1241-amino acid putative transmembrane protein of the immunoglobulin family of cell adhesion molecules. Nephrin forms paired molecules at the base of the podocytes and comprises the essential structural protein of the filtration slit diaphragm (39). At least 36 different mutations in the nephrin gene (*NPHS1*) have been identified, including deletions, insertions, splice-site mutations, and nonsense mutations, resulting in frameshifts or premature stop codons (20). Many of these mutations result in a truncated nephrin molecule that lacks the intracellular and transmembrane domains. In the Finnish population, two nonsense mutations account for 94 percent of the mutations in *NPHS1* (6). These mutations cause misfolding of the nephrin protein and its defective intracellular trafficking (24). Mutated nephrin protein mislocalizes to the endoplasmic reticulum, but fails to reach the plasma membrane.

There are rare cases of congenital nephrotic syndrome with focal segmental sclerosing phenotype in which tri-allelic mutations in *NPHS1* (the gene encoding nephrin) and *NPHS2* (the gene encoding podocin) have been identified (22).

Treatment and Prognosis. Patients with CNF pose enormous challenges for clinical management. The disease does not respond to steroids or any other immunosuppressive therapy. The prognosis is extremely poor: untreated, 75 percent of patients die before the age of 1 year, and only 3 percent live to the age of 2 years.

Modern therapy can be divided into short-term and long-range strategies. In the short-term, edema can be managed with oral diuretics and albumin infusions. Replacement of thyroid hormones, iron, and vitamin D is required to correct deficiencies. Prevention of thromboembolic complications is achieved by anticoagulation.

The most effective long-range strategy is double nephrectomy within the first year or two of life, followed by dialysis until the child is old enough for renal transplantation (usually between the ages of 2 and 3 years). This approach has the advantage of eliminating the risk of infection and growth retardation associated with unremitting severe nephrotic syndrome, and subsequently curing the nephrotic syndrome.

Patients may develop recurrences of CNF in the allograft, sometimes in the immediate post-transplant period (4,30). Recurrent disease in the allograft has been ascribed to "de novo minimal change disease," because the only identifiable morphologic abnormality is foot process effacement (17). Recurrence of nephrotic syndrome is mediated by formation of autoantibodies to nephrin, causing immunologic destruction of the slit diaphragm (30,44). Because it is antibody mediated, recurrence of nephrotic syndrome in the allograft may benefit from immunosuppressive (cyclophosphamide) therapy (30,44).

DIFFUSE MESANGIAL SCLEROSIS

Definition. First described by the French team of Habib and Bois in 1973 (10), diffuse mesangial sclerosis (DMS) is also known as *French-type congenital nephrotic syndrome* and manifests as severe, unremitting nephrotic syndrome within the first 9 months of life. Both familial and sporadic forms have been reported.

Clinical Features. Although some cases of DMS are identified as early as the first week of life, onset tends to be later than with CNF. Approximately half of the cases of DMS have delayed clinical onset until 3 to 9 months of age (11,12).

Unlike CNF, DMS is not associated with an enlarged placenta, low infant birth weight, or premature birth. This is because nephrotic syndrome does not develop in utero. Other distinguishing clinical features include prominent hypertension and a more accelerated course to renal failure, often within 1 to 3 months. Indeed, most patients have evidence of renal insufficiency at the time they present with nephrotic syndrome. At presentation, 75 percent of patients have edema, 66 percent have renal failure, and under 50 percent have microhematuria.

DMS occurs in males or females. Most cases are renal-limited, presenting with nephrotic syndrome. However, some patients have associated renal and extrarenal abnormalities. The combination of DMS, Wilms' tumor, and male pseudohermaphroditism is known as *Denys-Drash syndrome* or simply *Drash syndrome* (3,7, 12). Other associations include ocular anomalies such as cataracts, strabismus, nystagmus, myopia, and aniridia, as well as mental retardation, microcephaly, deafness, musculoskeletal abnormalities, and cleft palate.

Most cases of Denys-Drash syndrome occur in male pseudohermaphrodites with 46XY karyotype. The genitalia are typically ambiguous and include hypospadias, microphallus, cryptorchidism, partial labioscrotal fusion, clitoromegaly, or normal-appearing female external genitalia (26). The internal genital organs may be hypoplastic or normal-appearing, and may contain mixed mullerian and wolffian duct derivatives, purely mullerian duct derivatives, or purely wolffian duct derivatives. Gonadal development is extremely pleomorphic, including bilateral testes, unilateral testis, dysgenetic testes, hypoplastic testes, and streak gonads (26). There are rare associations with gonadoblastoma (known as *Frasier's syndrome*). In the setting of Denys-Drash syndrome, the onset of glomerulopathy (mean, 12 months; range, 0.5 to 24 months) generally predates the development of Wilms' tumor (mean, 22 months; range, 3 to 70 months) (26).

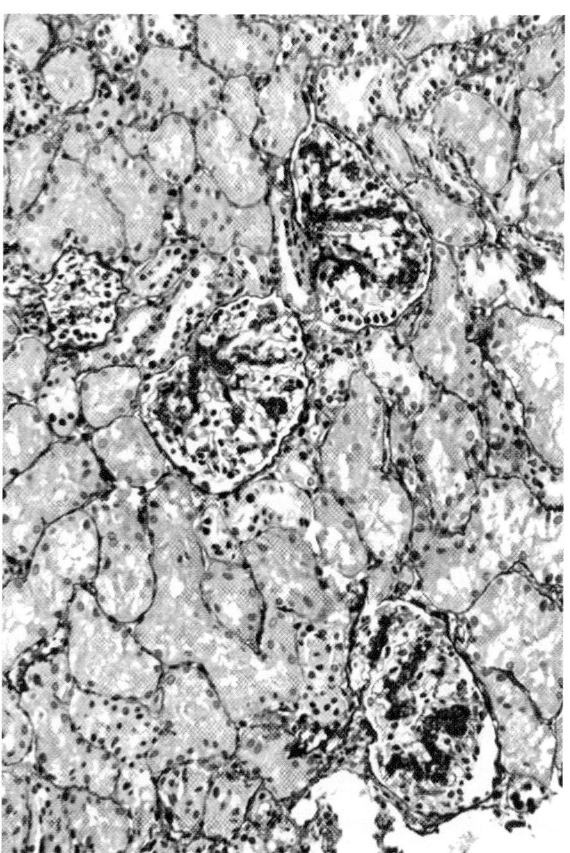

Figure 3-18

DIFFUSE MESANGIAL SCLEROSIS

An early stage shows mild diffuse and global mesangial sclerosis with preservation of the tubulointerstitial compartment (Jones methenamine [JMS] silver stain).

Light Microscopic Findings. The characteristic glomerular finding, even early in the disease, is the appearance of increased mesangial matrix in a relatively diffuse and global distribution (figs. 3-18, 3-19). Silver staining shows the mesangial sclerosis to have a somewhat reticulated, spongy texture (fig. 3-20). There may be associated mesangial hypercellularity. Other glomeruli may demonstrate focal segmental glomerulosclerosis or global glomerulosclerosis

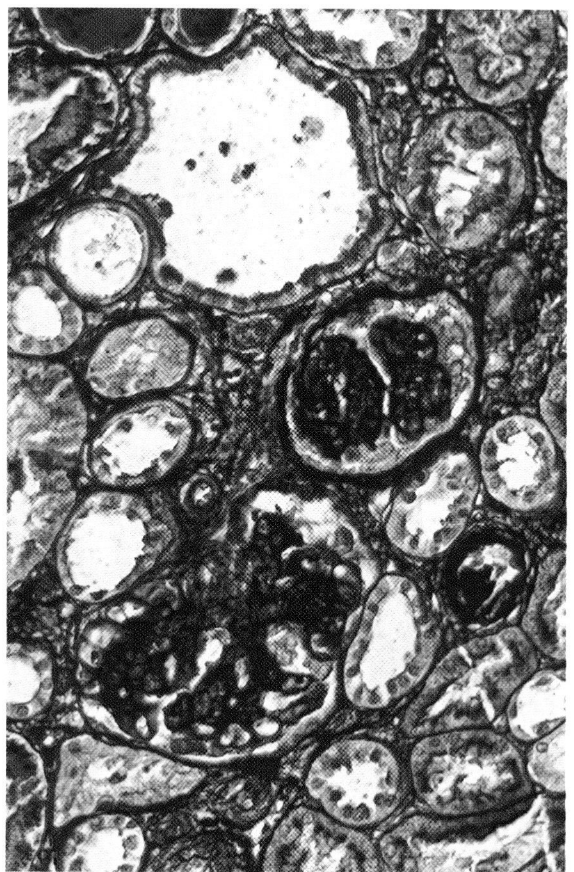

Figure 3-19

DIFFUSE MESANGIAL SCLEROSIS

A later stage shows more advanced diffuse and global mesangial sclerosis and focal tubular microcysts (JMS stain).

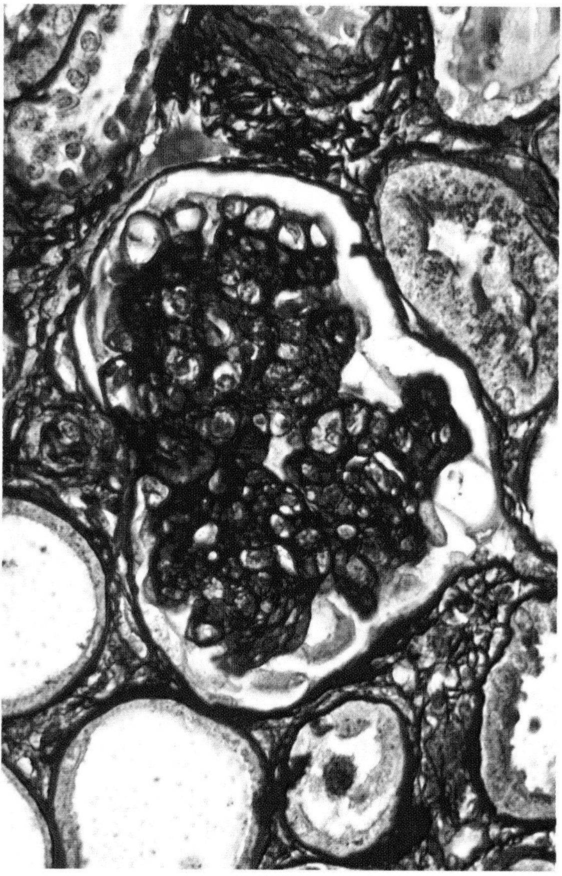

Figure 3-20

DIFFUSE MESANGIAL SCLEROSIS

The sclerotic mesangium has a reticulated matrix, with narrowing of most capillary lumens. The number of mesangial cells also appears to be increased (JMS stain).

(figs. 3-21, 3-22). There is often capping of swollen podocytes overlying the small, rounded, sclerotic tuft (fig. 3-21). The surrounding podocytes may display hypertrophy and hyperplasia, sometimes forming pseudocrescents. Glomerular hyalinosis is uncommon. Occasional endocapillary foam cells are seen.

Habib et al. (11) described a zonal distribution of the glomerular alterations from the capsular to the juxtamedullary cortex (figs. 3-23, 3-24). The outer cortex contains many shrunken, rounded, sclerotic glomeruli covered by a corona of hypertrophied podocytes as well as microglomeruli with immature features (figs. 3-23, 3-25). These glomerular abnormalities suggest arrested development in fetal life. There is a gradient of glomerular abnormalities that extends from the outer cortex (most severe) to inner cortex (least severe). In the outer cortex, the most severe chronic tubulointerstitial disease is found; the mid-cortical glomeruli display the full-blown findings of diffuse mesangial sclerosis (figs. 3-24, 3-26); in the inner cortex, milder diffuse mesangial sclerosis generally affects the larger juxtamedullary glomeruli.

The glomerular changes are accompanied by severe tubulointerstitial damage that includes tubular ectasia, simplification, and focal microcyst formation (figs. 3-25, 3-26). Some of these dilated tubules contain loose proteinaceous or waxy hyaline casts. Proximal tubular epithelial cells contain numerous intracytoplasmic protein resorption droplets. In the later stages, there

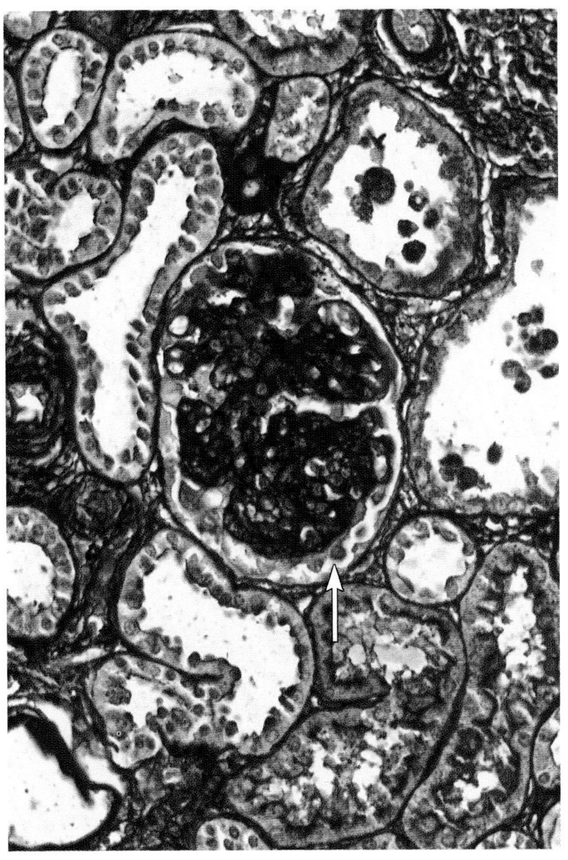

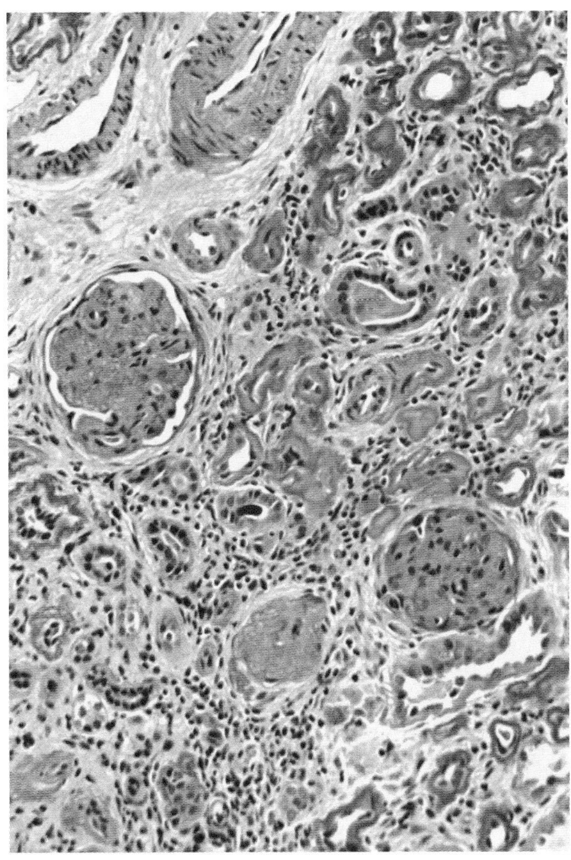

Figure 3-21

DIFFUSE MESANGIAL SCLEROSIS

A glomerulus displays a segmental lesion of sclerosis with podocyte capping (arrow); the adjacent lobules have mesangial sclerosis with patent lumens (JMS stain).

Figure 3-22

DIFFUSE MESANGIAL SCLEROSIS

An advanced stage shows diffuse and global solidification of the tuft by matrix material (PAS stain).

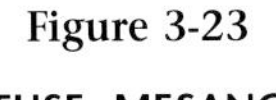

Figure 3-23

DIFFUSE MESANGIAL SCLEROSIS

Low-power view of a nephrectomy specimen shows zonation of the pathologic changes. The outer (subcapsular) cortex has a band of severe tubular atrophy and interstitial fibrosis (to the right). Some of the glomeruli in the outer cortex are approaching global sclerosis and some appear infantile. The midportion of cortex displays less severe changes (to the left) (Masson trichrome stain). (Figs. 3-23 and 3-24 are from the same patient.)

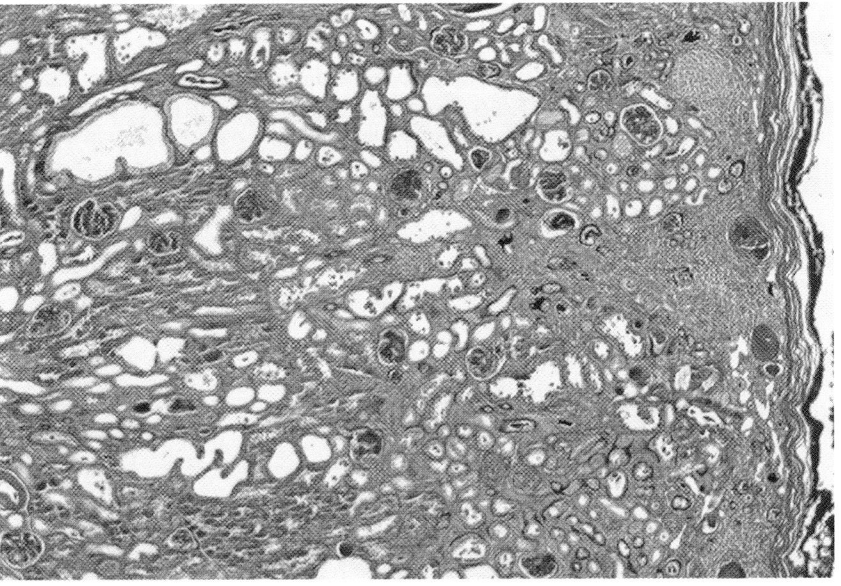

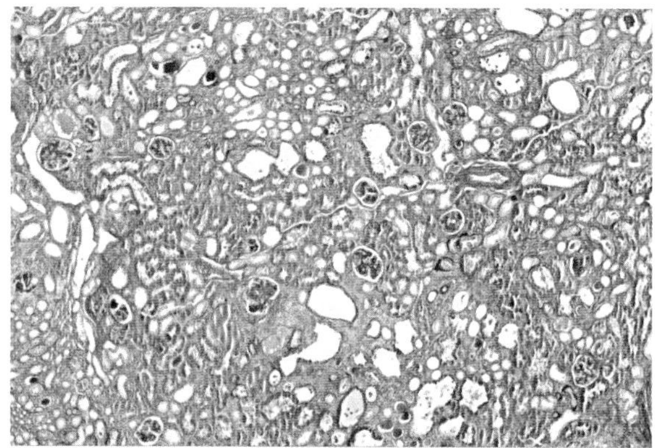

Figure 3-24

DIFFUSE MESANGIAL SCLEROSIS

Low-power view of the inner half of the cortex. The glomeruli in the inner cortex are larger, with well-developed diffuse mesangial sclerosis. In addition, the inner cortex has less severe tubular atrophy and interstitial fibrosis than the outer cortex seen in figure 3-23 (Masson trichrome stain).

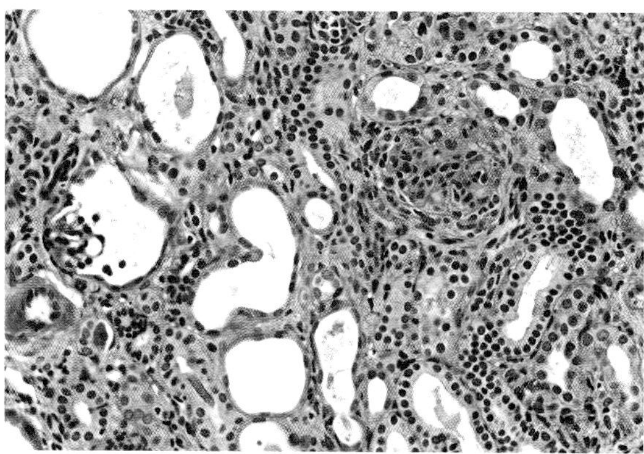

Figure 3-25

DIFFUSE MESANGIAL SCLEROSIS

The outer cortex contains some small infantile glomeruli and other glomeruli that are nearly globally sclerotic. The tubules are mildly and focally dilated (H&E stain).

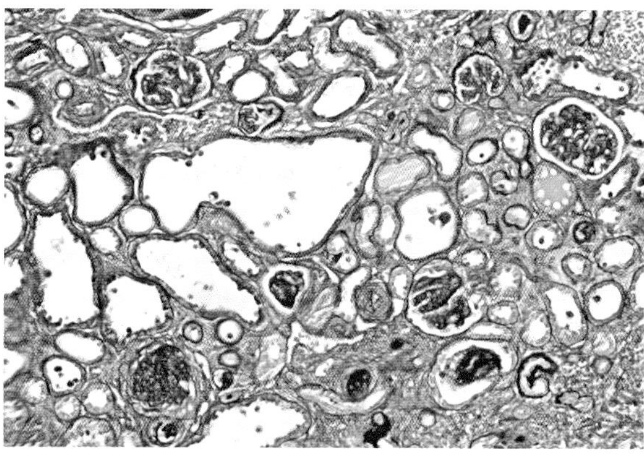

Figure 3-26

DIFFUSE MESANGIAL SCLEROSIS

The mid-cortex has the fully developed features of diffuse mesangial sclerosis, with focal tubular dilatation forming cysts (Masson trichrome stain).

is progression to tubular atrophy and interstitial fibrosis with associated interstitial inflammatory infiltrates.

In the setting of the Denys-Drash syndrome, diffuse mesangial sclerosis coexists with Wilms' tumor, which is bilateral in 25 percent of cases (fig. 3-27). There is also an increased incidence of nephrogenic rests that may be peripheral or intralobar, unilateral or bilateral, isolated or multifocal (14).

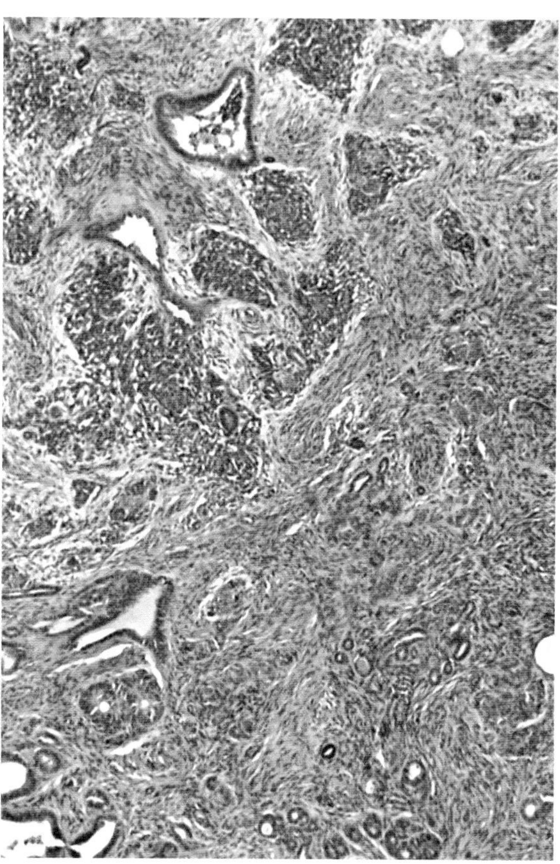

Figure 3-27

DENYS-DRASH SYNDROME

The Wilms' tumor is composed of metanephric blastema with primitive mesenchymal and epithelial differentiation, including formation of tubular structures (H&E stain).

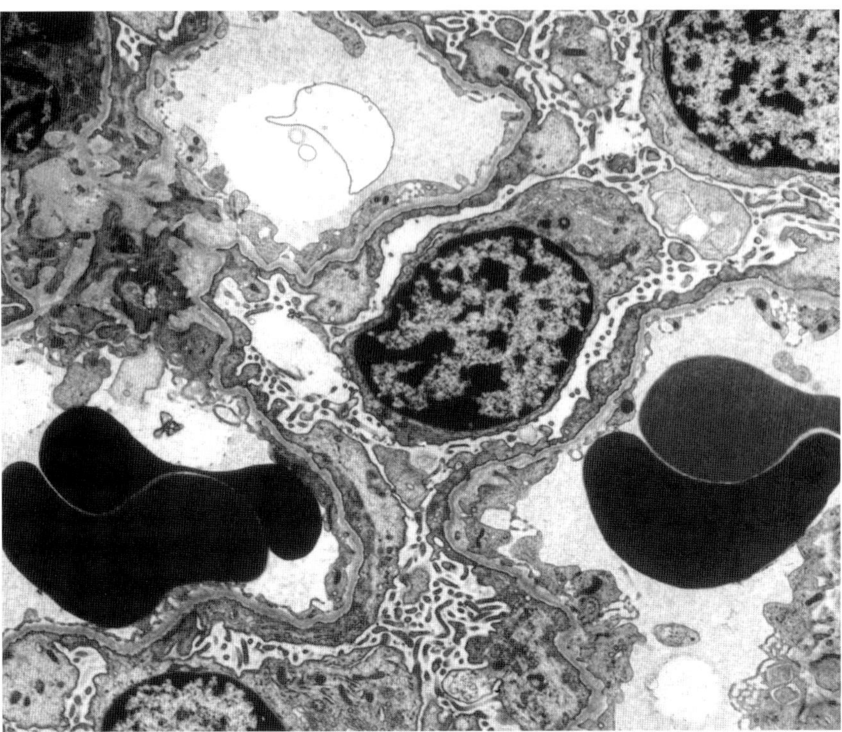

Figure 3-28

DIFFUSE MESANGIAL SCLEROSIS

Overlying patent capillaries, there is complete foot process effacement and microvillous transformation of the podocytes. The glomerular basement membranes appear thin, consistent with the patient's age (electron micrograph).

Immunofluorescence Findings. There are no glomerular immune deposits. Nonspecific staining of the glomerular mesangium or the sclerosing tuft for IgM, C3, and C1 may be identified in some glomeruli. Protein resorption droplets within the epithelial cells of the proximal tubule and the podocytes often stain conspicuously for albumin and immunoglobulins, particularly IgG and IgA.

Electron Microscopic Findings. There are no specific ultrastructural features. The major finding is extensive effacement of foot processes associated with prominent podocyte alterations, including intracytoplasmic transport vesicles, protein resorption droplets, and microvillous transformation (fig. 3-28). The mesangial matrix appears increased and narrows the capillary lumens. The glomerular basement membranes are often thickened and lamellated, with a basket-woven appearance (fig. 3-29). This is due primarily to layering of the outer portion of the glomerular basement membrane. In areas of segmental or global glomerulosclerosis, there is frequently detachment of the podocytes with intervening accumulation of loosely woven basement membrane material (fig. 3-30). Small electron densities, probably representing insuded plasma proteins, may be identified focally in the paramesangial, intramembranous, or inframembranous regions. In areas of sclerosis, larger hyaline deposits may occur. These ultrastructural findings are not unique but are similar to those seen in idiopathic focal segmental glomerulosclerosis and some cases of CNF.

Differential Diagnosis. The differential diagnosis of nephrotic syndrome occurring in the first 3 months of life primarily includes CNF (three fourths of cases) and diffuse mesangial sclerosis (about one tenth of cases) (see Table 3-1). Less common diagnostic considerations include minimal change disease and diffuse mesangial hypercellularity, as well as focal segmental glomerulosclerosis, membranous glomerulopathy, congenital syphilis, congenital toxoplasmosis, and congenital lupus nephritis (figs. 3-31–3-35) (37). Congenital focal segmental glomerulosclerosis has been linked to epidermolysis bullosa and mutations of the beta-4-integrin expressed on podocytes (figs. 3-36, 3-37) (19).

The differential diagnosis of infantile nephrotic syndrome (nephrotic syndrome occurring between 3 and 12 months of age) is more heterogeneous (see Table 3-2). Late-onset diffuse

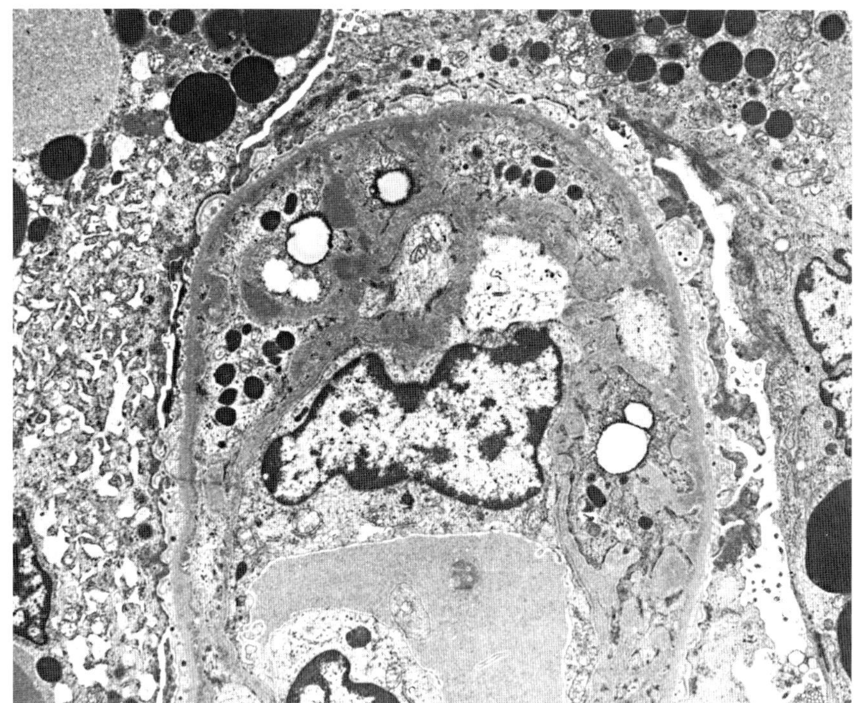

Figure 3-29

DIFFUSE MESANGIAL SCLEROSIS

In areas of sclerosis, there is detachment of podocytes from the glomerular basement membrane, with lamellation of basement membrane material. The podocytes are markedly hypertrophied and contain intracytoplasmic protein resorption droplets (electron micrograph).

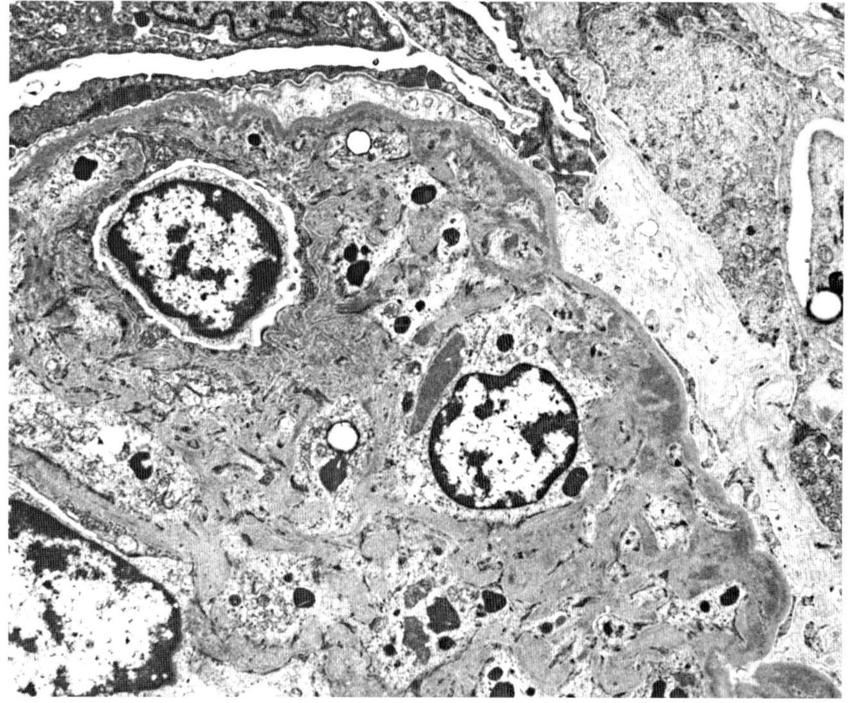

Figure 3-30

DIFFUSE MESANGIAL SCLEROSIS

Overlying a lesion of segmental sclerosis, there is podocyte detachment with woven neomembrane material. Electron densities suggestive of hyaline are present in the inframembranous region (electron micrograph).

mesangial sclerosis accounts for approximately one third of cases of infantile nephrotic syndrome. The remainder include diverse conditions that can cause nephrotic syndrome in older children (such as minimal change disease, focal segmental glomerulosclerosis, human immunodeficiency virus (HIV) nephropathy, hemolytic uremic syndrome, membranous

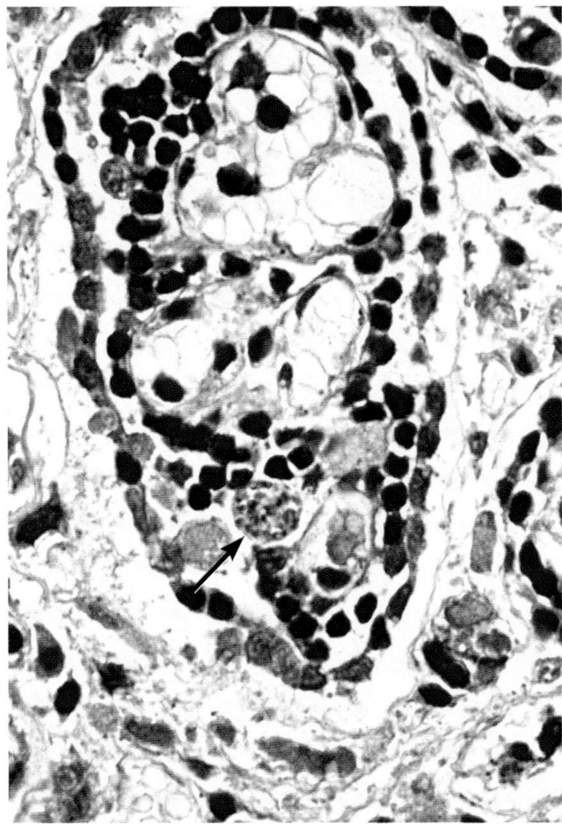

Figure 3-31

CONGENITAL TOXOPLASMOSIS WITH NEPHROTIC SYNDROME

Toxoplasma organisms are identified within a podocyte (arrow) (H&E stain).

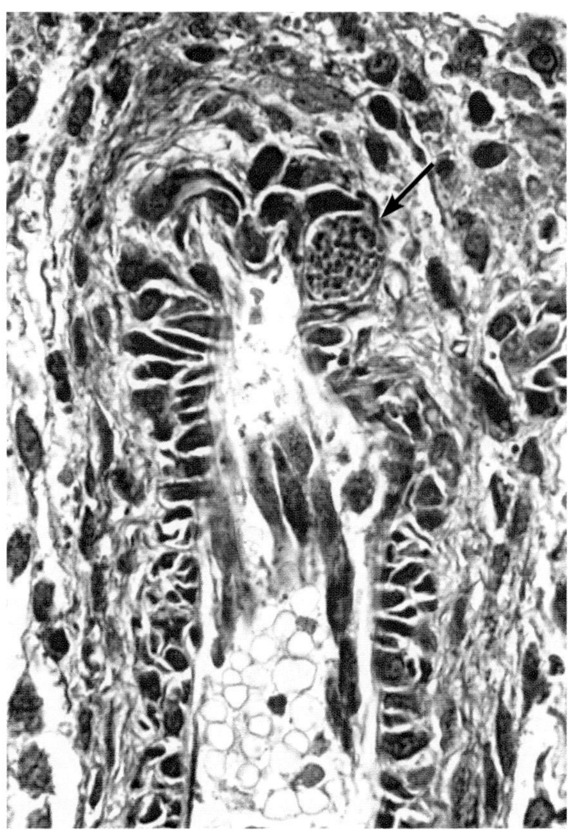

Figure 3-32

CONGENITAL TOXOPLASMOSIS WITH NEPHROTIC SYNDROME

Toxoplasma organisms are seen within a medial myocyte of an interlobular artery of the kidney (arrow) (Masson trichrome stain).

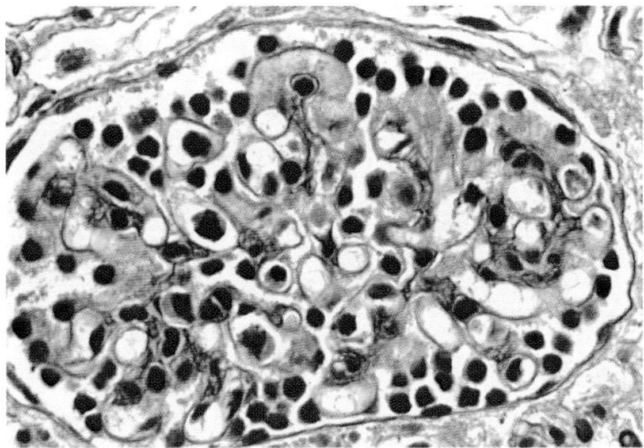

Figure 3-33

CONGENITAL LUPUS WITH MEMBRANOUS GLOMERULOPATHY

The glomerular capillary walls appear slightly thickened and rigid (H&E stain).

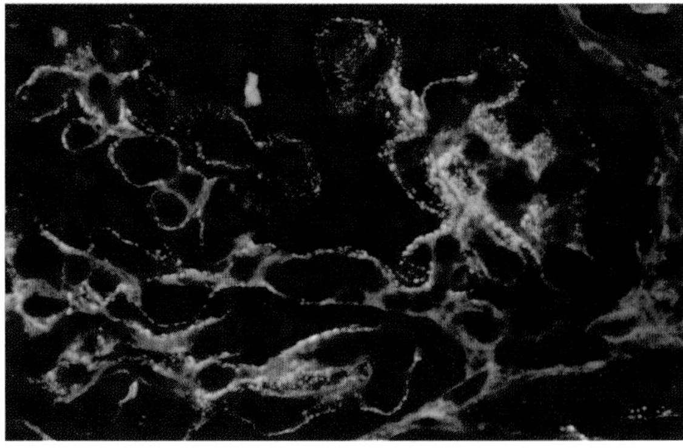

Figure 3-34

CONGENITAL LUPUS WITH MEMBRANOUS GLOMERULOPATHY

By immunofluorescence, there are finely granular deposits of IgG along the glomerular capillary walls, in a membranous pattern (immunofluorescence micrograph).

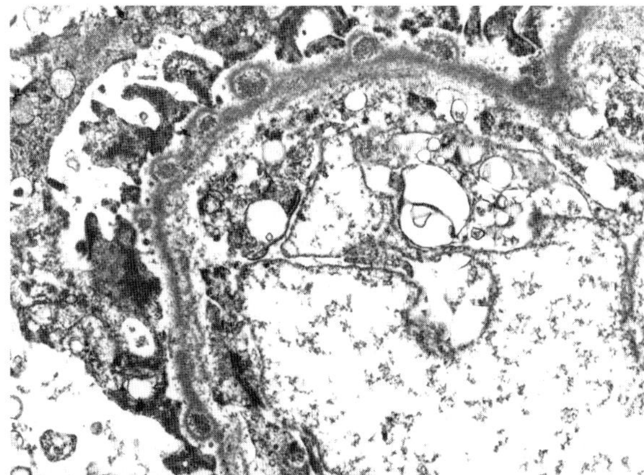

Figure 3-35

CONGENITAL LUPUS WITH MEMBRANOUS GLOMERULOPATHY

Minute, subepithelial, electron-dense deposits are overlaid by a delicate layer of neomembrane (electron microscopy; autolyzed necropsy specimen).

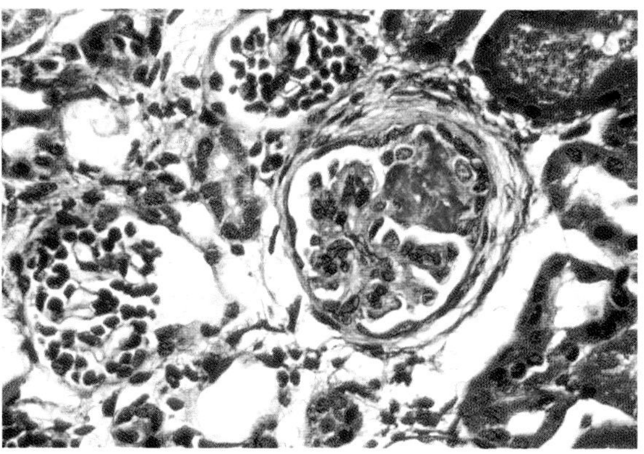

Figure 3-36

CONGENITAL FOCAL SEGMENTAL GLOMERULOSCLEROSIS

An example of focal segmental glomerulosclerosis with hyalinosis in a neonate with epidermolysis bullosa and nephrotic-range proteinuria (Masson trichrome stain).

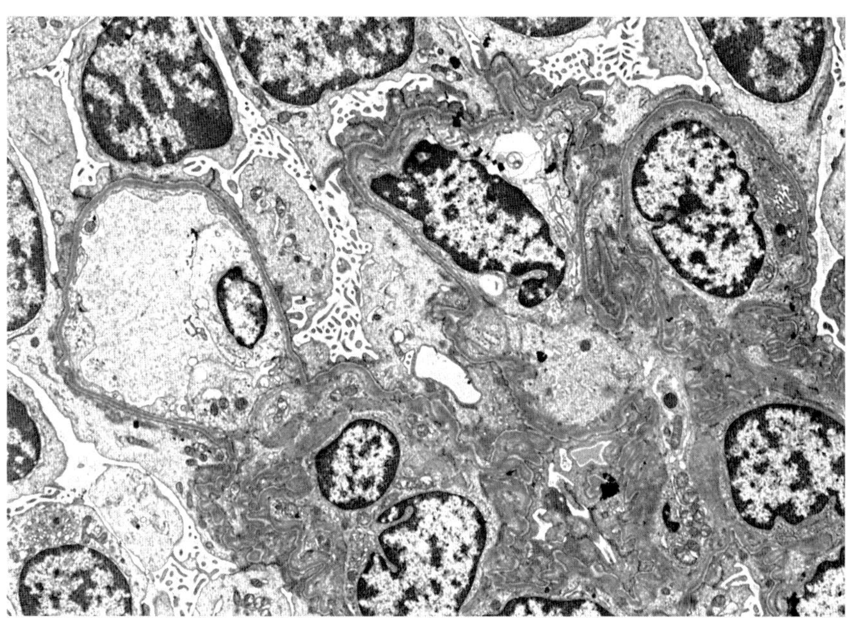

Figure 3-37

CONGENITAL FOCAL SEGMENTAL GLOMERULOSCLEROSIS

Nonsclerotic capillaries display complete foot process effacement and focal microvillous transformation (electron micrograph).

glomerulopathy, and lupus nephritis) (figs. 3-38, 3-39) (8,23). Also included are rare familial forms of steroid-resistant nephrotic syndrome (SRNS) with autosomal recessive transmission and manifesting a pattern of focal segmental glomerulosclerosis. The onset of SRNS is from 3 months to 5 years of age and progression to renal failure is generally rapid. The responsible gene is *NPHS2*, located on chromosome 1q25-31, which encodes the podocyte-specific protein, podocin (22).

In infantile nephrotic syndrome due to membranous glomerulopathy, the differential diagnosis includes secondary forms such as those related to congenital syphilis, congenital or infantile lupus nephritis (23), and membranous glomerulonephritis (MGN) with antitubular basement membrane (anti-TBM) nephritis and Fanconi's syndrome (see chapter 7). In the setting of MGN, the presence of mesangial proliferative features is more common with

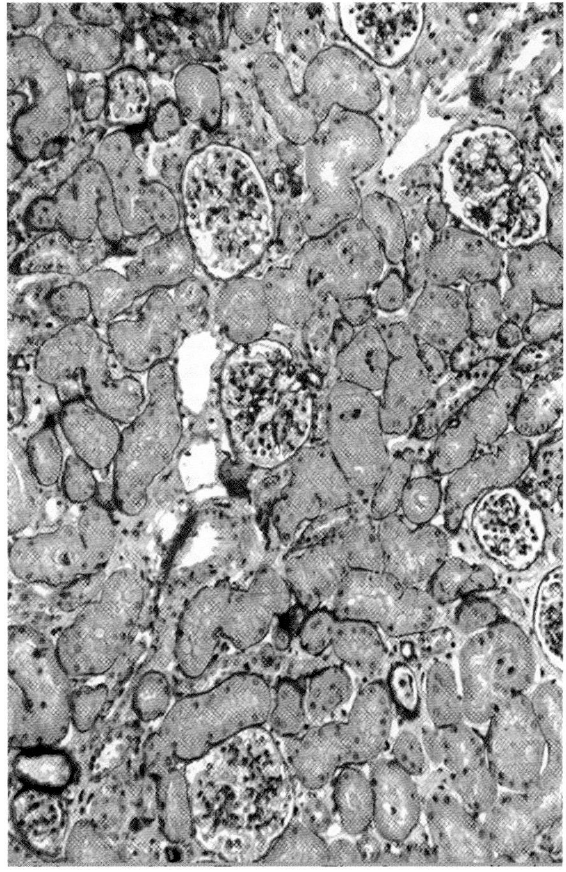

Figure 3-38

INFANTILE MINIMAL CHANGE DISEASE

An example from a 1-year-old child with congenital human immunodeficiency virus (HIV) infection. The glomeruli show no obvious abnormalities at the light microscopic level (JMS stain). (Figs. 3-38 and 3-39 are from the same patient.)

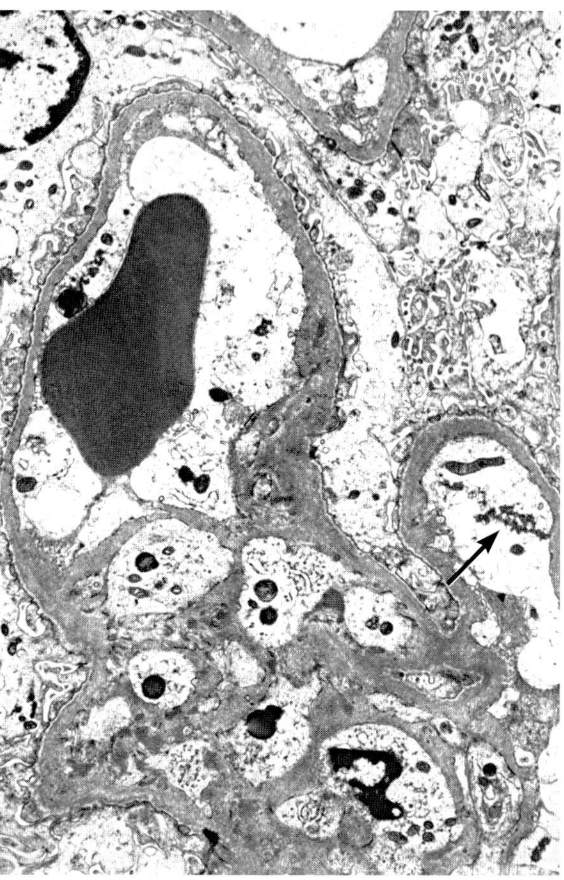

Figure 3-39

INFANTILE MINIMAL CHANGE DISEASE

Extensive foot process effacement and focal endothelial tubuloreticular inclusions (arrow) are seen in this HIV-infected baby. There are also a few small paramesangial electron densities, which correspond to mesangial deposits of IgM (electron micrograph).

syphilis-associated disease and membranous lupus nephritis than with idiopathic MGN.

Finally, DMS must be distinguished from Frasier's syndrome, which causes a later-onset glomerulopathy that resembles focal segmental glomerulosclerosis (FSGS) (5). Affected individuals have an XY genotype, complete feminization, and later onset and more slowly progressive glomerulopathy than patients with DMS. They may develop gonadoblastomas, but not Wilms' tumor. The genetic basis is a heterozygous mutation in a splicing region (intron) of *WT1*, leading to altered ratios of *WT1* isoforms, rather than a mutant product (5).

Etiology and Pathogenesis. Mutations in the Wilms' tumor gene (*WT1*) have been identified in over 90 percent of patients with Denys-Drash syndrome but only a small percentage of patients with isolated DMS (18,36). In Denys-Drash syndrome, there is a constitutional mutation of *WT1*, followed by a second somatic mutation, causing loss of heterozygosity in affected tissues.

The Wilms' tumor gene is a tumor suppressor gene that has been localized to chromosome 11p13 (33). It encodes a zinc finger transcription factor involved in renal and gonadal development (33). Two alternative splice sites produce four isoforms that are expressed at different levels in different tissue types. *WT1* is normally expressed in the condensing mesenchyme and glomerular vesicles of the developing kidney, but becomes restricted to the podocytes in the mature kidney. It is also expressed in the genital ridge and sex cord epithelium of the developing gonads.

In Denys-Drash syndrome, it has been postulated that two mutations in the *WT1* gene occur (31,32). The first is acquired by a prezygotic or postzygotic mutation. This first mutation is thought to mediate the development of dysgenetic gonads, glomerulopathy, and embryonic rests. The second mutation is postzygotic, resulting in loss of heterozygosity. Through this second hit, Wilms' tumor is postulated to arise in nephrogenic rests. More than 60 different mutations have been identified; the majority are missense mutations in exons 8 or 9, encoding zinc-fingers 2 and 3, with a hot spot at position 1180 (R394W) that interferes with DNA binding.

Normally, the *WT1* gene product switches off genes involved in maintaining cellular proliferation and switches on genes involved in blastemal differentiation. It has been proposed that mutations in *WT1* produce uncontrolled proliferation and abnormal differentiation by interfering with these downstream events. In the gonads, *WT1* regulates other genes such as *SRY* (the sex-determining region of the Y chromosome that promotes testicular differentiation), mullerian inhibiting substance, and *Dax-1* (located on the short arm of the X chromosome), which opposes testicular differentiation (21,29). By interfering with these downstream events, the mutant *WT1* gene product is thought to promote ambiguous and dysgenetic sexual differentiation.

The glomerular basement membrane in DMS has been shown to have altered composition of proteoglycans, with reduced heparan sulfate anionic sites and increased urinary excretion of heparan sulfate (41). These effects may be mediated by the aberrant synthesis of glomerular basement membrane on the part of the mature podocyte, which normally expresses WT1. In normal kidney development, WT1 represses PAX2, another transcription factor that is restricted to parietal cells in the mature kidney. Diminished WT1 expression and increased PAX2 expression have been demonstrated by immunohistochemistry in the podocytes of patients with isolated DMS and Denys-Drash syndrome (45).

Treatment and Prognosis. The therapeutic management of patients with nephrotic syndrome in isolated DMS is similar to that described above for CNF. Patients are not responsive to immunosuppressive therapy. Rather, the edema, hypoalbuminemia, and hypertension are treated medically until the only curative measure, bilateral nephrectomy followed by dialysis and renal transplantation, can be performed. Transplantation between the ages of 2 and 3 years has been most successful. Unlike CNF, recurrence of nephrotic syndrome has not been described following transplantation in DMS.

Karyotyping is recommended in all DMS patients to rule out pseudohermaphroditism. There should be periodic imaging/evaluation of the kidney and genitalia for early detection of possible Wilms' tumor and gonadoblastoma.

REFERENCES

1. Autio-Harmainen H. Renal pathology of fetuses with congenital nephrotic syndrome of the Finnish type. Acta Pathol Microbiol Scand 1981;89: 215–22.
2. Autio-Harmainen H, Rapola J. Renal pathology of fetuses with congenital nephrotic syndrome of the Finnish type. A qualitative and quantitative light microscopic study. Nephron 1981;29: 158–63.
3. Barakat AY, Papadopoulou ZL, Chandra RS, Hollerman CE, Calcagno PL. Pseudohermaphroditism, nephron disorder and Wilms' tumor: a unifying concept. Pediatrics 1974;54:366–9.
4. Barayan S, Al-Akash SI, Malekzadeh M, Marik JL, Cohen AH, Ettenger RB, Yadin O. Immediate post-transplant nephrosis in a patient with congenital nephrotic syndrome. Pediatr Nephrol 2001;16:547–9.
5. Barbosa AS, Hakjiathanasiou CG, Theodoris C, et al. The same mutation affecting the splicing of WT1 gene is present on Frasier syndrome patients with or without Wilms' tumor. Hum Mut 1999;13:146–53.
6. Beltcheva O, Martin P, Lenkkeri U, Trygvasson K. Mutation spectrum in the nephrin gene (NPHS1) in congenital nephrotic syndrome. Hum Mut 2001;17:368–73.
7. Drash A, Sherman F, Hartmann WH, Blizzard RM. A syndrome of pseudohermaphroditism, Wilms' tumor, hypertension and degenerative renal disease. J Pediatr 1970;76:585–93.
8. Dudley J, Fenton T, Unsworth J, Chambers T, Maclver A, Tizard L. Systemic lupus erythematosus presenting as congenital nephrotic syndrome. Pediatr Nephrol 1996;10:752–5.
9. Habib R. Nephrotic syndrome in the first year of life. Pediatr Nephrol 1993;7:347–53.
10. Habib R, Bois E. Congenital and infantile nephrotic syndrome. Pediatr Nephrol 1976;2:335–57.
11. Habib R, Gubler MC, Antignac C, Gagnadoux MF. Diffuse mesangial sclerosis: a congenital glomerulopathy with nephrotic syndrome. Adv Nephrol Necker Hosp 1993;22:43–57.
12. Habib R, Loirat C, Gubler MC, et al. The nephropathy associated with male pseudohermaphroditism and Wilms' tumor (Drash syndrome): a distinctive glomerular lesion—report of 10 cases. Clin Nephrol 1985;24:269–78.
13. Harris HW, Umetsu D, Geha R, Harmon WE. Altered immunoglobulin status in congenital nephrotic syndrome. Clin Nephrol 1986;25:308–13.
14. Heppe RK, Koyle MA, Beckwith JB. Nephrogenic rests in Wilms tumor patients with Drash syndrome. J Urol 1991;145:1225–8.
15. Huttunen NP. Congenital nephrotic syndrome of Finnish type. Study of 75 patients. Arch Dis Child 1976;41:344–8.
16. Jadresic L, Leake J, Gordon I, et al. Clinicopathologic review of twelve children with nephropathy, Wilms tumor and genital abnormalities (Drash syndrome). J Pediatr 1990;117:717–25.
17. Jarmo L, Jalanko H, Holthöfer H, et al. Post-transplantation nephrosis in congenital nephrotic syndrome of the Finnish type. Kidney Intern 1993;44:867–74.
18. Jeanpierre C, Denamur E, Henry I, et al. Identification of constitutional WT1 mutations in patients with isolated diffuse mesangial sclerosis, and analysis of genotype/phenotype correlations by use of a computerized mutation database. Am J Human Genet 1998;62:824–33.
19. Kambham N, Tanji N, Seigle RL, et al. Congenital focal segmental glomerulosclerosis associated with B4 integrin mutation and epidermolysis bullosa. Am J Kidney Dis 2000;36:190–6.
20. Kestila M, Lenkkeri U, Mannikko M, et al. Positionally cloned gene for a novel glomerular protein—nephrin—is mutated in congenital nephrotic syndrome. Mol Cell 1998;1:575–82.
21. Kim J, Prawitt D, Bardeesy N, et al. The Wilms' tumor suppressor gene (Wt1) product regulates Dax-1 gene expression during gonadal differentiation. Mol Cell Biol 1999;19:2289–99.
22. Koziell A, Grech V, Hussain S, et al. Genotype/phenotype correlations in NPHS1 and NPHS2 mutation in nephrotic syndrome advocate a functional inter-relationship in glomerular filtration. Hum Mol Genet 2002;11:379–88.
23. Lam C, Imundo L, Hirsch D, Yu Z, D'Agati V. Glomerulonephritis in a neonate with atypical congenital lupus and toxoplasmosis. Pediatr Nephrol 1999;13:850–3.
24. Liu L, Done SC, Khoshnoodi J, et al. Defective nephrin trafficking caused by missense mutation in the NPHS1 gene: insight into mechanisms of congenital nephrotic syndrome. Hum Mol Genet 2001;10:2637–44.
25. Mahieu P, Monnens L, van Haelst U. Chemical properties of glomerular basement membrane in congenital nephrotic syndrome. Clin Nephrol 1976;5:134–9.
26. Manivel C, Sibley RK, Dehner LP. Complete and incomplete Drash syndrome: a clinicopathologic study of five cases of a dysonotogenetic-neoplastic complex. Hum Pathol 1987;18:80–9.
27. Martul EV, Cuesta MG, Churg J. Histopathologic variability of the congenital nephrotic syndrome. Clin Nephrol 1987;28:161–8.

28. Morgan G, Postlethwaite RJ, Lendon M, Houston IB, Savage JM. Postural deformities in congenital nephrotic syndrome. Arch Dis Child 1981;56:959–66.
29. Nachtigal MW, Hirokawa Y, Enyeart-VanHouten DL, Flanagan JN, Hammer GD, Ingraham HA. Wilms' tumor 1 and Dax-1 modulate the orphan nuclear receptor SF-1 in sex-specific gene expression. Cell 1998;93:445–54.
30. Patrakka J, Ruotsalainen V, Reponen P, et al. Recurrence of nephrotic syndrome in kidney grafts of patients with congenital nephrotic syndrome of the Finnish type: role of nephrin. Transplantation 2002;73:394–403.
31. Pelletier J, Bruening W, Kashtan CE, et al. Germline mutations in the Wilms' tumor suppressor gene are associated with abnormal urogenital development in Denys-Drash syndrome. Cell 1991;67:437–47.
32. Pelletier J, Bruening W, Li FP, Haber DA, Glaser T, Housman ED. WT1 mutations contribute to abnormal genital system development and hereditary Wilms' tumor. Nature 1991;353:431–3.
33. Pritchard-Jones K, Fleming S, Davidson D, et al. The candidate Wilms' tumor gene is involved in genitourinary development. Nature 1990;346: 184–97.
34. Rapola J, Sariola H, Ekblom P. Pathology of fetal congenital nephrosis: immunohistochemical and ultrastructural studies. Kidney Int 1984;25: 701–7.
35. Ryynanen M, Seppala M, Kuusela P, et al. Antenatal screening for congenital nephrosis in Finland by maternal serum alpha-fetoprotein. Br J Obstet Gynecol 1983;90:437–42.
36. Schumacher V, Scharer K, Wuhl E, et al. Spectrum of early onset nephrotic syndrome associated with WT1 missense mutations. Kidney Int 1998;53:1594–600.
37. Sibley RK, Mahan J, Mauer SM, Vernier RL. A clinicopathologic study of forty-eight infants with nephrotic syndrome. Kidney Int 1985;27: 544–52.
38. Tryggvason K. Composition of the glomerular basement membrane in the congenital nephrotic syndrome of the Finnish type. Eur J Clin Invest 1977;7:177–80.
39. Tryggvason K. Unraveling the mechanisms of glomerular ultrafiltration: nephrin, a key component of the slit diaphragm. J Am Soc Nephrol 1999;10:2440–5.
40. Tryggvason K, Kouvalainen K. Number of nephrons in normal human kidneys and kidneys of patients with the congenital nephrotic syndrome. A study using a sieving method for counting of glomeruli. Nephron 1975;15:62–8.
41. Van den Heuvel LP, Westenend PJ, van den Born J, Assmannk J, Knoers N, Monnens LA. Aberrant proteoglycan composition of the glomerular basement membrane in a patient with Denys-Drash syndrome. Nephrol Dial Transplant 1995:10:2205–11.
42. Vermylen C, Levin M, Mossman J, Barratt TM. Glomerular and urinary heparan sulphate in congenital nephrotic syndrome. Pediatr Nephrol 1989;3:122–9.
43. Vernier RL, Klein DJ, Sisson SP, Mahan JD, Oegema TR, Brown DM. Heparan sulfate-rich anionic sites in the human glomerular basement membrane. Decreased concentration in congenital nephrotic syndrome. N Engl J Med 1983;309:1001–9.
44. Wang SX, Ahola H, Palmer T, Solin ML, Luimula P, Holthofer H. Recurrence of nephrotic syndrome after transplantation in CNF is due to autoantibodies to nephrin. Exp Nephrol 2001:9:327–31.
45. Yang T, Jeanpierre C, Dressler GR, Lacoste M, Niaudet P, Gubler MC. WT1 and PAX-2 podocyte expression in Denys-Drash syndrome and isolated diffuse mesangial sclerosis. Am J Pathol 1999;154:181–92.

4 HEREDITARY NEPHROPATHIES

HEREDITARY NEPHRITIS AND ALPORT'S SYNDROME

Definition. Hereditary nephritis is an inherited disorder of the glomerular basement membrane, manifesting with hematuria. It is caused by a mutation in one of the genes encoding the minor (alpha 3, 4, or 5) chains of collagen IV (15). In 1927, Alport described an association with hearing deficit in affected males. The combination of nephropathy and sensorineural hearing loss has since been designated Alport's syndrome.

As the molecular basis of the disease has been unraveled, it has become clear that its phenotypic expression is extremely diverse and includes patients with isolated nephropathy as well as those with abnormalities of other organs and cell types, including the ear, eye, skin, smooth muscle, platelets, and granulocytes (3). This has led to a revised understanding of the disease complex as one that includes as many, if not more, cases of isolated nephropathy (i.e., hereditary nephritis) as cases with associated hearing deficit (i.e., Alport's syndrome). This phenotypic diversity can be explained by the corresponding genetic heterogeneity of the disease, including X-linked (16), autosomal dominant (17,26,37), and autosomal recessive (8,25,26, 31) forms, as well as de novo mutations (27). Over 200 different mutations have been reported in association with hereditary nephritis.

Clinical Features. The frequency of the hereditary nephritis gene in the general population ranges from 1 in 5,000 to 10,000. The disease accounts for 0.2 to 5.0 percent of cases of end-stage renal failure in the United States and Europe. The severity of the renal manifestations depends on the type of genetic mutation and the sex of the patient (21).

In the X-linked form of hereditary nephritis, affected males may manifest hematuria in the first year of life, although the disease is usually not detected before 5 to 10 years of age. The major initial renal manifestation in males is persistent microhematuria (23). Episodes of intermittent gross hematuria are usually precipitated by upper respiratory tract infections or exercise. Flank pain or abdominal pain may accompany episodes of gross hematuria. Males usually develop progressive renal insufficiency, proteinuria, and hypertension in their second through fourth decades of life, although the rate of progression to renal failure varies considerably between kindreds. In some patients, there is proteinuria in the nephrotic range or full nephrotic syndrome in the later stages of the disease.

Females with the X-linked form of the disease generally have a milder clinical phenotype, with a later detection of hematuria (which may be intermittent), a lower incidence of renal insufficiency, and a slower course to renal failure (30). Because there is random inactivation of the mutated X chromosome in development, the severity of the disease varies widely in females; those with severe disease presumably have greater expression of the mutated X chromosome by the podocytes that synthesize glomerular basement membrane.

Extrarenal manifestations also vary in severity and type between kindreds. Hearing loss, which affects 30 to 50 percent of males with X-linked disease, can be detected at any time from early childhood to young adulthood. Hearing deficit is bilateral, sensorineural, and high tone (range, 2,000 to 8,000 Hz). Ocular lesions occur in 15 to 30 percent of patients and are seen exclusively in the juvenile form of Alport's syndrome, in those kindreds with hearing deficit. Abnormalities may involve the cornea, lens, and retina; these include anterior lenticonus, posterior subcapsular cataracts, posterior polymorphous dystrophy, and retinal flecks (18,36). Hematologic disorders are rare, and consist of macrothrombocytopenia (the presence of abnormally few, but large, platelets ranging from 5 to 15 μm in diameter) and cellular inclusions within the granulocytes and monocytes. Affected

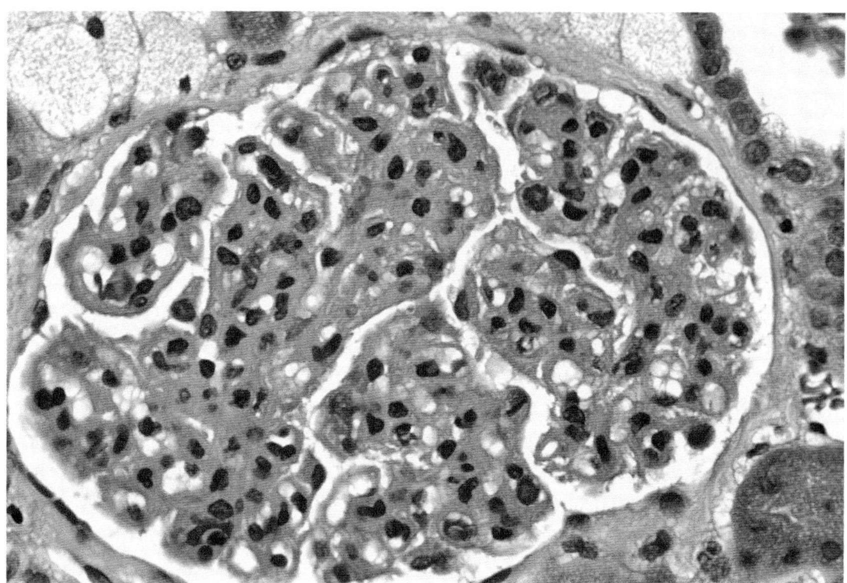

Figure 4-1

HEREDITARY NEPHRITIS

A glomerulus shows mild mesangial hypercellularity and irregular mild thickening of glomerular capillary walls (hematoxylin and eosin [H&E] stain).

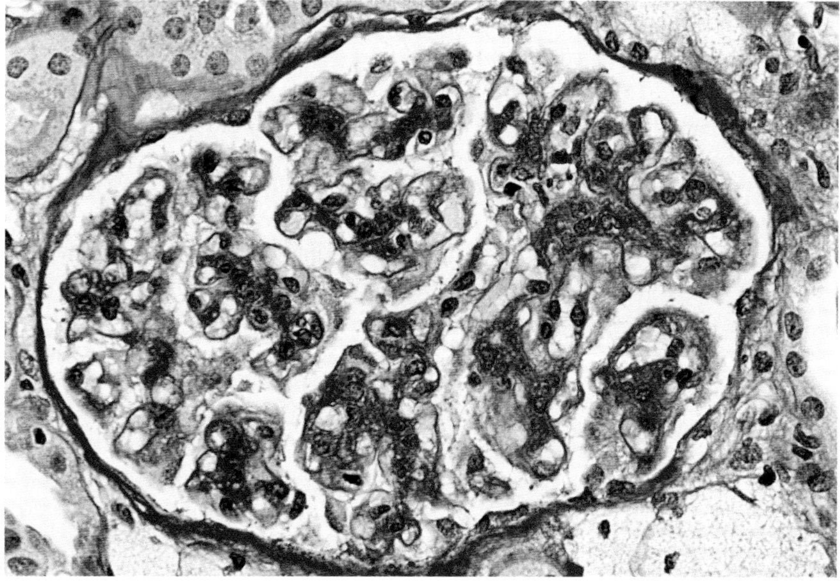

Figure 4-2

HEREDITARY NEPHRITIS

Some mesangial areas are mildly expanded by increased cells and matrix. There are mild textural irregularities of some glomerular basement membranes, which appear slightly vacuolated and duplicated over short segments (periodic acid–Schiff [PAS] stain).

patients may have prolonged bleeding times. Rare cases with associated mutations in the alpha 6 chain of collagen IV manifest diffuse leiomyomatosis of the esophagus, female genitalia, or both (1,32,38).

Light Microscopic Findings. There are no pathognomonic light microscopic findings (5). Early in the disease, the glomeruli usually appear normal. An increased number of fetal (immature) glomeruli has been observed in some biopsies taken during early childhood, suggesting a defect in glomerular maturation. Subtle glomerular abnormalities include mild focal mesangial widening (due to increased mesangial cell number, increased matrix, or both) (figs. 4-1, 4-2) and mild focal irregularities of glomerular basement membrane thickness and texture (uneven thinning and thickening, and segmental lamellation). The latter are detected with the Jones methenamine silver (JMS) or periodic acid–Schiff (PAS) stain (figs. 4-3–4-5). The thinned segments tend to take the basement membrane stains poorly. The podocytes often appear slightly hypertrophied, with prominent

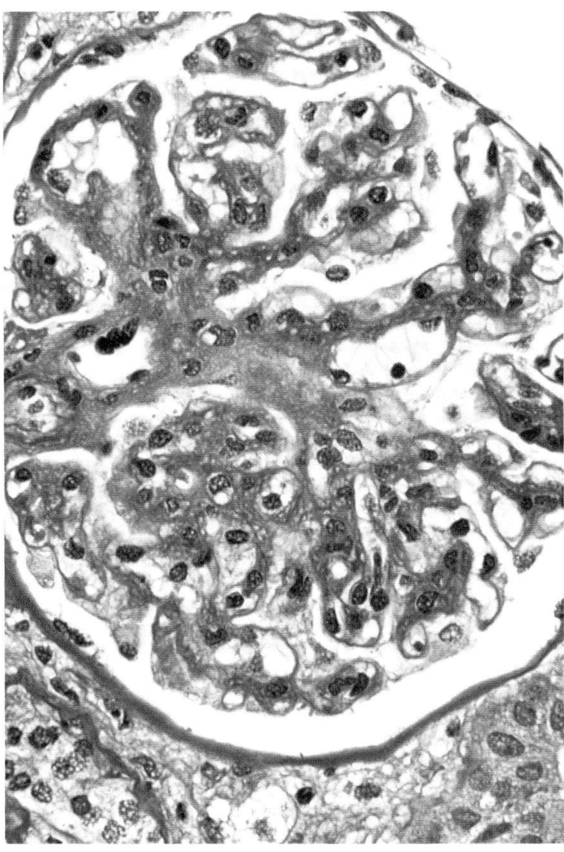

Figure 4-3

HEREDITARY NEPHRITIS

There is mild disturbance of the glomerular architecture, with segmental thickening and textural irregularities of the glomerular basement membranes (PAS stain).

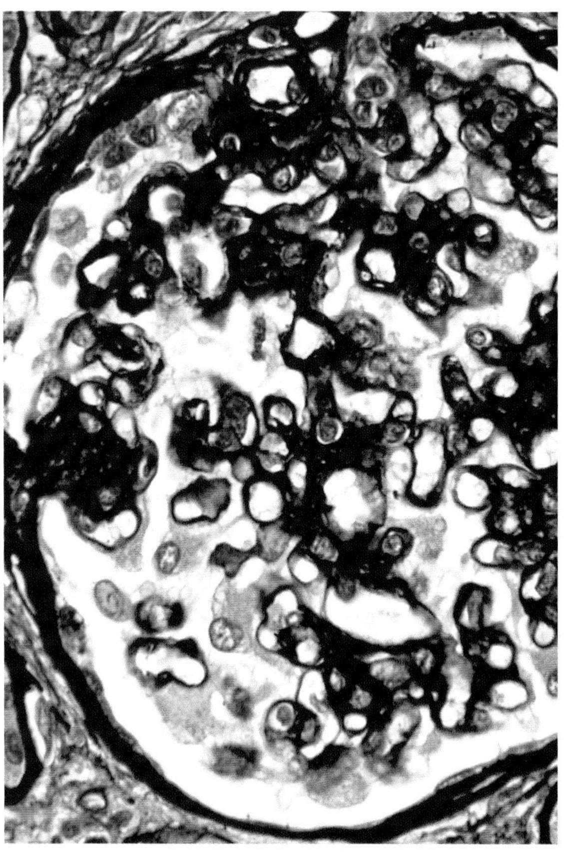

Figure 4-4

HEREDITARY NEPHRITIS

Some glomerular basement membranes appear reduplicated. There is a small synechia between the tuft and Bowman's capsule (Jones methenamine silver [JMS] stain).

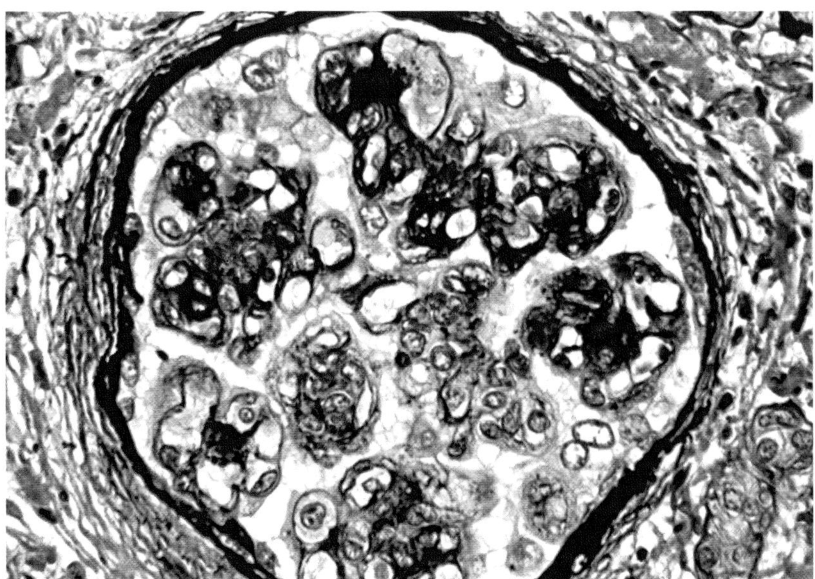

Figure 4-5

HEREDITARY NEPHRITIS

Some glomerular basement membranes fail to stain with the silver stain, probably owing to severe thinning, whereas others are thickened and reduplicated, mimicking membranoproliferative glomerulonephritis. There is diffuse swelling of the visceral epithelial cells (JMS stain).

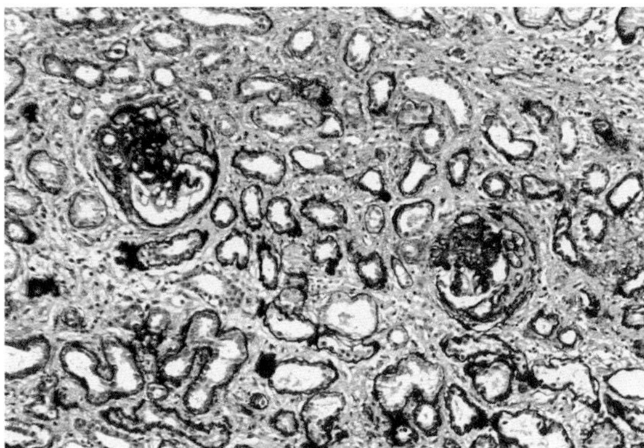

Figure 4-6

HEREDITARY NEPHRITIS

An advanced case of hereditary nephritis shows progression to segmental and global sclerosis with subcapsular fibrosis and severe chronic tubulointerstitial disease (JMS stain).

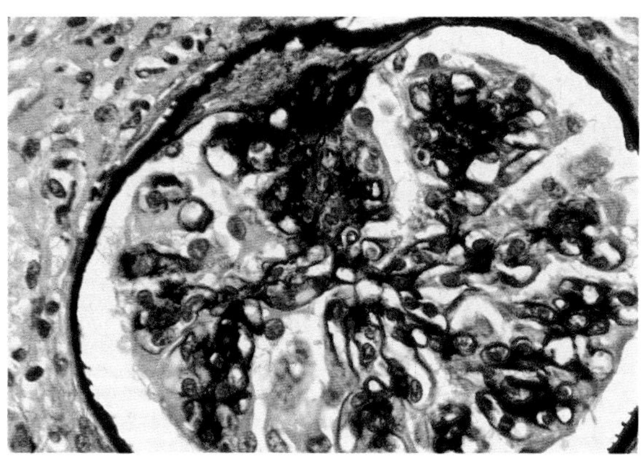

Figure 4-7

HEREDITARY NEPHRITIS

A glomerulus with a segmental scar produces a secondary pattern of focal segmental glomerulosclerosis (JMS stain).

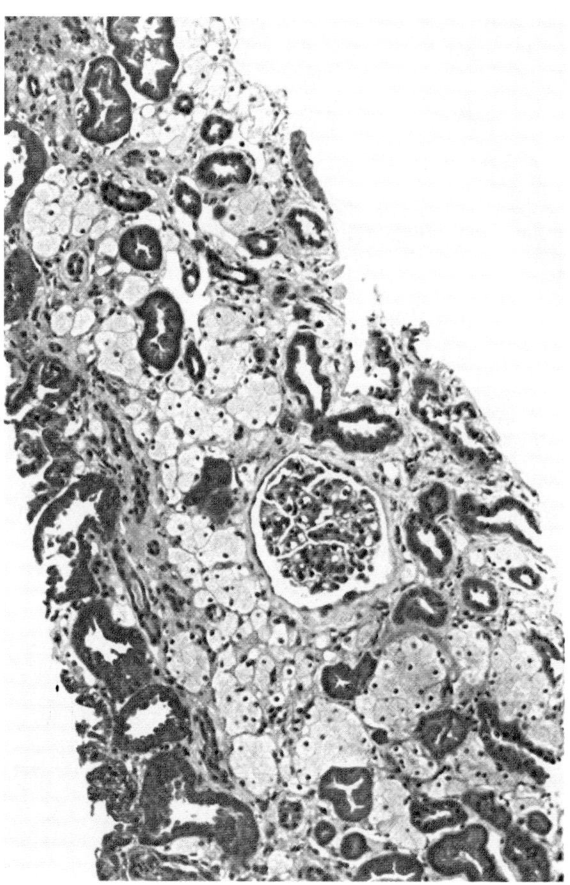

Figure 4-8

HEREDITARY NEPHRITIS

There are large interstitial aggregates of foam cells (Masson trichrome stain).

cell bodies (figs. 4-4, 4-5). As the disease progresses, there is evolution to a pattern of focal segmental and global glomerulosclerosis with focal synechiae (figs. 4-6, 4-7) (22). Crescents are rarely described.

Even early in the disease, erythrocytes and red blood cell casts may be found in the tubular lumens. Interstitial foam cells are common, although their presence does not correlate well with nephrotic proteinuria (fig. 4-8). Similarly, proximal tubular cells may contain numerous protein and lipid resorption droplets. With the development of focal segmental and global glomerulosclerosis, there is progressive tubular atrophy, interstitial fibrosis, and nonspecific arteriosclerosis (fig. 4-6).

Immunofluorescence Findings. Immunofluorescence studies are typically negative for immunoglobulin and complement. Thus, the major role of immunofluorescence in this disease is to exclude glomerular disease of the immune deposit type. Early in the disease, some patients display irregular, sparse glomerular basement membrane positivity for complement (C)3 only (fig. 4-9). This likely corresponds to nonspecific staining in areas of glomerular basement membrane thickening and lamellation. In the later stages of the disease, more coarsely granular positivity for immunoglobulin (Ig)M

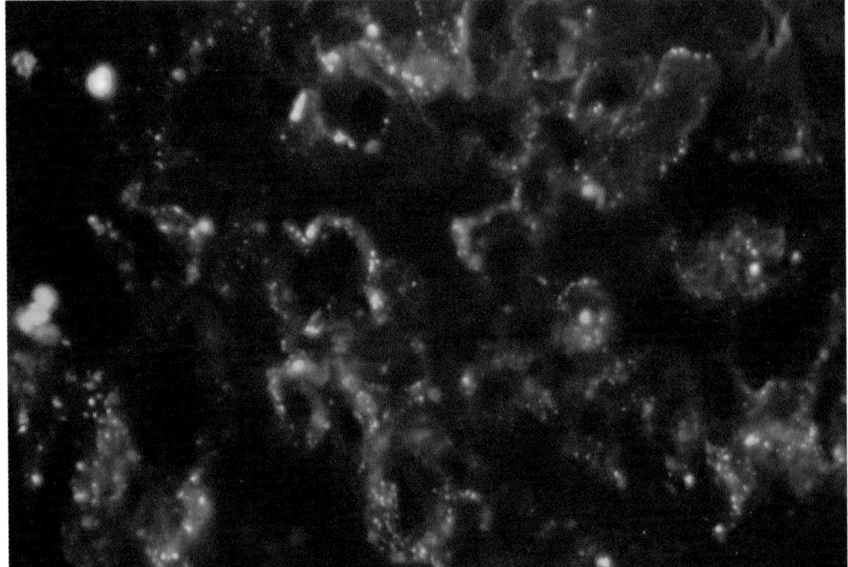

Figure 4-9

HEREDITARY NEPHRITIS

There is sparse granular staining of the glomerular basement membranes with antisera to C3 (immunofluorescence micrograph).

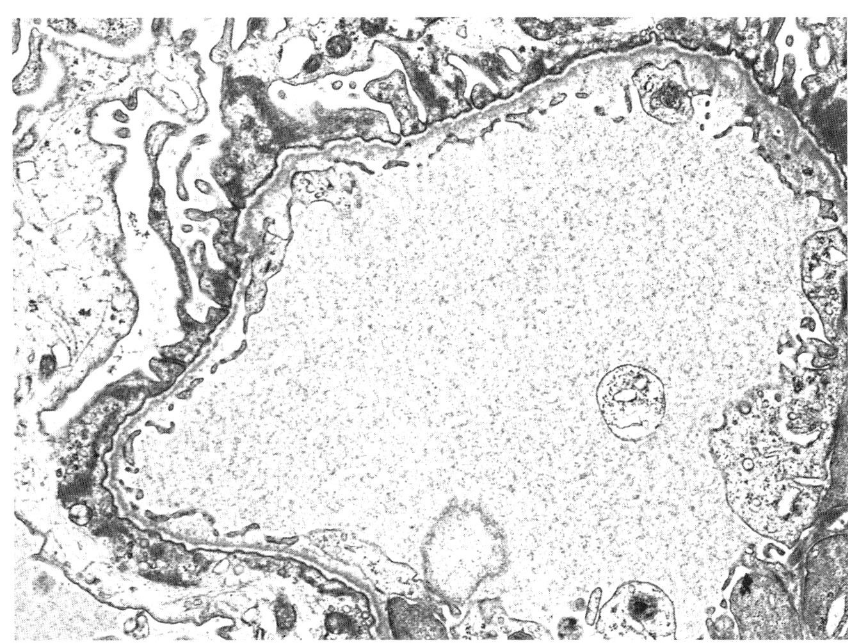

Figure 4-10

HEREDITARY NEPHRITIS

An early stage of hereditary nephritis in a young male shows diffuse thinning of glomerular basement membranes. There are mild textural irregularities of the lamina densa, but without evidence of lamellation. Although the disease is X-linked, the phenotype is one of thinning, resembling thin basement membrane disease (electron micrograph).

and/or C3 is commonly found in segmentally and globally sclerotic glomeruli.

Electron Microscopic Findings. The diagnostic lesions of hereditary nephritis are seen at the ultrastructural level (13,28). Early in the disease, the only abnormality may be diffuse thinning of the glomerular basement membrane to less than 150 nm (fig. 4-10) (20). Later in the disease, there is progressive thickening and lamellation of the glomerular basement membrane, producing a characteristic "split and splintered" appearance (figs. 4-11–4-13). The areas of lamellation may be segmental, affecting only some capillaries or a portion of the glomerular capillary circumference, often alternating with thinned stretches of glomerular basement membrane (fig. 4-13). The lamellations affect the lamina densa as well as the lamina rara interna and externa. In fully developed forms, the full thickness of the glomerular basement membrane

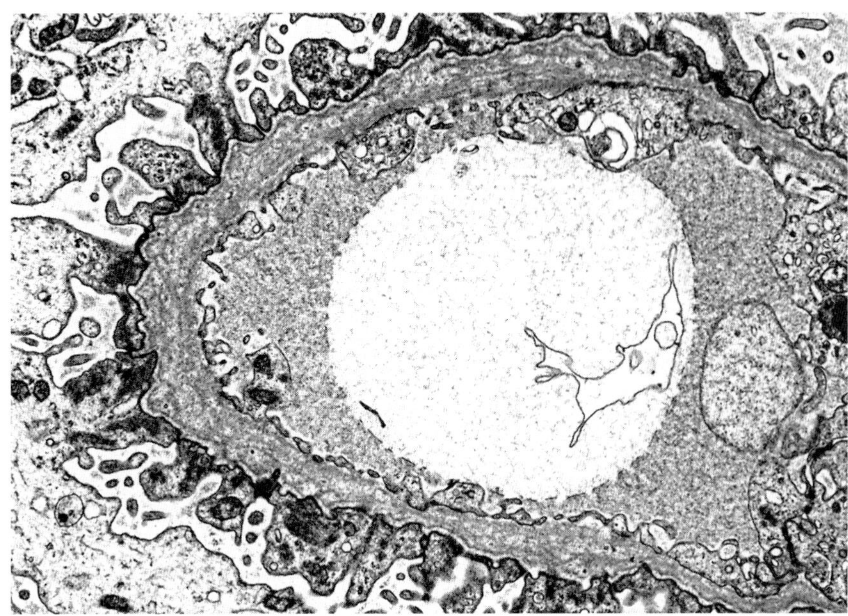

Figure 4-11

HEREDITARY NEPHRITIS

Lamellation of the lamina densa produces a basket-woven texture with internal lucencies, focal microspherical granules, and an irregular contour of the outer (epithelial) aspect of the glomerular basement membrane (electron micrograph).

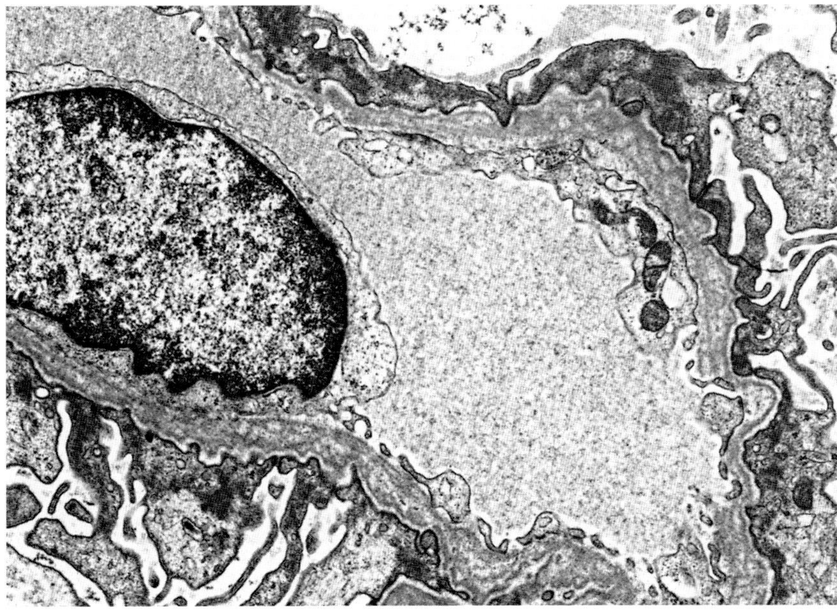

Figure 4-12

HEREDITARY NEPHRITIS

This specimen from a 10-year-old female shows extensive lamellation of the glomerular basement membrane associated with foot process effacement (electron micrograph).

is affected, often producing irregularities of the outer glomerular basement membrane contour. The lamellations of glomerular basement membrane material typically enclose relatively electron-lucent zones that may contain microspherical electron-dense granulations 20 to 90 nm in diameter (fig. 4-11). Focal ruptures of the glomerular basement membrane may be detected in the thinned or lamellated segments. These are typically plugged by invaginations of the podocyte and endothelial cell cytoplasm.

In general, these ultrastructural abnormalities are more severe and generalized in males with X-linked disease. In females, the areas of thinning and lamellation tend to be more focal and segmental, alternating with areas of normal-appearing glomerular basement membrane. Some female heterozygotes with X-linked

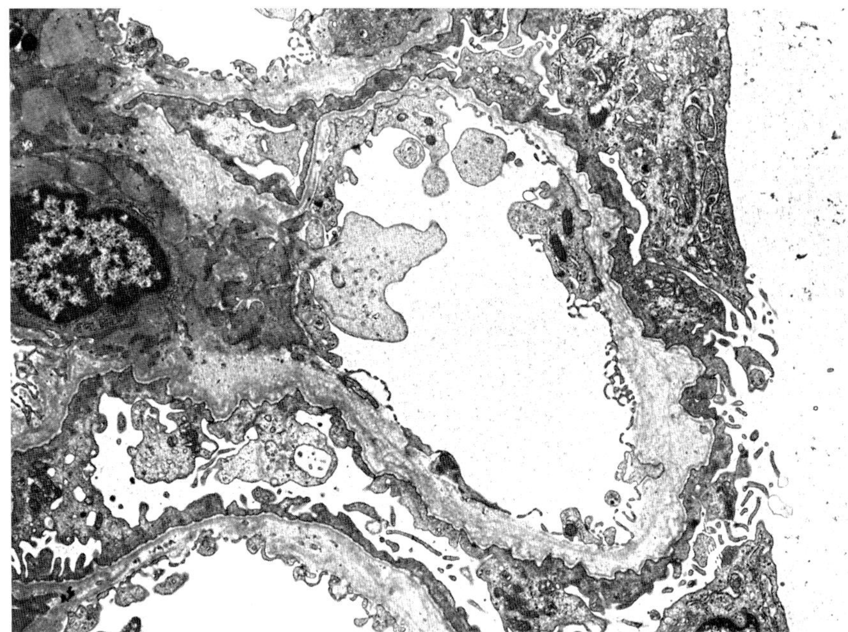

Figure 4-13

HEREDITARY NEPHRITIS

Thickened, lamellated segments alternate with thinned segments of glomerular basement membrane (electron micrograph).

disease have fairly diffuse thinning of glomerular basement membranes with very segmental and variable areas of lamellation. Foot process effacement commonly occurs overlying the thickened and lamellated segments. Sparse, small, paramesangial electron-dense deposits are occasionally identified; however, no typical immune deposits are detected involving the peripheral glomerular capillary walls. In rare cases, small intramembranous electron densities, likely corresponding to entrapped plasma proteins, are seen. In some kindreds with hereditary nephritis, thinning of the glomerular basement membrane (without lamellation) is the only ultrastructural finding.

Electron-lucent lipid resorption droplets and electron-dense protein resorption droplets may be detected in the proximal tubular cells. Interstitial foam cells contain abundant intracytoplasmic lipid vacuoles. Tubular basement membranes may be thickened and lamellated due to the intramembranous deposition of extracellular lipid deposits.

Special Studies for Collagen IV Subtypes. It was empirically observed the 1970s that glomeruli from patients with hereditary nephritis usually failed to stain with the sera of patients with Goodpasture's (or antiglomerular basement membrane) disease (29). It would be another 25 years before the molecular basis for this observation was elucidated. In that era, absence of staining of renal biopsies with Goodpasture's antisera as determined by indirect immunofluorescence was often used as an ancillary test to confirm the diagnosis of hereditary nephritis.

In recent years, the use of Goodpasture's antisera has been superceded by commercially available monospecific antibodies to the alpha subunits of collagen IV (33). These antibodies can be applied to frozen sections of renal or skin biopsies. The commercially available Wieslab kit includes antibodies to the alpha 1, 3, and 5 subunits of collagen IV. Antibodies to subunits alpha 1 and 2 (which comprise the major collagen IV network) normally stain all renal basement membranes including the mesangial matrix. Antibodies to subunits alpha 3, 4, and 5 (which comprise the minor collagen IV network) normally stain the entire thickness of the glomerular basement membrane as well as distal tubular basement membranes. Bowman's capsule and normal epidermal basement membrane have reactivity for alpha 1, 2, 5, and 6, but not alpha 3 or 4 (11,34). Staining for alpha 5 and 6 is also seen in distal tubular basement membranes.

Males with X-linked disease typically lack immunoreactivity for the alpha 5 subunit of collagen IV in their glomerular basement membranes and epidermal basement membranes (figs. 4-14, 4-15). Because mutations in the gene

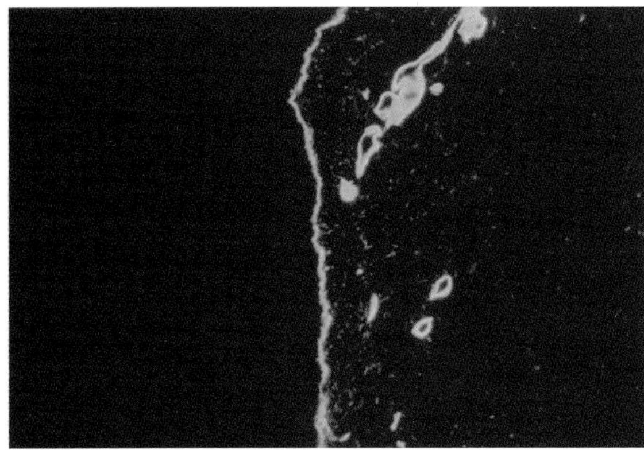

Figure 4-14

HEREDITARY NEPHRITIS

A punch skin biopsy from an 8-year-old boy with X-linked hereditary nephritis is stained with antisera to the alpha 1 subunit of collagen IV. Normal linear staining of the epidermal basement membrane is seen (immunofluorescence micrograph). (Figs. 4-14 and 4-15 are from the same patient.)

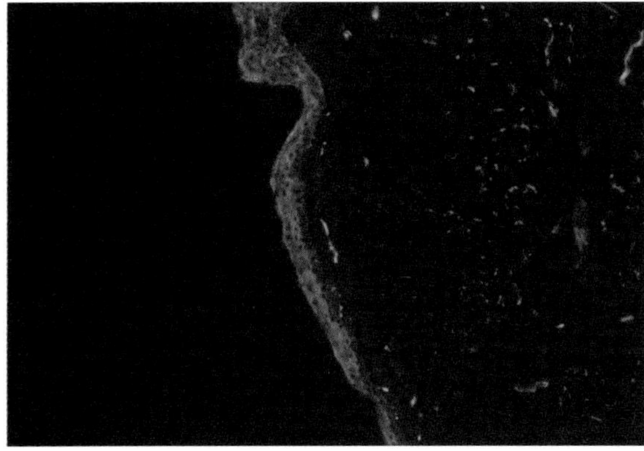

Figure 4-15

HEREDITARY NEPHRITIS

The epidermal basement membrane from a skin biopsy from the patient in figure 4-14 does not stain for the alpha 5 subunit of collagen IV (immunofluorescence micrograph).

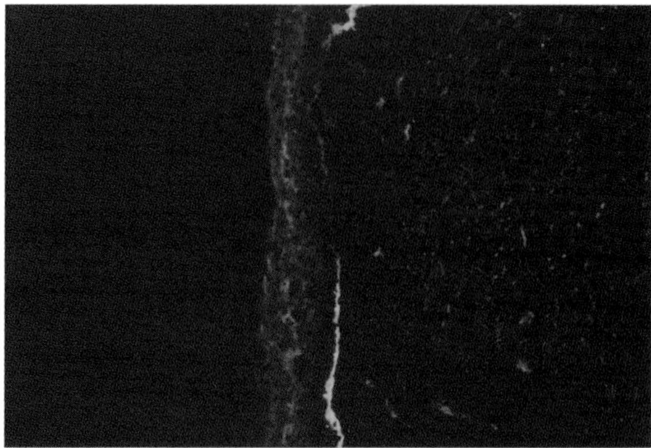

Figure 4-16

HEREDITARY NEPHRITIS

A skin biopsy (from a female with X-linked disease) shows weak and segmental (interrupted) positivity for the alpha 5 subunit of collagen IV in the epidermal basement membrane. This interrupted staining occurs because females are mosaics for the mutation in the alpha 5 subunit, with some epidermal epithelial cells expressing the normal allele, and others the mutated allele, according to random inactivation of one X chromosome (lyonization) (immunofluorescence micrograph). (Figs. 4-16 to 4-18 are from the same patient.)

encoding the alpha 5 subunit cause defective incorporation of alpha 3 and 4 into the supramolecular minor collagen IV network, lack of reactivity for alpha 3 and 4 usually accompanies the loss of alpha 5 in the glomerular basement membranes (9). Because alpha 3 and 4 are not normally expressed in epidermal basement membrane, however, immunostaining for these chains in skin biopsies is not diagnostically useful. In males with X-linked disease, there is also lack of staining of Bowman's capsule and the distal tubular basement membranes for alpha 5 and 6. Immunoreactivity for alpha 1 in glomerular basement membranes is normal or even increased, because this major collagen IV chain is part of a separate collagen IV network that does not form heterotrimers with the alpha 5 subunit (24,39).

Females with X-linked disease are mosaics exhibiting segmental (i.e., discontinuous) loss of alpha 3, 4, and 5 from their glomerular basement membranes and segmental loss of alpha 5 from their epidermal basement membranes (figs. 4-16–4-18).

In patients with the autosomal recessive or autosomal dominant form of Alport's disease, there is absent glomerular basement membrane staining for alpha 3, 4, and 5, but in contrast to X-linked cases, there is normal staining for alpha 5 in Bowman's capsule, distal tubular basement membranes, and skin.

As the application of these antibodies to renal biopsies has grown in recent years, greater practical experience with their sensitivity and specificity has become available. Unfortunately, not all cases of X-linked hereditary nephritis fail to stain with antibodies to the alpha 5 subunit of collagen IV; in fact, from 30 to 40 percent of

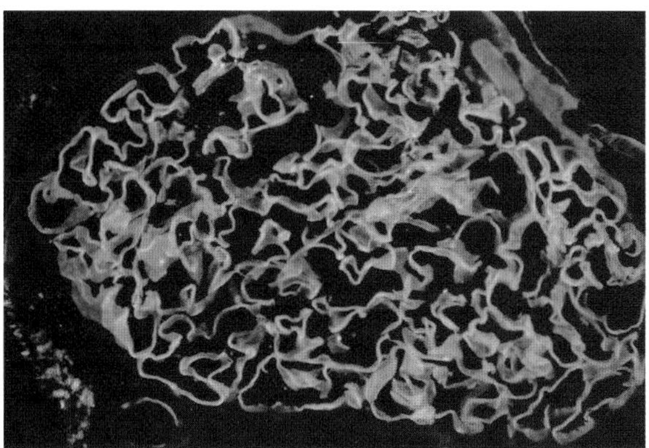

Figure 4-17

HEREDITARY NEPHRITIS

The glomerular basement membranes from a female with X-linked disease show normal linear staining with antisera to the alpha 1 subunit of collagen IV (immunofluorescence micrograph).

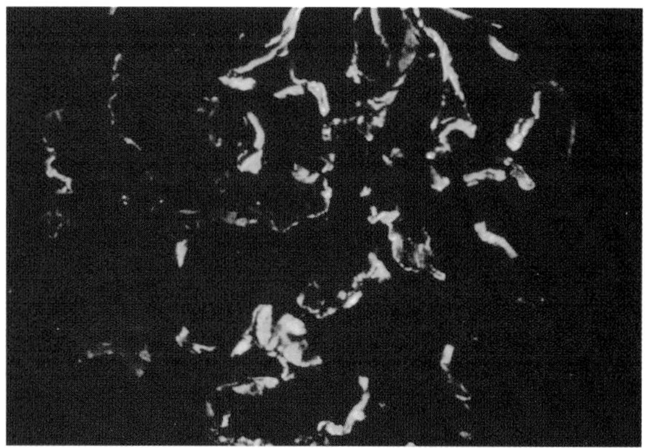

Figure 4-18

HEREDITARY NEPHRITIS

A glomerulus (in a female with X-linked disease) displays weak and segmental positivity for the alpha 5 subunit of collagen IV (immunofluorescence micrograph).

cases retain immunoreactivity for alpha 5. These cases likely have single amino acid substitutions or small deletions that cannot be detected with a monoclonal antibody directed to a single epitope within the large alpha 5 collagen chain. Thus, although a negative staining result provides confirmatory evidence of hereditary nephritis, positive staining for alpha 5 does not exclude the disease.

Differential Diagnosis. Abnormalities of glomerular basement membrane thickness and texture may occur secondarily in a variety of glomerular disorders (34). In hereditary nephritis, however, they occur in the absence of the other glomerular pathologic changes that are diagnostic of different glomerular diseases. In this sense, the diagnosis of hereditary nephritis can be considered a diagnosis of exclusion.

In those kindreds with X-linked hereditary nephritis that have exclusively thin basement membranes, the ultrastructural findings may be indistinguishable from those of thin basement membrane disease. In such cases, immunostaining for the alpha subunits of collagen IV is very helpful by showing loss of glomerular basement membrane staining for alpha 3, 4, and 5 in hereditary nephritis and retention of staining for all three isoforms in thin basement membrane disease.

Thinning of the glomerular basement membrane occurs commonly in IgA nephritis, where it may be quite diffuse (fig. 4-19). Segmental thinning of the glomerular basement membrane may also occur in a variety of other immune complex–mediated forms of glomerulonephritis or the thrombotic microangiopathies, especially in areas of glomerular basement membrane distention due to endocapillary proliferation or intracapillary thrombosis.

Thickening and lamellation of the glomerular basement membrane frequently occur secondarily in focal segmental glomerulosclerosis, particularly in areas of previous podocyte detachment with intervening layering of loosely formed neomembrane material (fig. 4-20). This may pose a difficult diagnostic dilemma, because hereditary nephritis frequently manifests focal segmental and global glomerular scarring and nephrotic-range proteinuria as it progresses. The degree of foot process fusion, however, is usually more marked in idiopathic focal segmental glomerulosclerosis and the extent of glomerular basement membrane lamellation is typically greater in hereditary nephritis. This lamellation tends to affect the lamina densa or full thickness glomerular basement membrane in hereditary nephritis but is more typically confined to the outer layer of the glomerular basement membrane in focal segmental glomerulosclerosis.

In a variety of immune complex–mediated glomerular diseases, thickening and lamellation of the glomerular basement membrane may

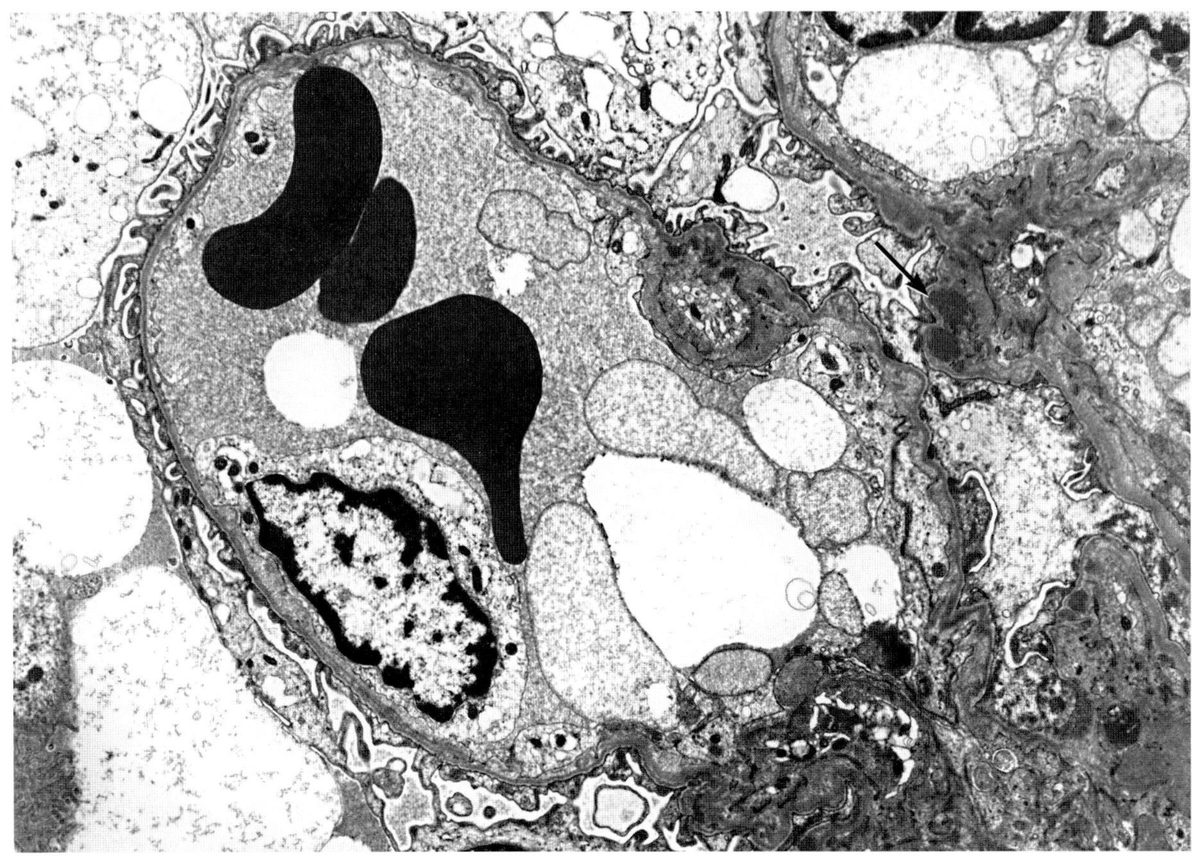

Figure 4-19

IgA NEPHROPATHY

There is marked thinning of the glomerular basement membrane, resembling the changes seen in thin basement membrane disease. Several electron-dense deposits are present in the paramesangial areas (arrow). The association of thin basement membrane disease and IgA nephropathy is common. It is uncertain whether this represents the chance coincidence of two unrelated glomerulopathies or an acquired abnormality in glomerular basement membrane synthesis secondary to IgA nephropathy (electron micrograph).

occur at sites of resorbed immune deposits, with subsequent reorganization of the glomerular basement membrane. This is particularly common in the resolving phase of acute postinfectious glomerulonephritis, IgA nephropathy (fig. 4-21), and the more advanced stages of membranous glomerulopathy.

There are a variety of nonimmune glomerular diseases that mimic hereditary nephritis at the ultrastructural level. In diabetic nephropathy, the glomerular basement membrane is typically thickened with a slightly lamellated texture. In addition to the clinical history, the pathologic findings of diffuse mesangial sclerosis and the regular nature of the glomerular basement membrane thickening help distinguish diabetic nephropathy from hereditary nephritis. In some heritable diseases, such as lecithin cholesterol acyltransferase (LCAT) deficiency and some forms of hepatic glomerulopathy, there is irregular thickening of the glomerular basement membrane with electron-lucent defects, corresponding to lipid inclusions that can mimic the glomerular basement membrane lamellations seen in hereditary nephritis. These conditions are typically distinguished by similar involvement of the mesangial matrix and by the presence of an electron-dense layer surrounding the rounded electron-lucent inclusions. Patients with the nail-patella syndrome may also have thickening and irregular lamellation of the glomerular basement membrane. The lucencies

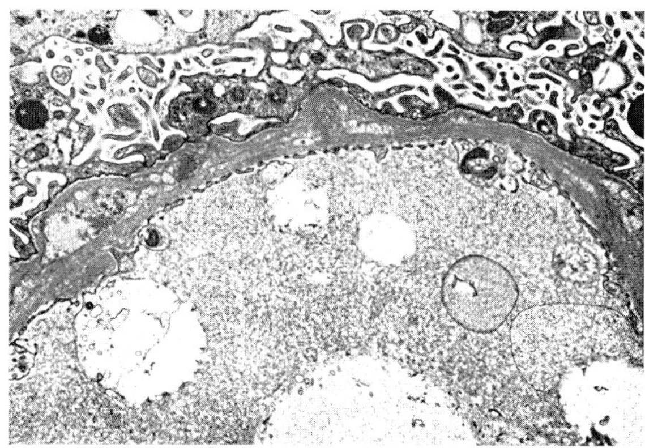

Figure 4-20

IDIOPATHIC FOCAL SEGMENTAL GLOMERULOSCLEROSIS

Lamellation of the glomerular basement membrane, mimicking hereditary nephritis, may result from foci of podocyte detachment and remodeling of the glomerular basement membrane (electron micrograph).

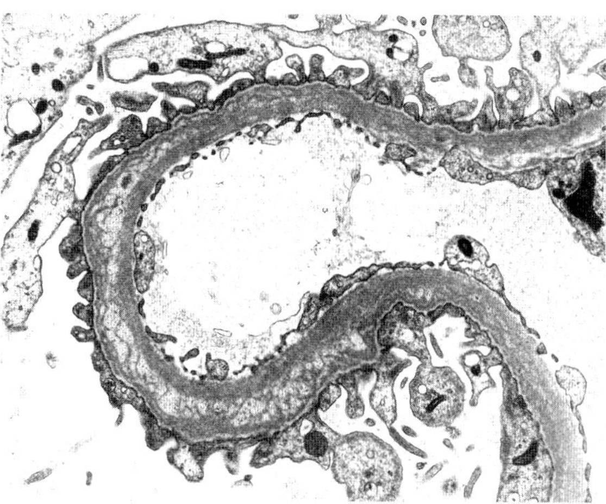

Figure 4-21

IgA NEPHROPATHY

Thickening and lamellation of the glomerular basement membrane in a patient with IgA nephropathy produce a basket-woven appearance that mimics the changes seen in hereditary nephritis. In this case, however, there were electron-dense mesangial deposits and strong immunofluorescent positivity for IgA, features diagnostic of IgA nephropathy (electron micrograph).

of the glomerular basement membrane in nail-patella syndrome are distinguished by their "moth-eaten" appearance and the ultrastructural demonstration of thickly banded collagen fibers within the lucent defects using a phosphotungstic acid counterstain (figs. 4-22, 4-23).

Etiology and Pathogenesis. The genetic basis of hereditary nephritis/Alport's syndrome has been elucidated in the last decade (2,14). Mutations affect the alpha 5 (and in some cases the alpha 6) subunits of collagen IV (encoded on the X chromosome), or the alpha 3 or 4 subunit (encoded on chromosome 2). The X-linked form accounts for approximately 80 percent of cases, with over 200 distinct mutations of the *COL4A5* gene described. Approximately 10 percent of these mutations are large deletions. Some of these cases cosegregate with leiomyomatosis of the esophageal tract, tracheobronchial tree, and female genital system. The latter cases have deletions of the 5′ end of *COL4A5* that extends to involve the first two exons of *COL4A6* (1). The remaining 20 percent of cases are autosomal-dominant or autosomal-recessive forms exhibiting mutations in the *COL4A3* or *COL4A4* gene.

Large deletions of *COL4A5* have been linked to earlier onset of nephropathy in childhood and the development of full Alport's syndrome (16). Involvement of the eye and ear is explained by the normal distribution of the alpha 3, 4, and 5 collagen IV network in the lens and cochlea. Most of the other mutations are missense, splice site, or small deletions. Missense mutations are more likely to result in late-onset nephropathy and clinical disease limited to the kidney. A common missense mutation is the replacement of the smallest amino acid, glycine (which comprises every third amino acid in the collagenous domain of collagen IV) with a larger amino acid. This causes defective folding of the mutant alpha 5 chain required for the formation of a tightly wound triple helix. Other common mutations involve the NC1 domain of collagen IV. These NC1 mutations prevent normal dimerization of the collagen IV molecules required for formation of the three-dimensional collagen network.

The abnormal alpha 5 subunit prevents incorporation of the alpha 3 and 4 chains into the normal triple helix that comprises the minor collagen IV network (4). In situ hybridization reveals normal mRNA transcription of alpha 3 and 4 chains, suggesting that they are synthesized by the podocytes but that post-transcriptional events cause their failure to be incorporated into the minor collagen IV network in patients with X-linked disease (9). The alpha 1

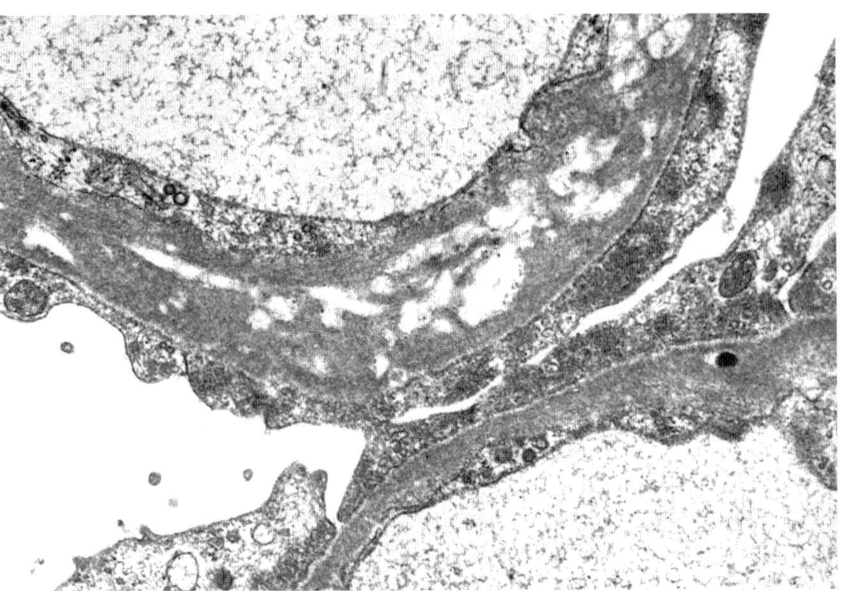

Figure 4-22

NAIL-PATELLA SYNDROME

The glomerular basement membranes are thickened with internal electron-lucent defects, mimicking the lamellations of hereditary nephritis (electron micrograph).

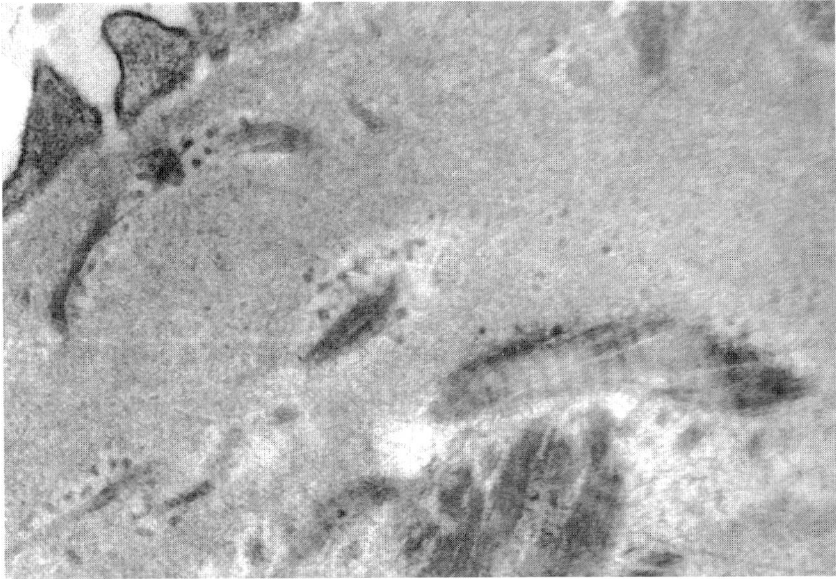

Figure 4-23

NAIL-PATELLA SYNDROME

Banded collagen fibers are demonstrated within the lacunae of the glomerular basement membrane using the phosphotungstic acid stain for collagen (electron micrograph).

and 2 subunits of collagen IV, which comprise the major collagen IV network, persist in the affected basement membranes and may even increase (presumably to compensate for the absence of a normal minor collagen IV network).

Females with X-linked disease are mosaics for the mutated alpha 5 chain due to random inactivation of the X chromosome during development (i.e., lyonization). Depending on the extent of expression of the mutated X chromosome in the podocytes, a range of mild to severe diseases may occur. In general, females have milder disease than males, with slower progression to renal failure.

Autosomal recessive forms of hereditary nephritis are due to homozygous or compound heterozygous mutations in either the *COL4A3* or *COL4A4* gene, including splice site, nonsense, missense, and frame shift mutations (10,15,26). These patients typically lack a family history of renal disease. Females are affected as frequently as males. Some cases of autosomal recessive Alport's syndrome arise from the intersection of two kindreds with benign familial hematuria.

In autosomal dominant Alport's syndrome, there may be mutations in either the *COL4A3* or the *COL4A4* genes, including splice site, missense, and inframe deletion mutations (6,10,15,26).

Treatment and Prognosis. Most males with X-linked disease progress to end-stage renal failure, although the rate of progression varies considerably between kindreds. Within a kindred, however, the rate tends to be fairly constant. Those with large deletions progress more rapidly to renal failure, as early as the second decade of life. Females with X-linked disease usually have a slower course, and many survive to old age without progression to renal failure. For those with autosomal recessive disease, progression to renal failure before the age of 30 years and deafness are common.

There is no specific treatment for hereditary nephritis. Proteinuria may respond to angiotensin-converting enzyme inhibitors (35). Transplantation is a successful therapy for those who progress to end-stage renal failure. Antiglomerular membrane disease develops in the allograft of 5 to 15 percent of patients with transplants, leading to graft failure (7,19). Due to defective incorporation of the alpha 3 chain in patients with hereditary nephritis, the immune system perceives the antigen as foreign when it is presented in the context of the renal transplant. Gene therapy holds promise for the future (12).

THIN BASEMENT MEMBRANE DISEASE

Definition. Thin basement membrane disease is a glomerular disorder characterized pathologically by diffuse thinning of the glomerular basement membrane and clinically by isolated hematuria (45–47). In contrast to hereditary nephritis, thin basement membrane disease is not associated with lamellation of the glomerular basement membrane, renal failure, or extrarenal manifestations. Because of the familial aggregation of the disease and absence of progression to renal failure, the clinical-pathologic syndrome has often been referred to as *benign familial hematuria* (57).

Clinical Features. The defining clinical manifestation of thin basement membrane disease is hematuria (56). Most patients have persistent microhematuria that is first detected in childhood. In some cases, however, the microhematuria is intermittent and is not detected until adulthood (54). Episodic gross hematuria has been reported, especially following upper respiratory tract infections. Significant proteinuria and renal insufficiency are not typical clinical features, although there are rare cases of purported thin basement membrane disease with proteinuria and progression to renal failure (44). Genetic analysis in such cases usually reveals mutations typical of hereditary nephritis, indicating that these cases represent atypical forms of hereditary nephritis with an exclusively thin basement membrane phenotype. The incidence of thin basement membranes may be as high as 5 percent in the general population.

Light Microscopic Findings. Microscopically, glomeruli usually appear normal (fig. 4-24). Delicate attenuated staining of the glomerular basement membranes with the JMS or PAS stain suggests the presence of thinning of the glomerular basement membrane, which can only be diagnosed definitively by electron microscopy. There may be focal global glomerulosclerosis consistent with age. Rarely, immature glomeruli have been reported. It is not uncommon to find erythrocytes in the tubular lumens.

Immunofluorescence Findings. Typically, there is no glomerular staining for immunoglobulins or complement components. In a few cases, sparse and nonspecific staining of the glomerular tuft for IgM and C3 may be identified. Vascular deposits of C3 may be observed.

Electron Microscopic Findings. The diagnostic finding is diffuse thinning of the glomerular basement membrane in the absence of other significant glomerular alterations (figs. 4-25, 4-26), (40). There are no standardized criteria for how thin or diffuse the glomerular basement membrane must be to qualify as thin basement membrane disease. Variability in reported findings depends to some degree on differences in the fixation, dehydration, and staining techniques employed by different laboratories.

Most definitions of thin basement membrane disease in adults require the thinning to be less than 250 nm (by World Health Organization [WHO] criteria) or less than 200 nm in over 50 percent of glomerular capillaries (43,53). In children, thinning below 200 nm is the diagnostic criterion used by Gubler et al. (46). Normally, the thickness of the glomerular basement membrane (as measured from endothelial to visceral

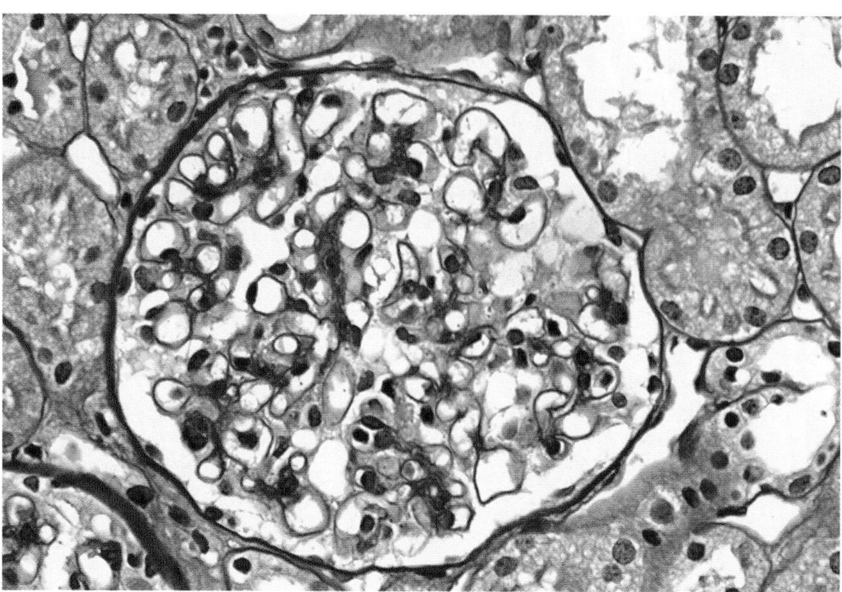

Figure 4-24

THIN BASEMENT MEMBRANE DISEASE

A glomerulus appears unremarkable by light microscopy, with very delicate but uniform basement membranes (PAS stain).

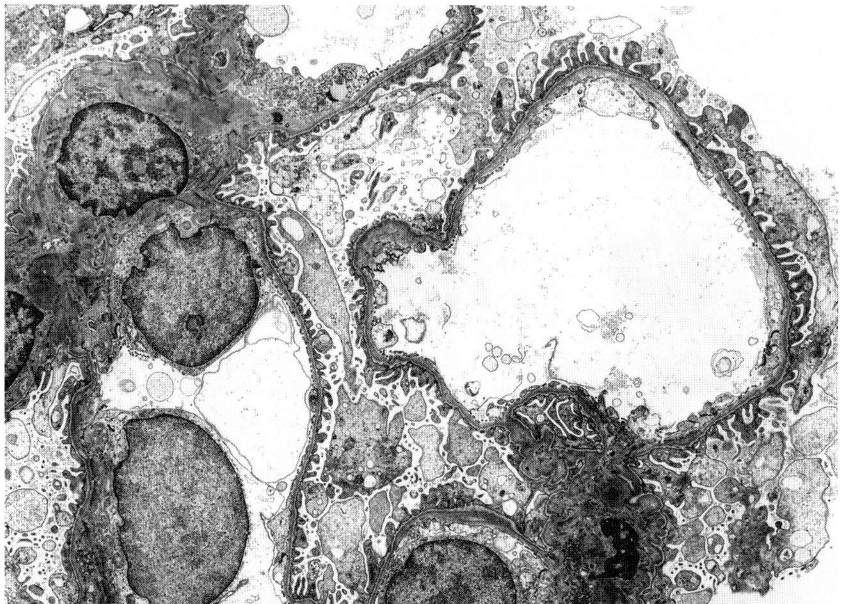

Figure 4-25

THIN BASEMENT MEMBRANE DISEASE

There is diffuse and uniform thinning of the glomerular basement membranes, which measure less than 150 nm in thickness. The texture of the glomerular basement membrane is uniform, without lamellation, and foot processes are preserved (electron micrograph).

epithelial cell) averages 169 +/- 30 nm at birth and increases rapidly to 245 +/- 49 nm by 2 years of age. It continues to increase gradually with age to reach its mature adult thickness of about 320 +/- 40 nm in females and 370 +/- 45 nm in males (53). Thus, thinning of the glomerular basement membrane can only be properly assessed in the context of the patient's age (55).

In some cases of thin basement membrane disease, the glomerular basement membranes are extremely attenuated, measuring less than 100 nm. Often the lamina rara interna and externa appear more conspicuous than usual because the thinning predominantly affects the lamina densa. The texture of the glomerular basement membrane tends to be uniform, without lamellation. Occasionally, however, mild irregularities of texture and contour are observed, including slight scalloping of the outer glomerular basement membrane.

Thinning is usually generalized, but may be focal and segmental in some cases. It is advisable to study more than one glomerulus by electron microscopy. Gaps in the glomerular basement membrane may be identified, with the

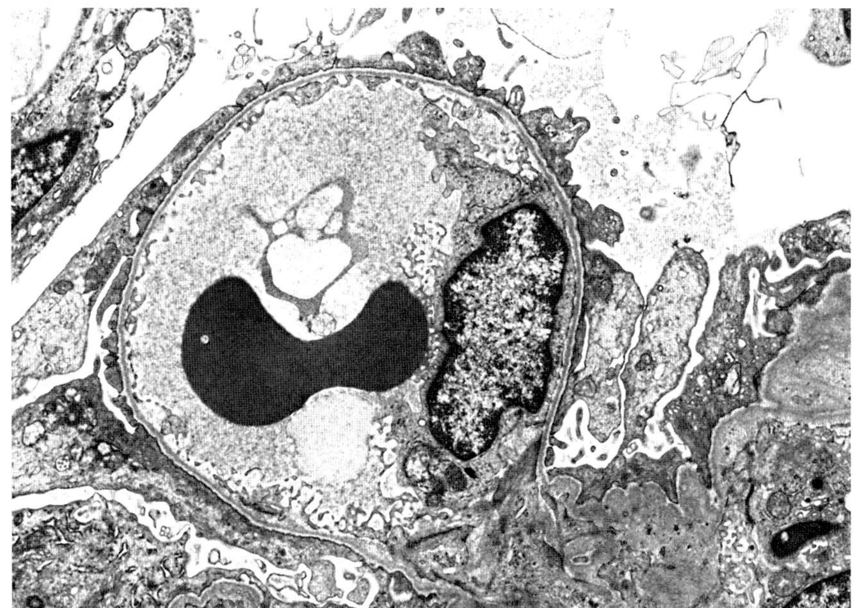

Figure 4-26

THIN BASEMENT MEMBRANE DISEASE

There is extreme regular thinning of the glomerular basement membrane. Foot processes are segmentally effaced (electron micrograph).

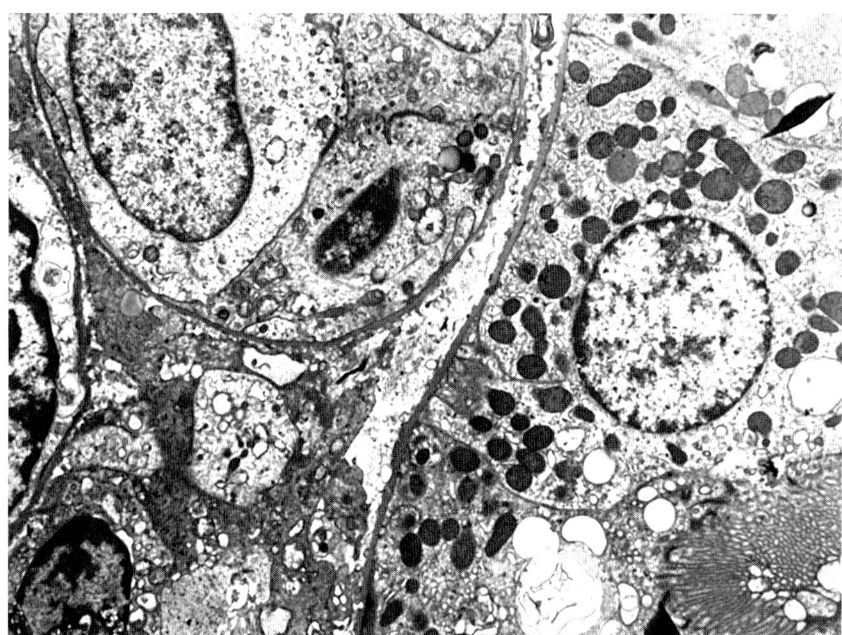

Figure 4-27

THIN BASEMENT MEMBRANE DISEASE

There is thinning of some of the basement membranes of cortical tubules (electron micrograph).

escape of erythrocytes into Bowman's space. There is often mild, focal effacement of foot processes, particularly those overlying the most highly attenuated glomerular basement membranes. No glomerular electron-dense deposits are identified. Mesangial areas are unremarkable. In some cases, the tubular basement membranes are also focally thinned (fig. 4-27).

Special Studies for Collagen IV Subtypes. In thin basement membrane disease, the glomeruli maintain their normal immunoreactivity for the alpha 1, 2, 3, 4, and 5 subunits of collagen IV, as well as for Goodpasture's antisera. However, due to the thinning of the glomerular basement membrane, the quality of the staining often appears attenuated, giving an impression of weaker positivity than normal.

Differential Diagnosis. The clinical-pathologic diagnosis of thin basement membrane disease is problematic because of the wide range of normal thickness of the glomerular basement membrane in the general population, the lack of uniformity of diagnostic criteria, and the fact that thinning may occur in other glomerular conditions as a preexisting or acquired process (42). Thus a diagnosis of thin basement membrane disease requires the systematic exclusion of other glomerular abnormalities that point to another disease process.

Thinning of the glomerular basement membrane, whether focal or diffuse, is particularly common in IgA nephropathy, suggesting an associated dysregulation of glomerular basement membrane synthesis or maintenance (see fig. 4-19) (50). It is not known whether the thinning in IgA nephropathy represents a chance concurrence of two unrelated diseases or a secondary phenomenon. In areas of glomerular capillary distension by endocapillary proliferation or thrombosis, the glomerular basement membrane may appear thinned. Thus, segmental thinning is also common in forms of endocapillary proliferative glomerulonephritis due to postinfectious glomerulonephritis or lupus nephritis, as well as in the thrombotic microangiopathies and necrotizing glomerulonephritides. Similarly, segmental thinning of the glomerular basement membrane is commonly observed as a nonspecific localized finding in a host of immune complex–mediated glomerular diseases, especially in foci of resorbed deposits with remodeled glomerular capillary walls.

Because thinning of the glomerular basement membrane may be the only detectable abnormality in some kindreds with hereditary nephritis/Alport's syndrome, especially early in the disease, the most difficult distinction is between thin basement membrane disease and atypical hereditary nephritis. In such cases, a full clinical history, including the mode of inheritance and a family history of renal failure and deafness, as well as the use of antibodies to the alpha subunits of collagen IV, are helpful. In thin basement membrane disease, the glomerular basement membranes retain normal immunoreactivity for the alpha 3, 4, and 5 chains of collagen IV, whereas reactivity for all three is typically lost in hereditary nephritis.

Etiology and Pathogenesis. The genetic basis of thin basement membrane disease is heterogeneous. Heterozygous mutations in either the *COL4A3* gene or the *COL4A4* gene have been reported (41,48,49,51). Mutations include missense, splice site, or frame shift. Most cases follow an autosomal dominant pattern of inheritance, although sporadic cases (possibly representing new mutations) have also been described. Because mutations in the same genetic loci can give rise to autosomal recessive Alport's syndrome when they occur as homozygous or compound heterozygous mutations, some investigators consider thin basement membrane disease to be a heterozygous form of autosomal recessive Alport's syndrome (47a). In this way, the distinction between thin basement membrane disease and hereditary nephritis has become less absolute. In thin basement membrane disease, there is a subtle reduction in the quantity of the alpha 3, 4, 5 (IV) network. Some kindreds with thin basement membrane disease lack linkage to *COL4A3* and *COL4A4*, suggesting the existence of other genetic loci that have not yet been assigned (52).

Treatment and Prognosis. The clinical course is benign and nonprogressive in most cases. There is no effective therapy. The main value of diagnosis is to ascertain a benign prognosis and exclude other conditions presenting with hematuria that may require specific therapy.

FABRY'S DISEASE

Definition. Fabry's disease, also known as *angiokeratoma corporis diffusum universale*, is an X-linked inherited disorder caused by a deficiency in the lysosomal hydrolase, alpha-galactosidase A (60).

Clinical Features. The disease is most often seen in Caucasians, but can affect any race. It is rare, with an estimated incidence of 1 in 40,000 population. The X-linked inheritance accounts for the complete clinical expression of disease in hemizygous males and the milder clinical phenotype in heterozygous females.

Deficiency of alpha-galactosidase A leads to the intracellular accumulation of glycosphingolipids in a variety of organs, including skin, kidney, heart, central nervous system, and cornea (62,66). Skin lesions, known as angiokeratomas, consist of dark red macules or papules that usually appear during the second decade of life and preferentially involve areas "below the belt," such as hips, buttocks, genitalia, and upper thighs

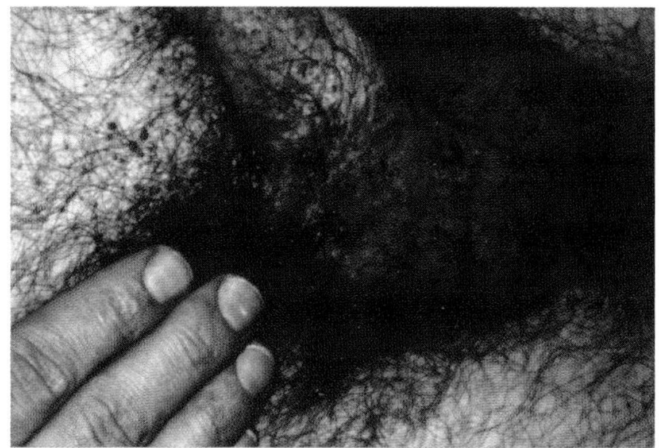

Figure 4-28

FABRY'S DISEASE

Angiokeratomas are visible on the skin of the penis and groin area of this 30-year-old man with a longstanding history of paresthesias and a recent onset of proteinuria.

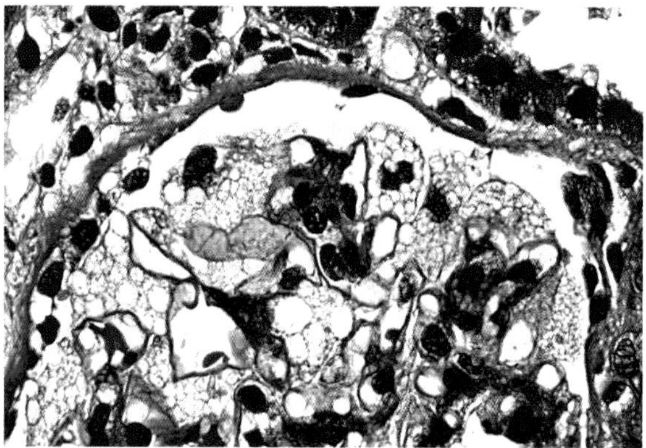

Figure 4-29

FABRY'S DISEASE

The podocytes are markedly enlarged with abundant, foamy, clear cytoplasm (Masson trichrome stain).

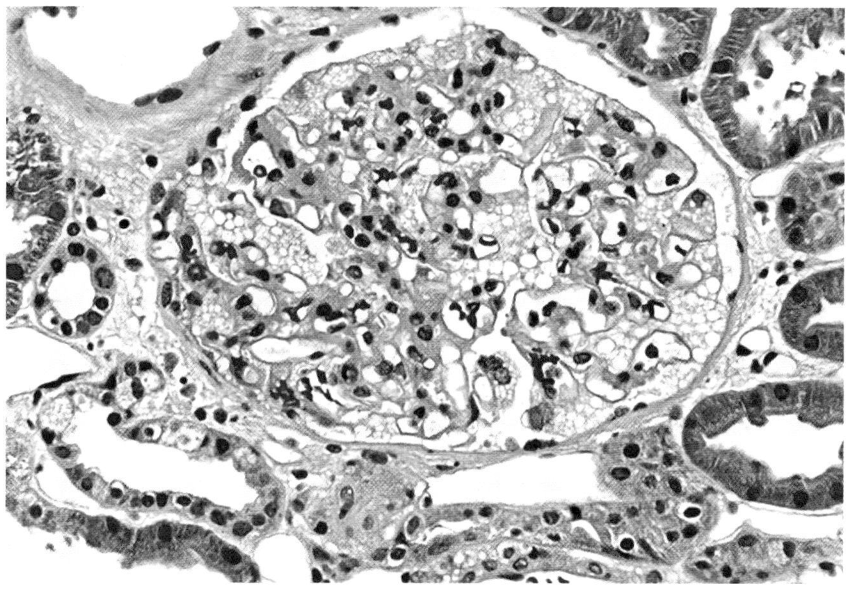

Figure 4-30

FABRY'S DISEASE

The glomerulus is normocellular. The podocytes have a bubbly appearance and fill the urinary space with their expanded cytoplasm (H&E stain).

(fig. 4-28). Involvement of the autonomic nervous system is characteristic, leading to painful paresthesias that are exacerbated by cold or exercise. Ischemic cardiovascular disease may produce cardiomyopathy or stroke. Corneal opacities consist of creamy-white discolorations that radiate towards the periphery of the cornea.

The renal presentation is usually in late adolescence or early adulthood with the appearance of proteinuria and slowly progressive renal insufficiency (65). Affected males often progress to end-stage renal failure in middle age. Some patients have an impaired ability to concentrate urine, resembling diabetes insipidus.

Light Microscopic Findings. The major findings involve the podocytes, which appear markedly enlarged, with a bubbly, clear, foamy cytoplasm that is best demonstrated with the trichrome stain (figs. 4-29, 4-30) (63,64). Although the glomeruli are normocellular, the swollen podocytes have a tendency to narrow the urinary space. Similar lipid vacuoles may be detected in tubular cells, vascular myocytes, and endothelial cells (fig. 4-31). With progression

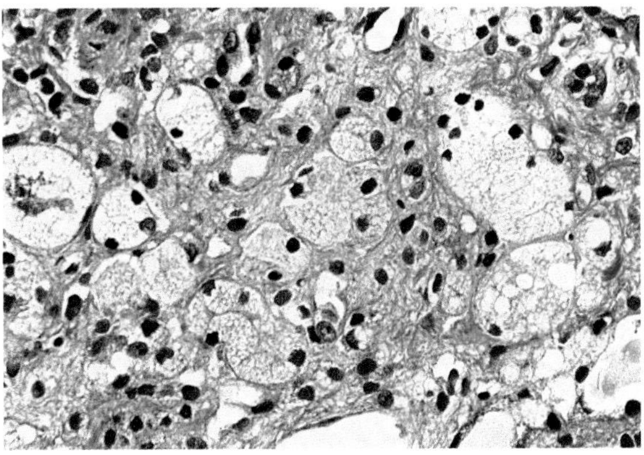

Figure 4-31

FABRY'S DISEASE

Foamy cells are identified in the tubules and interstitium in this paient with advanced, severe renal insufficiency (Masson trichrome stain).

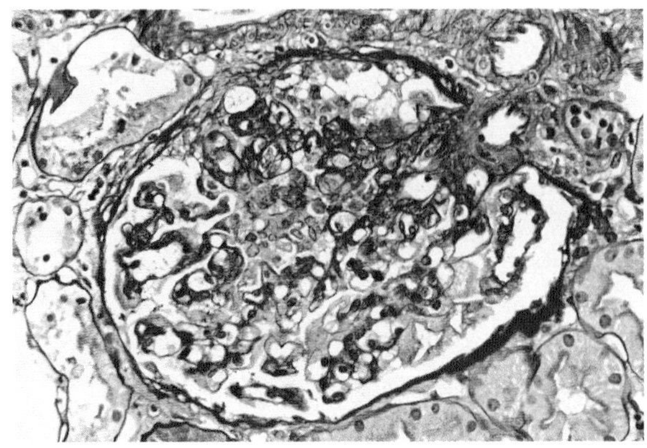

Figure 4-32

FABRY'S DISEASE

There is a secondary pattern of focal segmental sclerosis and adhesion to Bowman's capsule (PAS stain).

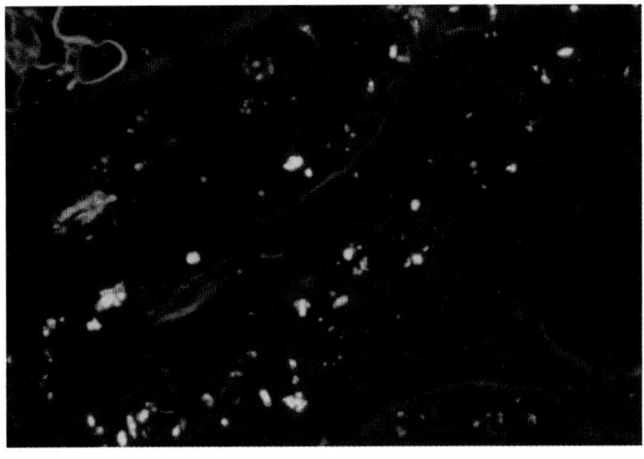

Figure 4-33

FABRY'S DISEASE

By immunofluorescence, staining for IgG is negative, however, there is orange autofluorescence of the medial myocytes of a small artery, corresponding to lipid deposits (immunofluorescence micrograph).

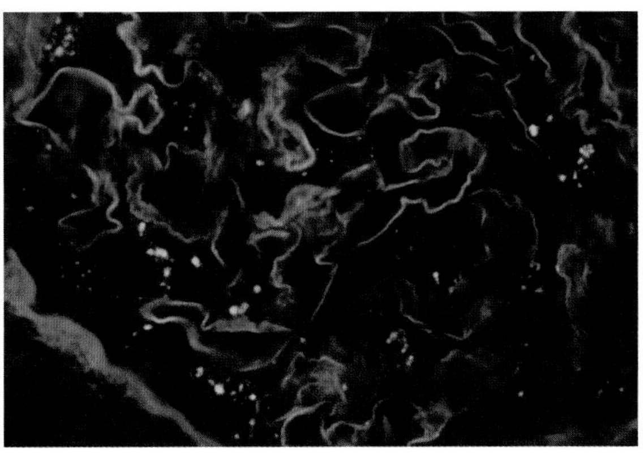

Figure 4-34

FABRY'S DISEASE

Autofluorescent orange pigment consistent with intracellular lipid is identified in the podocyte cytoplasm in this cryostat section stained with antisera to IgG. There is also nonspecific linear staining of the glomerular capillary walls (immunofluorescence micrograph).

of disease, evolution to a pattern of focal segmental and global glomerulosclerosis is common. There is corresponding patchy tubular atrophy, interstitial fibrosis, and nonspecific interstitial inflammation (fig. 4-32). The walls of arterioles and small arteries become thickened.

Immunofluorescence Findings. No specific immune staining for immunoglobulins or complement is identified. The careful observer will note, however, the presence of orange autofluorescence, corresponding to intracellular inclusions in the cytoplasm of podocytes, tubular epithelial cells, and arterial endothelial cells and medial myocytes (figs. 4-33, 4-34). Frozen sections stained with Sudan black or oil red-O show extensive lipid inclusions in these cell types. Because the lipid inclusions are removed in the course of tissue processing for light microscopy, they are best demonstrated as osmiophilic inclusions in plastic-embedded survey sections for electron microscopy (fig. 4-35).

Electron Microscopic Findings. Diagnostic myelin figures are identified diffusely in the

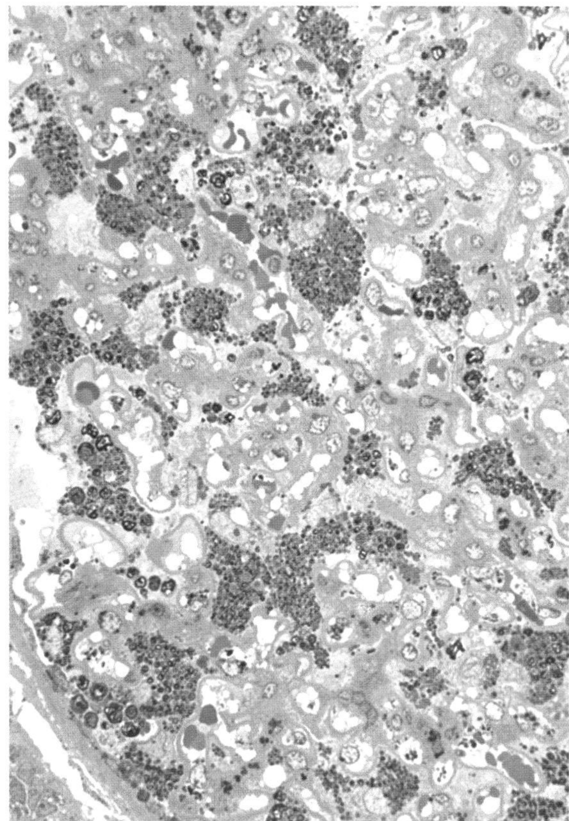

Figure 4-35

FABRY'S DISEASE

A semithin survey section stained with toluidine blue for electron microscopy retains the osmiophilic inclusions within the podocyte cytoplasm.

cytoplasm of the podocytes, with variable and usually less conspicuous involvement of mesangial cells, glomerular endothelial cells, tubular epithelial cells (particularly distal), and arterial myocytes and endothelial cells (fig. 4-36) (69). The whorled myelin figures form intracellular inclusions that are composed of concentrically arranged lamellae of electron-dense material with a periodicity of 4 to 10 nm. In the more advanced stages of the disease, mesangial sclerosis and glomerular basement membrane thickening may occur.

Differential Diagnosis. Diffuse podocyte involvement by myelin figures is most characteristic of Fabry's disease. The finding of an isolated podocyte containing abundant myelin figures has on rare occasion been described as a nonspecific ultrastructural curiosity in renal biopsies from patients with other renal conditions.

Ballooning and foaminess of the podocytes, as seen by light microscopy, may occur in other lysosomal storage diseases (62), including infantile nephrosialidosis, gangliosidosis, I-cell disease (mucolipidosis type 2), Hurler's syndrome, Niemann-Pick disease, Farber's disease (ceramidase deficiency), and fucosidosis, among others (fig. 4-37). These entities can be distinguished from Fabry's disease at the ultrastructural level because they lack electron-dense myeloid bodies. Instead, they contain a variety of other types of intracellular inclusions. In nephrosialidosis and I-cell disease (an autosomal recessive storage disease due to the deficiency of lysosomal enzyme N-acetylglucosaminylphosphotransferase encoded on chromosome 4q21-23), for example, the vacuoles correspond ultrastructurally to empty membrane-bound intracellular vesicles within the podocyte cytoplasm (fig. 4-38). In Hurler's syndrome, the intracellular vacuoles contain granular material. In Gaucher's disease, the storage material produces an appearance of pale, wrinkled cytoplasm within glomerular endocapillary cells (of possible endothelial or macrophage origin) and interstitial cells, but not podocytes (figs. 4-39–4-42).

In patients with biopsy findings suggestive of Fabry's disease, demonstration of reduced alpha-galactosidase A activity in plasma or in cells confirms the diagnosis.

Etiology and Pathogenesis. A deficiency in alpha-galactosidase A causes the accumulation of glycosphingolipids in many tissues. The responsible gene is located on the long arm of the X chromosome (Xq22-24). Multiple unique mutations have been detected in the alpha-galactosidase A gene, including missense mutations, nonsense mutations, and small insertions or deletions that lead to premature translational termination (58).

Treatment and Prognosis. Renal failure, cardiovascular disease, and cerebrovascular disease cause premature mortality in untreated patients (60). There was initial enthusiasm for renal transplantation as a means of reconstituting the deficient alpha-galactosidase A enzyme, however, renal transplantation has resulted in little, if any, improvement in the systemic disease. In the past few years, novel treatment strategies have turned to enzyme replacement

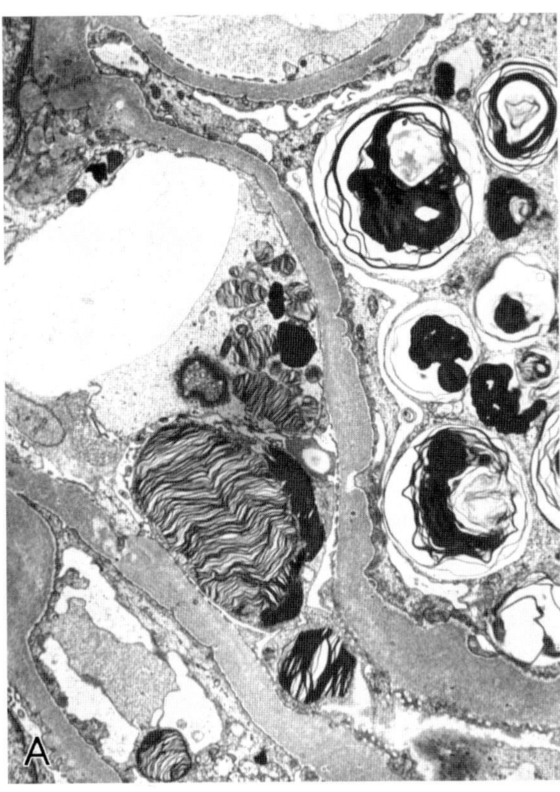

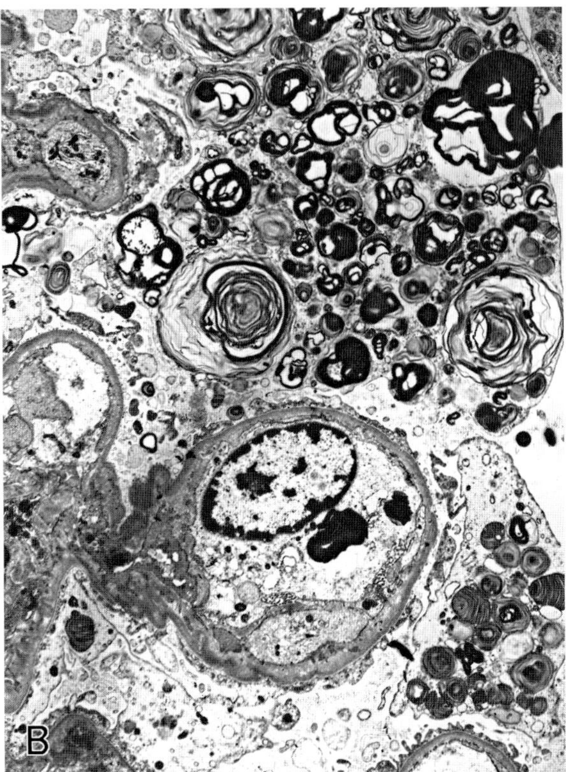

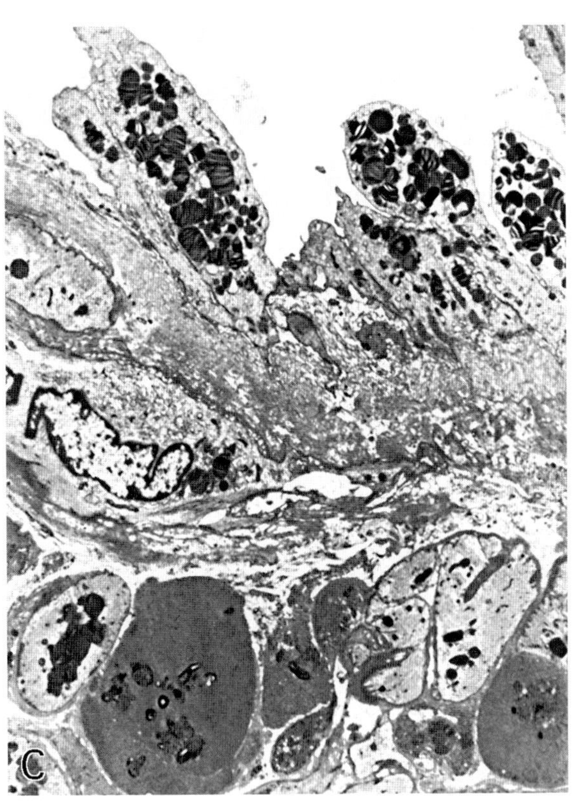

Figure 4-36

FABRY'S DISEASE

A: Whorled zebra bodies are identified in the cytoplasm of the podocytes and the glomerular endothelial cells (electron micrograph).

B: There are abundant myelin figures of varying size within the podocyte cytoplasm, and to a lesser extent, in the cytoplasm of glomerular endothelial cells (electron micrograph).

C: Abundant myelin inclusions are present in the cytoplasm of arterial endothelial cells and medial myocytes of a small interlobular artery (electron micrograph).

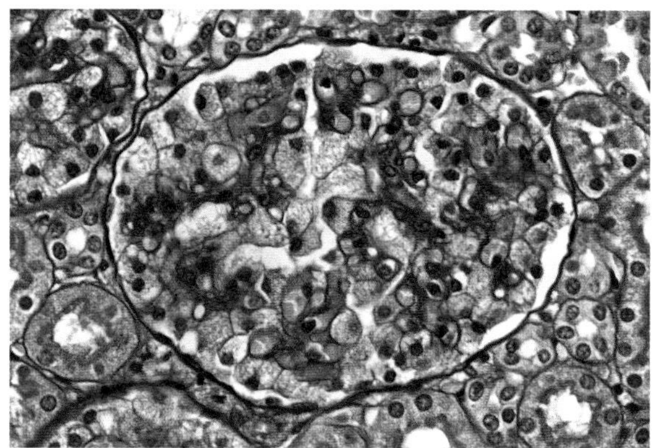

Figure 4-37

MUCOLIPIDOSIS TYPE 2 (I-CELL DISEASE)

By light microscopy, the podocytes are vacuolated, resembling the foamy podocytes seen in Fabry's disease. Unlike the case in Fabry's disease, however, the storage material in the podocytes of this 10-month-old girl with mucolipidosis type 2 stains with the alcian blue-PAS stain (pH 2.5).

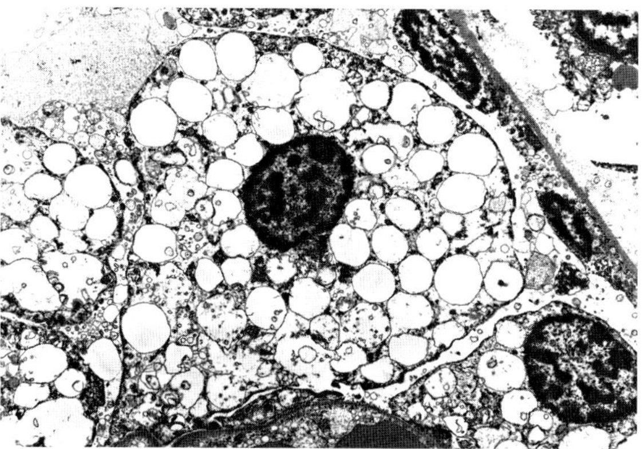

Figure 4-38

MUCOLIPIDOSIS TYPE 2 (I-CELL DISEASE)

By electron microscopy, the foamy podocytes contain intracytoplasmic membrane-bound vacuoles of electron-lucent, clear storage material. The underlying glomerular basement membrane is intact (electron micrograph).

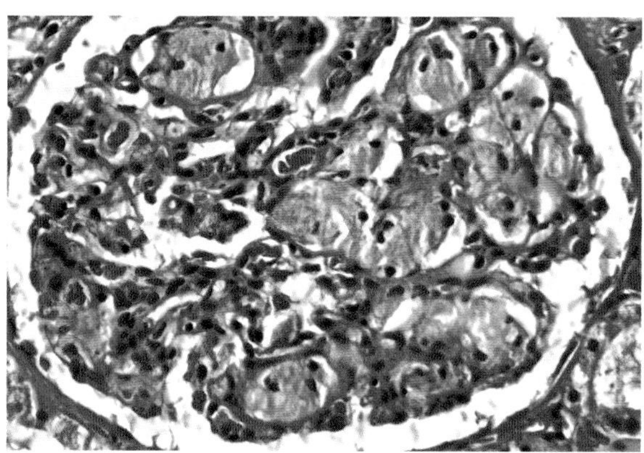

Figure 4-39

GAUCHER'S DISEASE

There are fluffy cells with cellophane-like, wrinkled cytoplasm occluding the glomerular capillary lumens in this woman who developed Gaucher's disease of the kidney several years following splenectomy. The podocytes are uninvolved (H&E stain).

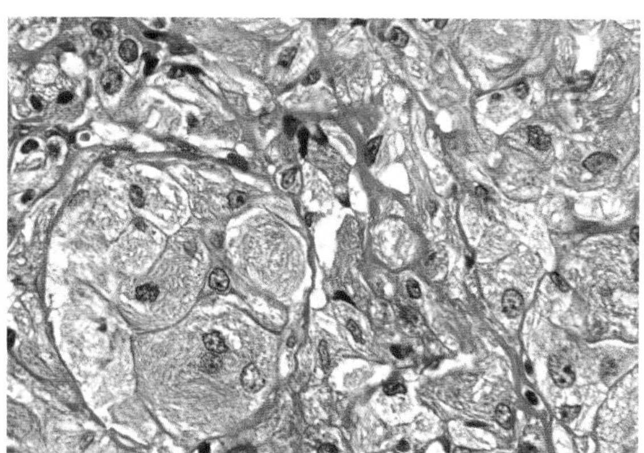

Figure 4-40

GAUCHER'S DISEASE

The endocapillary cells seen in figure 4-39 resemble the splenic cells shown here. Splenectomy was performed several years prior to renal biopsy (H&E stain).

therapy using recombinant human alpha-Gal A infusions (59,61,67,68). Clinical studies indicate a reduction in glomerular mesangial sclerosis and greater preservation of the glomerular filtration rate in patients with Fabry's disease treated with recombinant enzyme versus placebo, together with a 50 percent reduction in plasma glycosphingolipid levels and improved cardiac conduction. Gene therapy holds promise for the future (70).

LECITHIN CHOLESTEROL ACYLTRANSFERASE DEFICIENCY

Definition. Lecithin cholesterol acyltransferase (LCAT) deficiency is an autosomal recessive disorder of cholesterol esterification that causes increased levels of unesterified cholesterol, triglycerides, and phosphatidylcholine (73).

Clinical Features. Although originally described in Scandinavia, LCAT deficiency has been reported subsequently in patients of diverse ethnic and geographic origins. Total cholesterol

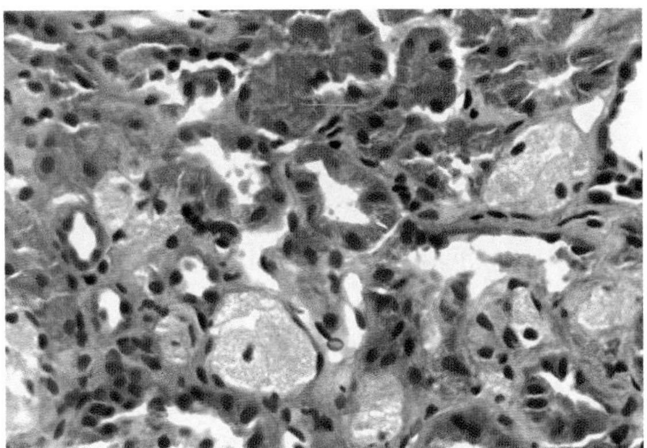

Figure 4-41

GAUCHER'S DISEASE

Pale cells with fluffy, wrinkled cytoplasm are identified within the interstitium, probably corresponding to interstitial macrophages (H&E stain).

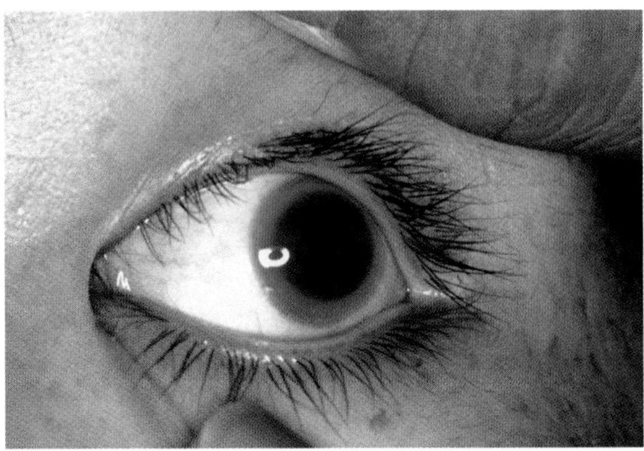

Figure 4-43

LECITHIN CHOLESTEROL ACYLTRANSFERASE DEFICIENCY

A typical corneal opacity is seen at the limbus of this 28-year-old woman with renal involvement.

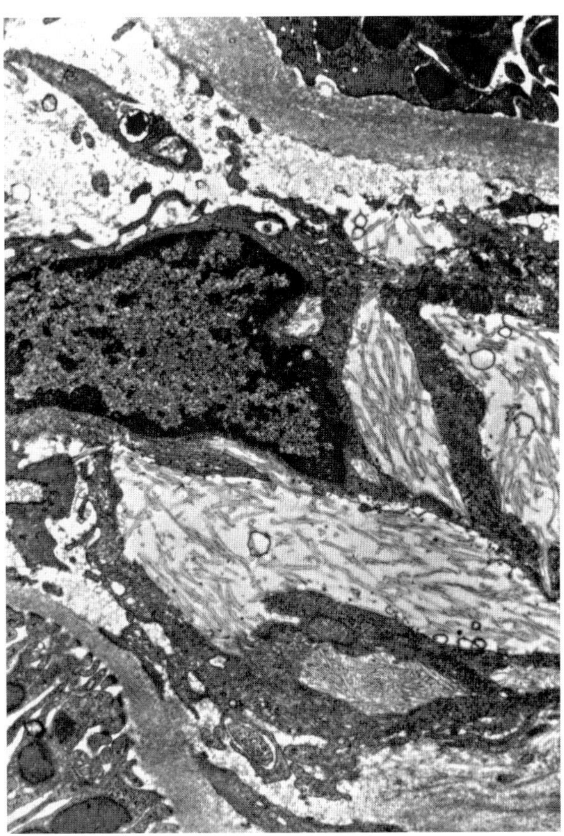

Figure 4-42

GAUCHER'S DISEASE

The interstitial cells contain inclusions of linear, electron-dense material with a branch-like appearance (electron micrograph).

levels range from low to high, however, levels of free cholesterol and lecithin are generally increased. The concentration of high-density lipoprotein (HDL) cholesterol is usually reduced. Plasma triglyceride levels are elevated and an increased component of free cholesterol can be found in virtually all lipoprotein fractions.

Lipid accumulates in a variety of tissues, leading to corneal opacities, accelerated atherosclerosis, and nephropathy characterized by proteinuria, nephrotic syndrome, and progressive renal insufficiency. Corneal opacities appear in childhood and are characterized by a lipoid arcus containing grayish spots (fig. 4-43).

Light Microscopic Findings. There is mesangial sclerosis and irregular thickening of the glomerular basement membrane. With the JMS and PAS stains, the glomerular basement membranes exhibit an irregular vacuolated appearance, mimicking stage 3 membranous alterations (figs. 4-44, 4-45). The mesangial matrix may exhibit a similar reticulated quality. Rarely are glomerular endocapillary foam cells seen. Over time, there is progression to focal segmental and global glomerulosclerosis, with nonspecific tubular atrophy, interstitial fibrosis, and arteriosclerosis.

Immunofluorescence Findings. Immunofluorescence is negative for immune reactants.

Electron Microscopic Findings. The characteristic glomerular lipid deposits are identified as irregularly distributed, rounded lacunae within

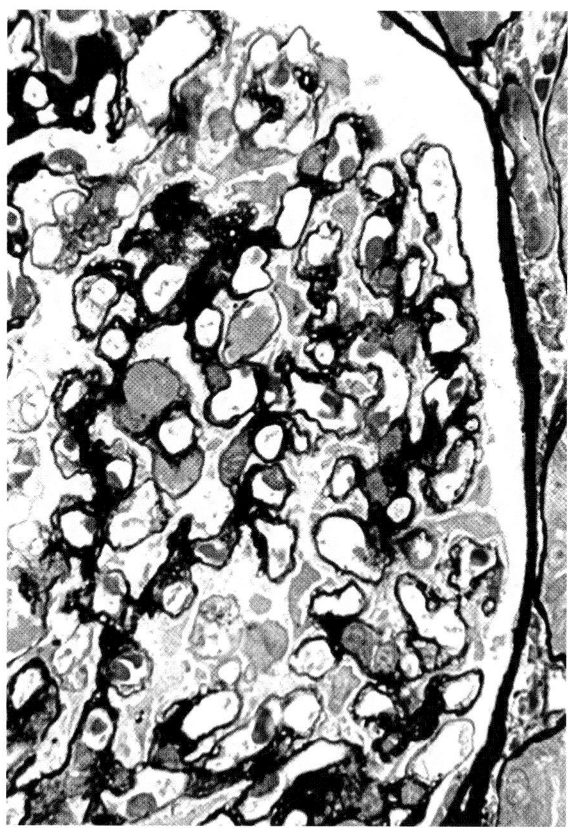

Figure 4-44

LECITHIN CHOLESTEROL ACYLTRANSFERASE DEFICIENCY

A renal biopsy from the patient pictured in figure 4-43 was performed for proteinuria. The glomerular basement membranes are focally vacuolated, with a bubbly texture. Pink hyaline deposits are noted in a few capillaries (JMS stain).

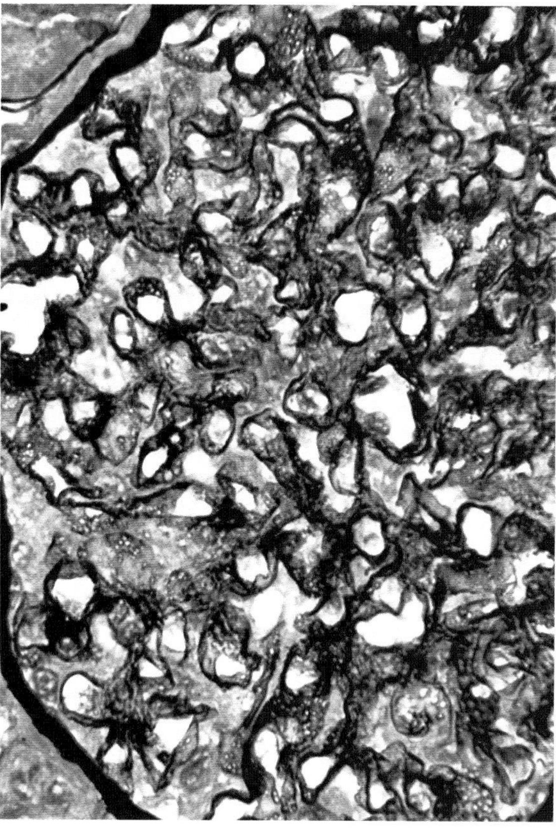

Figure 4-45

LECITHIN CHOLESTEROL ACYLTRANSFERASE DEFICIENCY

The extensive internal vacuolization of the glomerular basement membranes resembles the changes seen in stage 3 membranous glomerulopathy (JMS stain).

the mesangial matrix and the thickened glomerular basement membranes, extending from the subendothelial to the subepithelial aspect (figs. 4-46, 4-47) (75). These lipid accumulations are predominantly extracellular and resemble the lipid deposits seen in hepatic glomerulopathy. They are partially electron lucent and partially electron dense. The electron-dense component consists of lamellated curvilinear or lamellar densities of variable size, located at the center or the periphery of the electron-lucent deposits. Foam cells may be seen in the mesangium. Lipid deposits have also been reported in the vascular endothelial cells and medial myocytes.

Differential Diagnosis. The differential diagnosis of LCAT includes stage 3 membranous glomerulopathy and hepatic glomerulopathy. The absence of spikes or evidence of any immune complex deposits by immunofluorescence tends to eliminate membranous glomerulopathy. A history of cirrhosis, typically alcoholic, is usually found in patients with hepatic glomerulopathy. Of course, both these diagnostic considerations lack the systemic findings and family history characteristic of LCAT deficiency.

Etiology and Pathogenesis. The gene encoding LCAT has been mapped to chromosome 16. A number of different mutations have been identified in various families, including missense mutations leading to stop codons, and point mutations leading to amino acid substitutions, particularly in exons 4 and 5 of the *LCAT* gene (71,74). The former mutation leads to a nonsecreted protein whereas the latter produces a truncated protein lacking the enzyme's catalytic site (74). Due to a dysfunctional enzyme,

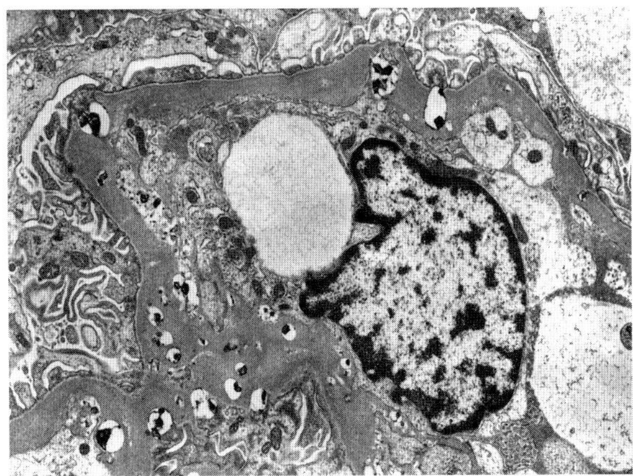

Figure 4-46

LECITHIN CHOLESTEROL ACYLTRANSFERASE DEFICIENCY

The glomerular basement membranes contain rounded inclusions with an electron-dense core surrounded by an electron-lucent zone (electron micrograph).

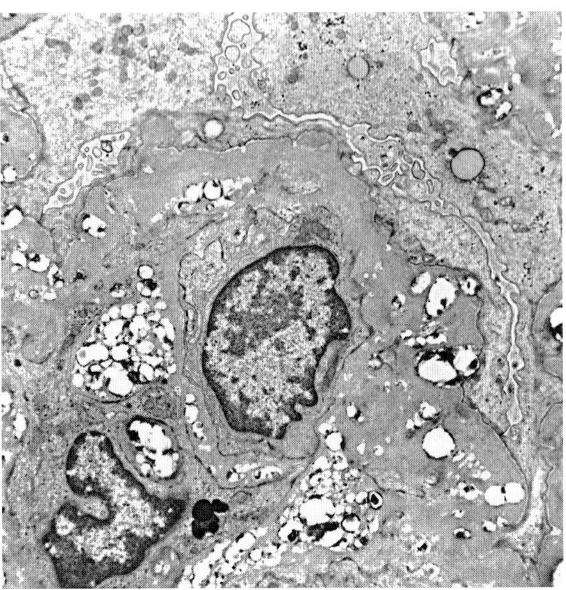

Figure 4-47

LECITHIN CHOLESTEROL ACYLTRANSFERASE DEFICIENCY

Abundant lacunae containing electron-lucent deposits with an electron-dense core stud the glomerular basement membranes and the mesangial matrix (electron micrograph).

there is injurious accumulation of unesterified cholesterol and oxidized phosphotidylcholine in the glomeruli (76).

Treatment and Prognosis. Untreated patients usually progress to renal failure by the fourth or fifth decade of life. The disease has been reported to recur in the transplanted kidney (77). Dietary therapy has not been effective in lowering lipid levels, nor have lipid-lowering drugs proven successful. In the future, gene therapy may hold promise for the treatment of this condition (78). Molecular diagnosis may allow identification of affected individuals prior to the clinical manifestations of disease (72).

CYSTINOSIS

Definition. Cystinosis is a rare autosomal recessive disease caused by a defect in the transport of cystine across lysosomal membranes. Intracellular accumulation of free cystine occurs in multiple organs, including kidney, brain, eye, thyroid, and pancreas.

Clinical Features. The incidence of cystinosis ranges from 1 in 20,000 to 1 in 326,000 and is geographically diverse. *Infantile cystinosis* presents between the ages of 3 and 6 months with Fanconi's syndrome and progresses to renal failure in the first decade of life. Corneal cystine crystals produce a painful photophobia by several years of age. In addition to retinal and renal involvement, generalized cystine deposition in multiple organs produces endocrinologic, hepatic, gastrointestinal, muscular, and neurologic disease. *Adolescent cystinosis* presents between 12 and 15 years of life with photophobia and a milder form of nephropathy that follows a slowly progressive course to renal failure. There is usually proteinuria and glomerular involvement, with less profound tubular dysfunction. Patients with *adult-onset cystinosis*, by comparison, usually have mild photophobia, but no evidence of renal involvement.

Clinical manifestations of Fanconi's syndrome, a defect in proximal tubular function, include polyuria, polydipsia, dehydration, aminoaciduria, glycosuria, and hyperphosphaturia. The resulting hypophosphatemia promotes growth retardation and vitamin D–resistant rickets. Urine potassium loss leads to hypokalemic, hyperchloremic metabolic acidosis. Involvement of other organ systems, such as eye, thyroid, and pancreas, may produce photophobia, retinal blindness, hypothyroidism, and diabetes mellitus. Cystine crystals can be demonstrated by slit lamp examination in the cornea, as well as

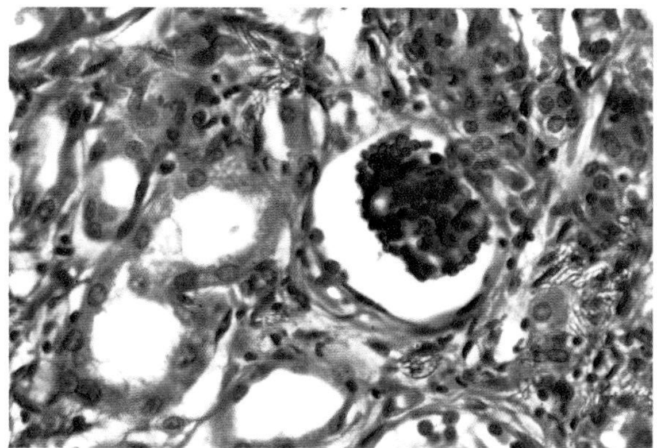

Figure 4-48

INFANTILE CYSTINOSIS

The glomerulus has a small globe with clustered podocytes. The surrounding tubules show mild tubular atrophy, interstitial fibrosis, and inflammation. There is a hint of some crystal deposition in the interstitium (H&E stain). (Courtesy of Dr. Jacob Churg, Paterson, NJ.) (Figs. 4-48 and 4-49 are from the same patient.)

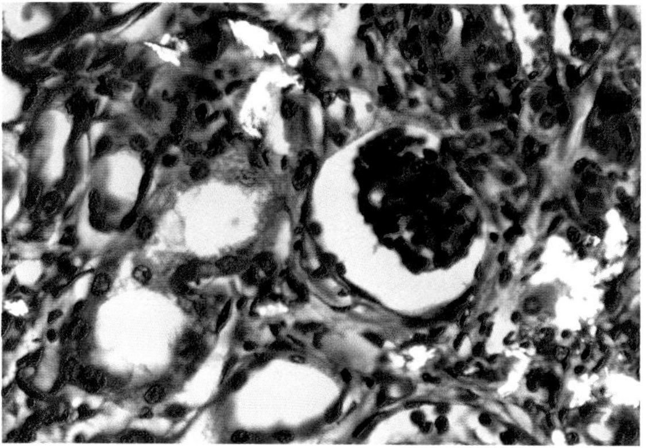

Figure 4-49

INFANTILE CYSTINOSIS

The field shows abundant birefringent crystals when this alcohol-fixed tissue is viewed under polarized light (H&E stain, polarized light). (Courtesy of Dr. Jacob Churg, Paterson, NJ.)

in the conjunctiva and retina, where they result in pigment degeneration.

Light Microscopic Findings. By light microscopy, the major findings are tubular atrophy, interstitial fibrosis, and variable degrees of interstitial inflammation. With disease progression, secondary glomerulosclerosis may occur. The tubular atrophy is most pronounced in the first portion (S1 segment) of the proximal tubule, causing tubular "swan neck" deformities on microdissection owing to thinning and shortening of this segment. This finding is not specific for cystinosis but can be found in other causes of Fanconi's syndrome. Deposition of cystine crystals is seen in tubular epithelial cells, interstitial macrophages, podocytes, and, to a lesser extent, mesangial cells (80,83). Affected podocytes may be multinucleated, which is a helpful, but not pathognomonic, finding (83). Because cystine is dissolved out of tissue by aqueous solutions, it is preferable to fix the specimen in alcohol for light microscopy. The cystine deposition may be relatively inconspicuous by routine light microscopy (fig. 4-48) and only fully appreciated using polarized light to demonstrate the birefringent needle-shaped crystals (figs. 4-48, 4-49). Cystine crystals can also be demonstrated as dark interstitial aggregates by phase microscopy (fig. 4-50).

Immunofluorescence Findings. Routine immunofluorescence shows no immune reactants. Refractile cystine crystals can be demonstrated by examination of the frozen tissue under polarized light.

Electron Microscopic Findings. Cystine crystals are well preserved by routine tissue processing for electron microscopy. Due to the formation of a reaction product between osmium tetroxide and cystine, the cells containing crystals may appear to have unusually dark or opaque cytoplasm against the clear crystals on light microscopic examination of toluidine blue–stained sections prepared from osmicated, plastic-embedded tissue (fig. 4-51) (82). On ultrastructural study, the intracellular crystals form clear, elongated, rectangular or rhomboidal clefts in the interstitium, interstitial leukocytes, tubular epithelial cells, and podocytes (figs. 4-52, 4-53).

Differential Diagnosis. Cystinosis is the most common cause of inherited renal Fanconi's syndrome. The differential diagnosis of Fanconi's syndrome includes other heritable diseases, such as Lowe's oculocerebrorenal syndrome (an X-linked disorder caused by a mutation in the gene *OCRL* encoding a protein homologous to phosphatidylinositol 4,5 bisphosphate 5 phosphatase, which is important in membrane trafficking and actin polymerization). Other diseases include Wilson's disease, mitochondriopathies,

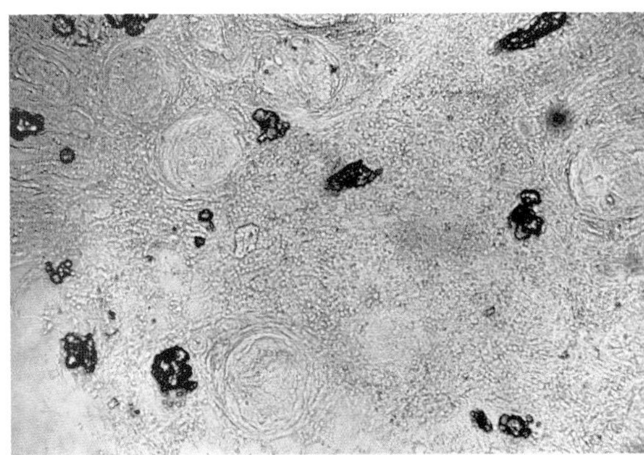

Figure 4-50

INFANTILE CYSTINOSIS

The crystals of cystine are seen as dark interstitial aggregates when viewed under phase microscopy. (Courtesy of Dr. Jacob Churg, Paterson, NJ.)

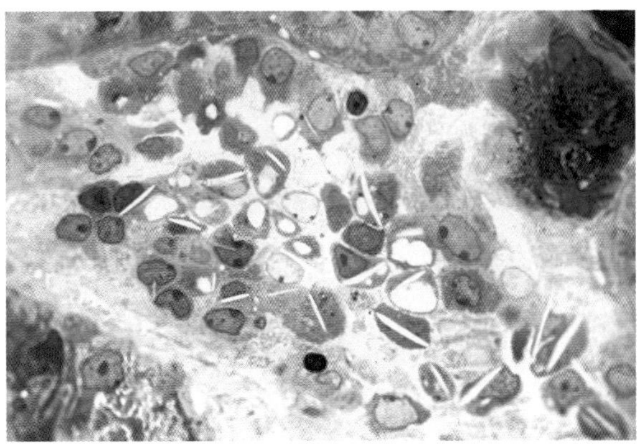

Figure 4-51

INFANTILE CYSTINOSIS

The toluidine blue–stained thick section reveals numerous clear clefts within the dark blue cytoplasm of interstitial macrophages. The crystals are thin and elongated, resembling needles. (Courtesy of Dr. Jacob Churg, Paterson, NJ.)

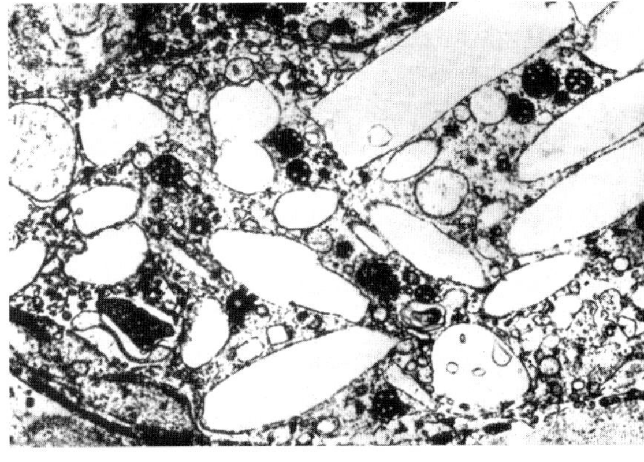

Figure 4-52

INFANTILE CYSTINOSIS

An interstitial macrophage contains multiple clear clefts that range from rectangular to elliptical to rounded, corresponding to intracellular cystine crystals (electron micrograph). (Courtesy of Dr. Jacob Churg, Paterson, NJ.)

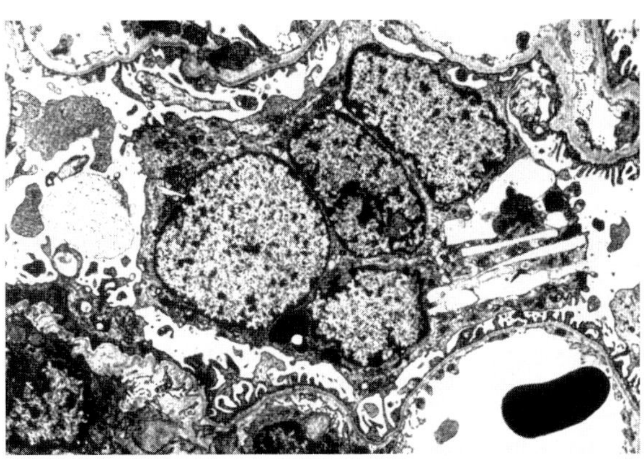

Figure 4-53

INFANTILE CYSTINOSIS

A multinucleated podocyte contains multiple rectangular clear intracytoplasmic crystals. The glomerular basement membrane is intact (electron micrograph). (Courtesy of Dr. Jacob Churg, Paterson, NJ.)

tyrosinemia, galactosemia, hereditary fructose intolerance, and hepatorenal glycogenosis (Fanconi-Bickel syndrome). Acquired causes of Fanconi's syndrome include heavy metal toxicity, childhood membranous glomerulopathy with antitubular basement membrane nephritis, and myeloma in adults. Cystinosis can be differentiated from all these entities by the presence of polarizable crystals in tissues. The diagnosis of cystinosis is confirmed by the demonstration of a markedly elevated cystine content in leukocytes or fibroblasts.

Etiology and Pathogenesis. Cystinosis is caused by mutations in *CTNS*, located on chromosome 17p13 (84). *CTNS* encodes a 367-amino acid protein called cystinosin, which functions as a H+ driven cystine transporter. Cystinosin is an integral lysosomal membrane protein with a 7-transmembrane domain, its C terminal tail predicted to lie in the cytosol, and its N terminus towards the lysosomal lumen (81). Over 20 different mutations have been identified, including a variety of missense mutations, in-frame deletions, and insertions, accounting for all the clinical phenotypes (79,81). A 57-kb deletion has been identified in the majority of European cases. Most mutations identified in the infantile form abolish cystine transport whereas most mutations associated with the adolescent or adult forms strongly reduce transport, consistent with their milder phenotype (79,81).

Treatment and Prognosis. Patients with the infantile form have the poorest prognosis and typically progress to renal failure. Renal transplantation has achieved success. Although there may be limited recurrence of cystinosis in the graft due to infiltration by host macrophages bearing crystals, cystine does not accumulate in the tubular epithelium and, therefore, graft function is not significantly impaired.

REFERENCES

Hereditary Nephritis and Alport's Syndrome

1. Antignac C, Zhou J, Sanak M, et al. Alport syndrome and diffuse leiomyomatosis: deletion in the 5' end of the COL4A5 gene. Kidney Int 1992;42:1178–83.
2. Atkin CL, Hasstedt SJ, Menlove L, et al. Mapping of Alport syndrome to the long arm of the X chromosome. Am J Hum Genet 1988;42:249–55.
3. Barker DF, Hostikka SL, Zhou J, et al. Identification of mutations in the COL4A5 collagen gene in Alport syndrome. Science 1990;248:1224–7.
4. Boutaud A, Borza DB, Bondar O, et al. Type IV collagen of the glomerular basement membrane. Evidence that the chain specificity of network assembly is encoded by the noncollagenous NC1 domains. J Biol Chem 2000;275:30716–24.
5. Churg J, Sherman RL. Pathologic characteristics of hereditary nephritis. Arch Pathol 1973;95: 374–9.
6. Ciccarese M, Casu D, Ki Wong F, et al. Identification of a new mutation in the alpha4(IV) collagen gene in a family with autosomal dominant Alport syndrome and hypercholesterolaemia. Nephrol Dial Transplant 2001:16:2008–12.
7. Ding J, Zhou J, Tryggvason K, Kashtan CE. COL4A5 deletions in three patients with Alport syndrome and posttransplant antiglomerular basement membrane nephritis. J Am Soc Nephrol 1994;4:161–8.
8. Gubler MC, Knebelmann B, Beziau A, et al. Autosomal recessive Alport syndrome: immunohistochemical study of type IV collagen chain distribution. Kidney Int 1995;47:1142–7.
9. Gunwar S, Ballester F, Noelken M, Sado Y, Ninomiya Y, Hudson BG. Glomerular basement membrane. Identification of a novel disulfide-cross-linked network of alpha3, alpha4, and alpha5 chains of type IV collagen and its implications for the pathogenesis of Alport syndrome. J Biol Chem 1998;273:8767–75.
10. Heidet L, Arrondel C, Forestier L, et al. Structure of the human type IV collagen gene COL4A3 and mutations in autosomal Alport syndrome. J Am Soc Nephrol 2001;12:97–106.
11. Heidet L, Cai Y, Guicharnaud L, Antignac C, Gubler MC. Glomerular expression of type IV collagen chains in normal and X-linked Alport syndrome kidneys. Am J Pathol 2000:156:1901–10.
12. Heikkila P, Tibell A, Morita T, et al. Adenovirus-mediated transfer of type IV collagen alpha5 chain cDNA into swine kidney in vivo: deposition of the protein into the glomerular basement membrane. Gene Therapy 2001;8:882–90.
13. Hinglais N, Grunfeld JP, Bois E. Characteristic ultrastructural lesion of the glomerular basement membrane in progressive hereditary nephritis (Alport's syndrome). Lab Invest 1972;27:473–87.
14. Hostikka SL, Eddy RL, Byers MG, Hoyhtya M, Shows TB, Tryggvason K. Identification of a distinct type IV collagen alpha chain with restricted kidney distribution and assignment of its gene to the locus of X chromosome-linked Alport syndrome. Proc Natl Acad Sci 1990;87:1606–10.
15. Hudson BG, Tryggvason K, Sundaramoorthy M, Neilson EG. Mechanisms of disease: Alport's syndrome, Goodpasture's syndrome and type IV collagen. N Engl J Med 2003;348:2543–56.

16. Jais JP, Knebelmann B, Giatras I, et al. X-linked Alport syndrome: natural history in195 families and genotype-phenotype correlations in males. J Am Soc Nephrol 2000;11:649–57.
17. Jefferson JA, Lemmink HH, Hughes AE, et al. Autosomal dominant Alport syndrome linked to the type IV collagen alpha3 and alpha4 genes (COL4A3 and COL4A4). Nephrol Dial Transplant 1997;12:1595–9.
18. Johnsson LG, Arenberg IK. Cochlear abnormalities in Alport's syndrome. Arch Otolaryngol 1981;107:340–9.
19. Kalluri R, Weber M, Netzer KO, Sun MJ, Neilson EG, Hudson BG. COL4A5 gene deletion and production of post-transplant anti-alpha 3(IV) collagen alloantibodies in Alport syndrome. Kidney Int 1994;45:721–6.
20. Kashtan CE. Alport syndrome and thin glomerular basement membrane disease. J Am Soc Nephrol 1998;9:1736–50.
21. Kashtan CE. Alport syndromes: phenotypic heterogeneity of progressive hereditary nephritis. Pediatr Nephrol 2000;14:502–12.
22. Kashtan CE, Gubler MC, Sisson-Ross S, Mauer M. Chronology of renal scarring in males with Alport syndrome. Pediatr Nephrol 1998;12:269–74.
23. Kim KH, Kim Y, Gubler MC, et al. Structure-functional relationships in Alport syndrome. J Am Soc Nephrol 1995;5:1659–68.
24. Kleppel MM, Fan WW, Cheong HI, Michael AF. Evidence for separate networks of classical and novel basement membrane collagen. Characterization of alpha 3(IV)-Alport antigen heterodimer. J Biol Chem 1992;267:4137–42.
25. Lemmink HH, Mochizuki T, van den Heuvel LP, et al. Mutations in the type IV collagen alpha 3 (COL4A3) gene in autosomal recessive Alport syndrome. Hum Mol Genet 1994;3:1269–73.
26. Longo I, Porcedda P, Mari F, et al. COL4A3/COL4A4 mutations: from familial hematuria to autosomal-dominant or recessive Alport syndrome. Kidney Int 2002;61:1947–56.
27. Massella L, Rizzoni G, De Blasis R, et al. De-novo COL4A5 gene mutations in Alport's syndrome. Nephrol Dial Transplant 1994;9:1408–11.
28. Mazzucco G, Barsotti P, Muda AO, et al. Ultrastructural and immunohistochemical findings in Alport's syndrome: a study of 108 patients from 97 Italian families with particular emphasis on COL4A5 gene mutation correlations. J Am Soc Nephrol 1998;9:1023–31.
29 McCoy RC, Johnson HK, Stone WJ, Wilson CB. Absence of nephritogenic GBM antigen(s) in some patients with hereditary nephritis. Kidney Int 1982;21:642–52.
30. Meleg-Smith S, Magliato S, Cheles M, Garola RE, Kashtan CE. X-linked Alport syndrome in females. Hum Pathol 1998;29:404–8.
31. Mochizuki T, Lemmink HH, Mariyama M, et al. Identification of mutations in the alpha 3(IV) and alpha 4(IV) collagen genes in autosomal recessive Alport syndrome. Nat Genet 1994;8:77–81.
32. Mothes H, Heidet L, Arrondel C, et al. Alport syndrome associated with diffuse leiomyomatosis: COL4A5-COL4A6 deletion associated with a mild form of Alport nephropathy. Nephrol Dial Transplant 2002;17:70–4.
33. Nakanishi K, Yoshikawa N, Iijima K, et al. Immunohistochemical study of alpha 1-5 chains of type IV collagen in hereditary nephritis. Kidney Int 1994;46:1413–21.
34. Pirson Y. Making the diagnosis of Alport's syndrome. Kidney Int 1999:56:760–75.
35. Proesmans W, Knockaert H, Trouet D. Enalapril in paediatric patients with Alport syndrome: 2 years' experience. Eur J Pediatr 2000;159:430–3.
36. Streeten BW, Robinson MR, Wallace R, Jones DB. Lens capsule abnormalities in Alport's syndrome. Arch Ophthalmol 1987;105:1693–7.
37. van der Loop FT, Heidet L, Timmer ED, et al. Autosomal dominant Alport syndrome caused by a COL4A3 splice site mutation. Kidney Int 2000;58:1870–5.
38. Zhou J, Mochizuki T, Smeets H, et al. Deletion of the paired alpha 5(IV) and alpha 6(IV) collagen genes in inherited smooth muscle tumors. Science 1993;261:1167–9.
39. Zhou J, Reeders ST. The alpha chains of type IV collagen. Contrib Nephrol 1996;117:80–104.

Thin Basement Membrane Disease

40. Abe S, Amagasaki Y, Iyori S, et al. Thin basement membrane syndrome in adults. J Clin Pathol 1987;40:318–22.
41. Badenas C, Praga M, Tazon B, et al. Mutations in the COL4A4 and COL4A3 genes cause familial benign hematuria. J Am Soc Nephrol 2002; 13:1248–54.
42. Cosio FG, Falkenhain ME, Sedmak DD. Association of thin glomerular basement membrane with other glomerulopathies. Kidney Int 1994;46:471–4.
43. Dische FE. Measurement of glomerular basement membrane thickness and its application to the diagnosis of thin-membrane nephropathy. Arch Pathol Lab Med 1992:116:43–9.
44. Dische FE, Weston MJ, Parsons V. Abnormally thin glomerular basement membranes associated with hematuria, proteinuria, or renal failure in adults. Am J Nephrol 1985;5:103–9.
45. Gauthier B, Trachtman H, Frank R, Valderrama E. Familial thin basement membrane nephropathy in children with asymptomatic microhematuria. Nephron 1989;51:502–8.

46. Gubler MC, Beaufils H, Noel LH, Habib R. Significance of thin glomerular basement membranes in hematuric children. Contrib Nephrol 1990;80:147–56.
47. Hisano S, Kwano M, Hatae K, et al. Asymptomatic isolated microhaematuria: natural history of 136 children. Pediatr Nephrol 1991;5:578–81.
47a. Hudson BG, Tryggvason K, Sundaramoorthy M, Neilson EG. Mechanisms of disease: Alport's syndrome, Goodpasture's syndrome and type IV collagen. N Engl J Med 2003;348:2543–56.
48. Lemmink HH, Nillesen WN, Mochizuki T, et al. Benign familial hematuria due to mutation of the type IV collagen alpha4 gene. J Clin Invest 1996;98:1114–8.
49. Longo I, Porcedda P, Mari F, et al. COL4A3/COL4A4 mutations: from familial hematuria to autosomal-dominant or recessive Alport syndrome. Kidney Int 2002;61:1947–56.
50. Monga G, Mazzucco G, Roccatello D. The association of IgA glomerulonephritis and thin glomerular basement membrane disease in a hematuric patient: light and electron microscopic and immunofluorescence investigation. Am J Kidney Dis 1991;18:409–12.
51. Ozen S, Ertoy D, Heidet L, et al. Benign familial hematuria associated with a novel COL4A4 mutation. Pediatr Nephrol 2001;16:874–7.
52. Piccini M, Casari G, Zhou J, et al. Evidence for genetic heterogeneity in benign familial hematuria. Am J Nephrol 1999;19:464–7.
53. Steffes MW, Barbosa J, Basgen JM, Sutherland DE, Najarian JS, Mauer SM. Quantitative glomerular morphology of the normal human kidney. Lab Invest 1983;49:82–6.
54. Tiebosch AT, Frederik PM, van Breda Vriesman PJ, et al. Thin-basement-membrane nephropathy in adults with persistent hematuria. N Engl J Med 1989;320:14–8.
55. Vogler C, McAdams AJ, Homan SM. Glomerular basement membrane and lamina densa in infants and children: An ultrastructural evaluation. Pediatr Pathol 1987;7:527–34.
56. Yoshikawa N, Hashimoto, Katayama Y, Yamada Y, Matsuo T, Okada S. The thin glomerular basement membrane in children with haematuria. J Pathol 1984;142:253–7.
57. Yoshiokawa N, Matsuyama S, Iijima K, Maehara K, Okada S, Matsuo T. Benign familial hematuria. Arch Pathol Lab Med 1988;112:794–7

Fabry's Disease

58. Altarescu GM, Goldfarb LG, Park KY, et al. Identification of fifteen novel mutations and genotype-phenotype relationship in Fabry disease. Clin Genet 2001;60:46–51.
59. Barngrover D. Fabrazyme—recombinant protein treatment for Fabry's disease. J Biotechnol 2002;95:280–2.
60. Branton MH, Schiffmann R, Sabnis SG, et al. Natural history of Fabry renal disease: influence of alpha-galactosidase A activity and genetic mutations on clinical course. Medicine 2002;81:122–38.
61. Desnick RJ, Wasserstein MP. Fabry disease: clinical features and recent advances in enzyme replacement therapy. Adv Nephol Necker Hosp 2001;31:317–39.
62. Faraggiana T, Churg J. Renal lipidoses: a review. Hum Pathol 1987;18:661–79.
63. Faraggiana T, Churg J, Grishman E, et al. Light- and electron-microscopic histochemistry of Fabry's disease. Am J Pathol 1981;103:247–62.
64. Farge D, Nadler S, Wolfe LS, Barre P, Jothy S. Diagnostic value of kidney biopsy in heterozygous Fabry's disease. Arch Pathol Lab Med 1985;109:85–8.
65. Grunfeld JP, Lidove O, Joly D, Barbey F. Renal disease in Fabry patients. J Inherit Metab Dis 2001;24(Suppl 2):71–4.
66. Lysosomal storage diseases. Fabry disease: new insights and future perspectives. Proceedings and abstracts of an international symposium, Seville, April 2001. J Inherit Metab Dis 2001;24(Suppl 2):1–185.
67. Schiffmann R, Brady RO. New prospects for the treatment of lysosomal storage diseases. Drugs 2002:62:733–42.
68. Schiffmann R, Kopp JB, Austin HA 3rd, et al. Enzyme replacement therapy in Fabry disease: a randomized controlled trial. JAMA 2001:285:2743–9.
69. Sessa A, Meroni M, Battini G, et al. Renal pathologic changes in Fabry disease. J Inherit Metab Dis 2001;24(Suppl 2):66–70.
70. Siatskas C, Medin JA. Gene therapy for Fabry disease. J Inherit Metab Dis 2001;24(Suppl 2):25–41.

Lecithin Cholesterol Acyltransferase Deficiency

71. Argyropoulos G, Jenkins A, Klein RL, et al. Transmission of two novel mutations in a pedigree with familial lecithin:cholesterol acyltransferase deficiency: structure-function relationships and studies in a compound heterozygous proband. J Lipid Res 1998;39:1870–6.
72. Cirera S, Julve J, Ferrer I, et al. Molecular diagnosis of lecithin: cholesterol acyltransferase deficiency in a presymptomatic proband. Clin Chem Lab Med 1998;36:443–8.
73. Gjone E. Familial lecithin: cholesterol acyltransferase deficiency—a new metabolic disease with renal involvement. Adv Nephrol Necker Hosp 1981:10:167–85.
74. Guerin M, Dachet C, Goulinet S, et al. Familial lecithin: cholesterol acyltransferase deficiency: molecular analysis of a compound heterozygote: LCAT (Arg147–> Trp) and LCAT (Tyr171–> Stop). Atherosclerosis 1997;131:85–95.

75. Imbasciati E, Paties C, Scarpioni L, Mihatsch MJ. Renal lesions in familial lecithin-cholesterol acyltransferase deficiency. Ultrastructural heterogeneity of glomerular changes. Am J Nephrol 1986;6:66–70.
76. Jimi S, Uesugi N, Saku K, et al. Possible induction of renal dysfunction in patients with lecithin: cholesterol acyltransferase deficiency by oxidized phosphatidylcholine in glomeruli. Arterioscler Thromb Vasc Biol 1999:19:794–801.
77. Panescu V, Grignon Y, Hestin D, et al. Recurrence of lecithin cholesterol acyltransferase deficiency after kidney transplantation. Nephrol Dial Transplant 1997;12:2430–2.
78. Rader DJ, Tietge UJ. Gene therapy for dyslipidemia: clinical prospects. Curr Atheroscler Rep 1999;1:58–69.

Cystinosis

79. Attard M, Jean G, Forestier L, et al. Severity of phenotype in cystinosis varies with mutations in the CTNS gene: predicted effect on the model of cystinosin. Hum Mol Genet 1999;13:2507–14.
80. Hory B, Billerey C, Royer J, Saint Hillier J. Glomerular lesions in juvenile cystinosis; report of 2 cases. Clin Nephrol 1994;42:327–30.
81. Kalatzis V, Nevo N, Cherqui S, et al. Molecular pathogenesis of cystinosis: effect of CTNS mutations on the transport activity and subcellular localization of cystinosin. Hum Mol Genet 2004; 13:1361–71.
82. Spear GS, Gubler MC, Habib R, Broyer M. Dark cells of cystinosis: occurrence in renal allografts. Hum Pathol 1989;20:472–6.
83. Spear GS, Slusser R, Schulman JD, Alexander F. Polykaryocytosis of the visceral glomerular epithelium in cystinosis with description of an unusual clinical variant. Johns Hopkins Med J 1971;129:83–99.
84. Town M, Jean G, Cherqui S, et al. A novel gene encoding an integral membrane protein is mutated in nephropathic cystinosis. Nature Genet 1998;18:319–24.

5 MINIMAL CHANGE DISEASE

MINIMAL CHANGE DISEASE

Definition. Minimal change disease (MCD) is a major cause of idiopathic nephrotic syndrome. It is defined pathologically as glomerular disease with minimal or no glomerular alterations (as detected by light microscopy), no glomerular immune deposits, and extensive effacement of foot processes (as detected by electron microscopy). The "minimal" light microscopic findings include visceral epithelial cell (i.e., podocyte) swelling and mild mesangial expansion. Because of the presence of severe podocyte abnormalities, in the absence of other glomerular alterations, this condition is considered the quintessential podocyte disease. MCD has been given numerous names through the years. *Lipoid nephrosis,* coined by Munk in 1913 (19) and used through the 1950s, referred to the light microscopic findings of fatty changes in the tubules and fatty casts in the urine. The synonym, *nil disease,* popular in the 1970s, referred to the absence of detectable glomerular abnormalities by light and fluorescence microscopy. Today, some clinicians and pathologists use *minimal change nephrotic syndrome, minimal lesion,* and *minimal change glomerulopathy* interchangeably with MCD.

Relationship of MCD to Focal Segmental Glomerulosclerosis (FSGS). Most investigators consider MCD and FSGS to be related entities that lie along a clinical-pathologic continuum. MCD represents a milder disease with a greater likelihood of steroid responsivity and a lack of progression to renal failure, whereas FSGS lies at the more severe end of the spectrum, manifesting a greater likelihood of steroid resistance and progression to end-stage renal failure. What remains unclear is whether MCD is a separate disease or whether it evolves into FSGS in some patients. Most renal pathologists have seen cases of apparent MCD on initial renal biopsy that developed steroid resistance and in which a second renal biopsy years later disclosed progression to FSGS. What cannot be proven without serially sectioning all glomeruli of the kidneys is whether these cases of apparent MCD on first biopsy actually represent unsampled FSGS or simply very early FSGS that has not yet developed diagnostic histologic lesions. The strongest evidence supporting the relatedness of the two lesions comes from experimental models of MCD and FSGS caused by different severities of injury by the same toxic factor (such as puromycin aminonucleoside or adriamycin) and the identification of a circulating "permeability factor" in both conditions (2,14,20). In addition, recurrence of FSGS in the transplant passes through an early phase that resembles MCD, followed by the progressive development of sclerotic lesions in serial biopsies.

Clinical Features. MCD may occur at any age, but is most common in children (12,15,22, 26). It accounts for approximately 90 percent of cases of primary nephrotic syndrome in preadolescent children, 50 percent in adolescents, and less than 25 percent in adults. In children, the median age of onset is 2.5 years, with a peak incidence between 24 and 36 months of age. In adults, there is a higher incidence in elderly than middle-aged adults. The male to female ratio is about 2 to 1 in children but approaches unity in adulthood.

MCD virtually always manifests nephrotic syndrome at the outset. Thus, the predominant findings are heavy proteinuria, hypoalbuminemia, edema, and elevated serum cholesterol. The chief complaint that brings the patient to medical attention is the development of edema, which is usually of abrupt onset and may involve the eyelids, scrotum, abdomen, hands, and lower extremities. The pathologist should hesitate to diagnose MCD in a patient with asymptomatic subnephrotic proteinuria, with the exception of cases that have undergone spontaneous partial remission. Nephrotic proteinuria in children is defined by the International Study of Kidney Disease in Children (ISKDC) as a protein excretion

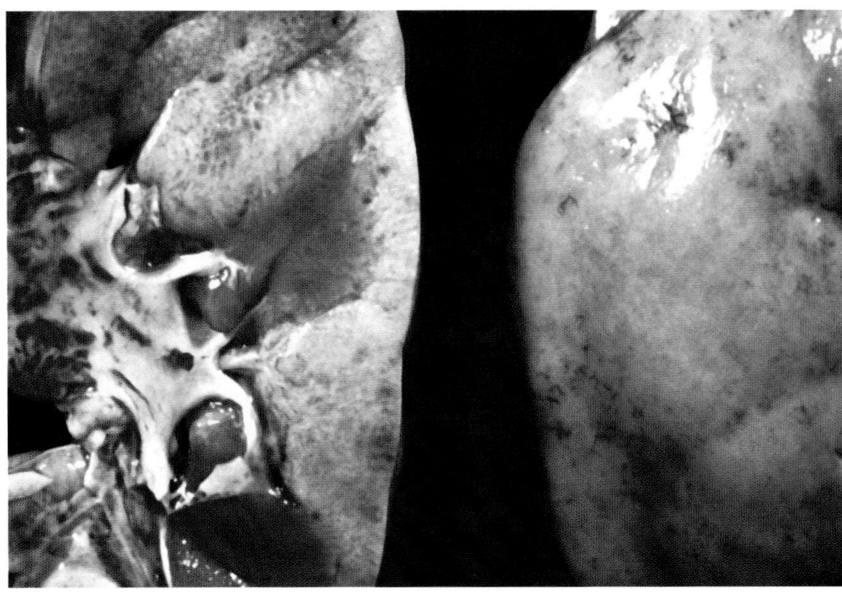

Figure 5-1

MINIMAL CHANGE DISEASE

Kidney at autopsy in a child with unremitting nephrotic syndrome complicated by peritonitis prior to the advent of steroid therapy. The kidney is slightly enlarged, with a smooth cortical surface and yellow, waxy discoloration of the cortical parenchyma owing to abundant lipid resorption by the proximal tubular cells.

rate of more than 40 mg/m^2/hour body surface area in an overnight collection of urine. In adults, a protein excretion rate of more than 3.5 g/1.73m^2/day body surface area is most widely used, although some accept a rate of more than 3.0 g/1.73 m^2/day. The proteinuria in MCD is usually highly selective, meaning that it consists predominantly of albumin. Hypoalbuminemia is defined as serum albumin of less than 2.5 g/dL in children and less than 3.5 g/dL in adults.

Most children with MCD have no evidence of renal insufficiency, hematuria, or hypertension. Mild renal insufficiency (elevated plasma creatinine over the 98th percentile) occurs in less than one third of children with MCD and results from the reduced glomerular hydraulic conductivity that is secondary to the obliteration of the filtration slit pores that maintain the extracellular route of filtration. Acute renal failure is unusual in children unless there is hypovolemic shock following the intravascular volume depletion that results from profound hypoalbuminemia or aggressive diuresis. A syndrome of acute renal failure is not uncommon, however, in older adults with MCD and hemodynamically-mediated acute tubular necrosis (14,17).

MCD may follow a remitting and relapsing course. Unlike FSGS, it is highly steroid responsive. Because of the markedly different incidence of MCD in children and adults, the clinical approach to idiopathic nephrotic syndrome depends on the age of the patient. Children presenting with idiopathic nephrotic syndrome are not subjected to diagnostic renal biopsy. Instead, they are treated empirically with an 8-week course of corticosteroids. The rationale for this approach is predicated on the fact that about 80 percent of childhood cases of nephrotic syndrome are caused by MCD and 95 percent of patients will enter remission following an 8-week course of therapy. In the event a child fails to respond to this therapeutic regimen, a renal biopsy is then performed to rule out other causes of nephrotic syndrome. Because the causes of idiopathic nephrotic syndrome in adults are much more diverse, it is not possible to predict the etiology based on statistical probability. Accordingly, renal biopsies are performed routinely on adults with idiopathic nephrotic syndrome at the time of presentation.

Gross Findings. Gross examination of the kidneys of patients with minimal change nephrotic syndrome is rare in the modern era owing to improved therapeutic management. Deaths were not uncommon prior to the advent of corticosteroid and antibiotic therapy and provided the material for early pathologic descriptions. Based on the study of autopsy material, the term lipoid nephrosis was coined. The kidneys are enlarged, pale, and waxy, with a yellowish, smooth cortical surface (fig. 5-1). The yellow discoloration is attributable to the abundant lipid resorption and accumulation by the proximal tubules.

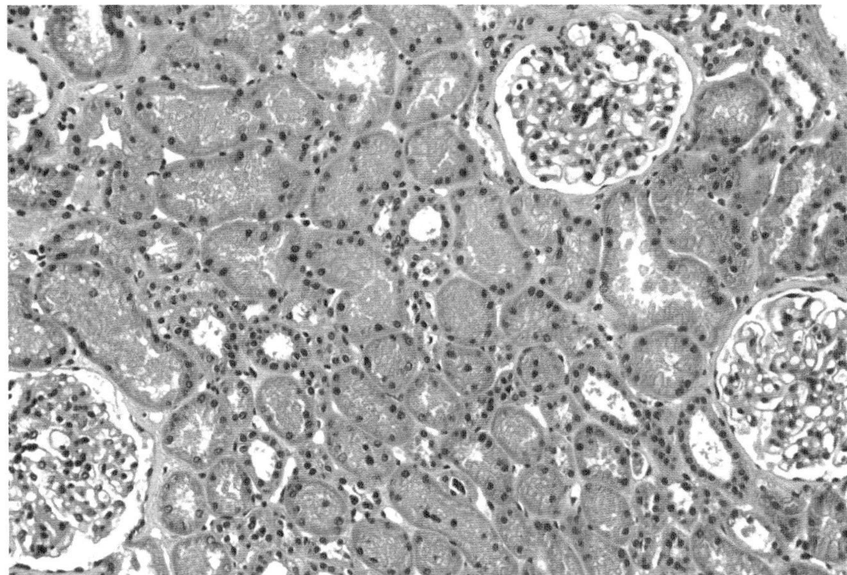

Figure 5-2

MINIMAL CHANGE DISEASE

Low-power view of the kidney shows no detectable histologic abnormalities (hematoxylin and eosin [H&E] stain).

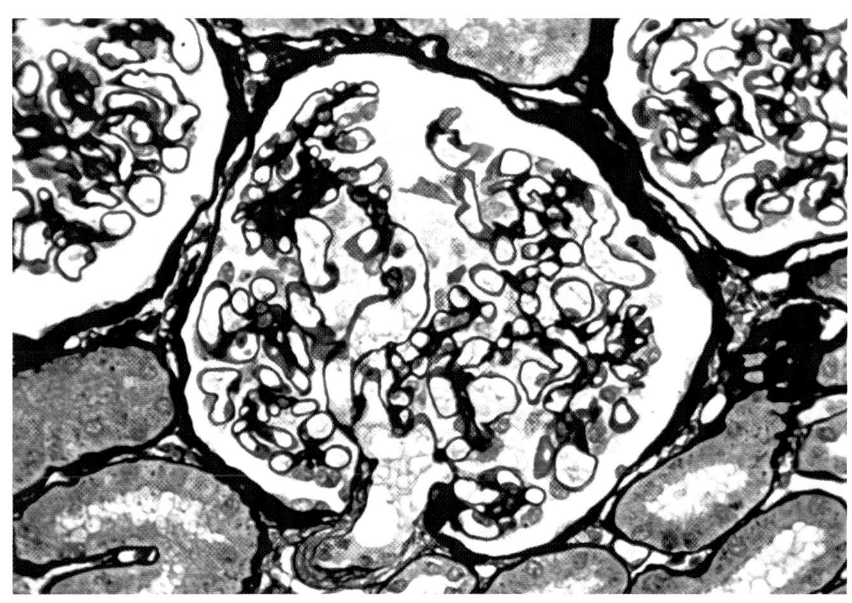

Figure 5-3

MINIMAL CHANGE DISEASE

High-power view shows glomeruli of normal size and cellularity, with fully patent capillaries. The glomerular basement membranes appear normal in thickness, with a regular smooth texture (Jones methenamine silver [JMS] stain).

Light Microscopic Findings. Glomeruli typically display little or no histologic abnormalities (figs. 5-2, 5-3) (5,12,26). The glomerular capillary lumens are fully patent and the glomerular tuft is usually normocellular. In a minority of cases, there may be mild mesangial prominence, typically in a focal distribution, and consisting of a slight increase in mesangial cellularity or matrix. The glomerular basement membranes appear normal in thickness, texture, and contour.

In some cases, the only detectable abnormality is mild swelling or prominence of the visceral epithelial cells (fig. 5-4). However, there is no evidence of the podocyte hyperplasia or capping frequently seen in FSGS. Unlike FSGS, intracytoplasmic protein resorption droplets are usually not discernable by light microscopy in the swollen podocytes of MCD. Endocapillary foam cells are so rare in MCD that their presence should raise the suspicion of unsampled FSGS.

In the patient with idiopathic nephrotic syndrome, the finding of a single glomerulus with segmental glomerular sclerosis, inframembranous hyalinosis, and/or synechiae to Bowman's

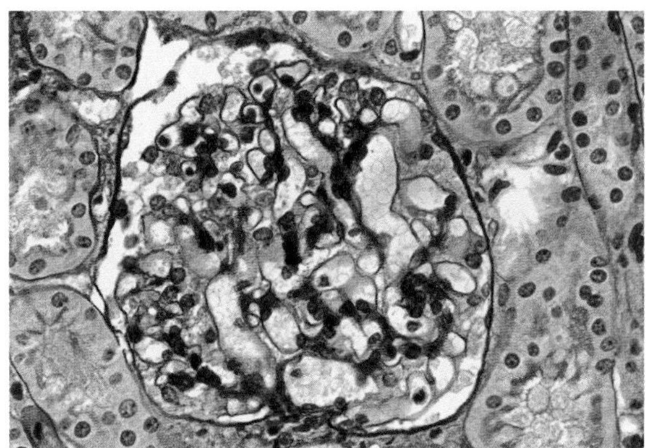

Figure 5-4

MINIMAL CHANGE DISEASE

There is slight swelling of the podocytes. This subtle finding may be the only light microscopic abnormality in minimal change disease (periodic acid–Schiff [PAS] stain).

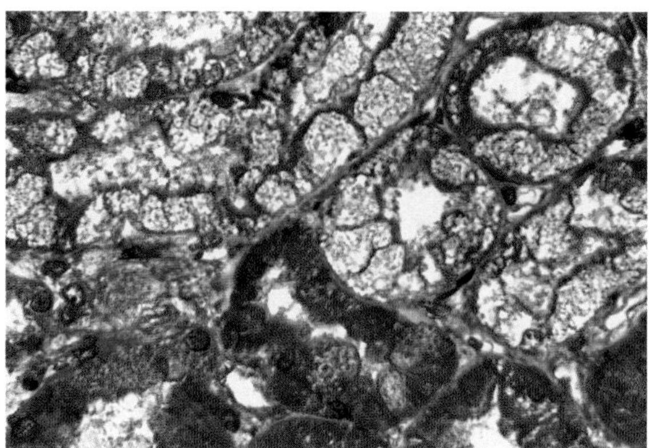

Figure 5-5

MINIMAL CHANGE DISEASE

The proximal tubules contain clear lipid resorption droplets (Masson trichrome stain).

capsule is sufficient for a diagnosis of FSGS, provided that immune complex–mediated processes, hereditary nephritis, and other glomerulopathies are ruled out by immunofluorescence and electron microscopy. The presence of globally sclerotic glomeruli does not have the same diagnostic specificity; such glomeruli are encountered at any age, even in infants. By the age of 40 years, up to 10 percent of glomeruli may be obsolescent in the course of aging, and the percentage increases to 30 percent by the age of 80.

The major tubular findings are intracytoplasmic protein and lipid resorption droplets within the proximal tubular epithelial cells. The protein resorption droplets, also referred to as hyaline droplets, appear eosinophilic, periodic acid–Schiff (PAS) positive and usually trichrome red. Lipid resorption droplets typically are clear in hematoxylin and eosin (H&E)-stained preparations and fail to stain with the PAS or trichrome stain (fig. 5-5). Lipid resorption droplets can be demonstrated in cryostat sections using stains for lipids, such as oil red-O. Tubular atrophy and interstitial fibrosis are usually absent. In older patients with arteriosclerosis and focal glomerular obsolescence, it is not uncommon to find focal tubular atrophy and interstitial fibrosis commensurate with the severity of the vascular disease. Adults with the syndrome of MCD and acute renal failure may display tubular degenerative and regenerative changes like those seen in ischemic acute tubular necrosis (see below).

The interstitium is usually unremarkable. Interstitial foam cells are rarely encountered, and usually occur as isolated cells, without formation of aggregates (fig. 5-6). Interstitial inflammation is not a feature of MCD. However, mild interstitial inflammation may be found with the tubular atrophy and interstitial fibrosis seen in older patients who have co-existent arterionephrosclerosis of aging or hypertension. The presence of a significant interstitial inflammatory infiltrate or tubulitis in the setting of MCD should suggest the possibility of acute interstitial nephritis in association with nonsteroidal anti-inflammatory drug (NSAID)-induced MCD (see below).

Immunofluorescence Findings. A defining feature of MCD is the absence of detectable glomerular immune deposits. In a minority of cases, there may be weak mesangial positivity for immunoglobulin (Ig)M, with or without complement (C)3 (usually not exceeding 1+ intensity) (fig. 5-7). Positivity for albumin is commonly seen in the distribution of proximal tubular epithelial cell protein resorption droplets (fig. 5-8). Activation of complement on tubular cells, due to increased protein trafficking, may result in tubular deposits of C3. Because the proteinuria in MCD is highly selective, it is less common to see tubular protein resorption droplets staining for immunoglobulins. Unlike FSGS,

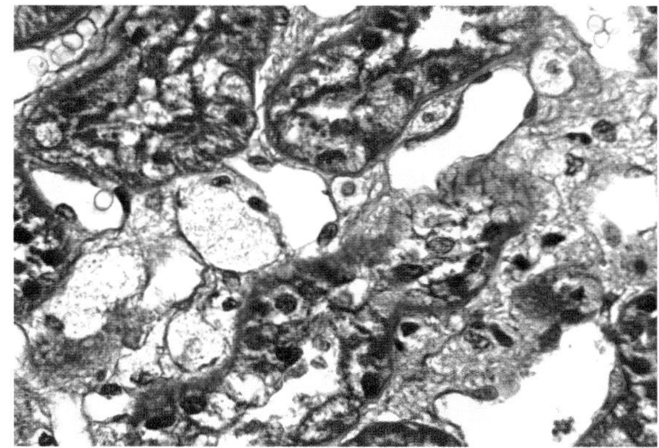

Figure 5-6

MINIMAL CHANGE DISEASE

There are rare isolated interstitial foam cells (Masson trichrome stain).

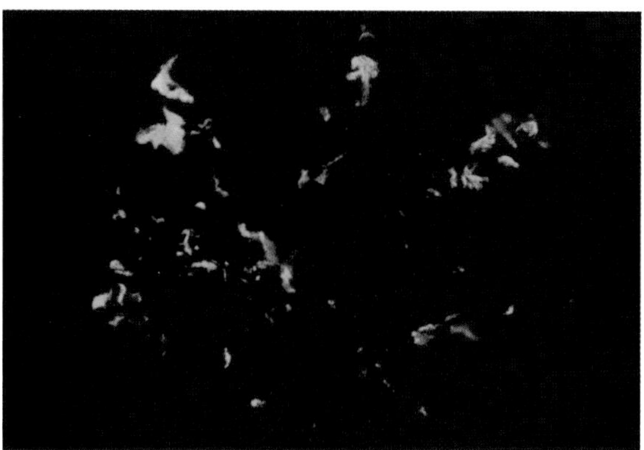

Figure 5-7

MINIMAL CHANGE DISEASE

An example with weak (1+) staining for IgM in a mesangial distribution. There are no deposits involving the peripheral glomerular capillary walls.

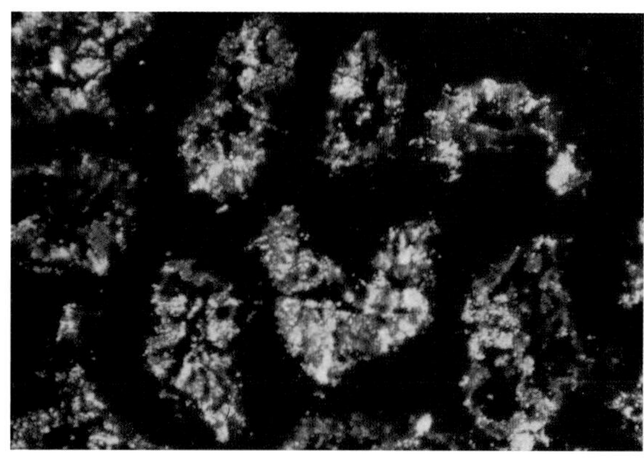

Figure 5-8

MINIMAL CHANGE DISEASE

Immunofluorescence reveals strong staining for albumin in the distribution of the protein resorption droplets within the proximal tubular cells. This finding reflects the severe albuminuria due to the defect in glomerular permselectivity.

it is rare to find positivity for albumin or immunoglobulins (usually IgG) in the distribution of visceral epithelial cell protein resorption droplets, and when present, such positivity is extremely fine and diffuse. By contrast, the protein resorption droplet staining seen in FSGS usually delineates larger and more segmentally distributed intracytoplasmic droplets.

In fewer than 5 percent of cases of apparent MCD, especially in children, there may be mesangial deposits of immunoglobulins (particularly IgG, as well as IgM and IgA) and complement components (C1q and C3), in the absence of corresponding electron-dense deposits. This unusual immunofluorescence finding may be associated with a worse prognosis and a greater likelihood of steroid resistance. The paramesangial staining pattern suggests a pathomechanism of nonspecific entrapment of circulating plasma proteins in the setting of glomerular proteinuria. The presence of substantial IgA-dominant mesangial deposits in a patient with severe nephrotic syndrome and complete foot process effacement should suggest a diagnosis of MCD with IgA nephropathy (see below). Alternatively, if the mesangial deposits contain dominant C1q, with or without IgG or other immunoglobulins, a diagnosis of C1q nephropathy should be considered (see chapter 6).

Electron Microscopic Findings. In MCD, the major pathologic abnormalities of the glomerulus are identified at the ultrastructural level and are typically limited to the podocyte. The hallmark of the disease is extensive effacement of foot processes in the absence of other abnormalities of the peripheral capillary walls. The term "effacement" of the podocyte is used synonymously with "fusion" of the foot processes, although effacement is more correct with respect to the subcellular changes of foot process retraction and spreading.

The extent of foot process effacement is variable from case to case. In general, it tends to be severe and diffuse, involving more than 75 percent of the total glomerular capillary surface area

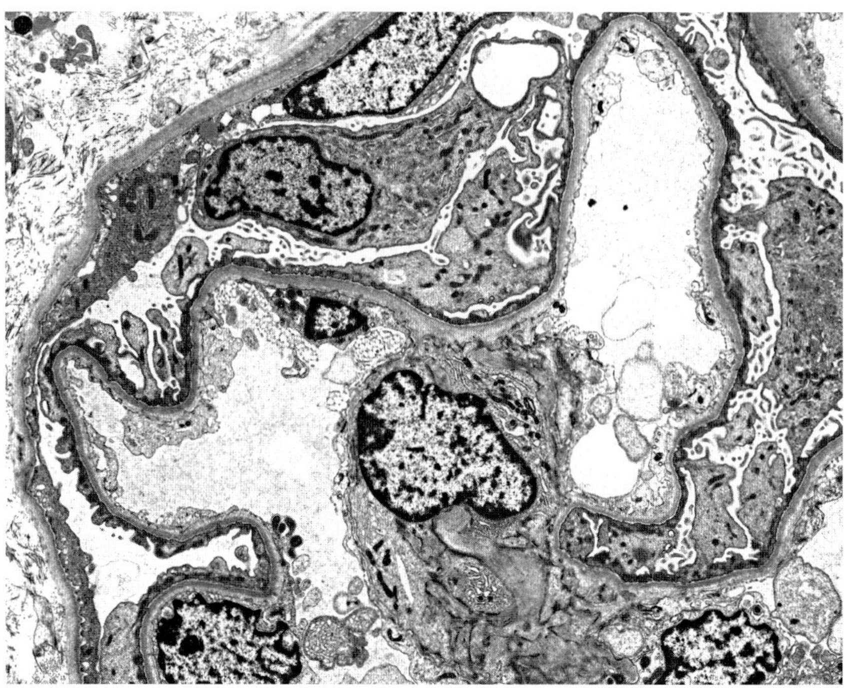

Figure 5-9

MINIMAL CHANGE DISEASE

By electron microscopy, there is extensive foot process effacement, with hypertrophy of the podocyte cell bodies. The primary processes are intact and slender cytoplasmic extensions form from the cell bodies to the foot processes. The glomerular basement membranes appear normal in thickness, without electron-dense deposits.

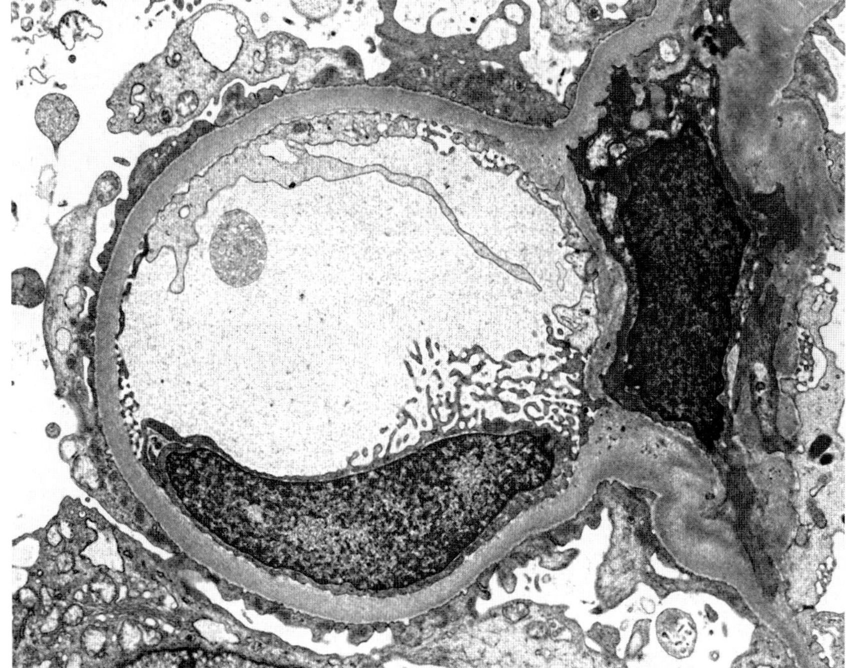

Figure 5-10

MINIMAL CHANGE DISEASE

The glomerular capillary lumens are fully patent, with well-preserved endothelial fenestrations. The glomerular basement membrane is of normal thickness and texture. The effaced foot processes form a sheet of undifferentiated podocyte cytoplasm over the capillary wall. The adjacent mesangium is unremarkable (electron micrograph).

(figs. 5-9, 5-10). If a biopsy is taken late in the course of the disease, however, when partial remission has occurred (either spontaneous or following therapy), there can be substantial restoration of foot processes (fig. 5-11). In general, the degree of foot process effacement correlates roughly with the severity of the proteinuria.

The podocyte cell body and primary processes are usually intact (fig. 5-9); however, the slender foot processes undergo progressive obliteration due to palm-like cytoplasmic expansion. Broadening and blunting of the highly ordered visceral epithelial pedicles produce a swath of undifferentiated podocyte cytoplasm

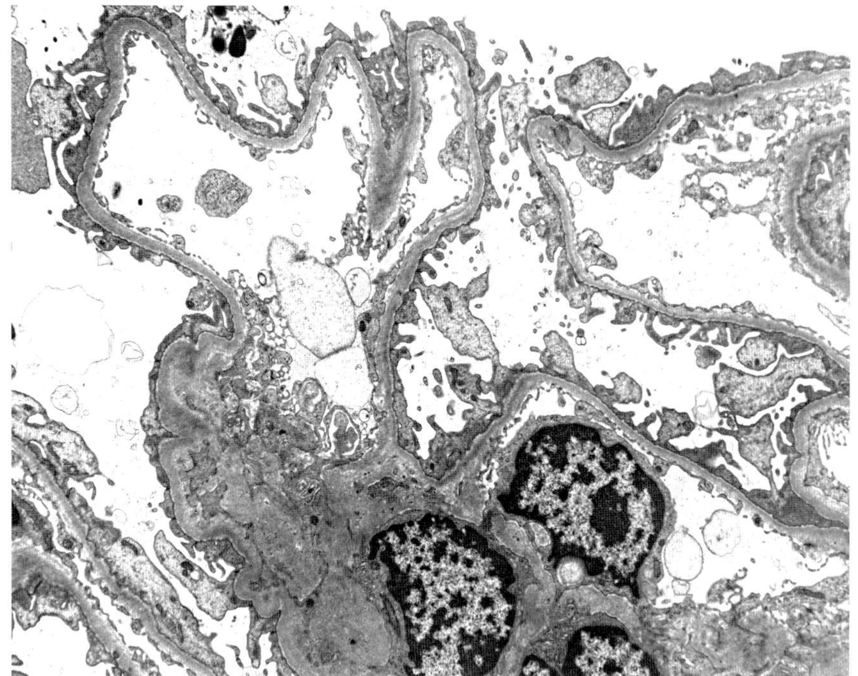

Figure 5-11

MINIMAL CHANGE DISEASE

Electron micrograph illustrates partial restoration of foot processes following steroid therapy. This biopsy was performed 3 weeks after initiation of steroid therapy, at which time proteinuria had fallen from 8.5 g/day to 2.3 g/day.

overlying the glomerular basement membranes (fig. 5-10). This cytoplasm displays mat-like condensations of actin cytoskeleton, oriented in the same axis as the glomerular basement membrane (fig. 5-12). On low-power microscopy, these cytoskeletal structures may be mistaken for electron-dense deposits. Higher resolution micrographs confirm their intracellular location by the demonstration of a surrounding plasma membrane. The filtration slit pores are largely obliterated. There is displacement and loss of the highly organized filtration slit diaphragms, with a corresponding loss of immunostaining for nephrin (13).

Other alterations of the podocytes include swelling of the cell bodies and an increased number of organelles, including rough endoplasmic reticulum, intracellular membrane-bound vesicles, and resorption droplets. Protein resorption droplets are typically electron dense, aqueous transport vesicles appear clear, and lipid resorption droplets are electron lucent, with a milky quality (fig. 5-13). A common finding is microvillous transformation of the podocyte cell bodies along the aspect that projects into the urinary space (fig. 5-14). All of these ultrastructural features are reversible upon remission of the nephrotic syndrome.

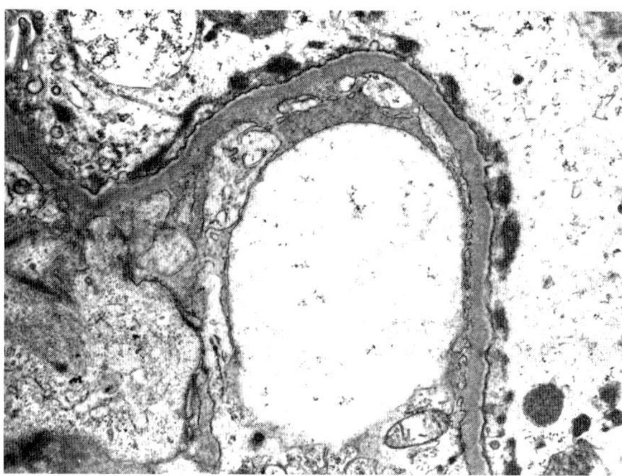

Figure 5-12

MINIMAL CHANGE DISEASE

Condensation of the actin cytoskeleton is seen at the base of the foot processes. These intracellular electron densities should not be mistaken for extracellular electron-dense deposits. The podocyte above is markedly swollen with pale cytoplasm.

The glomerular basement membrane is usually normal in thickness, texture, and contour. Foci of podocyte detachment from the glomerular basement membrane are extremely rare in MCD, in contrast to the frequent podocyte detachment and correspondingly higher incidence of nonselective proteinuria seen in FSGS.

Most cases have no mesangial abnormalities; however, a mild increase in mesangial cell number or matrix occurs in some patients. Small paramesangial electron densities are found segmentally in a minority of cases, corresponding to the mesangial staining for IgM seen by immunofluorescence (fig. 5-15). These mesangial densities probably represent plasma proteins trapped in the paramesangial region in the course of increased glomerular permeability (analogous to plasmatic insudation in arterioles) rather than true immune complex deposits. The finding of any immune deposits involving the peripheral glomerular capillary walls is incompatible with MCD.

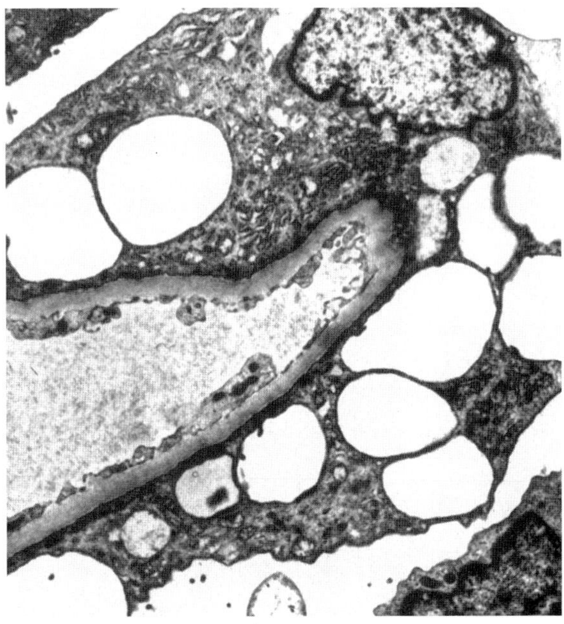

Figure 5-13

MINIMAL CHANGE DISEASE

The podocytes are engorged with clear transport vesicles, accompanied by complete foot process effacement.

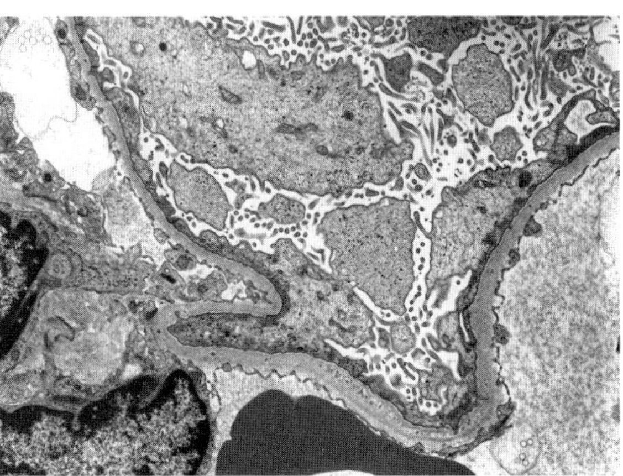

Figure 5-14

MINIMAL CHANGE DISEASE

There is extensive microvillous transformation of the podocytes. These finger-like cytoplasmic processes of the visceral epithelial cells project into the urinary space and resemble the microvillous brush border present on proximal tubular cells.

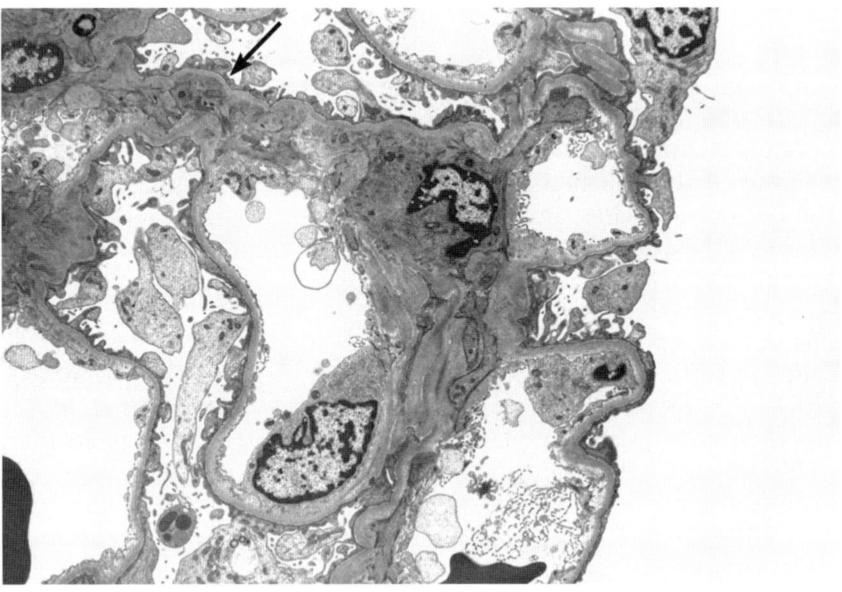

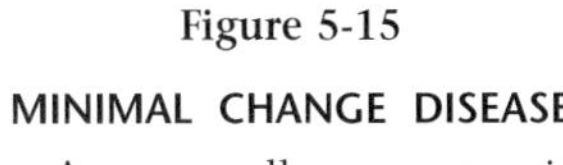

Figure 5-15

MINIMAL CHANGE DISEASE

A rare, small, paramesangial electron-dense deposit (arrow) corresponds to the weak mesangial positivity for IgM seen by immunofluorescence (not shown) (electron micrograph).

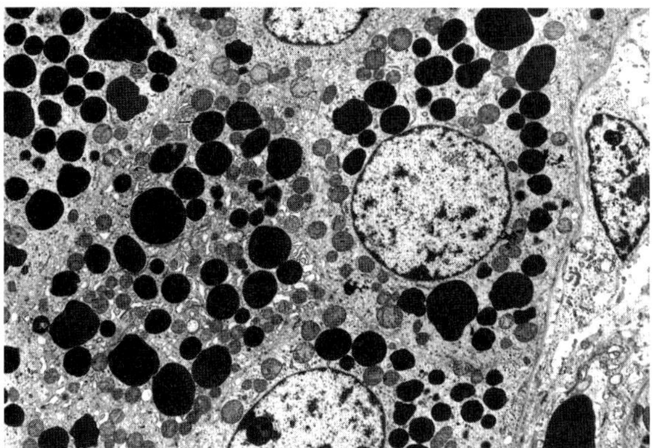

Figure 5-16

MINIMAL CHANGE DISEASE

Proximal tubular cells contain abundant intracytoplasmic protein resorption droplets, which appear electron dense and rounded (electron micrograph).

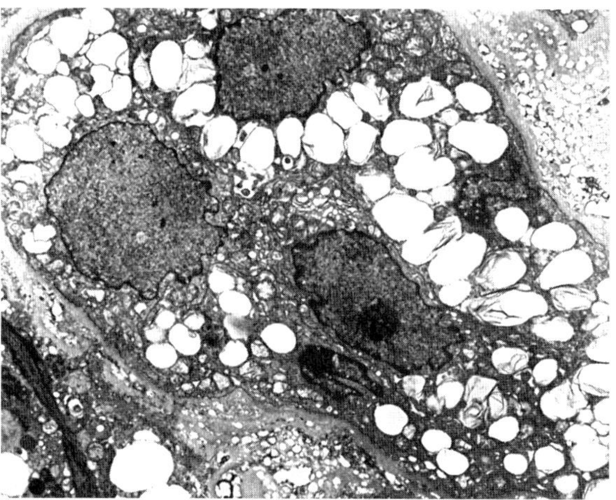

Figure 5-17

MINIMAL CHANGE DISEASE

The proximal tubules contain numerous electron-lucent lipid resorption droplets (electron micrograph).

The proximal tubules often contain intracellular electron-lucent lipid resorption droplets and electron-dense protein resorption droplets (figs. 5-16, 5-17). Shed lipid-laden tubular cells may be detected as "oval fat bodies" in the urine sediment (fig. 5-18).

Differential Diagnosis. The major differential diagnostic consideration is the distinction of MCD from FSGS. The ability of a percutaneous renal biopsy to discriminate between these entities is a function of the adequacy of the glomerular sampling. The possibility of FSGS should be considered in any biopsy of apparent MCD in which there is chronic tubulointerstitial disease. Serial sectioning of the biopsy and reprocessing of the frozen tissue for light microscopy increase the likelihood of sampling the diagnostic segmental lesions. It is important to remember that the presence of global glomerular sclerosis does not preclude a diagnosis of MCD, especially if there is underlying arterionephrosclerosis.

Foot process effacement is the sine qua non of MCD; however, foot process effacement is not specific for MCD. It can be seen in many forms of renal disease with substantial glomerular proteinuria. What distinguishes MCD is the presence of diffuse foot process effacement in the absence of any other significant glomerular alterations. In this sense, a diagnosis of MCD is a diagnosis of exclusion in which foot process effacement is identified after light, immunofluorescence, and electron microscopy have excluded other possible causes of proteinuria.

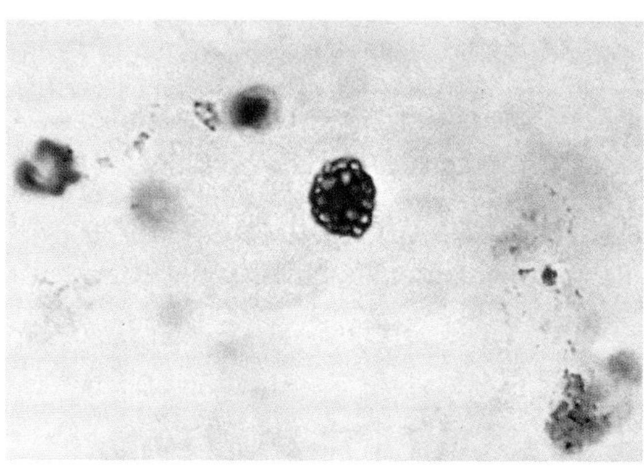

Figure 5-18

MINIMAL CHANGE DISEASE

A lipid-laden, shed tubular cell forms an "oval fat body" in the urine sediment (light microscopy of urine sediment).

MCD may occur superimposed on other conditions. We have seen this scenario in patients with mild mesangial proliferative lupus nephritis, for example (10). MCD with IgA nephropathy can be considered another example of such a dual glomerulopathy. The possibility of MCD as a superimposed disease should be suspected in a patient presenting with nephrotic syndrome who has mesangial pathology and complete foot process effacement in the absence of other peripheral capillary wall lesions that might explain the permeability defect. For example, a patient with systemic lupus erythematosus presenting with sudden onset of nephrotic syndrome may have mild class II lupus nephritis with immune deposits confined to the mesangium in the face of severe and diffuse foot process effacement, without associated subendothelial or subepithelial deposits.

Etiology and Pathogenesis. The etiology of MCD is unknown (23). Moreover, the issue of how it may be pathogenetically linked to FSGS has not been resolved. The high responsivity to steroids provides circumstantial evidence for the role of immunologic factors. Experimental models of MCD can be produced by administering podocyte toxins, such as puromycin aminonucleoside or adriamycin. More prolonged exposure to these agents can produce the more severe lesion of FSGS (2). Neutralization of the negative charge sites in the glomerular capillary wall by infusion of heparitinase or protamine sulfate in rats causes a reversible, highly selective proteinuria and foot process effacement resembling those of MCD.

Current emphasis has focused on the role of circulating "permeability factors" that may cause increased glomerular capillary wall permeability (19,23). Abnormal T-cell function was proposed as a possible pathogenetic factor as early as 1974 and is supported by the association of lymphoid malignancies with the development of MCD (8). Hybridomas made from the T cells of patients with MCD elaborate a factor that can produce foot process effacement and proteinuria in rats when injected intravenously (16). A variety of putative vascular permeability factors have been reported in MCD, although their nature and biochemical activity have not been fully characterized (23). These have been isolated from the serum, plasma, mononuclear cells, and urine of patients with MCD. They range in molecular weight from 12 to 160 kDa. Some have been reported to have kallikrein-like activity; others are cationic and may act by neutralization of fixed negative charges in the glomerular capillary wall; yet others may have a direct effect on podocyte cellular functions, including maintenance of foot process architecture, the synthesis and maintenance of glomerular basement membrane components, and cell adhesion (23).

Treatment and Prognosis. Both children and adults with MCD have an excellent prognosis. In the pre-steroid era, as many as 70 percent of cases of MCD underwent spontaneous remission over the course of months or years of follow-up. Today, corticosteroids are the mainstay of treatment (15): most children and adults achieve remission of nephrotic syndrome with corticosteroid therapy (20). Corticosteroids in doses of 60 mg/m^2/day produce remission of the nephrotic syndrome by 8 weeks in 90 to 95 percent of children with MCD. The response in adults is slower (20): only 75 to 85 percent of adults achieve remission by 8 weeks of daily or alternate day prednisone therapy. Therefore, adults are generally offered a longer course of therapy of up to 16 weeks before they are considered steroid resistant. Once remission is achieved, steroids are tapered over 1 to 2 months to prevent early relapse.

Relapses are common. Up to 50 percent of children and 30 percent of adults have a relapse within the first year. Relapses are generally treated with another course of steroids. Those patients who are steroid-dependent or frequent relapsers may respond to alkylating agents, such as chlorambucil or cyclophosphamide. Other steroid-sparing therapies include levamisole in children and cyclosporine in both children and adults. Cyclosporine has the disadvantage of potential nephrotoxicity and a high rate of relapse following discontinuation.

Some patients with biopsy-documented MCD appear to progress to FSGS in a subsequent biopsy, although there is debate as to whether this represents true evolution from one disease to another or a problem of sampling. In children with MCD, the presence of glomerular hypertrophy (glomerular area greater than 1.75 times that of age-matched controls) on initial biopsy may be a risk factor for subsequent evolution to FSGS on a later biopsy (11).

HISTOLOGIC VARIANTS OF MINIMAL CHANGE DISEASE

A number of histologic variants of MCD have been reported and are described below. These include diffuse mesangial hypercellularity, IgM nephropathy, and MCD disease with acute renal failure. For a discussion of C1q nephropathy and glomerular tip lesion, see chapter 6.

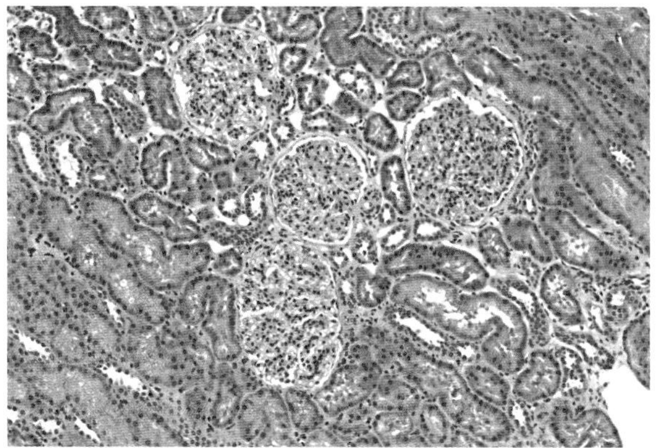

Figure 5-19

DIFFUSE MESANGIAL HYPERCELLULARITY

Low-power view shows diffuse and global mesangial hypercellularity, resembling proliferative glomerulonephritis (H&E stain).

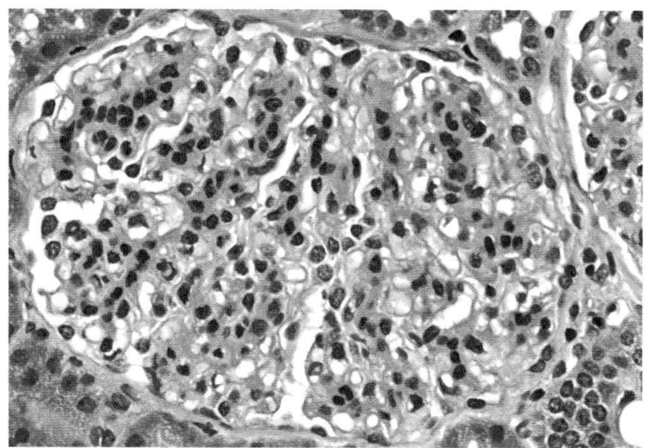

Figure 5-20

DIFFUSE MESANGIAL HYPERCELLULARITY

High-power view shows severe global mesangial hypercellularity, with more than 10 mesangial cells in some mesangial regions (H&E stain).

Diffuse Mesangial Hypercellularity

Definition. Diffuse mesangial hypercellularity (DMH) is a variant of MCD that primarily affects children (4,22); it accounts for approximately 3 percent of pediatric cases of idiopathic nephrotic syndrome. It is defined according to the ISKDC criteria as more than four mesangial cells per mesangial region affecting at least 80 percent of glomeruli in tissue sections of 2 to 3 µm in thickness (22). The Southwest Pediatric Nephrology Study Group (SPNSG) defines DMH as involvement of more than 75 percent of glomeruli by mesangial hypercellularity that can be graded as mild (three nuclei per mesangial area), moderate (four nuclei per mesangial area), or severe (five nuclei or more per mesangial area) (4).

Clinical Features. Patients with DMH present with nephrotic syndrome, but are more likely to have hematuria (89 percent) and hypertension (46 percent) than patients with MCD (22). In fact, some affected individuals develop gross hematuria.

Light Microscopic Findings. Glomerular hypercellularity is confined to the mesangium, without occlusion of the capillary lumens. Hypercellularity varies from mild to severe, but is not associated with membranoproliferative features (i.e., mesangial interposition or replication of glomerular basement membrane) (figs. 5-19–5-21).

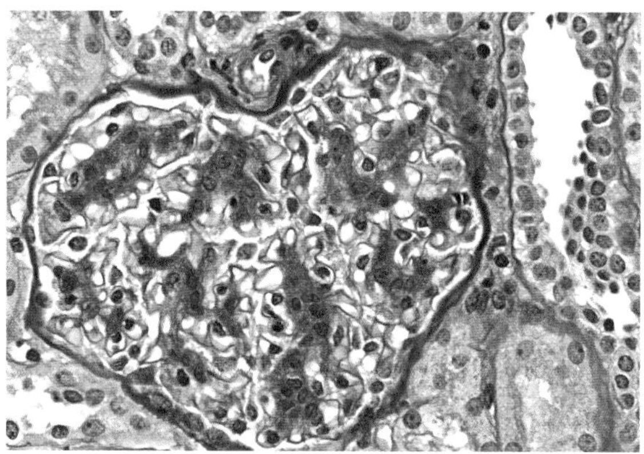

Figure 5-21

DIFFUSE MESANGIAL HYPERCELLULARITY

High-power view shows severe mesangial hypercellularity accompanied by a mild increase in mesangial matrix. Despite the mesangial hypercellularity, the glomerular capillary lumens remain patent. The glomerular basement membranes are of normal thickness and texture (PAS stain).

Immunofluorescence Findings. Immunofluorescence is usually negative. Some cases have mesangial positivity for IgM and C3, however (4).

Electron Microscopic Findings. There are diffuse podocyte alterations similar to those seen in MCD. Mesangial hypercellularity is less impressive by electron microscopy than by light microscopy because of the extreme thinness of the sections (fig. 5-22). Small, paramesangial, electron-dense deposits may be identified in up to 50 percent of cases.

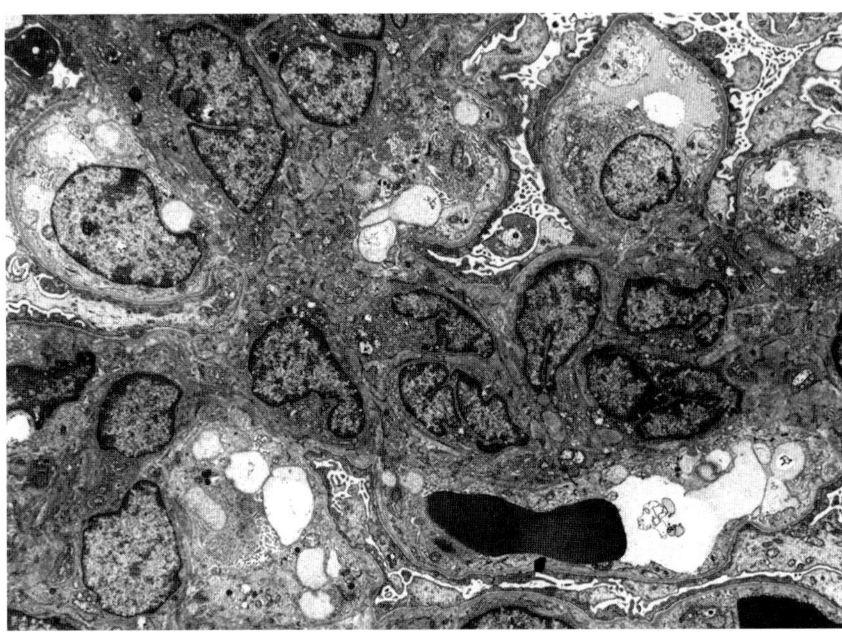

Figure 5-22

DIFFUSE MESANGIAL HYPERCELLULARITY

Electron micrograph shows the expansion of the mesangium by an increased number of mesangial cells, without electron-dense deposits. There is complete foot process effacement (electron micrograph).

Differential Diagnosis. DMH must be distinguished from mesangial proliferative forms of glomerulonephritis, such as mesangial proliferative lupus nephritis, mild membranoproliferative glomerulonephritis, IgA nephropathy, C1q nephropathy, and the resolving phase of acute postinfectious glomerulonephritis. Those cases of DMH with mesangial deposits usually stain for IgM and C3 only. If there are corresponding mesangial electron-dense deposits, they are confined to the paramesangial region, without involvement of the peripheral capillary wall. Careful analysis of the composition and distribution of glomerular immune deposits by immunofluorescence and electron microscopy can usually differentiate between these possibilities without difficulty. A complete clinical history, including serology and complement studies, is an essential adjunct. DMH should not be diagnosed in a patient who does not have or has not had full nephrotic syndrome. Even if the patient is biopsied in the course of spontaneous remission, a history of full nephrotic syndrome with edema at the time of clinical presentation can usually be elicited.

Treatment and Prognosis. According to an ISKDC study (22), patients with DMH had a higher rate of initial steroid resistance than those with MCD. By 52 weeks of follow-up, however, there was no statistical difference in remission rate between those with and without DMH. The presence of DMH did not correlate with the incidence of subsequent relapse or death. The SPNSG study (4) also found a higher rate of initial steroid resistance in the patients with DMH, and the response correlated with the severity of the mesangial hypercellularity. There were no significant differences, however, in long-term outcome.

IgM Nephropathy

Definition. IgM nephropathy was first described in 1978 by two independent investigators, Bhasin et al. (3) and Cohen et al. (7). It is defined as a clinical-pathologic variant of MCD with diffuse and global mesangial deposits of IgM (fig. 5-23). There is no general agreement on how intense and diffuse the deposits of IgM must be to qualify as this variant. This is particularly problematic, because low-intensity (trace to 1+) IgM deposition is extremely common in classic MCD. Most investigators reserve this term only for those cases in which the IgM deposition is 2+ or greater in intensity and is of diffuse and global distribution.

The patients described in the literature are heterogeneous with respect to the intensity and distribution of the IgM staining, as well as the presence of associated mesangial hypercellularity and mesangial electron-dense deposits. This lack of conformity in the defining criteria has hampered efforts to determine whether IgM nephropathy indeed represents a distinct clinicopathologic

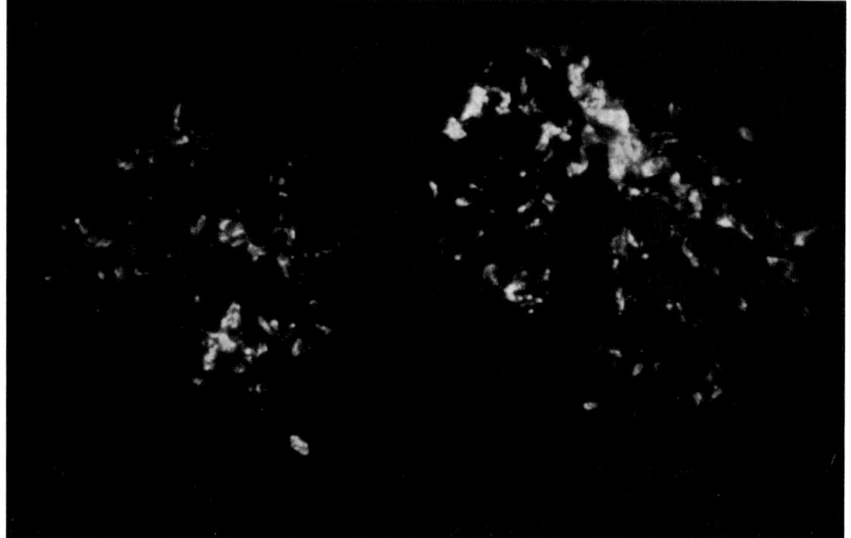

Figure 5-23

IgM NEPHROPATHY

By immunofluorescence, there is 2+ diffuse and global staining of mesangial areas for IgM, outlining the mesangial stalks of two glomeruli (immunofluorescence micrograph).

entity. We advocate that a diagnosis of IgM nephropathy be reserved for those variants of MCD with regular 2+ or stronger mesangial deposits of IgM, regardless of whether mesangial hypercellularity or mesangial electron-dense deposits are present.

Light Microscopic Findings. Glomeruli usually display no histologic abnormalities. Mild mesangial hypercellularity may be found in a minority of cases.

Immunofluorescence Findings. There are mesangial deposits of IgM exhibiting 2+ or stronger intensity. Co-deposits of C3 are identified in 30 to 100 percent of cases. Moreover, some reports of this entity describe low-intensity (trace to 1+) and relatively segmental mesangial codeposits of other immunoglobulins, including IgG and IgA, as well as C1. These mesangial deposits probably are not true immune complex deposits, but are thought to result from nonspecific entrapment of circulating plasma proteins due to impaired mesangial clearance.

Electron Microscopic Findings. There is extensive foot process effacement. Up to half of cases have small mesangial electron-dense deposits, predominantly in the paramesangial areas (fig. 5-24).

Differential Diagnosis. IgM nephropathy must be differentiated from other mild mesangial glomerulopathies, such as IgA nephropathy, mesangial proliferative lupus nephritis, and the resolving phase of acute postinfectious glomerulonephritis. IgM nephropathy is distinguished

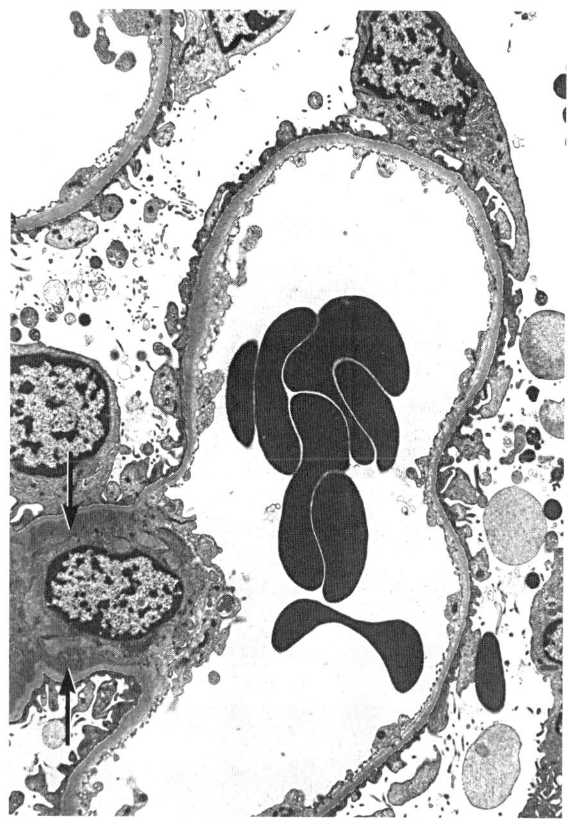

Figure 5-24

IgM NEPHROPATHY

An example with mesangial electron-dense deposits (arrows). Note the marked foot process effacement. There are no immune deposits involving the peripheral capillary walls (electron micrograph).

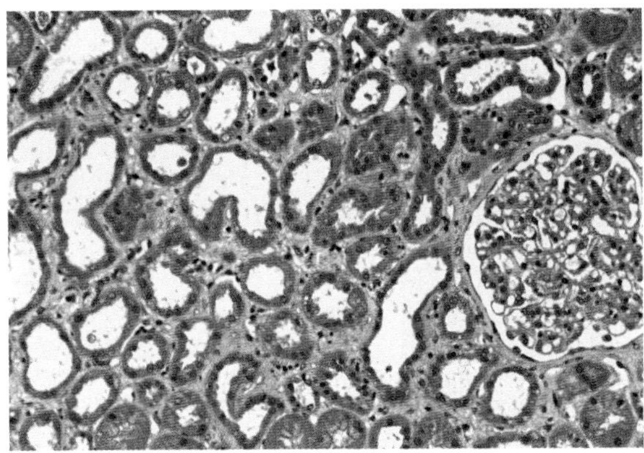

Figure 5-25

MINIMAL CHANGE DISEASE WITH ACUTE RENAL FAILURE

There is diffuse mild interstitial edema and simplification of the proximal tubules. The glomeruli appear normal by light microscopy (H&E stain).

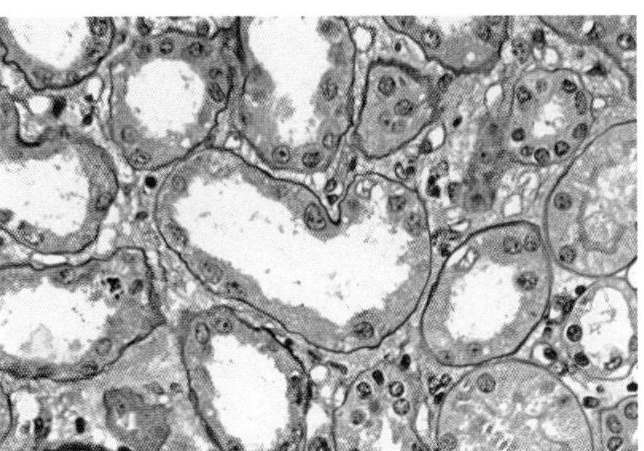

Figure 5-26

MINIMAL CHANGE DISEASE WITH ACUTE RENAL FAILURE

There are extensive tubular degenerative and regenerative changes, including flattened epithelial cells, loss of PAS-stained brush border, enlarged regenerative nuclei with nucleoli, and focal mitotic figures.

by the generally exclusive staining for IgM and C3 limited to the mesangium and the presence of severe foot process effacement in the setting of idiopathic nephrotic syndrome.

Treatment and Prognosis. Some investigators have reported that patients with IgM nephropathy have a greater likelihood of steroid resistance or dependence than patients with MCD. In a compilation of series, the incidence of steroid resistance ranged from 25 to 50 percent (25). Moreover, some cases of IgM nephropathy have been reported to evolve into FSGS on repeat biopsy (27). Nonetheless, not all renal pathologists recognize this variant as a distinct clinical-pathologic entity, but only mention in a note that the presence of IgM deposits may identify a subset of MCD patients with a greater likelihood of steroid resistance or dependence.

Minimal Change Disease with Acute Renal Failure

Definition. Acute renal failure is an under-recognized, reversible complication of MCD that predominantly affects older adults who have severe nephrotic syndrome, massive edema, and a history of systolic hypertension (14).

Clinical Features. Lowenstein et al. (17) first drew attention to this entity in 1981 in a report of renal failure occurring in 15 patients with minimal change nephrotic syndrome. Although one of the patients was as young as 15 years old, 9 of the 15 patients were over the age of 60. The peak serum creatinine level at presentation varied from 2.3 to 13.4 mg/dL (mean, 5.25 mg/dL). Most patients had severe markers of nephrotic syndrome: heavy proteinuria (range, 5.0 to 18.7 g/day; mean, 9.3 g/day), profound hypoalbuminemia (serum albumin range, 0.4 to 2.4 g/dL; mean, 1.5 g/dL), and anasarca.

Light Microscopic Findings. The glomeruli show typical features of MCD by light, fluorescence, and electron microscopy. The acute renal failure correlates with subtle tubulointerstitial findings of ischemic acute tubular necrosis. The most distinctive pathologic lesion is focal proximal tubular epithelial simplification, observed by light microscopy in about 70 percent of cases (14). The tubules appear ectatic, with irregular luminal profiles, flattened epithelium, attenuated or absent brush border, and enlarged regenerative nuclei with nucleoli (figs. 5-25, 5-26). In some cases, increased tubular epithelial mitotic figures and apoptotic bodies are seen (fig. 5-26). Cellular debris may shed into the tubular lumen; however, frank coagulation necrosis is not seen. Interstitial edema commonly accompanies the tubular injury. Arteriosclerosis is commonly identified in older individuals with a history of hypertension (fig. 5-27).

Immunofluorescence Findings. The glomeruli show no immune staining.

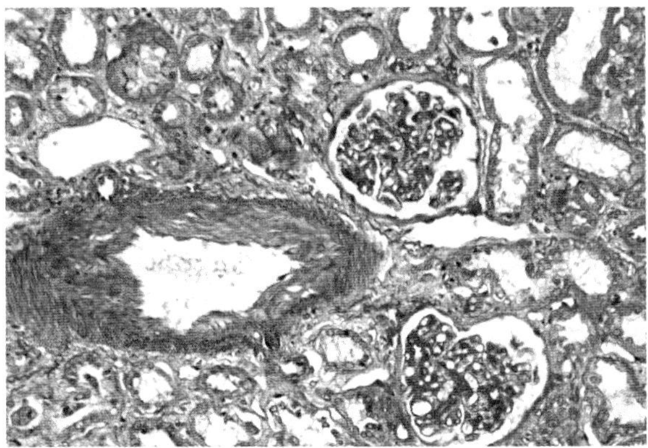

Figure 5-27

MINIMAL CHANGE DISEASE WITH ACUTE RENAL FAILURE

An example from a 68-year-old woman with moderate arteriosclerosis. There is diffuse interstitial edema and tubular simplification (Masson trichrome stain).

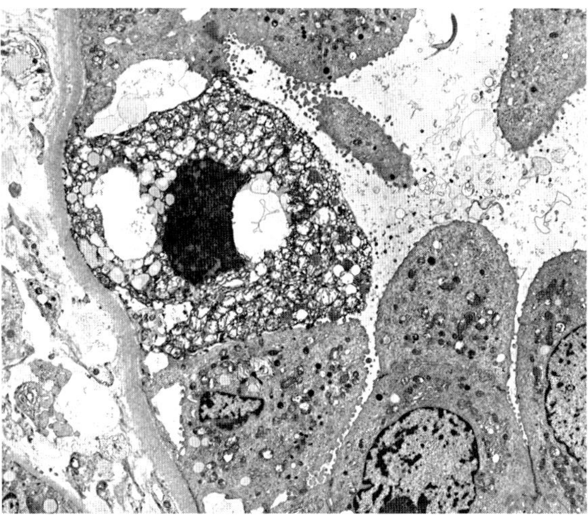

Figure 5-28

MINIMAL CHANGE DISEASE WITH ACUTE RENAL FAILURE

Shown is tubular simplification, including single cell apoptosis with swollen mitochondria, widening of the intercellular junctions, and complete loss of the brush border (electron micrograph).

Electron Microscopic Findings. The proximal tubular cells appear simplified, with reduced apical microvilli, widening of the intercellular junctions, reduced basolateral interdigitations, and fewer cytoplasmic organelles (fig. 5-28). In some cells, cytoplasmic fragments desquamate into the tubular lumen. There is mild interstitial edema and a scanty interstitial lymphocytic infiltrate, without tubulitis. These tubulointerstitial findings are indistinguishable from those of ischemic acute tubular necrosis occurring in patients in cardiogenic or hypovolemic shock.

Etiology and Pathogenesis. Calculation of the clearance rates of inulin and para-aminohippuric acid (PAH) revealed reduced filtration fractions due to a proportionately greater reduction in the glomerular filtration rate than the reduction in renal plasma flow (17). These data suggest that the pathophysiology of this condition involves disturbances in the glomerular hemodynamics related to fluid retention and reduced effective renal plasma flow. Indeed, Jennette et al. (14) noted an older age, heavier proteinuria, and more severe hypoalbuminemia to be risk factors for this complication of MCD. Affected individuals are also more likely to have systolic hypertension and arteriosclerosis than patients with MCD who do not develop acute renal failure. The underlying arteriosclerosis presumably predisposes to acute renal failure by reducing the patient's compensatory response to the hemodynamic stresses of severe nephrotic syndrome.

Treatment and Prognosis. This diagnosis is a gratifying one for the renal pathologist because the acute renal failure is highly reversible with combined management of the fluid overload with diuretics and the nephrotic syndrome with steroids. Most patients recover from the renal failure within 5 to 7 weeks, with the exception of some slower responders and rare patients with irreversible renal failure.

Minimal Change Disease and IgA Nephropathy

Definition. MCD occurring in association with IgA nephropathy is diagnosed in nephrotic patients by the presence of dominant mesangial IgA deposits and extensive foot process effacement in the absence of peripheral capillary wall deposits. The IgA deposits in this condition are confined to the mesangium and are inadequate to account for the severe proteinuria on the basis of immune complex load. Rather, the only peripheral capillary wall lesions are diffuse foot process effacement like that seen in MCD. In this respect, MCD and IgA nephropathy can be distinguished from pure IgA nephropathy that presents with nephrotic

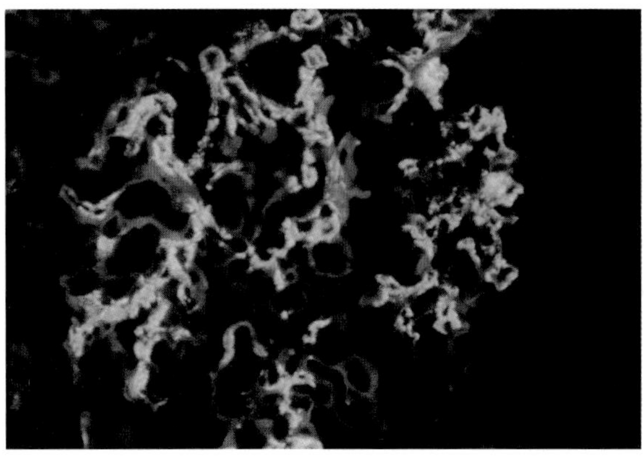

Figure 5-29

MINIMAL CHANGE DISEASE AND IgA NEPHROPATHY

By immunofluorescence, there is 2+ global mesangial positivity for IgA.

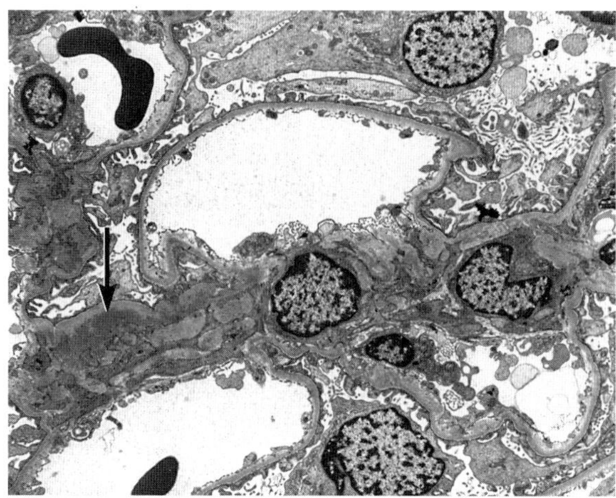

Figure 5-30

MINIMAL CHANGE DISEASE AND IgA NEPHROPATHY

By electron microscopy, there are paramesangial, electron-dense deposits (arrow), corresponding to the mesangial deposits of IgA. Although no electron-dense deposits are seen involving the peripheral capillary walls, there is extensive effacement of foot processes, consistent with superimposed minimal change disease in this patient with full nephrotic syndrome and urine protein excretion of 10 g/day.

syndrome and typically displays severe glomerular proliferative or sclerosing lesions with immune deposits involving the glomerular capillary walls. It is likely that this entity represents an overlap or superimposition of MCD on IgA nephropathy, because the nephrotic syndrome is often relapsing and responds to steroid therapy in a manner typical of MCD (1,6).

Clinical Features. MCD and IgA nephropathy is primarily a disease of childhood. Fifty percent of patients are under the age of 10 years, although the age range is wide (2 to 73 years) (5). The male to female ratio is 3 to 1. Nephrotic proteinuria is present in 100 percent of patients, hematuria in 50 percent, and episodes of gross hematuria (usually following upper respiratory tract infections) in 25 percent.

Light Microscopic Findings. The glomeruli display little or no mesangial hypercellularity. Glomerular capillary lumens are patent, without evidence of endocapillary proliferation or segmental sclerosis. Red blood cells may be identified in the tubular lumens, and proximal tubules contain intracytoplasmic protein resorption droplets.

Immunofluorescence Findings. There is dominant mesangial staining for IgA in a granular and diffuse pattern, with an intensity of 2+ or above (fig. 5-29). Variable but lower intensity mesangial deposits of IgG and IgM may also be seen. Characteristic of IgA nephropathy is the presence of mesangial deposits of C3, with negative to trace C1.

Electron Microscopic Findings. There are mesangial electron-dense deposits that correspond to the mesangial positivity for IgA (fig. 5-30). These deposits are most abundant in the paramesangial regions, subjacent to the reflection of the glomerular basement membrane over the mesangium. No regular immune deposits are found in the subendothelial or subepithelial regions. There is extensive effacement of foot processes, however, with frequent microvillous transformation of the podocytes (fig. 5-30).

Etiology and Pathogenesis. This entity probably represents a dual glomerulopathy caused by the chance concurrence of two relatively common diseases of childhood. This interpretation is supported by evidence from repeat biopsies that have shown that the MCD preceded the development of IgA nephropathy in some cases, whereas in others the reverse occurred.

Treatment and Prognosis. Steroid therapy should be directed to the component of MCD. Most patients have an early response to steroids and one quarter experience multiple relapses. Spontaneous remission of nephrotic syndrome has also been described.

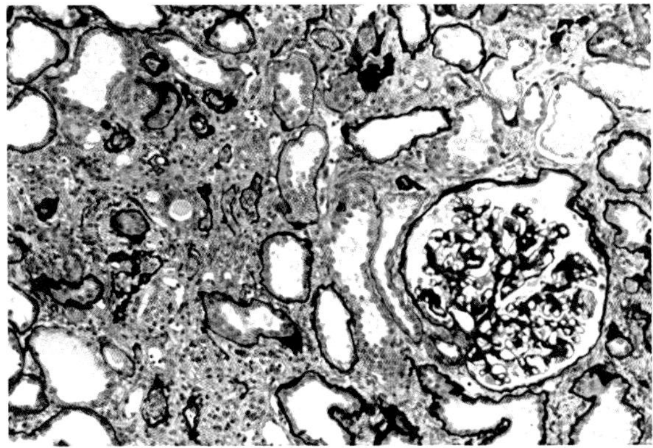

Figure 5-31

MINIMAL CHANGE DISEASE SECONDARY TO NON-STEROIDAL ANTI-INFLAMMATORY DRUG (NSAID) USE

A 58-year-old woman treated for 9 months with naproxen developed acute renal failure and nephrotic syndrome. Renal biopsy reveals normal-appearing glomeruli, consistent with minimal change disease. The prominent interstitial edema and inflammation indicate associated acute interstitial nephritis (JMS stain).

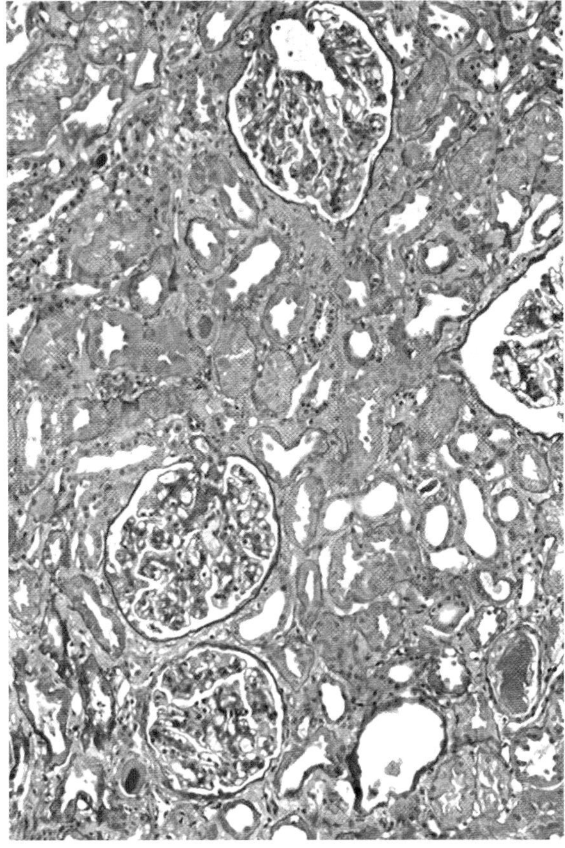

Figure 5-32

MINIMAL CHANGE DISEASE SECONDARY TO NSAID USE

A case of NSAID-induced minimal change disease with acute renal failure shows normal-appearing glomeruli by light microscopy. By electron microscopy (not shown), there was marked foot process effacement. The acute renal failure corresponds to associated acute tubular necrosis, featuring ectatic tubules, focal loss of brush border, and enlarged regenerative tubular nuclei (PAS stain).

SECONDARY FORMS OF MINIMAL CHANGE DISEASE

Associated with Therapeutic Agents

Definition. MCD may occur as a complication of certain forms of drug therapy (Table 5-1). The major drug association is with NSAIDs. MCD has also been associated, rarely, with lithium therapy. In both instances, the achievement of remission within weeks of withdrawal of the offending drug supports a pathogenetic role.

Clinical Features. Most patients who develop this toxicity have been on NSAID therapy for many months or years before the onset of the nephrotic syndrome. The average duration of drug exposure prior to the development of nephrotic syndrome is 11 months (21). Patients present with nephrotic syndrome alone, nephrotic syndrome with acute renal failure, or renal failure alone. These presentations correspond to the development of MCD alone, MCD with acute interstitial nephritis, or acute interstitial nephritis alone. Most patients are older adults (mean, 65 years). In those patients with associated acute interstitial nephritis, a hypersensitivity response (with fever, rash, and eosinophilia) is unusual, affecting fewer than 20 percent. The low incidence of hypersensitivity phenomena probably relates to the anti-inflammatory properties of the NSAID (21).

Pathologic Findings. In those patients with MCD alone, the only finding is diffuse foot process effacement, indistinguishable from that seen with idiopathic MCD. Patients with associated acute interstitial nephritis have interstitial edema and an inflammatory infiltrate that consists predominantly of lymphocytes (fig. 5-31). Eosinophils are sparse or absent, and tubulitis tends to be mild. Many cases of NSAID-induced MCD also have features of ischemic acute tubular necrosis related to the ability of this class of drugs to reduce the glomerular filtration rate through hemodynamic effects on renal blood flow (fig. 5-32).

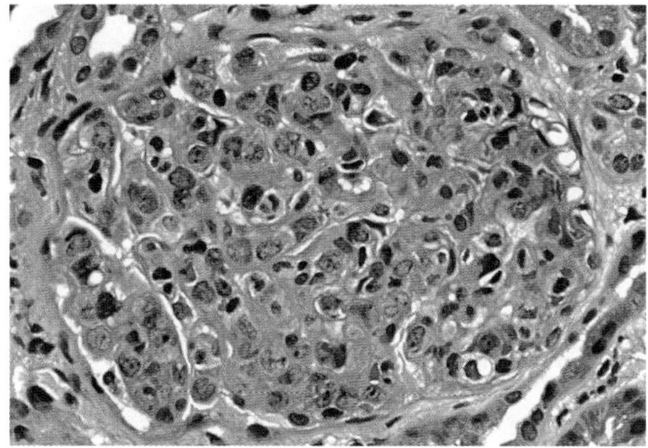

Figure 5-33

MINIMAL CHANGE DISEASE WITH ANGIOTROPIC (INTRAVASCULAR) LARGE CELL LYMPHOMA

Lymphoma cells with large atypical nuclei are marginated in the glomerular capillary lumens. The intracapillary cells are much more pleomorphic than the endocapillary cells typically seen in forms of proliferative glomerulonephritis (H&E stain).

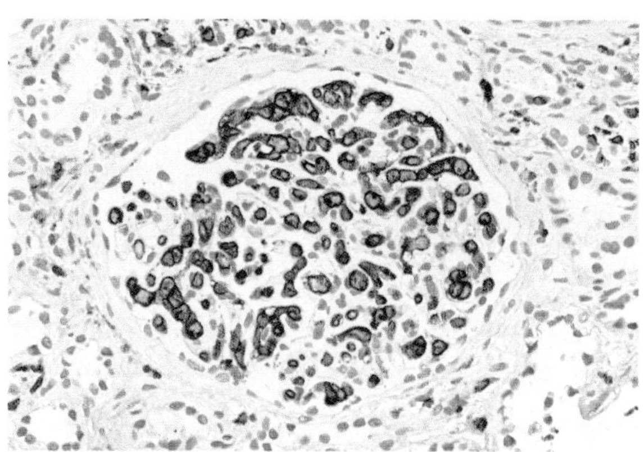

Figure 5-34

MINIMAL CHANGE DISEASE WITH ANGIOTROPIC (INTRAVASCULAR) LARGE CELL LYMPHOMA

Immunostain for common leukocyte antigen (CLA) highlights the atypical intracapillary cells, indicating that they represent malignant lymphocytes. The cells were also positive for CD20 (not shown), consistent with B cells (immunoperoxidase stain for CLA).

Differential Diagnosis. There are several major findings that distinguish this from most other forms of drug-induced allergic interstitial nephritis. Eosinophils are rarely identified, tubulitis is not prominent, and interstitial granulomas are rarely encountered.

Etiology and Pathogenesis. How NSAIDs produce MCD is unknown. Toxicity directed toward the podocyte has been proposed. The component of acute interstitial nephritis is presumably allergic in nature, although systemic allergic manifestations (such as eosinophilia, fever, and rash) are uncommon due to blunting of the allergic response by the drug's anti-inflammatory properties.

Treatment and Prognosis. The proteinuria and renal insufficiency usually resolve within 2 to 8 weeks after discontinuation of the offending NSAID. Although there have been no controlled studies, anecdotal evidence suggests that the use of steroids may hasten recovery. Future exposure to NSAID of any class should be avoided to prevent recurrence of MCD and/or acute interstitial nephritis.

Associated with Malignancies

Definition. The development of MCD has been associated with a variety of lymphoid malignancies. Most common is the association

Table 5-1

CLASSIFICATION OF MINIMAL CHANGE DISEASE AND VARIANTS

Idiopathic Forms
Minimal change disease (MCD)
Histologic variants of MCD
Diffuse mesangial hypercellularity
IgM nephropathy
Minimal change disease with acute renal failure
Dual glomerulopathies
Minimal change disease and IgA nephropathy
Minimal change disease and lupus nephritis
Secondary Forms
Secondary to therapeutic agents
Nonsteroidal anti-inflammatory drugs
Lithium
Secondary to malignancies
Hodgkin's disease
Non-Hodgkin's lymphoma
Acute myelogenous leukemia
Chronic myelogenous leukemia
Angioimmunoblastic lymphadenopathy
Angiotropic (intravascular) lymphoma
Mycosis fungoides
T-cell leukemias
Other associations
Bee stings
Food allergies
Viral infections (Epstein-Barr virus [EBV])
Human immunodeficiency virus (HIV)

with Hodgkin's disease. The development of MCD may precede or be simultaneous with the diagnosis of Hodgkin's disease. Evidence in favor of a pathogenic association is the response of the MCD to therapy directed to the Hodgkin's disease and the timing of recurrences of nephrotic syndrome with relapses of Hodgkin's disease. MCD has also been associated with a variety of other lymphoid lesions, including non-Hodgkin's lymphoma, chronic myelogenous leukemia, acute myelogenous leukemia, angioimmunoblastic lymphadenopathy, angiotropic (intravascular) large cell lymphoma, mycosis fungoides, and T-cell leukemias.

Pathologic Findings. The renal pathologic changes can be indistinguishable from those of idiopathic MCD. In patients with angiotropic (intravascular) large cell lymphoma, the glomerular capillaries are typically infiltrated by lymphoma cells with enlarged, hyperchromatic nuclei (fig. 5-33) (9,24). Immunostaining for lymphoid markers is helpful to prove that the intracapillary cells are of lymphoid origin (fig. 5-34). Foot process effacement has been reported to be most severe in capillaries containing the malignant cells (9), suggesting altered glomerular permeability related to the local elaboration of lymphokines or mechanical effects on glomerular hemodynamics.

Treatment and Prognosis. In lymphoma-associated MCD, antineoplastic therapy should be directed to the underlying malignancy.

Other Associations

MCD has also been reported to occur in association with bee stings, food allergies, and viral infections, including mononucleosis and human immunodeficiency virus (HIV) infection (Table 5-1). The onset of MCD may follow immunizations in childhood. Although it is difficult to prove direct causality, the association is strengthened by a close temporal relationship between the inciting agent and the development of the nephrotic syndrome.

REFERENCES

1. Association of IgA nephropathy with steroid-responsive nephrotic syndrome. A report of the Southwest Pediatric Nephrology Study Group. Am J Kidney Dis 1985;5:157–64.
2. Bertani T, Poggi A, Pozzoni R, et al. Adriamycin-induced nephrotic syndrome in rats: sequence of pathologic events. Lab Invest 1982;46:16–23.
3. Bhasin HK, Abuelo JG, Nayak R, Esparza AR. Mesangial proliferative glomerulonephritis. Lab Invest 1978;39:21–9.
4. Childhood nephrotic syndrome associated with diffuse mesangial hypercellularity. A report of the Southwest Pediatric Nephrology Study Group. Kidney Int 1983;24:87–94.
5. Churg J, Habib R, White RH. Pathology of the nephrotic syndrome in children: a report for the International Study of Kidney Disease in Children. Lancet 1970;1:1299–302.
6. Clive DM, Galvanek EG, Silva FG. Mesangial immunoglobulin A deposits in minimal change nephrotic syndrome: a report of an older patient and review of the literature. Am J Nephrol 1990;10:31–6.
7. Cohen AH, Border WA, Glassock RJ. Nephrotic syndrome with glomerular mesangial IgM deposits. Lab Invest 1978;38:610–9.
8. Cunard R, Kelly CJ. T cells and minimal change disease. J Am Soc Nephrol 2002;13:1409–11.
9. D'Agati V, Sablay LB, Knowles DM, Walter L. Angiotropic large cell lymphoma (intravascular malignant lymphomatosis) of the kidney: presentation as minimal change disease. Hum Pathol 1989;20:263–8.
10. Dube GK, Markowitz GS, Radhakrishnan J, Appel GB, D'Agati VD. Minimal change disease in systemic lupus erythematosus. Clin Nephrol 2002;57:120–6.
11. Fogo A, Hawkins EP, Berry PL, et al. Glomerular hypertrophy in minimal change disease predicts subsequent progression to focal glomerular sclerosis. Kidney Int 1990;38:115–23.
12. Habib R, Kleinknecht C. The primary nephrotic syndrome of childhood. Classification and clinicopathologic study of 406 cases. Pathol Annu 1971;6:417–74.
13. Huh W, Kim DJ, Kim MK, et al. Expression of nephrin in acquired human glomerular disease. Nephrol Dial Transplant 2002;17:478–84.
14. Jennette JC, Falk RJ. Adult minimal change glomerulopathy with acute renal failure. Am J Kidney Dis 1990;16:432–7.

15. Korbet SM, Schwartz MM, Lewis EJ. Minimal-change glomerulopathy of adulthood. Am J Nephrol 1988;8:291–7.
16. Koyama A, Fujisaki M, Kobayashi M, Igarashi M, Navita M. A glomerular permeability factor produced by human T cell hybridomas. Kidney Int 1991;40:453–60.
17. Lowenstein J, Schacht RG, Baldwin DS. Renal failure in minimal change nephrotic syndrome. Am J Med 1981;70:227–33.
18. Munk F. Klinische diagnostik der degenerativen Nierenerkrankungen. Z Klin Med 1913;78:1–52.
19. Musante L, Candiano G, Zennaro C, et al. Humoral permeability factors in the nephrotic syndrome: a compendium and prospectus. J Nephrol 2001;14(Suppl 4):S48–50.
20. Nolasco F, Cameron JS, Heywood EF, Hicks J, Ogg C, Williams DG. Adult-onset minimal change nephrotic syndrome: a long-term follow-up. Kidney Int 1986;29:1215–23.
21. Pirani CL, Valeri A, D'Agati V, Appel GB. Renal toxicity of nonsteroidal anti-inflammatory drugs. Contrib Nephrol 1987;55:159–75.
22. Primary nephrotic syndrome in children: clinical significance of histopathologic variants of minimal change and of diffuse mesangial hypercellularity. A report of the International Study of Kidney Disease in Children. Kidney Int 1981;20:765–71.
23. Savin VJ. Mechanisms of proteinuria in noninflammatory glomerular diseases. Am J Kidney Dis 1993;21:347–62.
24. Shaknovitch R, Francois DJ, Cattoretti G, D'Agati VD, Markowitz GS. A rare cause of nephrotic syndrome. Am J Kidney Dis 2002;39:892–5.
25. Tejani A, Nicastri AD. Mesangial IgM nephropathy. Nephron 1983;35:1–5.
26. White RH, Glasgow EF, Mills RJ. Clinicopathologic study of nephrotic syndrome in childhood. Lancet 1970;1:1353–9.
27. Zeis PM, Kavazarakis E, Nakopoulou L, et al. Glomerulopathy with mesangial IgM deposits: long-term follow up of 64 children. Pediatr Int 2001;43:287–92.

6 FOCAL SEGMENTAL GLOMERULOSCLEROSIS

Focal segmental glomerulosclerosis (FSGS) is a clinical-pathologic syndrome of proteinuria, usually of nephrotic range, associated with lesions of focal and segmental glomerular sclerosis and foot process effacement, without glomerular immune complex deposits (8,9,11). Early in the disease process, the pattern of glomerular sclerosis is focal, involving a subset of glomeruli, and segmental, involving a portion of the glomerular tuft. As the disease progresses, a more diffuse and global pattern of sclerosis evolves. Alterations of the podocyte cytoarchitecture are the major ultrastructural findings.

The approach to a diagnosis of FSGS is problematic because the morphologic features are nonspecific and can occur in a variety of other conditions or superimposed on other glomerular processes (9,11,42). In addition, because the defining glomerular lesion is focal, it may not be adequately sampled in small needle biopsies.

The diagnosis of FSGS is further complicated by the existence of a primary (or idiopathic) form and many secondary forms (Table 6-1) (8,9,11, 42). Before a diagnosis of primary FSGS can be reached, secondary forms must be carefully excluded. Primary FSGS must be distinguished from familial FSGS, human immunodeficiency virus (HIV)-associated nephropathy, and heroin nephropathy, as well as the large group of secondary FSGS caused by structural-functional adaptations mediated by intrarenal vasodilatation and by increased glomerular capillary pressures and plasma flow rates (42). Such maladaptive glomerular hemodynamic alterations can arise through: 1) a reduction in the number of functioning nephrons (such as following unilateral renal agenesis, surgical ablation, oligomeganephronia, or any advanced primary renal disease) or 2) mechanisms that place hemodynamic stress on an initially normal nephron population (as in morbid obesity, cyanotic congenital heart disease, and sickle cell anemia). Finally, primary and secondary FSGS must also be differentiated from the nonspecific pattern of focal and segmental glomerular scarring that can follow a variety of inflammatory, proliferative, thrombotic, and hereditary conditions.

Table 6-1

ETIOLOGIC CLASSIFICATION OF FOCAL SEGMENTAL GLOMERULOSCLEROSIS (FSGS)

1. Primary (Idiopathic) FSGS
2. Human Immunodeficiency Virus (HIV)-Associated Nephropathy
3. Heroin Nephropathy
4. Familial FSGS
   - Mutations in alpha-actinin-4 (autosomal dominant)
   - Mutations in podocin (autosomal recessive)
5. Drug Toxicity
   - Pamidronate
   - Lithium
   - Interferon
6. Secondary FSGS Mediated by Adaptive Structural-Functional Responses
   - Reduced renal mass
     - Oligomeganephronia
     - Unilateral renal agenesis
     - Renal dysplasia
     - Reflux nephropathy
     - Sequela to cortical necrosis
     - Surgical renal ablation
     - Any advanced renal disease with reduction in functioning nephrons
     - Chronic allograft nephropathy
   - Initially normal renal mass
     - Diabetes mellitus
     - Hypertension
     - Obesity
     - Cyanotic congenital heart disease
     - Sickle cell disease

Primary FSGS comprises a number of morphologic subtypes that have different prognostic and therapeutic implications (11). These morphologic variants are listed in Table 6-2. Primary FSGS, not otherwise specified (NOS), must be distinguished from the cellular variant, FSGS with diffuse mesangial hypercellularity, the collapsing variant, glomerular tip lesion, and C1q nephropathy. The pathologic features and

Table 6-2

MORPHOLOGIC VARIANTS OF PRIMARY (IDIOPATHIC) FOCAL SEGMENTAL GLOMERULOSCLEROSIS (FSGS)

FSGS, Not Otherwise Specified (Classic FSGS)
FSGS, Cellular Variant
FSGS with Diffuse Mesangial Hypercellularity
FSGS, Collapsing Variant
Glomerular Tip Lesion
C1q Nephropathy

clinical significance of each of these morphologic variants is discussed.

PRIMARY FSGS NOT OTHERWISE SPECIFIED (CLASSIC FSGS)

Definition. Primary FSGS, not otherwise specified (NOS), is a form of idiopathic nephrotic syndrome characterized by focal and segmental consolidation of the glomerular tuft by increased extracellular matrix, obliterating the capillary lumens. Synonyms include *classic FSGS* or *FSGS of the usual type*.

Clinical Features. In both children and adults, primary FSGS is slightly more common in males than females. It comprises 10 to 20 percent of the cases of idiopathic nephrotic syndrome in children. The incidence is higher in black than white children (26). In adults, several studies from New York and Chicago have suggested that the incidence of primary FSGS has increased over the past two decades (1,19, 20). From 1988 to 1993, the incidence of primary FSGS (8.8 percent of native kidney biopsies) actually superceded the incidence of membranous glomerulopathy (7.0 percent) at Columbia Presbyterian Medical Center (1). In some urban centers, FSGS is now the most common cause of idiopathic nephrotic syndrome in black adults (56 percent) and accounts for 25 percent of nephrotic syndrome in white adults (19,20). The reasons for these changing incidences likely reflect changing epidemiologic trends. Thus FSGS is becoming an increasingly prevalent and important disease, especially in the black population.

The major presenting clinical feature of primary FSGS is proteinuria, usually in the nephrotic range (defined as more than 3.5 g/day). This is often accompanied by full nephrotic syndrome (hypoalbuminemia, hypercholesterolemia, and edema). Subnephrotic proteinuria is not uncommon, however, especially in adults. Children with primary FSGS are more likely to present with full nephrotic syndrome (58). The incidence of nephrotic proteinuria is 90 percent in children and 70 percent in adults (32,58). Renal insufficiency is present at diagnosis in about 20 percent of children and 30 percent of adults; hypertension is identified in approximately 30 percent of children and 45 percent of adults; and microhematuria affects approximately 55 percent of children and 45 percent of adults with the disease (32).

Light Microscopic Findings. The classic lesion of primary FSGS is a discrete segmental solidification of the glomerular tuft (figs. 6-1–6-3). Early in the disease, the segmental lesions have a predilection for the juxtamedullary glomeruli (43). Lesions may involve the perihilar region or vascular pole (figs. 6-4, 6-5) or the periphery of the tuft (fig. 6-6). In some glomeruli, segmental lesions affect more than one lobule, involving both the perihilar and peripheral regions. According to one study using serial sections, peripheral lesions are more common in children than adults with FSGS (17).

Glomerular capillaries are segmentally occluded by relatively acellular matrix material, often associated with inframembranous hyalinosis, endocapillary foam cells, and wrinkling of the glomerular basement membrane (11,22). Hyalinosis, also known as plasmatic insudation, is the accumulation beneath the glomerular basement membrane of amorphous glassy material that is eosinophilic, periodic acid–Schiff (PAS) positive, nonargyrophilic, and trichrome red (fig. 6-7). Clear lipid vacuoles may be included in the hyaline material. There is often a continuity between the glomerular hyalinosis and the hyalinosis involving the contiguous afferent arteriole.

Adhesions or synechiae to Bowman's capsule are common (fig. 6-8). The overlying visceral epithelial cells often appear swollen and form a cellular "cap" over the sclerosing segment (fig. 6-9). Detachment of podocytes from the sclerosing segment, with the intervening accumulation of newly formed matrix material, may

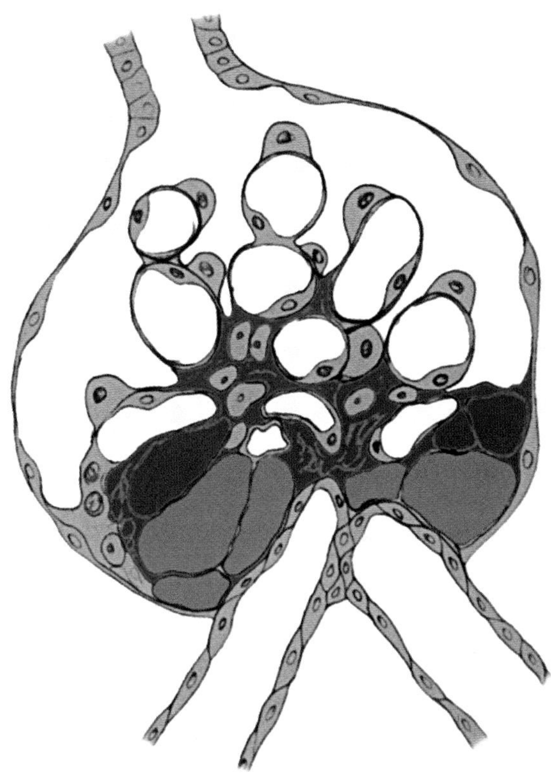

Figure 6-1

PRIMARY FOCAL SEGMENTAL GLOMERULOSCLEROSIS (FSGS) (NOS)

Illustration of the classic lesion of FSGS shows solidification of the segment of the glomerulus at the vascular pole by increased matrix (shown in blue) and hyalinosis (in orange).

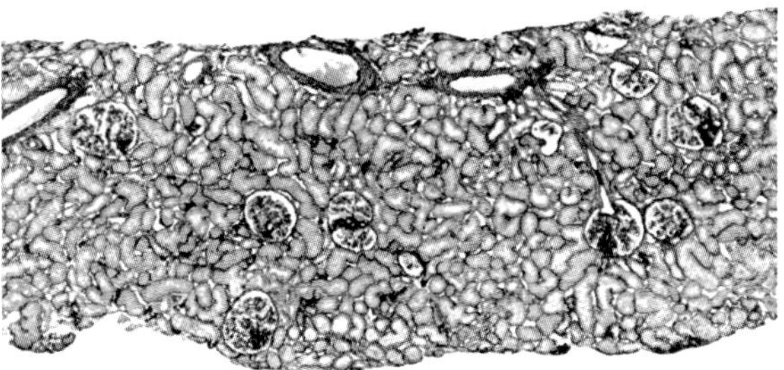

Figure 6-2

PRIMARY FSGS (NOS)

Low-power microscopic view shows segmental sclerosis involving many glomeruli. Uninvolved glomeruli appear histologically normal (Jones methenamine silver [JMS] stain).

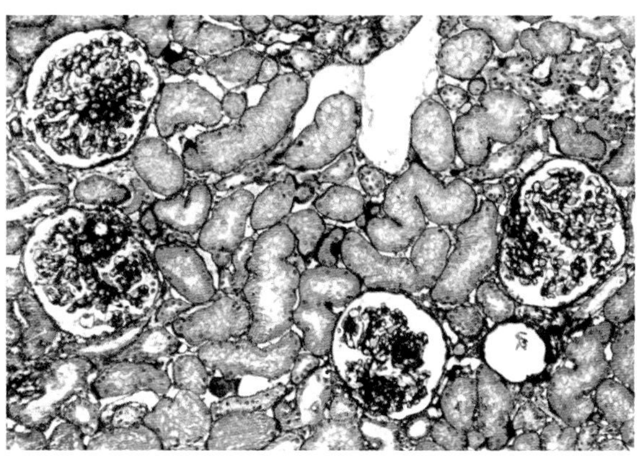

Figure 6-3

PRIMARY FSGS (NOS)

Lesions of segmental sclerosis are discrete, involving a portion of the tuft. The tubulointerstitial compartment is well preserved (JMS stain).

produce an apparent "halo" of weakly PAS-positive or weakly trichrome blue–positive matrix between the sclerosed segment and the detached visceral epithelial cells (fig. 6-9).

The number of glomeruli affected by segmental lesions depends on the severity of the disease process and the number of serial sections examined. As the lesions evolve globally, there is progression to complete glomerular obsolescence (fig. 6-10). Lobules unaffected by the segmental sclerosis usually appear normal by light microscopy but for mild swelling of the podocytes.

Typically, there is patchy tubular atrophy and interstitial fibrosis commensurate with the severity and distribution of the glomerular sclerosis (fig. 6-11). Proximal tubules frequently contain intracellular lipid and protein resorption droplets (fig. 6-12). The intracytoplasmic lipid vacuoles appear clear in hematoxylin and eosin (H&E)–stained sections. Protein resorption droplets are PAS positive and stain either orange or blue with the trichrome stain. In some cases, interstitial foam cells are identified, either as isolated cells or in aggregates (fig. 6-13).

In some cases, the tubulointerstitial damage is disproportionately severe relative to the degree of glomerular sclerosis (fig. 6-14). In such cases, the tubules may display degenerative and regenerative changes, including epithelial

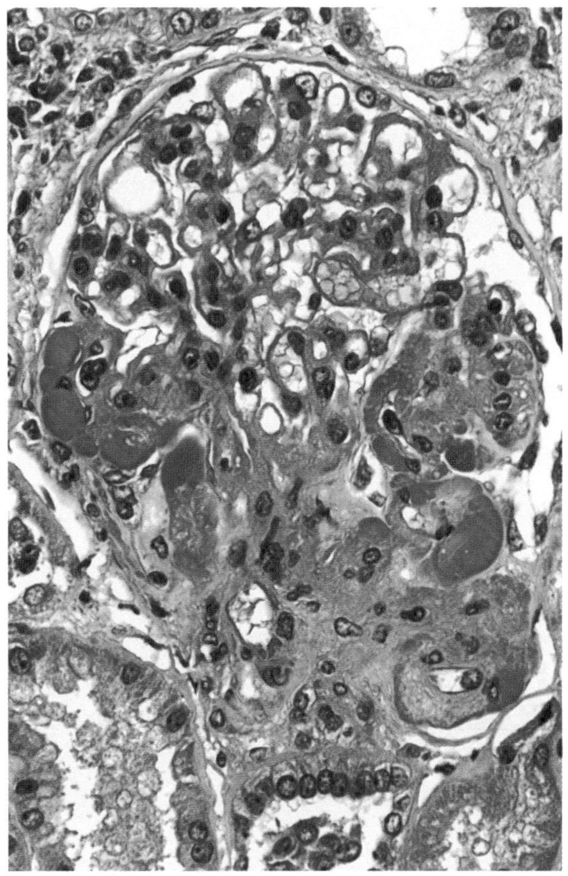

Figure 6-4

PRIMARY FSGS (NOS)

The perihilar segment is obliterated by increased matrix and hyalinosis (hematoxylin and eosin [H&E] stain).

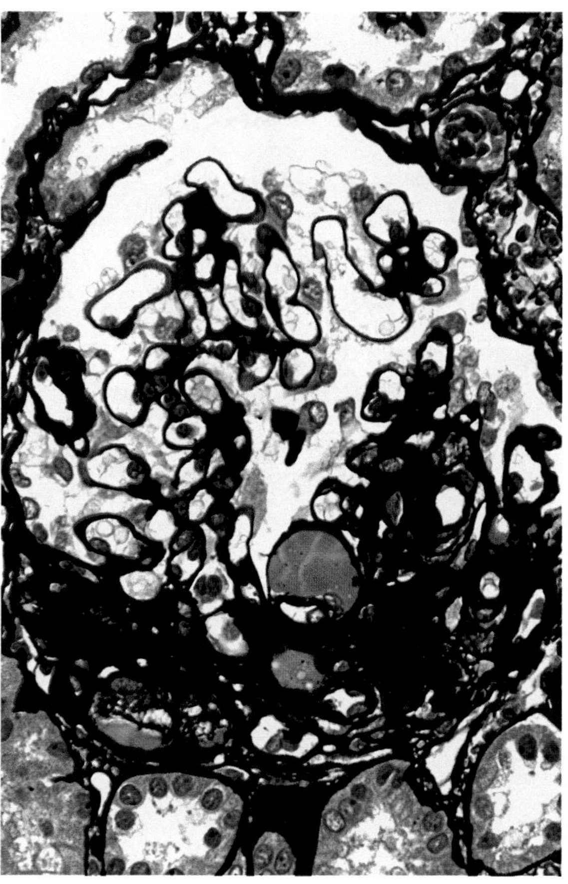

Figure 6-5

PRIMARY FSGS (NOS)

The JMS stain differentiates the argyrophilic matrix from the pink hyaline in the segmental lesions.

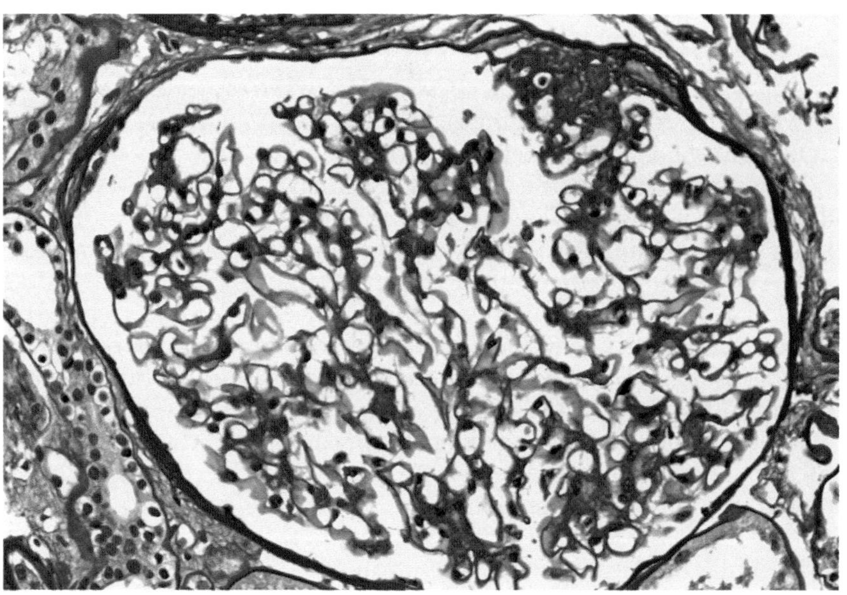

Figure 6-6

FSGS (NOS)

An example with segmental sclerosis involving a peripheral segment, associated with adhesion to Bowman's capsule (periodic acid–Schiff [PAS] stain).

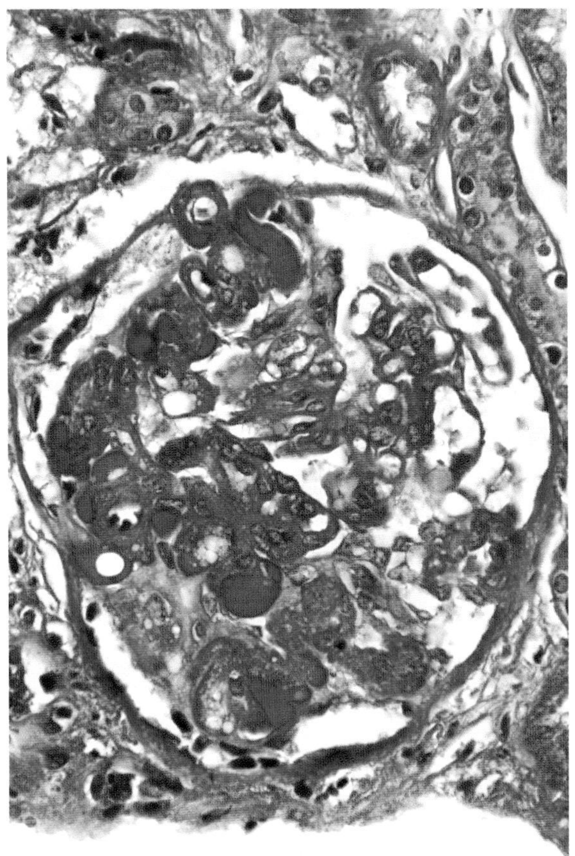

Figure 6-7

PRIMARY FSGS (NOS)

The trichrome stain differentiates the blue-staining matrix from the red-orange hyaline in the segmental lesions.

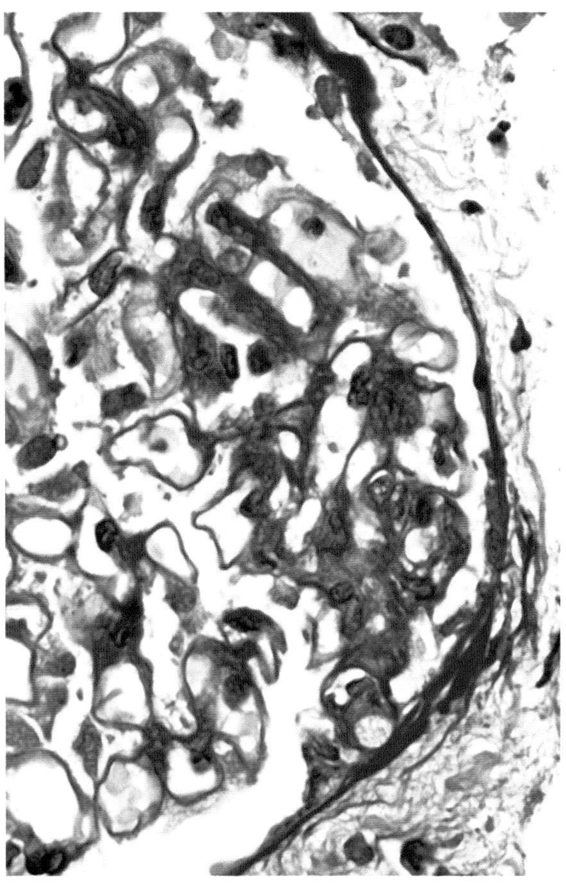

Figure 6-8

PRIMARY FSGS (NOS)

A minute segmental lesion forms a small synechia to Bowman's capsule (PAS stain).

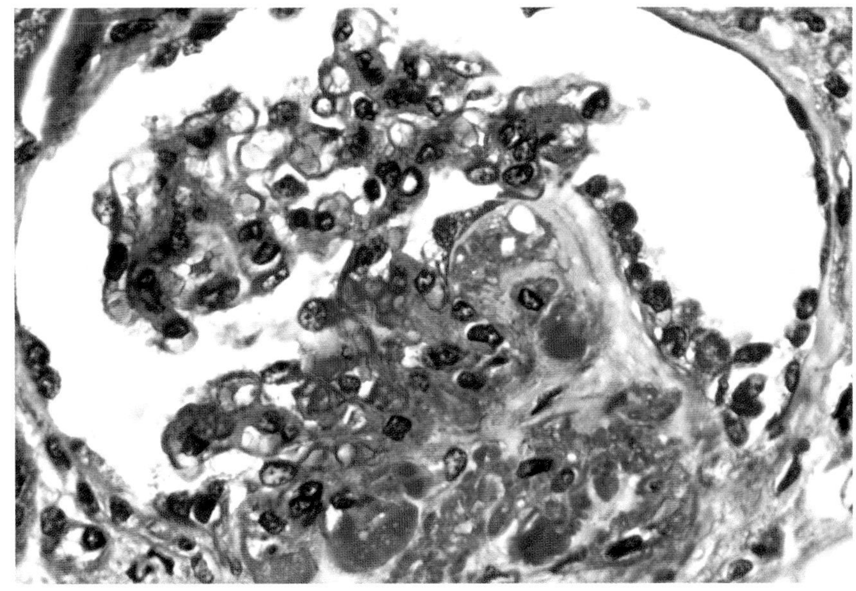

Figure 6-9

PRIMARY FSGS (NOS)

The segmental lesion is surrounded by a halo caused by the deposition of loose matrix overlying a focus of visceral epithelial cell detachment and capping (Masson trichrome stain).

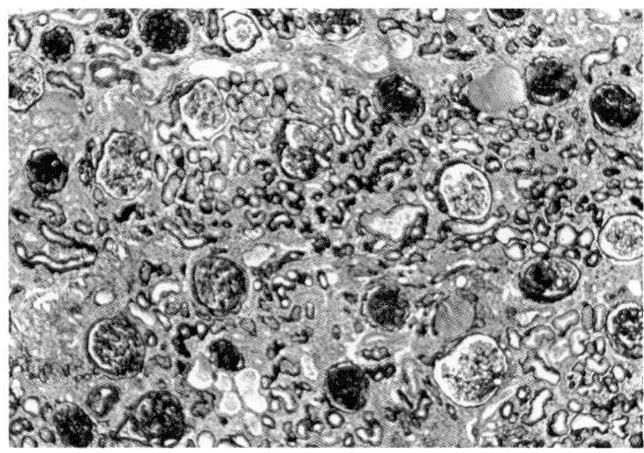

Figure 6-10

PRIMARY FSGS (NOS)

Advanced disease with progression to extensive global sclerosis, diffuse tubular atrophy, and interstitial fibrosis (JMS stain).

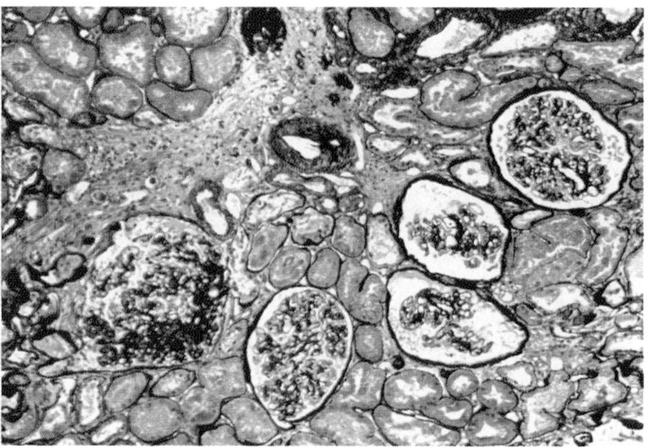

Figure 6-11

FSGS (NOS)

There is patchy tubulointerstitial disease in the distribution of the glomerulosclerosis (JMS stain).

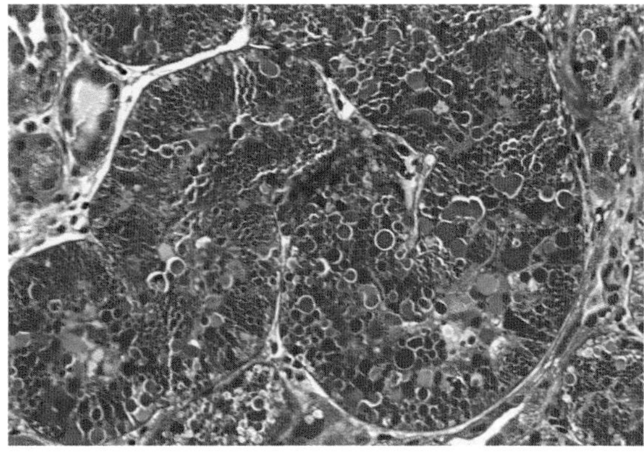

Figure 6-12

PRIMARY FSGS (NOS)

The tubules are engorged with numerous intracytoplasmic protein resorption droplets, which stain orange-red and blue with the Masson trichrome stain.

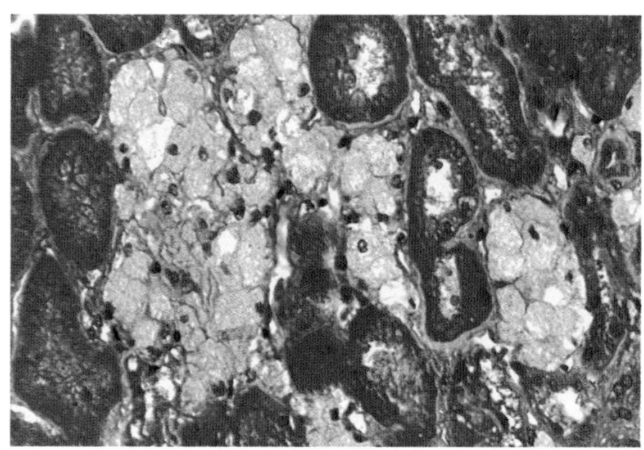

Figure 6-13

PRIMARY FSGS (NOS)

The patient had longstanding proteinuria of several years' duration. Numerous interstitial foam cells contain abundant lipid and appear clear with the trichrome stain.

simplification and enlarged hyperchromatic nuclei and nucleoli. Such damage tends to be more common in patients with severe unremitting nephrotic syndrome.

Immunofluorescence Findings. There is, typically, focal and segmental granular deposition of immunoglobulin (Ig)M, complement (C)3, and more variably, C1, in the distribution of the segmental glomerular sclerosis and hyalinosis (fig. 6-15). Not all glomeruli with segmental sclerosis contain these deposits. More generalized, weaker (less than 2+) mesangial deposition of IgM is also present in some cases.

Staining for albumin and some immunoglobulins (particularly IgA, as well as IgG) may be found within the podocytes, corresponding to intracytoplasmic protein resorption droplets (fig. 6-16). This intracellular staining should be distinguished from immune deposits within the glomerular tuft itself. Similarly, intracytoplasmic deposits of albumin, immunoglobulins, and sometimes C3 may be found involving proximal tubules that are engaged in active protein resorption (figs. 6-17, 6-18).

Electron Microscopic Findings. The lesions of segmental sclerosis cause wrinkling and

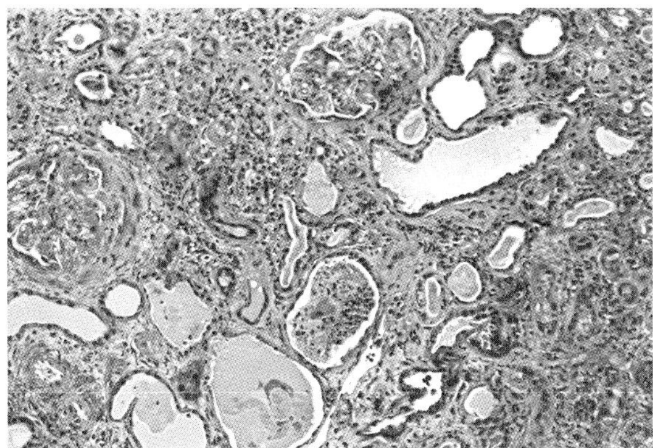

Figure 6-14

PRIMARY FSGS (NOS)

The severe tubulointerstitial disease is out of proportion to the degree of glomerulosclerosis. This disproportionate tubular damage is most often encountered in patients with severe unremitting nephrotic syndrome (Masson trichrome stain).

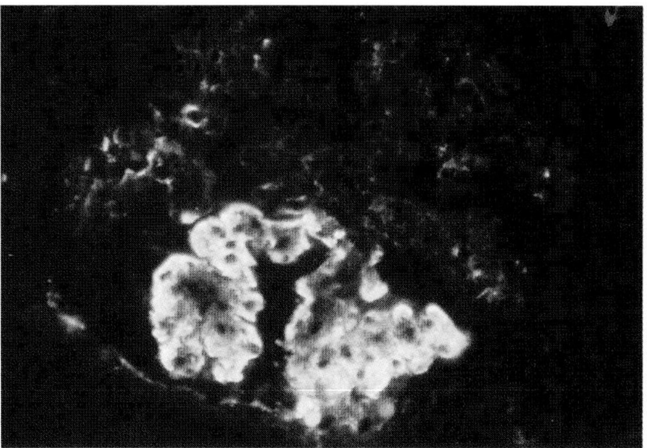

Figure 6-15

PRIMARY FSGS (NOS)

By immunofluorescence, there is segmental staining for IgM corresponding to a segmental lesion of sclerosis and hyalinosis.

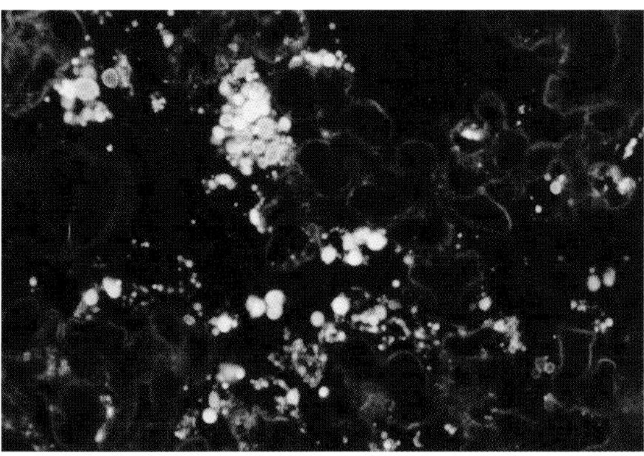

Figure 6-16

PRIMARY FSGS (NOS)

Protein resorption droplets within the podocytes stain with antisera to albumin (immunofluorescence micrograph).

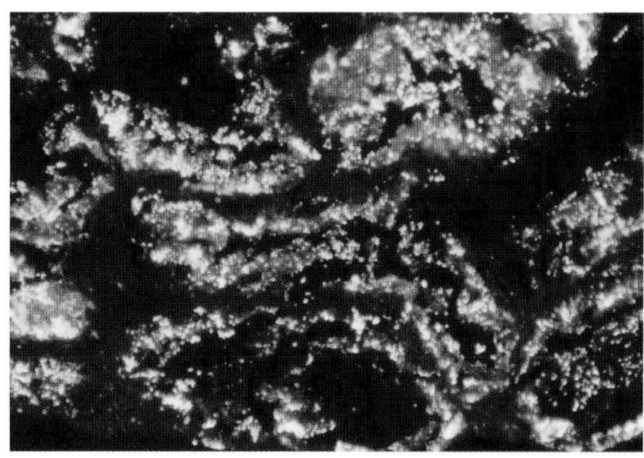

Figure 6-17

PRIMARY FSGS (NOS)

There is strong staining for albumin in the distribution of tubular protein resorption droplets (immunofluorescence micrograph).

retraction of the glomerular basement membrane and accumulation of inframembranous hyaline, with resulting narrowing or occlusion of the glomerular capillary lumens (fig. 6-19). The electron-dense hyaline material is usually more waxy in appearance than true immune complex deposits, and tends to pool beneath the glomerular basement membrane, conforming to the contours of the delimiting membrane. Hyaline deposits frequently contain curvilinear membranous particles or entrapped electron-lucent lipid globules. Endocapillary foam cells appear as large intracapillary cells containing abundant electron-lucent vacuoles (fig. 6-20).

Directly overlying the lesions of segmental sclerosis, there is usually complete effacement of foot processes, accompanied by podocyte alterations that include hypertrophy, increased organellar content, and focal microvillous transformation. The latter is due to the formation of slender cellular projections resembling villi along the surface of the podocytes facing the urinary space. The hypertrophied podocytes have rounded cell bodies that adhere smoothly

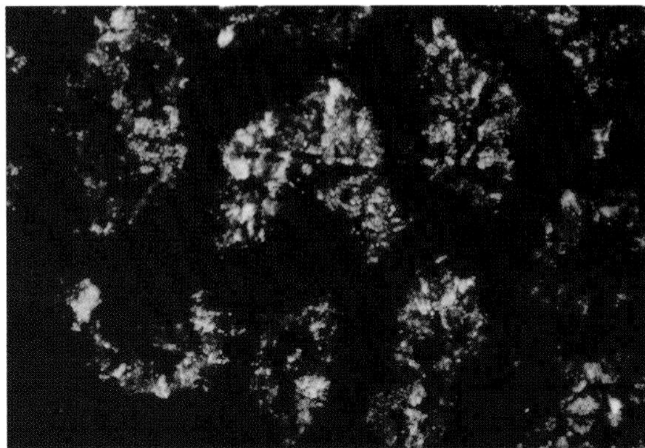

Figure 6-18

PRIMARY FSGS (NOS)

Staining for C3 is observed in areas of active protein resorption in the proximal tubular epithelial cells (immunofluorescence micrograph).

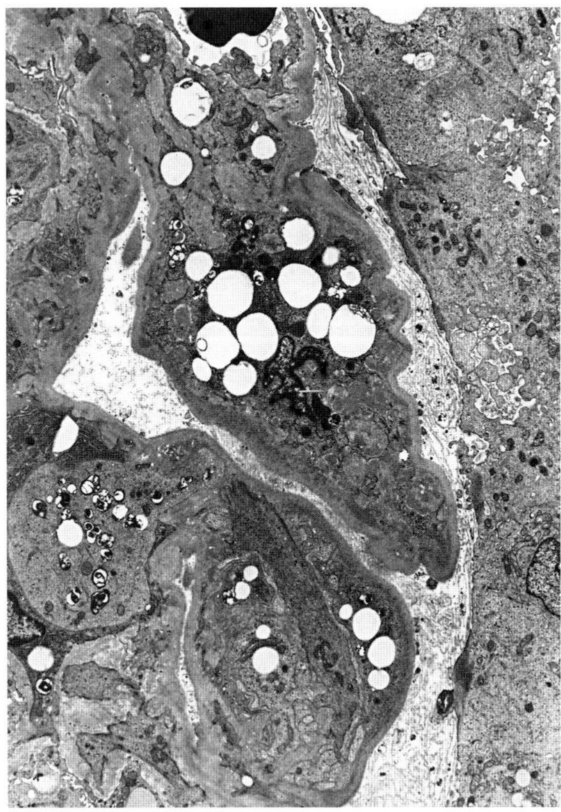

Figure 6-19

PRIMARY FSGS (NOS)

In the segmental area of sclerosis, there is solidification of the tuft by matrix, inframembranous hyaline, and endocapillary foam cells. The overlying foot processes are effaced and detached from the tuft, with intervening, loosely woven basement membrane material (electron micrograph).

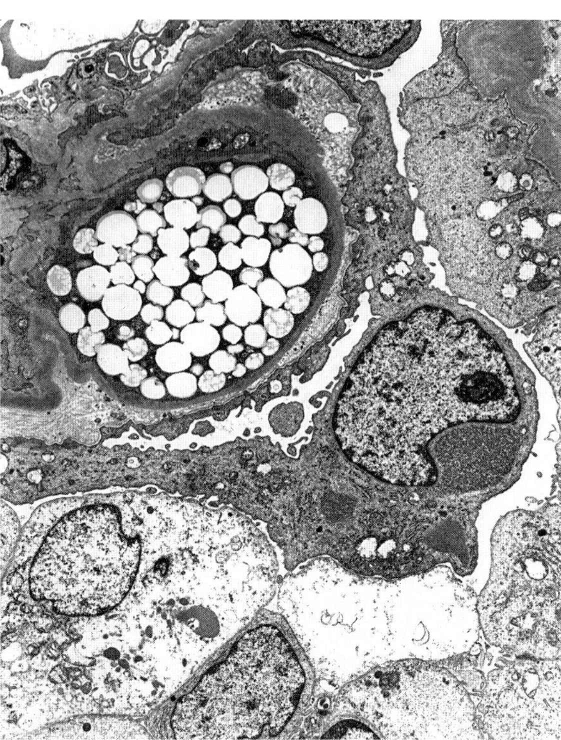

Figure 6-20

PRIMARY FSGS (NOS)

A lesion of segmental sclerosis with a prominent endocapillary foam cell shows detachment of the overlying podocytes, which are markedly hypertrophied (electron micrograph).

to the glomerular basement membrane, with frequent loss of primary processes.

In many cases, podocytes detach from the sclerosing segment. In these areas, an intervening accumulation of lamellated neomembrane material is commonly observed between the naked glomerular basement membrane and the retracted podocyte cell body (fig. 6-21). These foci of detachment correspond to the halos observed by light microscopy surrounding the sclerosing segments.

Synechiae between the sclerosed segment and Bowman's capsule are usually composed of loosely woven basement membrane material. They are lined by a continuous layer of parietal and visceral epithelial cells.

Adjacent nonsclerotic glomerular capillaries are usually remarkable only for foot process effacement (fig. 6-22). The degree of effacement observed overlying these open capillaries var-

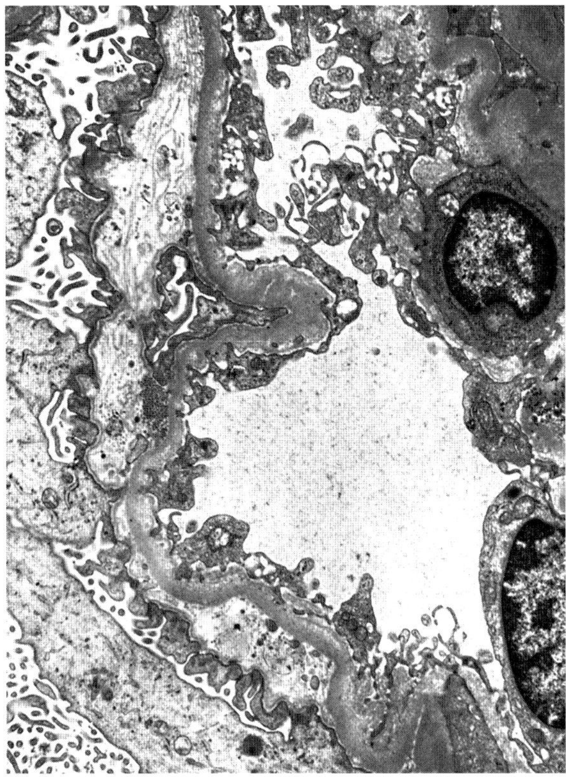

Figure 6-21

PRIMARY FSGS (NOS)

Podocyte detachment and basement membrane lamellation overlie nonsclerotic capillaries (electron micrograph).

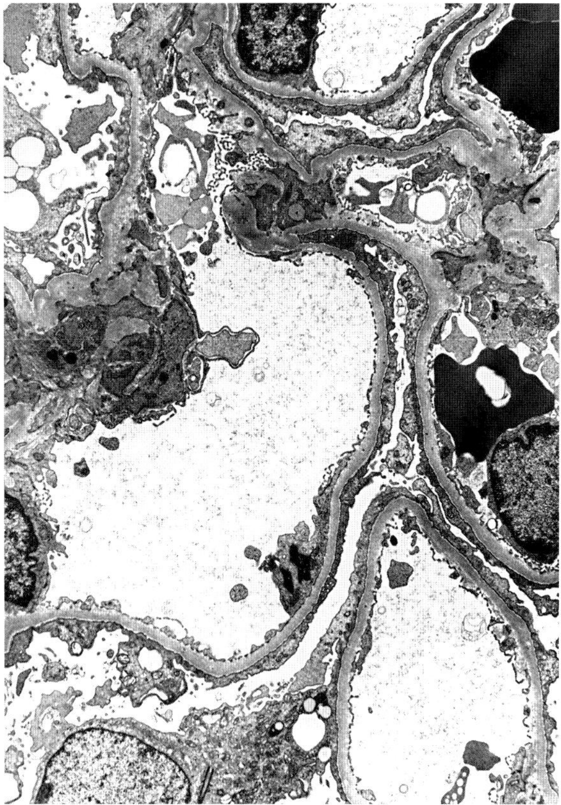

Figure 6-22

PRIMARY FSGS (NOS)

Nonsclerotic capillaries display marked foot process effacement, resembling that seen in minimal change disease. No electron-dense deposits are identified (electron micrograph).

ies from mild to severe. On average, greater than 50 percent of the total glomerular capillary surface area exhibits foot process effacement. The degree of effacement correlates roughly with the severity of the proteinuria, so that patients with subnephrotic proteinuria tend to have less foot process effacement than those who are fully nephrotic. In the effaced areas, there is usually loss of recognizable slit diaphragms and mat-like condensations of cytoskeletal filaments oriented parallel to the direction of the glomerular basement membrane. Thus, although the lesions of FSGS are focal at the light microscopic level, the podocyte alterations are relatively diffuse at the electron microscopic level.

Differential Diagnosis. Primary FSGS must be distinguished from minimal change disease (MCD). This differentiation is a common problem because being focal, the sclerosis may not be sampled in a small biopsy. Moreover, the nonsclerotic glomeruli in FSGS are indistinguishable from those of MCD, often manifesting extensive foot process effacement in the absence of other glomerular alterations. This is a particular problem in small biopsies that do not contain the corticomedullary junction, where the earliest lesions of segmental sclerosis arise.

The possibility of unsampled FSGS should be suspected if there is patchy tubulointerstitial disease (i.e., tubular atrophy and interstitial fibrosis) in a biopsy that looks otherwise like MCD, particularly in the absence of hypertensive vascular disease. In such cases, more extensive serial sectioning of the paraffin block may reveal the diagnostic segmental lesions. If immunofluorescence reveals segmental glomerular staining for IgM and C3 in a manner corresponding to a possible lesion of segmental sclerosis, reprocessing the cryostat sections for light microscopy may be rewarding. Similarly, the plastic-embedded tissue for electron microscopy may contain diagnostic lesions when the formalin-fixed tissue does not.

The finding of global glomerulosclerosis alone is not helpful in differentiating between MCD and FSGS. Global glomerulosclerosis may occur at any age and typically increases with age in otherwise normal kidneys or in those with the aging changes of arterionephrosclerosis. Even in infants, rare obsolescent glomeruli may be detected. Up to 10 percent of globally sclerotic glomeruli may be found by the age of 40 years, increasing to 30 percent by the age of 80 years. Smith (49) has suggested a formula for calculating the percentage of sclerotic glomeruli acceptable for age by halving the patient's age (in years) and subtracting ten.

Primary FSGS is distinguished from secondary FSGS by careful clinical-pathologic correlation. A detailed clinical history is essential to exclude the underlying renal conditions listed in Table 6-1. It is important to determine whether full nephrotic syndrome is present, because secondary FSGS caused by structural-functional adaptations usually lacks hypoalbuminemia.

Primary FSGS also must be distinguished from the nonspecific pattern of glomerular scarring that follows acute inflammatory glomerulonephritis. It is not uncommon for focal segmental and global glomerular sclerosis to supervene on chronic lupus nephritis, acute postinfectious glomerulonephritis, IgA nephropathy, or membranous glomerulonephritis. In such cases, immunofluorescence and electron microscopy usually reveal evidence of residual immune complex deposits in glomeruli with less advanced sclerosis; the proper diagnosis requires careful integration of the composition and distribution of the immune deposits as assessed by these techniques.

Pauci-immune focal segmental necrotizing and crescentic glomerulonephritis can be mistaken for primary FSGS if it is biopsied in the chronic scarred phase, especially because this condition lacks immune deposits. The findings of focal rupture of Bowman's capsule and subcapsular fibrous proliferations, best seen with the PAS or Jones methenamine silver (JMS) stain, are helpful in distinguishing scarred foci of previous necrotizing and crescentic glomerulonephritis from the synechiae of FSGS.

A pattern of segmental glomerulosclerosis may also develop in the course of a variety of hereditary conditions, including hereditary nephritis (Alport's syndrome), Fabry's disease, mitochondriopathies, and others. Because immunofluorescence is negative for immune deposits, electron microscopy is particularly important to differentiate these conditions from primary FSGS.

Etiology and Pathogenesis. The etiology of primary FSGS is unknown. In recent years, theories of the pathogenesis have focused on the podocyte (2). Direct podocyte damage caused by toxins such as puromycin and adriamycin is the basis of experimental models of FSGS. These substances injure the podocyte cytoskeleton, possibly through generation of reactive oxygen species. Lesions resembling MCD and FSGS can be produced experimentally using highly cationic compounds that neutralize the negative charges on the podocyte glycocalyx and by antibodies directed to podocyte membrane proteins or to alpha 3/beta 1 integrins that mediate attachment to the glomerular basement membrane. Analogous podocyte toxins or permeability factors have been proposed in human FSGS and steroid-resistant MCD, suggesting a relatedness of these entities (44). The identity of these permeability factors and their precise pathomechanism of podocyte injury remain to be elucidated.

In human FSGS, particularly the collapsing variant, the podocyte displays a dysregulated phenotype, with increased rates of proliferation and apoptosis (2). There is loss of mature podocyte markers (such as synaptopodin, podocalyxin, Wilms' tumor-1 protein [WT1], glomerular epithelial protein-1 [GLEPP1], C3b receptor, and common acute lymphoblastic leukemia antigen [CALLA]) (2). The podocytes also display altered expression of cyclin kinase inhibitors, with reduced p27 and p57, consistent with their role in permissive cellular proliferation (48). Podocytes lose their highly differentiated cytoarchitecture, probably through cellular activation of a genetic program that involves reentry into the cell cycle, disruption of the cytoskeleton, and cellular dedifferentiation.

In recent years, the existence of familial forms of FSGS with either autosomal dominant or autosomal recessive inheritance has been recognized. Although these familial forms were at one time considered idiopathic, they are now recognized as secondary forms of FSGS due to genetic mutations in podocyte-associated proteins. Autosomal dominant forms usually present in adulthood and are uniformly steroid resistant. The responsible gene has been mapped to chromosome 19q13 and encodes alpha-actinin-4, a cytoskeletal protein expressed in the podocyte (30,38). Autosomal recessive forms present in early childhood, are steroid resistant, and tend to progress rapidly to renal failure. The responsible gene has been mapped to chromosome 1q25 and encodes a novel podocyte protein, podocin (4). Mutations in podocin also have been identified in some spontaneous (nonfamilial) forms of steroid-resistant FSGS (56). Another podocyte-specific component of the slit diaphragm, nephrin, is known to be mutated in congenital nephrotic syndrome of the Finnish type (31). These recent advances point to the importance of integral podocyte proteins in the maintenance of the normal foot process architecture.

Unremitting proteinuria itself is also thought to play a role in progressive tubulointerstitial damage in FSGS. Evidence from human and animal studies indicates that increased protein trafficking through the tubular reabsorption of filtered protein promotes progressive tubulointerstitial damage (14,15). Protein overload of tubular cells leads to increased tubular expression of chemokines, such as monocyte chemoattractant protein-1 and osteopontin, which attract inflammatory cells to the interstitium. Enhanced secretion of tubular endothelin-1 may also promote interstitial macrophage infiltration and fibroblast proliferation (14). Infiltrating interstitial leukocytes in turn elaborate fibrogenic cytokines that eventuate in progressive interstitial fibrosis.

Treatment and Prognosis. The mainstay of treatment for primary FSGS is a prolonged course (3 to 9 months) of steroid therapy (40). Steroid-resistant patients are offered alternative therapy in the form of cyclophosphamide, cyclosporine, or newer immunosuppressive agents. Long-term cyclosporine therapy runs the risk of promoting chronic tubulointerstitial and vascular disease due to the nephrotoxicity of this agent. Angiotensin converting enzyme (ACE) inhibition or angiotensin II receptor antagonists are often given as adjuncts to reduce proteinuria and resulting tubular injury. ACE inhibition alone has been used as an alternative to steroid therapy in patients with subnephrotic proteinuria.

The most prognostically significant clinical features of FSGS are the level of serum creatinine and the severity of proteinuria at presentation (32). The presence of nephrotic proteinuria (more than 3.5 g/day) is associated with a worse outcome in patients with primary FSGS, with mean time to end-stage renal failure of 6 to 8 years (32). This is compared to an over 80 percent 10-year survival rate for patients with non-nephrotic proteinuria. Not surprisingly, severe proteinuria of over 10 g/day is associated with an even more rapid course to renal failure (less than 3 years). The prognosis is much better in those who undergo a remission of nephrotic syndrome than those with persistent nephrotic syndrome. Outcome is generally worse in blacks than whites. The best pathologic predictor of poor outcome is the degree of interstitial fibrosis. Interestingly, the percentage of glomeruli with segmental scars or global sclerosis has not been found to be independently predictive of outcome.

Primary FSGS recurs in the renal allograft in approximately 30 to 40 percent of patients. In the early stages of recurrence, the glomerular lesions resemble those of MCD, followed by the progressive development of segmental sclerosis. Recurrences may respond to plasmapheresis, presumably through the elimination of a circulating permeability factor.

PRIMARY FSGS, CELLULAR VARIANT

Definition. The cellular variant of primary FSGS is a histologic subtype characterized by focal and segmental endocapillary hypercellularity occluding lumens, typically with foam cells and karyorrhexis, often associated with podocyte hypertrophy and hyperplasia (11). The percentage of glomeruli with cellular lesions in a biopsy specimen is variable. Cellular lesions may coexist with other glomeruli that have classic lesions of sclerosis.

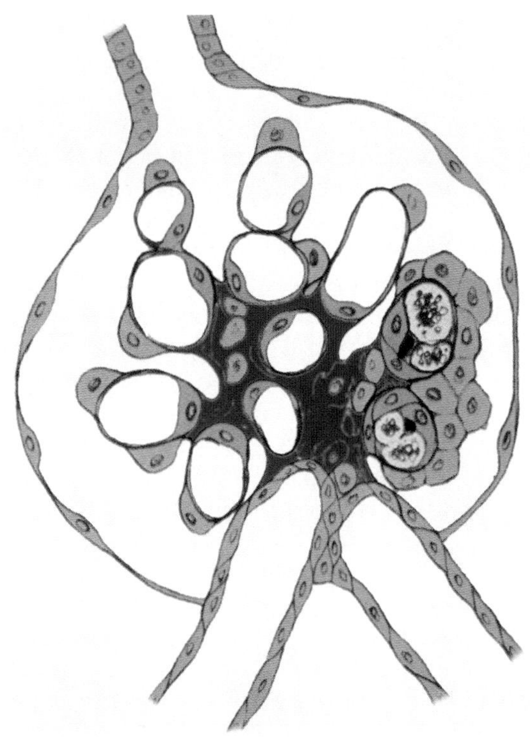

Figure 6-23

PRIMARY FSGS, CELLULAR VARIANT

An illustration shows segmental expansion of the tuft by endocapillary cells, including foam cells, with podocyte hyperplasia.

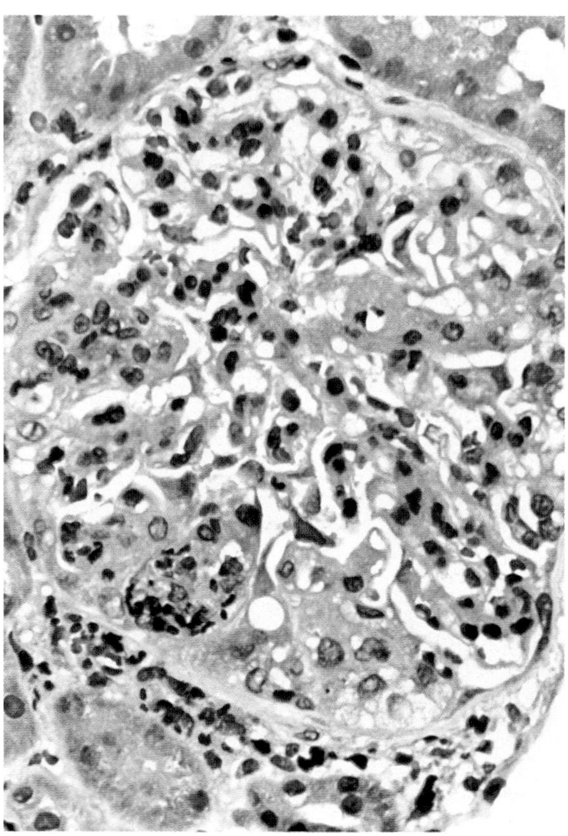

Figure 6-24

PRIMARY FSGS, CELLULAR VARIANT

An example with segmental infiltration of the tuft by leukocytes with karyorrhexis, resembling focal segmental proliferative glomerulonephritis. There is hypertrophy of the overlying podocytes (H&E stain).

Clinical Features. Compared to primary FSGS (NOS), the cellular variant is characterized by more severe proteinuria and a shorter course from clinical onset of renal disease to biopsy, suggesting an early phase in the evolution of the segmental sclerosis (47). Indeed, some of these patients have a very abrupt onset of severe nephrotic syndrome, resembling the presentation of MCD. Repeat biopsies in some cases have shown evolution to more typical segmental scars, supporting the concept that the hypercellularity is an early stage in the development of the segmental lesions. A similar evolution from cellular to more sclerosing lesions has been documented by repeat biopsy of recurrent FSGS in the transplant.

Light Microscopic Findings. The cellular variant of primary FSGS, first described by Schwartz and Lewis in 1985 (47), has focal and segmental glomerular hypercellularity that resembles a form of focal proliferative glomerulonephritis. The increased numbers of endocapillary cells include endothelial cells, foam cells, and infiltrating leukocytes, including monocytes and occasional neutrophils, often producing an expansile lesion (figs. 6-23–6-28). Some lesions are accompanied by foamy hyaline material, fibrin, and karyorrhexis, resembling segmental necrotizing lesions but without rupture of the glomerular basement membrane (fig. 6-28).

Many cases also have extracapillary hypercellularity due to hyperplasia of the podocytes. Podocytes may appear swollen and crowded, sometimes forming "pseudocrescents" (fig. 6-29). These pseudocrescents can usually be distinguished from true crescents by their lack of attachment to Bowman's capsule or continuity with the parietal epithelial cells. Moreover, the extracapillary cells tend to be plump, rounded, and poorly cohesive, with frequent intracellular

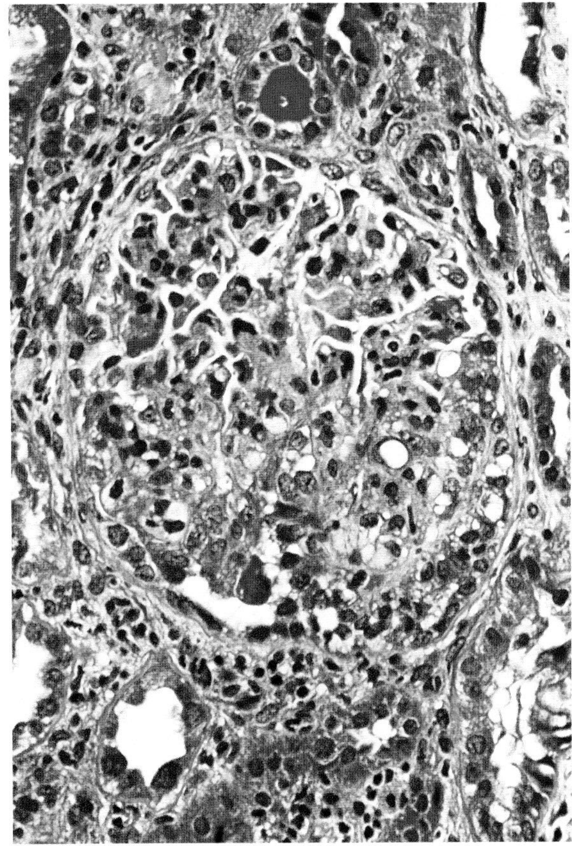

Figure 6-25

PRIMARY FSGS, CELLULAR VARIANT

Both endocapillary and extracapillary hypercellularity are seen, with several clear-staining endocapillary foam cells (Masson trichrome stain).

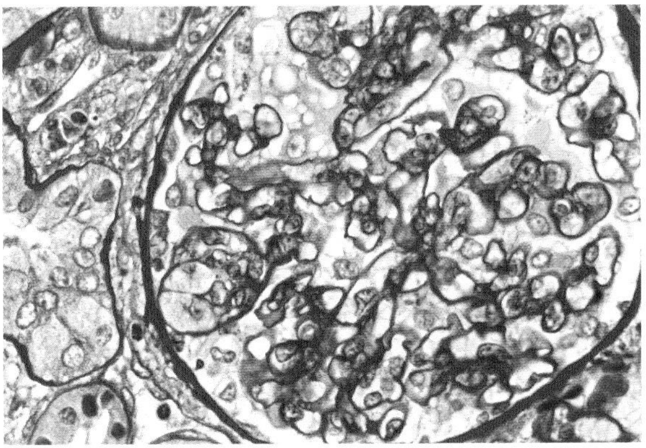

Figure 6-26

PRIMARY FSGS, CELLULAR VARIANT

An early cellular lesion affects a single capillary, which is engorged with foam cells (PAS stain).

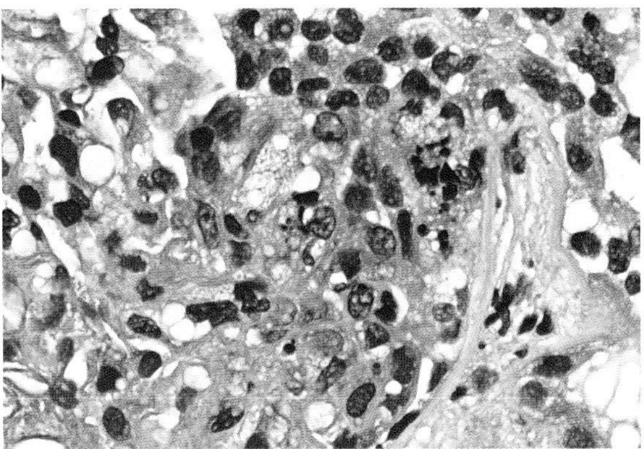

Figure 6-27

PRIMARY FSGS, CELLULAR VARIANT

Numerous infiltrating leukocytes and pyknotic debris segmentally obliterate the glomerular capillaries (H&E stain).

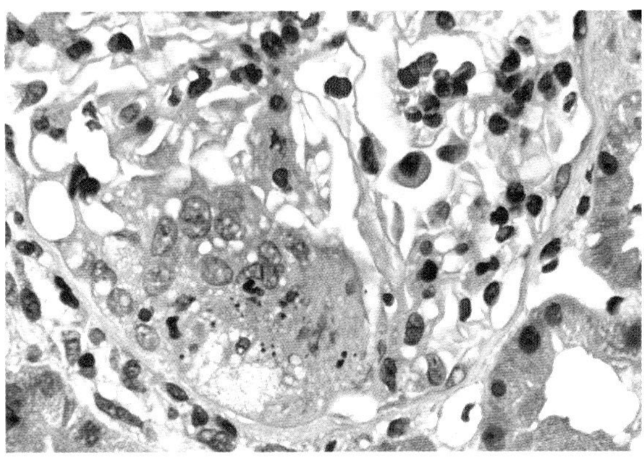

Figure 6-28

PRIMARY FSGS, CELLULAR VARIANT

The cellular lesion contains hyaline, foam cells, and infiltrating leukocytes with karyorrhexis (H&E stain).

protein resorption droplets. These extracapillary cells lack the spindled morphology or pericellular matrix typically observed in true crescents. Another distinguishing feature is that Bowman's capsule itself is intact, without the ruptures typical of cellular crescents of the inflammatory type.

Immunofluorescence Findings. There is focal and segmental glomerular positivity for IgM and C3.

Electron Microscopic Findings. The cellular variant usually displays severe foot process effacement, correlating with the generally high

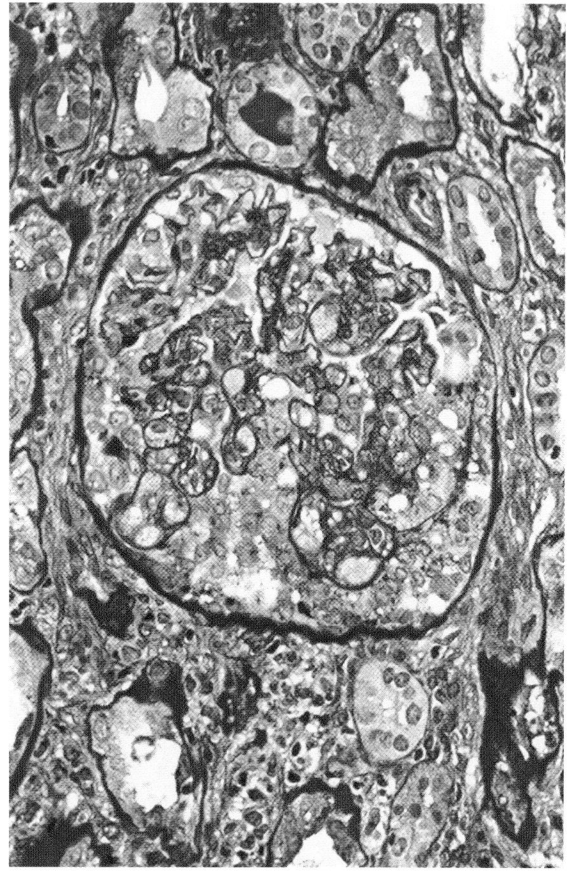

Figure 6-29

PRIMARY FSGS, CELLULAR VARIANT

The extracapillary cells mimic a cellular crescent, but lack spindling or pericellular matrix (PAS stain).

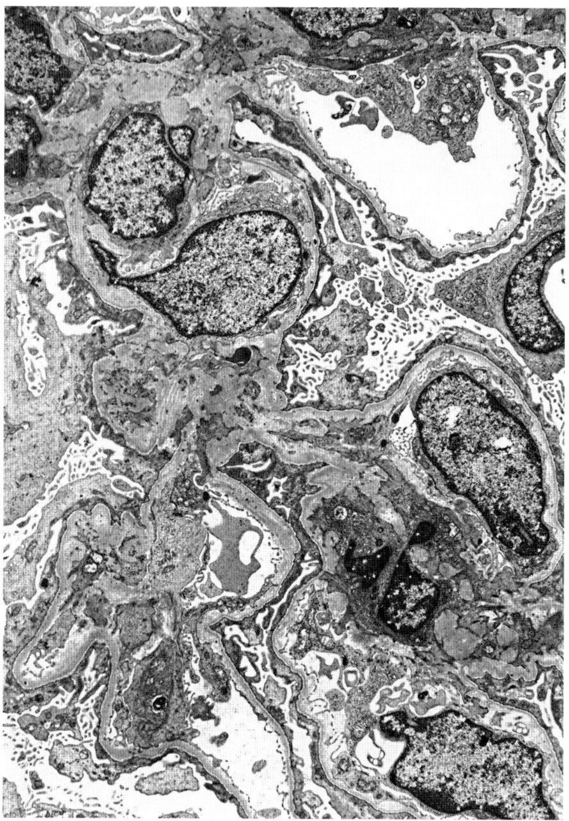

Figure 6-30

PRIMARY FSGS, CELLULAR VARIANT

Nonsclerotic capillaries have complete foot process effacement and focal microvillous transformation of the podocytes (electron micrograph).

levels of proteinuria (fig. 6-30). There is segmental occlusion of glomerular capillaries by endocapillary hypercellularity including foam cells and hyaline (figs. 6-31, 6-32). The glomerular basement membrane is intact, without evidence of rupture.

Differential Diagnosis. The cellular form of FSGS must be differentiated from focal and segmental proliferative glomerulonephritis, such as due to lupus nephritis, IgA nephropathy, or pauci-immune focal crescentic glomerulonephritis. The absence of glomerular immune deposits by immunofluorescence and electron microscopy, the severe foot process effacement, and the clinical findings of nephrotic syndrome help to differentiate this variant of FSGS from proliferative glomerulonephritis.

Treatment and Prognosis. Patients with the cellular variant may be responsive to immunosuppressive therapy (46). This favorable treatment response probably relates to the early and relatively active stage of glomerular injury in this variant of FSGS.

PRIMARY FSGS WITH DIFFUSE MESANGIAL HYPERCELLULARITY

Definition. As the name implies, this uncommon variant of FSGS has lesions of focal and segmental glomerular sclerosis and generalized mesangial hypercellularity which affect nonsclerotic glomeruli. Mesangial hypercellularity is defined as greater than three cells per mesangial region away from the vascular pole in 3-µm–thick sections.

Clinical Features. This form is much more common in children than adults.

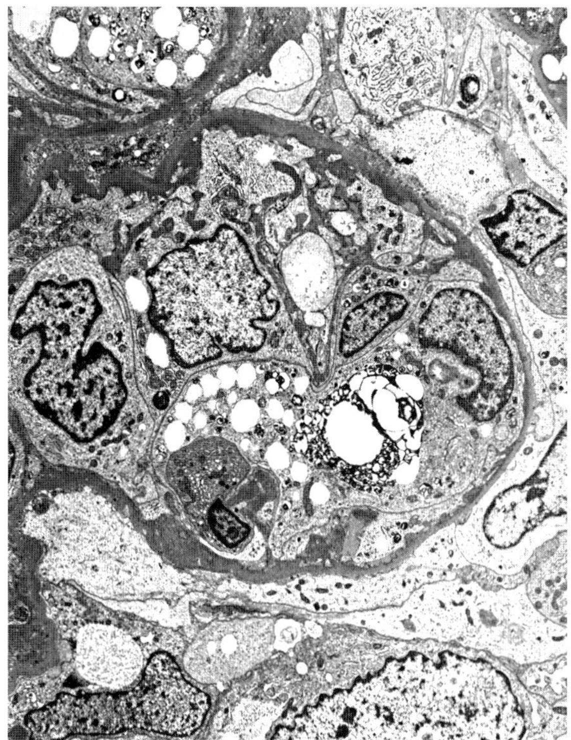

Figure 6-31

PRIMARY FSGS, CELLULAR VARIANT

The cellular lesion has endocapillary hypercellularity with foam cells, infiltrating monocytes, and a small amount of inframembranous hyaline. The overlying podocytes are hypertrophied, with complete foot process effacement (electron micrograph).

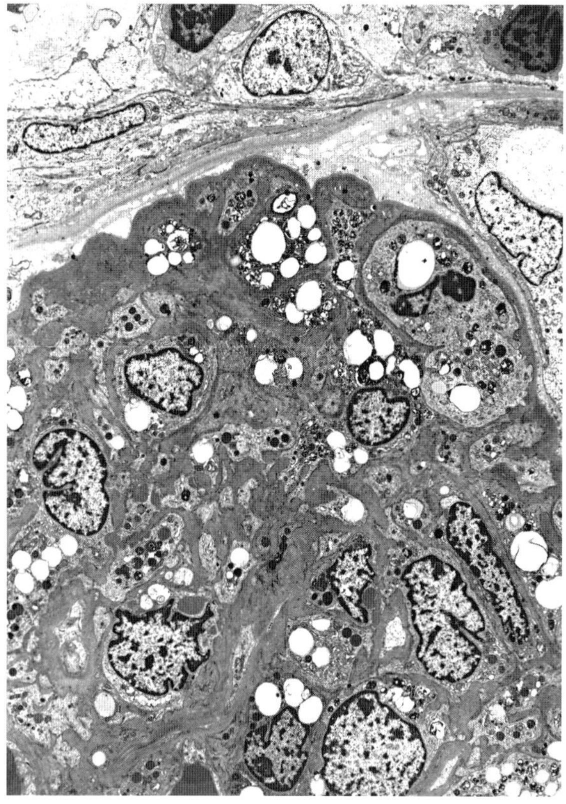

Figure 6-32

PRIMARY FSGS, CELLULAR VARIANT

An exuberant lesion with numerous foam cells, infiltrating monocytes, and detached overlying podocytes with intervening neomembrane material (electron micrograph).

Light Microscopic Findings. Lesions of focal and segmental glomerulosclerosis are present. Nonsclerotic glomeruli display diffuse and global mesangial hypercellularity (fig. 6-33).

Immunofluorescence Findings. There is diffuse mesangial positivity for IgM, with more variable mesangial staining for C3. The lesions of segmental sclerosis have coarser positivity for IgM and C3.

Electron Microscopic Findings. There is extensive foot process effacement. There are typically no identifiable glomerular electron-dense deposits.

Differential Diagnosis. The differential diagnosis includes a glomerulonephritis with focal sclerosing and mesangial proliferative features, such as chronic IgA nephropathy or lupus nephritis. In a setting of nephrotic syndrome, the absence of immune-type glomerular deposits and the presence of marked foot process effacement serve to differentiate this variant from immune-mediated forms of glomerulonephritis.

Treatment and Prognosis. The prognostic implications are controversial. Schoeneman and colleagues (45) compared 13 pediatric cases of FSGS with diffuse mesangial hypercellularity to cases of primary FSGS without mesangial hypercellularity and found a higher rate of progression to renal insufficiency in the former group. Two larger studies, however, failed to confirm these findings: 57 and 75 patients with this lesion studied by Yoshikawa et al. (58) and the Southwest Pediatric Nephrology Study Group (SPNSG) (16), respectively, did not show any prognostic difference. The only correlation reported by the SPNSG study was a shorter time course from clinical presentation to biopsy in the patients with FSGS and diffuse mesangial hypercellularity compared to FSGS without

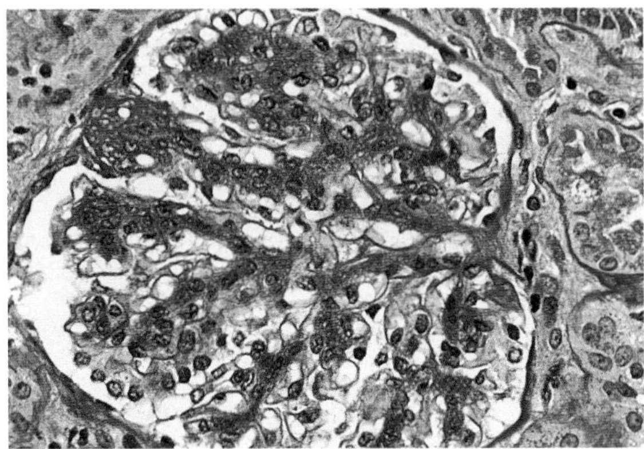

Figure 6-33

PRIMARY FSGS WITH DIFFUSE MESANGIAL HYPERCELLULARITY

A 9-year-old child with severe steroid-resistant nephrotic syndrome. The focal segmental glomerulosclerosis affected 10 percent of glomeruli on a background of diffuse mesangial hypercellularity affecting 100 percent of glomeruli. The glomerulus shown here appears enlarged and contains a small segmental lesion of sclerosis that adheres to Bowman's capsule. The nonsclerotic lobules display moderate mesangial hypercellularity (PAS stain).

mesangial hypercellularity. Thus, like cellular FSGS, this variant represents an early stage in the development of FSGS, but does not appear to correlate with outcome.

PRIMARY FSGS, COLLAPSING VARIANT (COLLAPSING GLOMERULOPATHY)

Definition. The designation, primary FSGS, collapsing variant, is applied to cases of primary FSGS in which the glomerular capillary lumens are segmentally or globally obliterated by the wrinkling and collapse of glomerular basement membranes associated with overlying podocyte hypertrophy and hyperplasia.

Clinical Features. The term glomerular collapse was first introduced by Weiss et al. in 1986 (55) to describe an unusual clinical-pathologic complex of severe nephrotic syndrome, rapidly progressive renal failure, and glomerular collapse occurring in six black patients. Two patients required dialysis within 10 weeks of clinical presentation and five had an ill-defined febrile illness. Although the clinical and pathologic findings suggested possible HIV-associated nephropathy, only one of these patients subsequently developed acquired immunodeficiency syndrome (AIDS).

Two subsequent series reported a similar malignant course to renal failure in patients with collapsing FSGS (NOS) without an associated HIV infection (13,52). When compared to patients with primary FSGS (NOS), patients with primary FSGS and collapsing features are more likely to be black and to present with more severe markers of nephrotic syndrome, including more severe proteinuria, hypoalbuminemia, and hypercholesterolemia. Moreover, the patients in these studies had a higher serum creatinine at presentation (3.5 versus 1.3 mg/dL and 4.2 versus 2.0 mg/dL) despite a shorter time period from clinical onset to biopsy.

The incidence of the collapsing variant is increasing. This variant comprised 11 percent of all cases of primary FSGS at the Columbia Presbyterian Medical Center from 1979 to 1985, 20 percent from 1986 to 1989, and 24 percent from 1990 to 1993 (1,52).

Light Microscopic Findings. Primary FSGS, collapsing variant, has a dramatic pattern of injury (fig. 6-34). Glomerular capillary lumens are occluded by an implosive wrinkling and collapse of the glomerular basement membranes that is more often global than segmental, without predilection for the perihilar segments (figs. 6-35–6-39). This glomerular basement membrane collapse is best delineated with the use of the PAS or Jones methenamine silver (JMS) stain. The acute nature of the glomerular injury is evidenced by the lack of an appreciable increase in intracapillary or mesangial matrix. The glomerular collapse is accompanied by striking hypertrophy and hyperplasia of the overlying podocytes, which have enlarged, open vesicular nuclei with frequent nucleoli; occasional binucleate forms; and rare mitotic figures (figs. 6-40, 6-41). The proliferation marker Ki-67 is frequently positive in the distribution of the podocytes, indicating that they are cell-cycle engaged (fig. 6-42) (2). Podocytes may be so crowded that they fill the urinary space, forming pseudocrescents; often, they contain prominent intracytoplasmic protein resorption droplets (figs. 6-36, 6-37, 6-39, 6-43).

Although the collapsing and cellular variants of FSGS share the feature of extracapillary hypercellularity owing to podocyte hyperplasia, primary FSGS with collapsing features is distinguished from the cellular variant by the absence of endocapillary hypercellularity. In fact, there

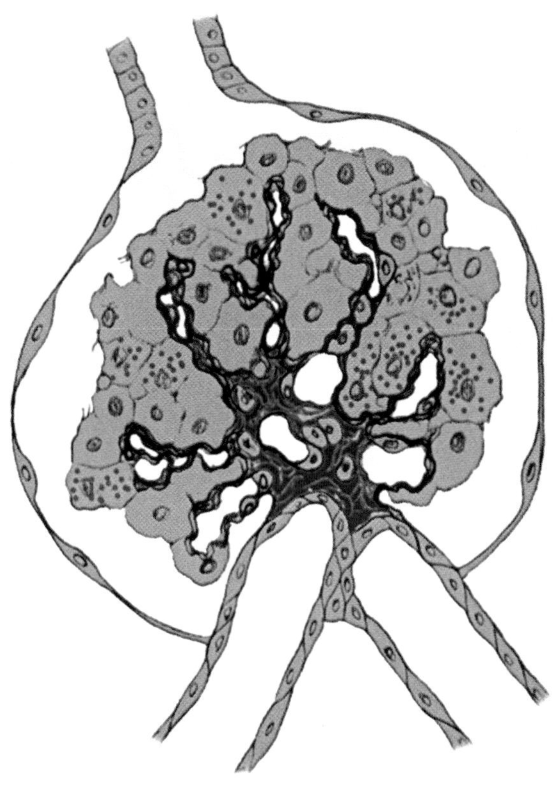

Figure 6-34

PRIMARY FSGS, COLLAPSING VARIANT

This illustration shows the defining features of glomerular basement membrane collapse with hypertrophy and hyperplasia of the overlying podocytes.

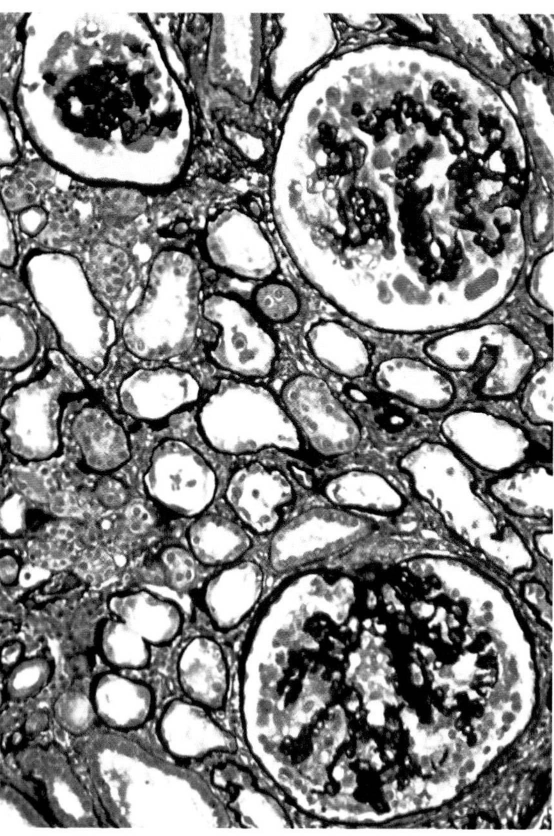

Figure 6-35

PRIMARY FSGS, COLLAPSING VARIANT

The collapse is diffuse and global in distribution, with associated severe tubular degenerative changes (JMS stain).

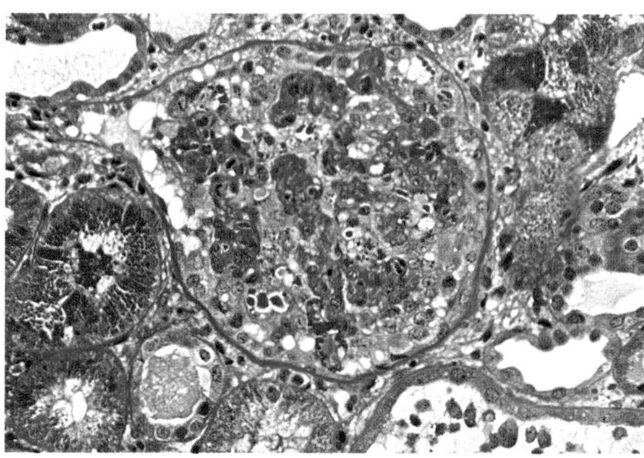

Figure 6-36

PRIMARY FSGS, COLLAPSING VARIANT

The hyperplastic podocytes are plump and rounded, forming a pseudocrescent that obliterates the urinary space (Masson trichrome stain).

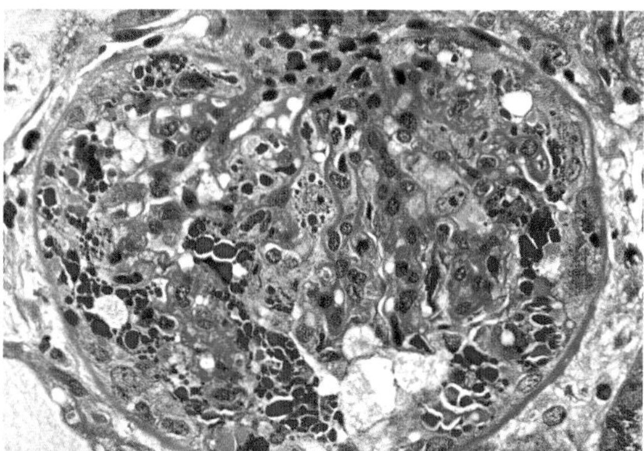

Figure 6-37

PRIMARY FSGS, COLLAPSING VARIANT

The hyperplastic podocytes contain numerous intracytoplasmic, red protein resorption droplets (Masson trichrome stain).

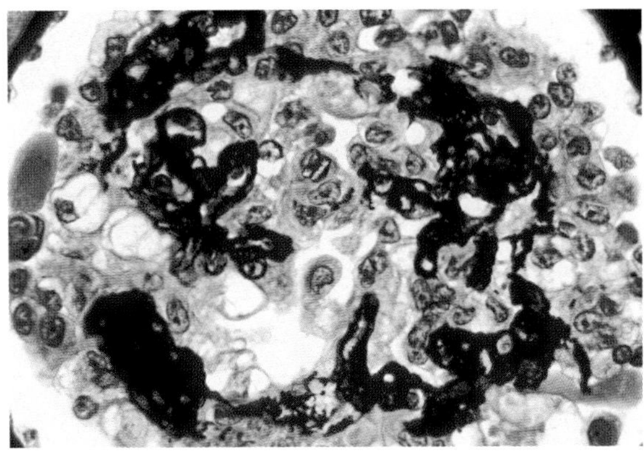

Figure 6-38

PRIMARY FSGS, COLLAPSING VARIANT

A severe example with implosive collapse of the tuft, no appreciable increase in endocapillary matrix, and poorly cohesive hyperplastic podocytes, some of which appear binucleated (JMS stain).

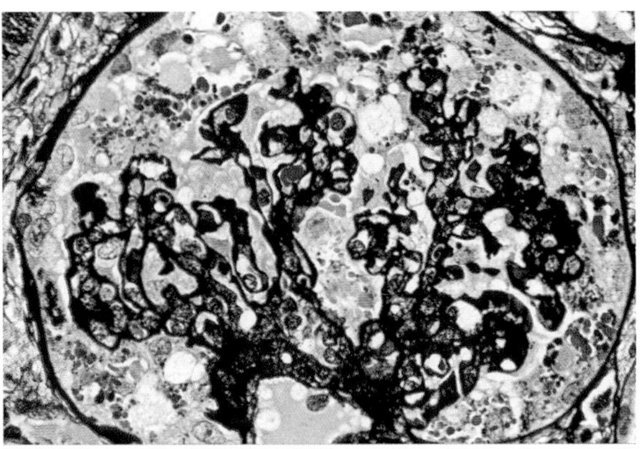

Figure 6-39

PRIMARY FSGS, COLLAPSING VARIANT

The hyperplastic podocytes contain many intracytoplasmic vesicles and resorption droplets. The parietal and visceral epithelial cells merge (JMS stain).

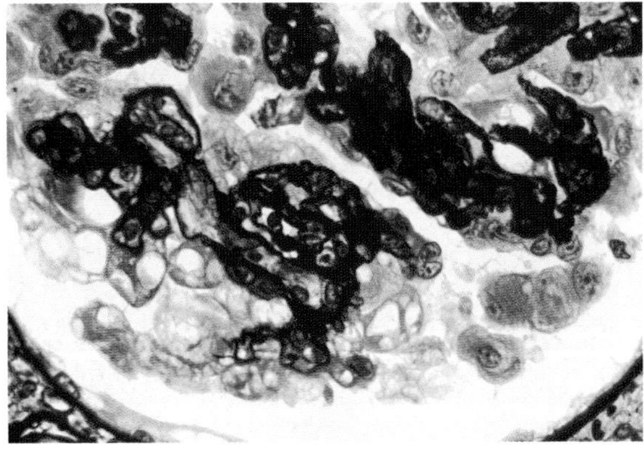

Figure 6-40

PRIMARY FSGS, COLLAPSING VARIANT

High-power microscopic view shows focal binucleated podocytes. Many podocytes do not adhere to the tuft, giving the impression that they are falling off into the urinary space (JMS stain).

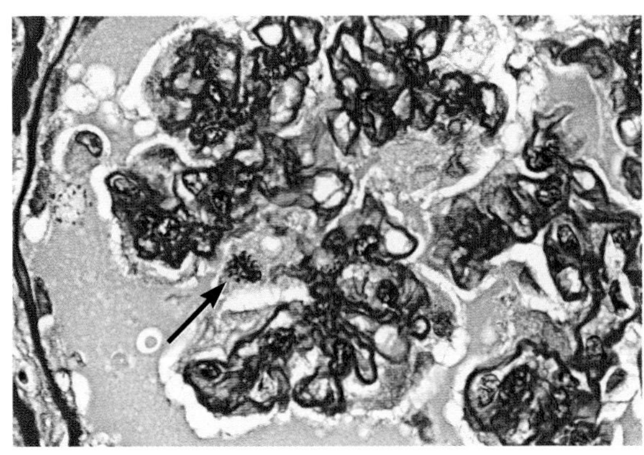

Figure 6-41

FSGS, COLLAPSING VARIANT

A mitotic figure (arrow) is identified in a visceral epithelial cell (PAS stain).

is often an apparent reduction in the number of glomerular endothelial cells in collapsed lobules. Unlike primary FSGS (NOS), glomeruli with collapsing sclerosis usually lack hyalinosis, endocapillary foam cells, and adhesions to Bowman's capsule. Collapsing lesions may exist side by side with glomeruli showing segmental and global sclerosis of the usual type, however.

Tubulointerstitial disease is an important component of this condition and often appears out of proportion to the degree of glomerular sclerosis. In addition to tubular atrophy, interstitial fibrosis, edema, and inflammation, there are widespread tubular degenerative and regenerative changes (52). These include tubular epithelial simplification with enlarged hyperchromatic nuclei, nucleoli, mitotic figures, and focal apoptosis. About 40 percent of cases have tubular microcysts that contain loose proteinaceous casts (fig. 6-44) (52).

Immunofluorescence Findings. There are segmental to global deposits of IgM and C3, and less commonly C1, in the collapsing segments (fig. 6-45). Visceral epithelial protein

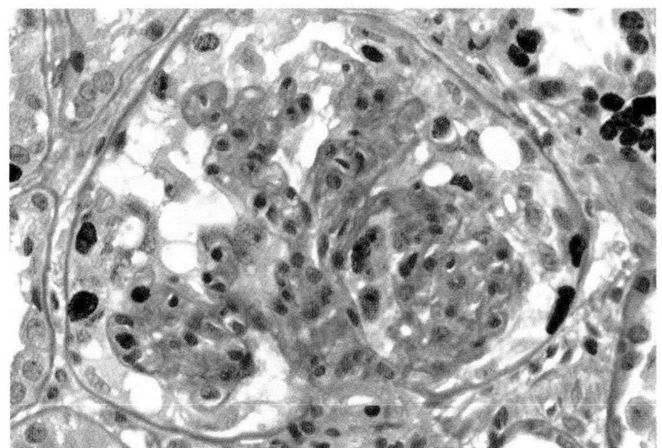

Figure 6-42

PRIMARY FSGS, COLLAPSING VARIANT

Immunostain for proliferation marker Ki-67 shows positivity in many podocytes, as well as some parietal epithelial cells and tubular epithelial cells (immunoperoxidase stain).

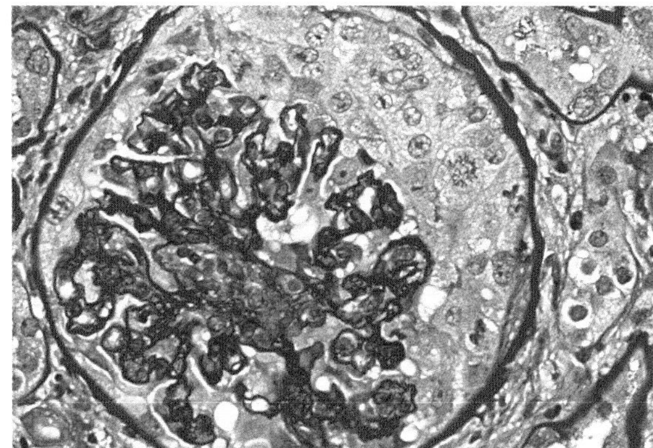

Figure 6-43

PRIMARY FSGS, COLLAPSING VARIANT

The extracapillary proliferation mimics a crescent and contains a mitotic figure. The extracapillary cells are plump and lack the spindled shape and pericellular matrix usually seen in true crescents (PAS stain).

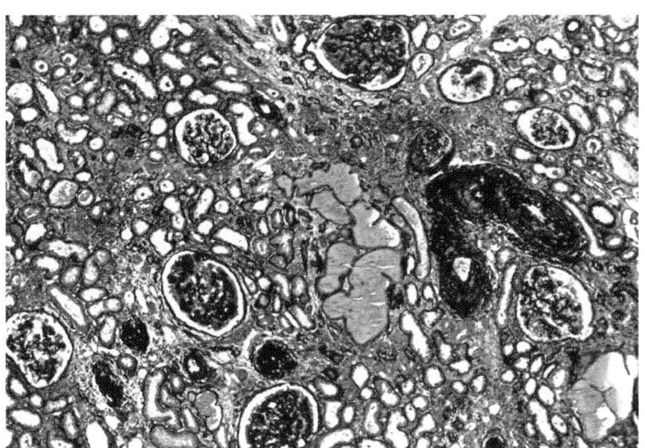

Figure 6-44

PRIMARY FSGS, COLLAPSING VARIANT

There is severe tubulointerstitial disease with focal tubular microcysts (JMS stain).

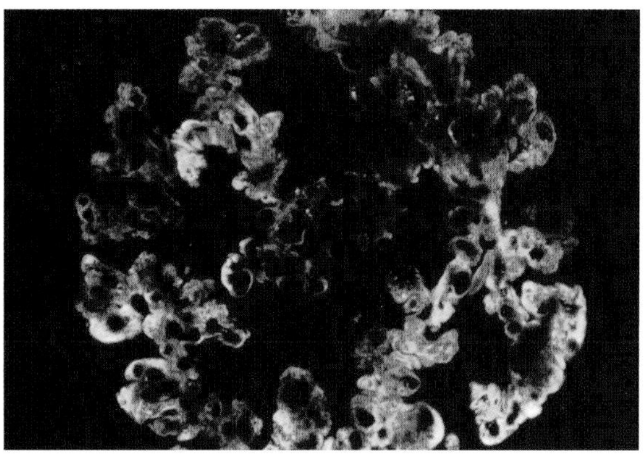

Figure 6-45

PRIMARY FSGS, COLLAPSING VARIANT

The collapsed tuft stains 1+ in a global distribution for IgM (immunofluorescence micrograph).

resorption droplets often stain for IgG, IgA, and albumin, with similar staining in the tubular epithelial protein droplets.

Electron Microscopic Findings. The collapsed lobules display wrinkling and little or no thickening of the glomerular basement membrane (fig. 6-46). The overlying podocytes are markedly hypertrophied, with severe foot process effacement, focal detachment, and increased numbers of organelles including electron-dense protein resorption droplets, electron-lucent transport vesicles, and rough endoplasmic reticulum (fig. 6-47). The actin cytoskeleton usually appears disrupted, giving the cells a relatively open appearing cytoplasm. Noncollapsed capillaries also display severe (mean, 80 percent) foot process effacement. No electron-dense deposits are observed, with the exception of rare, small, paramesangial electron densities corresponding to the mesangial deposits of IgM (fig. 6-48). In contrast to HIV-associated nephropathy, no tubuloreticular inclusions are identified.

Differential Diagnosis. Primary FSGS with collapsing features may be confused with forms

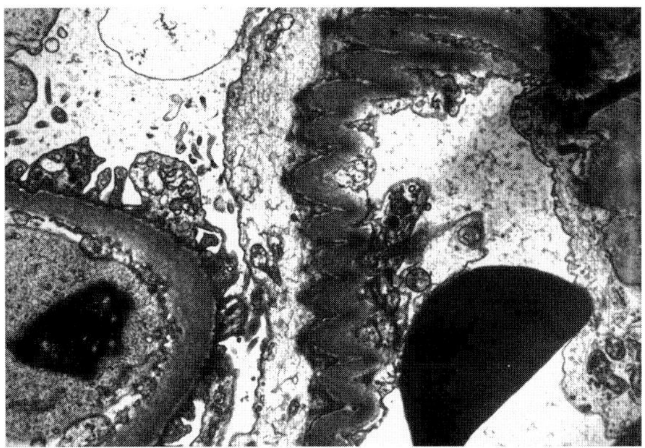

Figure 6-46

PRIMARY FSGS, COLLAPSING VARIANT

Early lesion with tight wrinkling and retraction of the glomerular basement membrane is accompanied by segmental foot process effacement (electron micrograph).

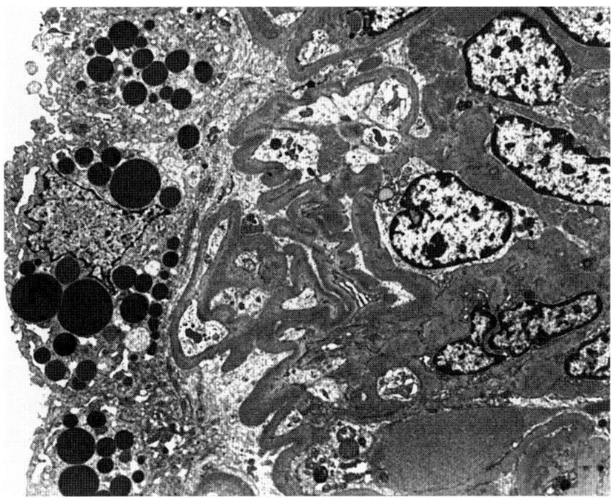

Figure 6-47

PRIMARY FSGS, COLLAPSING VARIANT

Well-established lesion with wrinkled glomerular basement membranes and hypertrophy of the podocytes, which contain intracellular protein resorption droplets (electron micrograph).

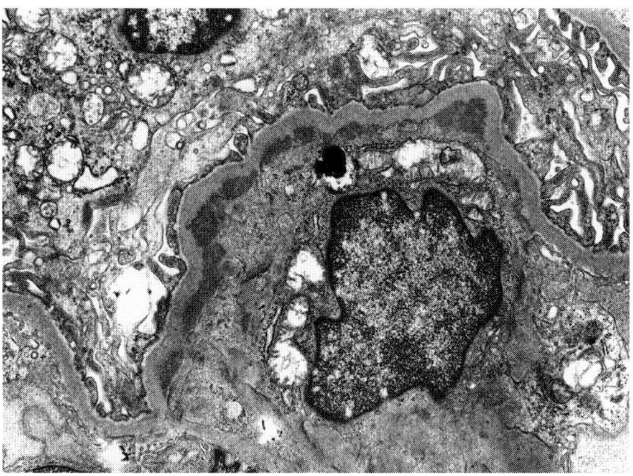

Figure 6-48

PRIMARY FSGS, COLLAPSING VARIANT

There is a small, paramesangial, electron-dense deposit (electron micrograph).

of crescentic glomerulonephritis. The hyperplastic podocytes in collapsing focal sclerosis lack the spindled morphology, extracapillary fibrin, and pericellular matrix that surrounds the proliferating parietal cells of true crescents. Crescentic glomerulonephritis is also distinguished by the presence of necrotizing lesions in the underlying tuft and breaks in the glomerular basement membrane.

Patients with the collapsing phenotype of FSGS may have primary FSGS or secondary FSGS caused by viral etiologies or drug toxicities. Exclusion of HIV-associated nephropathy is based on the demonstration of negative HIV serologies, as well as the absence of endothelial tubuloreticular inclusions. FSGS with collapsing features has been reported to occur in some patients with viral infections due to parvovirus B-19 or SV40. Recently, some cases of FSGS with collapsing features were identified as a form of drug nephrotoxicity in older patients treated with pamidronate (Aredia), an osteoclast inhibitor that reduces bone resorption, used for myeloma or carcinoma metastatic to bone (35). Reduction in proteinuria may be achieved following discontinuation of the offending agent.

Treatment and Prognosis. Patients with primary FSGS with collapsing features typically have a rapid course to renal failure and are usually unresponsive to steroid therapy. One group found a median survival period of 13.0 months compared to 62.5 months for controls with classic primary FSGS (52). Thus, this variant has also been considered the morphologic counterpart of the "malignant" FSGS proposed years earlier by Cameron (7).

GLOMERULAR TIP LESION

Definition. This controversial variant of primary FSGS is defined by the presence of segmental lesions in the periphery of the glomerular

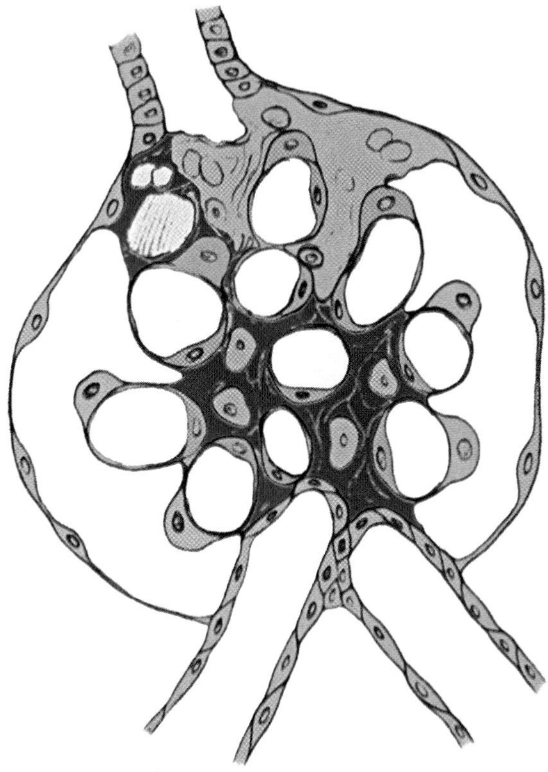

Figure 6-49

GLOMERULAR TIP LESION

This illustration shows a cellular lesion of sclerosis affecting the segment of the glomerulus at the tubular pole, with adhesion and confluence of the podocytes and the tubular epithelial cells.

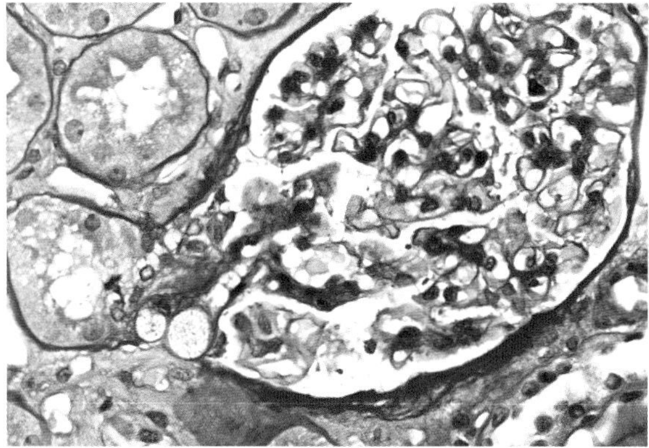

Figure 6-50

GLOMERULAR TIP LESION

A segment of the tuft containing endocapillary foam cells forms an adhesion to Bowman's capsule at the origin of the proximal tubule (PAS stain).

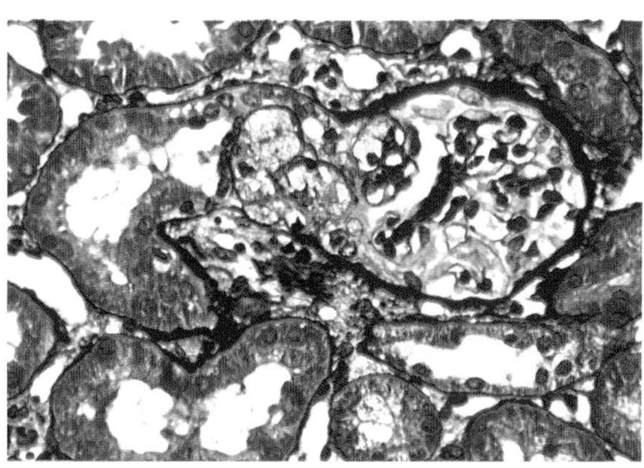

Figure 6-51

GLOMERULAR TIP LESION

A cellular lesion at the tip domain appears to prolapse into the tubular lumen and forms an adhesion to the tubular pole (JMS stain).

tuft, at the origin of the proximal tubule (figs. 6-49–6-54). There must be either confluence of podocytes with parietal epithelial or tubular epithelial cells at the tubular pole or synechia formation between the glomerular tuft and Bowman's capsule at the tubular pole (11).

Clinical Features. In the study by Stokes et al. (50), most cases of glomerular tip lesion occurred in adults: among 47 cases studied, 45 occurred in adults and 2 in children (mean age, 47.5 years; range, 12 to 79 years). Over three fourths of patients were Caucasians, without gender predominance. Most patients present with sudden onset of full nephrotic syndrome, which resembles the presentation of MCD. At presentation, 93.5 percent of patients had edema, 89.1 percent had nephrotic syndrome (with mean urine protein 8.31 g), and 34.8 percent had renal insufficiency. When compared to a control group of patients with MCD and idiopathic FSGS, patients with glomerular tip lesion more closely resembled those with MCD with respect to a high incidence of nephrotic syndrome, severity of proteinuria, short duration from clinical onset to biopsy, and the absence of chronic tubulointerstitial disease.

Light Microscopic Findings. As defined originally by Howie and Brewer (24), the early lesion is characterized by the confluence of swollen, hypertrophied, visceral epithelial cells with parietal or tubular epithelial cells at the tubular pole. The affected lobule may display

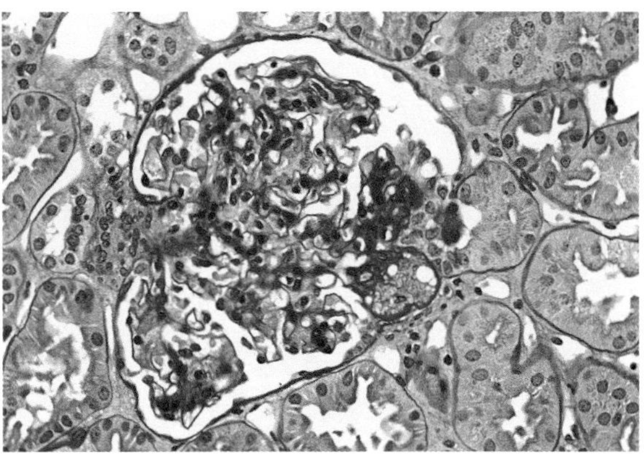

Figure 6-52

GLOMERULAR TIP LESION

Directly opposite the vascular pole, a discrete segmental lesion with endocapillary foam cells and inframembranous hyalinosis forms an adhesion to Bowman's capsule at the tubular pole. Confluent hypertrophied podocytes overlie this lesion, with tubular epithelial cells at the tubular neck (PAS stain).

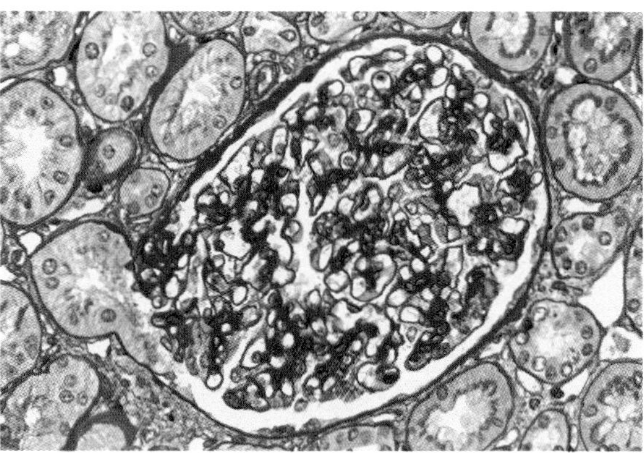

Figure 6-53

GLOMERULAR TIP LESION

There is a small synechia located at the origin of the proximal tubule (PAS stain).

endocapillary hypercellularity, with endocapillary foam cells and hyalinosis (figs. 6-50–6-52). As the lesion evolves, there is adhesion of the glomerular tuft to Bowman's capsule at the point of transition to the proximal tubular basement membrane (fig. 6-53) (24). Later lesions may form segmental scars (fig. 6-54). In the study by Stokes et al. (50), 26 percent of biopsies had glomerular tip lesions alone, 6 percent had glomerular tip lesions plus peripheral lesions, 36 percent had glomerular tip lesions plus indeterminate lesions, and 32 percent had glomerular tip lesions plus peripheral and indeterminate lesions. No initial biopsy contained perihilar sclerosis and most (81 percent) of glomerular tip lesions had cellular features. These findings support the distinctive peripheral phenotype of glomerular tip lesion.

Immunofluorescence Findings. The segmental lesions usually stain for IgM and C3.

Electron Microscopic Findings. But for their location at the tubular pole, the lesions resemble those of cellular FSGS at the ultrastructural level. There may be confluence of swollen podocytes, parietal epithelial cells, and tubular cells at the tubular pole.

Differential Diagnosis. Glomerular tip lesions occur in the setting of a variety of glomerular diseases, including membranous glomerulopathy, IgA nephropathy, diabetic glomerulosclerosis, and others (25). Thus Howie (24) advocates that the designation of glomerular tip lesion should be applied only to those cases with glomeruli that look otherwise like MCD (i.e., with extensive foot process effacement in the absence of other pathologic alterations). Others define the tip variant as a subtype of FSGS in which the lesion occurs alone or in association with segmental lesions that are peripheral or indeterminate in location. The presence of any perihilar sclerosis or collapsing sclerosis rules out the tip variant (11).

Etiology and Pathogenesis. It is uncertain how the pathogenesis of the tip lesion differs, if at all, from that of the more classic lesions of FSGS. A study of autopsied kidneys from children with MCD in the presteroid era revealed focal "tip lesions" in a small percentage of glomeruli (21). Studies such as this suggest that tip lesions may arise as a nonspecific response of the paratubular segment of the glomerular tuft to physical stress caused by the convergence of a protein-rich filtrate on the tubular pole in the setting of nephrotic syndrome. A role for prolapse of the paratubular segment into the tubular lumen has also been proposed.

Treatment and Prognosis. The relationship of glomerular tip lesion to MCD and FSGS has been hotly debated. Whereas some groups report a greater likelihood of steroid responsivity and excellent long-term prognosis, resembling

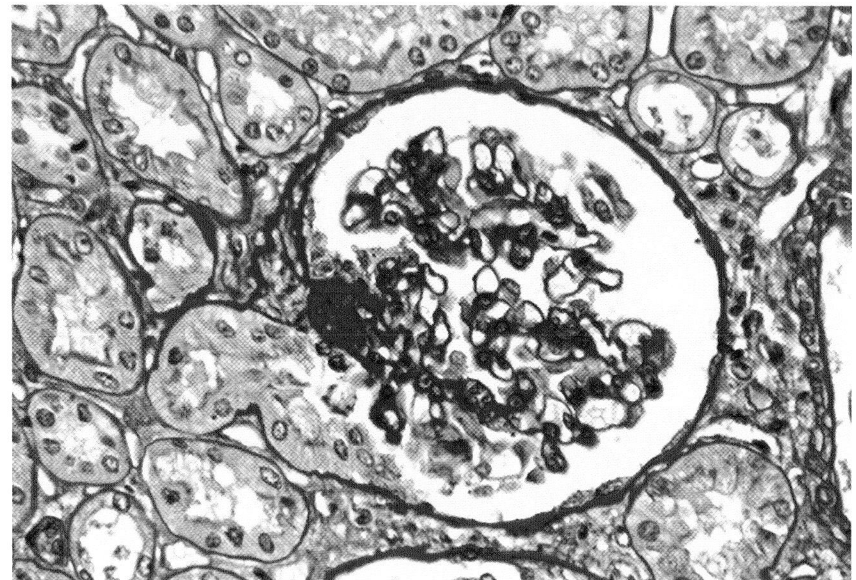

Figure 6-54

GLOMERULAR TIP LESION

A more advanced lesion forms a discrete segmental scar that adheres to the tubular origin (PAS stain).

that of patients with MCD, others describe an evolution towards more typical FSGS (3,24,50). Indeed, repeat biopsies in some of these patients have demonstrated progression to focal segmental and global glomerulosclerosis and the development of renal failure.

Recently, Hogan-Moulton et al. (23) described an 80 percent steroid responsivity in patients with glomerular tip lesion compared to 33 percent for those with FSGS, but with similar long-term survival rates (87 percent at 4 years in both groups). In a study by Stokes et al. (50), follow-up data were available in 29 patients, of whom 21 received steroids alone and 8 received sequential therapy with steroids and a cytotoxic agent. Of those 29 patients, 58.6 percent achieved complete remission of nephrotic syndrome, 13.8 percent had partial remission, and 27.6 percent had persistent nephrotic proteinuria. Only one patient progressed to end-stage renal disease (mean, 21 months of follow-up). Thus, the presenting features and outcome for patients with glomerular tip lesion more closely approximate those of MCD than FSGS, indicating a highly favorable histologic subtype.

C1q NEPHROPATHY

Definition. This controversial variant of primary FSGS was first described by Jennette et al. in 1985 (28). It is defined as a form of idiopathic nephrotic syndrome caused by a glomerulopathy with dominant paramesangial deposits of C1q (of at least 2+ intensity on a scale of 0 to 4+). In a study by Markowitz et al. (37), the disease was defined by dominant or co-dominant immunofluorescence staining for C1q, mesangial electron-dense deposits, and no clinical or serologic evidence of systemic lupus erythematosus (SLE). Using this definition, the biopsy incidence of disease is only 0.21 percent.

Clinical Features. Most patients present with idiopathic nephrotic syndrome, and some have renal insufficiency. In the study by Markowitz et al. (37), patients were predominantly black (73.7 percent), female (73.7 percent), young adults and children (range, 3 to 42 years; mean, 24.2 years). Presentation included nephrotic range proteinuria (78.9 percent), nephrotic syndrome (50.0 percent), renal insufficiency (27.8 percent), and hematuria (22.2 percent). Serologic tests for lupus and HIV were negative, serum complement levels were normal, and there was no clinical evidence of systemic, autoimmune, or infectious disease.

Light Microscopic Findings. The features seen by light microscopy are usually the same as those of FSGS with variable mesangial hypercellularity (fig. 6-55). Although early reports emphasized the mesangial proliferative features (28), subsequent reports have stressed the resemblance to FSGS or MCD (27,37). Among 19 cases reported by Markowitz et al. (37), 17 had a light microscopic appearance of FSGS (including 6 collapsing and 2 cellular) and 3 had a pattern of MCD.

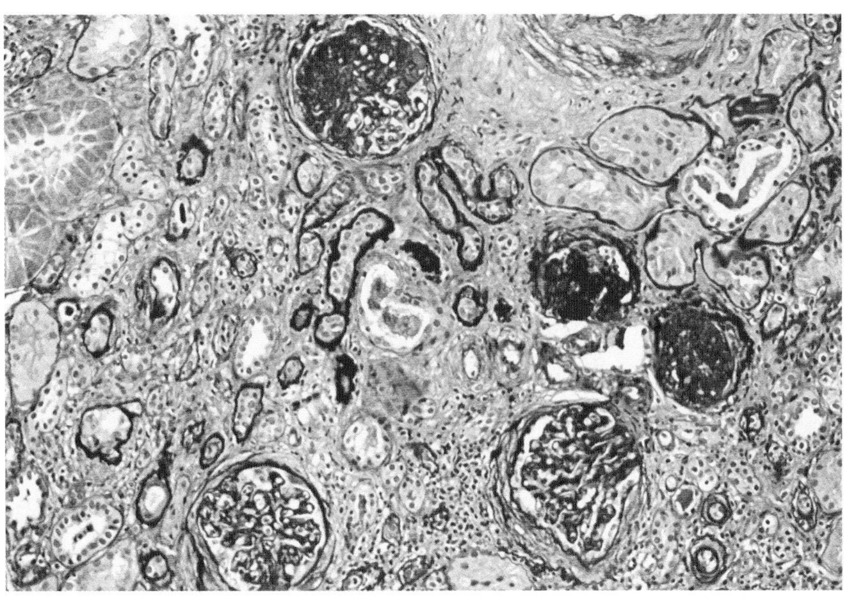

Figure 6-55

C1q NEPHROPATHY

The usual pattern by light microscopy is one of focal segmental and global glomerulosclerosis (PAS stain).

Immunofluorescence Findings. In addition to staining for C1q (of at least 2+ intensity), the study by Jennette et al. (28) showed most cases to have co-deposits of IgG (90 percent) of mean 1.6+ intensity or IgM (94 percent) of mean 1.1+ intensity, and C3 (90 percent) of mean 1.1+ intensity on a scale of 0 to 4+. Deposits of IgA were less common and were observed in 56 percent of biopsies, with a mean intensity 0.7+ (28). In the study by Markowitz et al. (36), all biopsies displayed co-deposits of IgG, with more variable IgM (84.2 percent), IgA (31.6 percent), and C3 (52.6 percent). In both studies, the mesangial deposits were often comma-shaped, owing to their paramesangial location and conformation to the overlying glomerular basement membrane reflection (figs. 6-56–6-58).

Electron Microscopic Findings. Electron-dense deposits are primarily or exclusively located in the mesangium. In over 90 percent of cases, electron microscopy reveals prominent, paramesangial, electron-dense deposits subjacent to the reflection of the glomerular basement membrane (fig. 6-59). In a minority of cases, rare subendothelial and subepithelial deposits are also seen (28). There is prominent, but variable, foot process effacement (range, 20 to 100 percent; mean, 51 percent) (37).

Differential Diagnosis. Diagnosis requires the exclusion of lupus nephritis and IgA nephropathy on clinical and pathologic grounds.

Etiology and Pathogenesis. The etiology is unknown. Some investigators believe that C1q nephropathy represents a morphologic variant of primary FSGS, with a similar pathogenesis and outcome. Because of the close clinical and pathologic resemblance to the FSGS/MCD spectrum, some have speculated that the paramesangial deposits of C1q and IgG may be a nonspecific marker of increased mesangial trafficking in the setting of glomerular proteinuria (37).

Treatment and Prognosis. Many patients are steroid resistant and some progress to end-stage renal failure. In the study by Markowitz (37), 12 of 16 patients with available follow-up received immunosuppressive therapy. One patient had complete remission of proteinuria and 6 had partial remission. Four patients with FSGS pattern had progressive renal insufficiency, including 2 who reached end-stage renal disease. Median time from biopsy to end-stage renal disease was 81 months. On multivariate analysis, the best correlate of renal insufficiency at biopsy and follow-up was the degree of tubular atrophy and interstitial fibrosis. Thus, the prognosis and outcome for patients with C1q nephropathy closely resemble those for idiopathic FSGS.

HIV-ASSOCIATED NEPHROPATHY

Definition. HIV-associated nephropathy (AN) is a secondary form of focal segmental glomerulosclerosis occurring in HIV-infected patients.

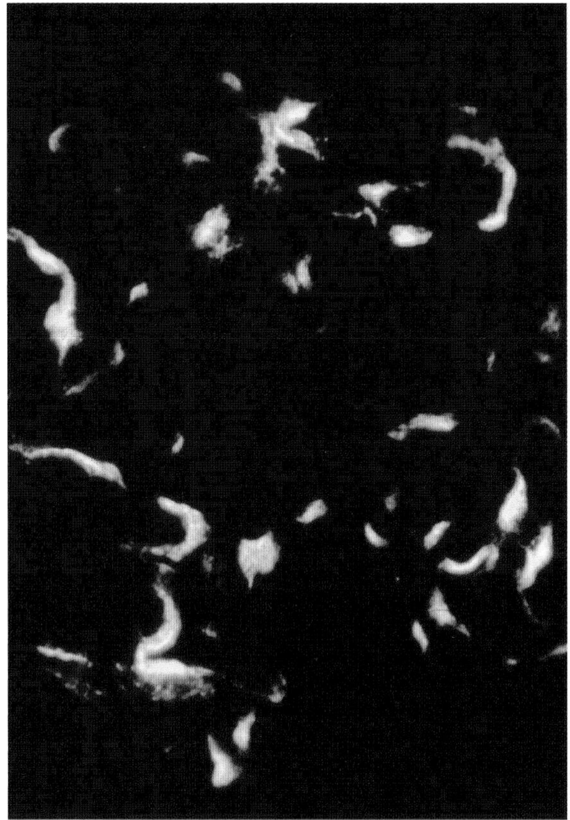

Figure 6-56

C1q NEPHROPATHY

By immunofluorescence, global comma-shaped deposits of C1q (2+) outline the paramesangial areas.

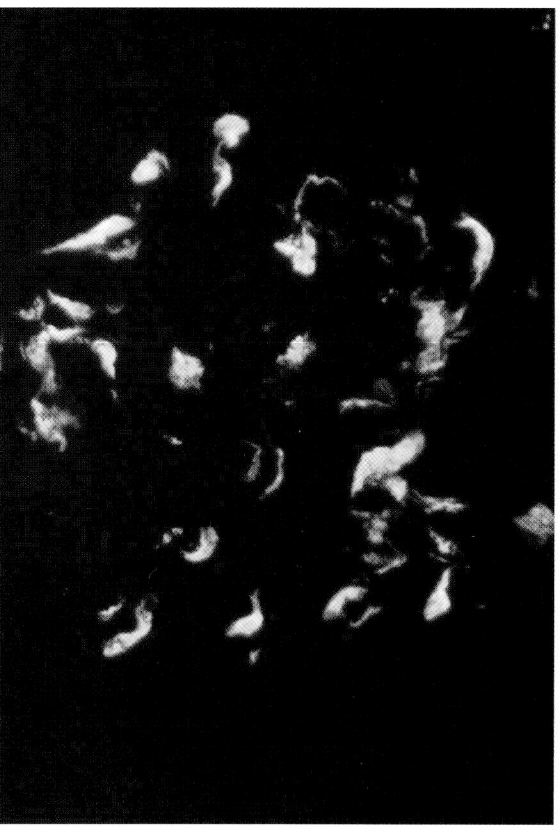

Figure 6-57

C1q NEPHROPATHY

The mesangial distribution of the C1q deposits is clearly seen (immunofluorescence micrograph).

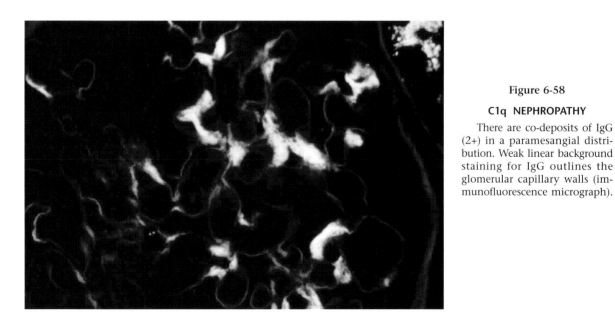

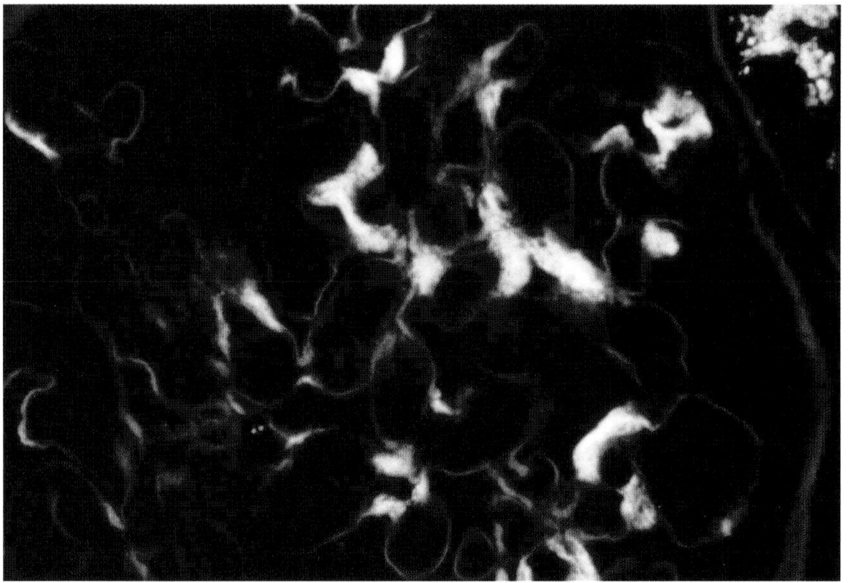

Figure 6-58

C1q NEPHROPATHY

There are co-deposits of IgG (2+) in a paramesangial distribution. Weak linear background staining for IgG outlines the glomerular capillary walls (immunofluorescence micrograph).

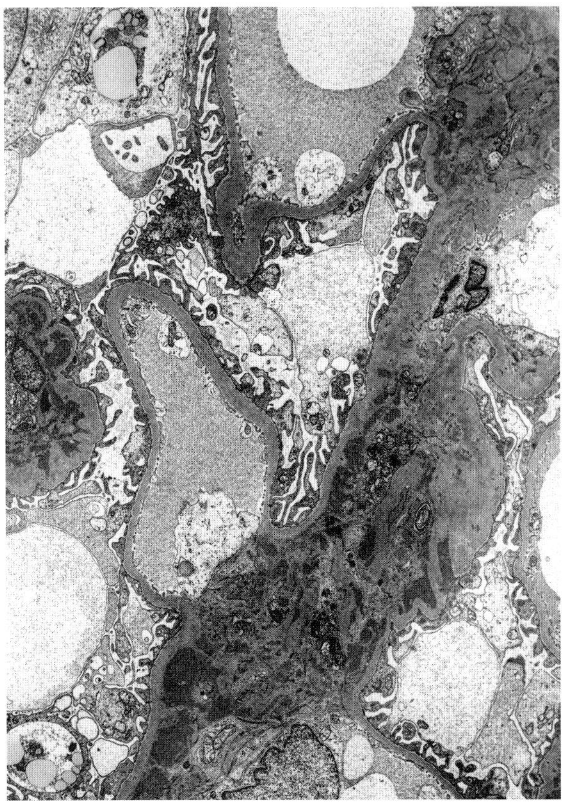

Figure 6-59

C1q NEPHROPATHY

Electron-dense deposits are confined to the paramesangial regions, subjacent to the reflection of the glomerular basement membrane over the mesangium (electron micrograph).

Clinical Features. The incidence of heroin nephropathy has fallen reciprocally with the advent of HIV-AN (1), a distinctive form of FSGS occurring in HIV-infected patients, first described at the Downstate Medical Center in New York City (41). HIV-AN is predominantly a disease of blacks (90 percent). Although it can occur in both sexes and with any HIV risk factor, it is most common in male intravenous drug abusers.

Presenting features include proteinuria, usually in the nephrotic range, and renal insufficiency. Despite the high frequency of nephrotic-range proteinuria and hypoalbuminemia, hypercholesterolemia and edema are uncommon. The absence of hypercholesterolemia likely reflects the reduced hepatic synthesis of lipoproteins in patients with AIDS. Hypertension is also relatively uncommon. Ultrasonography shows large and echogenic kidneys.

Light Microscopic Findings. The light microscopic findings in HIV-AN are qualitatively similar to those described above in primary FSGS with collapsing features (10,12). The characteristic glomerular lesion is a collapsing sclerosis with prominent podocyte alterations. As the lesion progresses, the glomerular tuft may be reduced to an acellular sclerotic ball, with crowning of the overlying podocytes and relative dilatation of the urinary space. A proteinaceous filtrate is frequently identified within the enlarged urinary space.

Tubular microcysts are common, found in approximately 30 to 40 percent of cases (fig. 6-60) (12). Some patients with advanced disease at autopsy have almost complete replacement of the cortical parenchyma by massive microcyst formation. This microcystic transformation likely contributes to the enlarged kidneys and increased echogenicity observed by ultrasound, even in patients with end-stage renal failure.

Immunofluorescence Findings. The findings are similar to those of primary FSGS with collapsing features.

Electron Microscopic Findings. Differences between HIV-AN and primary FSGS with collapsing features are seen only at the ultrastructural level (fig. 6-61). The major distinguishing feature is the abundance of tubuloreticular inclusions in the glomerular endothelial cells of HIV-AN (12). Tubuloreticular inclusions, also known as interferon footprints, consist of 24-nm interanastomosing tubular structures located within dilated cisternae of the endoplasmic reticulum (fig. 6-62). They may be large and multiple per cell. Although they are most readily identified in the glomerular endothelium, they also occur in arterial or interstitial capillary endothelial cells and infiltrating leukocytes.

Tubuloreticular inclusions were noted with frequency in the renal biopsies of HIV-infected patients in the 1980s. They are less frequent in the modern era of highly active antiretroviral therapy (HAART), probably due to the reduced viral burden (10).

Other characteristic, but relatively less frequent, ultrastructural findings include nuclear bodies within tubular and interstitial cells, granular-fibrillar transformation of the tubular nuclei, and confronting cylindrical cisternae (fig. 6-63) (12).

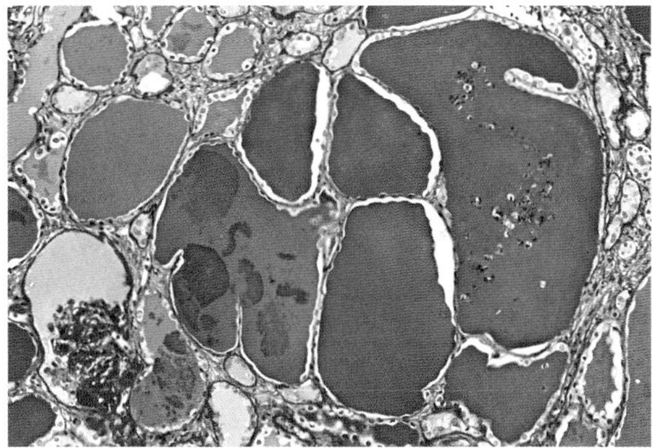

Figure 6-60

HUMAN IMMUNODEFICIENCY VIRUS (HIV)–ASSOCIATED NEPHROPATHY

There is glomerular collapse and prominent microcystic dilatation of the tubules (PAS stain).

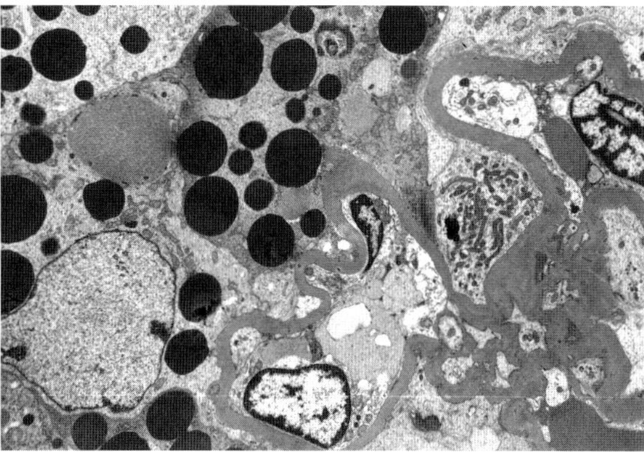

Figure 6-61

HIV-ASSOCIATED NEPHROPATHY

Overlying the collapsed capillaries, the hyperplastic podocytes contain numerous intracytoplasmic protein resorption droplets (electron micrograph).

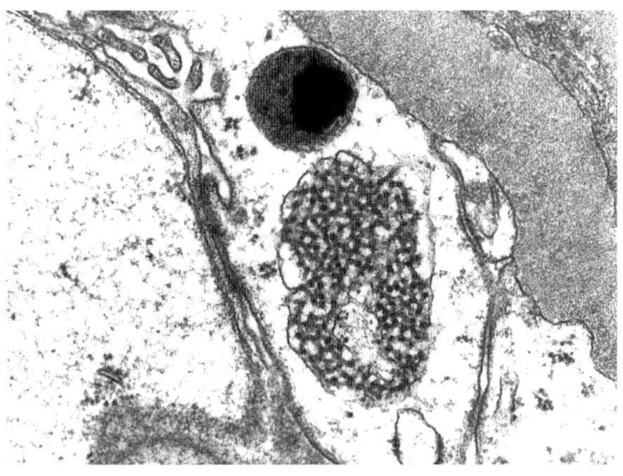

Figure 6-62

HIV-ASSOCIATED NEPHROPATHY

A tubuloreticular inclusion is present in a glomerular endothelial cell (electron micrograph).

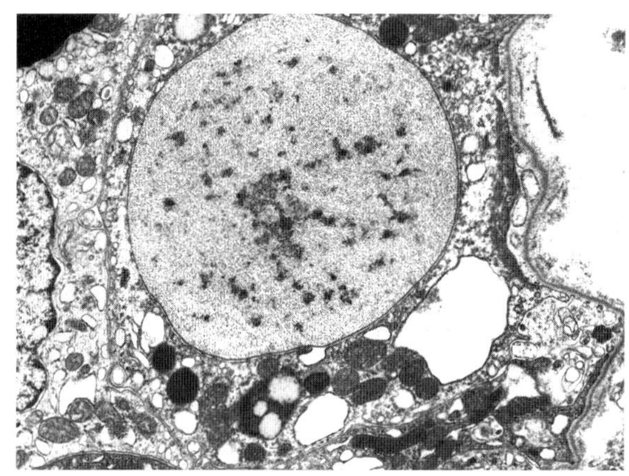

Figure 6-63

HIV-ASSOCIATED NEPHROPATHY

There is granular degeneration of the nucleus of a tubular cell (electron micrograph).

Differential Diagnosis. The major entity in the differential diagnosis is primary FSGS with collapsing features. HIV serologies are required for definitive distinction between these entities.

Included within the spectrum of HIV-AN are diffuse mesangial hypercellularity and MCD, which are more common in HIV-infected children than adults. These milder variants usually present with nephrotic syndrome and normal renal function, without the rapid course to renal failure that characterizes the collapsing form of HIV-AN.

HIV-AN must be differentiated from a variety of other glomerular and tubulointerstitial diseases that occur in HIV-infected patients (10). One of the most common immune complex–mediated glomerular lesions is membranoproliferative glomerulonephritis, particularly in HIV-infected patients co-infected with hepatitis C virus (HCV). These patients develop membranoproliferative glomerulonephritis type 1, with double contours and mesangial interposition, or membranoproliferative glomerulonephritis type 3, with mixed membranous features. Some of these patients have overlapping features of collapsing glomerulosclerosis and microcysts, suggesting superimposed HIV-AN.

Another common glomerular disease in the HIV population is IgA nephropathy, which may be associated with IgA-containing cryoglobulins. IgA nephropathy has been reported in both HIV-infected blacks and whites. Glomerular immune deposits eluted from the glomeruli of some of these patients have shown specificity for HIV envelope or core proteins.

Other glomerular lesions occurring in HIV-infected patients include membranous glomerulopathy, lupus-like glomerulonephritis, immunotactoid glomerulonephritis, acute postinfectious glomerulonephritis, and thrombotic microangiopathies.

Etiology and Pathogenesis. Recent advances suggest a role for direct viral infection of the kidney epithelial cells in the pathogenesis of HIV-AN, including tubular epithelial cells and podocytes (6). The kidney appears to be a reservoir for HIV infection in susceptible individuals (57).

The existence of an animal model of HIV-AN in mice transgenic for the noninfectious HIV genome (with a deletion of gag and pol, but expressing the HIV regulatory genes) also supports a role for viral gene expression in the kidney (5). Cross-renal transplantation experiments between transgenic mouse kidneys and nontransgenic litter mates have revealed that the renal phenotype is dictated by renal transgene expression (5). The failure of normal kidneys to develop nephropathy when transplanted into HIV transgenic mice argues strongly against a systemic cytokine effect.

Treatment and Prognosis. The course to renal failure is usually rapid. Early in the AIDS epidemic, the mean time to dialysis was less than 2 months (41). In the modern era, the use of HAART has reduced viral load and improved renal survival. Following HAART therapy, there may be dramatic improvement in the renal biopsy findings, with reversal of tubular microcysts (57).

SECONDARY FSGS MEDIATED BY ADAPTIVE STRUCTURAL-FUNCTIONAL RESPONSES

Definition. Secondary FSGS mediated by adaptive structural-functional responses denotes the pattern of focal and segmental glomerulosclerosis that develops in the course of a number of renal diseases in which there is either a reduced number of functioning nephrons or hemodynamic stress placed on an initially normal nephron population (see Table 6-1) (9,42).

Clinical Features. Secondary FSGS due to adaptive responses is most common in patients with obesity, the solitary kidney, hypertensive nephrosclerosis, sickle cell disease, reflux nephropathy, and any advanced renal process with significant loss of functioning nephrons. The particularly frequent problems of secondary FSGS associated with hypertensive nephrosclerosis and obesity will be covered in more depth in the sections below.

Knowledge of the presenting clinical features is essential to differentiate primary FSGS from secondary FSGS caused by structural-functional adaptations (42). Typically, patients with secondary FSGS manifest nephrotic or subnephrotic range proteinuria without full nephrotic syndrome. Thus they may have proteinuria of greater than 3.5 g/day, but usually without hypoalbuminemia, hypercholesterolemia, and edema. Because the development of FSGS is often a response to loss of functioning nephrons, most patients have a history of renal insufficiency (elevated serum creatinine, reduced glomerular filtration rate) preceding the development of nephrotic proteinuria. An exception is focal sclerosis secondary to morbid obesity. Obese patients often have a supernormal glomerular filtration rate that reflects the hyperfiltration/overwork state imposed by an increased ratio of body mass to renal mass (29).

Light Microscopic Findings. Glomerular hypertrophy, also known as glomerulomegaly, is a consistent finding (fig. 6-64). Although actual measurements of glomerular diameter are not performed routinely in clinical practice, an experienced renal pathologist can readily recognize hypertrophied glomeruli by light microscopy. As a simple rule of thumb, hypertrophied glomeruli usually do not fit into a 40X high-dry microscopic field. By measurement, the glomerular area is more than 1.5 times normal (11). Because the glomerular tuft is a sphere, glomerular hypertrophy is best assessed in a plane of section that transects the hilus of the glomerulus, at the epicenter of the glomerular tuft. The largest glomeruli recorded occur in oligomeganephronia, a

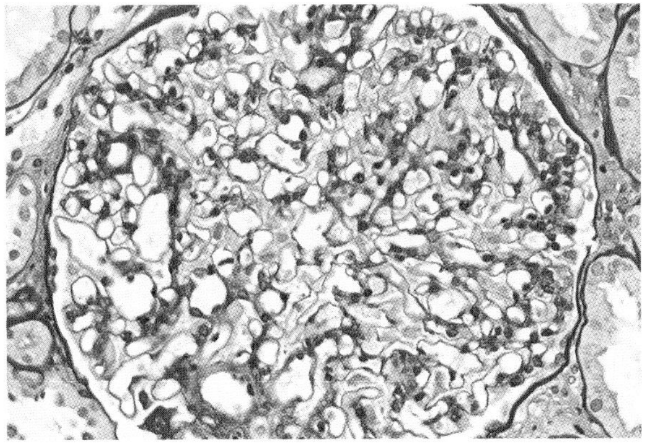

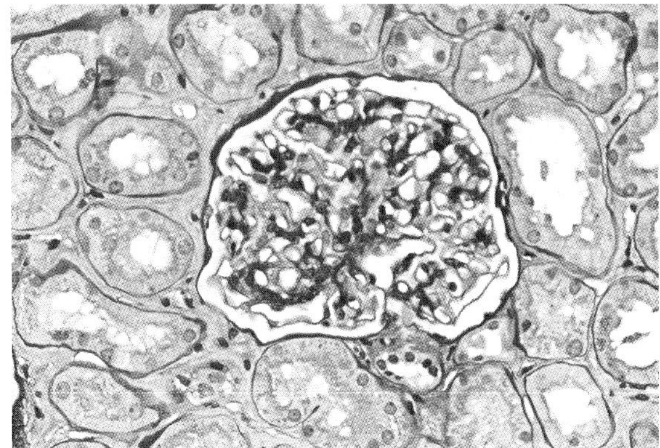

Figure 6-64

SECONDARY FSGS

Left: Glomerulomegaly is present in the nonsclerotic glomeruli of this patient with secondary FSGS due to obesity (a glomerulus from a normal age-matched control is shown on the right) (PAS stain).

Right: The glomerular diameter is approximately half that of the obese patient (PAS stain).

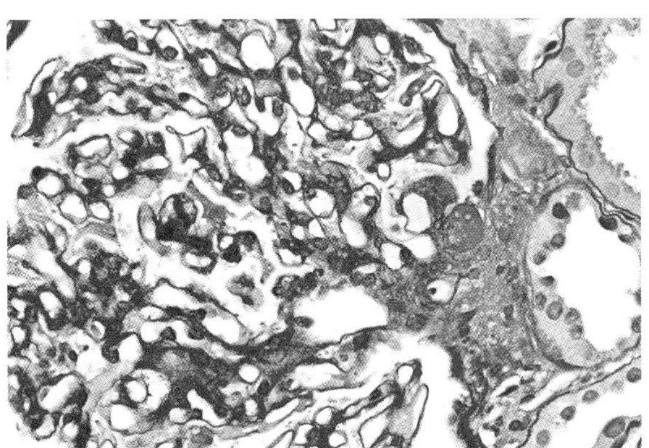

Figure 6-65

SECONDARY FSGS

An example from a patient with unilateral renal agenesis. The earliest lesion of sclerosis and hyalinosis arises from the vascular pole of this markedly hypertrophied glomerulus (PAS stain).

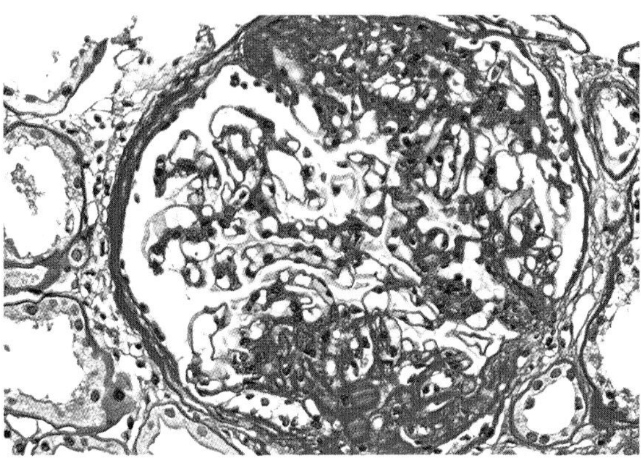

Figure 6-66

SECONDARY FSGS

Classic lesions of segmental sclerosis are present in this case of secondary FSGS related to obesity (PAS stain).

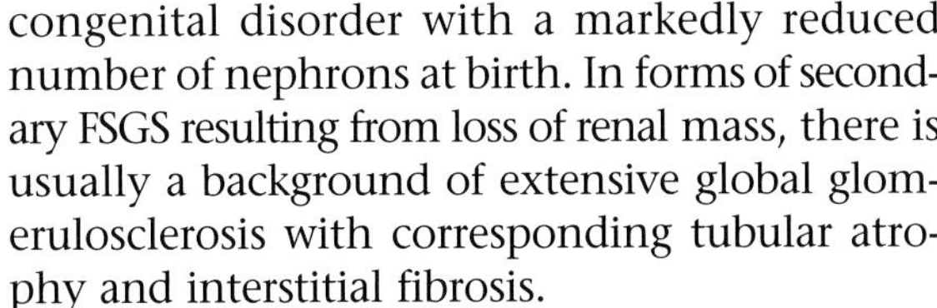

congenital disorder with a markedly reduced number of nephrons at birth. In forms of secondary FSGS resulting from loss of renal mass, there is usually a background of extensive global glomerulosclerosis with corresponding tubular atrophy and interstitial fibrosis.

Most forms of secondary FSGS have discrete segmental scars, often involving the perihilar regions of hypertrophied glomeruli (figs. 6-65, 6-66). Podocyte hypertrophy and hyperplasia are less frequent than in primary FSGS.

Secondary FSGS related to sickle cell disease usually displays distinctive morphologic features. There is often glomerular hypertrophy and glomerular capillary congestion by sickled erythrocytes. Glomerular capillaries that are not obliterated by the sclerotic lesions may display double contours resembling those seen in chronic thrombotic microangiopathy. These features likely reflect the unique pathogenesis of this lesion, which includes hyperfiltration and disturbed glomerular hemodynamics related to the intravascular sickling.

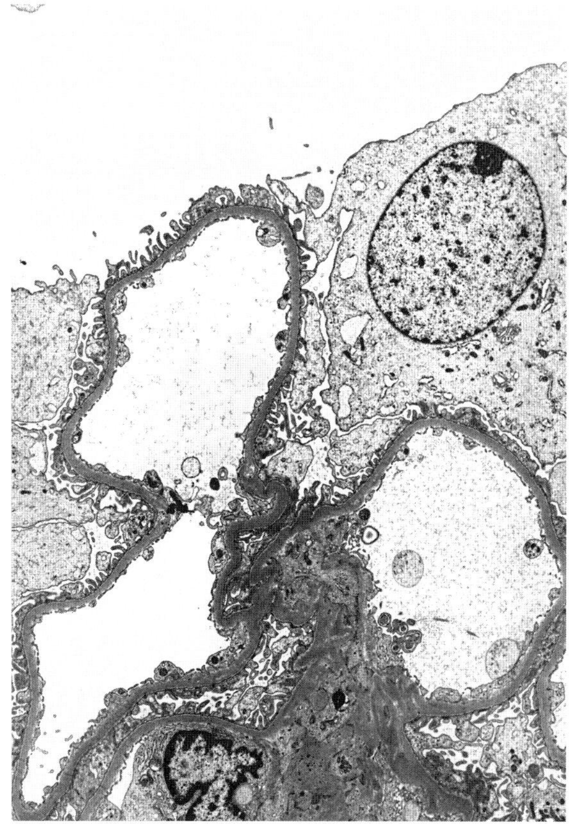

Figure 6-67

SECONDARY FSGS

Despite nephrotic-range proteinuria of over 5 g/day, there is minimal foot process effacement (involving approximately 10 percent of the glomerular capillary surface area) in this patient with secondary FSGS due to obesity (electron micrograph).

Immunofluorescence Findings. There is usually focal and segmental glomerular staining for IgM and C3 in lesions of segmental sclerosis.

Electron Microscopic Findings. The degree of foot process effacement is generally mild, affecting less than 50 percent of the total glomerular capillary surface area (fig. 6-67). Because of its variability, however, the percentage of foot processes that are effaced cannot be used as an absolute or specific criterion by which to distinguish primary from secondary FSGS.

Etiology and Pathogenesis. Secondary FSGS is thought to be mediated by increased glomerular capillary pressures and flow rates that occur as an adaptive response to the reduced number of functioning nephrons or other hemodynamic stresses (42). Increased wall tension causes mechanical strain on the connection between the podocyte foot process and the glomerular basement membrane, leading to local dilatation of capillaries and podocyte injury (33,34,39). If the tension on the podocyte is severe and prolonged, there is progressive cell body attenuation, pseudocyst formation, and ultimately, detachment from the glomerular basement membrane. Overload of the podocyte's lysosomal system with protein resorption droplets may promote cell autoinjury.

Podocyte detachment is the first committed lesion of segmental sclerosis, leaving bare patches of glomerular basement membrane. The concept of relative "podocyte insufficiency" proposed by Kriz (39) explains how these denuded segments come into contact with parietal epithelial cells, promoting synechiae to Bowman's capsule. If patent capillaries remain caught in the adhesion, a route of filtration into the periglomerular interstitium towards the tubular pole can lead to obliteration of the tubular pole and formation of atubular glomeruli, with microcystic dilatation of Bowman's capsule (35).

Treatment and Prognosis. Treatment of patients with secondary FSGS depends on the underlying condition. Correction of the underlying process, such as surgical repair for the patient with congenital heart disease, should be sought where appropriate. In patients with glomerular hyperfiltration due to reduction in functioning renal mass (such as following reflux nephropathy, surgical renal ablation, or renal agenesis), maneuvers to reduce glomerular capillary pressures are used. These include ACE inhibition, angiotensin II receptor antagonists, and a low protein diet. Steroids are uniformly ineffective in secondary FSGS and may even promote progressive sclerosis in patients with diabetes or obesity.

Secondary FSGS Due to Hypertensive Nephrosclerosis

Definition. This common cause of secondary FSGS in the older population is defined by the presence of lesions of focal and segmental glomerulosclerosis in the setting of hypertensive nephrosclerosis (51,54).

Clinical Features. Clinically, patients usually lack full nephrotic syndrome, although they may manifest modest or even high levels of nephrotic range proteinuria. A history of

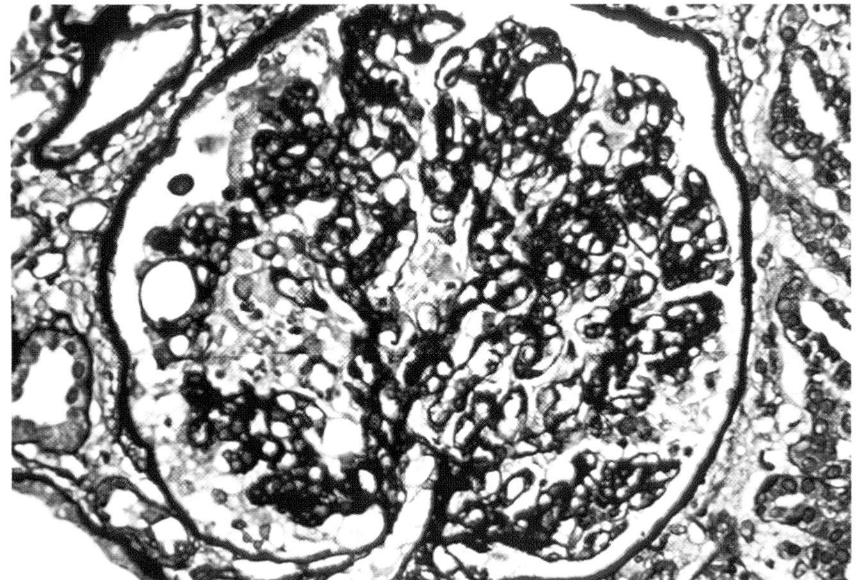

Figure 6-68

SECONDARY FSGS

A collapsing lesion of sclerosis is present in this patient with secondary FSGS related to renal artery stenosis and cholesterol embolization (JMS stain).

longstanding hypertension and atherosclerotic vascular disease can usually be elicited from the referring clinician. In cases with sequential measurements of renal function and urine protein excretion, it may be possible to document that the renal insufficiency predated the development of proteinuria by many months or even years.

Light Microscopic Findings. There is prominent arteriolosclerosis, arteriolar hyalinosis, and arteriosclerosis. The predilection for glomerular sclerosis to occur in the outer cortex, with formation of subcapsular scars, is readily appreciated in biopsies in which the renal capsule has been sampled. There is invariably prominent chronic tubulointerstitial disease and glomerular hypertrophy.

Lesions of segmental sclerosis and hyalinosis are often perihilar and develop in glomeruli that are also hypertrophied. Most lesions of segmental sclerosis are of the classic type, with solidification of the tuft by increased matrix and hyaline. In some cases there are also cellular or collapsing features that may mimic primary FSGS (fig. 6-68). This is especially the case in patients with secondary FSGS in the setting of cholesterol embolization or other acute vaso-occlusive events (18).

A common feature of secondary FSGS due to hypertensive nephrosclerosis is the development of atubular glomeruli, with cystic dilatation of Bowman's space (figs. 6-69, 6-70) (35). Atubular glomeruli are most abundant in the subcapsular region (fig. 6-69). The tuft is shrunken and partially resorbed into Bowman's capsule.

Immunofluorescence Findings. Nonspecific staining for IgM and C3 is usually seen in the sclerosing glomerular and vascular lesions.

Electron Microscopic Findings. Foot process effacement is usually relatively mild. There may be ischemic-type wrinkling and thickening of the glomerular basement membranes.

Differential Diagnosis. The presence of longstanding hypertension (preceding the development of proteinuria), prominent vascular disease, glomerular hypertrophy, predominantly perihilar distribution of the segmental lesions, and mild foot process effacement help to differentiate this entity from primary FSGS.

Etiology and Pathogenesis. A secondary pattern of FSGS results from both elevated glomerular capillary pressure attributable to systemic hypertension and the adaptive glomerular responses that follow loss of functioning nephrons due to progressive hypertensive nephrosclerosis.

Treatment and Prognosis. A proper diagnosis is essential to avoid inappropriate treatment with immunosuppressive therapy. Treatment should be directed at the hypertension. Angiotensin receptor blockade or ACE inhibitors may be helpful, not only to treat the systemic hypertension, but to lower glomerular intracapillary pressures.

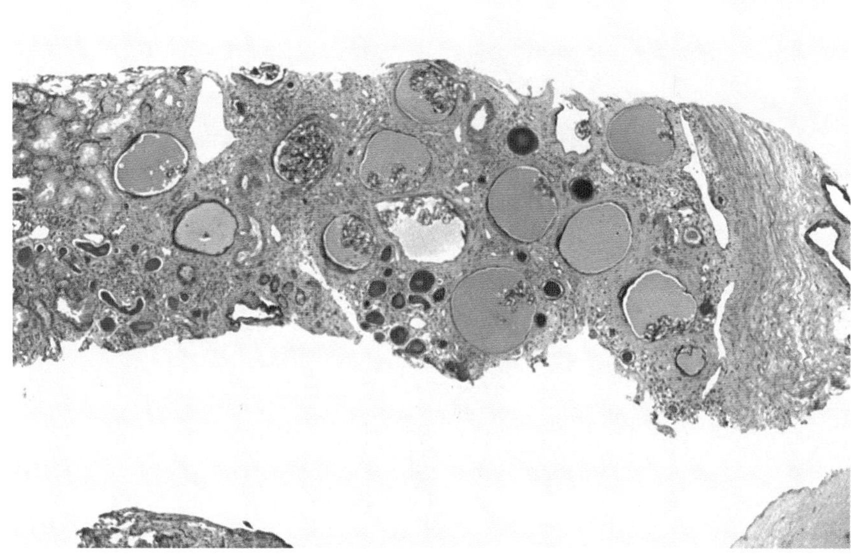

Figure 6-69

SECONDARY FSGS

A subcapsular scar containing many cystically dilated, atubular glomeruli is seen in this patient with secondary FSGS related to hypertensive arterionephrosclerosis (PAS stain).

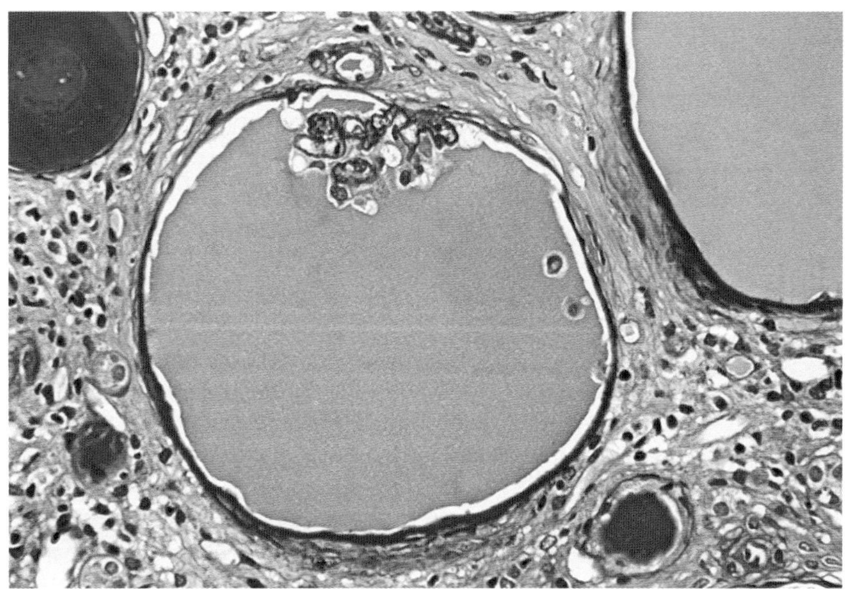

Figure 6-70

SECONDARY FSGS

High-power view of an atubular glomerulus with a shrunken tuft and dilated urinary space from the same case of hypertensive arterionephrosclerosis shown in figure 6-69 (PAS stain).

Secondary FSGS Related to Obesity (Obesity-Related Glomerulopathy)

Definition. Obesity-related glomerulopathy is defined as a secondary form of focal segmental glomerulosclerosis seen in obese patients (body mass index [BMI] over 30) with glomerulomegaly (29).

Clinical Features. Obesity-related glomerulopathy may develop in patients with grade 1 obesity (BMI, 30.0 to 34.9), grade 2 obesity (BMI, 35.0 to 39.9), and grade 3 or morbid obesity (BMI, 40 or higher). Early in the disease, there is often a supernormal glomerular filtration rate (more than 120 mL/min). There is typically subnephrotic or nephrotic range proteinuria, without full nephrotic syndrome. Even in patients with nephrotic range proteinuria, serum albumin is usually normal.

Light Microscopic Findings. Glomerular hypertrophy, also known as glomerulomegaly, is a consistent finding (29). The FSGS is usually mild, affecting a minority of hypertrophied glomeruli (29,53). Lesions are usually perihilar, with associated hyalinosis (fig. 6-66). There is little if any podocyte reactivity. FSGS usually develops in the absence of significant background tubulointerstitial disease. Mild mesangial sclerosis may be seen, resembling the changes of early diabetic glomerulosclerosis.

Electron Microscopic Findings. Foot process effacement is generally mild and usually does not exceed 50 percent of the glomerular capillary surface area (fig. 6-67).

Differential Diagnosis. The major entity in the differential diagnosis is primary FSGS. Primary FSGS occurring in the obese patient can usually be distinguished from obesity-related glomerulopathy by the presence of severe nephrotic range proteinuria with full nephrotic syndrome and, pathologically, by the presence of extensive foot process effacement with severe podocyte alterations as detected by electron microscopy (29).

Etiology and Pathogenesis. There is glomerular overwork imposed by increased body mass relative to kidney mass. Obesity increases renal plasma flow and the glomerular filtration rate. Hypoxia related to sleep apnea activates the sympathetic nervous system, thereby stimulating the renin-angiotensin system.

Treatment and Prognosis. It is rare for patients with obesity-related glomerulopathy to progress to end-stage renal disease. Steroid therapy is contraindicated and may actually promote weight gain and latent diabetes. Reductions of proteinuria can be achieved with weight loss, sleep apnea therapy, and angiotensin receptor blockade or ACE inhibitors.

REFERENCES

1. Barisoni L, D'Agati V. The changing epidemiology of focal segmental glomerulosclerosis in New York City. Mod Pathol 1994;7:156A.
2. Barisoni L, Kriz W, Mundel P, D'Agati V. The dysregulated podocyte phenotype: a novel concept in the pathogenesis of collapsing idiopathic focal segmental glomerulosclerosis and HIV-associated nephropathy. J Am Soc Nephrol 1999;10:51–61.
3. Beaman M, Howie AJ, Hardwicke J, Michael M, Adu D. The glomerular tip lesion: a steroid responsive nephrotic syndrome. Clin Nephrol 1987;27:217–21.
4. Boute N, GribouvaL O, Roselli S, et al. NPHS2, encoding the glomerular protein podocin, is mutated in autosomal recessive steroid-resistant nephrotic syndrome. Nat Genet 2000;24:349–54.
5. Bruggeman LA, Dikman S, Meng C, Quaggin SE, Coffman TM, Klotman PR. Nephropathy in human immunodeficiency virus-1 transgenic mice is due to renal transgene expression. J Clin Invest 1997;100:84–92.
6. Bruggeman LA, Ross MD, Tanji N, et al. Renal epithelium is a previously unrecognized site of HIV-1 infection. J Am Soc Nephrol 2000;11:2079–87.
7. Cameron JS, Turner DR, Ogg CS, Chantler C, Williams DS. The long-term prognosis of patients with focal segmental glomerulosclerosis. Clin Nephrol 1978;10:213–8.
8. D'Agati V. Pathologic classification of focal segmental glomerulosclerosis. Semin Nephrol 2003;23:117–34.
9. D'Agati V. The many masks of focal segmental glomerulosclerosis. Kidney Int 1994;46:1223–41
10. D'Agati V, Appel GB. Renal pathology of human immunodeficiency virus infection. Semin Nephrol 1998;18:406–21.
11. D'Agati VD, Fogo AB, Bruijn JA, Jennette JC. Pathologic classification of focal segmental glomerulosclerosis: a working proposal. Am J Kidney Dis 2004;43:368–82.
12. D'Agati VD, Suh JI, Carbone L, Cheng JT, Appel G. Pathology of HIV-associated nephropathy: a detailed morphologic and comparative study. Kidney Int 1989;35:1358–70.
13. Detwiler RK, Falk RJ, Hogan SL, Jennette JC. Collapsing glomerulopathy: a clinically and pathologically distinct variant of focal segmental glomerulosclerosis. Kidney Int 1994;45:1416–24.
14. Eddy AA. Expression of genes that promote renal interstitial fibrosis in rats with proteinuria. Kidney Int 1996;54(Suppl):S49–54.
15. Eddy AA. Interstitial nephritis induced by protein-overload proteinuria. Am J Pathol 1989;135:719–33.

16. Focal segmental glomerulosclerosis in children with idiopathic nephrotic syndrome. A report of the Southwest Pediatric Nephrology Study Group. Kidney Int 1985;27:442–9.
17. Fogo A, Glick AD, Horn SL, Horn RG. Is focal segmental glomerulosclerosis really focal? Distribution of lesions in adults and children. Kidney Int 1995;47:1690–6.
18. Greenberg A, Bastacky SI, Iqbal A, Borochovitz D, Johnson JP. Focal segmental glomerulosclerosis associated with nephrotic syndrome in cholesterol embolization: clinicopathologic correlations. Am J Kidney Dis 1997;29:334–44.
19. Haas M, Meehan SM, Karrison TG, Spargo BH. Changing etiologies of unexplained adult nephrotic syndrome: a comparison of renal biopsy findings from 1976-1979 and 1995-1997. Am J Kidney Dis 1997;30:621–31.
20. Haas M, Spargo BH, Coventry S. Increasing incidence of focal-segmental glomerulosclerosis among adult nephropathies: a 20-year renal biopsy study. Am J Kidney Dis 1995;26:740–50.
21. Haas M, Yousefzadeh N. Glomerular tip lesion in minimal change nephropathy: a study of autopsies before 1950. Am J Kidney Dis 2002;39: 1168–75.
22. Habib R. Focal glomerular sclerosis [Editorial]. Kidney Int 1973;4:355–61.
23. Hogan-Moulton AE, Hogan S, Falk R, Jennette JC. Glomerular tip lesion (GTL): clinical features, response to corticosteroids and comparison to focal segmental glomerulosclerosis (FSGS). J Am Soc Nephrol 1997;8:87A.
24. Howie AJ, Brewer DB. The glomerular tip lesion: a previously undescribed type of segmental glomerular abnormality. J Pathol 1984;142:205–20.
25. Huppes W, Hene RJ, Kooiker CJ. The glomerular tip lesion: a distinct entity or not? J Pathol 1988;154:187–90.
26. Ingulli E, Tejani A. Racial differences in the incidence and renal outcome of idiopathic focal segmental glomerulosclerosis in children. Pediatr Nephrol 1991;5:393–7.
27. Iskandar SS, Browning MC, Lorentz WB. C1q nephropathy: a pediatric clinicopathologic study. Am J Kidney Dis 1991;18:459–65.
28. Jennette JC, Hipp CG. C1q nephropathy: a distinct pathologic entity usually causing nephrotic syndrome. Am J Kidney Dis 1985;6:103–10.
29. Kambham N, Markowitz GS, Valeri AM, Lin J, D'Agati VD. Obesity-related glomerulopathy: an emerging epidemic. Kidney Int 2001;59:1498–509.
30. Kaplan JM, Kim SH, North KN, et al. Mutations in ACTN4, encoding alpha-actinin-4, cause familial focal segmental glomerulosclerosis. Nat Genet 2000;24:251–6.
31. Kestila M, Lenkkeri U, Mannikko M, et al. Positionally cloned gene for a novel glomerular protein—nephrin—is mutated in congenital nephrotic syndrome. Mol Cell 1998;1:575–82.
32. Korbet SM. Primary focal segmental glomerulosclerosis. J Am Soc Nephrol 1998;9:1333–40.
33. Kriz W, Elger M, Nagata M, et al. The role of podocytes in the development of glomerular sclerosis. Kidney Int 1994;45(Suppl):S64–72.
34. Kriz W, Gretz N, Lemley KV. Progression of glomerular diseases: is the podocyte the culprit? 1998;54:687–97.
35. Kriz W, Hosser H, Hahnel B, Gretz N, Provoost AP. From segmental glomerulosclerosis to total nephron degeneration and interstitial fibrosis: a histopathologic study in rat models and human glomerulopathies. Nephrol Dial Transplant 1998;13:2781–98.
36. Markowitz GS, Appel GB, Fine PL, et al. Collapsing focal segmental glomerulosclerosis following high dose pamidronate. J Am Soc Nephrol 2001;12:1164–72.
37. Markowitz GS, Schwimmer JA, Stokes MB, et al. C1q nephropathy: a variant of focal segmental glomerulosclerosis. Kidney Int 2003;64:1232–40.
38. Mathis BJ, Kim SH, Calabrese K, et al. A locus for inherited focal segmental glomerulosclerosis maps to chromosome 19q13. Kidney Intern 1998;53:282–6.
39. Nagata M, Kriz W. Glomerular damage after uninephrectomy in young rats. II. Mechanical stress on podocytes as a pathway to sclerosis. Kidney Int 1992;42:148–60.
40. Pei Y, Cattran D, Delmore T, Katz A, Lang A, Rance P. Evidence suggesting under-treatment in adults with idiopathic focal segmental glomerulosclerosis. Regional Glomerulonephritis Registry Study. Am J Med 1987;82:938–44.
41. Rao TK, Filippone EJ, Nicastri AD, et al. Associated focal and segmental glomerulosclerosis in the acquired immunodeficiency syndrome. N Engl J Med 1984;310:669–73.
42. Rennke HG, Klein PS. Pathogenesis and significance of nonprimary focal and segmental glomerulosclerosis. Am J Kidney Dis 1989;13:443–56.
43. Rich AR. A hitherto undescribed vulnerability of the juxta-medullary glomeruli in lipoid nephrosis. Bull Johns Hopkins Hosp 1957;100:173–86.
44. Savin VJ, Sharma R, Sharma M, et al. Circulating factor associated with increased glomerular permeability to albumin in recurrent focal segmental glomerulosclerosis. N Engl J Med 1996;334:878–83.
45. Schoeneman MJ, Bennett B, Greifer I. The natural history of focal segmental glomerulosclerosis with and without mesangial hypercellularity in children. Clin Nephrol 1978;9:45–54.

46. Schwartz MM, Evans J, Bain R, Korbet SM. Focal segmental glomerulosclerosis: prognostic implication of the cellular lesion. J Am Soc Nephrol 1999;10:1900–7.
47. Schwartz MM, Lewis EJ. Focal segmental glomerular sclerosis: the cellular lesion. Kidney Int 1985;28:968–74.
48. Shankland SJ, Eitner F, Hudkins KL, Goodpaster T, D'Agati V, Alpers CE. Differential expression of cyclin-dependent kinase inhibitors in human glomerular disease: role in podocyte proliferation and maturation. Kidney Int 2000;58:674–83.
49. Smith SM, Hoy WE, Cobb L. Low incidence of glomerulosclerosis in normal kidneys. Arch Pathol Lab Med 1989;113:1253–5.
50. Stokes MB, Markowitz GS, Lin J, Valeri AM, D'Agati VD. Glomerular tip lesion: a distinct entity within the minimal change disease/focal segmental glomerulosclerosis spectrum. Kidney Int 2004;65:1690–702.
51. Thadhani R, Pascual M, Nickeleit V, Tolkoff-Rubin N, Colvin R. Preliminary description of focal segmental glomerulosclerosis in patients with renovascular disease. Lancet 1996;347:231–3.
52. Valeri A, Barisoni L, Appel GB, Seigle R, D'Agati V. Idiopathic collapsing focal segmental glomerulosclerosis: a clinicopathologic study. Kidney Int 1996;50:1734–46.
53. Verani RR. Obesity-associated focal segmental glomerulosclerosis: pathologic features of the lesion and relationship with cardiomegaly and hyperlipidemia. Am J Kidney Dis 1992;20:629–34.
54. Wehrmann M, Bohle A. The long-term prognosis of benign nephrosclerosis accompanied by focal glomerulosclerosis and renal cortical interstitial fibrosis, designated so-called decompensated benign nephrosclerosis by Fahr, Bohle and Ratscheck. Pathol Res Pract 1998;194:571–6.
55. Weiss MA, Daquioag E, Margolin EG, Pollack VE. Nephrotic syndrome, progressive irreversible renal failure, and glomerular "collapse." A new clinicopathologic entity? Am J Kidney Dis 1986; 7:20–8.
56. Winn MP. Not all in the family: mutations of podocin in sporadic steroid-resistant nephrotic syndrome. J Am Soc Nephrol 2002:13:577–9.
57. Winston JA, Bruggeman LA, Ross MD, et al. Nephropathy and establishment of a renal reservoir of HIV type 1 during primary infection. N Engl J Med 2001;344:1979–84.
58. Yoshikawa N, Ito H, Akamatsu R, et al. Focal segmental glomerulosclerosis with and without nephrotic syndrome in children. J Pediatr 1986;109:65–70.

7 MEMBRANOUS GLOMERULOPATHY

PRIMARY (IDIOPATHIC) MEMBRANOUS GLOMERULOPATHY

Definition. Membranous glomerulopathy (MGN), also known as *membranous glomerulonephritis* or *membranous nephropathy*, is defined pathologically as a spectrum of glomerular capillary wall abnormalities resulting from the formation of subepithelial immune deposits. The term membranous glomerulopathy emphasizes the major light microscopic finding of diffuse glomerular capillary wall thickening seen in the fully developed forms of the disease. Because significant glomerular hypercellularity and inflammatory cell infiltration are not characteristic features of this disease, most pathologists prefer the term membranous glomerulopathy over glomerulonephritis.

Four major stages have been defined based primarily on histologic and ultrastructural features (Table 7-1) (16). Although the presence of subepithelial deposits is the initiating factor that gives rise to the glomerular capillary wall changes, these deposits may not be identifiable in all stages. Conversely, because subepithelial immune deposits are not specific to MGN, the diagnosis requires careful exclusion of other entities that manifest such deposits. The clinical course is usually dominated by proteinuria, often associated with the nephrotic syndrome. However, because there are no specific clinical features, a proper diagnosis can only be made by the pathologic examination of renal tissue.

Approximately 60 to 80 percent of cases are primary (idiopathic); the remainder develop as a secondary glomerular disease in the setting of a variety of autoimmune, infectious, neoplastic, and other systemic diseases, or following exposure to certain medications (Table 7-2) (20). Because the clinical approach to MGN is tailored to the stage of the disease and knowledge of whether it is primary or secondary, proper management requires a systematic exclusion of secondary forms.

Clinical Features. The incidence of primary MGN varies depending on patient age and the population. Although it occurs at all ages, it is much more common in adults than children, with a peak incidence in the fourth and fifth decades (7). MGN comprises less than 2 percent of all cases of idiopathic nephrotic syndrome in children under the age of 5 years, but the incidence increases progressively through adolescence and into adulthood; by adulthood it is the most common cause of idiopathic nephrotic syndrome in white adults, accounting for 40 to

Table 7-1

STAGES OF MEMBRANOUS GLOMERULOPATHY

Stage	LM[a]	IF	EM
1	GBM normal thickness or slightly thickened, slight GBM vacuolization	IgG, C3, finely granular	Small focal subepi deposits, no spikes, focal foot process effacement
2	GBM moderately thickened, spikes and vacuolizations	IgG, C3, moderate size, granular	Diffuse subepi deposits, well-developed spikes, diffuse foot process effacement
3	GBM markedly thickened, chain-like appearance, residual spikes, vacuoles	IgG, C3, coarsely granular	Intramembranous deposits, resorbed deposits, lacunae, spikes, neomembrane, diffuse foot process effacement
4	GBM markedly thickened, few spikes, vacuoles, sclerotic glomeruli	IgG, C3 sparse; IgM, C3 in sclerotic segments	Few deposits, lacunae, thickened sclerotic GBM, some restored foot processes

[a]LM = light microscopy; IF = immunofluorescence microscopy; EM = electron microscopy; GBM = glomerular basement membrane; Subepi = subepithelial.

Table 7-2

CONDITIONS ASSOCIATED WITH MEMBRANOUS GLOMERULOPATHY

Autoimmune/Collagen Vascular Diseases
Systemic lupus erythematosus
Rheumatoid arthritis
Mixed connective tissue disease
Sjögren's syndrome
Autoimmune thyroiditis
Primary biliary cirrhosis
Ankylosing spondylitis
Crohn's disease
Infections
Hepatitis B
Hepatitis C
Syphilis (congenital or latent)
Schistosomiasis
Malaria
Filariasis
Medications
Gold salts
Penicillamine
Captopril
Mercury
Trimethadione
Bucillamine
Neoplasms
Carcinomas of colon, lung, breast, stomach, pancreas, kidney, prostate, cervix
Melanoma
Wilms' tumor
Lymphocytic leukemia
Hodgkin's disease
Non-Hodgkin's lymphoma
Miscellaneous
Sarcoidosis
Sickle cell disease
Guillain-Barre syndrome
Angiofollicular lymph node hyperplasia (Castleman's disease)

50 percent of cases. This disease incidence is influenced by both sex and race. MGN is about 1.5 to 2.0 times more common in males than females. It is also more common in whites than blacks. Among black adults, primary focal segmental glomerulosclerosis has surpassed MGN as the most common cause of idiopathic nephrotic syndrome in the past decade.

The clinical presentation of patients with primary MGN is dominated by heavy proteinuria. Nephrotic range proteinuria (more than 3.5 g/day) is detectable at clinical outset in 50 to 80 percent of patients, and many have full nephrotic syndrome. The remainder have subnephrotic, often asymptomatic proteinuria that may be detected as an incidental finding during a routine physical examination. Proteinuria exceeds 10 g in approximately 30 percent of patients. Features of nephrotic syndrome, including edema, hypoalbuminemia, hypercholesterolemia, and thrombotic tendency, are severe presenting manifestations in some cases. The proteinuria is predominantly nonselective, as determined by studies that measure the immunoglobulin (Ig)G/transferrin clearance ratio. Microhematuria is detectable in up to half of patients at presentation, although red blood cell casts are rarely seen. Gross hematuria is exceedingly rare and may herald the development of superimposed acute renal vein thrombosis. Approximately half of patients have an elevated serum creatinine level at the time of presentation, but renal failure is rarely a major presenting feature. Hypertension is present in one quarter to half of cases. Complement membrane attack complex (C5b-9) may be detected in the urine and appears to correlate with disease activity, but is not used as a general diagnostic tool in clinical practice.

Pathologic Findings by Stage. Four major stages of MGN have been defined by Ehrenreich and Churg (16) according to the histologic and ultrastructural findings. These stages give an approximate indication of the duration and evolution of the disease process, but they do not represent a choreographed sequence in all patients. MGN must be envisioned as a dynamic process in which there may be new waves of immune deposition superimposed on more chronic basement membrane changes, resulting in multiple generations of immune deposits. Moreover, not all patients pass from stage 1 through to stage 4, and some undergo spontaneous resolution at early stages. Finally, several stages of disease may be present simultaneously in different glomeruli or adjacent glomerular capillaries, in the same biopsy. In such cases, the stage may be designated as 2 to 3 or 3 to 4, for example, or as the dominant stage.

Light Microscopic Findings. In stage 1, thickening of the glomerular capillary walls is usually not detected by light microscopy using the hematoxylin and eosin (H&E) or periodic acid–Schiff (PAS) stains, although subepithelial deposits are readily detected at this early stage by immunofluorescence and electron microscopy

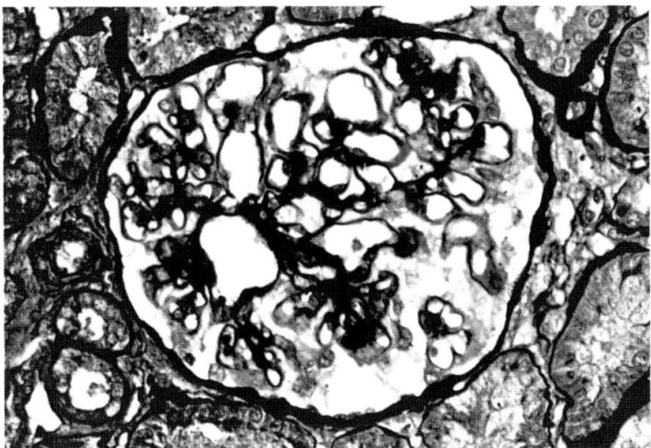

Figure 7-1

MEMBRANOUS GLOMERULOPATHY (MGN) STAGE 1

The glomerulus is normocellular, with basement membranes of normal thickness and texture. There is slight dilatation of the glomerular capillary lumens (Jones methenamine silver [JMS] stain).

(fig. 7-1). Trichrome-stained specimens viewed under 100X oil immersion may reveal minute subepithelial fuchsinophilic deposits contrasting with the blue-staining glomerular basement membranes. With the Jones methenamine silver (JMS) stain, the glomerular basement membranes either show no abnormalities or contain subtle vacuolizations, corresponding to indentations made by the nonargyrophilic subepithelial deposits (fig. 7-2). The glomerular tuft is usually normocellular, without mesangial widening. A clue to the diagnosis of MGN, even in early disease, is an enlarged, patulous appearance of the glomerular capillary lumens. This is probably due to effacement of the foot processes, which causes increased compliance of the glomerular capillary walls. Visceral epithelial cells appear swollen. But for the presence of intracytoplasmic lipid and protein resorption droplets within tubular epithelial cells, the tubulointerstitial compartment may appear unremarkable. Interstitial foam cells, a feature of chronic lipiduria, are rare in stage 1 disease. Vessels show no characteristic features.

In stage 2, MGN reaches its most fully expressed form. There is usually obvious thickening and rigidity of the glomerular capillary walls in a diffuse and regular distribution, visible with all the histologic stains (figs. 7-3–7-10). The apparently uniform thickening seen by the H&E stain can be resolved, with special stains, into

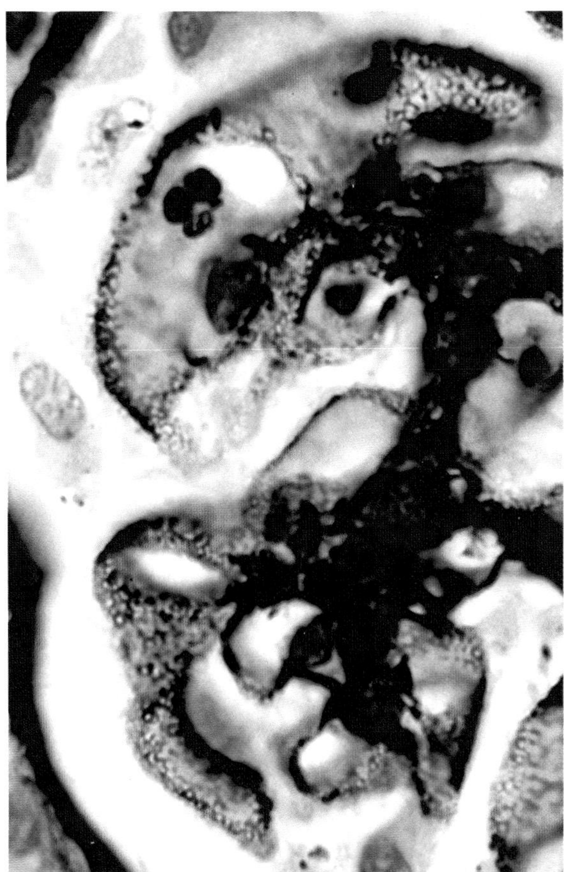

Figure 7-2

MGN STAGE 1

Vacuolization of the glomerular basement membranes is seen where cut obliquely, owing to indentation by deposits. No spikes are identified (JMS stain).

basement membrane spikes separating subepithelial deposits. Spikes consist of perpendicular projections of basement membrane material along the outer aspect of the glomerular basement membrane, resembling the bristles on a fine-tooth comb whose backbone corresponds to the glomerular basement membrane. Spikes are most readily discerned with the JMS stain at 100X magnification, but can also be seen with a good quality PAS stain in most cases (figs. 7-5–7-9). A well-differentiated trichrome stain delimits large subepithelial fuchsinophilic deposits separated by blue-staining basement membrane spikes (fig. 7-10). Where the glomerular basement membrane is cut en face, vacuolizations or reticulations impart a "Swiss-cheese" appearance to the glomerular basement

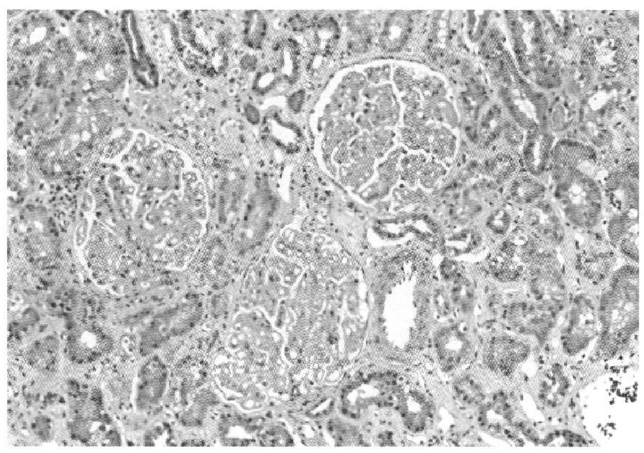

Figure 7-3

MGN STAGE 2

There is diffuse and regular thickening of the glomerular capillary walls. Proximal tubules contain focal intracytoplasmic lipid resorption droplets (hematoxylin and eosin [H&E] stain).

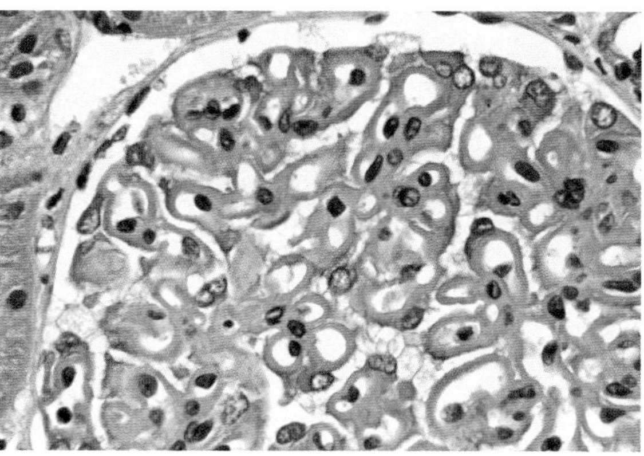

Figure 7-4

MGN STAGE 2

The glomerular capillary walls are uniformly thickened and have a rigid aspect (H&E stain).

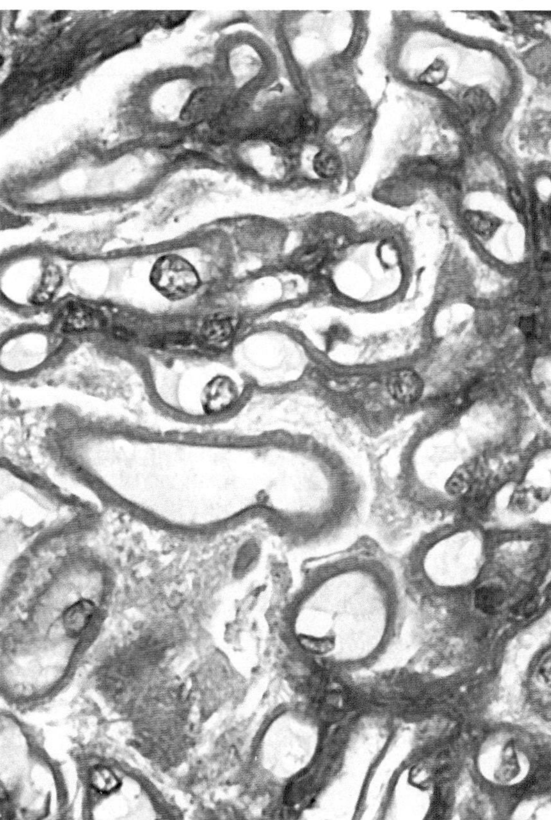

Figure 7-5

MGN STAGE 2

The periodic acid–Schiff (PAS) stain reveals delicate spiking of the glomerular basement membranes.

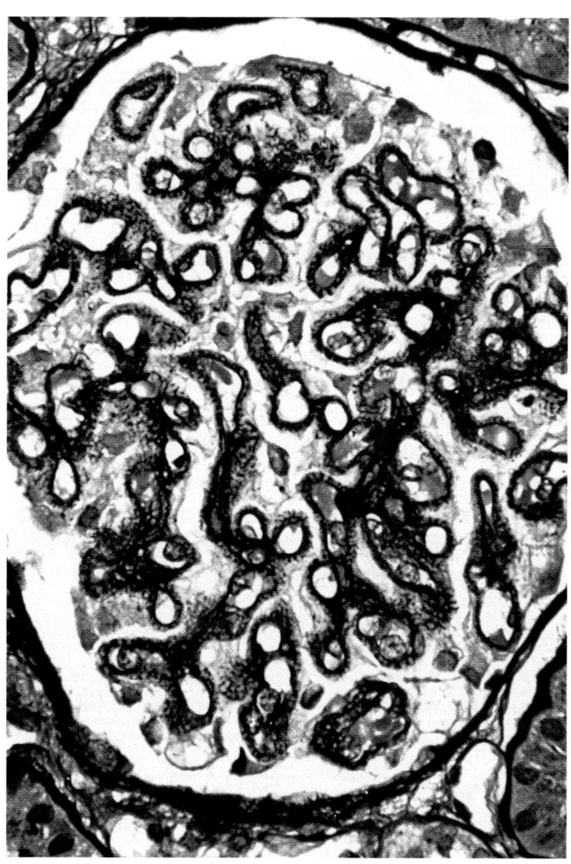

Figure 7-6

MGN STAGE 2

The glomerular basement membrane spikes are best delineated with the JMS stain. There is diffuse swelling of the podocytes.

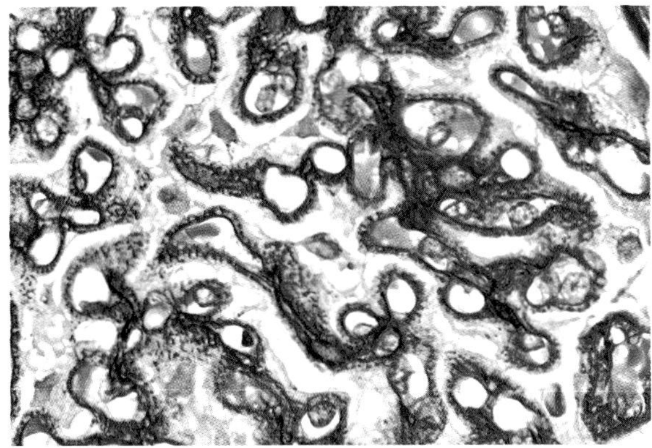

Figure 7-7

MGN STAGE 2

The spikes project at right angles from the glomerular basement membrane and resemble the bristles on a comb. The immune deposits located between the spikes are nonargyrophilic and therefore are seen as clear apparent spaces between the individual spikes. All glomerular capillary walls are affected uniformly (JMS stain).

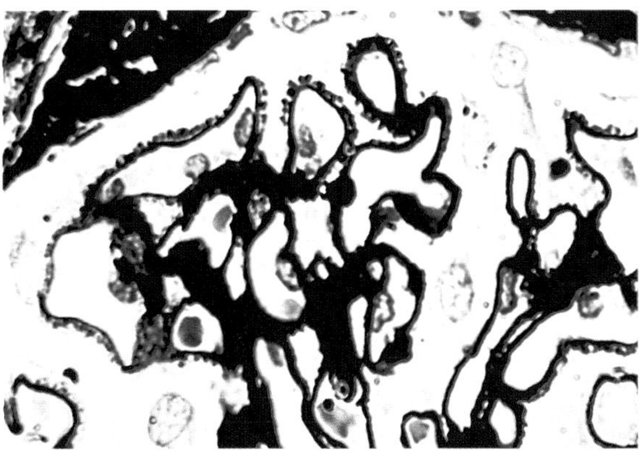

Figure 7-8

MGN STAGE 2

Spikes are detected in only those capillaries that are cut in cross section. In practice, spikes may be difficult to demonstrate, depending on the plane of section (JMS stain).

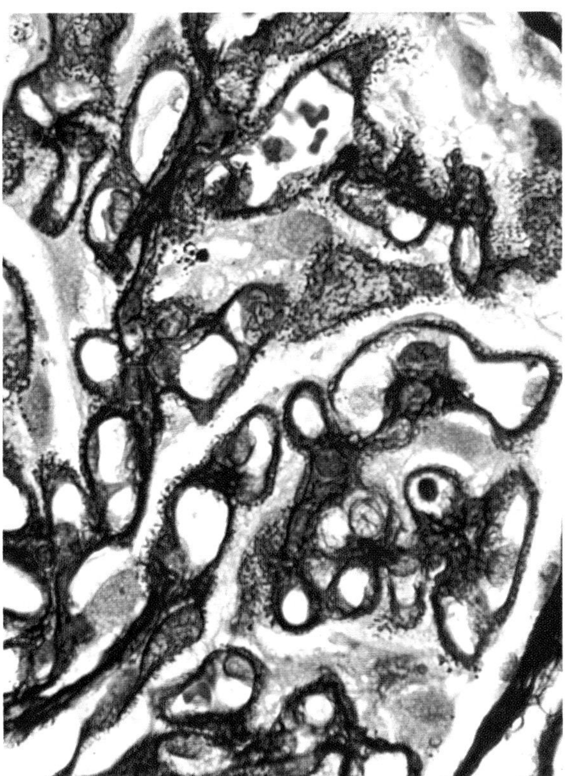

Figure 7-9

MGN STAGE 2

Where the glomerular basement membranes are cut en face, the spikes produce a reticulated network (JMS stain).

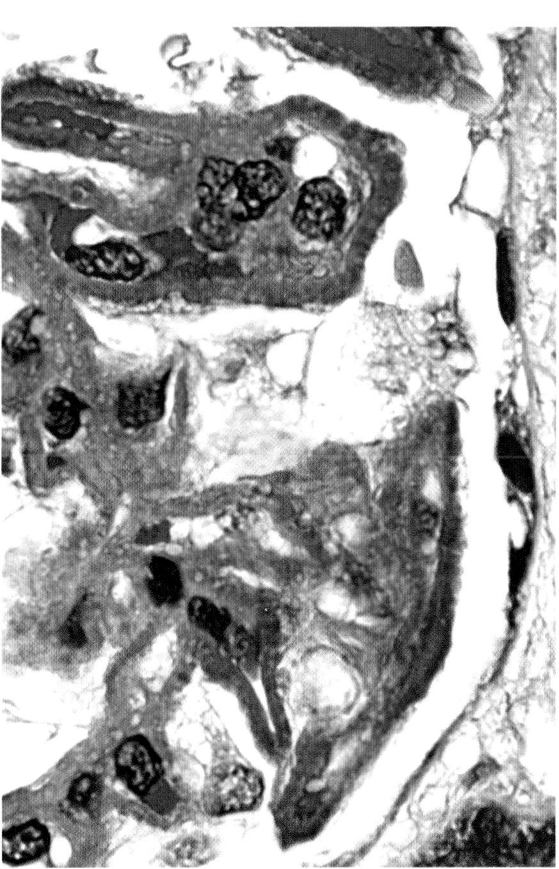

Figure 7-10

MGN STAGE 2

The subepithelial deposits stain red and the basement membrane spikes stain blue with the trichrome stain.

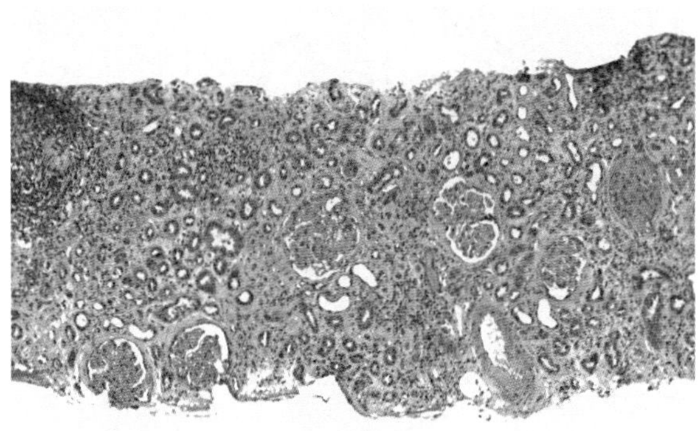

Figure 7-11

MGN STAGE 2

There is severe interstitial fibrosis, inflammation, and tubular atrophy that appears out of proportion to the glomerular disease in a patient with severe unremitting nephrotic syndrome of 3 years' duration (H&E stain).

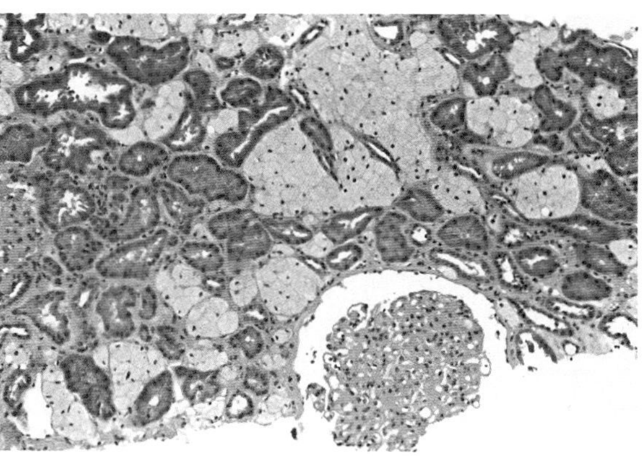

Figure 7-12

MGN STAGE 2

There are numerous interstitial foam cells in this patient with MGN developing in the solitary kidney, with associated glomerular hypertrophy (H&E stain).

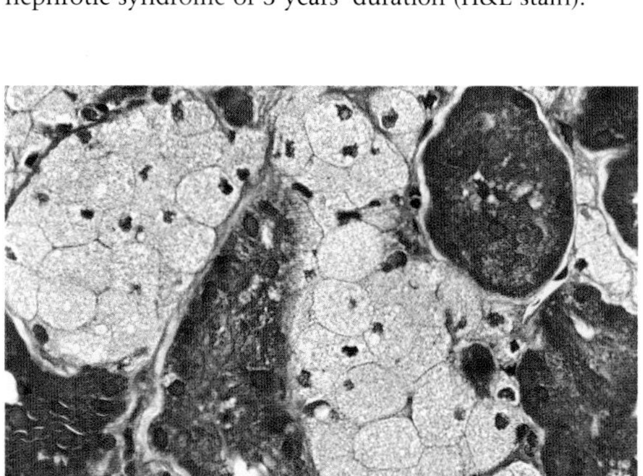

Figure 7-13

MGN STAGE 2

The interstitial foam cells have a bubbly cytoplasm and form large interstitial aggregates between the tubules (Masson trichrome stain).

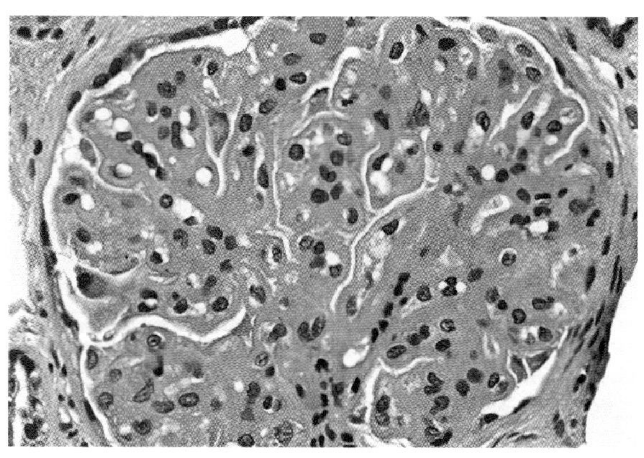

Figure 7-14

MGN STAGE 3

The marked glomerular capillary wall thickening encroaches on the glomerular capillary lumens, and is associated with mesangial sclerosis and focal adhesion to Bowman's capsule (H&E stain).

membrane (fig. 7-9). This helpful finding results from the three-dimensional extension of basement membrane material (JMS positive) around and between the subepithelial deposits (JMS negative), as revealed by grazing cuts of the glomerular capillary wall. Focal tubular atrophy and interstitial fibrosis may occur. In some cases, there is disproportionate injury to the tubulointerstitial compartment, with prominent tubular degenerative and regenerative changes (fig. 7-11). This tubular damage is more commonly observed in patients with severe unremitting proteinuria and may be mediated in part by protein trafficking through the tubules. Interstitial foam cells are readily identified in some cases (figs. 7-12, 7-13).

In stage 3, the glomerular capillary walls become progressively thickened, with some narrowing of the capillary lumens (fig. 7-14). The deposits are now predominantly intramembranous, with residual intervening spikes and the formation of an overlying layer of neomembrane (figs.

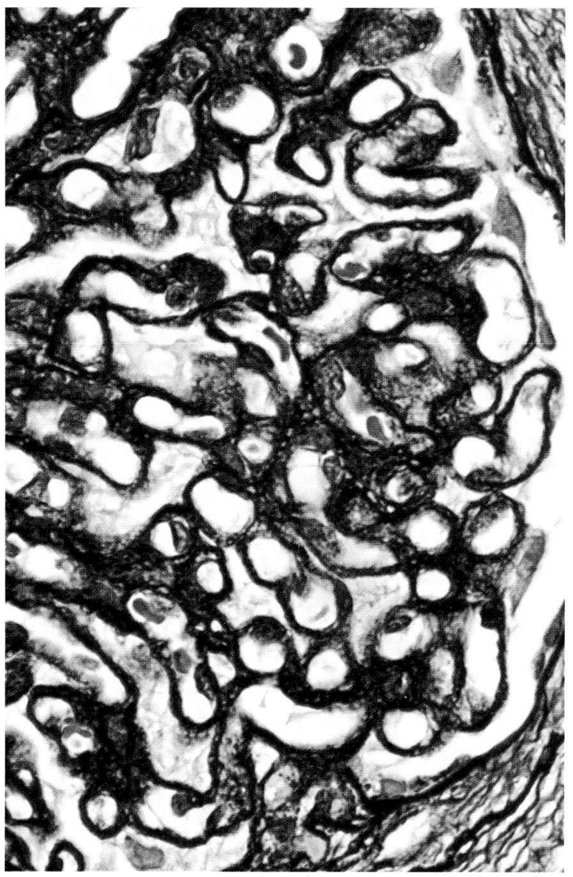

Figure 7-15

MGN STAGE 3

The JMS stain delineates a complex, woven, chain-like thickening of the glomerular capillary walls. Because the deposits have been incorporated into the glomerular capillary wall by an overlying layer of newly formed basement membrane material, some capillaries appear to have narrow double contours.

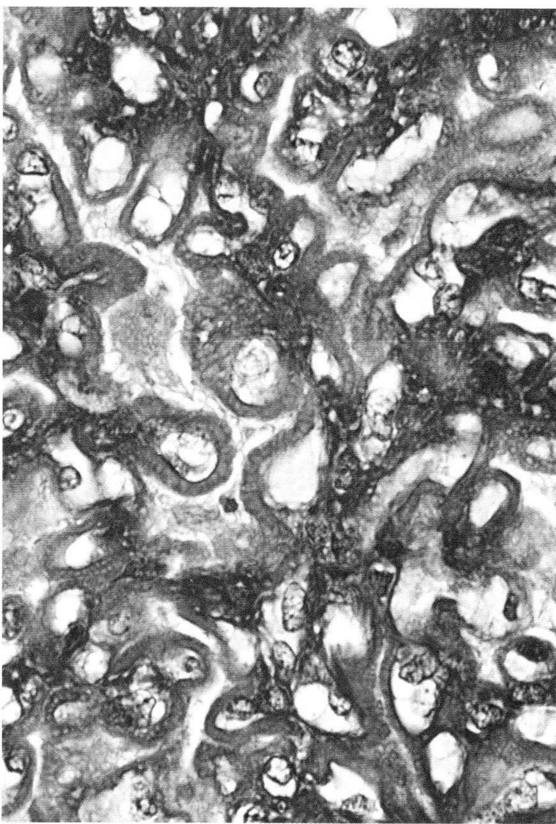

Figure 7-16

MGN STAGE 3

The PAS stain shows weakly positive deposits encircled by more strongly PAS-positive matrix.

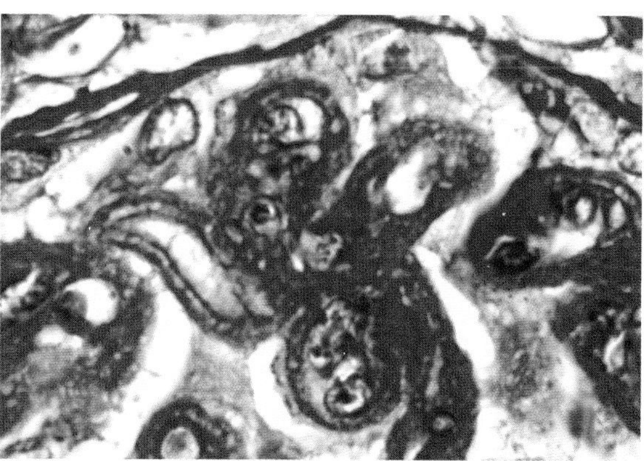

Figure 7-17

MGN STAGE 3

There is extensive resorption of deposits, producing a train-track appearance on the glomerular capillary wall. The PAS-positive spikes and neomembrane completely enclose the clear intramembranous lacunae that correspond to the resorbed deposits.

7-15–7-17). This gives the impression of a chain-like or railroad track–like thickening of the glomerular capillary wall in JMS-stained sections. The intramembranous deposits are often partially resorbed so that they appear variably fuchsinophilic or clear in trichrome-stained sections (figs. 7-18, 7-19). With the PAS and JMS stains, the glomerular basement membrane displays a complex texture, with numerous internal vacuolizations (figs. 7-15–7-17). Partial mesangial interposition may be seen. There is frequently mild mesangial sclerosis, with little or no mesangial hypercellularity. Visceral epithelial cells appear swollen. It is not uncommon to see some glomeruli that have progressed

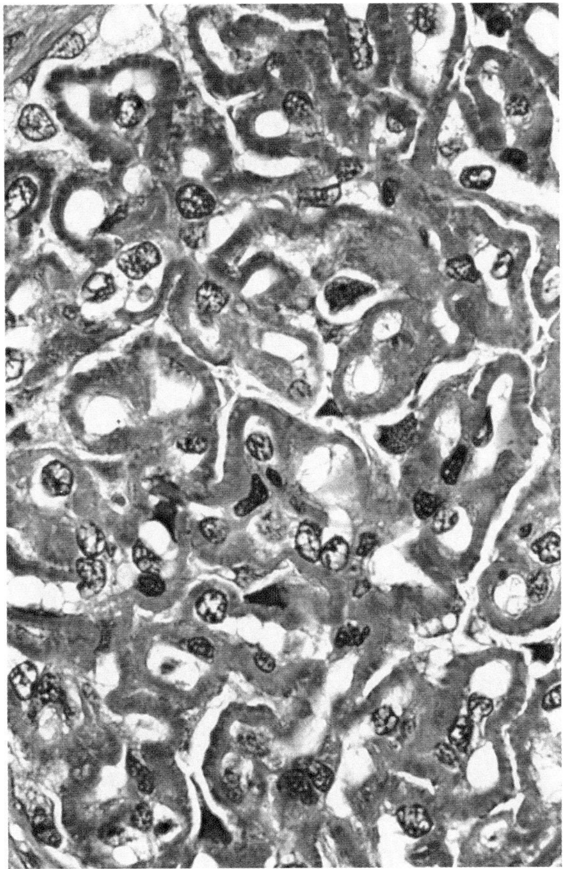

Figure 7-18

MGN STAGE 3

The thickened glomerular capillary walls contain residual intramembranous fuchsinophilic deposits. Blue basement membrane material completely encircles some of the intramembranous deposits (Masson trichrome stain).

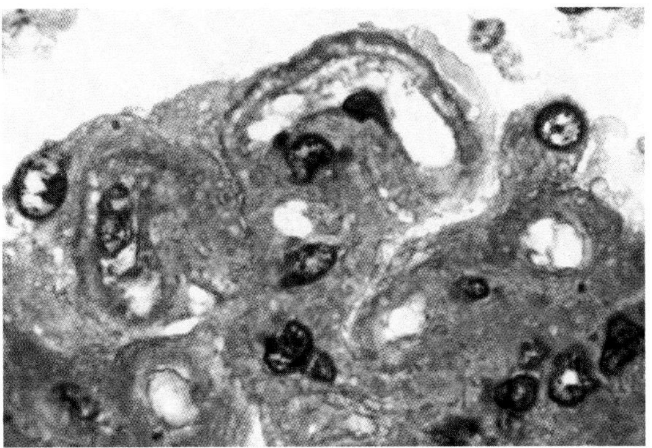

Figure 7-19

MGN STAGE 3

Extensive resorption of deposits leaves clear spaces between the blue-staining spikes. A thin layer of overlying neomembrane covers the clear lacunae, giving the impression of a double contour or train track (Masson trichrome stain).

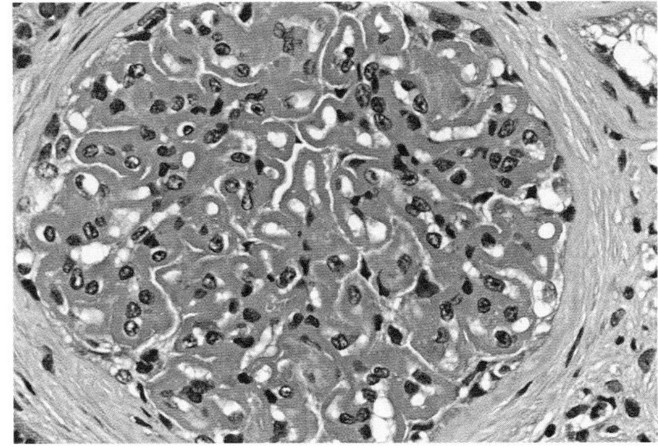

Figure 7-20

MGN STAGE 4

The glomerular capillary lumens are compromised by the massively thickened glomerular capillary walls (H&E stain).

to segmental or global glomerulosclerosis. There is corresponding patchy tubular atrophy and interstitial fibrosis. Intersitial foam cells are more common in stage 3 than in the earlier stages, reflecting the longstanding proteinuria and lipiduria.

In stage 4, there is marked thickening of the glomerular capillary walls, with widespread segmental and global glomerulosclerosis (figs. 7-20–7-22). Even with the special stains, spikes and vacuolizations of the glomerular basement membrane are more difficult to identify. Deposits are rarely identifiable with the trichrome stain because of their extensive resorption and replacement by basement membrane material. Mesangial sclerosis is common. There is usually advanced tubular atrophy and interstitial fibrosis in the distribution of the obsolescent glomeruli.

Immunofluorescence Findings. The characteristic immunofluorescence feature of primary MGN is the presence of subepithelial immune deposits involving the glomerular capillary walls, in a diffuse and global, generally uniform pattern. In primary MGN, mesangial immune deposits are not identified. Because the subepithelial deposits also involve the reflection of the glomerular basement membrane over the

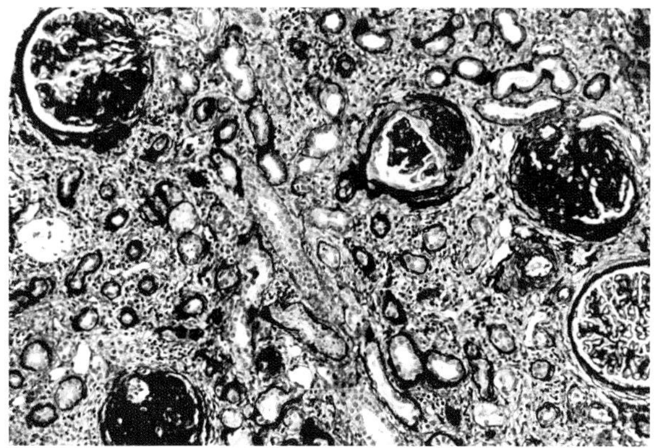

Figure 7-21

MGN STAGE 4

There is advanced segmental and global glomerulosclerosis and chronic tubulointerstitial disease (JMS stain).

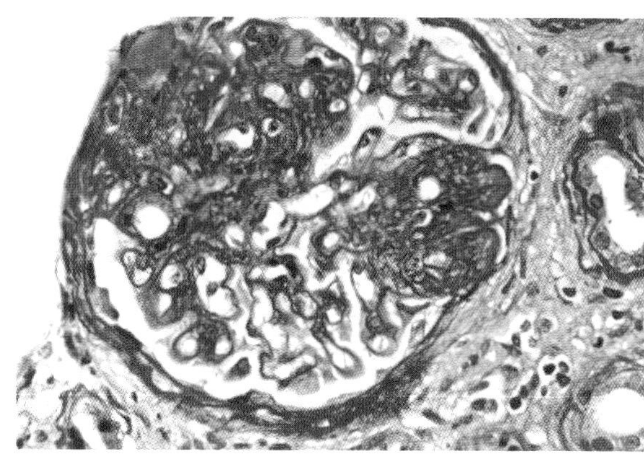

Figure 7-22

MGN STAGE 4

A glomerulus has irregularly thickened glomerular capillary walls and segmental glomerulosclerosis (PAS stain).

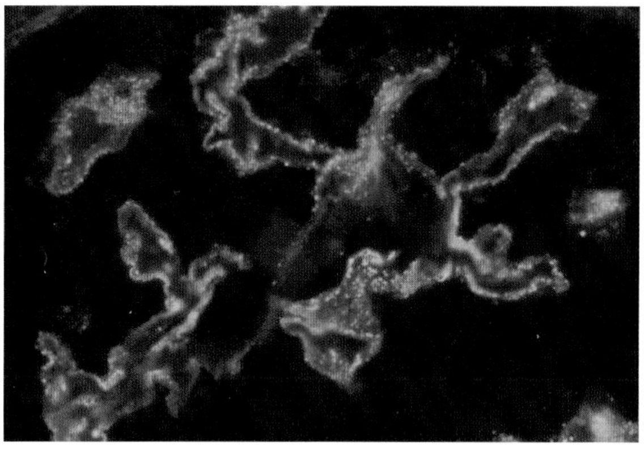

Figure 7-23

MGN STAGE 1

Immunofluorescence reveals minute, finely granular deposits of IgG along the outer aspect of the glomerular capillary walls (immunofluorescence micrograph).

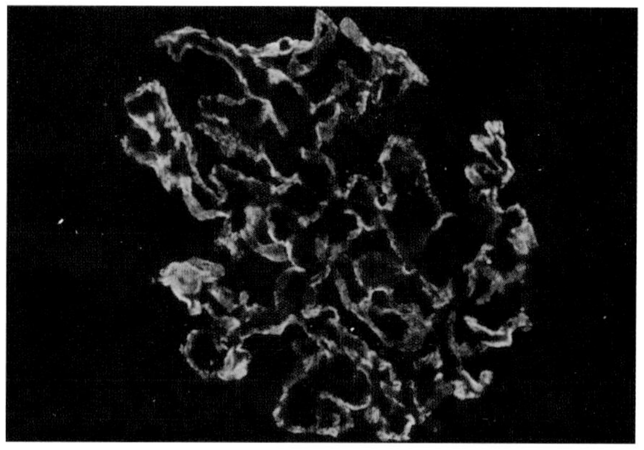

Figure 7-24

MGN STAGE 1

A case of early recurrence of MGN in the transplant. The subepithelial deposits of IgG are so finely granular and confluent that they appear pseudolinear. The fine granularity is best seen where the glomerular basement membrane is cut obliquely (immunofluorescence micrograph).

mesangium, it may be difficult to determine whether mesangial deposits are present.

Subepithelial deposits contain IgG in virtually 100 percent of cases, and complement (C) 3 in about 80 percent. The intensity of staining for IgG is generally stronger than that for C3. Deposits of IgM, IgA, and C1 are rarely identified (less than 30 percent of cases) and are of low intensity. Although not studied in routine diagnostic practice, deposits show strong staining for C5b-9 (membrane attack complex).

The quality, size, and intensity of the subepithelial immune deposits vary with the stage of the disease. In stage 1, deposits tend to be minute and finely granular (fig. 7-23). Sometimes they are so closely aggregated that they appear pseudolinear (fig. 7-24). Careful high-power microscopic inspection, however, usually reveals irregularities and minute granularities that distinguish these deposits from true linear staining. In stage 2, deposits are usually larger, coarser, and of stronger intensity (figs. 7-25–7-27). In

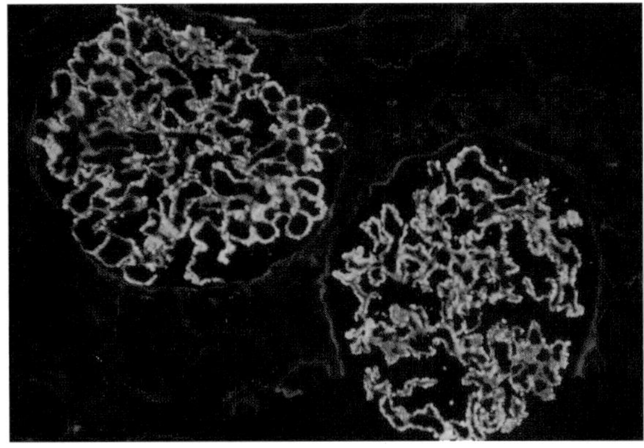

Figure 7-25

MGN STAGE 2

Granular deposits of IgG are regularly distributed throughout the glomerular capillary walls. The two glomeruli pictured here are affected uniformly and diffusely (immunofluorescence micrograph).

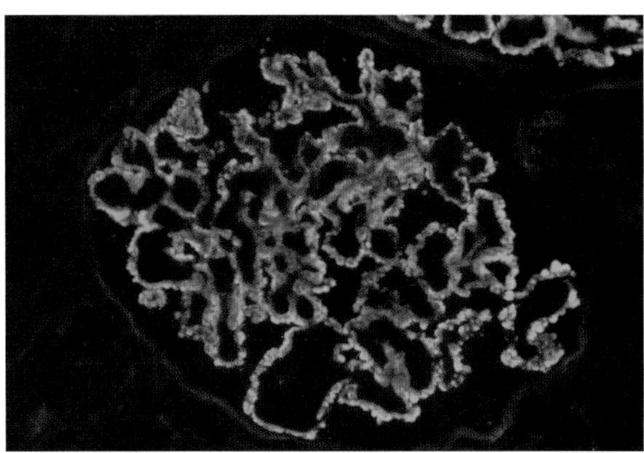

Figure 7-26

MGN STAGE 2

The deposits of IgG are large, with a "lumpy-bumpy" appearance (immunofluorescence micrograph).

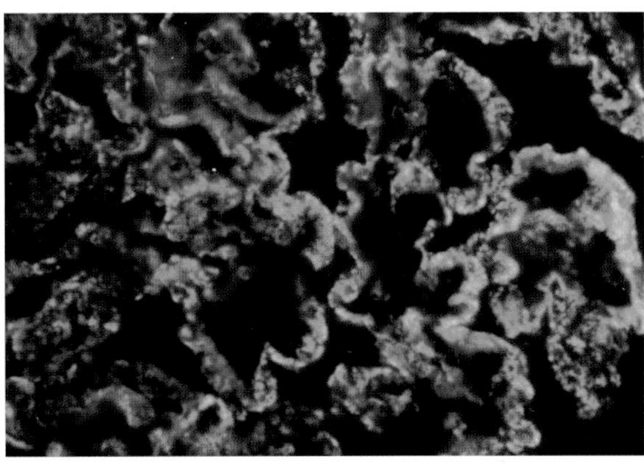

Figure 7-27

MGN STAGE 2

The subepithelial deposits of IgG have a fluffy appearance where the glomerular basement membranes are cut en face (immunofluorescence micrograph).

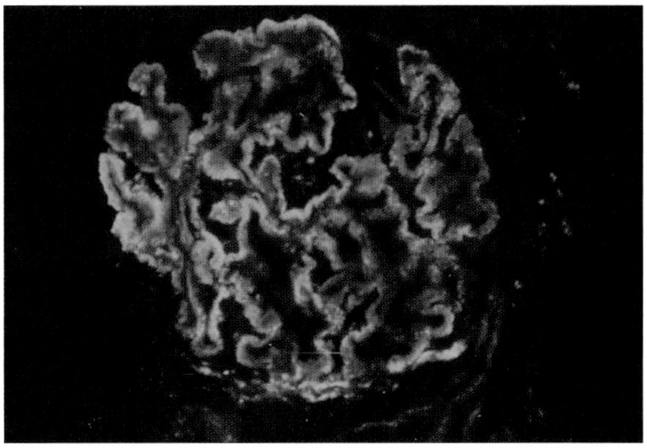

Figure 7-28

MGN STAGE 3

The deposits of IgG are more coarsely granular and less sharply defined than in stage 2 disease (immunofluorescence micrograph).

stage 3, the deposits remain coarsely granular and large, but are often of weaker intensity than in stage 2 due to ongoing resorption (figs. 7-28, 7-29). In stage 4, where deposits are typically extensively resorbed and the glomerular basement membranes very thickened, it may be difficult to identify residual deposits. At this stage, the deposits may be more sparse, less uniformly distributed, and of weak intensity (fig. 7-30). Sclerotic glomeruli commonly contain nonspecific deposits of IgM, C3, and C1 in the sclerosing tuft. In some patients, deposits are relatively focal and segmental in distribution; thus they involve some glomeruli but not others and outline a subset of capillaries.

Albumin and immunoglobulin may be identified in the cytoplasm of visceral epithelial cells and tubular epithelial cells, corresponding to intracytoplasmic protein resorption droplets. Similarly, it is common to find activation of C3 on tubular epithelial cells, as may be seen in other conditions with heavy glomerular proteinuria.

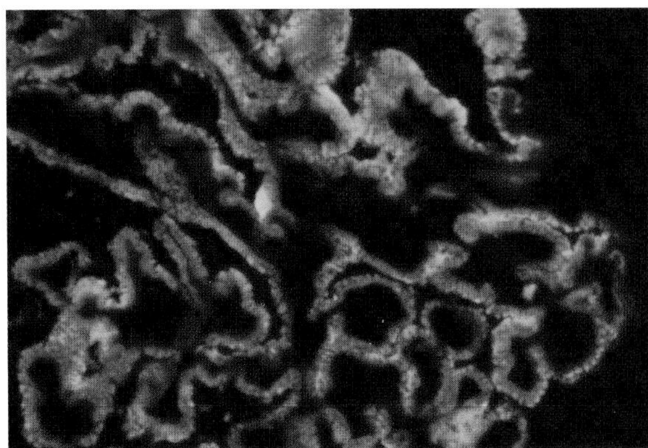

Figure 7-29

MGN STAGE 3

Staining for C3 is similar in texture and distribution to that of IgG shown in figure 7-28 (immunofluorescence micrograph).

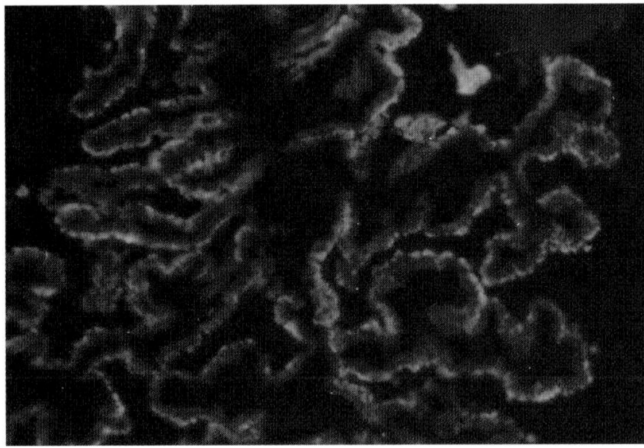

Figure 7-30

MGN STAGE 4

The deposits of IgG are weakly stained although the glomerular capillary walls are markedly thickened. This weak immunofluorescence staining in stage 4 disease is due to the extensive resorption of the intramembranous deposits (immunofluorescence micrograph).

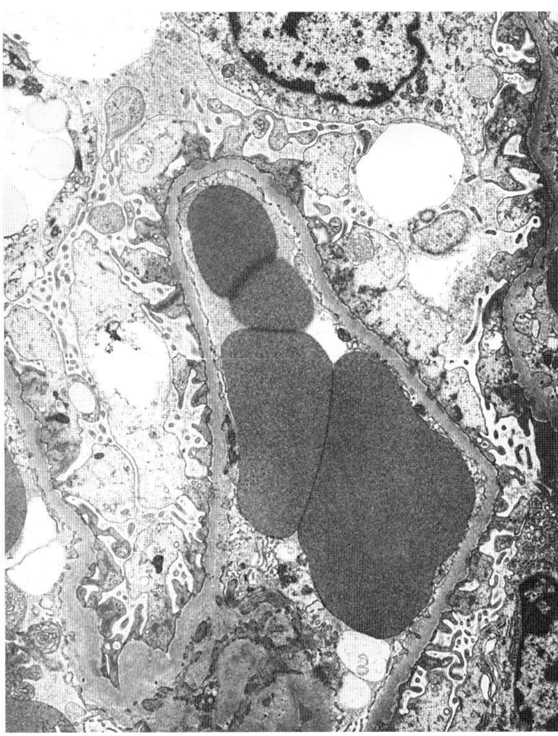

Figure 7-31

MGN STAGE 1

There are sparse, minute, subepithelial deposits, without well-developed spikes. Foot process effacement is seen directly overlying the deposits (electron micrograph).

Electron Microscopic Findings. The stages of MGN were originally defined at the ultrastructural level by Ehrenreich and Churg (16). In stage 1, subepithelial deposits tend to be small and sparse, and may not involve all glomerular capillaries (figs. 7-31, 7-32). The deposits are not closely aggregated and lack intervening spikes, although they may indent the glomerular basement membrane. Foot process effacement is generally restricted to the segments of glomerular basement membrane directly overlying the subepithelial deposits.

In stage 2, subepithelial deposits are abundant, larger, and closely aggregated (figs. 7-33, 7-34). What distinguishes stage 2 is the presence of intervening spikes that project at right angles from the glomerular basement membranes, between the subepithelial deposits. In the two-dimensional images obtained by routine transmission electron microscopy, spikes resemble pegs; however, by three-dimensional scanning, the spikes actually form a complex lattice of interconnecting basement membrane material that encircles individual deposits (4). At this stage, there is widespread, if not complete, foot process effacement. The podocytes are markedly hypertrophied and may contain intracellular transport vesicles and resorption droplets (fig. 7-35).

Stage 3 MGN is characterized by predominantly intramembranous deposits that range from electron dense to electron lucent, consistent with partial resorption (figs. 7-36–7-39).

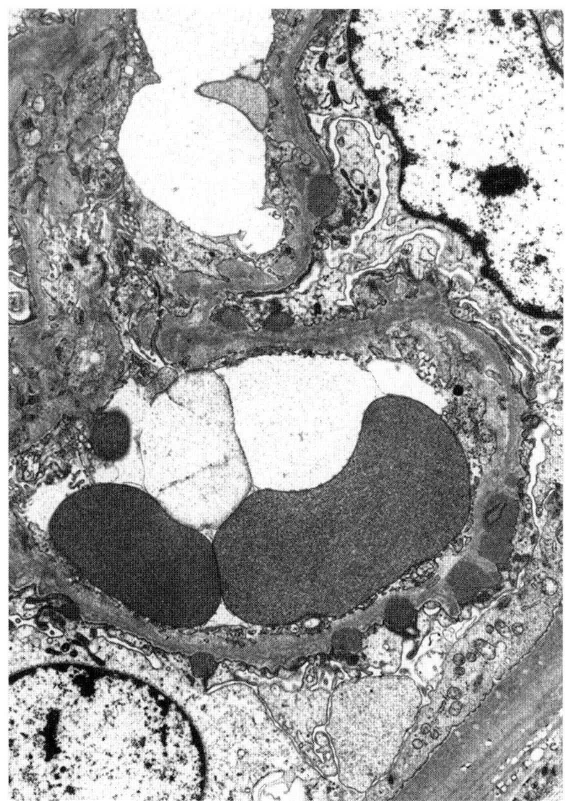

Figure 7-32

MGN STAGE 1 TO 2

The subepithelial deposits are sparse but larger than those in figure 7-31. A few of the deposits are surrounded by basement membrane spikes (electron micrograph).

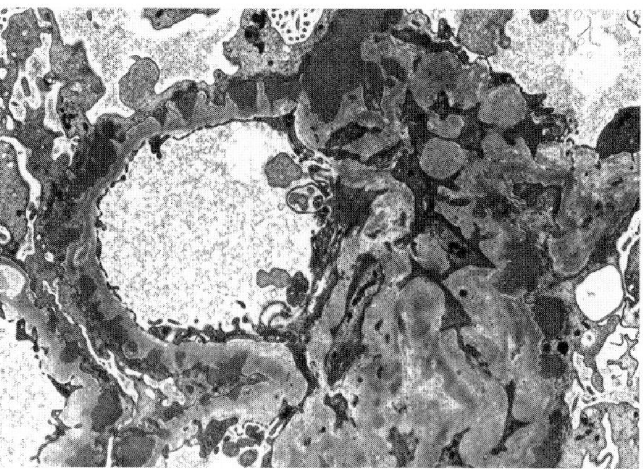

Figure 7-33

MGN STAGE 2

The subepithelial deposits are close to each other, with intervening tall spikes. No deposits are identified in the mesangium (electron micrograph).

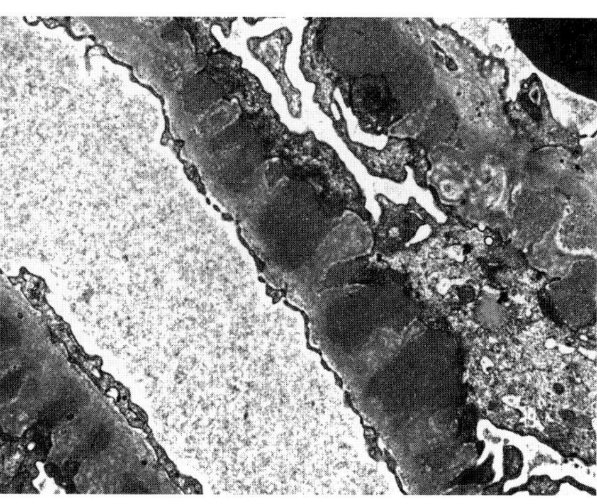

Figure 7-34

MGN STAGE 2

The basement membrane spikes and deposits are uniform and regularly distributed (electron micrograph).

The resorbing deposits appear relatively electron lucent and may contain curvilinear membranous particles and microspherical granulations (fig. 7-39). At this stage, the basement membrane has grown up around the deposits, incorporating them into the thickened glomerular capillary wall. Spikes become linked to each other by a layer of overlying neomembrane formed above the deposits. This encapsulation of the deposits by basement membrane material imparts a complex, lamellated texture to the glomerular capillary wall. Foot processes are extensively effaced. In some cases, fresh electron-dense deposits form a new generation of immune deposits on top of the older resorbing deposits, consistent with immunologic reactivation of disease (fig. 7-40). Such cases may be difficult to classify according to the Ehrenreich and Churg scheme (16).

In stage 4, the glomerular capillary walls are markedly thickened, with textural irregularities consisting of lacunae and irregular lamellations of glomerular basement membrane, imparting a woven appearance (fig. 7-41). At this stage, there has been extensive resorption of immune deposits, and only few residual electron-dense deposits may be discernible (fig. 7-42). Thus, it is the basement membrane changes, rather than the deposits, that define this stage of disease. Because

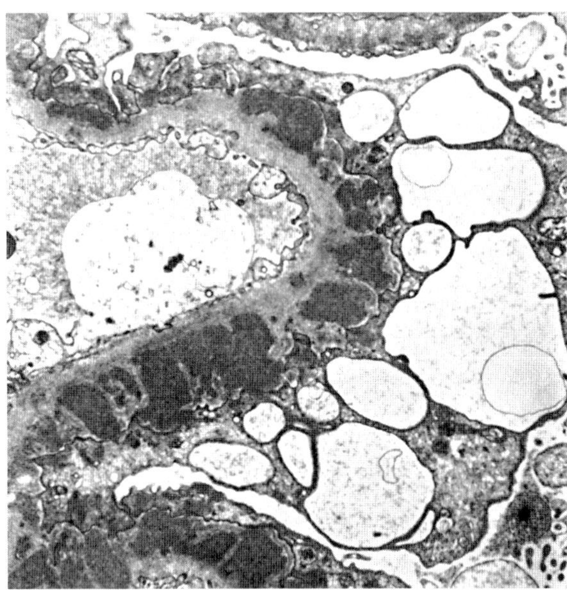

Figure 7-35

MGN STAGE 2

Overlying the deposits, complete foot process effacement and podocyte hypertrophy are seen, with intracytoplasmic electron-lucent transport vesicles (electron micrograph).

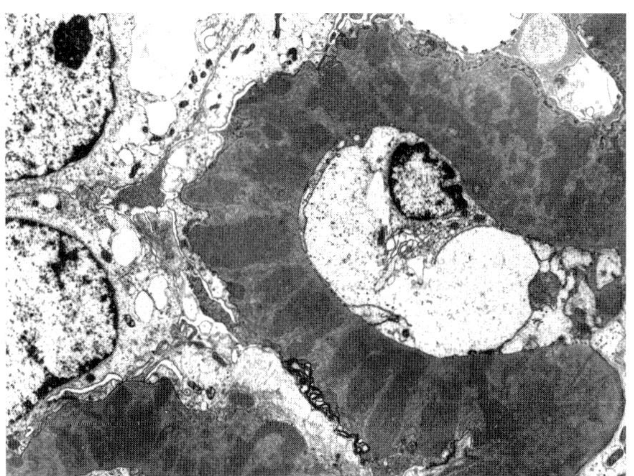

Figure 7-36

MGN STAGE 3

Early stage 3 in which deposits are still electron dense. A delicate layer of neomembrane covers the deposits and bridges the intervening spikes. The glomerular capillary lumen appears narrowed by the massive thickening of the glomerular capillary wall. The foot processes are completely effaced (electron micrograph).

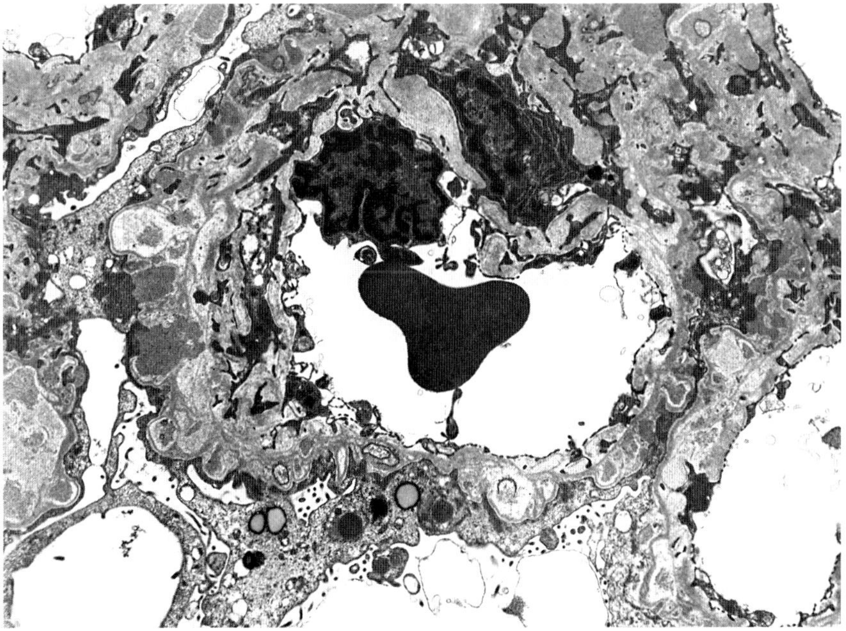

Figure 7-37

MGN STAGE 3

Electron-dense deposits are adjacent to variably electron-lucent, partially resorbed deposits. The glomerular capillary wall has a complex texture owing to the varying stages of deposit resorption and neomembrane formation over the deposits. There is also some irregularity of the subendothelial aspect of the glomerular basement membrane, consistent with remodeling of the glomerular capillary wall (electron micrograph).

the major direction of glomerular basement membrane synthesis is from the epithelial aspect, the greatest irregularities of the glomerular capillary wall may be present along the older, subendothelial aspect. Subendothelial electron-lucent zones represent sites of resorption of originally subepithelial electron-dense deposits. There may be considerable restoration of foot processes.

Differential Diagnosis. The first task in the differential diagnosis of MGN is to distinguish

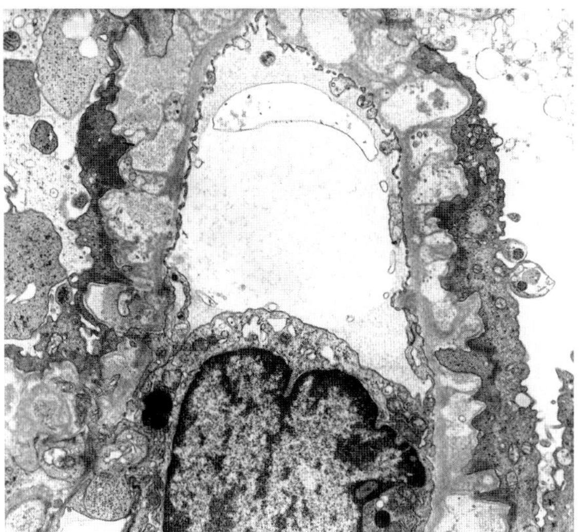

Figure 7-38

MGN STAGE 3

Widespread resorption of deposits produces electron-lucent defects between the spikes (electron micrograph).

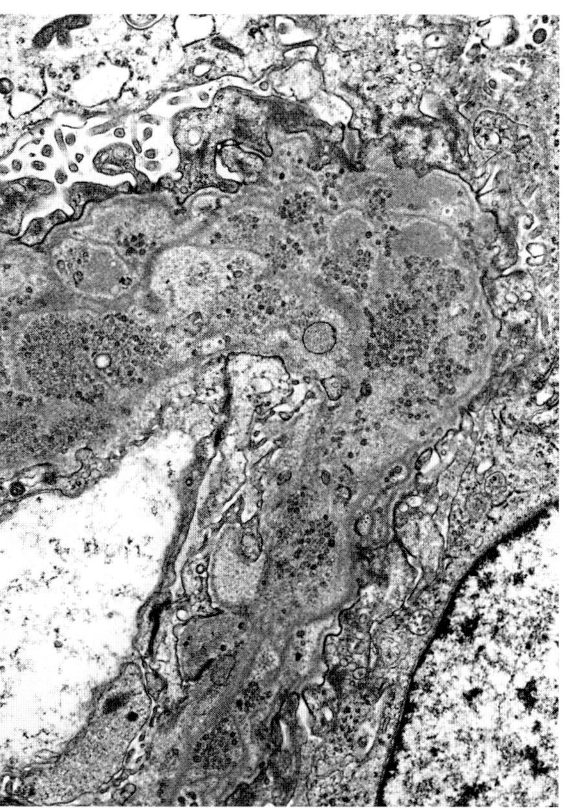

Figure 7-39

MGN STAGE 3

In a minority of cases, numerous microspherical particles are admixed with the granular intramembranous deposits. The microspherical particles are most often observed in stage 3 MGN, when the deposits are being resorbed. They are of unknown composition and may represent cellular debris caught in the remodeled basement membranes (electron micrograph).

it from other conditions in which subepithelial or intramembranous deposits and basement membrane lamellation may occur. Acute postinfectious glomerulonephritis, like MGN, has abundant subepithelial deposits. However, these typically have a hump shape, are unassociated with basement membrane spikes, number no more than 4 or 5 per capillary, and stain more intensely for C3 than IgG. Examples of postinfectious glomerulonephritis with florid endocapillary proliferation do not usually pose a diagnostic problem; however, cases that are biopsied during the resolving phase, when endocapillary proliferation and neutrophil infiltration have subsided and the humps are undergoing resorption, may be confused with MGN. In such cases, a history of previous infection, nephritic (rather than nephrotic) syndrome, and hypocomplementemia are helpful distinguishing clinical features. Also, cases of resolving acute postinfectious glomerulonephritis usually stain for C3 (and not IgG), often have mesangial deposits, and have a tendency to show subepithelial deposits at the mesangial waist or angle.

Membranoproliferative glomerulonephritis (MPGN) may be confused with MGN, particularly stage 3 MGN. This diagnostic dilemma arises in stage 3 MGN because the deposits are predominantly intramembranous, the glomerular basement membranes may appear duplicated, and there may even be focal partial mesangial interposition. This distinction is particularly problematic in cases of MPGN with only mild mesangial proliferative features and little mesangial interposition. Most helpful in the recognition of MPGN is the demonstration of mesangial and subendothelial deposits at the ultrastructural level. In MPGN, the mesangial interposition is more widespread and regular. Spikes are typically not identified unless there are associated membranous features (consistent with MPGN type 3). Clinically, 75 percent of patients with MPGN have hypocomplementemia, whereas serum complements are normal in patients with primary MGN.

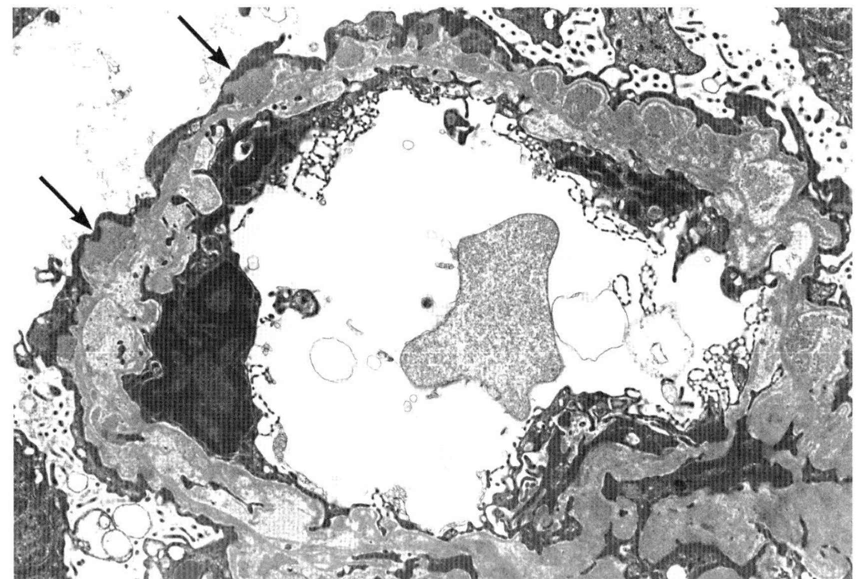

Figure 7-40

MGN STAGE 3

There are several generations of deposits, with an outer layer of fresh electron-dense deposits (arrows) superimposed on older, partially resorbed, intramembranous deposits. The subendothelial layers of the basement membrane are irregular, due to extensive matrix remodeling (electron micrograph).

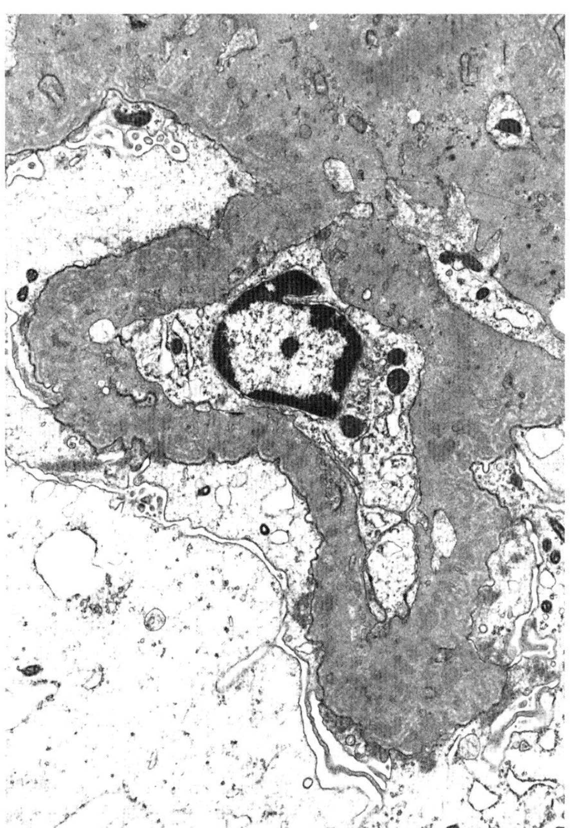

Figure 7-41

MGN STAGE 4

The glomerular capillary walls are massively thickened by indistinct deposits that merge with the matrix material (electron micrograph).

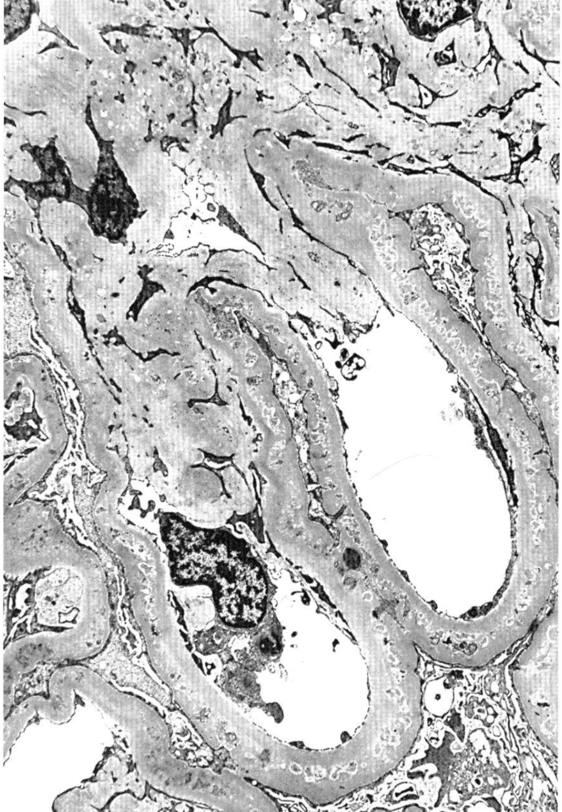

Figure 7-42

MGN STAGE 4

Markedly thickened glomerular capillary walls contain poorly defined intramembranous deposits that are almost completely resorbed. There is also prominent mesangial sclerosis (electron micrograph).

The light and electron microscopic features of the late stages (3 and 4) of MGN can mimic hereditary nephritis due to the extensive lamellation of the glomerular basement membrane enclosing electron-lucent zones, representing resorbed deposits. Immunofluorescence demonstrates residual but sparse glomerular capillary wall deposits of IgG in the cases of advanced MGN. Electron microscopy delineates the thinning of the glomerular basement membrane common in hereditary nephritis but not advanced MGN. Clinically, patients with hereditary nephritis usually have a longstanding history of hematuria (gross or microscopic) preceding the development of the proteinuria and renal insufficiency seen in the late stages of the disease. By contrast, the clinical presentation of MGN is typically dominated by severe proteinuria, although microhematuria is not uncommon. A helpful diagnostic test in difficult cases is to stain the frozen or fixed tissue with antisera to the alpha subunits of collagen IV, now available commercially. Most cases of hereditary nephritis lack glomerular basement membrane reactivity for the alpha 5 and alpha 3 subunits of collagen IV; both subunits are retained in the glomerular basement membranes of MGN.

The next step in the differential diagnosis of MGN is to differentiate primary MGN from secondary forms. This requires a complete clinical history with knowledge of underlying medical conditions, medications, serologies, and serum complement levels. Morphologically, the findings of mesangial proliferative features; membranoproliferative features; deposits in mesangial, subendothelial, or extraglomerular locations; endothelial tubuloreticular inclusions; and strong glomerular staining for IgA and C1 (as well as IgG and C3) and tissue antinuclear antigen (ANA) should be noted (29). The presence of any of these atypical findings, alone or in combination, raises the suspicion of a secondary form of MGN (see Secondary MGN below). Careful clinical-pathologic correlation usually leads to a correct diagnosis. In some patients, however, a secondary form of MGN is suspected but cannot be further characterized due to an incomplete clinical workup or lack of diagnostic specificity of the clinical and laboratory findings.

Etiology and Pathogenesis. The etiology of primary MGN in man is unknown. The experimental prototype of human MGN is Heymann's nephritis in the rat, where in situ formation of immune deposits in the subepithelial zone follows binding of antibody to a locally produced or intrinsic glomerular capillary wall antigen (9). In Heymann's nephritis, MGN results from autoantibodies to the gp330/megalin complex, a glycoprotein component of the clathrin-coated pits located on the soles of the podocyte foot processes. The same antigen is located on the microvillous brush border of the proximal epithelial cells (FX1A fraction). MGN is produced in this model by immunization of rats with homogenates of kidney containing this brush border antigen (active Heymann's nephritis). The disease can also be transferred to naive animals by passive administration of serum from immunized rats (passive Heymann's nephritis). Subepithelial immune deposits are generated when circulating antibody to gp330/megalin binds in situ to the podocyte membrane antigen. Antigen-antibody complexes are then capped and shed off the clathrin-coated pits into the subepithelial space.

The development of proteinuria requires the activation of complement, probably through the alternative pathway. The podocytes are able to scavenge membrane attack complex by uptake of C5b-9 in endocytotic vesicles followed by exocytosis into the urinary space (9). Depletion of C6 can prevent the development of proteinuria, despite the presence of immune deposits, indicating the importance of membrane attack complex in the mediation of proteinuria (3). The podocytes undergo cellular activation, with the generation of toxic oxygen radicals and proteases that can damage the glomerular basement membrane by lipid peroxidation. Thus, both podocyte injury resulting from membrane attack complex and secondary damage to the glomerular basement membrane itself may promote proteinuria in this condition (17).

The human counterpart of Heymann's antigen remains to be identified. It is likely to be a glomerular epithelial antigen that is membrane-associated or secreted into the glomerular capillary wall. Recently, a rare case of membranous glomerulopathy in a neonate was demonstrated to be mediated by maternal antibodies to neutral endopeptidase, an antigen expressed by both podocytes and proximal tubular cells (13). Neutral endopeptidase is the first human podocyte antigen identified as an antigenic target in human membranous glomerulopathy.

Treatment and Prognosis. The natural history of untreated primary MGN is highly variable (12,15). This unpredictable course has made it difficult to evaluate the efficacy of treatment regimens (49). Approximately one third of untreated patients undergo spontaneous remission; one third have persistent proteinuria without the development of renal failure; the final third progress to end-stage renal failure over 5 to 10 years of follow-up. The overall 5-year renal survival rate is about 85 percent and 10-year renal survival ranges from 75 to 80 percent.

Multiple pathologic and clinical features have been linked to a worse prognosis. Pathologic features include a more advanced stage (3 or 4) of the glomerular lesions, more extensive segmental and global glomerulosclerosis, and chronic tubulointerstitial disease. The development of lesions of segmental sclerosis in this setting are best interpreted as an evolution to chronicity, rather than a superimposed disease (48). Clinical features linked to poor prognosis include an elevated serum creatinine level at presentation, more advanced age, male sex, hypertension, and nephrotic proteinuria. Remission of proteinuria, either spontaneously or following therapy, is more likely to occur in patients with a lower stage of MGN.

Three major treatment approaches have been used in primary MGN. These include no specific therapy, steroids alone, or steroids alternating with a cytotoxic or alkylating agent such as cyclophosphamide or chlorambucil (6,8,19, 42). Because of the significant rate of spontaneous remission and the equivocal value of long-term steroid therapy in meta-analyses (23, 38), most nephrologists opt to treat only those patients who are at high risk for progression to renal failure (particularly older patients, males, and those with heavy proteinuria, hypertension, or renal insufficiency). The addition of an ACE inhibitor may reduce the proteinuria and allay progression to renal failure (45).

VARIANTS OF MGN

MGN with Crescents

Cellular crescents are identified in a small percentage of cases of primary MGN (fig. 7-43). These patients are usually distinguished clinically by a more rapidly progressive course to renal failure. Three subgroups of patients develop crescents in apparently primary MGN. The first group of patients develop antiglomerular basement membrane (anti-GBM) antibodies and appear to have anti-GBM nephritis superimposed on the MGN (32,41). By immunofluorescence, they usually display granular subepithelial deposits of IgG and C3 overlying linear glomerular basement membrane deposits of IgG. The second group has associated antineutrophil cytoplasmic antibodies (ANCAs) consistent with pauci-immune focal crescentic glomerulonephritis superimposed on primary MGN. Indeed, the presence of circulating ANCAs may promote the development of a crescentic phenotype in a variety of immune complex–mediated glomerular diseases (30). In the third group, neither anti-GBM antibody nor ANCA can be demonstrated. In these patients, the formation of crescents is thought to represent an unusual morphologic evolution of primary MGN, without an identifiable superimposed disease.

Childhood MGN with Antitubular Basement Membrane Nephritis

Primary MGN is extremely rare in young children; however, an unusual subtype is identified almost exclusively in young children, namely MGN associated with antitubular basement membrane (anti-TBM) nephritis (37). Onset is between the ages of 2 months and 5 years of age. There is a strong male predominance. Occurrence of this condition in siblings and the demonstration of certain human leukocyte antigen (HLA) associations (DRW8 and B7) suggest the importance of predisposing genetic factors. Patients present with Fanconi's syndrome (glycosuria, aminoaciduria, hypophosphatemia, and metabolic acidosis) due to proximal tubular dysfunction as well as heavy glomerular proteinuria leading to nephrotic syndrome due to the glomerular lesion.

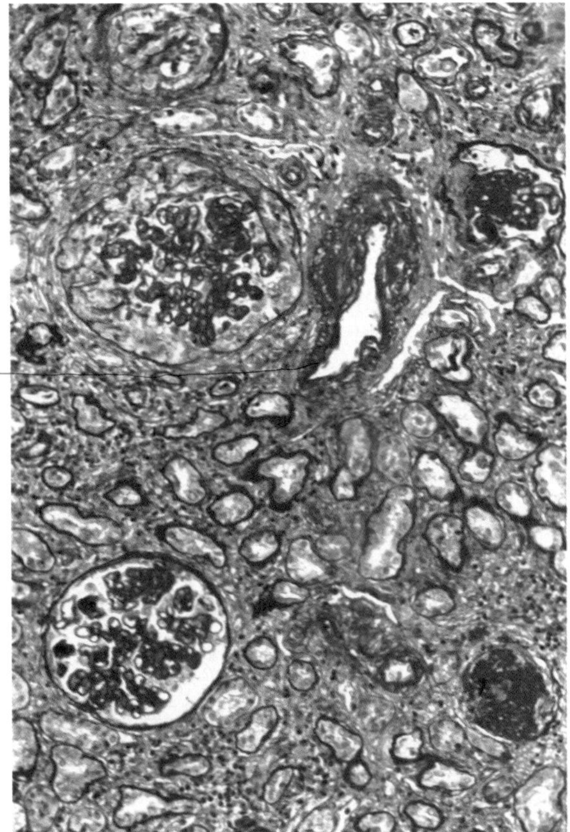

Figure 7-43

MGN WITH CRESCENTS

In this case, there was no evidence of either anti-glomerular basement membrane (anti-GBM) antibody or antineutrophil cytoplasmic antibody (ANCA). Crescentic transformation such as this is rarely encountered in primary MGN (PAS stain).

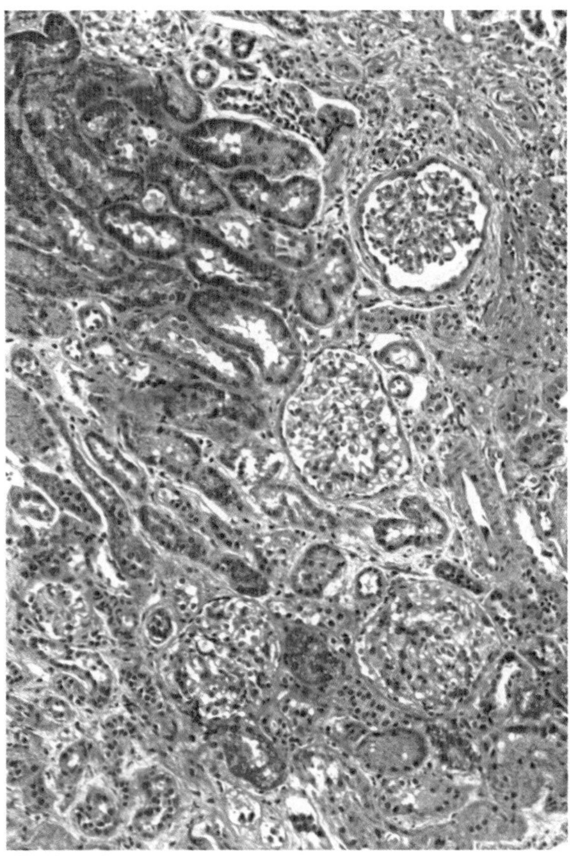

Figure 7-44

CHILDHOOD MGN WITH ANTITUBULAR BASEMENT MEMBRANE NEPHRITIS

Specimen from a 2-year-old child with nephrotic syndrome and progressive renal insufficiency. There is moderate tubular atrophy, interstitial fibrosis, and inflammation (Masson trichrome stain).

Pathologically, these patients have typical MGN associated with a tubulointerstitial nephropathy that includes varying degrees of tubular atrophy, interstitial fibrosis, and inflammation (fig. 7-44). The diagnostic feature by immunofluorescence is the presence of linear deposits of IgG along tubular basement membranes and Bowman's capsule, but not in the glomerular basement membranes (fig. 7-45). Rather, the glomerular basement membranes display the typical, granular, subepithelial deposits of IgG and C3 characteristic of MGN (fig. 7-46). By electron microscopy, subepithelial electron-dense deposits are identified in the glomerular capillary walls. However, the tubular basement membranes typically display no electron-dense deposits, despite the linear staining for IgG demonstrated by immunofluorescence.

The presence of anti-TBM deposits can be demonstrated by applying patient serum to cryostat sections of normal kidney, followed by the addition of fluoresceinated rabbit anti-human IgG (37). This indirect immunofluorescence technique yields the same linear staining of tubular basement membranes and Bowman's capsule that is demonstrated by direct immunofluorescence (fig. 7-47).

The nature of the tubular basement membrane autoantigen is unknown. It appears to be a 58-kDa noncollagenous glycoprotein (40). Some patients have extrarenal manifestations, including autoimmune enteropathy, ocular abnormalities,

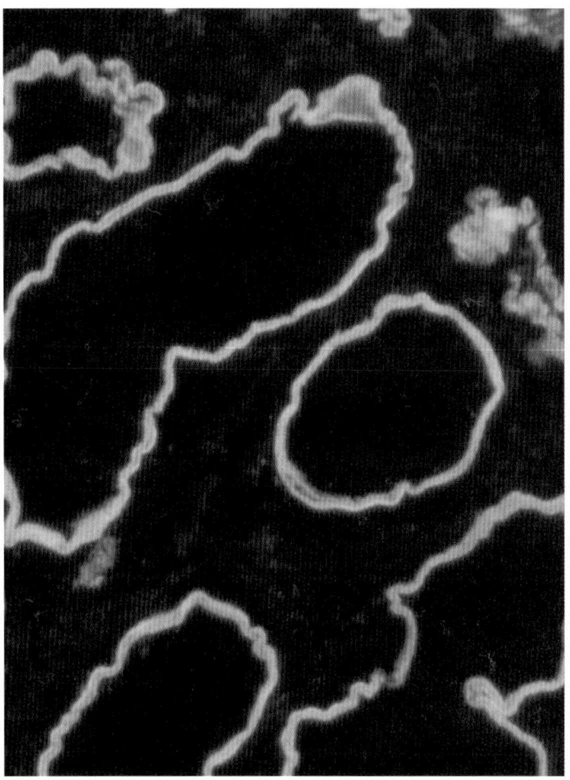

Figure 7-45

CHILDHOOD MGN WITH ANTITUBULAR BASEMENT MEMBRANE NEPHRITIS

Direct immunofluorescence reveals diffuse strong linear staining for IgG along the tubular basement membranes (immunofluorescence micrograph).

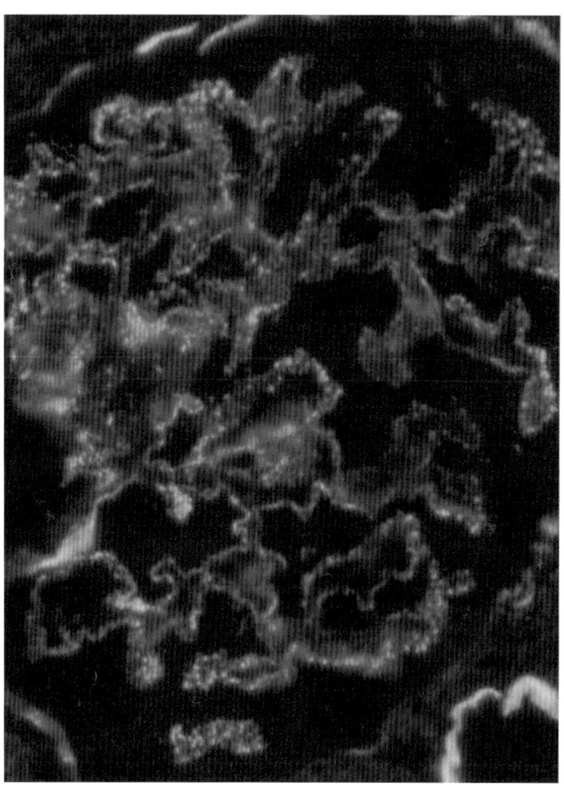

Figure 7-46

CHILDHOOD MGN WITH ANTITUBULAR BASEMENT MEMBRANE NEPHRITIS

There is finely granular staining of the glomerular capillary walls for IgG in a membranous distribution; however, linear staining is present in Bowman's capsule and the adjacent tubular basement membranes (immunofluorescence micrograph).

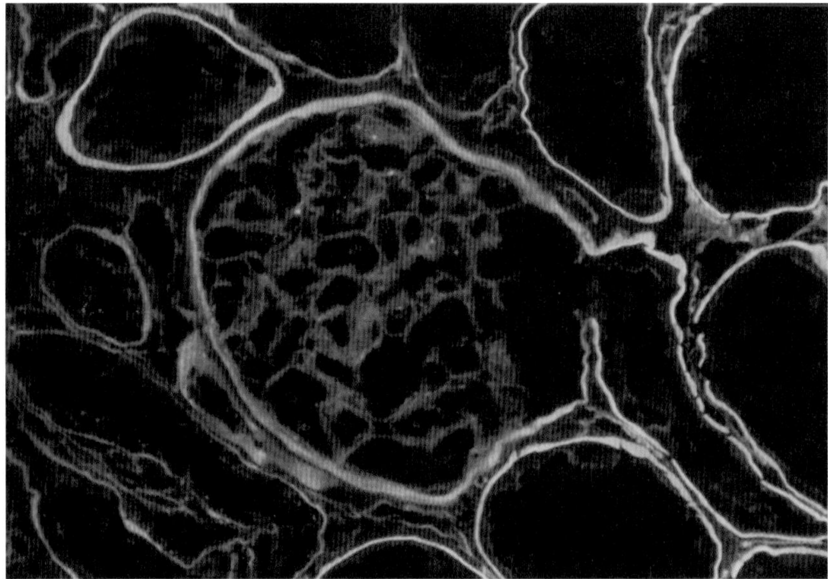

Figure 7-47

CHILDHOOD MGN WITH ANTITUBULAR BASEMENT MEMBRANE NEPHRITIS

When a cryostat section of normal kidney is overlaid with the patient's serum, followed by rabbit antihuman IgG, linear staining is obtained in the distribution of Bowman's capsule and tubular basement membranes, but not glomerular basement membranes. These findings demonstrate the presence of a circulating antitubular basement membrane antibody (indirect immunofluorescence micrograph).

eczematoid dermatitis, and diabetes. Although some patients experience improvement in renal function and proteinuria with plasmapheresis, prognosis is poor and most cases progress to end-stage renal disease in childhood. Anti-TBM nephritis has been reported to recur in the transplant.

MGN in the Transplant

The majority of cases of MGN seen in the allograft represent de novo disease (see chapter 26); approximately 25 percent represent recurrence of disease. Among patients whose original disease was MGN and who undergo transplantation, fewer than 20 percent will develop recurrence of disease in the allograft, usually within the first 6 months post transplantation (43). There are rare cases of donor-transmitted MGN due to inadvertent transplantation of a kidney with previously undetected MGN (39). Sequential biopsies have shown partial resolution of donor-transmitted MGN within 7 weeks post transplant, indicating the importance of host factors in the mediation of the disease (39).

Secondary MGN

Definition. Secondary MGN, as opposed to primary MGN, is a form that can be attributed to a particular underlying disease or pathogenetic mechanism, such as autoimmune diseases, infections, drugs, and neoplasms (see Table 7-2) (20,35). Some of these conditions, such as MGN related to drug therapy and neoplasia, are indistinguishable morphologically from primary MGN. In such cases, the association with an underlying condition is only possible by clinical correlation. There are other forms of secondary MGN, particularly due to autoimmune diseases or infections, in which there are helpful morphologic clues to suggest that the MGN is secondary.

The possibility of secondary MGN related to collagen vascular disease or infectious processes should be suspected in any case of MGN in which the immune deposits are not restricted to the subepithelial region (such as in mesangial, subendothelial, or extraglomerular locations). Mesangial electron-dense deposits are not a feature of primary MGN; in fact, less than 10 percent of cases of primary MGN have demonstrable mesangial deposits at the ultrastructural level (11,24). It is likely that many cases of apparently "primary" MGN with mesangial deposits represent unrecognized forms of secondary MGN. Similarly, tubular basement membrane deposits have only rarely been identified in primary MGN (36), possibly due to the rare presence of an autoantibody to a shared antigen secreted by both the podocytes and the tubular epithelial cells. Deposits in these atypical locations are so rare in primary MGN that they should be a red flag alerting the pathologist to the possibility of associated systemic conditions.

MGN Secondary to Autoimmune Diseases. MGN secondary to systemic lupus erythematosus (SLE) is one of the most common forms of secondary MGN encountered in clinical practice. Many of these patients present with MGN before the serologic or extrarenal features of SLE manifest clinically (1). Thus, the renal biopsy assumes a particularly important diagnostic role in these cases. Morphologic clues that the MGN is likely to be secondary to SLE include the presence of endothelial tubuloreticular inclusions, mesangial immune deposits, sparse subendothelial deposits, and tubulointerstitial deposits, as detected by immunofluorescence and electron microscopy (figs. 7-48, 7-49) (29). By light microscopy, there are often mesangial proliferative features. By immunofluorescence, the composition of the deposits is more likely to be "full house," consisting of all three classes of immunoglobulins, as well as C3 and C1. The presence of tissue ANA (staining of nuclei in the cryostat sections of kidney using fluoresceinated anti-IgG) reflects the presence of a circulating antinuclear antibody. Endothelial tubuloreticular inclusions ("interferon footprints") are particularly common. The presence of any of these atypical features in combination increases the likelihood that the MGN is secondary to SLE (29). MGN has also been linked to rheumatoid arthritis in patients not receiving therapeutic drugs (such as gold or penicillamine) (25). There are rare associations of MGN with autoimmune thyroiditis, and antithyroglobulin antibodies have been localized to the immune deposits (27).

MGN Secondary to Infections. MGN associated with hepatitis B or hepatitis C infection is one of the most common forms of MGN related to infection (28,31,33,47). Many of these cases have associated mesangial hypercellularity and mesangial immune deposits (figs. 7-50, 7-51).

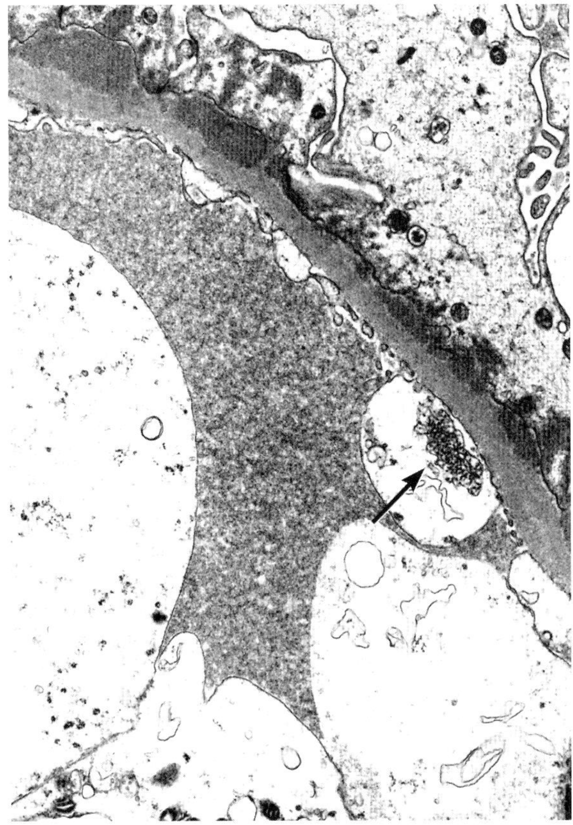

Figure 7-48

SECONDARY MGN DUE TO LUPUS NEPHRITIS CLASS V

There are small subepithelial electron-dense deposits and an endothelial tubuloreticular inclusion (arrow) (electron micrograph).

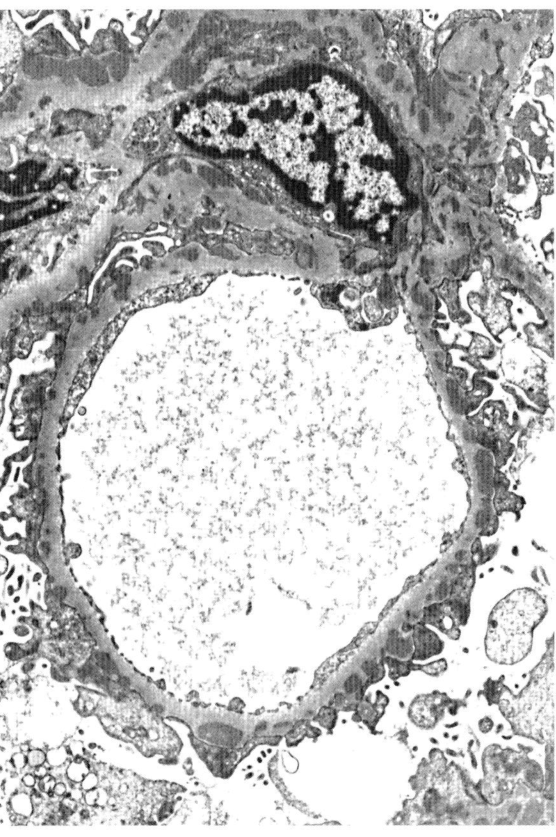

Figure 7-49

SECONDARY MGN DUE TO LUPUS NEPHRITIS CLASS V

There are mesangial electron-dense deposits in addition to the subepithelial deposits (electron micrograph).

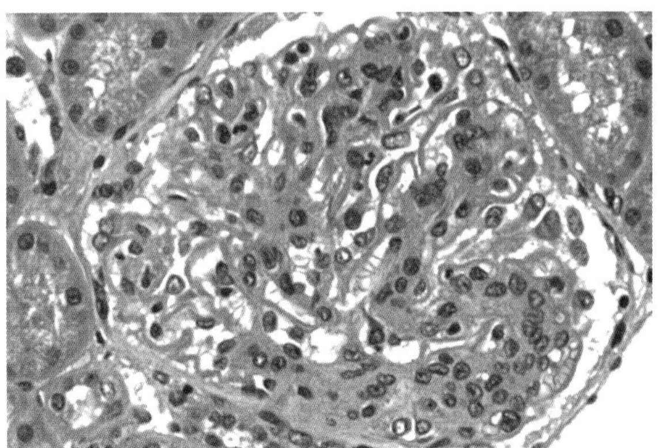

Figure 7-50

MGN ASSOCIATED WITH HEPATITIS B INFECTION IN A 10-YEAR-OLD CHILD

There is mild mesangial proliferation in addition to diffuse thickening of the glomerular capillary walls (H&E stain).

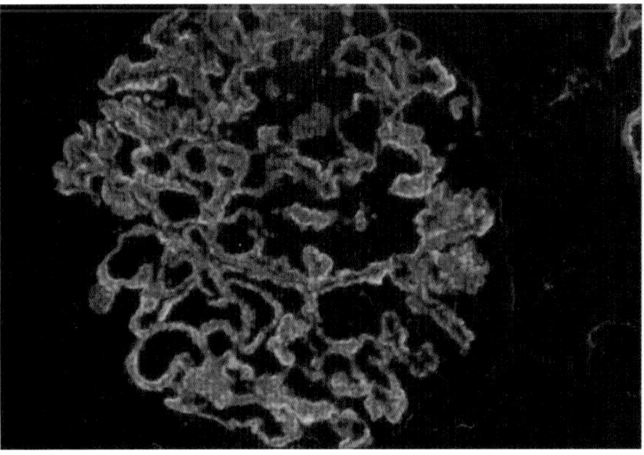

Figure 7-51

MGN ASSOCIATED WITH HEPATITIS B INFECTION

Granular deposits of IgG are present in a combined subepithelial and mesangial distribution (immunofluorescence micrograph).

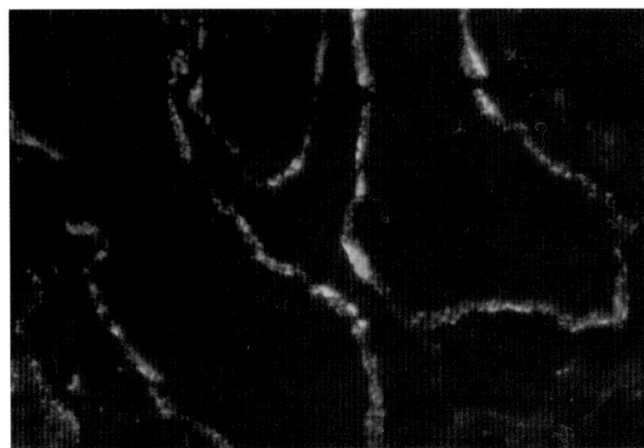

Figure 7-52

MGN ASSOCIATED WITH HEPATITIS B INFECTION

Granular deposits of IgG are present along some tubular basement membranes. Tubular basement membrane deposits are not generally seen in idiopathic MGN and should lead to a search for secondary causes (particularly autoimmune diseases such as systemic lupus erythematosus or infectious diseases such as hepatitis B) (immunofluorescence micrograph).

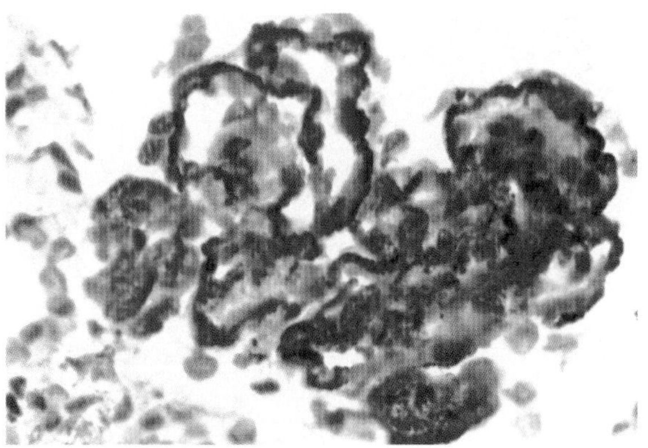

Figure 7-53

MGN ASSOCIATED WITH HEPATITIS B INFECTION

Hepatitis B core antigen can be demonstrated in the distribution of the subepithelial deposits by immunoperoxidase performed on cryostat sections.

It is not uncommon to find segmental membranoproliferative features in some glomeruli, with corresponding subendothelial deposits and mesangial interposition. If the associated membranoproliferative features are well-developed, such cases of mixed membranous and membranoproliferative glomerulonephritis can be termed membranoproliferative glomerulonephritis type 3. Rarely have cases of hepatitis B-associated MGN been associated with TBM deposits (fig. 7-52). MGN secondary to hepatitis B is one of the few secondary forms of MGN in which viral antigens (including hepatitis B surface, core, and e antigens) have been demonstrated in the glomerular deposits (fig. 7-53) (33,47). MGN secondary to hepatitis B may occur in both children and adults, and is frequently associated with hypocomplementemia and abnormal liver function tests. By contrast, MGN secondary to hepatitis C is usually a late manifestation of the infection and thus is primarily diagnosed in adulthood (31). There may be associated hypocomplementemia and/or cryoglobulinemia. Attempts to localize hepatitis C viral antigens to the glomerular deposits have been unsuccessful.

In some parts of the world, other infectious causes of MGN are common (listed in Table 7-2), including MGN related to syphilis (congenital or latent), filariasis, schistosomiasis, and malaria. Treponemal antigens have been localized to the subepithelial deposits in some cases of MGN associated with syphilis.

MGN Secondary to Drugs. MGN related to therapeutic drugs, such as gold, penicillamine, and captopril, usually presents in an early stage of disease (typically stage 1 or 2) (21,22,26). Mesangial deposits or proliferative features are not identified. The glomerular disease is readily reversible within 2 to 6 months upon discontinuation of the inciting therapeutic agent (21,22). MGN related to gold therapy may contain curvilinear particles consistent with gold within the phagosomes of the proximal tubules (figs. 7-54, 7-55).

MGN Secondary to Neoplasms. Secondary MGN has been reported in association with a number of neoplasms, such as carcinomas of the gastrointestinal tract, lung, and breast (2,5,10). These cases are morphologically indistinguishable from primary MGN. Tumor antigens, such as carcinoembryonic antigen, may be detected in the glomerular immune deposits (10).

Etiology and Pathogenesis. Secondary MGN may be caused by the deposition of preformed circulating immune complexes, as well as by the in-situ formation of immune complexes. Formation of deposits in the subepithelial space is promoted by small, low-avidity, low-affinity immune complexes that can dissociate at the level of the capillary lumen and reform on the

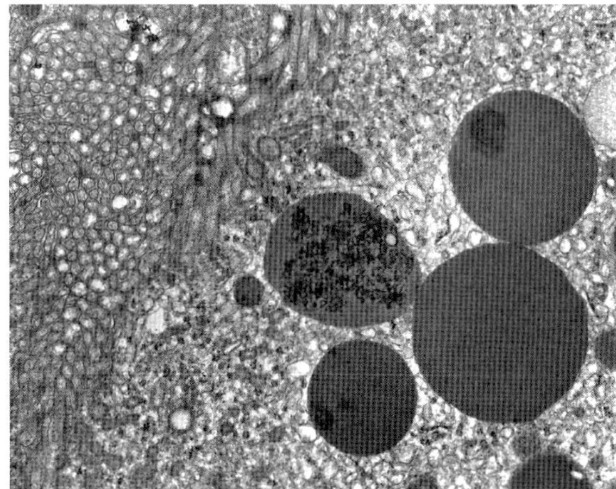

Figure 7-54

MGN ASSOCIATED WITH GOLD THERAPY

Gold particles are present in phagolysosomes of the proximal tubules, which can be recognized by their brush border (at left) (electron micrograph).

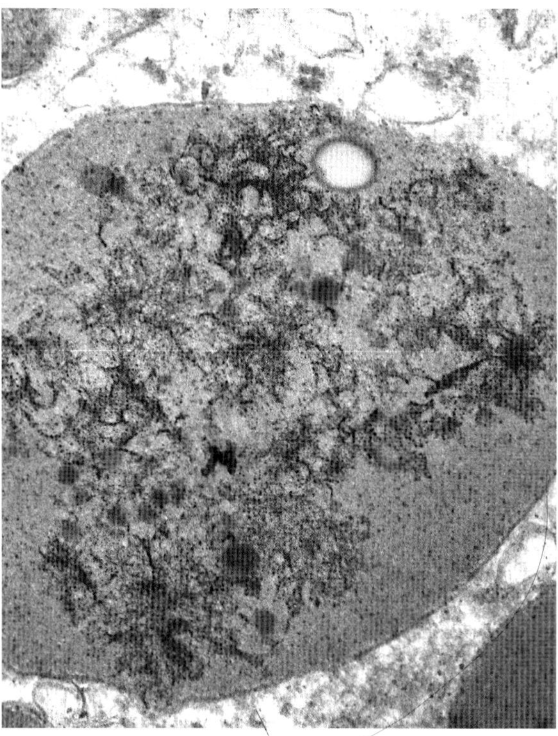

Figure 7-55

MGN ASSOCIATED WITH GOLD THERAPY

High-power view of a tubular phagolysosome containing curvilinear delicate filamentous particles consistent with gold (electron micrograph).

subepithelial side. Experimental evidence in membranous lupus nephritis suggests that subepithelial immune complex formation is favored by the presence of cationic immune complexes that interact with negative charge sites in the lamina rara externa. In secondary forms of MGN, it is likely that the antigen is nonglomerular. Putative antigens include viral antigens in hepatitis B and C, treponemal antigen in syphilis, carcinoembryonic antigen in carcinoma, nuclear antigens in SLE, and thyroglobulin in autoimmune thyroiditis. In most cases, the nature of the antigenic stimulus is unknown.

Treatment and Prognosis. Treatment of patients with secondary forms of MGN depends on the associated disease. Patients with hepatitis B- or C-associated MGN may be offered interferon or ribavirin therapy. Steroids are contraindicated because they can promote viral replication and reactivation of the hepatitis. Syphilis-associated MGN responds promptly to penicillin. Drug-induced forms of MGN are usually reversible within 2 to 6 months after withdrawal of the inciting agent, without other specific therapy. Patients with forms of MGN related to autoimmune diseases, such as SLE, rheumatoid arthritis, or autoimmune thyroiditis, are generally offered a trial of steroid therapy for up to 6 months. In the case of MGN related to neoplasia, surgical resection of tumor may be followed by resolution of the MGN (2). These variable approaches to treatment underscore the importance of accurate recognition of the secondary forms of MGN.

MGN Superimposed on Other Diseases

MGN is a common disease; therefore, it is not surprising that it may occur superimposed on other common glomerular diseases. Some have suggested that this association is merely co-incidental whereas others believe that the presence of one glomerular disease may predispose to the development of MGN. As a superimposed disease, MGN is particularly common with diabetic nephropathy (fig. 7-56). In some diabetic patients with superimposed MGN, anti-insulin antibodies have been identified in the glomerular deposits (18). MGN has also been reported to occur superimposed on IgA nephropathy, amyloidosis, and anti-GBM disease, among others. In the case of underlying IgA

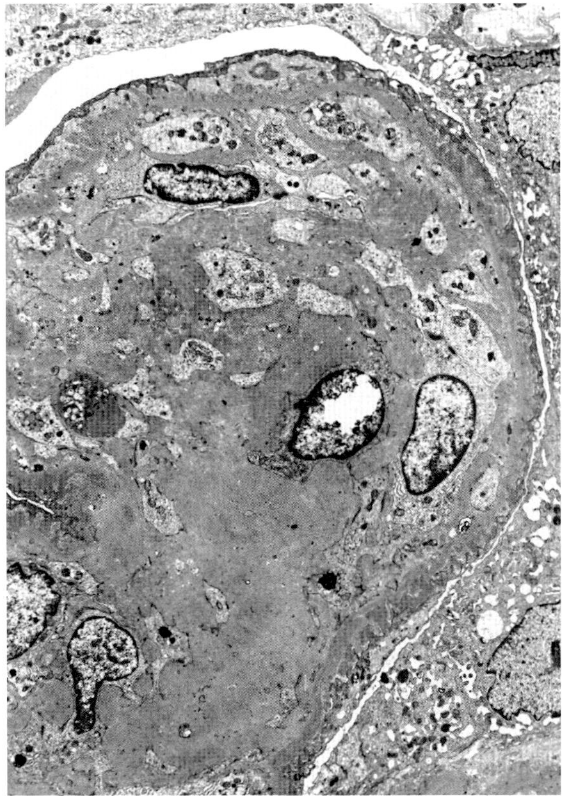

Figure 7-56

MGN SUPERIMPOSED ON DIABETIC NEPHROPATHY

There is marked nodular mesangial sclerosis, typical of diabetic nephropathy. Subepithelial deposits have formed on the thickened glomerular basement membranes of diabetic glomerulosclerosis. The membranous changes are of stage 2 to 3, with a focal overlying neomembrane. The foot processes are completely effaced (electron micrograph).

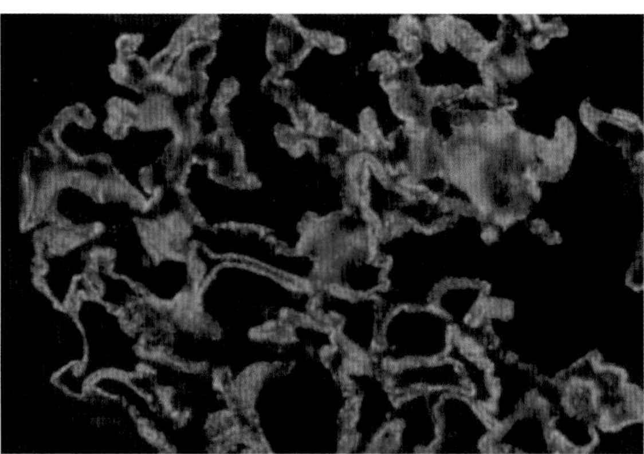

Figure 7-57

MGN SUPERIMPOSED ON IgA NEPHROPATHY

There is granular staining for IgG in the distribution of the subepithelial deposits. No staining for IgG is seen in the mesangium (immunofluorescence micrograph). (Figs. 7-57 and 7-58 are from the same patient.)

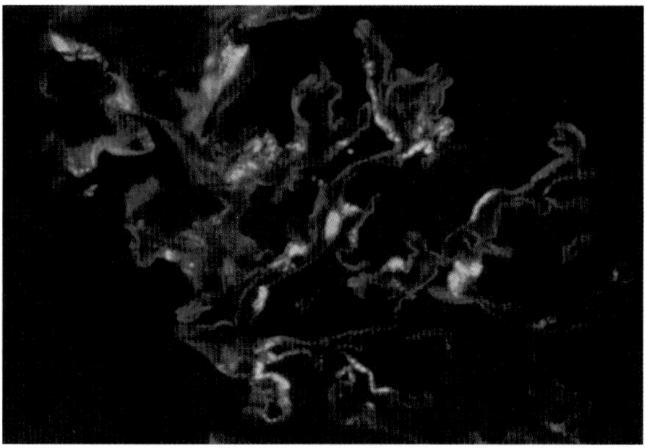

Figure 7-58

MGN SUPERIMPOSED ON IgA NEPHROPATHY

Deposits of IgA are confined to the mesangium, without involvement of the peripheral capillary walls (immunofluorescence micrograph).

nephropathy, the IgA deposits are confined to the mesangium, whereas the subepithelial deposits consist of IgG (figs. 7-57, 7-58) (14,46).

MGN with Superimposed Renal Vein Thrombosis

Renal vein thrombosis (RVT) is a common complication of MGN, whether primary or secondary (fig. 7-59) (34). Patients with a serum albumin level below 2.5 g/dL are particularly at risk. Flank pain and hematuria may herald the development of RVT in patients with sudden and complete venous thrombosis. In others, the development of RVT is more insidious, without localizing signs or symptoms. The incidence of RVT in patients with MGN may be as high as 50 percent, depending on how aggressively a diagnosis is sought using the sensitive tests of renal venogram, Doppler ultrasonogram, and magnetic resonance imaging. In some patients, the possibility of complicating RVT is first suspected at renal biopsy (44).

Morphologic clues to the diagnosis may be found in both the acute and chronic forms of RVT. In acute RVT, there is often diffuse interstitial edema, sometimes associated with interstitial

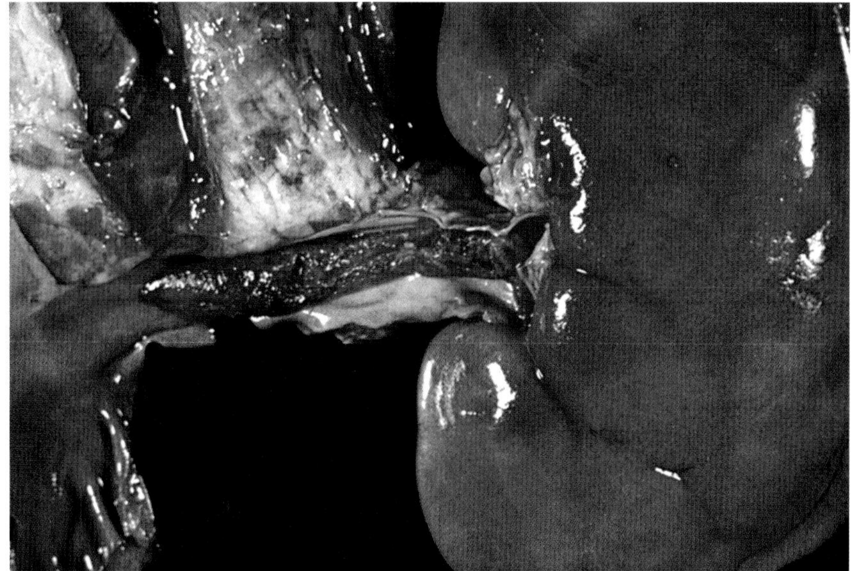

Figure 7-59

MGN WITH RENAL VEIN THROMBOSIS

There is complete occlusion of the renal vein by a thrombus that extends into the inferior vena cava.

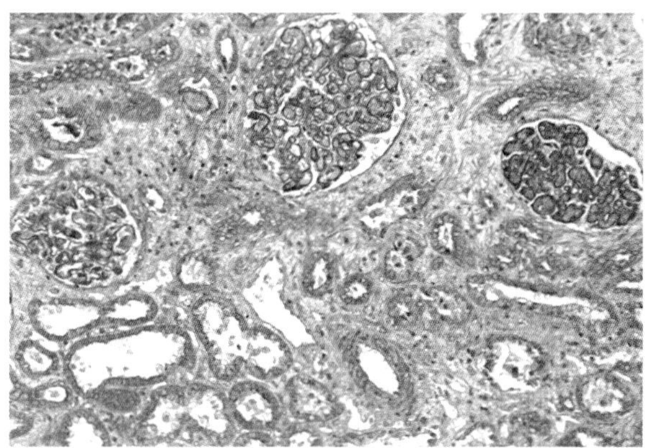

Figure 7-60

MGN WITH ACUTE RENAL VEIN THROMBOSIS

There is severe diffuse interstitial edema and glomerular capillary congestion (Masson trichrome stain).

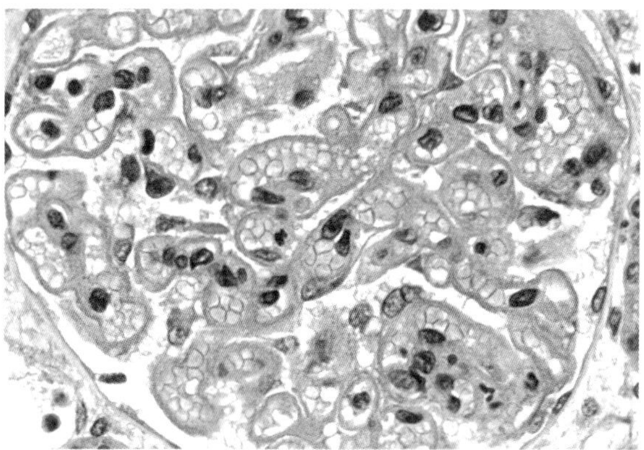

Figure 7-61

MGN WITH ACUTE RENAL VEIN THROMBOSIS

The glomerular capillary lumens are congested with erythrocytes and marginated neutrophils. The glomerular capillary walls are diffusely thickened, typical of stage 2 membranous glomerulopathy (H&E stain).

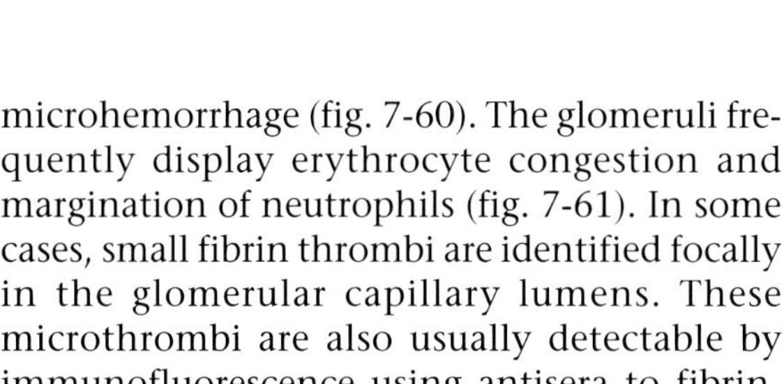

microhemorrhage (fig. 7-60). The glomeruli frequently display erythrocyte congestion and margination of neutrophils (fig. 7-61). In some cases, small fibrin thrombi are identified focally in the glomerular capillary lumens. These microthrombi are also usually detectable by immunofluorescence using antisera to fibrin-related antigens. In chronic RVT, there is typically diffuse interstitial fibrosis and tubular atrophy out of proportion to the severity of the glomerular sclerosis (fig. 7-62). The possibility of RVT should be promptly reported to the clinician because of the need for immediate anticoagulation therapy to prevent a life-threatening pulmonary embolus.

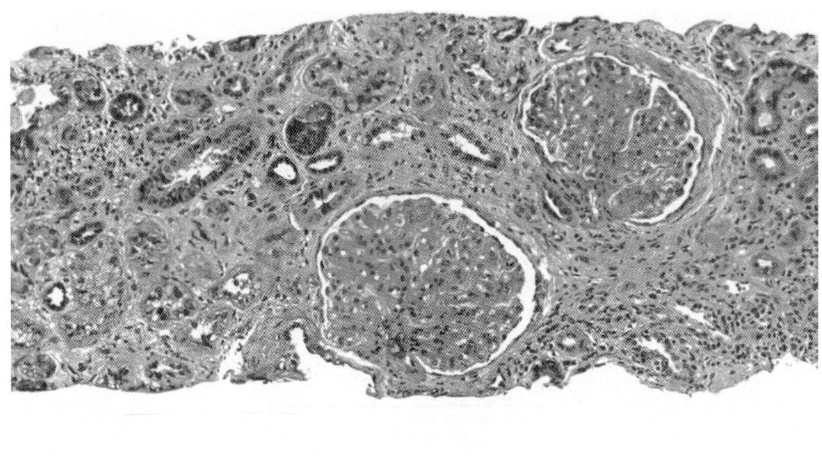

Figure 7-62

MGN WITH CHRONIC RENAL VEIN THROMBOSIS

The patient had a history of nephrotic syndrome for several months and an occlusive renal vein thrombus was identified by venogram. There is severe and diffuse tubular atrophy and interstitial fibrosis out of proportion to the degree of glomerulosclerosis (Masson trichrome stain).

REFERENCES

1. Adu D, Williams DG, Taube D, et al. Late onset systemic lupus erythematosus and lupus-like disease in patients with apparent idiopathic glomerulonephritis. Q J Med 1983;52:471–87.
2. Alpers CE, Cotran RS. Neoplasia and glomerular injury. Kidney Int 1986;30:465–73.
3. Baker PJ, Ochi RF, Schulze M, Johnson RJ, Campbell C, Couser WG. Depletion of C6 prevents development of proteinuria in experimental membranous nephropathy in rats. Am J Pathol 1989;135:185–94.
4. Bonsib SM. Scanning electron microscopy of acellular glomeruli in nephrotic syndrome. Kidney Int 1985;27:678–84.
5. Burstein DM, Korbet SM, Schwartz MM. Membranous glomerulonephritis and malignancy. Am J Kidney Dis 1993;22:5–10.
6. Cattran DC, Delmore T, Roscoe J, et al. A randomized controlled trial of prednisone in patients with idiopathic membranous nephropathy. N Engl J Med 1989;320:210–5.
7. Cattran DC, Pei Y, Greenwood CM, Ponticelli C, Passerini P, Honkanen E. Validation of a predictive model of idiopathic membranous nephropathy: its clinical and research implications. Kidney Int 1997;51:901–7.
8. A controlled study of short-term prednisone treatment in adults with membranous nephropathy. Collaborative Study of the Adult Idiopathic Nephrotic Syndrome. N Engl J Med 1979;301:1301–6.
9. Couser WG. Mediation of immune glomerular injury. J Am Soc Nephrol 1990;1:13–29.
10. Couser WG, Wagonfeld JB, Spargo BH, Lewis EJ. Glomerular deposition of tumor antigen in membranous nephropathy associated with colonic carcinoma. Am J Med 1974;57:962–70.
11. Davenport A, MacIver AG, Hall CL, MacKenzie JC. Do mesangial immune complex deposits affect the renal prognosis in membranous glomerulonephritis? Clin Nephrol 1994;41:271–6.
12. Davison AM, Cameron JS, Kerr DN, Ogg CS, Wilkinson RW. The natural history of renal function in untreated idiopathic membranous glomerulonephritis in adults. Clin Nephrol 1984;22:61–7.
13. Debiec H, Guigonis V, Mougenot B, et al. Antenatal membranous glomerulonephritis due to anti-neutral endopeptidase antibodies. N Engl J Med 2002;346:2053–60.
14. Doi T, Kanatsu K, Nagai H, Kohrogi N, Hamashima Y. An overlapping syndrome of IgA nephropathy and membranous nephropathy? Nephron 1983;35:24–30.
15. Donadio JV Jr, Torres VE, Velosa JA, et al. Idiopathic membranous nephropathy: the natural history of untreated patients. Kidney Int 1988;33:708–15.
16. Ehrenreich T, Churg J. Pathology of membranous nephropathy. In: Sommers SC, Rosen P, eds. Pathology annual. New York: Appleton-Century-Crofts; 1968;3:145.
17. Exner M, Susani M, Witzum JL, et al. Lipoproteins accumulate in immune deposits and are modified by lipid peroxidation in passive Heymann nephritis. Am J Pathol 1996;149:1313–20.
18. Furuta T, Seino J, Saito T, et al. Insulin deposits in membranous nephropathy associated with diabetes mellitus. Clin Nephrol 1992;37:65–9.

19. Geddes CC, Cattran D. The treatment of idiopathic membranous nephropathy. Semin Nephrol 2000;20:299–308.
20. Glassock RJ. Secondary membranous glomerulonephritis. Nephrol Dial Transplant 1992;7 (Suppl 1):64–71.
21. Hall CL, Fothergill NJ, Blackwell MM, Harrison PR, MacKenzie JC, MacIver AG. The natural course of gold nephropathy: long-term study of 21 patients. Br Med J 1987;295:745–8.
22. Hall CL, Jawad S, Harrison PR, et al. Natural course of penicillamine nephropathy: a long-term study of 33 patients. Br Med J 1988;296:1083–6.
23. Hogan S, Muller KE, Jennette JC, Falk RJ. A review of therapeutic studies in idiopathic membranous glomerulopathy. Am J Kidney Dis 1995;25:862–75.
24. Honig C, Mouradian JA, Montoliu J, Susin M, Sherman RL. Mesangial electron-dense deposits in membranous nephropathy. Lab Invest 1980; 42:427–32.
25. Honkanen E, Tornroth T, Pettersson E, Skrifvars B. Membranous glomerulonephritis in rheumatoid arthritis not related to gold or D-penicillamine therapy: a report of four cases and review of the literature. Clin Nephrol 1987;27:87–93.
26. Hoorntje SJ, Kallenberg CG, Weening JJ, Donker AJ, The TH, Hoedemaeker PJ. Immune-complex glomerulopathy in patients treated with captopril. Lancet 1980;1:1212–5.
27. Horvath F Jr, Teague P, Gaffney EF, Mars DR, Fuller TJ. Thyroid antigen associated immune complex glomerulonpheritis in Graves' disease. Am J Med 1979;67:901–4.
28. Hsu HC, Wu CY, Lin CY, Lin GJ, Chen CH, Huang FY. Membranous nephropathy in 52 hepatitis B surface antigen (HbsAg) carrier children in Taiwan. Kidney Int 1989;36:1103–7.
29. Jennette JC, Iskandar SS, Dalldorf FG. Pathologic differentiation between lupus and nonlupus membranous glomerulopathy. Kidney Int 1983; 24:377–85.
30. Jennette JC, Wilkman AS, Tuttle RH, Falk RJ. Frequency and pathologic significance of anti-proteinase 3 and anti-myeloperoxidase antineutrophil cytoplasmic autoantibodies in immune complex glomerulonephritis. Lab Invest 1996;74:167.
31. Johnson RJ, Willson R, Yamabe H, et al. Renal manifestations of hepatitis C infection. Kidney Int 1994;46:1255–63.
32. Klassen J, Elwood C, Grossberg AL, et al. Evolution of membranous nephropathy into anti-glomerular-basement-membrane glomerulonephritis. N Engl J Med 1974;290:1340–4.
33. Lai FM, Lai KN, Tam JS, Lui SF, To KF, Li PK. Primary glomerulonephritis with detectable hepatitis B virus antigens. Am J Surg Pathol 1994;18:175–6.
34. Llach F, Papper S, Massry SG. The clinical spectrum of renal vein thrombosis: acute and chronic. Am J Med 1980;69:819–27.
35. Markowitz GS. Membranous glomerulopathy: emphasis on secondary forms and disease variants. Adv Anat Pathol 2001;8:119–25.
36. Markowitz GS, Kambham N, Maruyama S, et al. Membranous glomerulopathy with Bowman's capsular and tubular basement membrane deposits. Clin Nephrol 2000;54:478–86.
37. Markowitz GS, Seigle RL, D'Agati VD. Three-year-old boy with partial Fanconi syndrome. Am J Kidney Dis 1999;34:184–8.
38. Muirhead N. Management of idiopathic membranous nephropathy: evidence-based recommendations. Kidney Int 1999;155(Suppl 70):S47–55.
39. Nakazawa K, Shimojo H, Komiyama Y, et al. Preexisting membranous nephropathy in allograft kidney. Nephron 1999;81:76–80.
40. Nelson TR, Charonis AS, McIvor RS, Butkowski RJ. Identification of a cDNA encoding tubulointerstitial nephritis antigen. J Biol Chem 1995;270:16265–70.
41. Pettersson E, Tornroth T, Miettinen A. Simultaneous anti-glomerular basement membrane and membranous glomerulonephritis: case report and literature review. Clin Immunol Immunopathol 1984;31:171–80.
42. Ponticelli C, Zucchelli P, Passerini P, et al. A 10-year follow-up of a randomized study with methylprednisolone and chlorambucil in membranous nephropathy. Kidney Int 1995;48:1600–4.
43. Ramos EL. Recurrent disease in the renal allograft. J Am Soc Nephrol 1991;2:109–21.
44. Rosenmann E, Pollak VE, Pirani CL. Renal vein thrombosis in the adult: a clinical and pathologic study based on renal biopsies. Medicine 1968;47:269–335.
45. Ruggenenti P, Mosconi L, Vendramin G, et al. ACE inhibition improves glomerular size selectivity in patients with idiopathic membranous nephropathy and persistent nephrotic syndrome. Am J Kidney Dis 2000:35:381–91.
46. Stokes MB, Alpers CE. Combined membranous nephropathy and IgA nephropathy. Am J Kidney Dis 1998;32:649–56.
47. Venkataseshan VS, Lieberman K, Kim DU, et al. Hepatitis-B associated glomerulonephritis: pathology, pathogenesis, and clinical course. Medicine 1990;69:200–16.
48. Wakai S, Magil AB. Focal glomerulosclerosis in idiopathic membranous glomerulonephritis. Kidney Int 1992;41:428–34.
49. Wehrmann M, Bohle A, Bogenschutz O, et al. Long-term prognosis of chronic idiopathic membranous glomerulonephritis. An analysis of 334 cases with particular regard to tubulo-interstitial changes. Clin Nephrol 1989;31:67–76.

8 AN APPROACH TO THE PATHOLOGIC DIAGNOSIS OF GLOMERULONEPHRITIS

INTRODUCTION

Inflammatory glomerular lesions (i.e., various forms of glomerulonephritis) are the primary lesions identified in approximately a third of all native kidney biopsy specimens (1,2). The pathologic diagnosis of glomerulonephritis is challenging because it requires the knowledgeable and careful integration of observations made by light, immunofluorescence, and electron microscopy with clinical and laboratory data for optimum diagnostic accuracy and precision. Specific details about the pathology of various forms of glomerulonephritis are discussed in depth in many chapters of this book, especially chapters 9 through 15. In this chapter, we propose an approach to the overall evaluation of glomerulonephritis that provides a basis for reaching an informative diagnosis that is most valuable for patient management.

The pathologic diagnosis of a specific category of glomerulonephritis is made in the context of ruling out other categories. Thus, an organized approach to diagnosis should consider all the possibilities first. The diagnostic line for glomerulonephritis usually includes two components (Table 8-1). One component describes the morphologic expression of the disease (terms in group A) and another designates a particular

Table 8-1

PATHOLOGIC DIAGNOSIS OF GLOMERULONEPHRITIS[a]

A. Morphologic Categories in the Spectrum of Proliferative and Necrotizing Glomerulonephritis
Mesangiopathy with no lesion by light microscopy
Focal or diffuse mesangioproliferative (mesangial proliferative) glomerulonephritis
Focal or diffuse proliferative (endocapillary proliferative) glomerulonephritis
Acute diffuse proliferative glomerulonephritis (exudative glomerulonephritis)
Focal or diffuse necrotizing glomerulonephritis
Crescentic glomerulonephritis (extracapillary glomerulonephritis)
Focal or diffuse sclerosing glomerulonephritis (chronic glomerulonephritis)
Type 1 membranoproliferative glomerulonephritis (mesangiocapillary glomerulonephritis)
Type 2 membranoproliferative glomerulonephritis (dense deposit disease)
B. Disease Modifiers Based on Data in Addition to Light Microscopy (e.g., Immunohistology, Electron Microscopy, Serology, and Extrarenal Manifestations)
Immune Complex Glomerulonephritis
IgA nephropathy
Henoch-Schönlein purpura nephritis
Lupus glomerulonephritis
IgM mesangial nephropathy
C1q nephropathy
Cryoglobulinemic glomerulonephritis
Postinfectious/infectious glomerulonephritis
Anti-glomerular basement membrane (GBM) glomerulonephritis
Goodpasture's syndrome
Pauci-immune Glomerulonephritis (usually antineutrophil cytoplasmic antibody [ANCA] associated)
Renal-limited vasculitis
Microscopic polyangiitis
Wegener's granulomatosis
Churg-Strauss syndrome

[a]A complete pathologic diagnosis of glomerulonephritis should include both a descriptive morphologic designation (from group A) and, whenever possible, a more specific indicator of the disease process (from group B). For example, the diagnostic designations "IgA nephropathy with focal mesangioproliferative glomerulonephritis" and "focal proliferative lupus glomerulonephritis" include indicators of categories in both groups A and B.

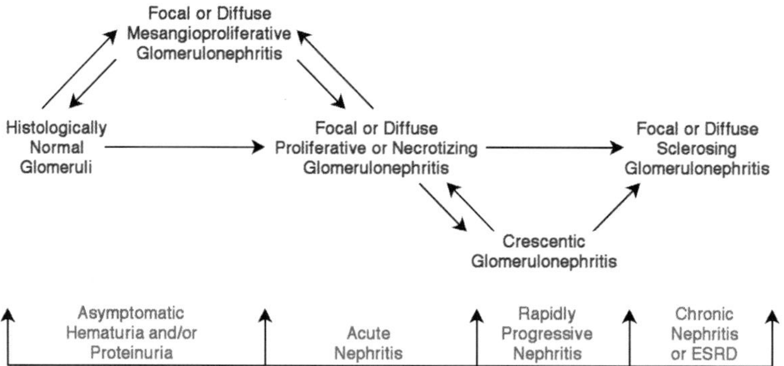

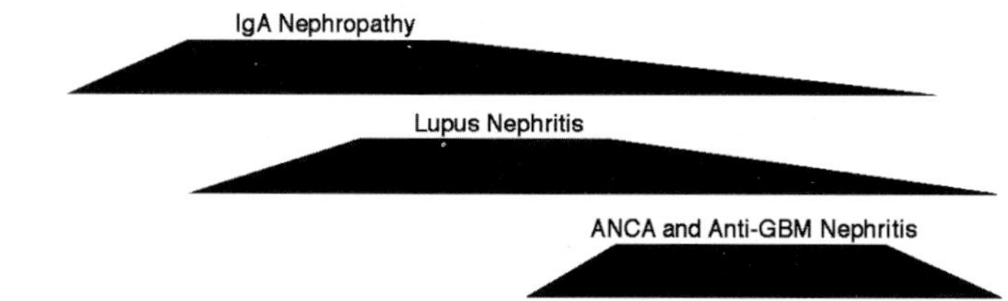

Figure 8-1

THE CORRELATION BETWEEN THE LIGHT MICROSCOPIC MORPHOLOGY OF GLOMERULONEPHRITIS AND RESULTANT CLINICAL MANIFESTATIONS

The top (blue) and middle (red) portions of the diagram illustrate the histologic and clinical spectrums of glomerulonephritis, respectively. Mesangioproliferative glomerulonephritis, for example, usually causes relatively mild clinical abnormalities whereas crescentic glomerulonephritis usually causes rapidly progressive nephritis. The lower portion of the diagram illustrates that different pathogenic categories of glomerulonephritis have different predilections for manifesting certain patterns of injury at the time of renal biopsy. For example, IgA nephropathy most often presents as a focal mesangioproliferative or proliferative glomerulonephritis, whereas antineutrophil cytoplasmic antibody (ANCA) and antiglomerular basement membrane (anti-GBM) glomerulonephritis usually present as crescentic nephritis (modified from fig. 5 from reference 1.)

pathogenic or clinicopathologic category of disease (terms in group B). This approach is complicated by the fact that a given morphologic expression (e.g., focal proliferative glomerulonephritis or crescentic glomerulonephritis) can be caused by many different disease processes with different prognoses and appropriate treatments (e.g., immunoglobulin [Ig]A nephropathy, lupus nephritis, antiglomerular basement membrane [anti-GBM] glomerulonephritis, antineutrophil cytoplasmic antibody [ANCA] glomerulonephritis); also a given relatively specific disease process (e.g., IgA nephropathy or lupus glomerulonephritis) has many different morphologic expressions.

AN APPROACH TO THE LIGHT MICROSCOPIC EVALUATION OF GLOMERULONEPHRITIS

Each category of glomerulonephritis has a spectrum of histologic expressions that vary relative to the duration, severity, activity, and chronicity of the disease process at the time of evaluation (fig. 8-1) (1,2). The observed histologic abnormalities are a "snap shot" of only one point in time within a continuum of injury. Based on the pathologic changes at this one point in time, the pathologist should try to envision what has gone before and what is likely to occur later. This will help not only in arriving at the appropriate diagnosis but also in providing useful prognostic information to the clinician. The arrows in the upper portion of figure 8-1 indicate the potential for the evolution over time of histologic expressions of glomerulonephritis.

A frequent histologic indicator of glomerulonephritis is glomerular hypercellularity (fig. 8-2). The major categories of glomerular hypercellularity are mesangial, endocapillary, and extracapillary. Mesangial hypercellularity is defined as the presence of three or more mononuclear cells in at least one mesangial region (i.e., in one contiguous peripheral zone of mesangial matrix) in a section that is approximately 3 μm in thickness (fig. 8-2B). Ultrastructural evaluation reveals that isolated mesangial hypercellularity in the setting of histologically unremarkable capillary loops is caused predominantly by an increase in mesangial cells, with only rare leukocytes (predominantly macrophages).

Endocapillary hypercellularity usually includes mesangial hypercellularity but also encompasses the increased cellularity in the glomerular capillaries that is caused by the proliferation

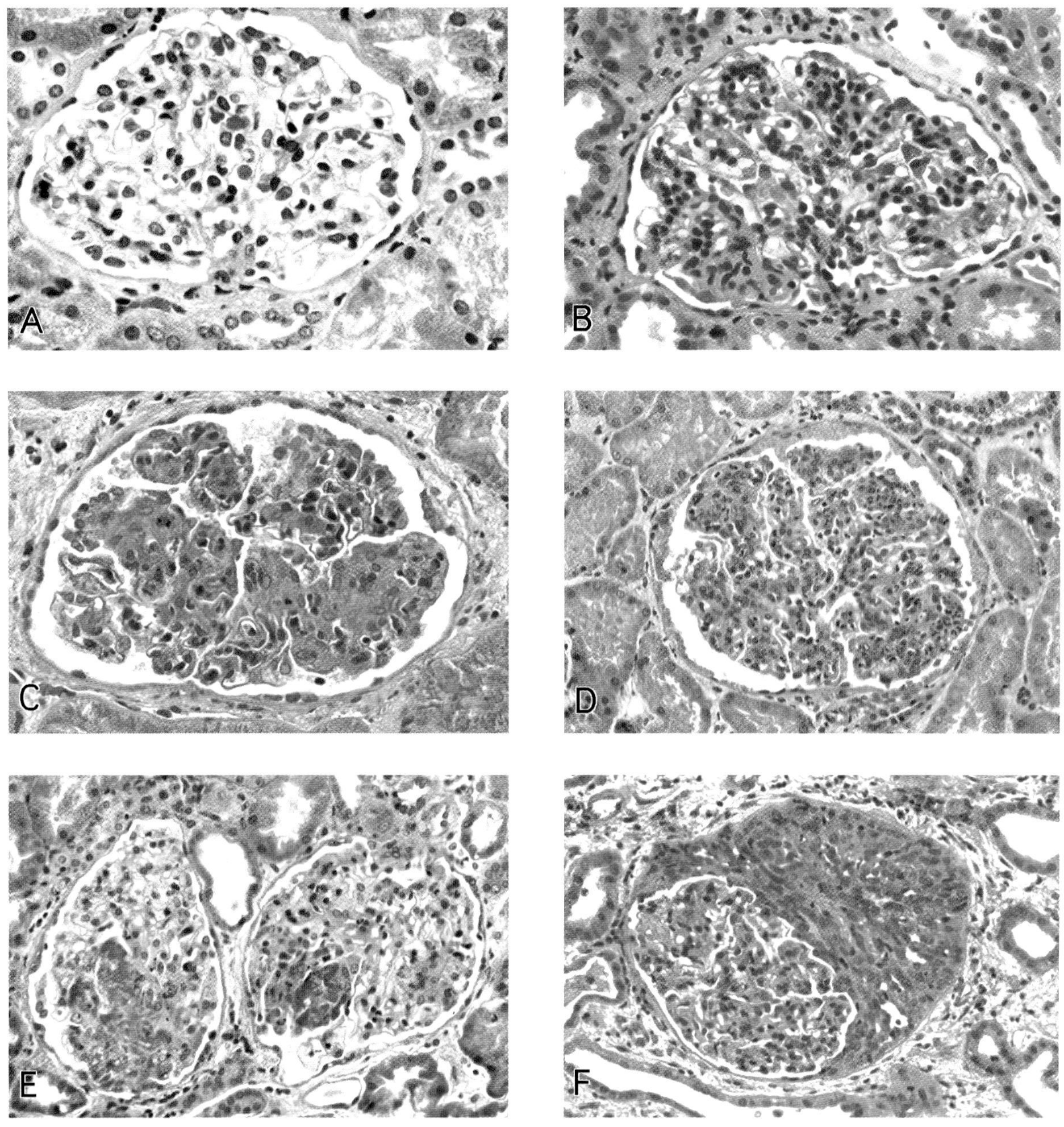

Figure 8-2

LIGHT MICROSCOPIC APPEARANCE OF DIFFERENT EXPRESSIONS OF GLOMERULONEPHRITIS IN HEMATOXYLIN AND EOSIN–STAINED SECTIONS

A: No lesion by light microscopy. There is normal cellularity, with no clustering of cells, as well as open capillary lumens and thin capillary walls.

B: Mesangioproliferative glomerulonephritis. There is segmentally variable mesangial hypercellularity, with three or more nuclei in individual mesangial zones, as well as patent capillary lumens and thin capillary walls.

C: Proliferative glomerulonephritis. There is complex endocapillary hypercellularity and obliteration or narrowing of many capillary lumens.

D: Acute proliferative glomerulonephritis. There is marked global hypercellularity with numerous segmented neutrophils.

E: Necrotizing glomerulonephritis. Both glomeruli have segmental fibrinoid necrosis with slight adjacent karyorrhexis and leukocyte infiltration.

F: Crescentic glomerulonephritis. There is a large crescent-shaped zone of extracapillary hypercellularity on the right.

of endothelial cells, influx of leukocytes, or both (fig. 8-2C). Endocapillary hypercellularity results in narrowing or occlusion of capillary lumens. When endocapillary hypercellularity includes numerous neutrophils (fig. 8-2D), it is sometimes called "exudative" but this is a misnomer because most of the neutrophils are marginated along the capillary walls and thus are not an exudate.

Extracapillary hypercellularity is an increase in cells within Bowman's space. Normally, there is a single layer of parietal epithelial cells lining Bowman's capsule and a single layer of visceral epithelial cells (podocytes) on the outer surface of the glomerular tuft. Two or more layers of cells at either site is extracapillary hypercellularity (fig. 8-2F). Extracapillary hypercellularity usually is described as crescent formation, however, one exception is the epithelial hyperplasia of the collapsing variant of focal segmental glomerulosclerosis, which, by convention, is not called crescent formation (see chapter 6). The extracapillary cellularity of collapsing focal segmental glomerulosclerosis is predominantly produced by podocyte hyperplasia whereas the extracapillary hypercellularity of glomerulonephritis (crescents) is caused predominantly by hyperplasia of parietal epithelial cells and influx of macrophages.

Glomerulonephritis also causes reduced cellularity in glomeruli. An acute loss of cells results from necrosis and typically is accompanied by fibrin formation, resulting in the pattern of injury called fibrinoid necrosis (fig. 8-2E). Inflammatory or necrotizing injury to a glomerulus may result in scarring (sclerosis) that appears as a consolidated zone with a dense collagenous matrix and few cells. Sclerotic zones may have adhesions to Bowman's capsule or adjacent fibrotic crescents. As is illustrated and discussed in detail in other chapters, special stains are valuable for identifying and differentiating between sclerosis and necrosis. For example, a Masson trichrome stain stains sclerosis blue (or green) and fibrinoid necrosis red.

As with other glomerular lesions, glomerular hypercellularity, necrosis, and sclerosis are either diffuse (affecting 50 percent or more of glomeruli) or focal (affecting fewer than 50 percent of glomeruli), and either global (affecting the entire glomerular tuft) or segmental (affecting only a portion of the glomerular tuft).

Each indicator of glomerulonephritis (i.e., mesangial hypercellularity, endocapillary hypercellularity, extracapillary hypercellularity, necrosis, and sclerosis) should be sought and described in the pathology report. The nature and distribution of these lesions will allow assignment of most examples of glomerulonephritis to one of the morphologic categories in group A of Table 8-1. *Mesangioproliferative glomerulonephritis*, or *mesangial proliferative glomerulonephritis*, is an appropriate morphologic designation if the glomeruli have mesangial hypercellularity in the absence of endocapillary or extracapillary hypercellularity (fig. 8-2B). *Proliferative glomerulonephritis* is the term often used for lesions characterized by endocapillary hypercellularity (e.g., diffuse proliferative lupus glomerulonephritis) (fig. 8-2C). An alternative term is *endocapillary glomerulonephritis*, or *endocapillary proliferative glomerulonephritis*. When a proliferative glomerulonephritis has very conspicuous glomerular neutrophils, this may be referred to as *acute proliferative glomerulonephritis*, or *exudative glomerulonephritis* (fig. 8-2D). This pattern of injury most often is an expression of acute postinfectious, especially poststreptococcal, glomerulonephritis.

Crescentic glomerulonephritis is the appropriate term when 50 percent or more of glomeruli have extracapillary hypercellularity (fig. 8-2F). When less than 50 percent of glomeruli have crescents (extracapillary hypercellularity), this should be indicated in the diagnostic line as a percentage (e.g., proliferative glomerulonephritis with 15 percent crescents), but it may be misleading to refer to the glomerulonephritis as crescentic glomerulonephritis when most glomeruli do not have crescents. Effectively communicating the extent of crescent formation to clinicians is important because this has prognostic implications and may influence the use of toxic therapeutic agents.

The pathologic accumulation of immune complexes may occur in the mesangium of glomeruli but not be detectable by light microscopy (e.g., in very mild IgA nephropathy or lupus glomerulonephritis). A pathologic diagnosis of a "mesangiopathy with no lesion by light microscopy" requires the identification of mesangial immune deposits by immunohistology or electron microscopy.

There are a number of special variants of glomerulonephritis that have distinct structural features that warrant specific designations. Type 1 membranoproliferative glomerulonephritis (mesangiocapillary glomerulonephritis) and type 2 membranoproliferative glomerulonephritis (dense deposit disease) have very distinctive abnormalities that are revealed best by electron microscopy, as discussed in detail in chapter 10 and briefly later in this chapter. Fibrillary glomerulonephritis and immunotactoid glomerulopathy, which are discussed in chapter 9, manifest histologically with varying patterns of glomerular hypercellularity and sclerosis that are shared by other forms of glomerulonephritis.

Glomerular sclerosis or necrosis (fig. 8-2E) may occur as the only histologic manifestation of glomerulonephritis (i.e., sclerosing glomerulonephritis or necrotizing glomerulonephritis) or may be combined with other lesions. For example, a specimen may have endocapillary hypercellularity and sclerosis that would warrant a morphologic diagnosis of proliferative and sclerosing glomerulonephritis, or a specimen may have necrosis and extracapillary hypercellularity in most glomeruli warranting a diagnosis of necrotizing and crescentic glomerulonephritis.

Light microscopic categorization of glomerulonephritis is only one step in the pathologic evaluation. This must be supplemented at least with immunohistology, and preferably with both immunohistology and electron microscopy.

AN APPROACH TO THE IMMUNOHISTOLOGIC EVALUATION OF GLOMERULONEPHRITIS

For an adequate pathologic evaluation of glomerulonephritis, specimens must be examined by immunohistology for glomerular localization of immunoglobulins (Ig) and complement (C) components. Immunofluorescence microscopy or immunoenzyme microscopy can be used. Staining of snap-frozen tissue provides the best sensitivity for antigen detection, however, satisfactory results can be obtained with fixed tissue if antigen-retrieval strategies are employed. Staining for fibrin also is useful. An acceptable set of reagents includes antibodies specific for IgG, IgA, IgM, C3, C1q, kappa light chains, lambda light chains, and fibrin or fibrinogen. Antialbumin can be added to assess nonspecific plasma protein entrapment. Based on immunohistologic findings, glomerulonephritis is classified into three immunohistologic categories that relate to the pathogenesis of the inflammation (fig. 8-3): 1) granular glomerular localization of immunoglobulin and complement, indicative of immune complex–mediated injury; 2) linear glomerular basement membrane localization of immunoglobulin, indicative of anti-GBM antibody-mediated injury; and 3) no or scanty glomerular immunoglobulin localization, which is referred to as pauci-immune glomerulonephritis in the appropriate setting (e.g., when there is glomerular necrosis or crescent formation).

Immune complex glomerulonephritis is divided into more specific categories based on the composition and distribution of immune deposits and additional information about pathogenic factors, such as etiologic infections or autoimmune diseases (figs. 8-3, 8-4). These specific categories are discussed in detail in other chapters, and include infectious and postinfectious glomerulonephritis (chapter 11), IgA nephropathy and Henoch-Schönlein purpura nephritis (chapter 12), lupus nephritis (chapter 13), cryoglobulinemic glomerulonephritis and other forms of membranoproliferative glomerulonephritis (chapter 10), and fibrillary glomerulonephritis and immunotactoid glomerulopathy (chapter 9).

Anti-GBM glomerulonephritis, which is discussed in detail in chapter 14, is a special form of immune complex glomerulonephritis with in situ formation of immune complexes along the glomerular basement membranes as a result of anti-GBM antibodies binding to epitopes in type IV collagen. This results in a very distinctive pattern of linear immunostaining for IgG along the glomerular basement membranes (fig. 8-3). The immune complex deposits are not detectable by electron microscopy and thus anti-GBM glomerulonephritis cannot be distinguished from pauci-immune (ANCA) glomerulonephritis by electron microscopy. In addition, both anti-GBM glomerulonephritis and ANCA-associated glomerulonephritis cause a histologically indistinguishable necrotizing and crescentic glomerulonephritis. Thus, immunohistology is required to pathologically differentiate the two.

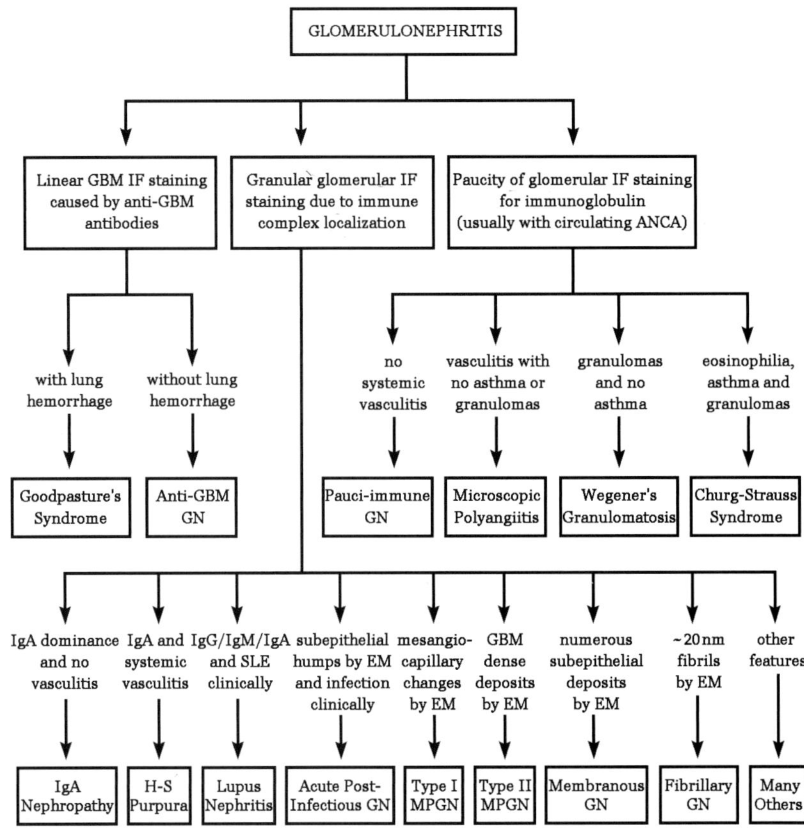

Figure 8-3

ALGORITHM FOR CATEGORIZING SOME FORMS OF GLOMERULONEPHRITIS

The first level of arborization is based on findings by immunohistology, such as immunofluorescence microscopic findings. Subsequent categorization requires an integration of additional pathologic data, laboratory data, and clinical data. GN = glomerulonephritis; IF = immunofluorescence microscopy; EM = electron microscopy; MPGN = membranoproliferative glomerulonephritis; GMB = glomerular basement membrane; and H-S = Henoch-Schönlein. (Modified from fig. 4 from reference 1.)

The term pauci-immune glomerulonephritis typically is applied to lesions that have little or no staining for immunoglobulin and also have evidence of active fibrinoid necrosis or crescent formation, or chronic sclerotic lesions that indicate earlier necrosis or crescent formation. Although some patients with pauci-immune necrotizing and crescentic glomerulonephritis have renal-limited disease, most have evidence of systemic vasculitis that can be categorized as microscopic polyangiitis, Wegener's granulomatosis, or Churg-Strauss syndrome. When the presence of ANCA is documented serologically, a diagnosis of ANCA glomerulonephritis is appropriate, e.g., ANCA necrotizing and crescentic glomerulonephritis. Data in addition to renal pathology are required to determine if the glomerulonephritis is a renal-limited process or a component of microscopic polyangiitis, Wegener's granulomatosis, or Churg-Strauss syndrome (fig. 8-3). Pauci-immune (ANCA) glomerulonephritis is discussed in depth in chapter 15.

AN APPROACH TO THE ELECTRON MICROSCOPIC EVALUATION OF GLOMERULONEPHRITIS

The inflammatory changes seen by light microscopy are observed in greater detail by transmission electron microscopy (figs. 8-5, 8-6). The cell types producing glomerular hypercellularity are more readily identified. Increased numbers of mesangial cells, with their typical smooth muscle features (e.g., subplasmalemmal dense bodies), are identified in the mesangial regions in specimens with mesangial hypercellularity. When endocapillary hypercellularity is present by light microscopy, electron microscopy reveals the influx of leukocytes into capillary lumens and mesangial regions, and varying degrees of endothelial proliferation. Mitotic figures may be observed. When crescent formation is observed by light microscopy, breaks in glomerular basement membranes usually can be found by electron microscopy, although this may require a diligent search. Bundles of polymerized fibrin (fibrin

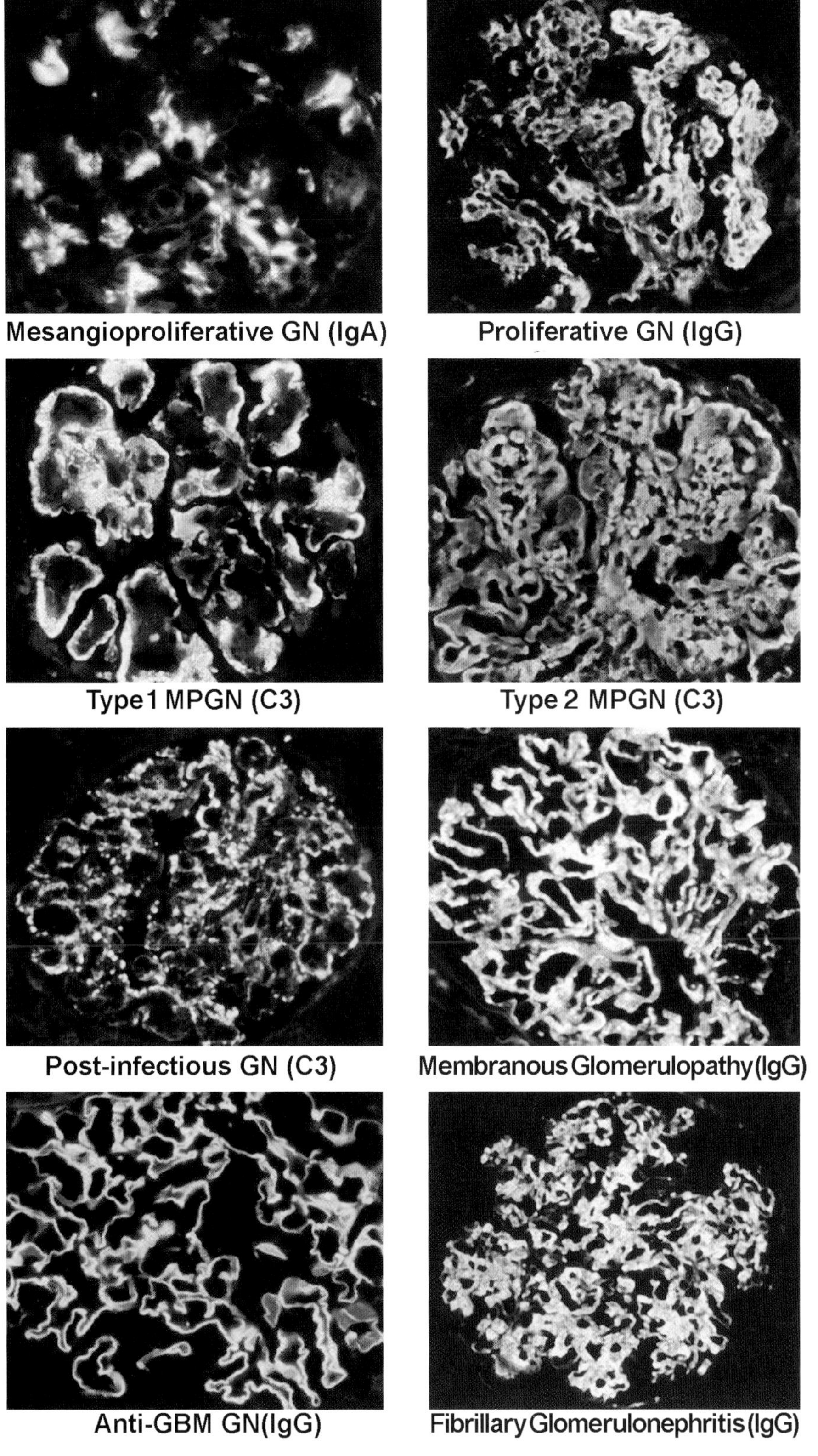

Figure 8-4

IMMUNOFLUORESCENCE MICROSCOPIC APPEARANCE OF DIFFERENT FORMS OF GLOMERULONEPHRITIS

These differences can be used to contribute to diagnostic categorization. The specificities of the antibodies used for each stain are in parenthesis. There is mesangial localization of immunoglobulin in mesangioproliferative glomerulonephritis (GN) compared to the mesangial and capillary wall granular staining in proliferative glomerulonephritis. There is band-like peripheral staining of the capillary wall for C3 in both categories of membranoproliferative glomerulonephritis (MPGN). The very coarsely granular staining of postinfectious glomerulonephritis is compared to the more finely granular staining of membranous glomerulopathy. Similarities and differences between the staining in fibrillary glomerulonephritis are compared to other forms of proliferative immune complex glomerulonephritis. The linear staining in anti-GBM glomerulonephritis is compared to the granular staining in other forms of glomerulonephritis.

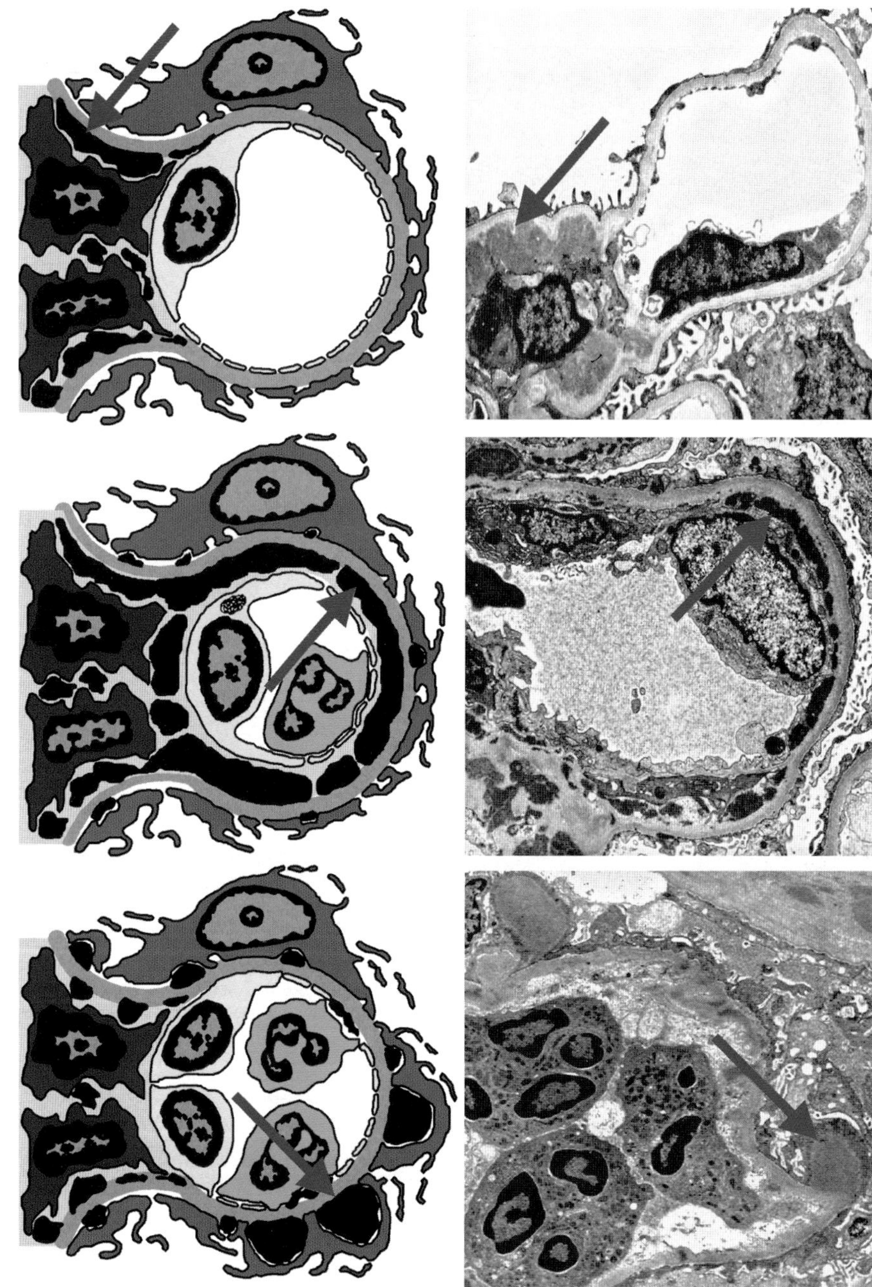

Figure 8-5

DIAGRAMS AND ELECTRON MICROGRAPHS THAT ILLUSTRATE THE ULTRASTRUCTURAL DIFFERENCES BETWEEN MESANGIOPROLIFERATIVE GLOMERULONEPHRITIS, PROLIFERATIVE GLOMERULONEPHRITIS, AND ACUTE PROLIFERATIVE POSTINFECTIOUS GLOMERULONEPHRITIS

Top: The mesangioproliferative glomerulonephritis has mesangial dense deposits beneath the paramesangial glomerular basement membrane (arrows) but no capillary wall deposits.

Middle: The proliferative glomerulonephritis has subendothelial deposits (arrows) as well as mesangial and a few subepithelial deposits.

Bottom: The postinfectious glomerulonephritis has subepithelial hump-like deposits (arrows) and numerous neutrophils in the lumen.

tactoids) are present between crescent cells, in thrombosed capillaries, and within sites of fibrinoid necrosis. Crescents are composed of varying mixtures of epithelial cells and macrophages.

Electron-dense deposits correspond to the sites of immune complex localization in immune complex–mediated glomerulonephritis. The configuration and distribution of electron-dense deposits are useful in categorization of different types of immune complex–mediated glomerulonephritis (figs. 8-5, 8-6). The pathology report should indicate the location of dense deposits as mesangial, subendothelial, intramembranous, or subepithelial. The presence of mesangial immune complex dense deposits, in the absence of capillary wall deposits, most often corresponds to mesangioproliferative or very mild proliferative glomerulonephritis by light micros-

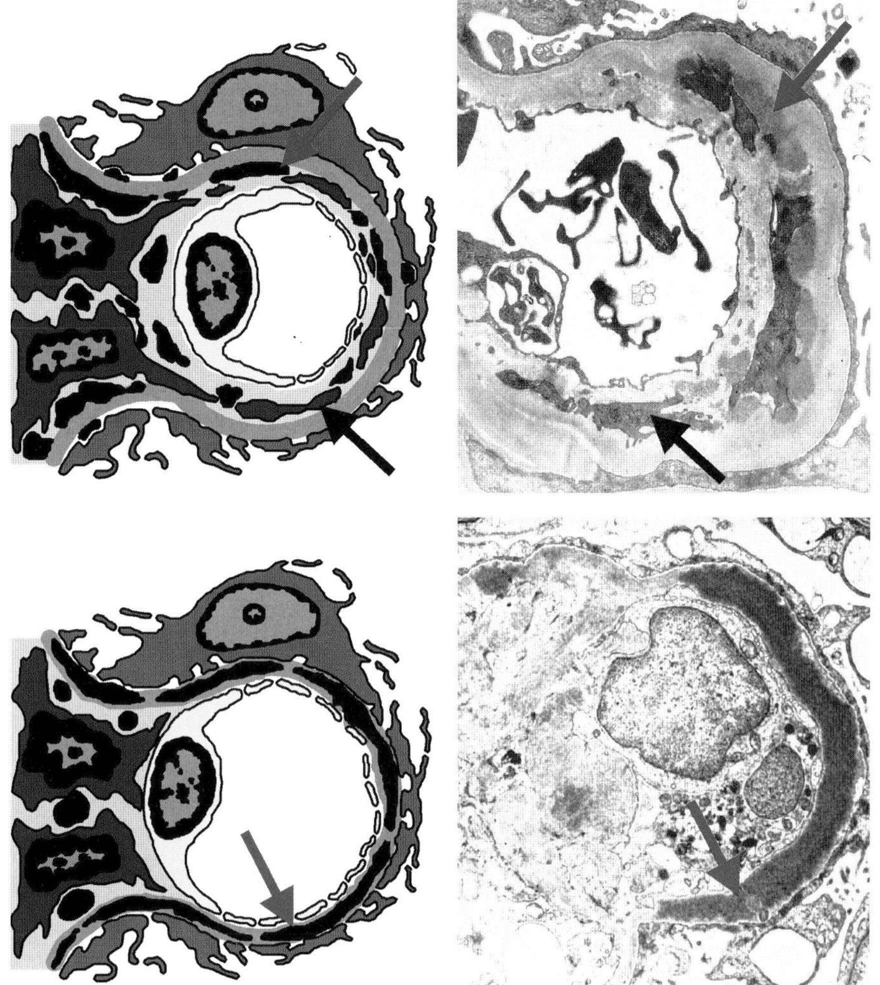

Figure 8-6

DIAGRAMS AND ELECTRON MICROGRAPHS THAT ILLUSTRATE THE ULTRASTRUCTURAL DIFFERENCES BETWEEN TYPE 1 AND TYPE 2 MEMBRANOPROLIFERATIVE GLOMERULONEPHRITIS

Top: Type 1 membranoproliferative glomerulonephritis (MPGN) has subendothelial deposits (blue arrows) and subendothelial mesangial interposition (black arrows).

Bottom: Type 2 MPGN has intramembranous dense deposits (arrows).

copy (e.g., IgA nephropathy with focal mesangioproliferative glomerulonephritis) (fig. 8-5, top). Numerous large subendothelial immune complex dense deposits usually correspond to active proliferative glomerulonephritis by light microscopy (e.g., diffuse proliferative lupus glomerulonephritis) (fig. 8-5, middle). Scattered large subepithelial dense deposits (often called humps), along with scattered mesangial and small subendothelial deposits, raise the possibility of acute postinfectious glomerulonephritis, especially poststreptococcal glomerulonephritis (fig. 8-5, bottom). The two major types of membranoproliferative glomerulonephritis have distinctive electron microscopic features. Type 1 has subendothelial dense deposits accompanied by subendothelial interposition of projections of mesangial cytoplasm (fig. 8-6, top). This extension of mesangium into the capillary walls is sometimes referred to as mesangiocapillary change. Thus, a synonym for type 1 membranoproliferative glomerulonephritis is mesangiocapillary glomerulonephritis. Type 2 membranoproliferative glomerulonephritis has pathognomonic dense bands within glomerular basement membranes (fig. 8-6, bottom), and a synonym based on this distinctive feature is dense deposit disease.

In addition to the distribution of the deposits, their texture should be assessed ultrastructurally. Most immune complex deposits are finely granular or amorphous. Organized deposits with a particular substructure (e.g., fibrils or microtubules) are seen in such diseases as cryoglobulinemic glomerulonephritis, fibrillary glomerulonephritis, immunotactoid glomerulopathy, and some examples of lupus glomerulonephritis. Diseases with organized textured deposits are discussed in detail in chapter 9.

Anti-GBM glomerulonephritis and pauci-immune (ANCA) glomerulonephritis do not have specific electron microscopic features. When pauci-immune glomerulonephritis has low intensity immunostaining for immunoglobulins or complement, a few scattered immune complex–type electron-dense deposits may be identified by electron microscopy. The likelihood of positive ANCA serology in a patient with glomerulonephritis is inversely proportional to the amount of dense deposits seen by electron microscopy and immunoglobulin seen by immunohistology. A minority of patients with typical pathologic findings of immune complex glomerulonephritis and crescent formation are ANCA positive, indicating concurrent immune complex and ANCA glomerulonephritis.

In some specimens, electron microscopy merely confirms the diagnosis that was rendered by light microscopy and immunohistology. However, in other specimens, findings by electron microscopy provide new information that substantially clarifies the diagnosis and is valuable for patient management. For example, the finding of endothelial tubuloreticular inclusions in a patient with immune complex proliferative glomerulonephritis raises the possibility of unrecognized or latent lupus nephritis; the presence of microtubular configurations in the immune deposits of membranoproliferative glomerulonephritis raises the possibility of cryoglobulinemia and hepatitis C infection. In a few specimens, electron microscopy corrects an erroneous conclusion that would be made based on light microscopy and immunohistology alone. For example, what appears to be a sclerosing glomerulonephritis by light microscopy can be shown by electron microscopy to be in fact hereditary nephritis with glomerular basement membrane laminations. This correction in the diagnosis would have important consequences not only for the patient but also the family. A few glomerular diseases that have light microscopic and immunohistologic features that are shared with many forms of glomerulonephritis can only be conclusively diagnosed by electron microscopy, for example, fibrillary glomerulonephritis, immunotactoid glomerulopathy, and collagenofibrotic glomerulopathy (all of which are discussed in chapter 9).

SUMMARY

Optimum pathologic evaluation of glomerulonephritis requires light microscopy, immunohistology, and electron microscopy. A methodical diagnostic approach should be followed that takes into consideration all categories of glomerulonephritis. This allows the confident exclusion of incompatible categories of glomerulonephritis and should provide evidence for the most appropriate category. The pathologic diagnostic line should always contain terms that define the morphologic expression of glomerulonephritis (terms in group A of Table 8-1). Whenever possible, the diagnostic line also should include designations that indicate a more specific pathogenic or clinicopathologic category of glomerulonephritis (terms in group B of Table 8-1). Formulating the most useful diagnosis often requires integrating information not only from light microscopy, immunohistology, and electron microscopy, but also from laboratory data and clinical manifestations.

REFERENCES

1. Jennette JC, Falk RJ. Diagnosis and management of glomerular diseases. Med Clin North Am 1997;81:653–77.
2. Jennette JC, Falk RJ. Glomerular clinicopathologic syndromes. In: Greenberg A, Cheung AK, Coffman TM, Falk RJ, Jennette JC, eds. National Kidney Foundation primer on kidney diseases, 3rd ed. San Diego: Academic Press; 2001:129–43.

9 GLOMERULAR DISEASES WITH PARAPROTEINEMIA OR ORGANIZED DEPOSITS

A number of renal diseases are distinguished by abnormal renal deposits that have distinctive ultrastructural patterns (fig. 9-1). These deposits may be composed of a variety of proteins, such as whole or truncated immunoglobulin molecules, amyloid A protein, fibronectin, or collagen. The most common components of the organized deposits of renal disease are monoclonal immunoglobulin molecules. Table 9-1 lists a number of clinically and pathologically distinct types of renal disease caused by these molecules. The diseases that usually have extensive glomerular involvement are discussed in this chapter. The tubulointerstitial diseases are discussed in chapter 22. More than one type of glomerular or tubulointerstitial disease can be produced in the same kidney by a monoclonal gammopathy. Therefore, once one disease caused by monoclonal immunoglobulin is identified in a kidney specimen, others should be sought. The precise diagnosis of glomerular diseases caused by monoclonal immunoglobulin molecules requires integration of findings by light, immunofluorescence, and electron microscopy (Table 9-2).

Table 9-1

RENAL DISEASES INDUCED BY MONOCLONAL IMMUNOGLOBULIN MOLECULES

Glomerular/Vascular Diseases (Tubules and Interstitium May Be Involved)
- AL amyloidosis
- AH amyloidosis
- Light chain deposition disease (LCDD)
- Heavy chain deposition disease (HCDD)
- Light and heavy chain deposition disease (LHCDD)
- Cryoglobulinemia (types 1 and 2)
- Monoclonal immunotactoid glomerulopathy

Tubulointerstitial Disease
- Light chain (myeloma) cast nephropathy
- Tubular epithelial cell dysfunction (e.g., Fanconi's syndrome)
- Acute tubular necrosis

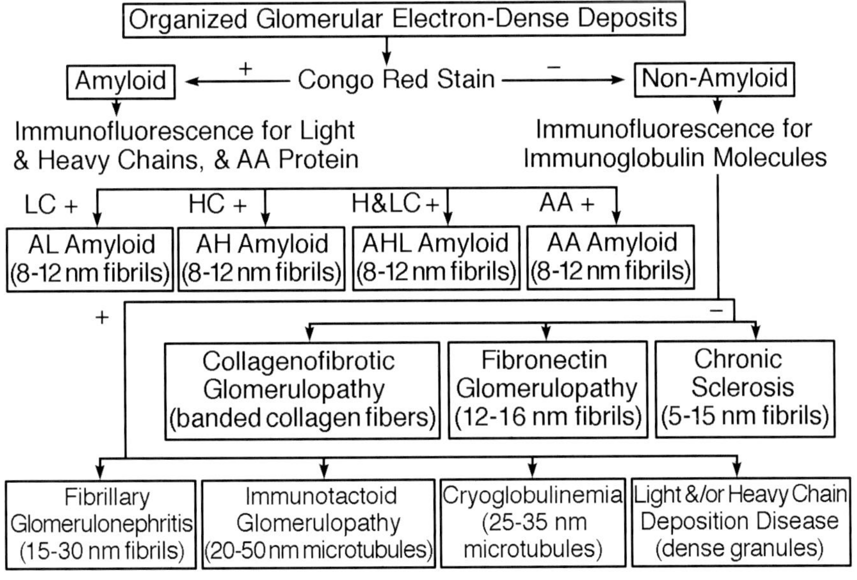

Figure 9-1

ALGORITHM

Algorithm for identifying glomerular diseases with deposits that have an organized appearance by electron microscopy.

Table 9-2

DIFFERENTIAL PATHOLOGIC GLOMERULAR FEATURES OF DISEASES WITH GLOMERULAR MONOCLONAL IMMUNOGLOBULIN DEPOSITS AND THEIR MIMICS

	AA Amyloidosis	AL Amyloidosis	AH Amyloidosis	LCDD[a]	HCDD	LHCDD	Diabetic GS	Fibrillary GN	Immunotactoid GN	Cyroglobulinemia	MPGN
Usual LM[b] Pattern	fluffy acidophilic deposits	fluffy acidophilic deposits	fluffy acidophilic deposits	nodular sclerosis	nodular sclerosis	nodular sclerosis	nodular sclerosis, thick GBM[c]	thick capillaries, expanded mesangium	thick capillaries, expanded mesangium	thick capillaries, expanded mesangium	thick capillaries, expanded mesangium
Deposit Staining											
PAS	weak/–	weak/–	weak/–	+	+	+	+	mottled	mottled	double GBM	double GBM
JMS	weak/–	weak/–	weak/–	weak/+	weak/+	weak/+	+	mottled	mottled	double GBM	double GBM
Congo red	+	+	+	–	–	–	–	–	–	–	–
IM Staining											
Ig	–	one LC, usually λ	one HC, usually γ	one LC, usually κ	one HC, usually γ	one LC, one HC	polyclonal HC and LC	oligoclonal HC and LC	monoclonal > polyclonal	polyclonal >> monoclonal	poly clonal HC and LC
C3	–	–	weak/–	weak/–	+	+	–	strong +	strong +	strong +	strong +
EM Pattern	fibrils, 8-12 nm	fibrils, 8-12 nm	fibrils, 8-12 nm	dense granules	dense granules	dense granules	thickened GBM and mesangium	fibrils, 15-30 nm	microtubules, 20-50 nm	dense deposits, often 25-35 nm microtubules	homogeneous dense deposits

[a]LCDD = light chain deposition disease; HCDD = heavy chain deposition disease; LHCDD = light and heavy chain deposition disease; GS = glomerulosclerosis; GN = glomerulonephritis; MPGN = membranoproliferative glomerulonephritis.

[b]LM = light microscopy; IM = immunofluorescence microscopy; EM = electron microscopy; PAS = periodic acid–Schiff stain; JMS = Jones methenamine silver stain; Ig = immunoglobulin; C = complement.

[c]GBM = glomerular basement membrane; LC = light chain; HC = heavy chain.

AMYLOIDOSIS

Definition. Amyloidosis is defined by the extracellular accumulation of proteins in a characteristic form that results in positive staining with Congo red, as detected by light microscopy, and the formation of approximately 10-nm, randomly oriented, nonbranching fibrils that can be seen by standard transmission electron microscopy (4,5,15,19). The molecular configuration of amyloid is as an antiparallel, beta-pleated sheet. Amyloid can be composed of a variety of different monotypic polypeptides, including immunoglobulin light chains (AL amyloid), immunoglobulin heavy chains (AH amyloid), amyloid A protein (AA amyloid), beta-2-microglobulin, prealbumin (transthyretin), procalcitonin, islet amyloid polypeptide, atrial natriuretic peptides, beta-amyloid protein, cystatin C, gelsolin, apolipoprotein AI or AII, lysozyme, and others (5). No matter what the molecular composition, however, amyloid always has the same characteristic histologic and ultrastructural appearance. Immunohistology or some other assay that can identify the molecular composition is required to differentiate between the different types of amyloid. Of the many types of amyloid, AL and AA most often affect the kidneys.

Clinical Features. *AA amyloidosis*, also called *secondary amyloidosis*, often occurs with an identifiable chronic inflammatory disease that is the presumed cause of the amyloidosis. Such diseases include chronic autoimmune diseases

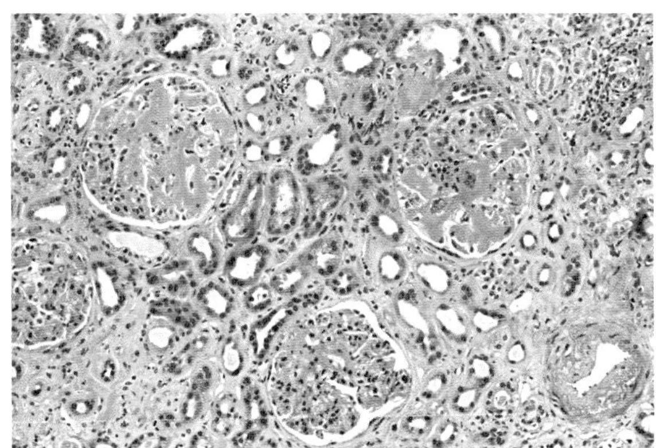

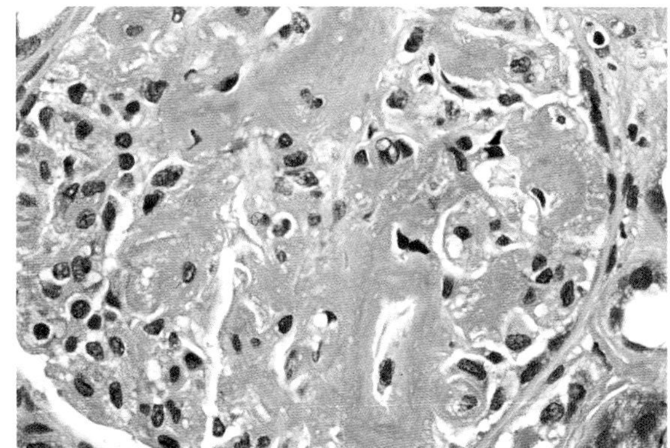

Figure 9-2

AMYLOIDOSIS

Left: The low-power magnification demonstrates focally and segmentally variable glomerular deposition of pale acidophilic material. There is also interstitial fibrosis and tubular atrophy.

Right: The higher magnification shows segmentally variable involvement of the capillary walls and mesangium, with obliteration of some capillary lumens (hematoxylin and eosin [H&E] stain).

(e.g., rheumatoid arthritis) and chronic infectious diseases (e.g., tuberculosis, osteomyelitis, and chronic suppurative skin infections caused by "skin popping" by drug abusers) (5,19). AA amyloidosis also occurs as a major complication of familial Mediterranean fever, which is an autosomal recessive disease characterized by recurrent attacks of fever and peritonitis, pleuritis, arthritis, or erythema (13).

Patients with *AL amyloidosis* always have a B-cell dyscrasia of some type that is the source of the amyloidogenic light chains, although this may not be identifiable when the AL amyloid is first identified in the kidney. Careful evaluation reveals monoclonal immunoglobulin light chains in the blood or urine in more than 90 percent of patients with AL amyloidosis, and most of the remaining patients have abnormal monoclonal populations of plasma cells in bone marrow biopsy specimens. Only about 20 percent of patients meet the diagnostic criteria for multiple myeloma or B-cell lymphoma/leukemia at the time AL amyloidosis is diagnosed (4); some B-cell neoplasms do not become apparent until 15 or more years after the initial diagnosis of AL amyloidosis (9).

Extrarenal manifestations of amyloidosis include congestive heart failure caused by myocardial infiltration by amyloid, orthostatic hypertension, bladder dysfunction, dysesthesias caused by infiltration of amyloid into autonomic and peripheral nerves, hepatomegaly, splenomegaly, and macroglossia.

At the time of diagnosis of renal amyloidosis, virtually all patients have proteinuria, often in the nephrotic range. Approximately two thirds have renal insufficiency at the time of diagnosis. Hematuria may be present but is rarely a prominent feature.

Gross Findings. Kidneys typically are enlarged, pale, firm, and sometimes waxy. The cut surfaces of the kidney are firm and remain very flat, which differs from the normal kidney, which bulges slightly resulting in slight curvature of the cut surfaces.

Light Microscopic Findings. AA and AL amyloid have the same pathologic features when viewed by light microscopy. As in other tissues, amyloid in the kidney is amorphous and acidophilic (fig. 9-2) (15,19). The acidophilia usually is less dense than the acidophilia of the mesangial matrix or zones of glomerular sclerosis or interstitial fibrosis. Thus, the amyloid deposits have a "softer" (paler) appearance than the sclerosis of diabetic glomerulosclerosis, light chain deposition disease, and many other forms of glomerular sclerosis. Usually, amyloid deposits are only weakly positive for periodic acid–Schiff (PAS) (figs. 9-3; 9-4, left). Thus, in glomeruli, PAS staining demarcates amyloid deposits as pale zones within the more deeply staining mesangial matrix or interrupting darker staining basement

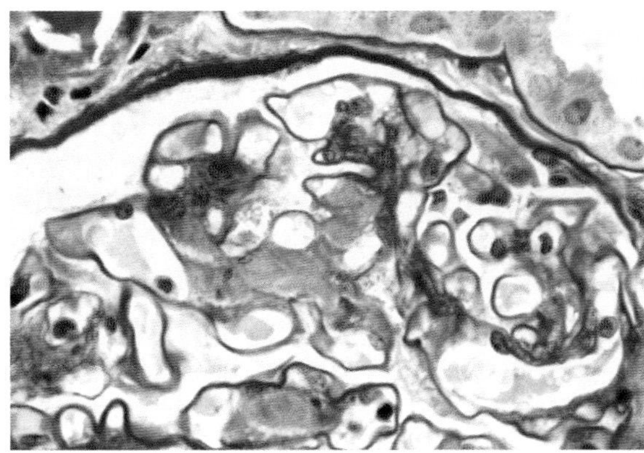

Figure 9-3

AMYLOIDOSIS

Periodic acid–Schiff (PAS) stain shows focal, predominantly mesangial accumulations of amyloid that stain less strongly than uninvolved mesangial matrix areas, glomerular basement membranes, and Bowman's capsule.

membranes. In the same way, amyloid deposits stain weakly or not at all with Jones methenamine silver (JMS) stain, and thus appear as negative defects in the expanded glomerular mesangium and thickened basement membranes (fig. 9-4, right). In other words, the replacement of basement membrane and mesangial matrix by amyloid causes a loss of argyrophilia (19). There may be delicate argyrophilic new basement membrane material formed internal to subendothelial amyloid and external to subepithelial amyloid.

Occasional examples of amyloidosis have focal, parallel alignment of amyloid fibrils in the subepithelial zone that results in focal capillary wall spikes that have enough adjacent matrix to be seen with PAS and JMS staining (fig. 9-4). These spikes are more focal, closely clustered, and longer than the typical spikes of membranous

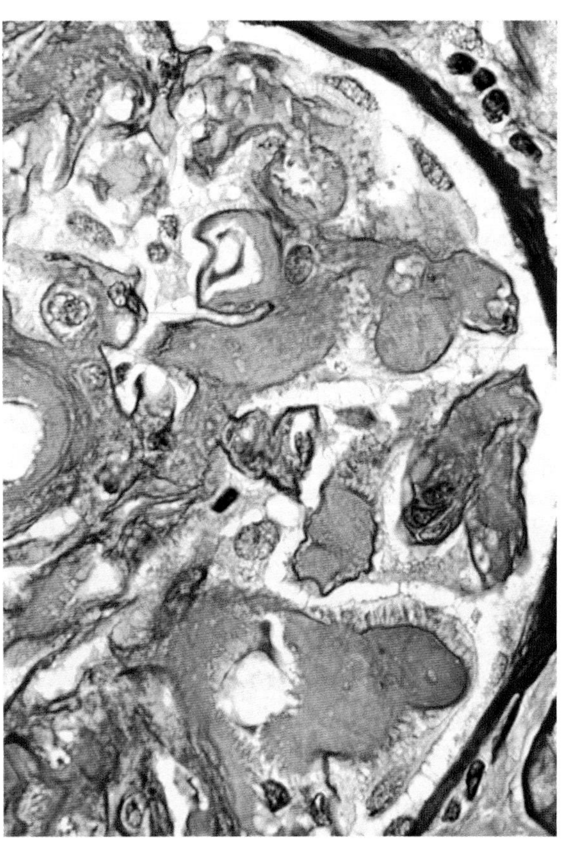

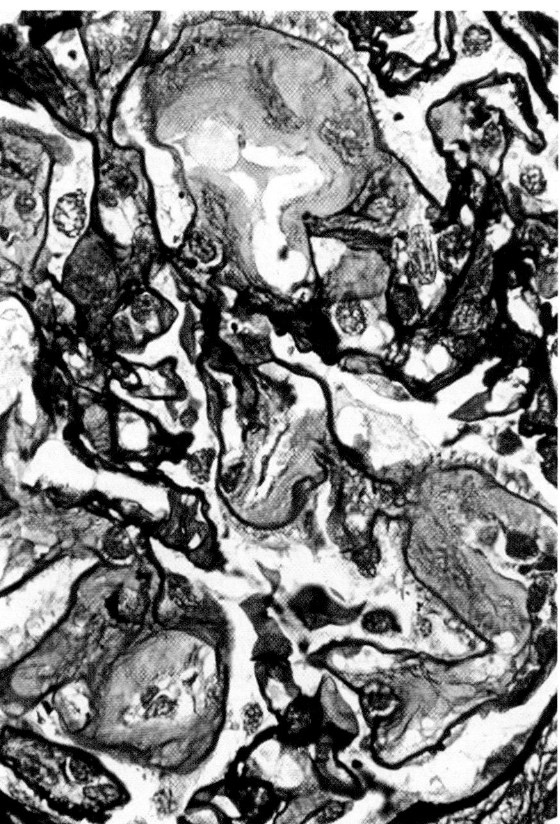

Figure 9-4

AMYLOIDOSIS

The PAS (left) and Jones methenamine silver (JMS, right) stains delineate poorly staining areas in expanded mesangial regions and thickened capillary walls that correspond to amyloid deposits. Some capillary walls have delicate spikes projecting from the outer surface of the glomerular capillaries ("cock's combs").

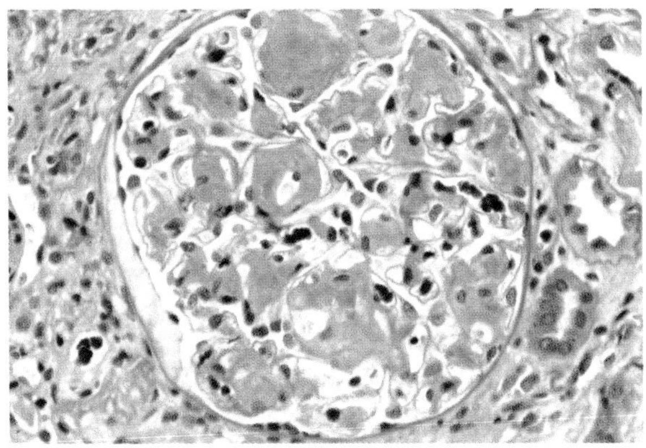

Figure 9-5

AMYLOIDOSIS

The extensive glomerular deposition of amyloid stains in a similar manner to collagen with the Masson trichrome stain.

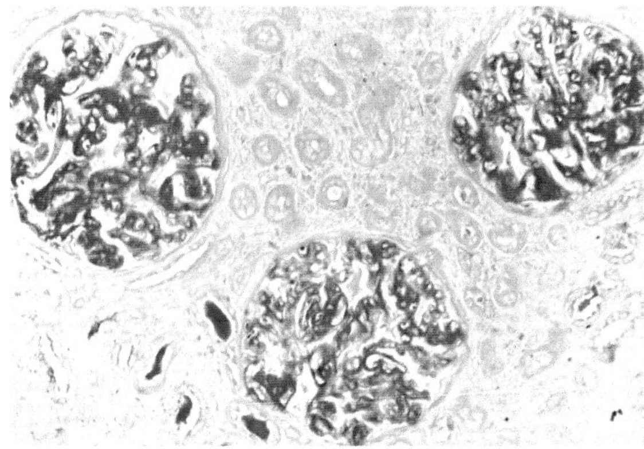

Figure 9-6

AMYLOIDOSIS

The amyloid within the glomeruli is clearly demarcated by this crystal violet stain.

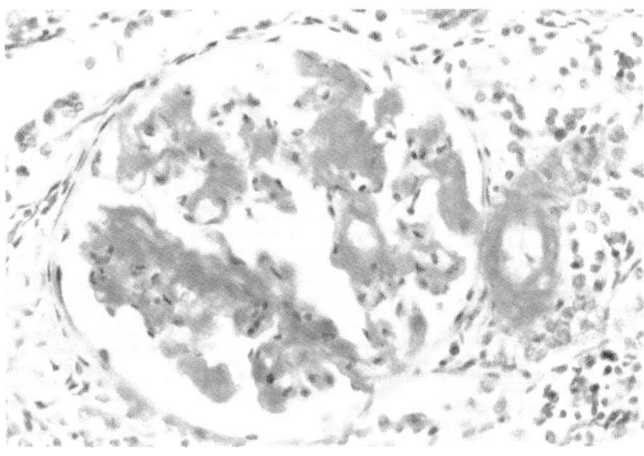

Figure 9-7

AMYLOIDOSIS

The glomerulus and arteriole stain with Congo red.

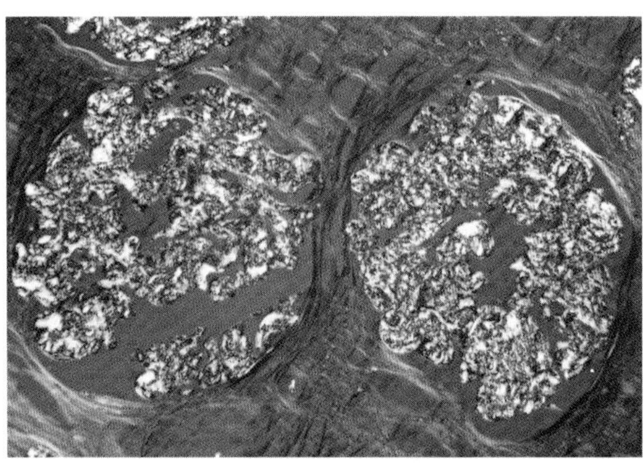

Figure 9-8

AMYLOIDOSIS

Polarized microscopy of renal tissue stained with Congo red shows extensive staining of the glomeruli. The slight yellow lighting in the interstitium is nonspecific birefringence induced by interstitial collagen.

glomerulopathy. The focal clusters of spikes may resemble a "cock's" comb. Amyloid usually stains similarly to collagen with the Masson trichrome stain, but may be paler (fig. 9-5). Although not used often in routine diagnostic work, the metachromatic stain, crystal violet, has a strong affinity for amyloid (fig. 9-6).

The definitive light microscopic staining reaction is with Congo red (figs. 9-7–9-9). Amyloid deposits appear red when stained with Congo red and viewed by standard bright field microscopy (fig. 9-7). This is referred to as congophilia, or congophilic staining. If thick sections are stained with Congo red (8 to 10 μm), amyloid displays apple green birefringence when view by polarized light microscopy (figs. 9-8; 9-9, left). Potassium permanganate treatment prior to Congo red staining can be used to discriminate between AA and AL amyloid: after this treatment, birefringent Congo red staining is lost by AA amyloid but retained by AL amyloid. A sensitive but less specific way to view Congo red staining is with fluorescence microscopy: green excitation results in red fluorescence of the Congo red stain (fig. 9-9, right).

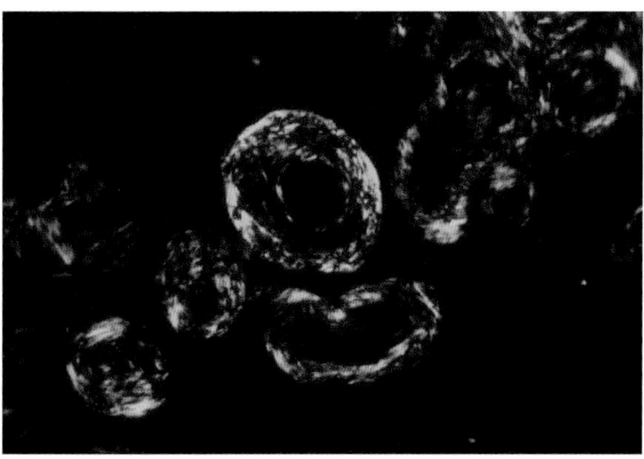
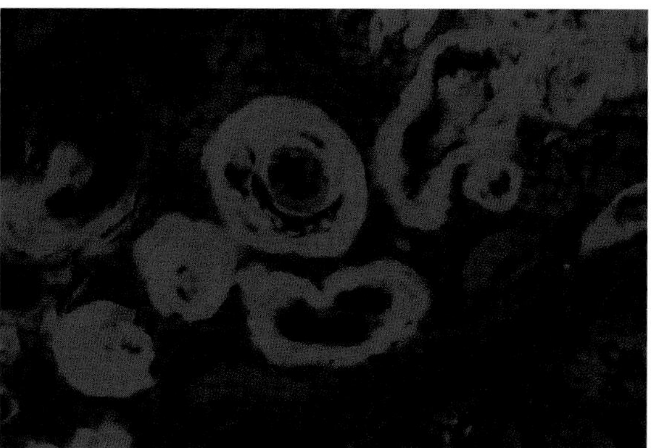

Figure 9-9

AMYLOIDOSIS

Amyloid in the renal arteries is revealed by staining the tissue with Congo red and viewing it by polarized microscopy (left) to demonstrate the birefringence of the amyloid and immunofluorescence microscopy (right) using green light excitation to stimulate red light emission by the Congo red stain.

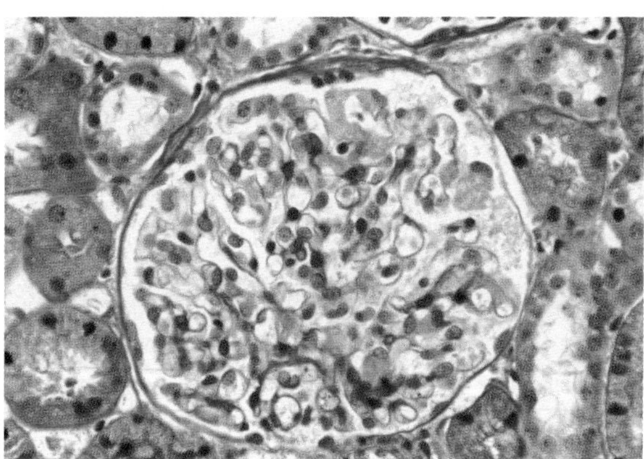
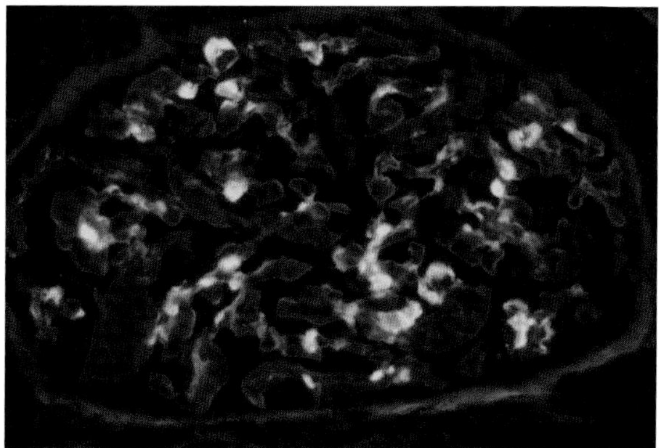

Figure 9-10

MILD AMYLOIDOSIS

Left: Masson trichrome staining shows predominantly mesangial, slightly focal accumulations of amyloid that appear as small foci of pale blue (e.g., at the very top of the tuft). These are so inconspicuous that they could be overlooked by hasty examination.

Right: Immunofluorescence microscopy of the same specimen shows small but conspicuous segmental mesangial accumulations of AL amyloid that stain brightly with an antiserum specific for immunoglobulin lambda light chains.

A similar sensitive but nonspecific fluorescent stain for amyloid uses thioflavin T, which is activated by blue light to emit yellow fluorescence. If fluorescence microscopy of Congo red– or thioflavin T–stained sections detects no staining, amyloid probably is not present. However, if staining is seen with these methods, the presence of amyloid should be confirmed by a more specific technique, such as Congo red birefringence, electron microscopy, or specific immunohistochemistry for immunoglobulin light chains or amyloid A protein.

In glomeruli, the mesangium typically is involved before the peripheral capillary walls (see fig. 9-3) (19). In early or mild renal amyloidosis, there may be only a few very small mesangial foci of amyloid in a few glomerular segments (fig. 9-10). These can be overlooked by routine light microscopy, and may result in an erroneous diagnosis of minimal change glomerulopathy

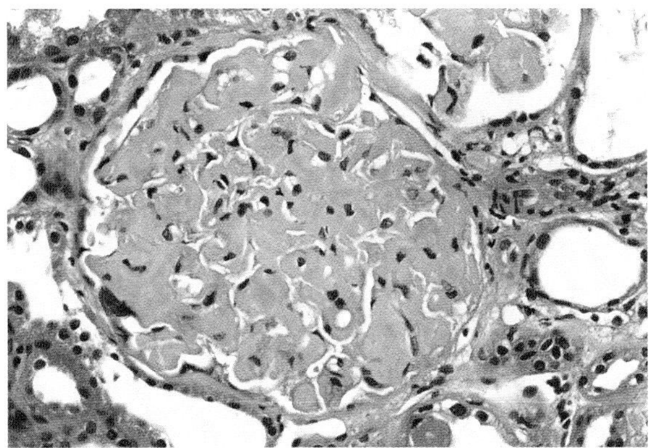

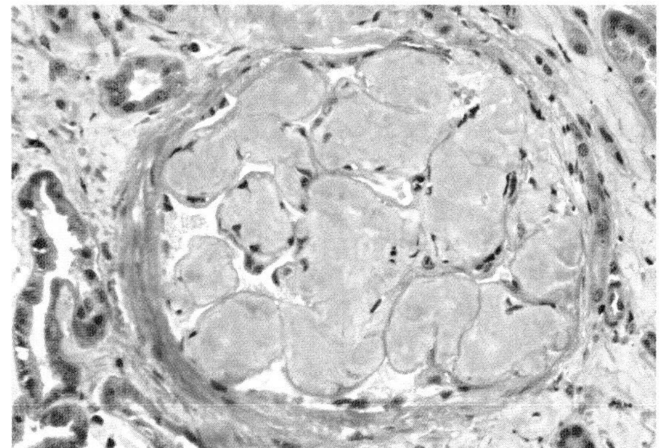

Figure 9-11

ADVANCED AMYLOIDOSIS

H&E (left) and Masson trichrome (right) stains show extensive effacement of the glomerular architecture by amorphous amyloid. Lumens are obliterated and many cells have disappeared.

(12). If the amyloid is AL amyloid, this error usually is corrected by immunofluorescence microscopy because even small scattered mesangial deposits of fluorescing monoclonal light chains are easy to see against the dark background (fig. 9-10, right).

As the glomerular amyloid deposits increase in size, they efface progressively more glomerular architecture until the entire glomerulus becomes a mass of amorphous material with no patent capillaries and few intact cells (fig. 9-11). PAS or JMS staining is helpful for determining the extent of glomerular sclerosis versus amyloid deposition in kidneys with advanced disease. The pale-staining foci of amyloid may be the only hint of amyloidosis during routine examination of an end-stage kidney specimen (fig. 9-12).

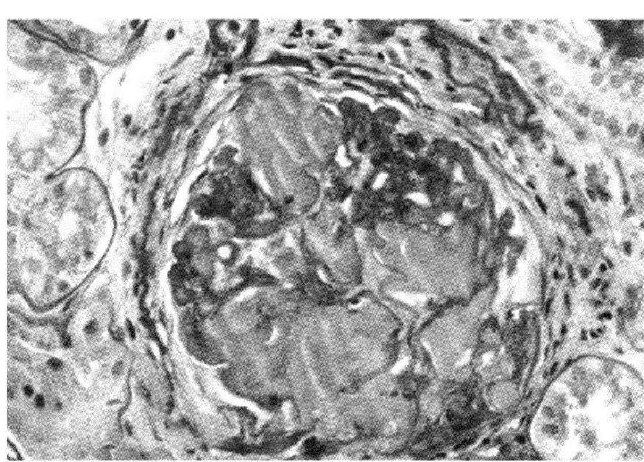

Figure 9-12

ADVANCED AMYLOIDOSIS

A glomerulus with partial sclerosis and partial effacement by amyloid. The residual basement membranes, mesangial matrix, and sclerosis are more PAS positive than the amyloid.

The glomerulus is the renal structure most frequently involved by amyloidosis, however, the renal vasculature and interstitium usually also are involved, and, rarely, are the only sites of involvement. Amyloid deposits usually develop in the extraglomerular renal vessels, tubules, and interstitium in parallel with the glomerular deposits (figs. 9-9, 9-13–9-15). Congo red staining is useful for determining the distribution of vascular and tubulointerstitial amyloid (fig. 9-14). Occasional specimens have only glomerular deposits, and rare specimens have only extraglomerular deposits. The most frequently involved vessels are the interlobular arteries and arterioles, although any renal vessel can be affected, including the vasa recta in the medulla. Interlobular arteries and hilar arterioles are involved in over 95 percent of renal biopsy specimens that have glomerular involvement (19). Interstitial involvement often is contiguous with involvement of vessels or tubular basement membranes. As the amyloidosis progresses in the renal parenchyma, nonspecific chronic interstitial fibrosis, tubular atrophy, and chronic interstitial inflammation develop. With advanced chronic tubulointerstitial injury, Congo red staining or immunohistochemistry may be required to distinguish interstitial amyloid from interstitial fibrosis.

Immunofluorescence Findings. Immunohistology is useful for confirming the presence of amyloid and for demonstrating its specific composition (figs. 9-10, 9-16–9-20) (15). All native renal biopsy specimens should be stained routinely for kappa and lambda light chains. This identifies the composition of AL amyloid and increases the likelihood that subtle renal involvement by AL amyloid is not overlooked (fig. 9-10). Staining for light chains also facilitates the diagnosis of a number of other renal diseases, thus justifying its routine use. About three quarters of AL amyloidosis is caused by lambda light chains rather than kappa light chains (Table 9-3). The reverse is true for light chain deposition disease. Rare examples of amyloid do not stain for immunoglobulin light chains but are positive for heavy chains, usually truncated gamma chains, indicating AH amyloidosis (3,18). AH amyloidosis is distinguished from heavy chain deposition disease by having the distinctive light microscopic and ultrastructural features that are diagnostic for amyloid. Rare examples of amyloid stain intensely for one heavy chain (usually gamma) and one light chain, suggesting that the amyloid contains portions of both a heavy and a light chain.

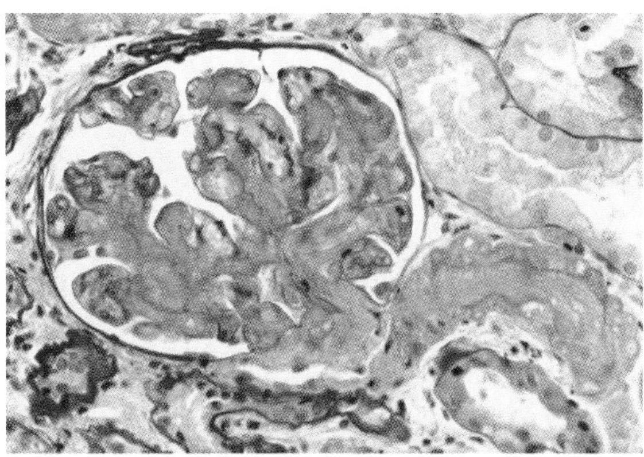

Figure 9-13

AMYLOIDOSIS

Extensive effacement of a hilar arteriole and most of a glomerular tuft by amyloid that stains weakly with PAS.

Immunostaining for AA protein is used in specific specimens to document AA amyloidosis (figs. 9-17–9-19). Amyloid also stains intensely for amyloid P component, but this does not distinguish among different types of amyloid. Amyloid P component is a normal plasma protein that binds to all forms of amyloid (5). Lesser amounts of P component are present in normal renal tissue and may be accentuated in a variety of renal diseases.

In addition to specific staining for proteins that comprise the amyloid, amyloid deposits often have low levels of nonspecific staining with many different reagent antibodies, including antibodies against complement components and immunoglobulins. This varies with different reagents and different specimens, and is more common with AA than AL amyloid. The basis for this low level of staining is unknown but may result from a charge interaction between

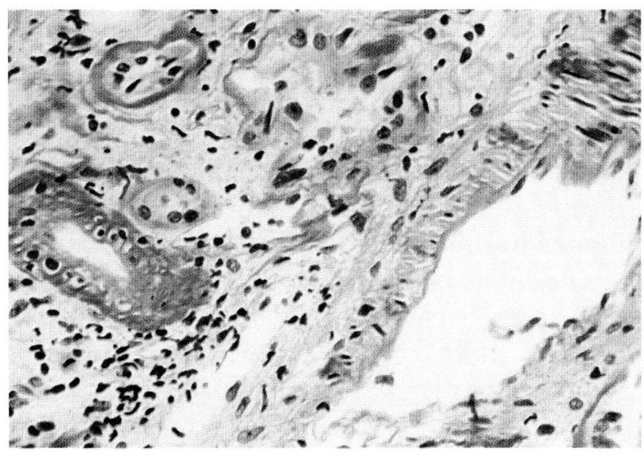

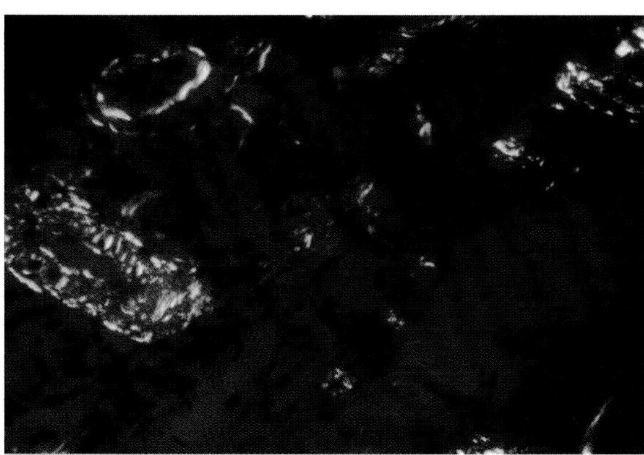

Figure 9-14

AMYLOIDOSIS

The focal accumulation of amyloid in renal arteries, tubular basement membranes, and interstitium is demonstrated with a Congo red stain viewed by standard light microscopy (left) and polarized light microscopy (right).

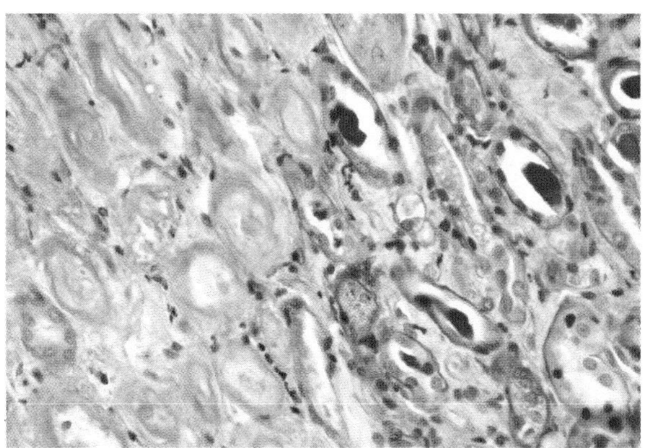

Figure 9-15

AMYLOIDOSIS

Focal tubulointerstitial involvement of the renal medulla by amyloid. Note the pale staining with PAS.

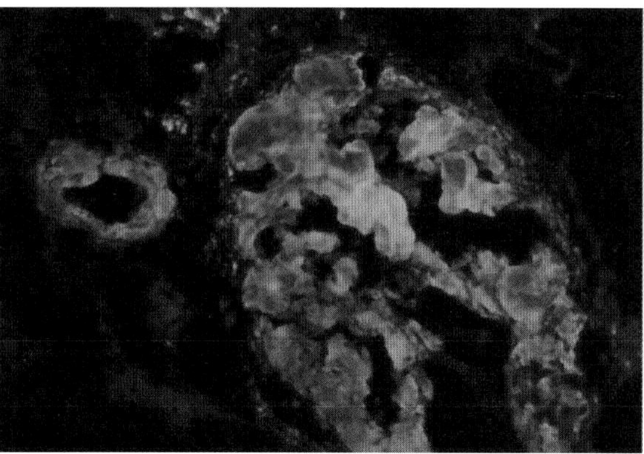

Figure 9-16

AL AMYLOIDOSIS

The extensive involvement of a glomerulus and arteriole by AL amyloid is revealed by immunofluorescence microscopy using antilambda light chain antiserum. Compare this advanced involvement with the mild involvement seen in figure 9-10.

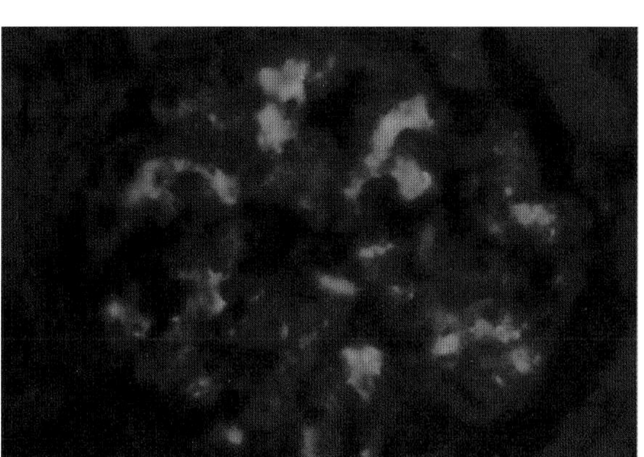

Figure 9-17

AA AMYLOIDOSIS

The involvement of a glomerulus by AA amyloid is revealed by immunofluorescence microscopy using antiserum specific for amyloid A protein.

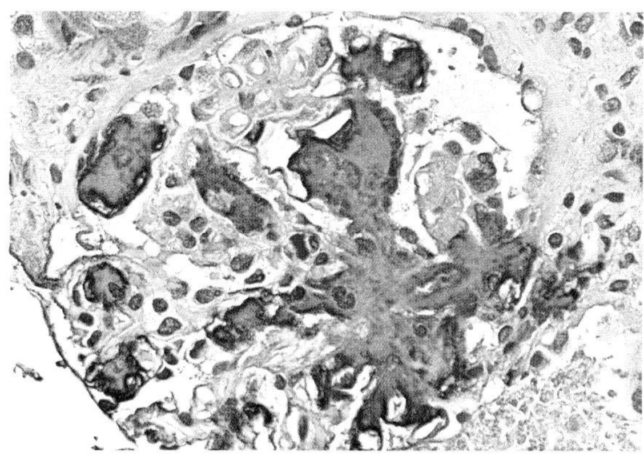

Figure 9-18

AA AMYLOIDOSIS

The involvement of a glomerulus by AA amyloid is revealed by immunoenzyme microscopy using antiserum specific for amyloid A protein.

the amyloid and the reagent antibodies. Usually, the more intense staining produced by a specific antibody reaction is more apparent above the nonspecific background staining produced by other antibodies. If multiple antibodies are staining the amyloid equally, additional dilution of the antibodies may improve the signal to noise ratio and allow recognition of specific staining.

The immunostaining of amyloid for immunoglobulin chains or AA protein reveals a pattern of distribution matching that seen by light microscopy. The foci of amyloid often have fuzzy borders that are less demarcated than the borders of immune complex deposits or the deposits of monoclonal immunoglobulin chain deposition disease. Early scanty glomerular deposits may be exclusively in the mesangium (see fig. 9-10). More extensive glomerular deposits extend into or obliterate capillary walls (fig. 9-16). Immunostaining of extraglomerular vascular deposits often shows a circumferential transmural distribution (figs. 9-16, 9-19), however, slight

Table 9-3

CHARACTERISTICS OF AL AMYLOIDOSIS, MONOCLONAL IMMUNOGLOBULIN DEPOSITION DISEASE, AND FIBRILLARY GLOMERULONEPHRITIS IDENTIFIED IN RENAL BIOPSY SPECIMENS EVALUATED IN THE UNIVERSITY OF NORTH CAROLINA NEPHROPATHOLOGY LABORATORY[a]

	AL Amyloidosis	Light or Heavy Chain Deposition Disease	Fibrillary Glomerulonephritis
	n=80	n=25	n=74
Frequency in kidney biopsy specimens	15/1000	4/1000	8/1000
Mean age (range)	63 (38-82)	60 (35-79)	52 (21-75)
Sex (male:female)	1:1.1	1:0.6	1:1.2
Race (black:white)[b]	1:3.5	1:4.6	1:13.0
Mean proteinuria	7.2	3.7	6.0
Mean creatinine	1.9	5.1	3.8
Light chain staining	23% kappa 75% lambda	76% kappa 20% lambda	98% kappa 92% lambda

[a]Unpublished data.

[b]Expected black to white ratio in the renal biopsy population is approximately 1 to 3.

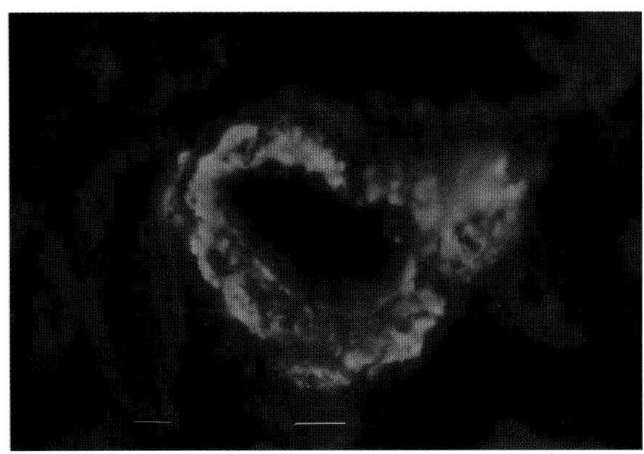

Figure 9-19

AA AMYLOIDOSIS

The involvement of an artery by AA amyloid is revealed by immunofluorescence microscopy using antiserum specific for amyloid A protein.

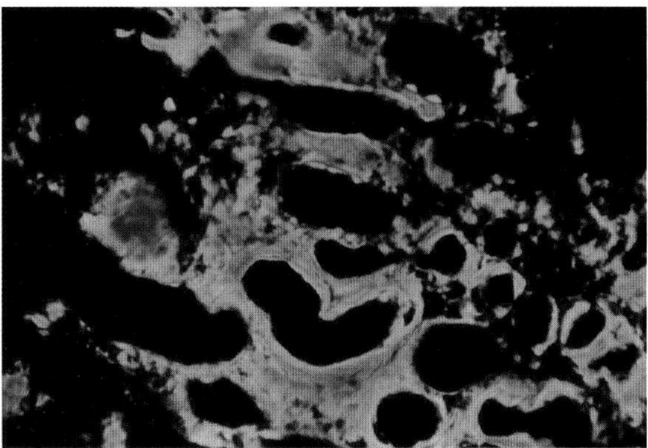

Figure 9-20

AL AMYLOIDOSIS

The focal involvement of tubular basement membranes and interstitium by AL amyloid is revealed by immunofluorescence microscopy using antiserum specific for kappa light chains.

focal involvement may occur, including small isolated foci in the muscularis of arteries or arterioles. Interstitial staining usually is multifocal rather than uniform, and often is contiguous with vascular or peritubular staining (fig. 9-20).

Electron Microscopic Findings. The fibrillary ultrastructural architecture of amyloid is very distinctive but not absolutely specific (11, 15,16). All types of amyloid have the same ultrastructure. The fibrils are approximately 10 nm in diameter (rarely outside the range of 8 to 12 nm), relatively straight, nonbranching, and arranged randomly (fig. 9-21). At high magnification (100,000X), the fibrils show an electron-lucent core. At low magnification (5,000X), the individual fibrils cannot be resolved but the amyloid deposits have a characteristic cottony appearance (figs. 9-21–9-23) that should alert the electron microscopist to investigate at higher magnification the possibility of amyloidosis.

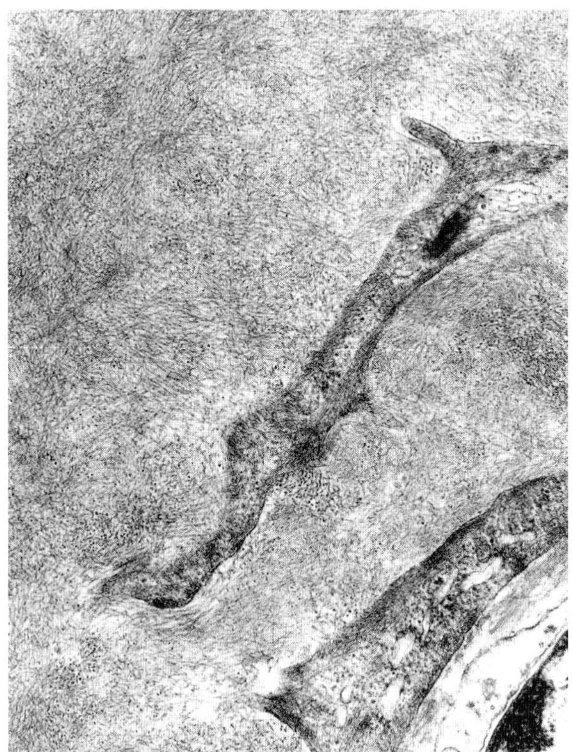

Figure 9-21

AMYLOIDOSIS

This transmission electron micrograph demonstrates relatively straight, nonbranching, randomly arranged amyloid fibrils in the mesangium of a glomerulus.

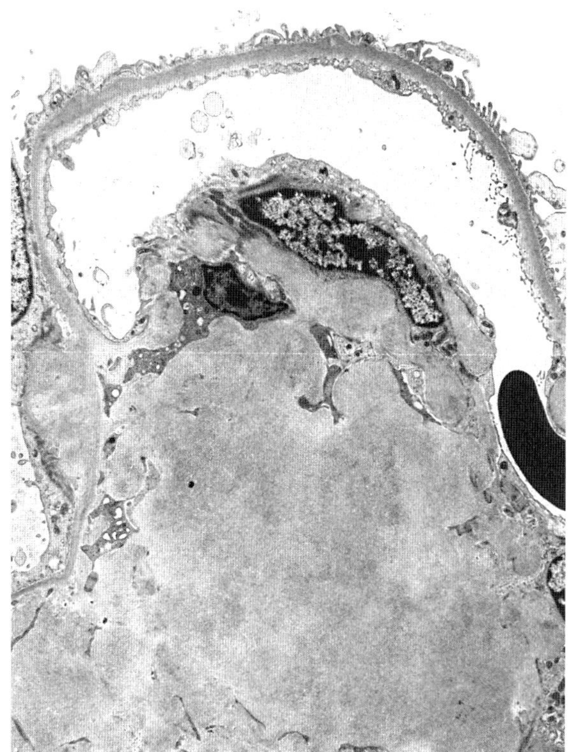

Figure 9-22

AMYLOIDOSIS

This low-power magnification electron micrograph shows the extensive expansion of the mesangium by amyloid that appears as a cottony material.

In mild renal amyloidosis, the fibrillary deposits often are confined to the mesangium (fig. 9-22). With more extensive glomerular involvement, they extend into the capillary walls (fig. 9-23). Capillary wall amyloid deposits often infiltrate through glomerular paramesangial and capillary basement membranes rather than accumulating beneath them. There is effacement of visceral epithelial foot processes at sites of capillary wall involvement by amyloid (figs. 9-23, 9-24). The podocyte cytoplasm adjacent to the amyloid deposits often has extensive electron-dense condensations of actin.

An unusual divergence from the random orientation of amyloid fibrils occurs in the subepithelial zone when the fibrils align in roughly parallel arrays perpendicular to the glomerular basement membrane (fig. 9-24). This produces a focal cock's comb appearance that also can be seen by light microscopy using a PAS or silver stain (see fig. 9-4).

Amyloid deposits in extraglomerular vessels and interstitium have the same ultrastructural features as those in the glomeruli.

Differential Diagnosis. By light microscopy, the pathologic differential diagnosis includes any process that results in an accumulation of acidophilic material in glomeruli, vessels, and interstitium. Accumulations of collagenous matrix, as in diabetic glomerulosclerosis or sclerosis secondary to glomerulonephritis, usually can be readily distinguished from amyloid by routine staining. As mentioned earlier, amyloid stains weakly with PAS and very little with JMS stains, whereas sclerotic matrix is intensely PAS and JMS positive. Massive glomerular deposits of immune complex glomerular diseases, fibrillary glomerulonephritis, immunotactoid glomerulopathy, fibronectin glomerulopathy, and collagenofibrotic glomerulopathy also may mimic amyloidosis on hematoxylin and eosin (H&E)–stained sections, but special stains,

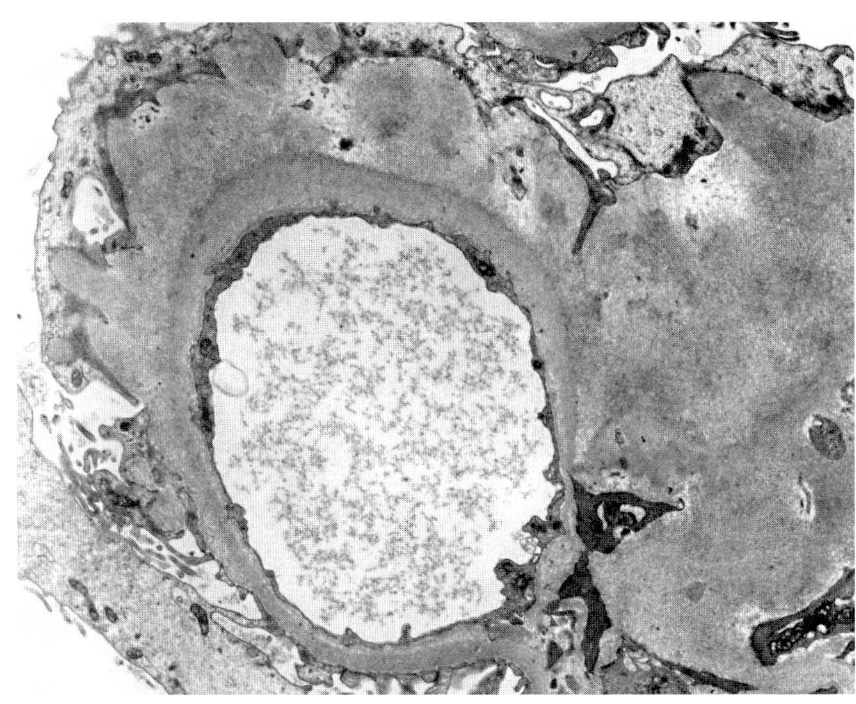

Figure 9-23

AMYLOIDOSIS

The extensive mesangial and focal transmembranous and subepithelial accumulation of amyloid appears as cottony material in this low-power magnification electron micrograph. Note the effacement of podocyte foot processes over the capillary wall deposits and condensation of actin adjacent to the deposits.

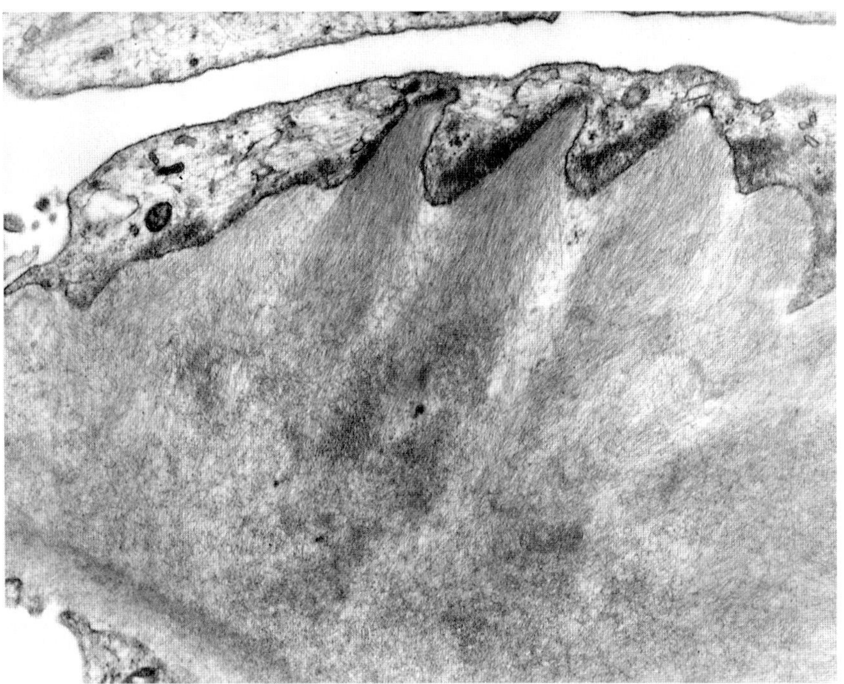

Figure 9-24

AMYLOIDOSIS

Parallel alignment of amyloid fibrils in the subepithelial zone of a glomerular capillary. This is the basis for the JMS-positive spikes that may be seen by light microscopy (see figure 9-4).

immunohistology, and electron microscopy demonstrate the distinctive features of each of these diseases. Congo red staining, of course, is always an option to confirm a diagnosis of amyloidosis. The sections must be cut thick enough (8 to 10 µm) to detect the birefringence of Congo red–stained amyloid.

In developed countries, most renal amyloidosis is of AL amyloid and thus is detectable by routine immunofluorescence microscopy if antisera against immunoglobulin light chains are used. In less developed countries, AA amyloid is more frequent because of the higher prevalence of chronic infectious diseases.

The pattern of fluorescence for amyloid is very distinctive. AL amyloidosis is diagnosed with great accuracy from the immunofluorescence microscopy findings alone. In fact, when deposits are scanty, amyloidosis may initially be overlooked by light and electron microscopy but unequivocally identified by immunofluorescence microscopy (12). Once seen by immunofluorescence microscopy, however, a review of the specimen by light and electron microscopy reveals the amyloid in retrospect. Amyloidosis with scanty deposits should always be considered in an older adult who on first examination appears to have minimal change glomerulopathy.

Light chain deposition disease (LCDD) shares monoclonal immunoglobulin light chain staining with AL amyloidosis but the pattern of staining is very different. LCDD typically has a more diffuse and regular distribution of staining that appears linear in glomerular and tubular basement membranes. Expanded mesangial regions also show staining, but it is a "harder" pattern of staining compared to the "softer" or fluffy pattern of amyloid staining with fuzzy borders. Low intensity, nonspecific, increased background staining for immunoglobulin molecules, including light chains, frequently is seen in sclerotic glomeruli, but this rarely is intense enough to falsely suggest AL amyloidosis.

By electron microscopy, the differential diagnosis includes other renal diseases that have deposits with an organized fibrillar or microtubular ultrastructure. The most problematic of these is fibrillary glomerulonephritis. Immunotactoid glomerulopathy is not a problem because the parallel arrays of microtubules have a very different appearance than amyloid. As is discussed in more detail later in this chapter, fibrillary glomerulonephritis is characterized by glomerular deposits composed of randomly oriented, nonbranching filaments that usually are approximately 20 nm in diameter, although the fibril size varies from 10 to 30 nm in some patients. If fibrils are clearly 20 nm or larger, a diagnosis of amyloidosis is unlikely and fibrillary glomerulonephritis or some other disease with organized deposits should be considered. An internal point of reference for fibril size is the filamentous cytoskeleton of cells that are adjacent to organized fibrillary or microtubular deposits. Most intracellular filaments range from 5 to 10 nm in diameter (5 nm, actin; 10 nm, myosin; 10 nm, vimentin; 10 nm, tubulin). Thus extracellular amyloid fibrils are similar in diameter to intracellular filaments, whereas the fibrils of fibrillary glomerulonephritis typically are distinctly larger. Of course, the only definitive way to determine fibril diameter is by morphometry. This usually is not necessary to resolve the differential diagnosis because the diagnosis of amyloidosis can be made definitively when the ultrastructural finding of fibrillary deposits matches with light microscopic identification of congophilic deposits and the immunofluorescence finding of deposits of immunoglobulin light chains, AA protein, or other monotypic amyloidogenic protein.

The possibility of amyloidosis occasionally arises during the electron microscopic examination of glomeruli with sclerosis, including diabetic glomerulosclerosis, ischemic sclerosis, and postnephritic sclerosis. In scarred glomeruli, ultrastructurally identifiable fibrils (usually 12 to 16 nm in diameter) form within the expanded collagenous extracellular matrix. When they are prominent, they can raise the possibility of amyloidosis, which is resolved by considering the findings by light and immunofluorescence microscopy. The fibrils arising in collagenous mesangial matrix usually are less numerous at a given site than amyloid fibers, tend to be more often aligned in parallel, and may be slightly curved. These fibrils sometimes are oriented at right angels to mesangial cell surfaces and may touch the plasma membrane.

Etiology and Pathogenesis. The formation of AA amyloid often is associated with chronic inflammatory processes, such as rheumatoid arthritis, ankylosing spondylitis, or longstanding infection (5,15). AA amyloid deposition also occurs in patients with familial Mediterranean fever. The precursor to AA amyloid, serum amyloid A protein, is an apolipoprotein that is increased in the circulation during inflammatory diseases. The genetic defect in familial Mediterranean fever causes dysregulation of inflammation, which secondarily causes AA amyloidosis (13).

The precursor to AL amyloid is monoclonal immunoglobulin light chain molecules, which usually includes the N-terminal variable region (1,10). Many patients with AL amyloidosis have an identifiable B-cell neoplasm, most often multiple myeloma, but the majority do not. Even patients without an identifiable neoplasm are thought to have an occult B-cell dyscrasia that is producing the amyloidogenic light chains.

AH amyloid is composed of immunoglobulin heavy chains (3,18). These chains must be abnormally truncated to be amyloidogenic (3), which makes them structurally more like amyloidogenic light chains.

The tropism of amyloidogenic monoclonal immunoglobulin molecules for the kidney and the capacity to form amyloid fibrils are determined by their molecular composition (1,2,8, 10,17). Amyloidogenesis requires a proteolytic step that cleaves precursor immunoglobulin light chain molecules to produce molecules that self aggregate and become insoluble and resistant to further proteolysis (e.g., light chain variable region fragments). This may be facilitated by destabilizing the amino acid replacements that cause the molecules to unfold and aggregate (1,10).

The major pathologic effects of amyloid deposition probably result from the distortion of tissue composition and architecture, however, there may also be direct cytotoxic effects (5).

Treatment and Prognosis. The prognosis for patients with AL amyloidosis is not good but can be prolonged with treatment. The most common cause of death is cardiac failure (4). AL amyloidosis is treated with chemotherapeutic regimens appropriate for B-cell or plasma cell neoplasms (1,4,5,7). The median survival period of patients who respond to Melphalan-based chemotherapy can be extended from approximately 1 year to more than 5 years (4). This treatment also ameliorates the renal disease in many patients (5). Bone marrow ablation followed by bone marrow or stem cell transplantation may be more effective than chemotherapy alone (1,4,5,7). The clinical course of AL amyloidosis may be dominated by the external manifestations of the B-cell neoplasm.

Patients with AA amyloidosis have a better prognosis than those with AL amyloidosis. Nevertheless, without treatment, the 5- and 15-year survival rates for patients with AA amyloidosis are 50 percent and 25 percent, respectively (5). AA amyloidosis caused by familial Mediterranean fever responds to treatment with Colchicine (13). The effectiveness of Colchicine for AA amyloidosis not caused by familial Mediterranean fever is less clear. Treatment of the underlying chronic inflammatory disease, such as immunosuppressive agents for rheumatoid arthritis, is beneficial for patients with secondary AA amyloidosis (5).

AA and AL amyloidoses may recur in renal transplants. In one study, amyloidosis recurred in 10 percent of renal transplants after an average of 5 years and contributed to graft loss in about a third of the transplants with recurrence (6). Another study determined a risk of 20 percent for recurrent amyloidosis in renal transplants of more than 1 year duration (14).

MONOCLONAL IMMUNOGLOBULIN DEPOSITION DISEASE

Definition. Monoclonal immunoglobulin deposition disease (MIDD) includes *light chain deposition disease (LCDD), heavy chain deposition disease (HCDD),* and *light and heavy chain deposition disease (LHCDD)* (20–24). All are characterized by the pathologic accumulation of abnormally truncated monoclonal immunoglobulin molecules in vascular and tubular basement membranes without a fibrillary or microtubular appearance by electron microscopy. This distinguishes MIDD from AL amyloidosis, which is fibrillary when viewed by electron microscopy, and from immunotactoid glomerulopathy, which may contain monoclonal immunoglobulin but has microtubular deposits when viewed by electron microscopy. The tissue distribution of MIDD distinguishes it from light chain cast nephropathy, which is defined by the presence of distinctive casts in the lumens of renal tubules (this is discussed in detail in chapter 22).

The pathogenic monoclonal immunoglobulin chain in LCDD is a kappa light chain in approximately three quarters of patients (Table 9-3). Approximately 10 percent of patients with a LCDD pattern have a similarly distributed heavy chain and thus have LHCDD. Gamma, mu, and alpha HCDD are rare (20–23).

The term monoclonal immunoglobulin deposition disease has been used by some in the past as a generic term for all diseases caused by monoclonal immunoglobulin localization in tissues, including AL amyloidosis, light chain cast nephropathy, LCDD, HCDD, LHCDD, and others. In this text, in line with current usage trends, the term MIDD will be used specifically for LCDD, HCDD, and LHCDD.

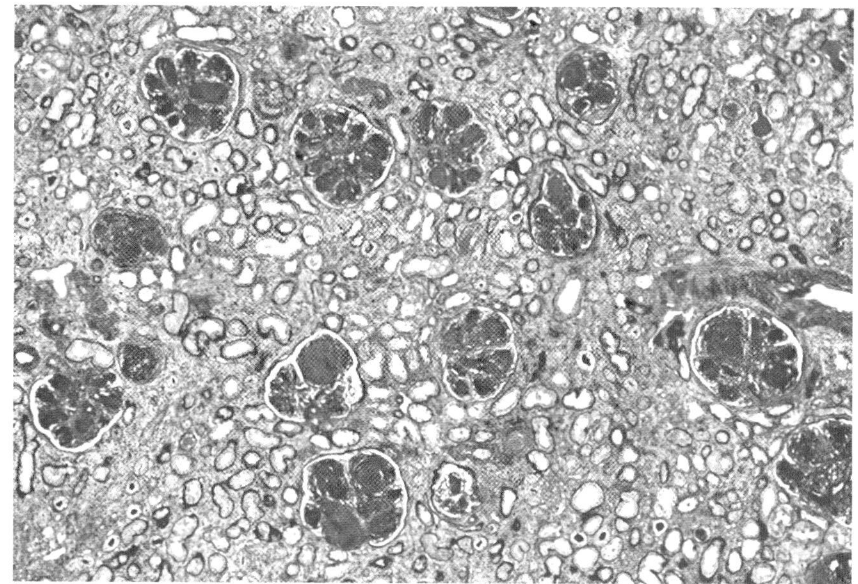

Figure 9-25

LIGHT CHAIN DEPOSITION DISEASE

The nodular glomerular sclerosis could not be distinguished from nodular diabetic glomerulosclerosis by light microscopy alone with this PAS stain.

Clinical Features. The most common clinical manifestation of MIDD is proteinuria, often with nephrotic syndrome, and renal insufficiency (21–24). Hematuria and hypertension are frequent. Hypocomplementemia may occur, especially in patients with gamma HCDD (21,22). Patients with HCDD often have positive serology for hepatitis C virus (22). Severe renal insufficiency is more common when MIDD is concurrent with light chain cast nephropathy (22). Monoclonal immunoglobulin is detectable in the plasma or urine of most, but not all, patients. Bone marrow biopsy usually reveals an increase in monoclonal plasma cells. Over half the patients have overt multiple myeloma and a few have B-cell lymphomas (22–24).

MIDD is a systemic process that can affect many organs. Symptomatic involvement is most common in the kidneys. Next in frequency are the liver and heart (23). The presence of liver deposits, primarily beneath sinusoidal endothelial cells, is a frequent pathologic finding. Hepatomegaly and mildly elevated circulating liver enzymes are the most common clinical manifestations of liver involvement. The most common cardiac manifestations are arrhythmias, conduction abnormalities, and congestive heart failure.

Light Microscopic Findings. LCDD, HCDD, and LHCDD share the same histologic features (15,21–24). The most frequent and most distinctive expression is nodular glomerular sclerosis that can be histologically indistinguishable from diabetic glomerulosclerosis using H&E or PAS stains (figs. 9-25, 9-26). In general, the nodules are more diffusely distributed among glomeruli and glomerular segments than the nodules of diabetic glomerulosclerosis, which tend to be more asymmetrically distributed. The light microscopic features are variable and thus the absence of nodules does not rule out MIDD. Examples of MIDD that lack mesangial nodules usually have focal or diffuse expansion of the mesangial matrix (fig. 9-27), occasionally with slight mesangial hypercellularity. Nodules are least frequently seen when LCDD is concurrent with light chain cast nephropathy.

Small mesangial nodules often have mesangial hypercellularity. Larger nodules typically have an acellular eosinophilic center with residual cells at the periphery. Nodules can be either amorphous or have concentric laminations. Nodular lesions often have some degree of mesangiolysis, resulting in aneurysmal dilation of the peripheral capillaries (fig. 9-26B). Glomerular basement membranes may be thickened, but usually this is less pronounced than in diabetic glomerulosclerosis. On the other hand, focal replication of glomerular basement membranes is more frequent than in diabetic glomerulosclerosis. Crescent formation is uncommon but may occur, especially with HCDD (fig. 9-28) (20,21).

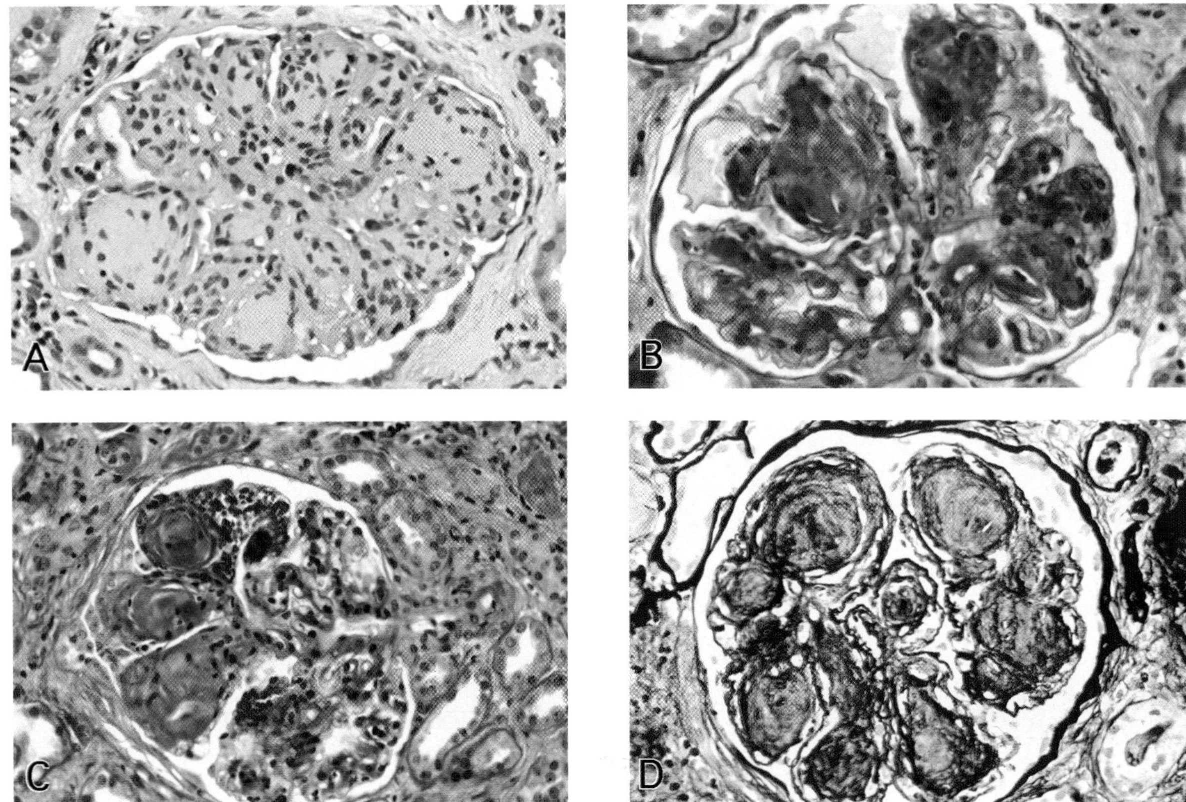

Figure 9-26

MONOCLONAL IMMUNOGLOBULIN DEPOSITION DISEASE

Nodular sclerosing light and heavy chain deposition disease (LHCDD) is stained with H&E (A), light chain deposition disease (LCDD) with PAS (B), LCDD with Masson trichrome (C), and LCDD with JMS (D). Unlike amyloid deposits, but identical to those of diabetic glomerulosclerosis, the nodules are very PAS positive; however, they are less JMS positive than the nodules of diabetic glomerulosclerosis. Also like diabetic glomerulosclerosis, there is segmental mesangiolysis causing peripheral capillary aneurysm formation that is seen best in B and C. Glomerular basement membranes are not as thickened as would usually be the case for full-blown diabetic glomerulosclerosis.

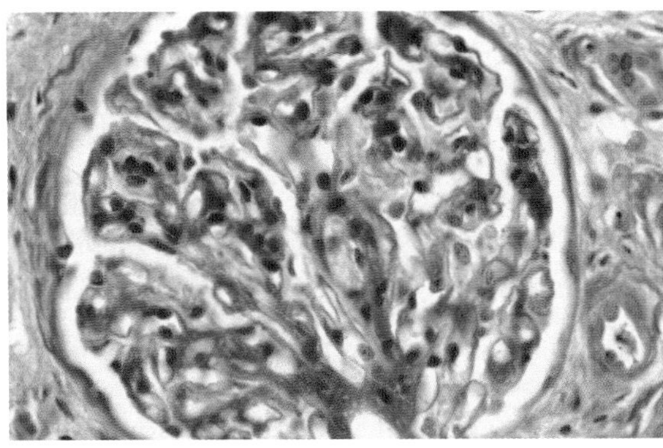

Figure 9-27

LIGHT CHAIN DEPOSITION DISEASE

Well-defined mesangial nodules are not seen by light microscopy, however, there is a segmentally variable slight increase in coarse PAS-positive material in the mesangium.

Unlike amyloidosis, but identical to diabetic glomerulosclerosis, the matrix of the nodules stains intensely with PAS (figs. 9-25, 9-26B) but does not stain with Congo red. Special stains demonstrate variable thickening of the glomerular basement membranes. Cortical and medullary tubular basement membranes usually have more extensive alterations than glomerular basement membranes. Typically, there is marked hyaline thickening of the tubular basement membranes (fig. 9-29). Arteries and arterioles occasionally have increased mural extracellular matrix caused by the accumulation of monoclonal immunoglobulins. The material usually is PAS positive and vaguely granular, with a tendency to surround (outline) individual medial myocytes (fig. 9-30).

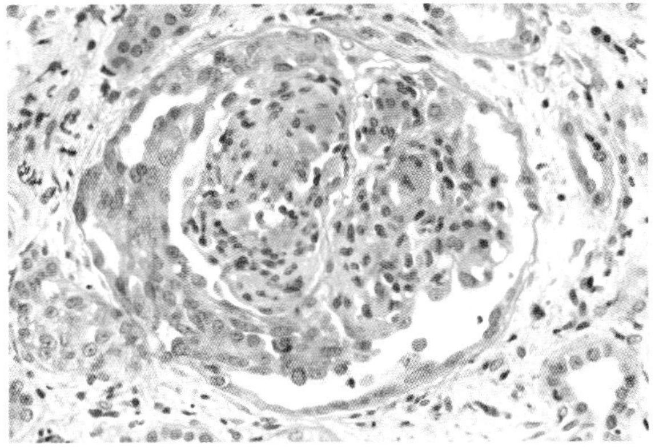

Figure 9-28

HEAVY CHAIN DEPOSITION DISEASE

Crescents were found in 40 percent of glomeruli of this gamma HCDD specimen. Immunofluorescence microscopy revealed only truncated gamma heavy chains in the glomeruli. There was no staining for complement.

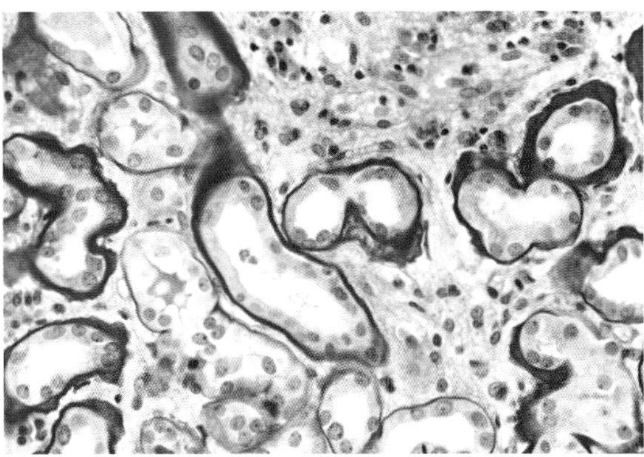

Figure 9-29

LIGHT CHAIN DEPOSITION DISEASE

The marked PAS-positive thickening of tubular basement membranes is caused by LCDD.

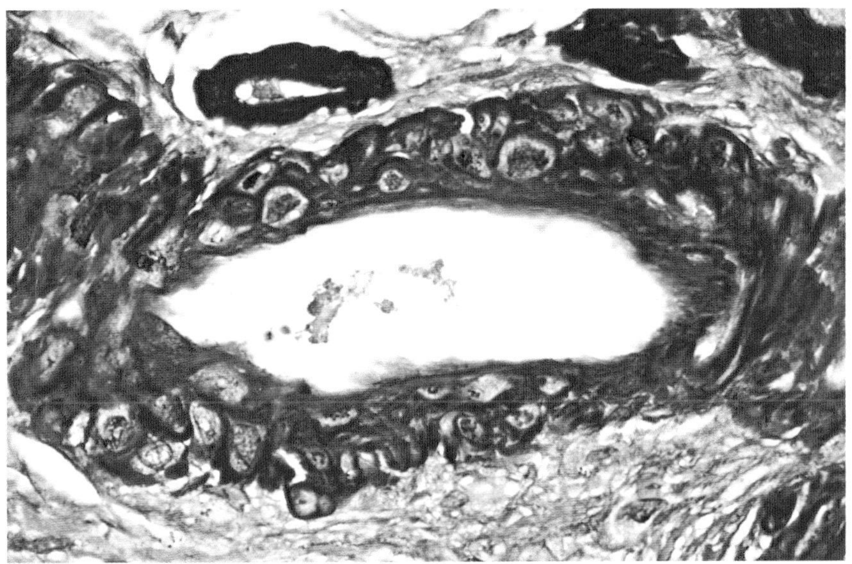

Figure 9-30

LIGHT CHAIN DEPOSITION DISEASE

Extensive thickening of arterial walls by coarse PAS-positive material that surrounds myocytes.

As the disease progresses, there is a corresponding increase in interstitial fibrosis, tubular atrophy, and interstitial infiltration by chronic inflammatory cells.

Immunofluorescence Findings. The sine qua non of MIDD is positive immunostaining of renal tissue for monoclonal immunoglobulin molecules (figs. 9-31–9-34) (15,21–24). The staining usually involves many different types of basement membranes, including glomerular basement membranes, Bowman's capsule, and cortical and medullary tubular basement membranes (figs. 9-31, 9-32). Glomeruli often have expanded mesangial areas that stain for monoclonal immunoglobulin molecules (fig. 9-32). In arteries, the staining may be predominantly in the outer muscularis just beneath the adventitia, or may be transmural in the interstices between smooth muscle cells (figs. 9-31, 9-34). Interstitial staining is variable and may be undetectable or extensive. In addition to the immunostaining for the monoclonal immunoglobulin chain, there may be glomerular staining for complement components, especially with

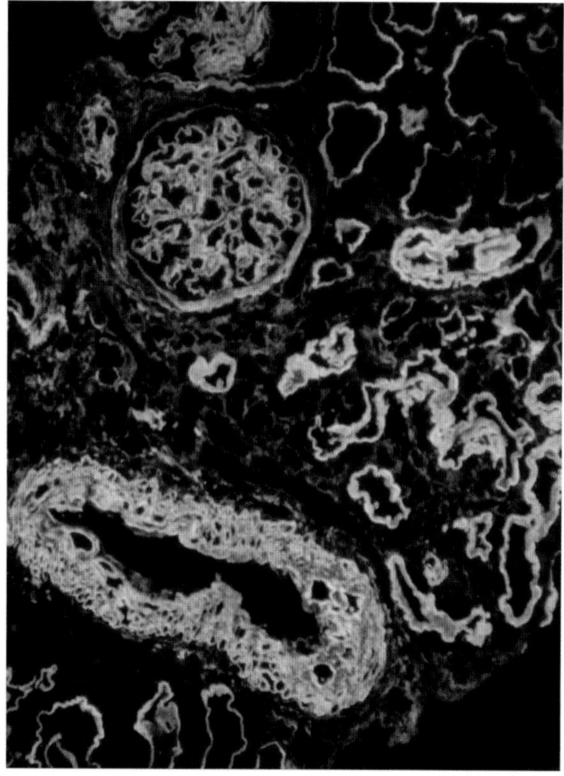

Figure 9-31

LIGHT CHAIN DEPOSITION DISEASE

Immunofluorescence microscopy demonstrates staining with an antiserum for gamma heavy chains in a specimen of gamma HCDD. There is extensive staining of glomeruli, arterioles, arteries, and tubular basement membranes.

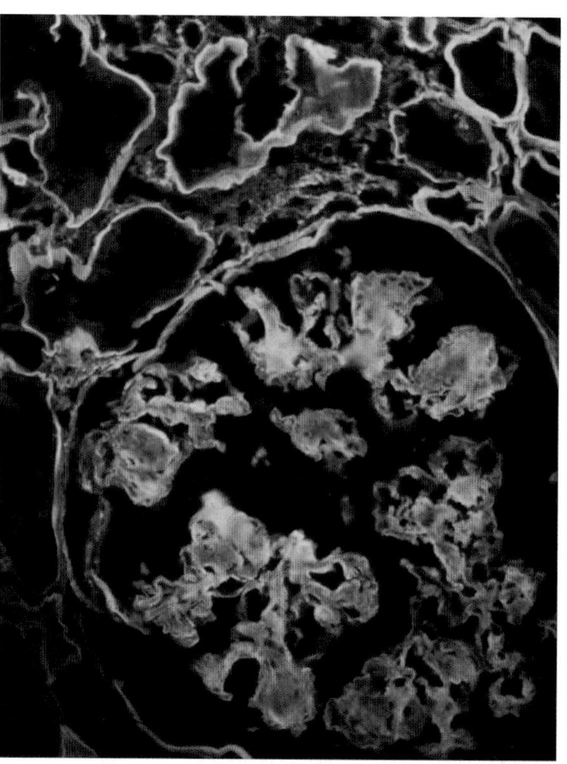

Figure 9-32

LIGHT CHAIN DEPOSITION DISEASE

Immunofluorescence microscopy demonstrates staining with an antiserum for kappa light chains in a specimen of kappa LCDD. There is extensive staining of the expanded mesangial regions, glomerular basement membranes, Bowman's capsule, and tubular basement membranes.

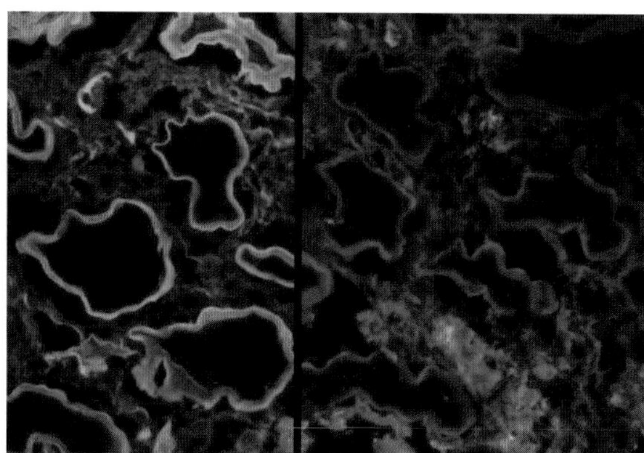

Figure 9-33

LIGHT CHAIN DEPOSITION DISEASE

Immunofluorescence microscopy using antisera against kappa light chains (left) and lambda light chains (right) shows linear staining of the tubular basement membranes, with the former but not the latter indicative of kappa LCDD.

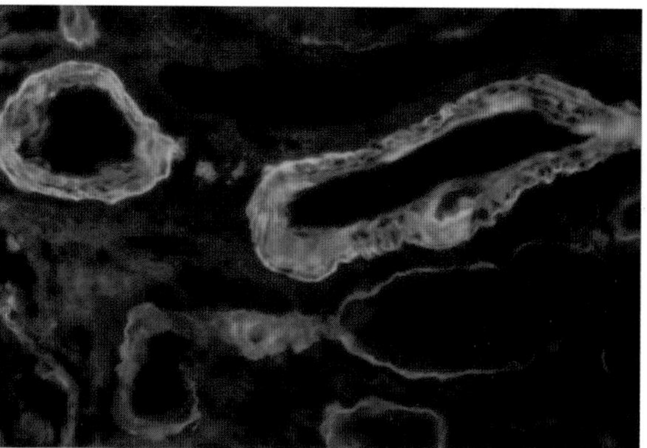

Figure 9-34

HEAVY CHAIN DEPOSITION DISEASE

Immunofluorescence microscopy using an antiserum specific for gamma heavy chains shows extensive transmural staining of the walls of two arteries in a patient with gamma HCDD. Note also the linear staining of the tubular basement membranes.

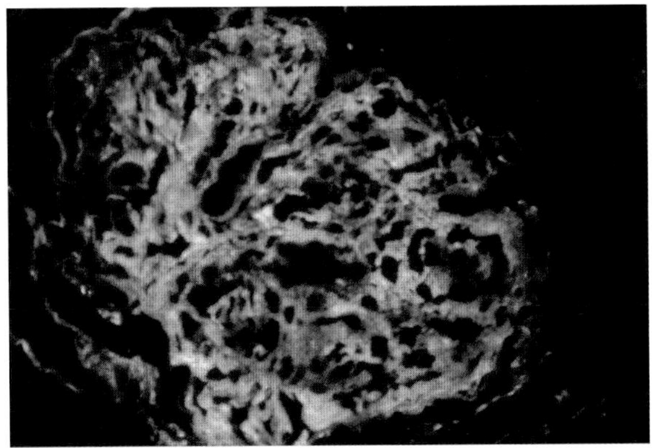

Figure 9-35

HEAVY CHAIN DEPOSITION DISEASE

Immunofluorescence microscopy of a specimen of gamma HCDD using an antiserum specific for C3 shows extensive glomerular staining.

HCDD (fig. 9-35). Antibodies that are specific for specific sites on immunoglobulin molecules can be used to identify abnormal truncation of the pathogenic immunoglobulin molecules (20–22). For example, the monoclonal gamma chains of gamma HCDD typically have a deletion of the CH1 domain (22).

Electron Microscopic Findings. The ultrastructural features of MIDD are distinctive, but are absent in a minority of specimens of otherwise typical MIDD (15,21–24). The characteristic finding is a band of dense granules within the basement membranes (figs. 9-26–9-41). These are seen most often in the portion of the glomerular basement membrane that is adjacent to endothelial cells or mesangium (i.e., lamina lucida interna and inner portion of lamina densa) (figs. 9-26, 9-38), and the portion of tubular basement membrane that is adjacent to the interstitium (fig. 9-41), which are the sites that are most heavily exposed to proteins in the circulation or interstitial fluid, respectively. Some specimens, however, have granular deposits throughout the full thickness of lamina densa (fig. 9-37).

The mesangial matrix is expanded, especially in segments with nodule formation (figs. 9-38–9-40). Freely dispersed or clustered dense granules are scattered throughout the mesangial matrix, especially in the matrix of mesangial nodules. Dense granules also occur in the extraglomerular vasculature, including peritubular capillaries and arteries. In arteries, the granules may accumulate predominantly in the extracellular matrix in the outer muscularis (fig. 9-42), or may permeate the entire muscularis. The distribution suggests that the abnormal monoclonal immunoglobulins enter the muscularis of arteries from the interstitial fluid rather than from the blood.

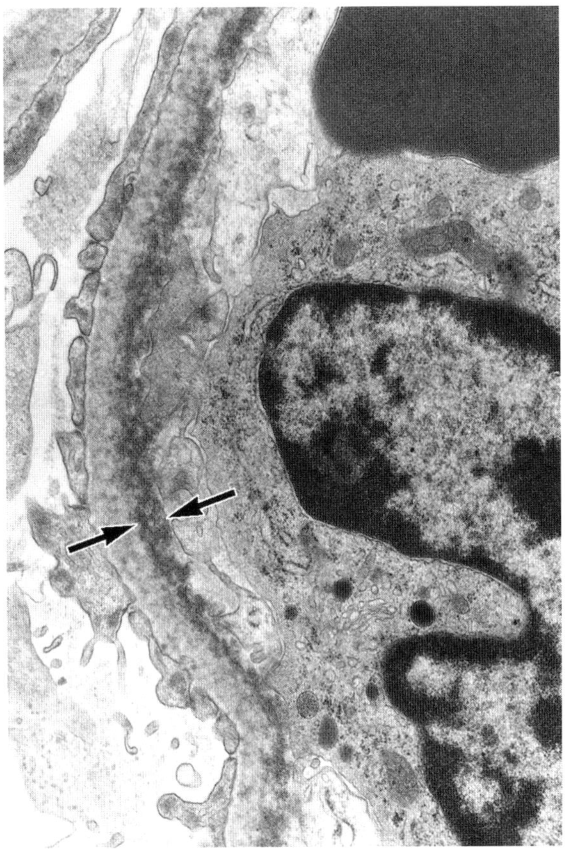

Figure 9-36

HEAVY CHAIN DEPOSITION DISEASE

Electron micrographs of gamma HCDD show granular electron-dense material predominantly in the lamina lucida interna and inner portion of the lamina densa of the capillary wall basement membrane (between arrows).

Differential Diagnosis. The light microscopic pathologic differential diagnosis for MIDD is very broad because of the varied histologic phenotypes that MIDD can produce. Frequent considerations include diabetic glomerulosclerosis, idiopathic nodular glomerulosclerosis, membranoproliferative glomerulonephritis, amyloidosis, and fibrillary glomerulonephritis. Immunofluorescence microscopy usually resolves the differential diagnosis by

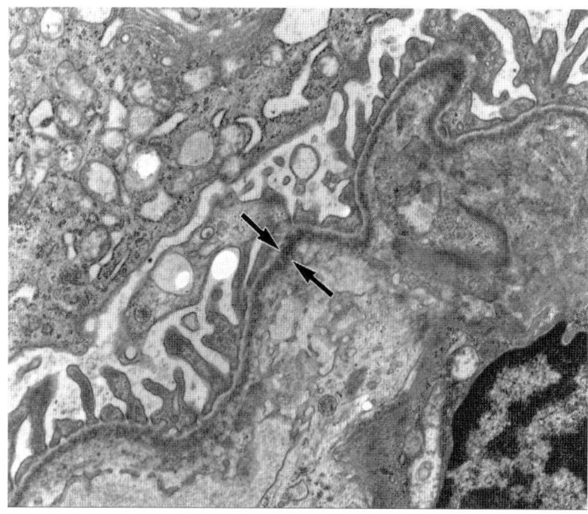

Figure 9-37

LIGHT CHAIN DEPOSITION DISEASE

Electron micrograph of kappa LCDD shows granular electron-dense material permeating the full thickness of the lamina densa but sparing the lamina lucida externa (between arrows).

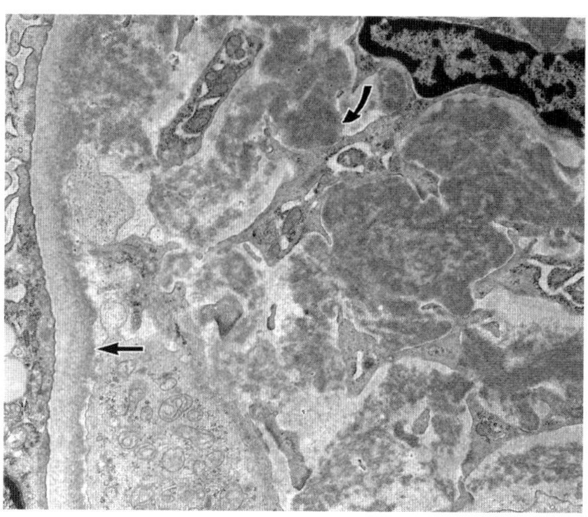

Figure 9-38

LIGHT CHAIN DEPOSITION DISEASE

Electron micrograph of kappa LCDD shows granular deposits along the inner aspect of the paramesangial basement membrane (straight arrow) and within the expanded mesangial matrix (curved arrow).

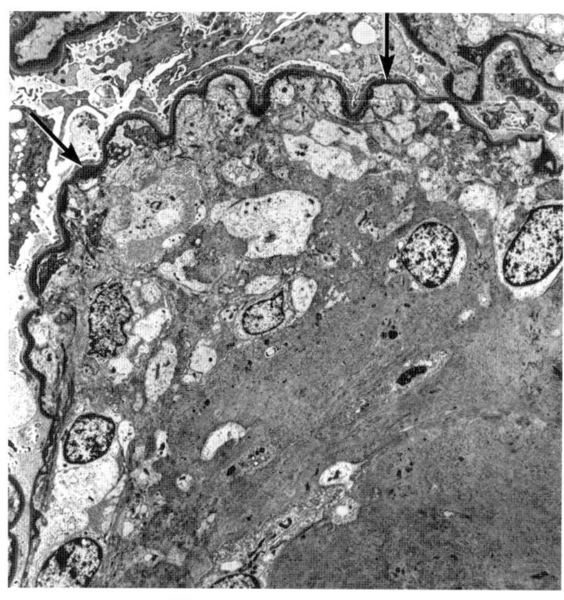

Figure 9-39

LIGHT AND HEAVY CHAIN DEPOSITION DISEASE

Electron micrograph of a mesangial nodule from a patient with gamma kappa LHCDD. The center of the nodule is at the bottom right, with granular densities scattered throughout the expanded matrix. The glomerular basement membrane is at the periphery of the segment and is permeated by more densely packed granules (arrows).

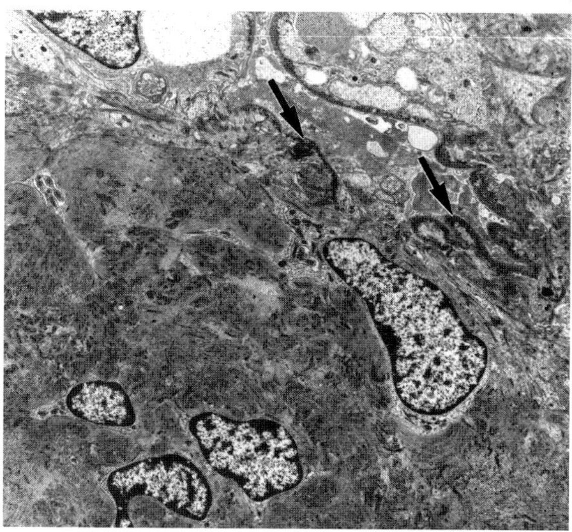

Figure 9-40

LIGHT AND HEAVY CHAIN DEPOSITION DISEASE

Higher magnification electron micrograph of the same specimen shown in figure 9-39. The mesangium has numerous dense granules, some of which appear to be aggregated into larger clusters. Bands of dense granules also are in the paramesangial basement membrane (arrows).

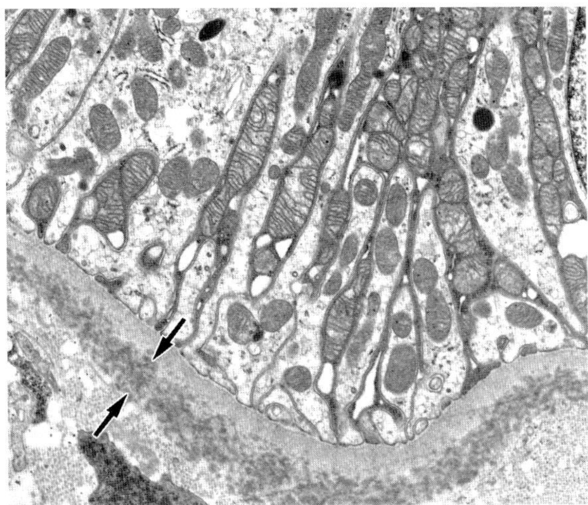

Figure 9-41

LIGHT CHAIN DEPOSITION DISEASE

Electron micrograph shows granular electron-dense material (arrows) accruing on the outer aspect of the basement membrane of a proximal tubule from a patient with kappa LCDD.

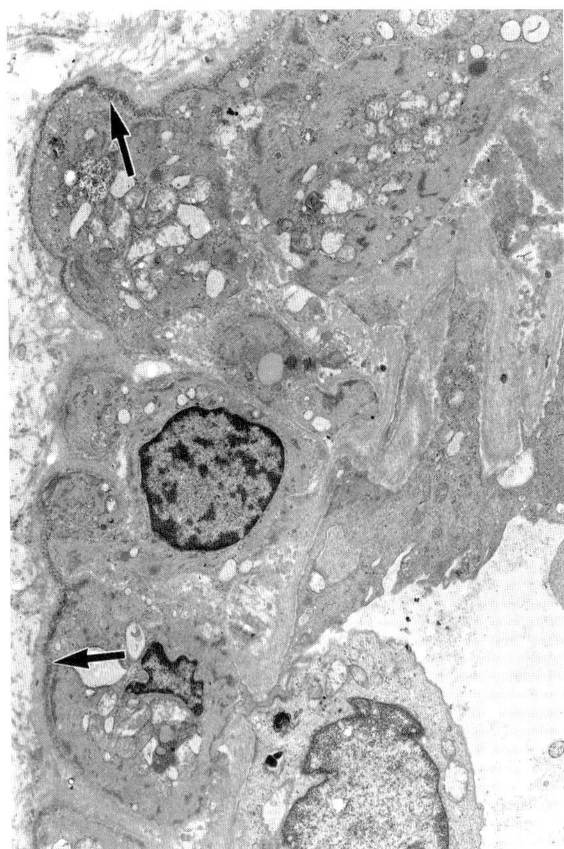

Figure 9-42

LIGHT CHAIN DEPOSITION DISEASE

Electron micrograph of an interlobular artery from a patient with kappa LCDD shows a band of dense granules on the outer side of the outer row of myocytes (arrows). There are no granules on the inner aspect of the elastica (i.e., beneath the endothelial cell).

demonstrating the monoclonal immunoglobulin in glomerular basement membranes and mesangium, and in tubular basement membranes. Somewhat problematic is gamma HCDD and HLCDD, which may be confused with diabetic glomerulosclerosis, because there is also linear staining for IgG in the glomerular and tubular basement membranes. The immunoglobulin deposits in diabetic glomerulosclerosis, however, are polyclonal, with both kappa and lambda light chains, which rules out MIDD. Also, if albumin staining if evaluated, this is conspicuous in diabetic glomerulosclerosis but not MIDD.

Amyloidosis can be a diagnostic consideration because it results in the accumulation of acellular acidophilic material in glomeruli, which can mimic the nodules of MIDD. In the amyloidosis, the eosinophilic material has a softer appearance when stained with H&E than the harder appearance of MIDD nodules. In addition, the deposits of MIDD are not congophilic and stain intensely with PAS. Electron microscopy also readily distinguishes between the fibrillar deposits of amyloidosis and the distinctive granular deposits of MIDD. However, the granular deposits may be indistinct or absent in some specimens of MIDD. Thus, the absence of granular deposits does not rule out a diagnosis of MIDD. There also are rare specimens that have features of both LCDD and AL amyloidosis (24). These warrant both diagnoses. A more frequent concurrence is LCDD with light chain cast nephropathy. When both are present, the LCDD often lacks nodular sclerosing glomerular lesions (24).

Etiology and Pathogenesis. MIDD is caused by the deposition of abnormally truncated monoclonal immunoglobulin molecules in renal tissue, and the subsequent increase in basement membrane and matrix material. The abnormal truncation appears to be the basis for the pattern of tissue localization that distinguishes MIDD from AL amyloidosis (20,23). In vitro studies suggest that the pathogenic immunoglobulin molecules are able to stimulate mesangial cells to produce more type IV collagen and fibronectin, and to decrease the production of collagenase (20a,20b). This is mediated through the activation of transforming growth factor-beta, which also stimulates other cells to produce more extracellular matrix in vivo. Thus, the structural changes in the kidney with MIDD are a combined effect of physical accumulation of monoclonal immunoglobulin molecules and an increased synthesis of extracellular matrix material stimulated by the monoclonal immunoglobulin molecules.

Treatment and Prognosis. The prognosis of patients with MIDD is more variable than the uniformly bad prognosis for those with AL amyloidosis (23). The 5-year patient and renal survival rates are approximately 70 percent and 37 percent, respectively (23). Patients with combined MIDD and light chain cast nephropathy have worse outcomes than patients with MIDD alone (22). Treatment is chemotherapy (with or without bone marrow transplantation) directed at eliminating the B-cell or plasma cell clone that is producing the pathogenic truncated immunoglobulin molecules. Successful treatment can result in termination of tissue deposition of monoclonal immunoglobulins, and improvement in sclerotic lesions.

FIBRILLARY GLOMERULONEPHRITIS

Definition. Fibrillary glomerulonephritis is defined by the electron microscopic finding of randomly arranged, straight, nonbranching fibrils ranging in diameter from 10 to 30 nm (averaging approximately 20 nm in most patients) (26–29,32,35,36,40). The deposits do not stain with Congo red. Fibrillary glomerulonephritis differs from amyloidosis not only by the lack of congophilia, but also by the composition of the deposits, which usually contain polyclonal immunoglobulins and complement. Fibrillary glomerulonephritis differs from immunotactoid glomerulopathy by the ultrastructural pattern of the deposits. Unlike the fibrils in fibrillary glomerulonephritis, by electron microscopy, the microtubules of immunotactoid glomerulopathy have an overt tubular appearance at 5,000 to 10,000X magnification, have focal parallel alignment, and usually are more than 30 nm in diameter. Some investigators prefer to group both fibrillary glomerulonephritis and immunotactoid glomerulopathy into one disease category designated *immunotactoid glomerulopathy* (37,40,42–44), however, we conclude that the pathologic and clinical features of these two patterns of injury are so distinct that they warrant separation into different pathologic categories.

Clinical Features. Fibrillary glomerulonephritis is identified in about 1 percent of patients who undergo native kidney biopsy; it is found approximately half as often as amyloidosis and twice as often as MIDD (33,35). It is more common in older adults and rare in children. There is no sex predilection. The disease is rare in blacks (35).

Patients with fibrillary glomerulonephritis can manifest any of the signs and symptoms that are caused by glomerular injury, including asymptomatic proteinuria, nephrotic syndrome, acute nephritis, rapidly progressive nephritis, and chronic nephritis (28,32,33,35,40). Proteinuria occurs in essentially all patients; over two thirds have nephrotic syndrome. The degree of hematuria, renal insufficiency, and hypertension is variable among patients and depends on the nature of the underlying glomerulonephritis. For example, patients who present with nephrotic syndrome usually have extensive capillary wall deposits and those who present with rapidly progressive nephritis typically have active proliferative glomerulonephritis with crescent formation. Hypocomplementemia is rare but has been observed (25). Unlike immunotactoid glomerulopathy, fibrillary glomerulonephritis is only rarely associated with B-cell neoplasms (27,34).

Light Microscopic Findings. The most common light microscopic abnormality in fibrillary glomerulonephritis is the accumulation of amorphous acidophilic extracellular material in the mesangium, capillary walls, or, most often, both (fig. 9-43) (26-29,32,35,36,40,43). This results in capillary wall thickening and mesangial matrix expansion. The degree of mesangial, endocapillary, and extracapillary hypercellularity is variable among patients. Crescent formation is uncommon. Of the last 101 cases of fibrillary glomerulonephritis evaluated in the University of North Carolina Nephropathology Laboratory, 23 percent had crescent formation but only 5 percent had crescents in greater than 50 percent of glomeruli. The light microscopic appearance

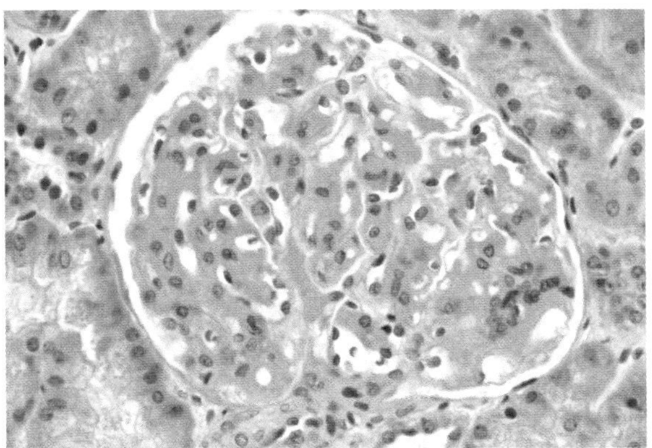

Figure 9-43

FIBRILLARY GLOMERULONEPHRITIS

H&E-stained section shows prominent global mesangial matrix expansion and focal thickening of capillary walls by amorphous acidophilic material. There is mild segmental hypercellularity.

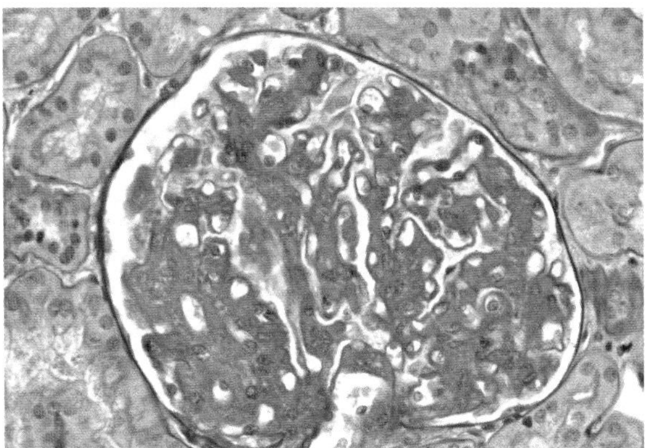

Figure 9-44

FIBRILLARY GLOMERULONEPHRITIS

PAS-stained section shows prominent global mesangial matrix expansion and focal thickening of capillary walls by material that stains well with PAS but has a degree of coarseness or irregularity. There is slight segmental hypercellularity.

of fibrillary glomerulonephritis is extremely variable and can mimic most other forms of glomerular disease, especially in H&E-stained sections. For example, a predominance of capillary wall thickening in the absence of significant hypercellularity resembles membranous glomerulopathy, a predominance of mesangial matrix expansion and hypercellularity with little or no capillary wall thickening resembles mesangioproliferative glomerulonephritis, and combined mesangial hypercellularity and capillary wall thickening resembles membranoproliferative glomerulonephritis. Electron microscopy, however, readily distinguishes fibrillary glomerulonephritis from other glomerular diseases.

Routine stains other than H&E are helpful in raising the suspicion of fibrillary glomerulonephritis. The deposits are more PAS-positive than amyloid, but may have a slightly uneven texture (fig. 9-44); staining with the Masson trichrome stain is variable, probably depending on the ratio of deposits to collagenous matrix. Some specimens have blue/green staining similar to collagen, whereas others have an admixture of fuchsinophilic (red) staining. The Jones methenamine silver (JMS) stain is most useful because the expanded mesangial matrix and thickened capillary walls have a distinctive "moth-eaten" appearance because of silver-negative deposits admixed with the remains of silver-positive collagenous matrix (fig. 9-45).

Immunofluorescence Findings. In all but rare cases, fibrillary glomerulonephritis has a characteristic pattern and composition of deposits as revealed by immunofluorescence microscopy (figs. 9-46, 9-47) (26–29,32,35,36,40). Over 90 percent of specimens have immunostaining indicative of polyclonal immunoglobulin (Ig)G and complement (C)3 in the glomerular deposits. Less than 10 percent of specimens stain for monoclonal immunoglobulin (usually IgG kappa); only rare specimens do not stain for immunoglobulins (31). The finding of no staining for immunoglobulins is so rare that it should raise the level of suspicion for another process with immunoglobulin-negative organized deposits, such as AA amyloidosis or fibronectin glomerulopathy.

The mesangium almost always stains for the immune deposits, and the capillary walls usually are positive as well. The pattern of capillary wall staining is very distinctive and is characterized by irregular, flocculent staining (fig. 9-46); by band-like or pseudolinear staining (fig. 9-47); or a mixture of the two. With experience, fibrillary glomerulonephritis can be predicted with substantial accuracy from the immunofluorescence microscopy findings alone. Unlike amyloidosis and MIDD, staining of renal structures other than the glomeruli is rare.

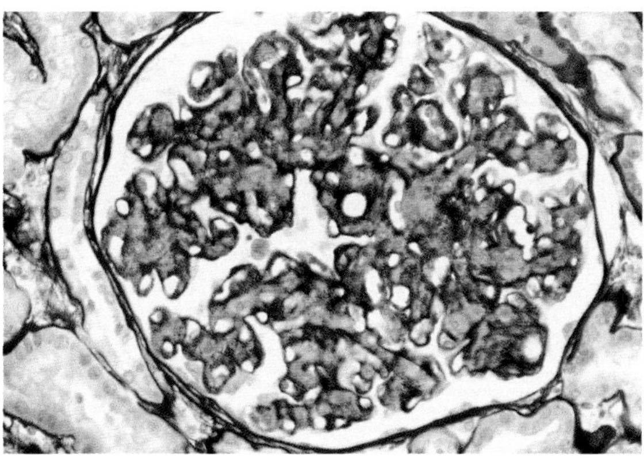

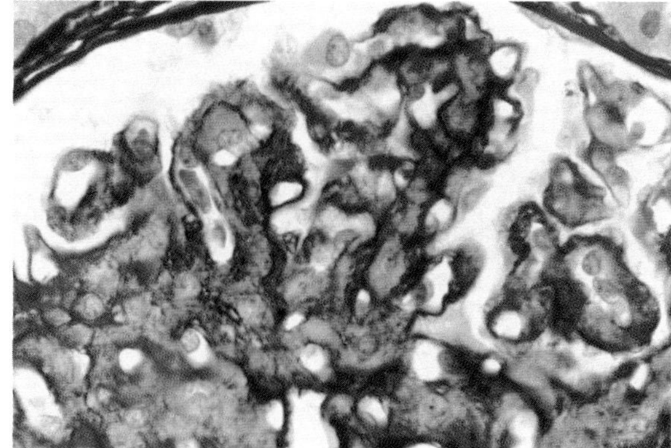

Figure 9-45

FIBRILLARY GLOMERULONEPHRITIS

Lower (top) and higher (bottom) magnification photomicrographs of JMS-stained sections show prominent global mesangial matrix expansion and focal thickening of capillary walls by material that has a distinctive motheaten appearance.

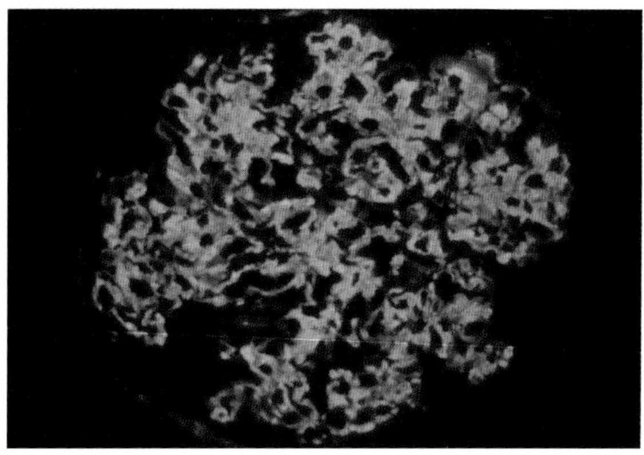

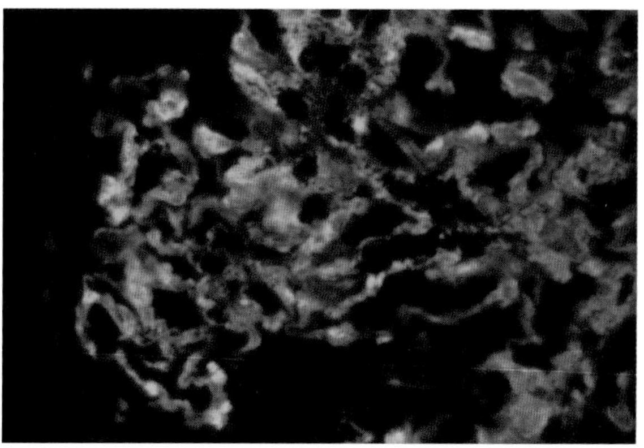

Figure 9-46

FIBRILLARY GLOMERULONEPHRITIS

Lower (left) and higher (right) magnification immunofluorescence photomicrographs show irregular, flocculent staining of capillary walls and mesangium with an antiserum specific for IgG.

Electron Microscopic Findings. As mentioned, the sine qua non of fibrillary glomerulonephritis is the finding of glomerular deposits of randomly arranged, straight, nonbranching fibrils, ranging in diameter from 10 to 30 nm (figs. 9-48, 9-49) (26–29,32,35,36,40). In most patients the fibrils average around 20 nm in diameter. The fibrils can be seen distinctly at 5,000 to 10,000X magnification (fig. 9-48). At this magnification, the fibrils of amyloidosis appear as a cottony mass with individual fibrils poorly defined (see fig. 9-22) and the microtubules of immunotactoid glomerulopathy have clearly defined electron-lucent cores. The fibrils of fibrillary glomerulonephritis may be in the mesangium (fig. 9-48, left), the capillary walls (figs. 9-48, right; 9-49), or both. Unlike most immune complex deposits and more like amyloid deposits, the deposits of fibrillary glomerulonephritis often infiltrate through the glomerular basement membrane rather than heaping up on the subendothelial or subepithelial side of the basement membrane (fig. 9-49). A frequent and very distinctive feature of fibrillary glomerulonephritis deposits is the admixture of smudgy, electron-dense material with the fibrillary material (fig. 9-48, right). This probably represents more conventional immune complex dense deposits mixed with the fibrillary immune deposits. Fibrillary deposits in tubular basement membranes are rare.

Differential Diagnosis. As noted earlier, fibrillary glomerulonephritis can mimic many other forms of glomerular disease because of the varied histologic appearance. The findings by electron microscopy usually provide definitive support for the diagnosis. The glomerular sclerosis (scarring) caused by some disease processes may have a poorly defined fibrillary texture that should not be confused with fibrillary glomerulonephritis (38). The other pathologic findings by light, immunofluorescence, and electron microscopy should be factored in to conclude whether the fibrils are indicative of fibrillary glomerulonephritis or glomerular scarring.

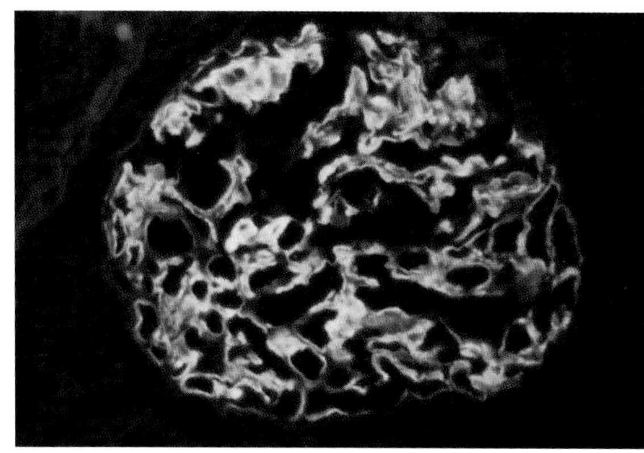

Figure 9-47

FIBRILLARY GLOMERULONEPHRITIS

Band-like or pseudolinear staining of capillary walls and contiguous mesangial staining with an antiserum specific for IgG.

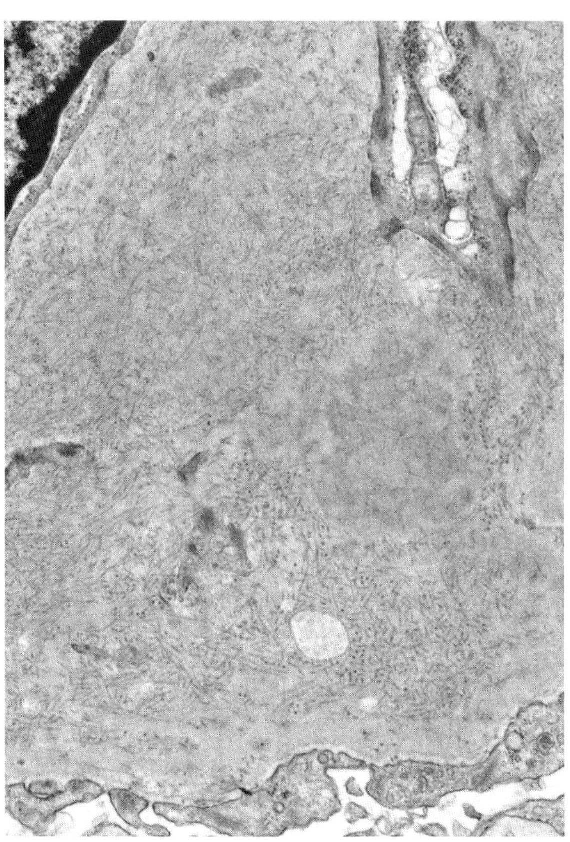

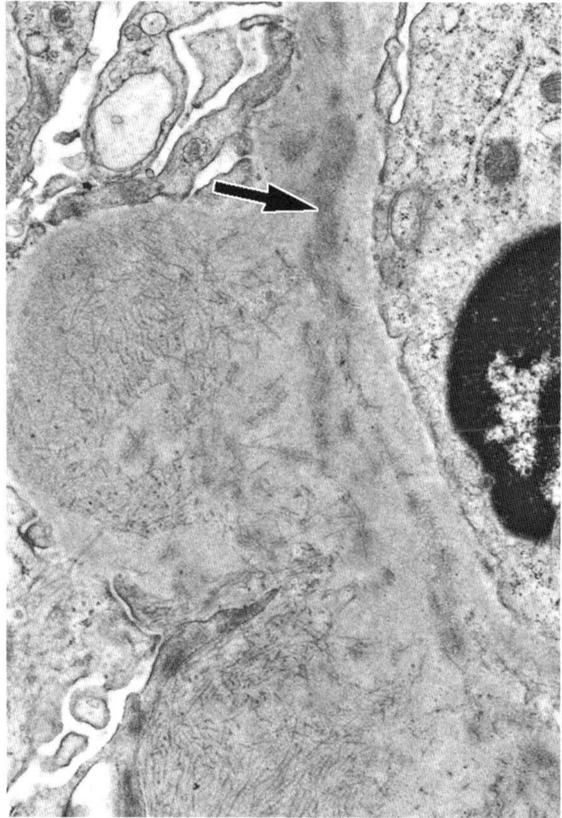

Figure 9-48

FIBRILLARY GLOMERULONEPHRITIS

Electron micrographs demonstrate fibrillary deposits predominantly in the mesangium (left) and subepithelial zone of a capillary wall (right). Note the random orientation of the fibrils. The right figure demonstrates admixed, smudgy, electron-dense material (arrow).

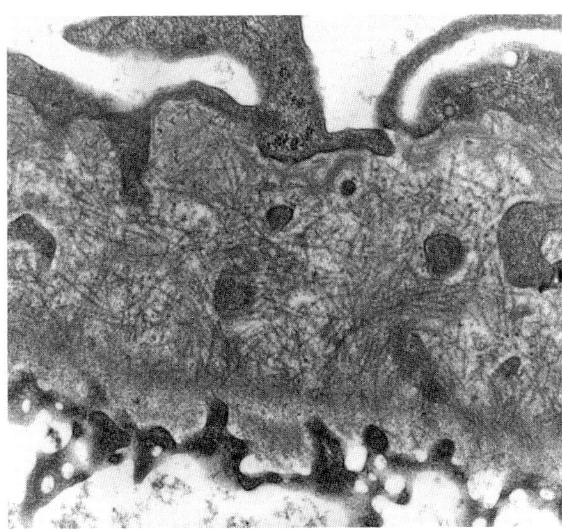

Figure 9-49

FIBRILLARY GLOMERULONEPHRITIS

Electron micrograph demonstrates fibrillary deposits disrupting the glomerular basement membrane and expanding the subepithelial space. The podocyte is at the top and the fenestrated endothelial cell is at the bottom of the figure.

By electron microscopy, amyloidosis resembles fibrillary glomerulonephritis. The fibrils in rare examples of fibrillary glomerulonephritis are similar in diameter to those of amyloidosis. Other pathologic features, such as staining with Congo red and the composition of the deposits revealed by immunohistology, allow differentiation of fibrillary glomerulonephritis from amyloidosis even when the fibrils are relatively thin.

Fibrillary glomerulonephritis is distinguished from immunotactoid glomerulopathy by the electron microscopic findings. Unlike the fibrils of fibrillary glomerulonephritis, the microtubules of immunotactoid glomerulopathy have an overt tubular appearance at 5,000 to 10,000X magnification, have focal parallel alignment, often are curved, and usually are more 30 nm in diameter.

Etiology and Pathogenesis. Based on the presence of IgG and C3 in the fibrillary deposits of almost all patients with fibrillary glomerulonephritis, the deposits probably are caused by immune complex localization. Only rare familial occurrences have been reported (30). A few cases of fibrillary glomerulonephritis have been identified in patients with hepatitis C virus infection, suggesting that the immune complex disease caused by hepatitis C virus can have a fibrillary glomerulonephritis phenotype (39). In addition, some patients with hepatitis C virus infection have pathologic features consistent with immunotactoid glomerulopathy (39). The most common pattern of glomerular injury caused by hepatitis C is membranoproliferative glomerulonephritis, often with microtubular structures in the immune deposits. Thus, looking at the spectrum of immune complex deposits in glomeruli caused by hepatitis C virus infection, it seems that some qualitative characteristics of the immune deposits causes them to align into either fibrillary or microtubular (immunotactoid) configurations. A homogeneous component may be required for deposits of immunoglobulins to have a patterned ultrastructural appearance. The fibrils of AL amyloidosis contain homogeneous fragments of monoclonal immunoglobulin light chains. Microtubular cryoglobulin deposits usually contain a monoclonal anti-immunoglobulin component, and microtubular immunotactoid deposits often contain monoclonal immunoglobulins (27). Thus, homogeneous or partially homogeneous accumulations of immunoglobulin molecules are prone to develop ultrastructural organized patterns. The homogeneous immunoglobulin component of the fibrils of fibrillary glomerulonephritis may be IgG4, which is the exclusive or predominant immunoglobulin subclass in the fibrillary deposits (35). IgG1 may be present but IgG2 and IgG3 are consistently absent. Although not monoclonal, the immunoglobulin in the deposits of fibrillary glomerulonephritis is at least more homogeneous than most immune complex deposits that do not have an organized ultrastructure.

Treatment and Prognosis. Most patients with fibrillary glomerulonephritis have persistent and progressive disease that often results in end-stage renal disease. In one study, 44 percent of patients progressed to end-stage renal disease after an average of 10 1/2 months (33). No effective therapy has been documented, although patients often are treated with corticosteroids, with or without other immunosuppressive agents. Fibrillary glomerulonephritis recurs in renal transplants (40,41). Although prolonged graft function is possible, recurrence may happen quickly and result in graft loss.

IMMUNOTACTOID GLOMERULOPATHY

Definition. Immunotactoid glomerulopathy is defined by the electron microscopic finding of glomerular deposits of microtubules that have an overt tubular appearance at 5,000 to 10,000X magnification, focal parallel alignment, and a diameter that usually is more than 30 nm (range, 20 to 90 nm) (27,33,42). The size of the microtubules of immunotactoid glomerulopathy overlaps with that of the fibrils of fibrillary glomerulonephritis, however, the ultrastructural appearance of these two diseases is very different. Unlike the microtubules of immunotactoid glomerulopathy, the fibrils of fibrillary glomerulonephritis have no apparent lucent cores at 5,000 to 10,000X magnification, are randomly arranged rather than having focal parallel organization, and usually are smaller with diameters ranging from 10 to 30 nm (averaging approximately 20 nm in most patients). As noted earlier, some investigators prefer to group fibrillary glomerulonephritis with immunotactoid glomerulopathy, however, we consider these to be pathologically and clinically distinct processes.

Clinical Features. Immunotactoid glomerulopathy is more frequent in older individuals, usually those over 60 years of age (33). Most patients have proteinuria, often accompanied by hematuria and renal insufficiency. Patients with immunotactoid glomerulopathy are at increased risk of having an associated B-cell neoplasm and paraproteinemia (27,33).

Light Microscopic Findings. As with fibrillary glomerulonephritis, the light microscopic appearance of immunotactoid glomerulopathy is varied (27,33,42). For example, some specimens have only capillary wall thickening, others only mesangial expansion, and others both. The most frequent appearance, however, is marked combined capillary wall thickening and mesangial expansion with endocapillary hypercellularity (figs. 9-50–9-52). Thus, by light microscopy, immunotactoid glomerulopathy often has a lobular pattern of injury that resembles membranoproliferative glomerulonephritis. Crescents and necrosis are uncommon. The acidophilic material in the capillary walls and mesangium does not stain with Congo red. Many specimens have very extensive capillary wall thickening and mesangial expansion that results in narrowing or obliteration of capillary lumens. Hyaline thrombi, which are in fact large accumulations of the immunotactoid deposits in capillary lumens, occasionally occur. Even larger deposits may cause confluent areas of hyalinosis within glomeruli (fig. 9-51). The expanded mesangial regions typically have a mottled or moth-eaten appearance with the Masson trichrome and JMS stains (fig. 9-52), similar to fibrillary glomerulonephritis and different from amyloidosis.

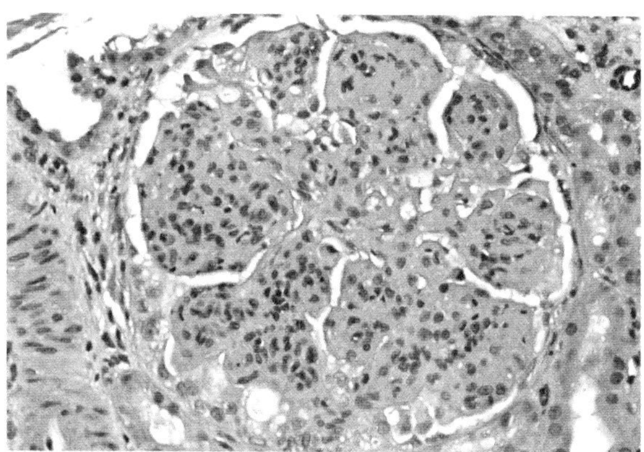

Figure 9-50

IMMUNOTACTOID GLOMERULOPATHY

Light microscopy shows a lobular pattern, with marked endocapillary hypercellularity, thickening of capillary walls, and obliteration of most capillary lumens. There is slight segmental extracapillary proliferation (crescent formation) at the bottom of the field (H&E stain).

Immunofluorescence Findings. Immunofluorescence microscopy demonstrates varying patterns of diffuse immunoglobulin deposition, usually with at least segmental and usually global capillary wall and mesangial involvement (figs. 9-53, 9-54). Capillary wall deposits may be granular or band-like. Globular deposits may occur in capillary lumens but are less frequent than in cryoglobulinemic glomerulonephritis. Deposits most often stain predominantly for IgG (33). When the deposits are monoclonal, staining for kappa light chains is more frequent than for lambda light chains. Complement staining is variable, but often is of relatively low intensity, which differs from membranoproliferative glomerulonephritis.

Electron Microscopic Findings. The necessary ultrastructural finding that allows a diagnosis of immunotactoid glomerulopathy is glomerular deposits of microtubules with an overt

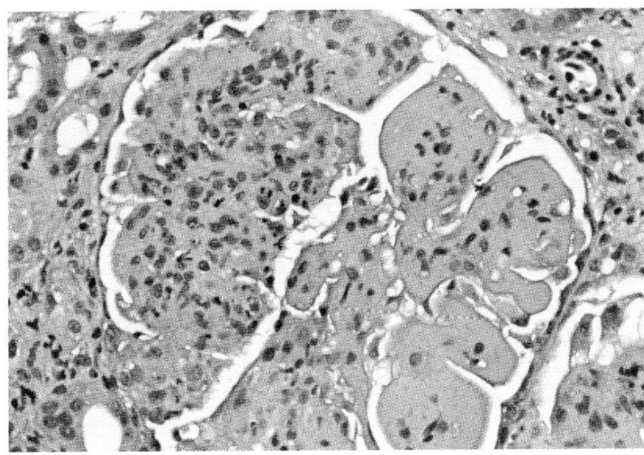

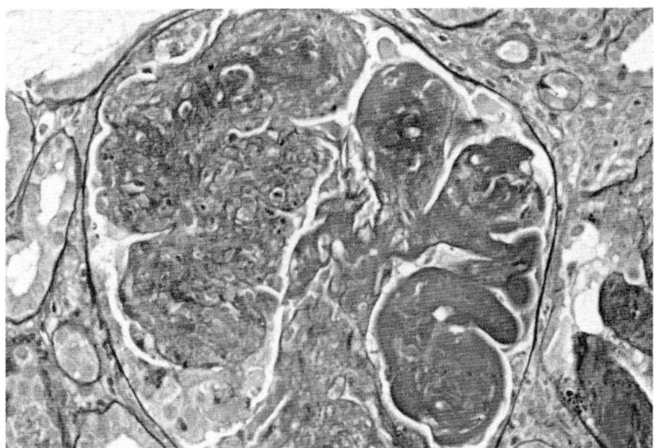

Figure 9-51

IMMUNOTACTOID GLOMERULOPATHY

H&E (left) and PAS (right) staining of the same glomerulus show a zone on the right side of the tuft with massive accumulation of immunotactoid deposits, resulting in hyalinosis. The other segments show marked endocapillary hypercellularity and extensive replication of basement membranes. There is a small focus of extracapillary hypercellularity.

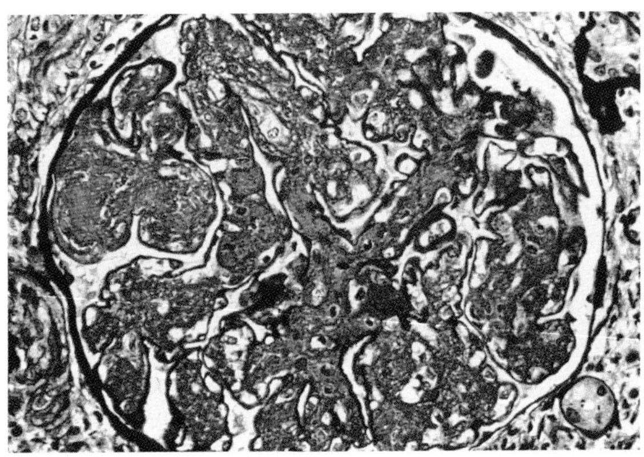

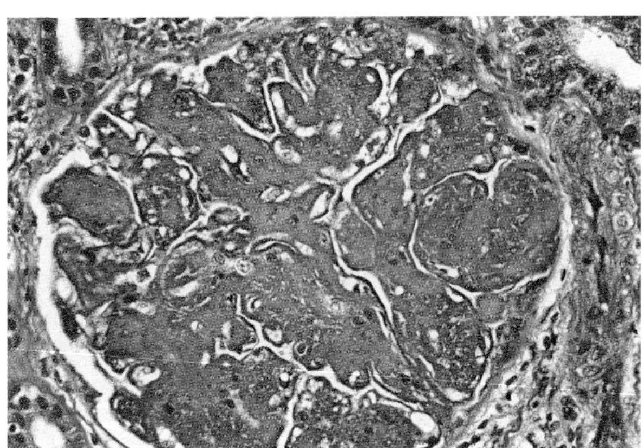

Figure 9-52

IMMUNOTACTOID GLOMERULOPATHY

JMS (left) and Masson trichrome (right) stains show marked mesangial expansion by material with a mottled staining pattern because most of the material is JMS negative.

tubular appearance at 5,000 to 10,000X magnification (figs. 9-55–9-57). These microtubules may be straight but often are slightly curved. There is essentially always focal parallel alignment of the microtubules, which appears as grouped hollow cylinders when cut in cross section, or as stacks of microtubules when viewed longitudinally (fig. 9-57). The diameter of the microtubules varies substantially among different specimens, ranging from 20 to 90 nm; however, in most specimens the microtubules range from 25 to 35 nm.

The deposits of immunotactoid glomerulopathy may be composed almost exclusively of organized microtubules or may have a varying density of microtubules on a background of unorganized electron-dense material. When the electron-dense background material is conspicuous or the microtubules are very short or poorly defined, there is a greater likelihood of cryoglobulinemic glomerulonephritis (fig. 9-58). The microtubules of immunotactoid glomerulopathy may be located predominately in the mesangium and subendothelial zones, where they

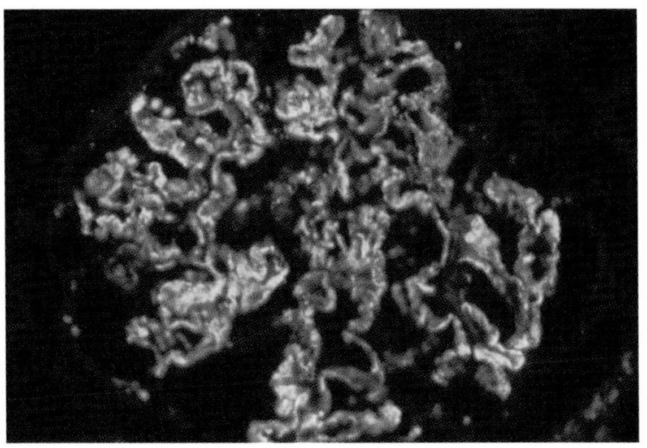

Figure 9-53

IMMUNOTACTOID GLOMERULOPATHY

Granular capillary wall and mesangial staining for IgG.

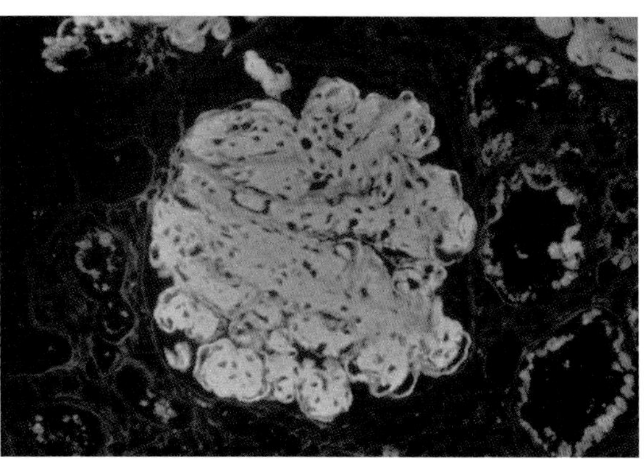

Figure 9-54

IMMUNOTACTOID GLOMERULOPATHY

Very dense, confluent capillary wall and mesangial staining for IgG in glomeruli as well as cytoplasmic staining of some tubular epithelial cells.

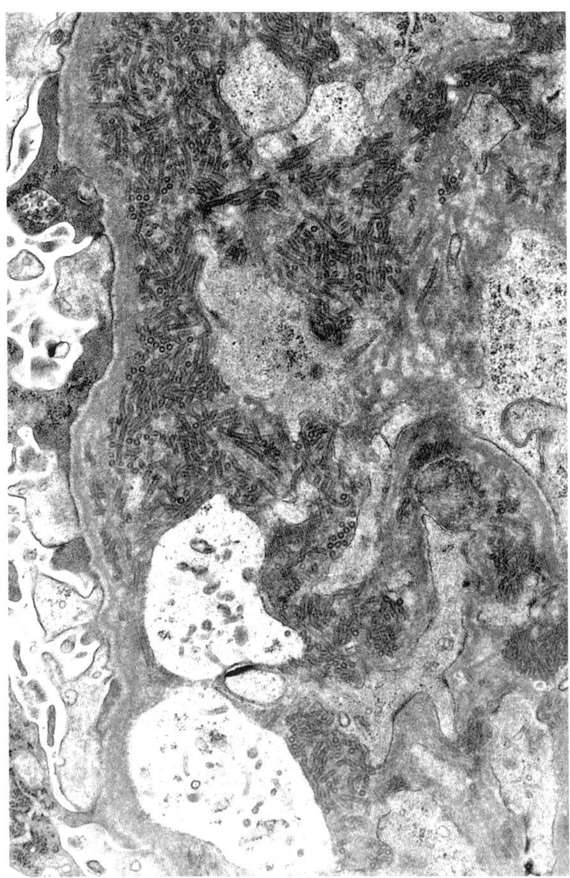

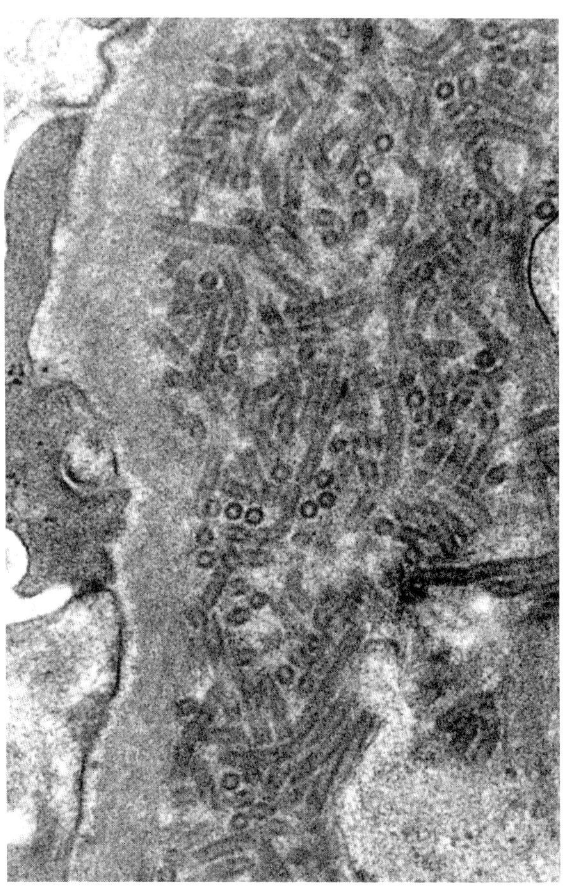

Figure 9-55

IMMUNOTACTOID GLOMERULOPATHY

Electron micrograph demonstrates numerous microtubular structures beneath the glomerular basement membrane at approximately 10,000X (left) and 25,000X (right) magnification. (Courtesy of Dr. Charles Alpers, Seattle, WA.)

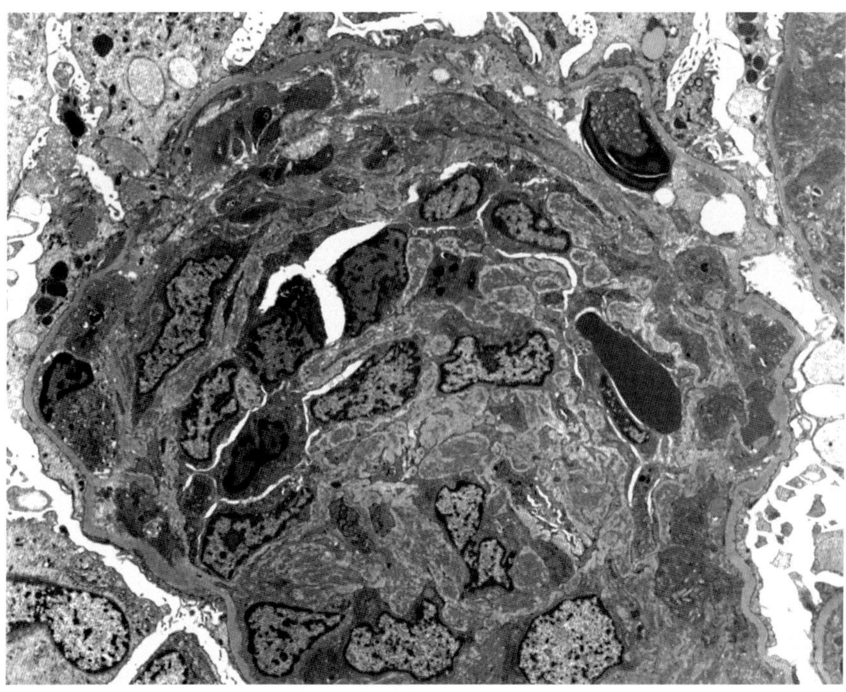

Figure 9-56

IMMUNOTACTOID GLOMERULOPATHY

On low-power electron microscopy, features include marked endocapillary hypercellularity, mesangial interposition into the subendothelial zone, mesangial matrix expansion and basement membrane replication, and scattered densities within the mesangial and subendothelial areas.

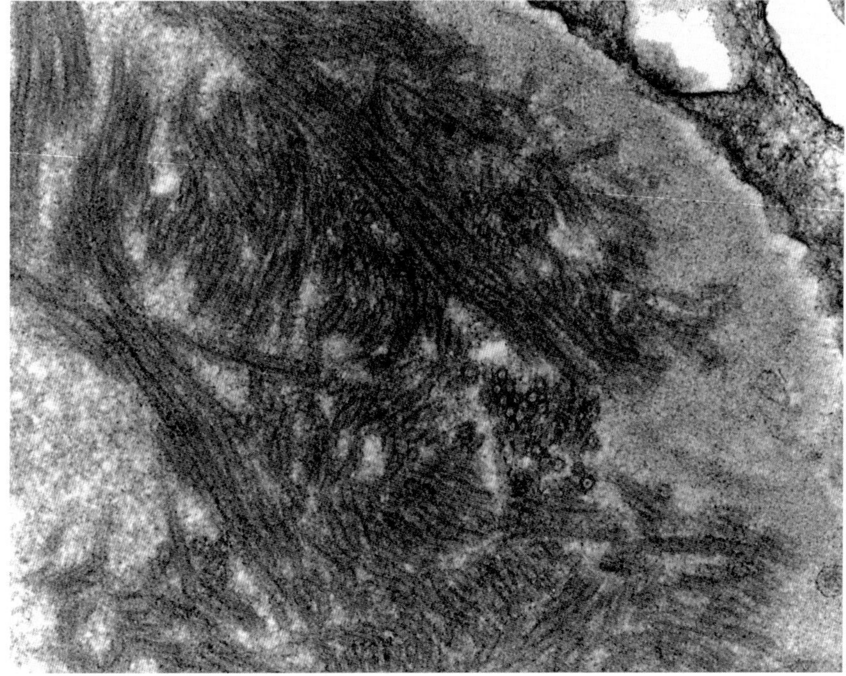

Figure 9-57

IMMUNOTACTOID GLOMERULOPATHY

A higher magnification of the specimen in figure 9-56 shows immunotactoid deposits composed of slightly curved, microtubular structures that have a tendency for parallel alignment.

stimulate mesangial proliferation and subendothelial interposition that can mimic membranoproliferative glomerulonephritis (fig. 9-56). Less commonly, there may be conspicuous subepithelial clusters of immunotactoid microtubules that mimic the distribution of deposits of membranous glomerulopathy.

Differential Diagnosis. Cryoglobulinemic glomerulonephritis is a major pathologic differential diagnostic consideration. Essentially by definition, if a patient fulfills the clinical or laboratory criteria for cryoglobulinemia, glomerulonephritis that otherwise would be called immunotactoid glomerulopathy is diagnosed as

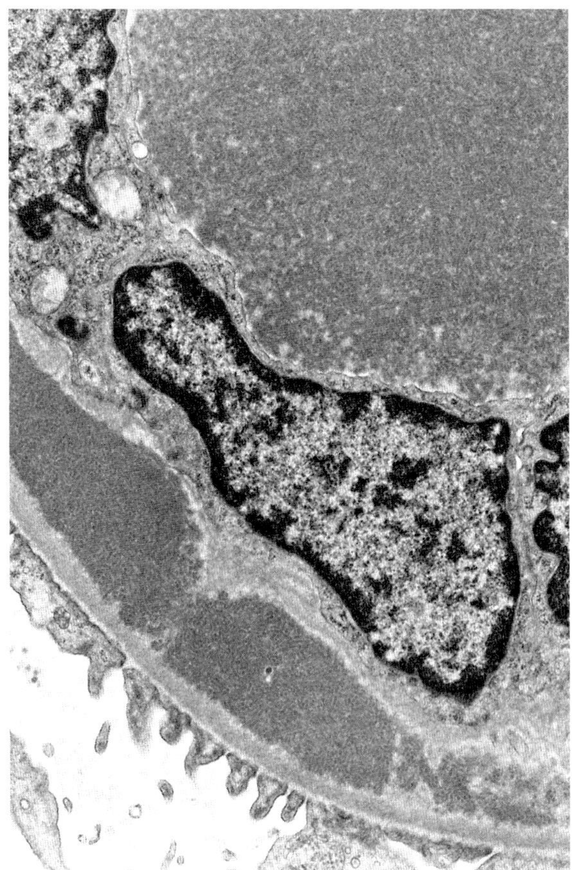

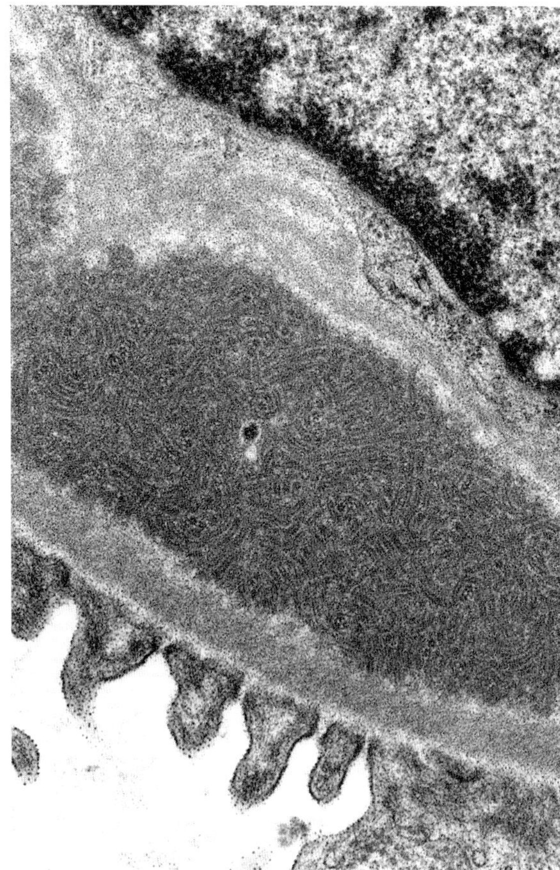

Figure 9-58

CRYOGLOBULINEMIC GLOMERULONEPHRITIS

Left: Large subendothelial deposits are between the endothelial cell and the glomerular basement membrane. An aggregate of cryoglobulins in the lumen corresponds to a hyaline thrombus by light microscopy.

Right: At higher magnification, the microtubular organization within the subendothelial deposits is seen. The overall electron density of the cryoglobulin deposits is greater and the microtubule length is less than that of the immunotactoid deposits in figures 9-55 to 9-57.

cryoglobulinemic glomerulonephritis. Most but not all examples of cryoglobulinemic glomerulonephritis have immune deposits containing organized microtubular structures; the remainder have amorphous electron-dense immune deposits. The organized deposits of cryoglobulinemic glomerulonephritis often have a different appearance than most specimens of immunotactoid glomerulopathy. In particular, the microtubular configurations in cryoglobulinemic glomerulonephritis frequently are only vaguely apparent within a predominantly amorphous or granular electron-dense background, and the microtubules tend to be shorter (fig. 9-58). This tendency, however, is not consistent enough to accurately distinguish cryoglobulinemic glomerulonephritis from immunotactoid glomerulopathy.

By light microscopy, immunotactoid glomerulopathy can mimic most forms of glomerular disease, depending upon the relative degree of glomerular capillary wall thickening, mesangial matrix expansion, and hypercellularity; the disease most similar is membranoproliferative glomerulonephritis. Electron microscopy is the ultimate basis for differentiating the two.

Based on light microscopy alone, immunotactoid glomerulopathy also resembles diffuse proliferative lupus glomerulonephritis, including the presence of wire loops and hyaline thrombi. However, the electron microscopic features of immunotactoid glomerulopathy are

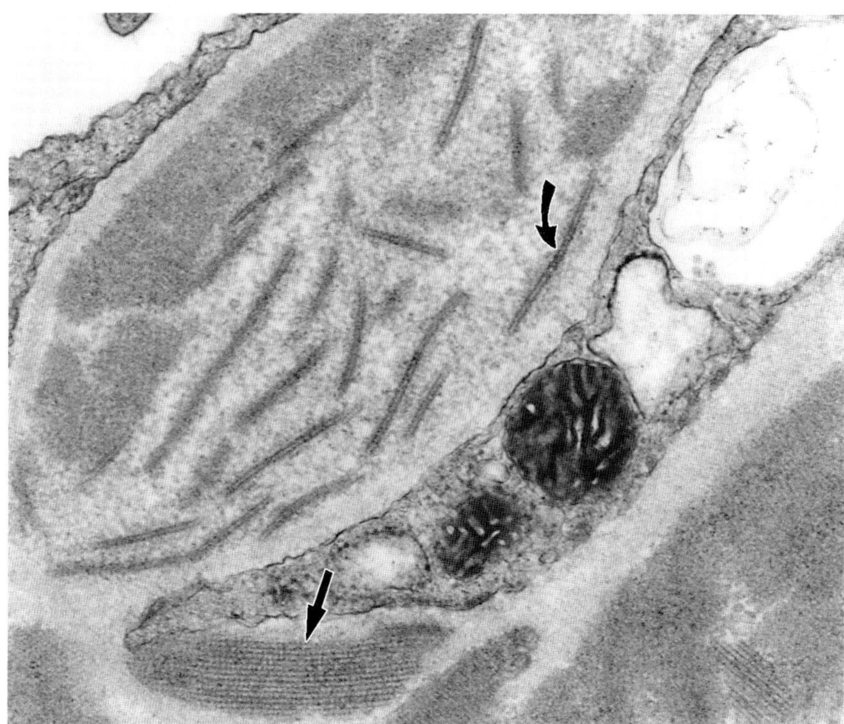

Figure 9-59

LUPUS GLOMERULONEPHRITIS

Electron micrograph shows glomerular organized deposits in a patient with lupus glomerulonephritis. These include scattered microtubules (curved arrow) and fingerprint patterns (straight arrow).

distinct from those of lupus nephritis. This is complicated by the fact that electron microscopy occasionally reveals organized microtubular deposits in lupus nephritis. Unlike immunotactoid glomerulopathy, these typically are very focal and often have a "fingerprint" configuration (fig. 9-59). In addition, clinical findings help differentiate patients with lupus nephritis with organized deposits from patients with immunotactoid glomerulopathy.

Etiology and Pathogenesis. Deposits of monoclonal immunoglobulins are the apparent cause of immunotactoid glomerulopathy in some patients (28). Because of this, all patients with a diagnosis of immunotactoid glomerulopathy should be evaluated carefully for an underlying B-cell dyscrasia. As discussed in the section on fibrillary glomerulonephritis, the occurrence of microtubules in immunoglobulin deposits may be caused by a homogeneous component. In those patients with monoclonal immunoglobulin–immunotactoid deposits, the homogeneous component is obvious. There may be an as yet unrecognized homogeneous component in other cases.

Treatment and Prognosis. Those patients with an identifiable underlying B-cell neoplasm should be treated with the appropriate chemotherapy. Patients with idiopathic immunotactoid glomerulopathy usually are treated with high-dose corticosteroids, cytotoxic drugs (e.g., cyclophosphamide), or both. Immunotactoid glomerulopathy is so rare, however, that there are no controlled studies of therapeutic efficacy.

FIBRONECTIN GLOMERULOPATHY

Definition. Fibronectin glomerulopathy is an autosomal dominant familial disease defined by the presence of massive fibronectin deposits in glomeruli (45–49).

Clinical Features. Patients present during the third or fourth decade of life with proteinuria and varying degrees of hematuria, renal insufficiency, and hypertension (45,46).

Light Microscopic Findings. The characteristic finding is massive, homogeneous, pale eosinophilic deposits in glomeruli, expanding mesangial and subendothelial areas (fig. 9-60) (45). This often produces a lobular pattern of glomerular consolidation. The massive subendothelial deposits frequently cause narrowing or obliteration of capillary lumens. Hypercellularity is mild or absent. The deposits stain diffusely with PAS (fig. 9-61) but only weakly with the JMS stain (fig. 9-

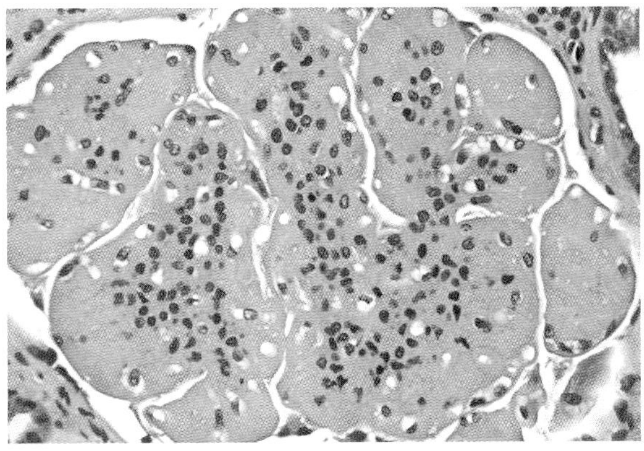

Figure 9-60

FIBRONECTIN GLOMERULOPATHY

H&E-stained section shows massive accumulation of amorphous, pale, acidophilic material in the capillary walls and mesangium. Most capillary lumens are obliterated. Note the hyaline appearance of some deposits.

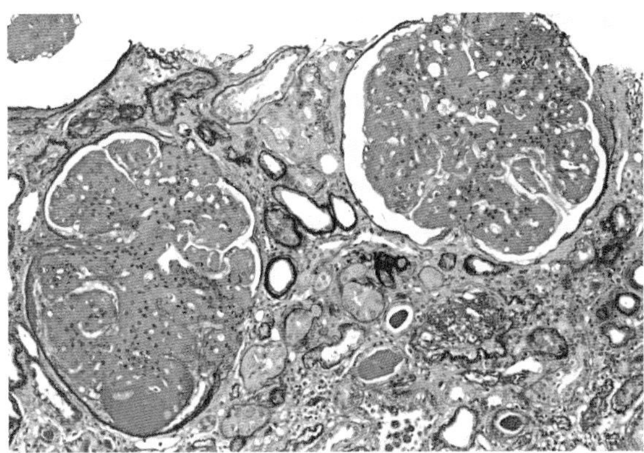

Figure 9-61

FIBRONECTIN GLOMERULOPATHY

The massive fibronectin deposits are weakly PAS positive.

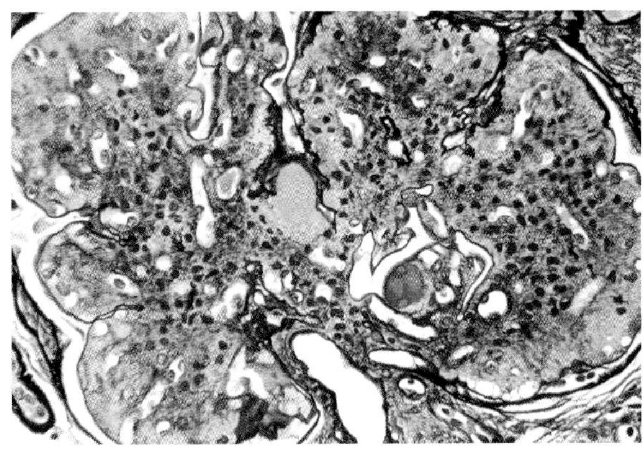

Figure 9-62

FIBRONECTIN GLOMERULOPATHY

The fibronectin deposits stain poorly with the JMS stain.

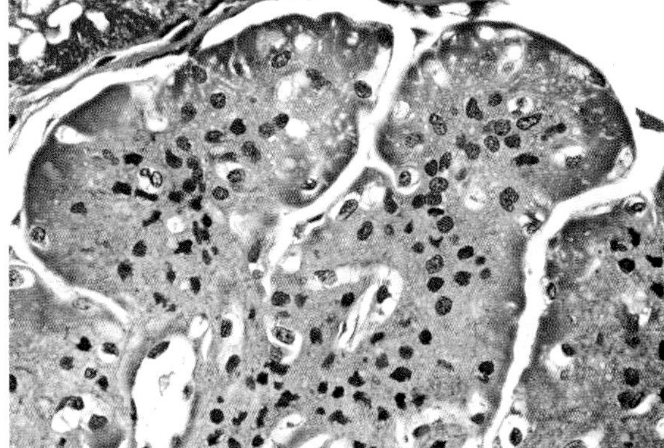

Figure 9-63

FIBRONECTIN GLOMERULOPATHY

The fibronectin deposits show focal fuchsinophilia (red staining) with the Masson trichrome stain.

62). The deposits stain variably with Masson trichrome, but may be fuchsinophilic (red) (fig. 9-63). The deposits are negative with Congo red stain.

Immunofluorescence Findings. By definition, the deposits stain predominantly for fibronectin (fig. 9-64), and specifically for plasma fibronectin rather than cell-derived fibronectin (45,49). There may be scanty staining for immunoglobulins and complement, but not to the degree that is typical for immune complex glomerulonephritis. The deposits stain minimally with antisera specific for type IV collagen or laminin (45,49).

Electron Microscopic Findings. The abnormal deposits are electron dense, and are in the mesangium and subendothelial zone (fig. 9-65). They can be so massive that capillary lumens are obliterated. The deposits may be finely granular or have a fibrillary substructure, with randomly arranged, 12- to 16-nm fibrils (48). The deposits often appear more granular than fibrillar at 5,000 to 10,000X, and even at more than 20,000X the fibrillary texture may be focal rather than diffuse and the fibers are shorter than those typically seen with amyloidosis or fibrillary glomerulonephritis.

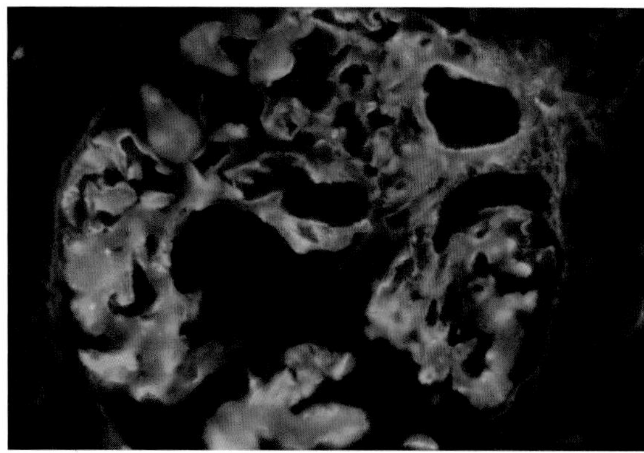

Figure 9-64

FIBRONECTIN GLOMERULOPATHY

Immunofluorescence microscopy using antiserum specific for fibronectin reveals extensive mesangial and capillary wall staining that typically has a homogeneous or cottony appearance.

Differential Diagnosis. By light microscopy, fibronectin glomerulopathy most often resembles membranoproliferative glomerulonephritis, nodular MIDD, fibrillary glomerulonephritis, immunotactoid glomerulopathy, or cryoglobulinemic glomerulonephritis. The distinctive findings by immunofluorescence microscopy, such as extensive immunoglobulin deposits, rule out fibronectin glomerulopathy; if there is no staining for immunoglobulins or complement, fibronectin glomerulopathy is a more likely diagnosis. The fibrillary pattern that is usually seen by electron microscopy in fibronectin glomerulopathy, such as more granular than fibrillar deposits at 5,000 to 10,000X, is relatively distinct from that seen with fibrillary glomerulonephritis, immunotactoid glomerulopathy, and cryoglobulinemic glomerulonephritis.

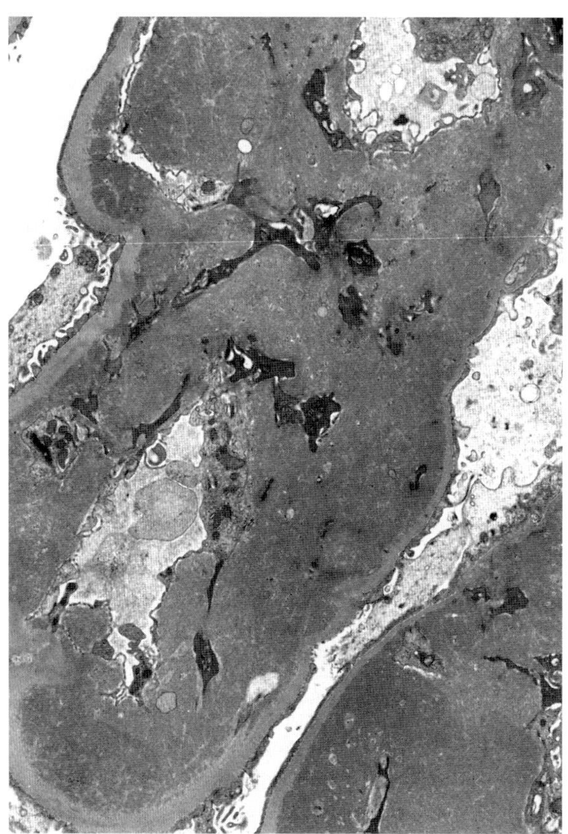

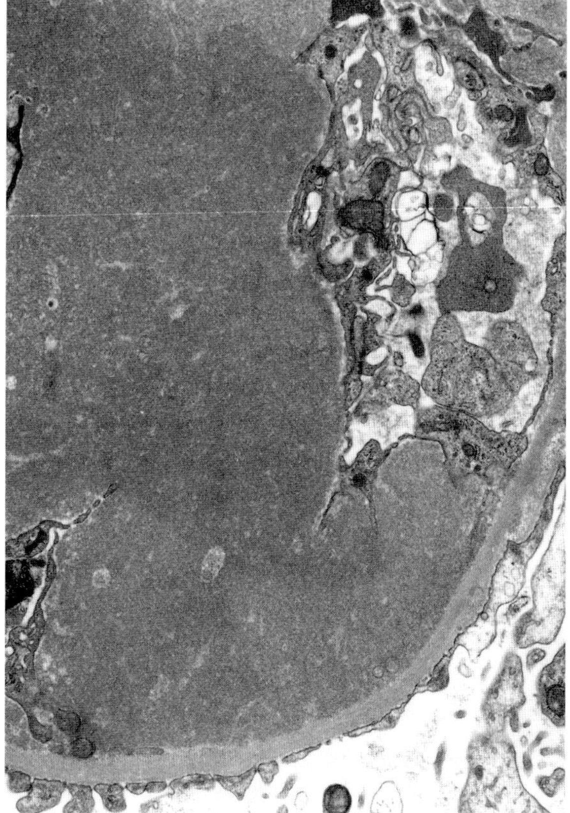

Figure 9-65

FIBRONECTIN GLOMERULOPATHY

Electron micrograph shows massive subendothelial and mesangial electron-dense fibronectin deposits.
Left: At low-power magnification (3,000X) the deposits appear relatively homogeneous.
Right: At 6,000X, a fine granularity becomes apparent.

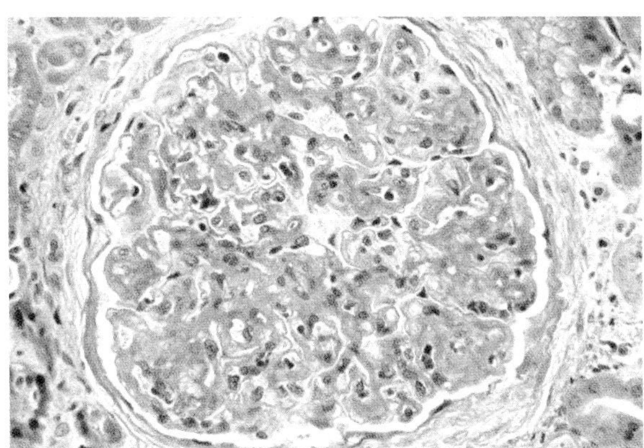
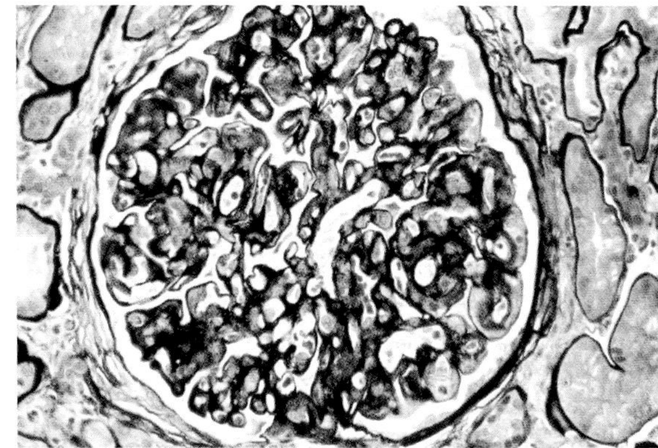

Figure 9-66

COLLAGENOFIBROTIC GLOMERULOPATHY

Masson trichrome (left) and JMS (right) stains show global capillary wall thickening and mesangial matrix expansion. The thickening of capillary walls narrows most capillary lumens.

Immunofluorescence microscopy, especially when staining for fibronectin is included, readily resolves the differential diagnosis.

Etiology and Pathogenesis. The abnormal accumulation of fibronectin in the kidney is an autosomal dominant genetic abnormality; however, the nature of this lesion has not been identified. It does not appear to be an abnormality in the genes for fibronectin, villin, or desmin (48). The abnormal gene maps to chromosome 1q32 in a region involved in the regulation of a complement activation gene cluster.

Treatment and Prognosis. Fibronectin glomerulopathy usually becomes clinically apparent as proteinuria during the third to fourth decade of life and often progresses to end-stage renal disease within 15 to 20 years of the onset of proteinuria (46). The disease may recur in renal transplants.

COLLAGENOFIBROTIC GLOMERULOPATHY

Definition. Collagenofibrotic glomerulopathy is an autosomal recessive familial disease defined pathologically by the presence of extensive accumulations of banded collagen in glomeruli (50,51,54,55,57). Alternative names include *primary glomerular fibrosis* and *collagen III glomerulopathy*.

Clinical Features. The initial clinical manifestation usually is proteinuria, which may be of nephrotic range with edema. The onset may be in childhood or adulthood. Approximately a third of patients have hypertension and a minority have hematuria. Most patients initially have normal renal function but progress to renal insufficiency over a number of years. Hemolytic uremic syndrome may develop in patients and their siblings (50). Extrarenal involvement may occur (59), for example, liver disease caused by type III collagen deposits in the perisinusoidal spaces of the liver (55). Collagenofibrotic glomerulopathy has been reported in patients with hypocomplementemia caused by an inherited factor H deficiency (58).

Light Microscopic Findings. There is marked thickening of capillary walls and expansion of mesangial areas in the glomeruli, which may impart a lobular appearance (figs. 9-66, 9-67) (50–53). The thick walls and expanded mesangium are eosinophilic and stain poorly or irregularly with PAS, trichrome, and JMS stains. A portion of the deposits may stain more intensely, however, possibly because of greater maturity of the collagen in these areas or, more likely, because of deposition of new basement membrane material (fig. 9-67). The deposits do not stain with Congo red. Capillary lumens often are narrowed or obliterated by the thickened walls and expanded mesangium. Hypercellularity is minimal or absent.

Immunofluorescence Findings. The collagen deposits do not stain for immunoglobulin or complement. Immunohistochemistry with antisera specific for collagen types reveals

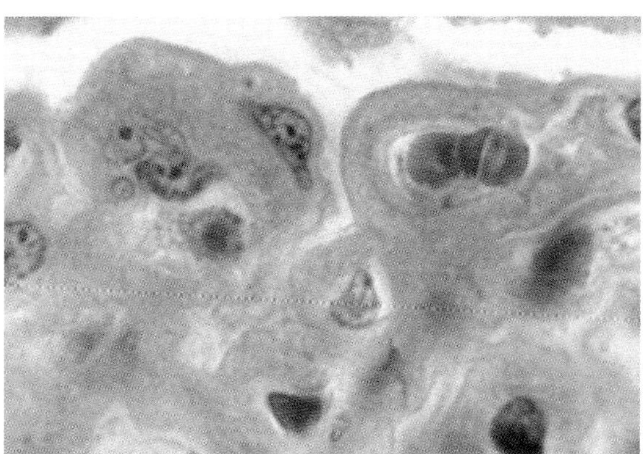

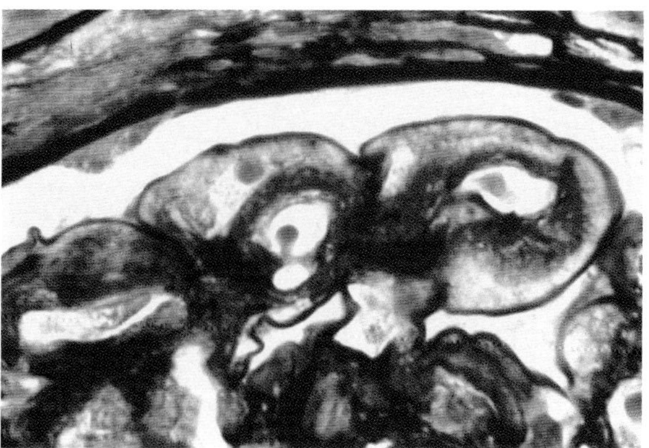

Figure 9-67

COLLAGENOFIBROTIC GLOMERULOPATHY

High-power magnification of glomerular segments stained with Masson trichrome (left) and JMS (right). Much of the expanded subendothelial zone does not stain well with the silver or trichrome stains but there is an inner, better staining band that could be newly formed basement membrane material or better organized abnormal collagen deposits.

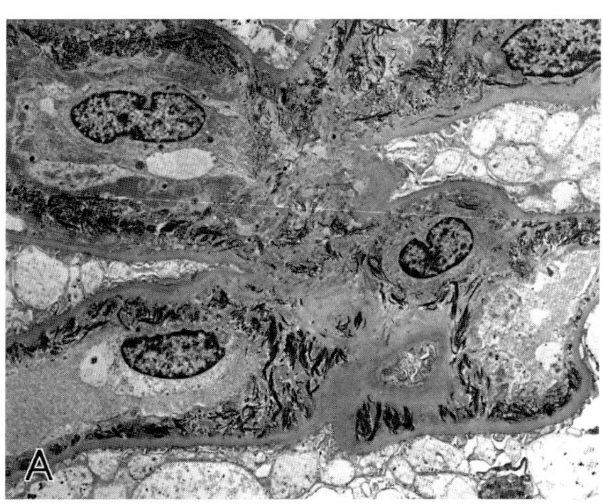

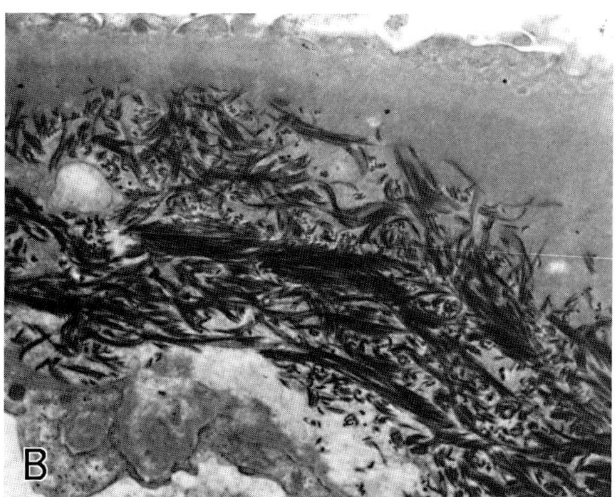

Figure 9-68

COLLAGENOFIBROTIC GLOMERULOPATHY

Low- (A), medium- (B), and high-powered (C) magnification electron micrographs of a glomerulus from a patient with collagenofibrotic glomerulopathy. The deposits are in subendothelial and mesangial areas but not in the subepithelial zone (A,B). The fibrils are curved and often have a frayed appearance at their ends (B,C). At high magnification, the typical periodicity of banded collagen can be discerned (C).

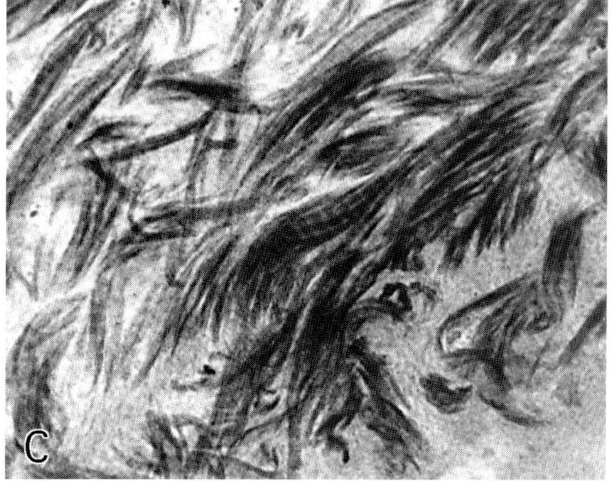

predominant or exclusive staining for type III collagen. Weaker staining for type I collagen may occur.

Electron Microscopic Findings. The diagnostic finding is numerous curved and often frayed electron-dense fibers of banded collagen, with a periodicity of 45 to 65 nm, predominantly in the mesangium and subendothelial zone of capillary walls (fig. 9-68). Subepithelial banded collagen deposits typically are absent. Visceral epithelial foot processes usually are extensively effaced.

Differential Diagnosis. The light microscopic appearance of collagenofibrotic glomerulopathy often resembles membranoproliferative glomerulonephritis, however, the distinctive findings by electron microscopy readily distinguish the two processes. The major differential diagnostic consideration based on the ultrastructural findings is autosomal dominant nail-patella syndrome, in which glomerular deposits of curved fragments of banded collagen also occur (50). In nail-patella syndrome, the abnormal fibers are sparsely located primarily in the lamina densa of the glomerular basement membrane, whereas in collagenofibrotic glomerulopathy, the fibers are massively deposited primarily in the subendothelial zone and mesangium (52).

Etiology and Pathogenesis. Studies indicate that collagenofibrotic glomerulopathy is a familial autosomal recessive disease (57). Increased levels of circulating procollagen III peptides (51, 52,55,57) are found in patients with collagenofibrotic glomerulopathy. This raises the possibility that the abnormal synthesis of type III collagen may be occurring outside the kidney, with secondary accumulation of procollagen molecules in the kidney and in situ assembly into type III collagen fibers. Alternatively, the type III collagen may be synthesized by endogenous glomerular cells, such as endothelial cells and mesangial cells (56).

Treatment and Prognosis. The usual course is one of progressive renal failure. There is no specific treatment.

REFERENCES

Amyloidosis

1. Bellotti V, Mangione P, Merlini G. Review: immunoglobulin light chain amyloidosis—the archetype of structural and pathogenic variability. J Struct Biol 2000;130:280–9.
2. Comenzo RL, Zhang Y, Martinez C, Osman K, Herrera GA. The tropism of organ involvement in primary systemic amyloidosis: contributions of Ig V(L) germ line gene use and clonal plasma cell burden. Blood 2001;98:714–20.
3. Eulitz M, Weiss DT, Solomon A. Immunoglobulin heavy-chain-associated amyloidosis. Proc Natl Acad Sci U S A 1990;87:6542–6.
4. Gertz MA, Lacy MQ, Dispenzieri A. Immunoglobulin light chain amyloidosis and the kidney. Kidney Int 2002;61:1–9.
5. Gillmore JD, Hawkins PN, Pepys MB. Amyloidosis: a review of recent diagnostic and therapeutic developments. Br J Haematol 1997;99: 245–56.
6. Hartmann A, Holdaas H, Fauchald P, et al. Fifteen years' experience with renal transplantation in systemic amyloidosis. Transpl Int 1992;5:15–8.
7. Herrera GA. Renal manifestations of plasma cell dyscrasias: an appraisal from the patients' bedside to the research laboratory. Ann Diagn Pathol 2000;4:174–200.
8. Herrera GA, Russell WJ, Isaac J, et al. Glomerulopathic light chain-mesangial cell interactions modulate in vitro extracellular matrix remodeling and reproduce mesangiopathic findings documented in vivo. Ultrastruct Pathol 1999;23: 107–26.
9. Herrera GA, Sanders PW, Reddy BV, Hasbargen JA, Hammond WS, Brooke JD. Ultrastructural immunolabeling: a unique diagnostic tool in monoclonal light chain-related renal diseases. Ultrastruct Pathol 1994;18:401–16.
10. Hurle MR, Helms LR, Li L, Chan W, Wetzel R. A role for destabilizing amino acid replacements in light-chain amyloidosis. Proc Natl Acad Sci U S A 1994;91:5446–50.
11. Jao W, Pirani CL. Renal amyloidosis: electron microscopic observations. Acta Pathol Microbiol Scand [A] 1972;233:217–27.

12. Jones BA, Shapiro HS, Rosenberg BF, Bernstein J. Minimal renal amyloidosis with nephrotic syndrome. Arch Pathol Lab Med 1986;110:889–92.
13. Orbach H, Ben-Chetrit E. Familial Mediterranean fever—a review and update. Minerva Medica 2001;92:421–30.
14. Pasternack A, Ahonen J, Kuhlback B. Renal transplantation in 45 patients with amyloidosis. Transplantation 1986;42:598–601.
15. Schwartz MM. The dysproteinemias and amyloidosis. In: Jennette JC, Olson JL, Schwartz MM, Silva FG, eds. Heptinstall's pathology of the kidney, 5th ed. Philadelphia: Lippincott-Raven; 1998:1321–69.
16. Shirahama T, Cohen AS. Fine structure of the glomerulus in human and experimental renal amyloidosis. Am J Pathol 1967;51:869–911.
17. Solomon A, Weiss DT, Kattine AA. Nephrotoxic potential of Bence Jones proteins. N Engl J Med 1991;324:1845–51.
18. Solomon A, Weiss DT, Murphy C. Primary amyloidosis associated with a novel heavy-chain fragment (AH amyloidosis). Am J Hematol 1994;45:171–6.
19. Watanabe T, Saniter T. Morphological and clinical features of renal amyloidosis. Virchows Arch A Pathol Anat Histol 1975;366:125–35.

Monoclonal Immunoglobulin Deposition Disease

20. Cheng IK, Ho SK, Chan DT, Ng WK, Chan KW. Crescentic nodular glomerulosclerosis secondary to truncated immunoglobulin alpha heavy chain deposition. Am J Kidney Dis 1996;28:283–8.
20a. Herrera GA. Renal manifestations of plasma cell dyscrasias: an appraisal from the patients' bedside to the research laboratory. Ann Diagn Pathol 2000;4:174–200.
20b. Herrera GA, Russell WJ, Isaac J, et al. Glomerulopathic light chain-mesangial cell interactions modulate in vitro extracellular matrix remodeling and reproduce mesangiopathic findings documented in vivo. Ultrastruct Pathol 1999;23:107–26.
21. Kambham N, Markowitz GS, Appel GB, Kleiner MJ, Aucouturier P, D'Agati VD. Heavy chain deposition disease: the disease spectrum. Am J Kidney Dis 1999;33:954–62.
22. Lin J, Markowitz GS, Valeri AM, et al. Renal monoclonal immunoglobulin deposition disease: the disease spectrum. J Am Soc Nephrol 2001;12:1482–92.
23. Ronco PM, Alyanakian MA, Mougenot B, Aucouturier P. Light chain deposition disease: a model of glomerulosclerosis defined at the molecular level. J Am Soc Nephrol 2001;12:1558–65.
23a. Schwartz MM. The dysproteinemias and amyloidosis. In: Jennette JC, Olson JL, Schwartz MM, Silva FG, eds. Heptinstall's pathology of the kidney, 5th ed. Philadelphia: Lippincott-Raven; 1998:1321–69.
24. Strom EH, Fogazzi GB, Banfi G, Pozzi C, Mihatsch MJ. Light chain deposition disease of the kidney. Morphological aspects in 24 patients. Virchows Arch 1994;425:271–80.

Fibrillary and Immunotactoid Glomerulopathies

25. Adey DB, MacPherson BR, Groggel GC. Glomerulonephritis with associated hypocomplementemia and crescents: an unusual case of fibrillary glomerulonephritis. J Am Soc Nephrol 1995;6:171–6.
26. Alpers CE. Glomerulopathies of dysproteinemias, abnormal immunoglobulin deposition, and lymphoproliferative disorders. Curr Opin Nephrol Hypertens 1994;3:349–55.
27. Alpers CE. Immunotactoid (microtubular) glomerulopathy: an entity distinct from fibrillary glomerulonephritis? Am J Kidney Dis 1992;19:185–91.
28. Alpers CE, Rennke HG, Hopper J Jr, Biava CG. Fibrillary glomerulonephritis: an entity with unusual immunofluorescence features. Kidney Int 1987;31:781–9.
29. Brady HR. Fibrillary glomerulopathy. Kidney Int 1998;53:1421–29.
30. Chan TM, Chan KW. Fibrillary glomerulonephritis in siblings. Am J Kidney Dis 1998;31:E4.
31. Churg J, Venkataseshan VS. Fibrillary glomerulonephritis without immunoglobulin deposits in the kidney. Kidney Int 1993;44:837–42.
32. Duffy JL, Khurana E, Susin M, Gomez-Leon G, Churg J. Fibrillary renal deposits and nephritis. Am J Pathol 1983;113:279–90.
33. Fogo A, Qureshi N, Horn RG. Morphologic and clinical features of fibrillary glomerulonephritis versus immunotactoid glomerulopathy. Am J Kidney Dis 1993;22:367–77.
34. Grove P, Neale PH, Peck M, Schiller B, Haas M. Monoclonal immunoglobulin G1-kappa fibrillary glomerulonephritis. Mod Pathol 1998;11:103–9.
35. Iskandar SS, Falk RJ, Jennette JC. Clinical and pathologic features of fibrillary glomerulonephritis. Kidney Int 1992;42:1401–7.
36. Jennette JC, Iskandar SS, Falk RJ. Fibrillary glomerulonephritis. In: Tisher CC, Brenner BM, eds. Renal pathology with clinical and functional correlations, 2nd ed. Philadelphia: J.B. Lippincott Co.; 1994:553–63.
37. Korbet SM, Schwartz MM, Lewis EJ. The fibrillary glomerulopathies. Am J Kidney Dis 1994;23:751–65.

38. Kronz JD, Neu AM, Nadasdy T. When noncongophilic glomerular fibrils do not represent fibrillary glomerulonephritis: nonspecific mesangial fibrils in sclerosing glomeruli. Clin Nephrol 1998;50:218–23.
39. Markowitz GS, Cheng JT, Colvin RB, Trebbin WM, D'Agati VD. Hepatitis C viral infection is associated with fibrillary glomerulonephritis and immunotactoid glomerulopathy. J Am Soc Nephrol 1998;9:2244–52.
40. Pronovost PH, Brady HR, Gunning ME, Espinoza O, Rennke HG. Clinical features, predictors of disease progression and results of renal transplantation in fibrillary/immunotactoid glomerulopathy. Nephrol Dial Transplant 1996;11:837–42.
41. Samaniego M, Nadasdy GM, Laszik Z, Nadasdy T. Outcome of renal transplantation in fibrillary glomerulonephritis. Clin Nephrol 2001;55:159–66.
42. Schwartz MM. Glomerular diseases with organized deposits. In: Jennette JC, Olson JL, Schwartz MM, Silva FG, eds. Heptinstall's pathology of the kidney, 5th ed. Philadelphia: Lippincott-Raven; 1998:369–88.
43. Schwartz MM. Renal amyloidosis and other fibrillar glomerular diseases. Curr Opin Nephrol Hypertens 1993;2:238–45.
44. Strom EH, Banfi G, Krapf R, et al. Glomerulopathy associated with predominant fibronectin deposits: a newly recognized hereditary disease. Kidney Int 1995;48:163–70.

Fibronectin Glomerulopathy

45. Assmann KJ, Koene RA, Wetzels JF. Familial glomerulonephritis characterized by massive deposits of fibronectin. Am J Kidney Dis 1995;25:781–91.
46. Gemperle O, Neuweiler J, Reutter FW, Hildebrandt F, Krapf R. Familial glomerulopathy with giant fibrillar (fibronectin-positive) deposits: 15-year follow-up in a large kindred. Am J Kidney Dis 1996;28:668–75.
47. Gibson IW, More IA. Glomerular pathology: recent advances. J Pathol 1998;184:123–9.
48. Hildebrandt F, Strahm B, Prochoroff A, et al. Glomerulopathy associated with predominant fibronectin deposits: exclusion of the genes for fibronectin, villin and desmin as causative genes. Am J Med Genet 1996;63:323–7.
49. Mazzucco G, Maran E, Rollino C, Monga G. Glomerulonephritis with organized deposits: a mesangiopathic, not immune complex-mediated disease? A pathologic study of two cases in the same family. Hum Pathol 1992;23:63–8.

Collagenofibrotic Glomerulopathy

50. Gubler MC, Dommergues JP, Foulard M, et al. Collagen type III glomerulopathy: a new type of hereditary nephropathy. Pediatr Nephrol 1993;7:354–60.
51. Hisakawa N, Yasuoka N, Nishiya K, et al. Collagenofibrotic glomerulonephropathy associated with immune complex deposits. Am J Nephrol 1998;18:134–41.
52. Ikeda K, Yokoyama H, Tomosugi N, Kida H, Ooshima A, Kobayashi K. Primary glomerular fibrosis: a new nephropathy caused by diffuse intraglomerular increase in atypical type III collagen fibers. Clin Nephrol 1990;33:155–9.
53. Imbasciati E, Gherardi G, Morozumi K, et al. Collagen type III glomerulopathy: a new idiopathic glomerular disease. Am J Nephrol 1991;11:422–29.
54. Komatsuda A, Imai H, Yasuda T. [Collagenofibrotic glomerulonephropathy, collagen deposition disease.] Ryoikibetsu Shokogun Shirizu 1997;16(Pt. 1):140–3.
55. Mizuiri S, Hasegawa A, Kikuchi A, Amagasaki Y, Nakamura N, Sakaguchi H. A case of collagenofibrotic glomerulopathy associated with hepatic perisinusoidal fibrosis. Nephron 1993;63:183–7.
56. Naruse K, Ito H, Moriki T, et al. Mesangial cell activation in the collagenofibrotic glomerulonephropathy. Case report and review of the literature. Virchows Arch 1998;433:183–8.
57. Tamura H, Matsuda A, Kidoguchi N, Matsumura O, Mitarai T, Isoda K. A family with two sisters with collagenofibrotic glomerulonephropathy. Am J Kidney Dis 1996;27:588–95.
58. Vogt BA, Wyatt RJ, Burke BA, Simonton SC, Kashtan CE. Inherited factor H deficiency and collagen type III glomerulopathy. Pediatr Nephrol 1995;9:11–5.
59. Yasuda T, Imai H, Nakamoto Y, et al. Collagenofibrotic glomerulopathy: a systemic disease. Am J Kidney Dis 1999;33:123–7.

10 MEMBRANOPROLIFERATIVE GLOMERULONEPHRITIS

Membranoproliferative glomerulonephritis (MPGN) is a morphologic entity that is defined primarily at the light microscopic level (7,19). The membranoproliferative pattern of injury is characterized by mesangial proliferation and thickening of the glomerular capillary walls due to mesangial interposition and double contours of the glomerular basement membrane. In most cases, these glomerular changes occur in response to immune deposition in the glomerular capillary walls. Although the process tends to be diffuse and global in distribution, each of the morphologic features described above may vary in severity from glomerulus to glomerulus, or even in adjacent lobules of individual glomeruli. Because MPGN manifests mesangial proliferation and extension of cells into the peripheral capillaries, thereby causing accentuation of the glomerular lobularity, the terms *mesangiocapillary glomerulonephritis* and *lobular glomerulonephritis* have been used synonymously.

The membranoproliferative pattern of glomerular injury is nonspecific, occurring in either primary (idiopathic) forms or secondary forms related to a variety of underlying conditions and systemic processes (35). The primary forms are in turn subdivided into three major types based on their combined light microscopic, immunofluorescence, and ultrastructural appearance (outlined in Table 10-1). The secondary conditions are actually more common than the primary forms and include a variety of autoimmune, infectious, neoplastic, and thrombotic disorders (listed in Table 10-2). Differentiation of primary from secondary MPGN requires careful integration of the clinical and renal histologic, immunofluorescence, and electron microscopic findings. Most cases of MPGN occurring

Table 10-1

SUBTYPES OF PRIMARY MEMBRANOPROLIFERATIVE GLOMERULONEPHRITIS

Type	LM[a]	IF	EM Deposits
1 Mesangiocapillary	Diffuse and uniform mesangial proliferation and sclerosis, mesangial interposition, double contours	IgG and C3 or C3 alone, +/–IgM, IgA, C1, mesangial and subendothelial	Mesangial, subendothelial
2 Dense deposit disease	Mild and variable mesangial proliferation and sclerosis, GBM[b] thickening (silver positive or negative), rare mesangial interposition and double contours	C3 only, linear GCW, mesangial rings	Intramembranous dense deposits, mesangial nodular deposits
3 Burkholder subtype (MPGN1 and MGN)[c]	Diffuse and uniform mesangial proliferation and sclerosis, mesangial interposition, double contours, spikes	IgG and C3 or C3 alone, +/– IgM, IgA, C1, mesangial, subendothelial, and subepithelial	Mesangial, subendothelial, subepithelial
3 Strife and Anders subtype (complex intramembranous deposits	Diffuse and uniform mesangial proliferation and sclerosis, marked GBM thickening (silver negative), variable mesangial interposition and double contours	IgG and C3 or C3 alone, +/– IgM, IgA, C1, mesangial and transmembranous	Mesangial, intramembranous, +/– subendothelial, +/– subepithelial

[a]LM = light microscopy; IF = immunofluorescence microscopy; EM = electron microscopy.
[b]GBM = glomerular basement membrane; Ig = immunoglobulin; C = complement; GCW = glomerular capillary wall.
[c]MPGN = membranoproliferative glomerulonephritis; MGN = membranous glomerulonephritis.

Table 10-2

CAUSES OF SECONDARY MEMBRANOPROLIFERATIVE GLOMERULONEPHRITIS

With Immune Deposits
Infections
Cryoglobulinemia (predominantly type 2, also type 3)
Hepatitis B
Hepatitis C
Endocarditis
Visceral abscesses
Infected ventriculoatrial shunts
Malaria
Schistosomiasis
Mycoplasma
Ebstein-Barr virus
Human immunodeficiency virus (HIV)
Autoimmune Diseases
Systemic lupus erythematosus
Mixed connective tissue disease
Rheumatoid arthritis
Sjögren's syndrome
Dysproteinemias
Cryoglobulinemia (types 1 or 2)
Light chain deposition disease (LCDD)
Light and heavy chain deposition disease (LHCDD)
Heavy chain deposition disease (HCDD)
Waldenström's macroglobulinemia
Fibrillary glomerulonephritis
Immunotactoid glomerulonephritis
Without Immune Deposits
Chronic Liver Disease
Cirrhosis
Alpha-1-antitrypsin deficiency
Thrombotic Microangiopathy
Hemolytic uremic syndrome
Thrombotic thrombocytopenic purpura
Antiphospholipid antibody syndrome
Radiation nephritis
Sickle cell anemia
Transplant glomerulopathy
Systemic sclerosis

in children are primary, while secondary forms predominate in adults.

PRIMARY MPGN (TYPES 1, 2, AND 3)

Definition. Primary (idiopathic) MPGN is a glomerulonephritis with a membranoproliferative pattern for which there is no known underlying cause or disease association. It is subdivided into three clinical-pathologic entities, designated MPGN types 1 to 3.

Clinical Features. Primary MPGN is most common in older children, adolescents, and young adults (ages 7 to 30 years). Rarely does the disease occur in children as young as age 2 or in adults over the age of 50 years (18). The disease occurs with equal prevalence in males and females. There is a white racial predominance.

The most common form of primary MPGN is type 1. Type 2 is extremely rare, comprising less than 5 percent of all cases of primary MPGN. The incidence of type 3 varies with the pathologic definition. Most series suggest it is far less common than type 1, but more common than type 2.

Patients with primary MPGN often present with mixed nephrotic and nephritic syndromes. In roughly two thirds of patients, nephrotic manifestations (heavy proteinuria, hypoalbuminemia, hyperlipidemia, and edema) predominate. Other presentations include acute nephritic syndrome, subnephrotic proteinuria with stable or slowly progressive renal insufficiency, recurrent episodes of gross hematuria, or asymptomatic hematuria with erythrocyte casts. An upper respiratory tract infection commonly precedes the first clinical recognition of renal disease. In some patients, there is a documented preceding streptococcal pharyngitis with elevated antistreptolysin-O (ASLO) titers. These patients usually present with acute nephritic syndrome and hypocomplementemia that mimics acute poststreptococcal glomerulonephritis. The failure of the hematuria, proteinuria, and hypocomplementemia to resolve within 6 weeks is an ominous clue that the disease may represent MPGN, which must then be confirmed by renal biopsy. Primary MPGN type 1 usually has a chronic, slowly progressive course that may be punctuated by periods of remission or exacerbation. Over time, the clinical features evolve from an initially nephritic presentation to a predominantly nephrotic picture.

The major serologic finding in all three forms of primary MPGN is hypocomplementemia (43). In fact, the designation "hypocomplementemic glomerulonephritis" was commonly applied in the past. Hypocomplementemia is identified in about 80 percent of cases of MPGN type 1, nearly 100 percent of cases of type 2, and about 50 percent of cases of type 3. Although there is considerable overlap, the patterns of complement activation tend to differ in the three subtypes.

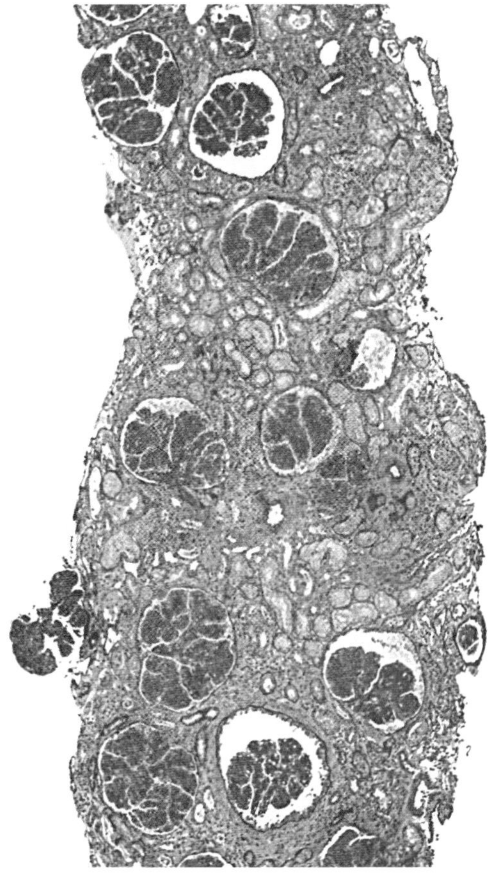

Figure 10-1

MEMBRANOPROLIFERATIVE GLOMERULONEPHRITIS (MPGN) TYPE 1

Low-power view shows the uniform diffuse and global glomerular hypercellularity affecting all glomeruli (periodic acid–Schiff [PAS] stain).

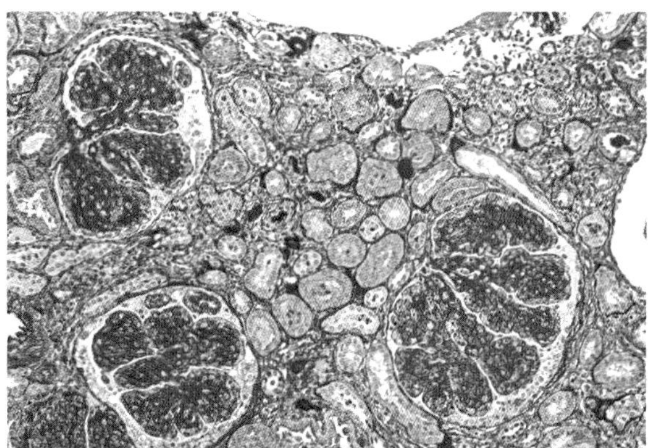

Figure 10-2

MPGN TYPE 1

There is prominent lobular accentuation of the glomerular tuft due to expansion of the endocapillary zones by cells and matrix, producing a floral pattern (Jones methenamine silver [JMS] stain).

In type 1, serum complement (C)3 and total hemolytic complement (CH) 50 levels are reduced in up to half of patients; concentrations of C1q, C4, properdin, and factor B are borderline or reduced in less than half of patients. These findings are consistent with the hypothesis that there is both classic complement pathway activation by immune complexes, as well as alternative complement pathway activation. Inherited complement deficiencies (including C2, C3, C6, C7, and C8) are also common in MPGN type 1 and may influence the levels of individual complement components. There is also evidence that reduced hepatic synthesis of complement may contribute to the complement deficiencies in types 1 and 3 MPGN.

In type 2 MPGN, there is persistent and often profound depression of C3, with normal levels of early complement components C1q and C4. This reduced C3 is linked to the presence of C3 nephritic factor. C3 nephritic factor is an autoantibody directed to C3bBb, the C3 convertase of the alternative pathway. Once bound to C3bBb, this autoantibody stabilizes the convertase and maintains it in an active state by preventing the action of C3b inactivator. Although C3 nephritic factor is most common in type 2 MPGN, it has also been identified in about a quarter of patients with type 1 disease (43).

Type 3 MPGN is typically associated with reduced C3 levels, normal C4 levels, and the absence of C3 nephritic factor. The presence of reduced C5, C6, C7, and C9 levels in some patients with type 3 disease has been linked to a separate terminal pathway nephritic factor that activates complement more distally in the complement cascade.

MPGN Type 1: Pathologic Features. *Light Microscopic Findings*. There are pathologic alterations of both the mesangium and the peripheral glomerular capillary walls (18). The changes tend to be diffuse and global, but may be more focal and segmental in mild cases (fig. 10-1). At low-power, the glomeruli often display accentuated lobularity (fig. 10-2).

Mesangial changes include expansion due to an increased number of mesangial cells and

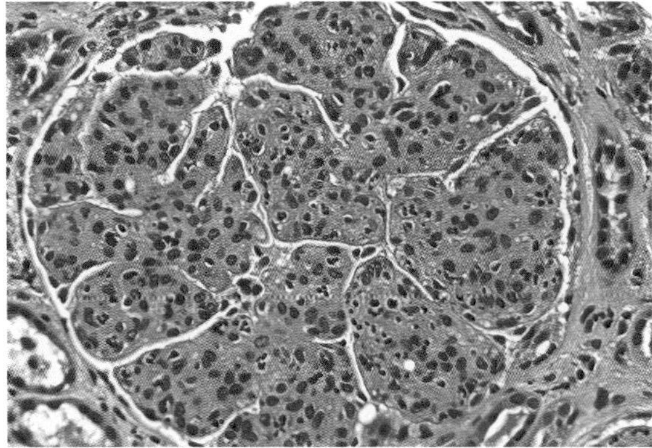

Figure 10-3

MPGN TYPE 1

The glomerular capillary lumens are narrowed or occluded by the proliferation of mesangial and endothelial cells, with numerous infiltrating leukocytes (hematoxylin and eosin [H&E] stain).

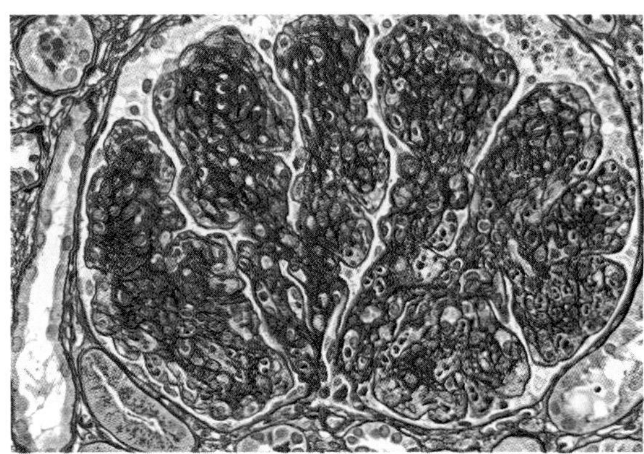

Figure 10-4

MPGN TYPE 1

High-power microscopy shows the severe expansion of the mesangial areas by mesangial cells and matrix, which encroach on the capillary lumens (JMS stain).

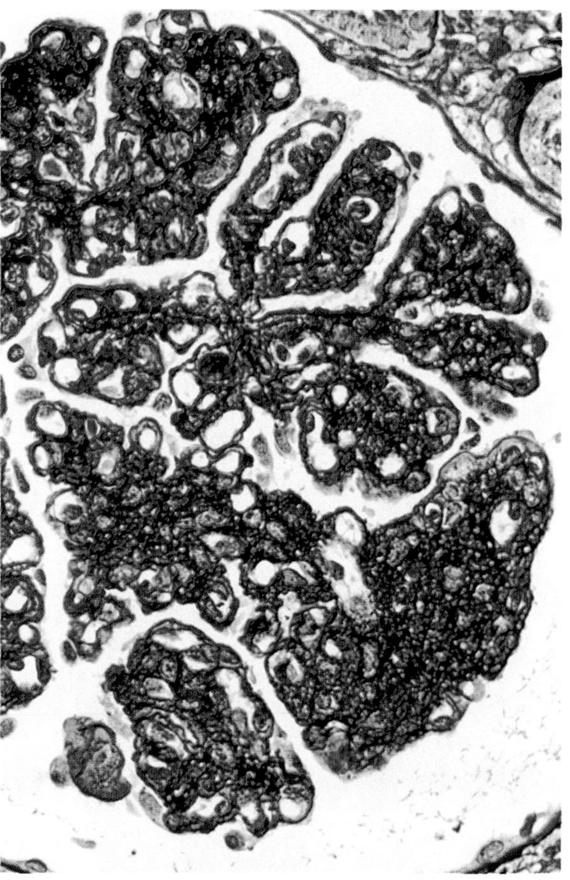

Figure 10-5

MPGN TYPE 1

Only modest mesangial hypercellularity is present. Glomerular capillary lumens are patent but narrowed by double contours enclosing silver-negative subendothelial deposits (JMS stain).

amount of matrix accompanied by mesangial immune deposits (figs. 10-3, 10-4). The extent of these mesangial changes varies widely from case to case, but tends to be relatively uniform from glomerulus to glomerulus (fig. 10-5). Where pronounced, the mesangial expansion may assume a nodular appearance (fig. 10-6). Mesangial hypercellularity typically gives way to increasing mesangial sclerosis as the disease progresses. The presence of mesangial immune deposits may impart a glassy, hypereosinophilic, strongly periodic acid–Schiff (PAS)-positive appearance to the glomerular mesangium. In some cases, the glomerular mesangium contains worm-like eosinophilic material corresponding to immune aggregates (fig. 10-7).

The glomerular capillary walls are thickened by varying degrees of mesangial interposition and duplication of glomerular basement membrane (figs. 10-8, 10-9). Mesangial interposition refers to the migration of mesangial cells into the peripheral glomerular capillary walls by insinuating themselves between the glomerular endothelium and the glomerular basement membrane. Mesangial interposition is described as circumferential if it involves the entire circumference of an individual capillary, or partial if only

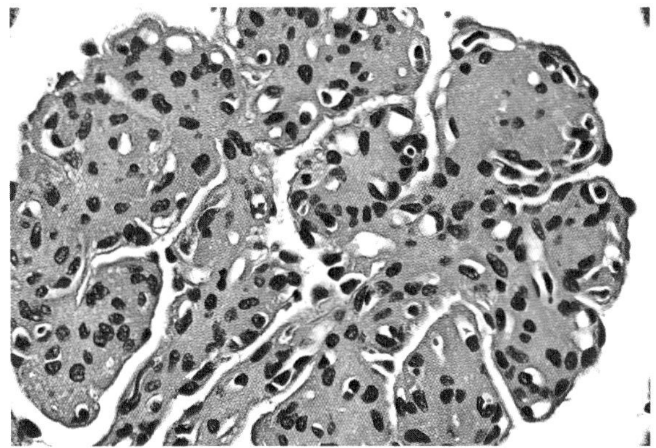

Figure 10-6

MPGN TYPE 1

Some mesangial areas display nodular mesangial sclerosis (H&E stain).

a segment of the peripheral capillary wall is involved. Once mesangial cells become located in the peripheral capillaries, they synthesize new basement membrane material, producing a double contour (or "tram-track") of the glomerular capillary wall. This new layer of basement membrane material is produced internal to the original glomerular basement membrane, just beneath the glomerular endothelium. Double contours are best delineated with the Jones methenamine silver (JMS) stain. They can usually be recognized with the PAS and trichrome stains, but may not be evident in hematoxylin and eosin (H&E)-stained preparations. Between the double layers of the glomerular basement membrane are subendothelial immune deposits that may be large enough to be identified by light microscopy. These subendothelial deposits appear strongly PAS positive, fuchsinophilic with the trichrome stain, and nonargyrophilic with the JMS stain (fig. 10-10).

In some cases, neutrophils and monocytes contribute to the glomerular hypercellularity. In fact, the exudative component can be so severe that it mimics acute postinfectious glomerulonephritis (fig. 10-11). Crescents are present in some cases (fig. 10-12).

The tubulointerstitial and vascular changes are nonspecific. Varying degrees of tubular atrophy, interstitial fibrosis, edema, and inflammation may be present. In cases with heavy proteinuria, there are frequently intracytoplasmic

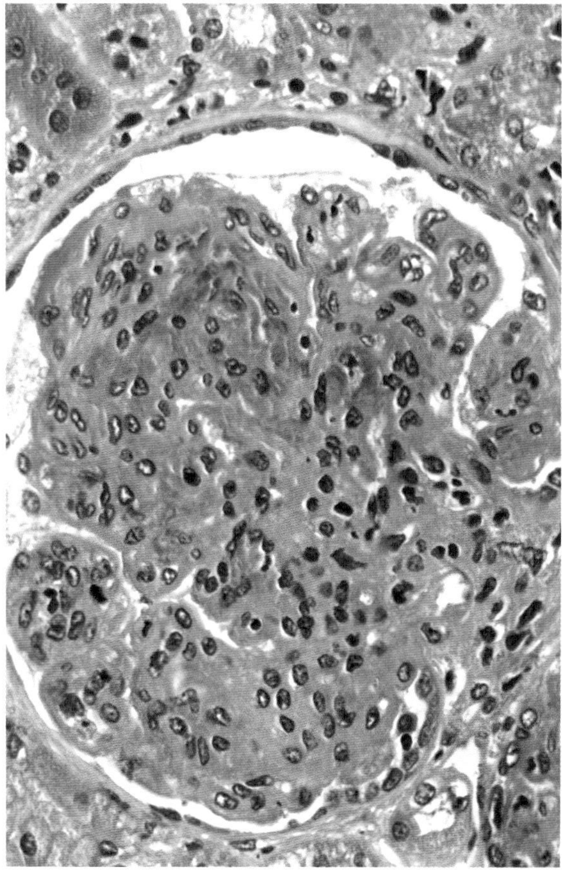

Figure 10-7

MPGN TYPE 1

Vermiform hypereosinophilic deposits are identified in the mesangial areas (H&E stain).

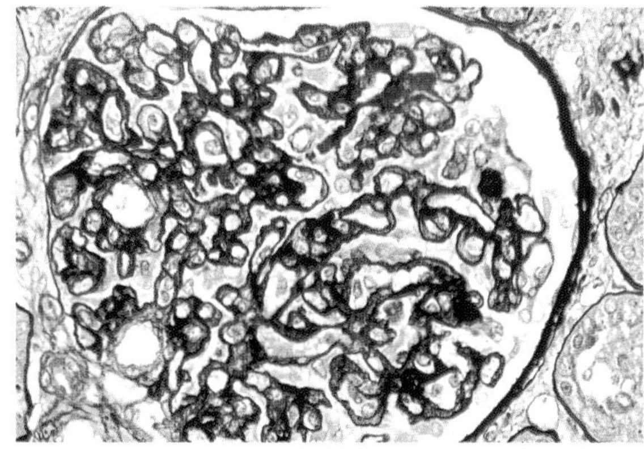

Figure 10-8

MPGN TYPE 1

Relatively mild hypercellularity, but extensive double contours and mesangial interposition, in a patient with hepatitis B infection (JMS stain).

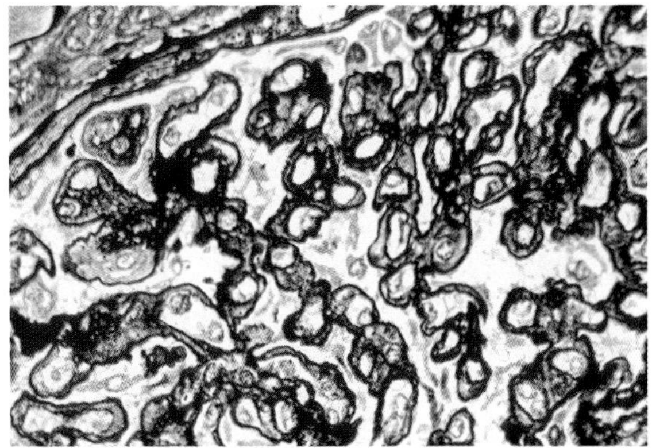

Figure 10-9

MPGN TYPE 1

This high-power microscopic view of the glomerular capillaries illustrates the regular double contours with intervening subendothelial deposits and interposed mesangial cells (JMS stain).

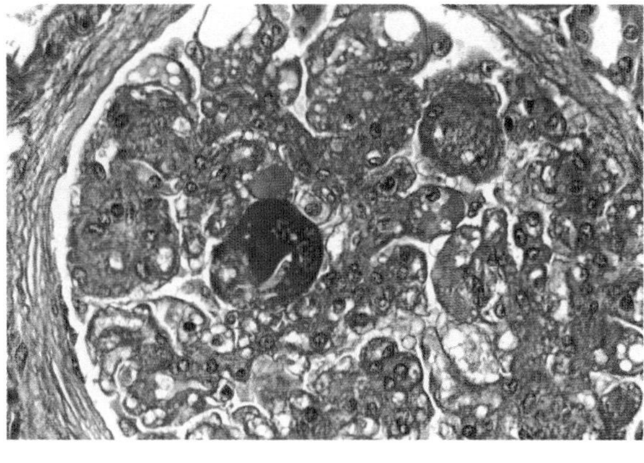

Figure 10-10

MPGN TYPE 1

A large subendothelial deposit stains red (fuchsinophilic) with the trichrome stain.

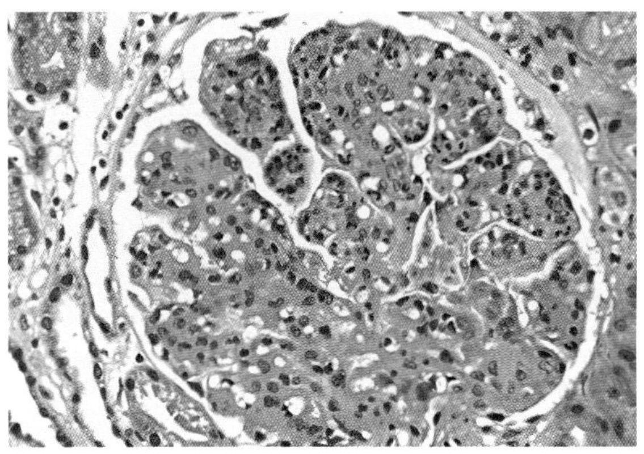

Figure 10-11

MPGN TYPE 1

There are numerous infiltrating neutrophils, resembling acute postinfectious glomerulonephritis (H&E stain).

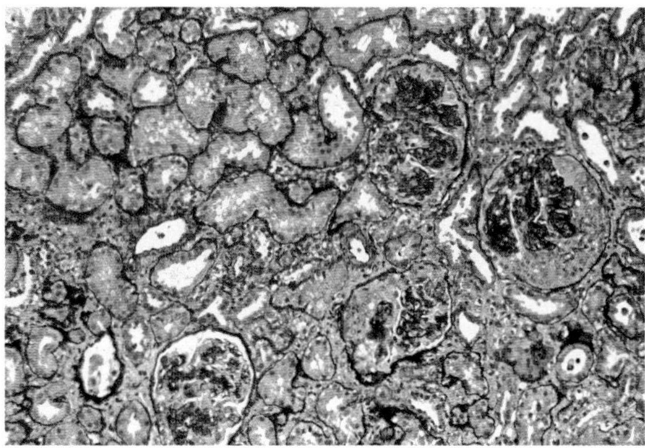

Figure 10-12

MPGN TYPE 1

Recurrent MPGN in the transplant shows numerous crescents, recapitulating the pattern of crescentic MPGN diagnosed in the native kidney 10 years before (JMS stain).

lipid and protein resorption droplets within the proximal tubular epithelial cells. Intersitial foam cells are common. There may be red blood cell casts (fig. 10-13).

Immunofluorescence Findings. The glomerular immune deposits are usually distributed in the mesangium and in the peripheral capillary walls, in a granular to semilinear subendothelial pattern that outlines the glomerular lobules. In some cases, the major deposition is in the peripheral capillary walls, whereas in other cases it is more abundant in the mesangium (figs. 10-14–10-16). A helpful clue that the peripheral capillary wall deposits are subendothelial comes from their smooth outer contour, owing to their conformation to the delimiting outer glomerular basement membrane. The glomerular deposits are usually composed of both immunoglobulins (predominantly IgG) and complement (predominantly C3). However, in a up to a quarter of cases, there may be staining for C3 only. Usually the intensity of the C3 staining is greater than that of IgG. Weaker and more variable positivity for IgM,

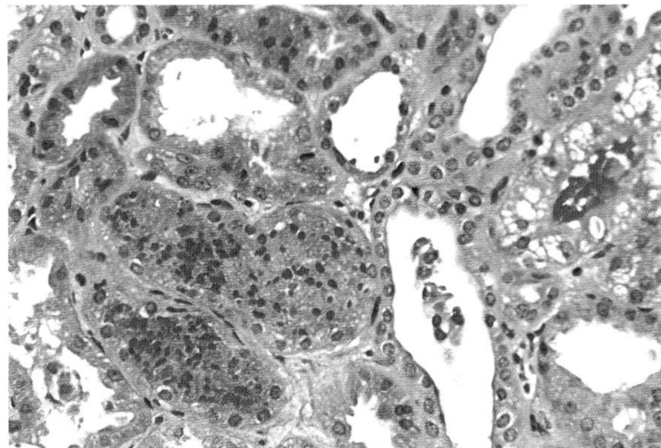

Figure 10-13

MPGN TYPE 1

There are scattered red blood cell casts, a morphologic correlate of the nephritic component. The intratubular clear lipid resorption droplets are a reflection of the nephrotic component, which causes hyperlipidemia and lipiduria (H&E stain).

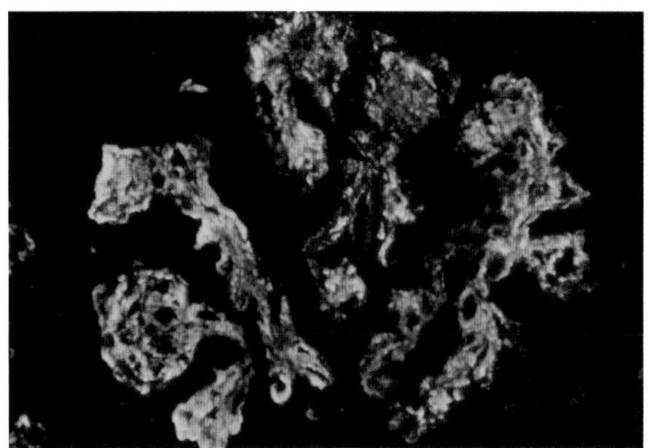

Figure 10-14

MPGN TYPE 1

Intense, predominantly mesangial deposition of C3, with less prominent involvement of the peripheral capillary walls (immunofluorescence micrograph).

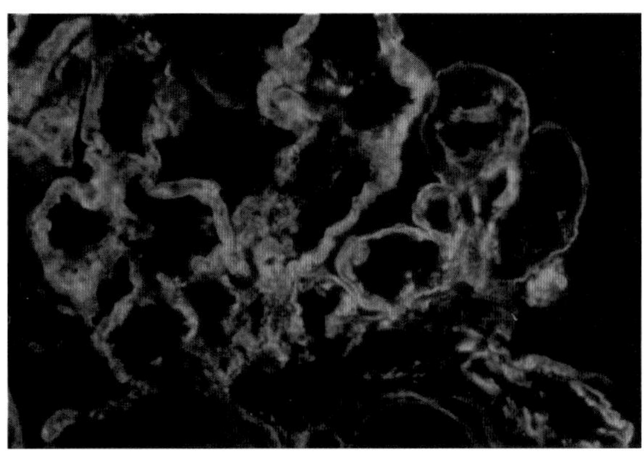

Figure 10-15

MPGN TYPE 1

Predominantly peripheral capillary wall deposits of IgG, in areas outlining the double contours, have a semilinear to granular texture (immunofluorescence micrograph).

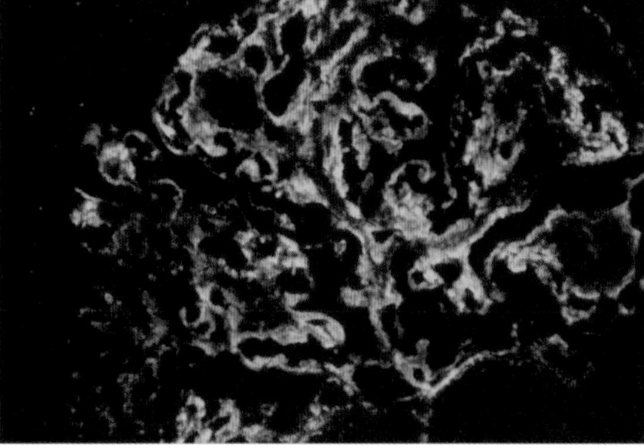

Figure 10-16

MPGN TYPE 1

Relatively intense deposits of C3 in both the mesangium and the peripheral capillary walls (immunofluorescence micrograph).

IgA, and C1q may be identified in some cases. Focal tubular basement membrane deposits of C3 with a granular or semilinear texture are seen in a few cases.

Electron Microscopic Findings. The mesangium is hypercellular, with variable amounts of electron-dense deposits. The extension of mesangial cells into the peripheral glomerular capillaries narrows the glomerular capillary lumens (fig. 10-17). In some cases, cells with the appearance of monocytes are interposed between the endothelial cells and the glomerular basement membrane (fig. 10-18). The double contours of glomerular basement membrane correspond to the original outer glomerular basement membrane and the newly formed inner neomembrane (fig. 10-19). This newly synthesized inner layer is typically more irregular in texture and contour than the original glomerular basement membrane. By electron microscopy, it is continuous with the subendothelial extension of the mesangial matrix into the peripheral capillary

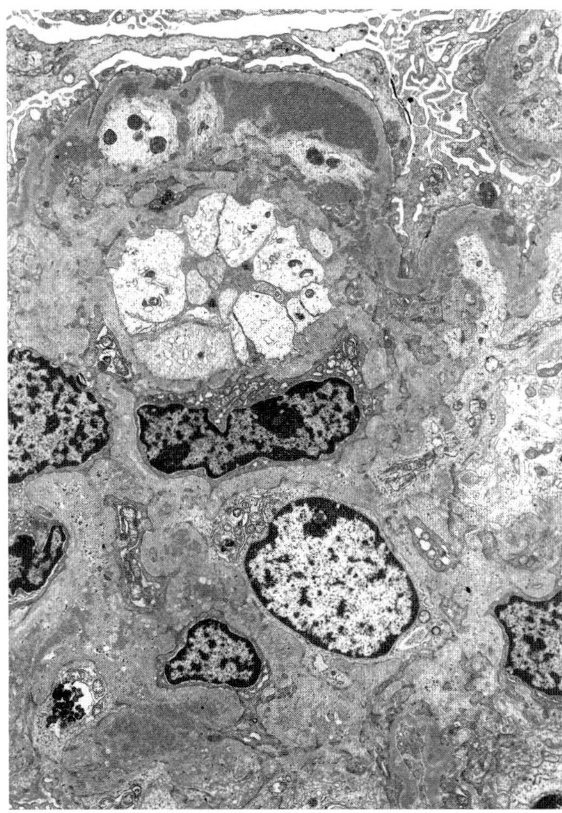

Figure 10-17

MPGN TYPE 1

The mesangium is expanded by increased cells and matrix containing electron-dense deposits. The glomerular capillary lumen is narrowed by circumferential mesangial interposition, double contoured glomerular basement membrane, and subendothelial electron-dense deposits. There is severe foot process effacement (electron micrograph).

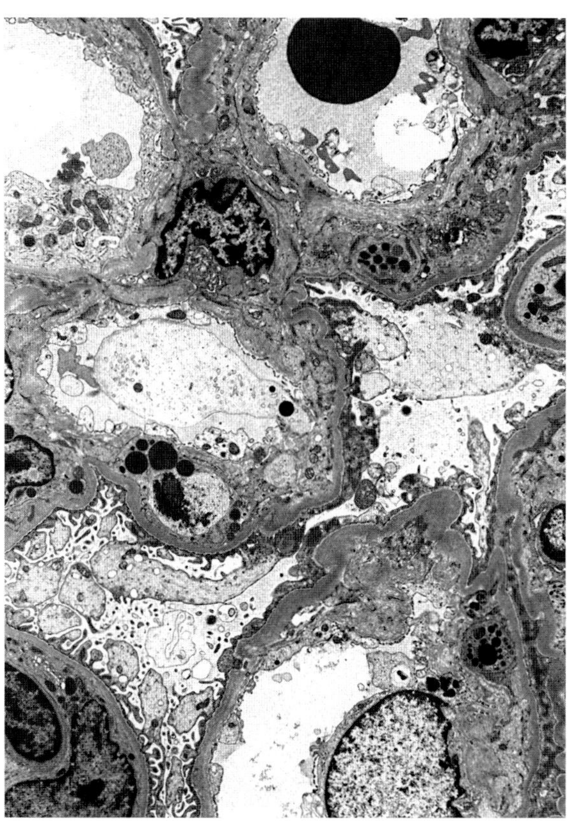

Figure 10-18

MPGN TYPE 1

Monocytes containing prominent phagolysosomes are located between the double contours. In this case, the subendothelial deposits are small and scant (electron micrograph).

walls. Between the layers of glomerular basement membrane, variable amounts of electron-dense deposits are seen (fig. 10-20). In some cases, the subendothelial deposits are sparse whereas in others they are abundant. Although occasional subepithelial electron-dense deposits may be seen in type 1, the presence of numerous, regularly distributed subepithelial deposits is best classified as MPGN type 3. There is usually extensive effacement of foot processes, accompanied by podocyte hypertrophy and focal microvillous transformation.

MPGN Type 2 (Dense Deposit Disease): Pathologic Features. *Light Microscopic Findings.* In MPGN type 2, the degree of mesangial hypercellularity is highly variable and less uniform than in type 1. In most cases, the mesangial hypercellularity is relatively mild, although it can be severe and accompanied by neutrophil infiltration (figs. 10-21–10-23). The double contours of the glomerular basement membrane are often less developed than in type 1 (fig. 10-24); in some cases, it is difficult to identify any double contours (fig. 10-25).

By light microscopy, the most distinctive feature is ribbon-like thickening of the glomerular basement membranes by intramembranous deposits that are typically highly eosinophilic and glassy in appearance (17). These intramembranous deposits are generally PAS positive and stain red with the trichrome stain (fig. 10-26). The intramembranous deposits usually fail to take the JMS stain well, producing a grayish black, brown, or pink reaction (fig. 10-27). The

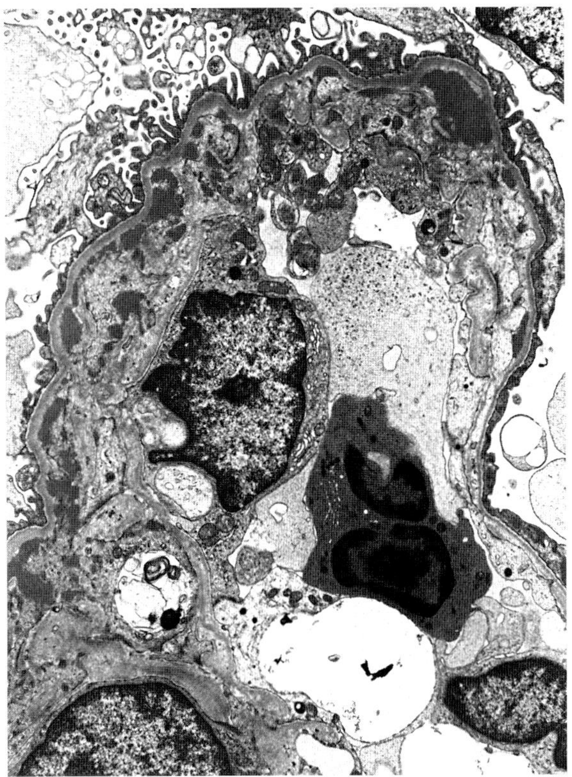

Figure 10-19

MPGN TYPE 1

The glomerular capillary lumen is narrowed by circumferential mesangial interposition associated with subendothelial electron-dense deposits and an irregular subendothelial layer of neomembrane. A neutrophil is present in the lumen (electron micrograph).

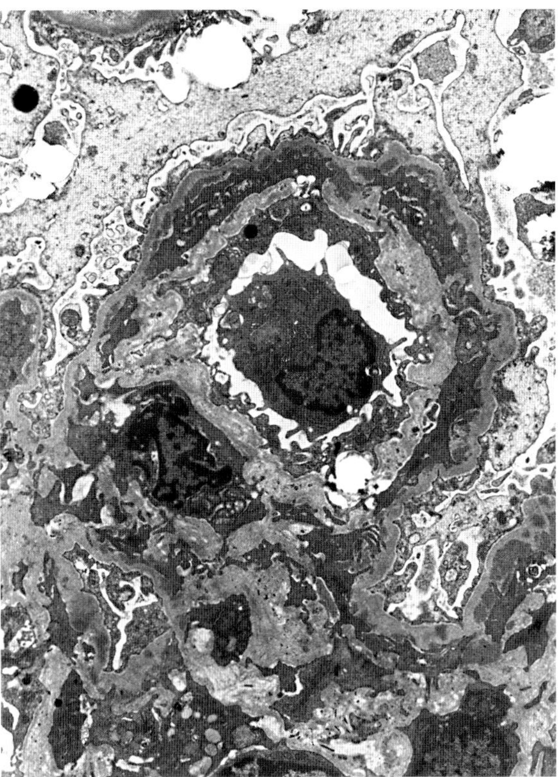

Figure 10-20

MPGN TYPE 1

There is circumferential mesangial interposition, a thick but irregular layer of neomembrane beneath the endothelium, and relatively small subendothelial electron-dense deposits. A monocyte is marginated in the glomerular capillary lumen (electron micrograph).

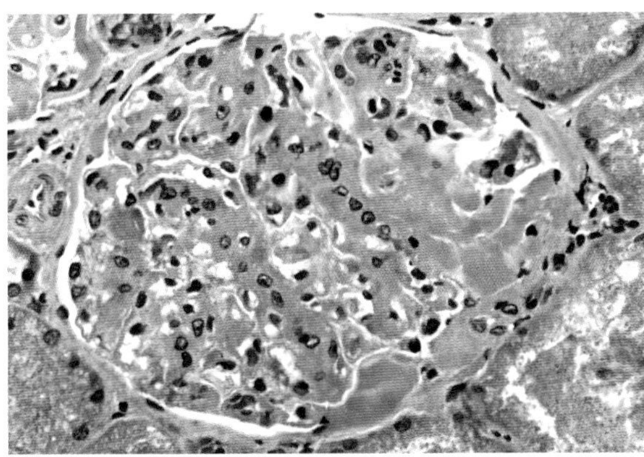

Figure 10-21

MPGN TYPE 2

The glomerulus displays only mild mesangial hypercellularity. Glassy eosinophilic material expands the mesangial matrix and irregularly thickens some glomerular capillary walls (H&E stain).

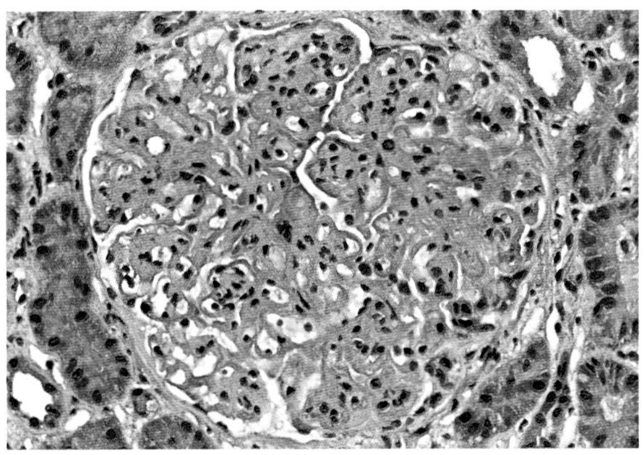

Figure 10-22

MPGN TYPE 2

Moderate mesangial hypercellularity and global ribbon-like thickening of the glomerular capillary walls are shown (H&E stain).

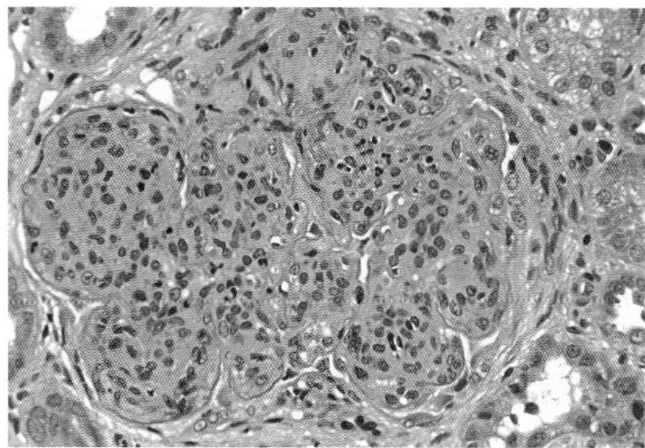

Figure 10-23

MPGN TYPE 2

A severe example with an exuberant mesangial proliferation that occludes most glomerular capillaries. The glomerular basement membranes have a hypereosinophilic appearance (H&E stain).

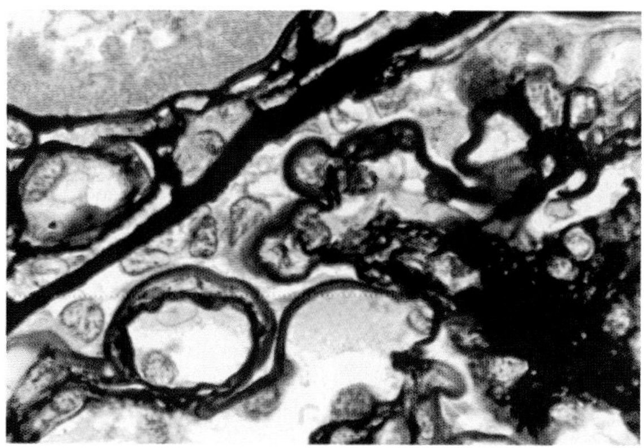

Figure 10-24

MPGN TYPE 2

The rare double contour stains brown with the JMS stain.

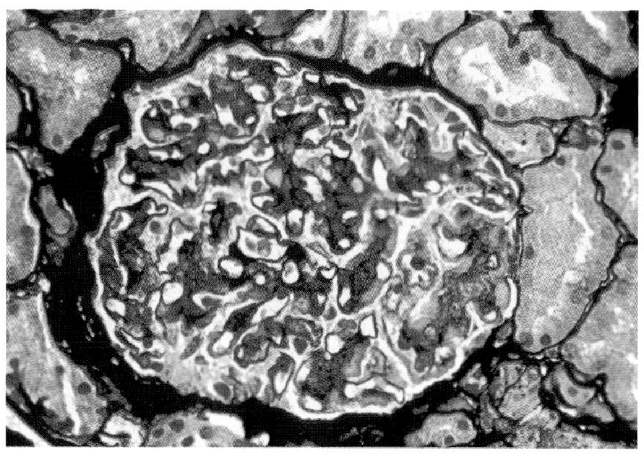

Figure 10-25

MPGN TYPE 2

Glomerular capillary walls are segmentally thickened by pink-staining material that fails to take the JMS stain.

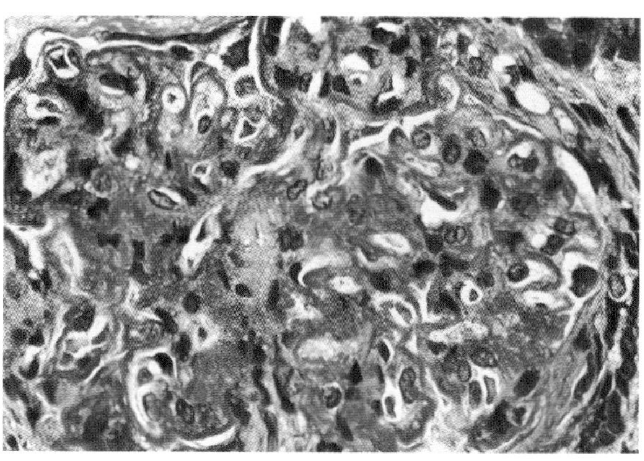

Figure 10-26

MPGN TYPE 2

The glomerular capillary walls and mesangium stain red with the trichrome stain, owing to the massive replacement by deposits.

deposits are also positive for the thioflavin T and alcian blue–PAS stains (figs. 10-28, 10-29). Similar band-like deposits thicken the basal lamina of Bowman's capsule and some tubular basement membranes (figs. 10-30, 10-31). These thickenings of the glomerular basement membrane, Bowman's capsule, and tubular basement membranes are often irregular, involving segments of the entire circumference of these structures. In the glomerular basement membranes, the relatively segmental fusiform thickening has been likened to a "sausage-string" appearance (19,37).

Some atypical cases have been described with focal segmental glomerular proliferation and necrosis. Crescents may be present.

Immunofluorescence Findings. The immunofluorescence appearance of MPGN type 2 is highly distinctive. In most cases there is positivity for C3 only, without associated immunoglobulins or C1q. The C3 staining is usually intense (2+ to 3+), involving the mesangium as well as the peripheral capillary walls, Bowman's capsule, and focal tubular basement membranes (figs. 10-32, 10-33). In the mesangium, C3

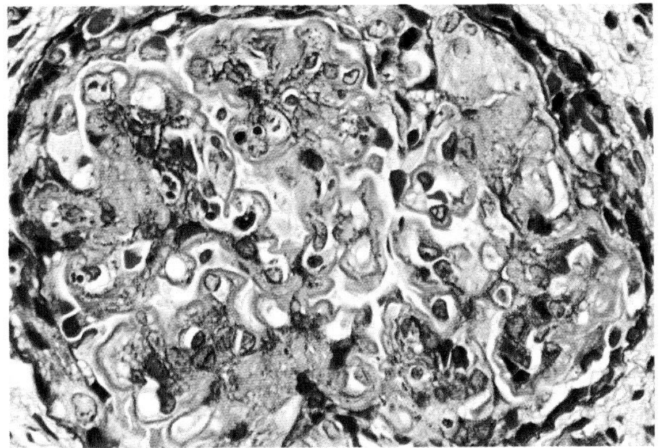

Figure 10-27

MPGN TYPE 2

The thickened glomerular capillary walls and mesangial matrix do not stain with the JMS stain, giving a pink reaction that contrasts with the argyrophilia of Bowman's capsule.

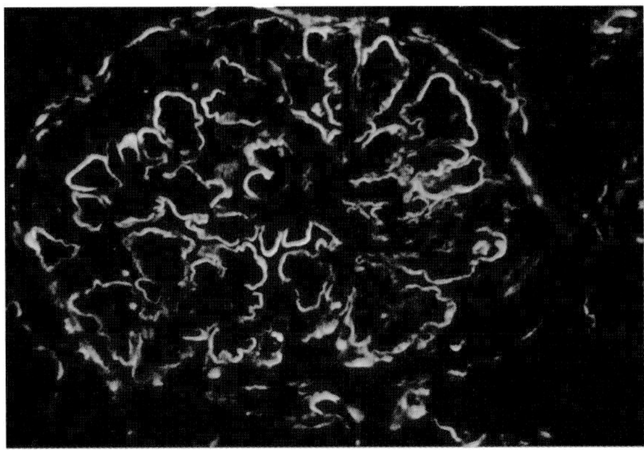

Figure 10-28

MPGN TYPE 2

Linear staining with thioflavin T involves the glomerular basement membranes and Bowman's capsule. (Courtesy of Dr. Jacob Churg, Paterson, NJ.)

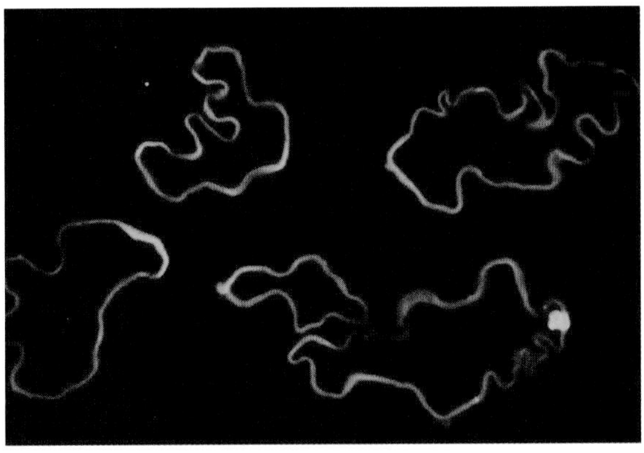

Figure 10-29

MPGN TYPE 2

Linear staining of the tubular basement membranes with thioflavin T viewed under immunofluorescence microscopy. (Courtesy of Dr. Jacob Churg, Paterson, NJ.)

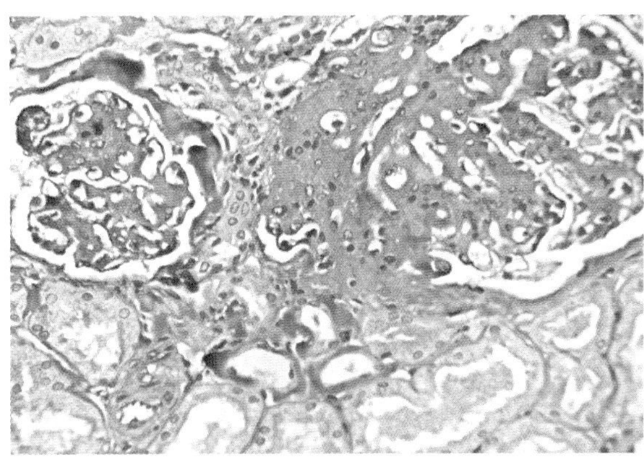

Figure 10-30

MPGN TYPE 2

Prominent ribbon-like deposits are present in Bowman's capsule and some tubular basement membranes, as well as the glomerular mesangium and capillary walls (alcian blue-PAS stain).

staining outlines "ring forms" that correspond to the nodular mesangial deposits seen by electron microscopy (fig. 10-34). The texture of the C3 staining of the glomerular basement membrane varies from semilinear to linear. On high-power microscopic examination, the staining of the linear peripheral capillary wall for C3 may be resolved into a narrow double line that corresponds to the inner and outer margins of the intramembranous deposits, but not the center of the deposits (37). Staining for properdin and C4 has also been demonstrated in some cases.

Electron Microscopic Findings. Electron microscopy is required for a definitive diagnosis of MPGN type 2. The defining lesion is a transformation of the lamina densa by ribbon-like, highly electron-dense material with a uniform waxy texture (figs. 10-35–10-37) (19). These intramembranous deposits frequently thicken the lamina densa itself. They may be discontinuous, alternating with segments of relatively well-preserved or even thinned glomerular basement membrane. This interrupted deposition often imparts a "sausage-string" or fusiform appearance

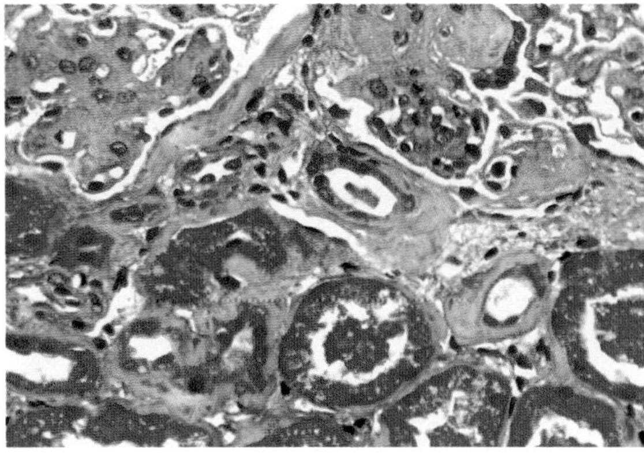

Figure 10-31

MPGN TYPE 2

Irregular pink-red deposits thicken Bowman's capsule and some tubular basement membranes (Masson trichrome stain).

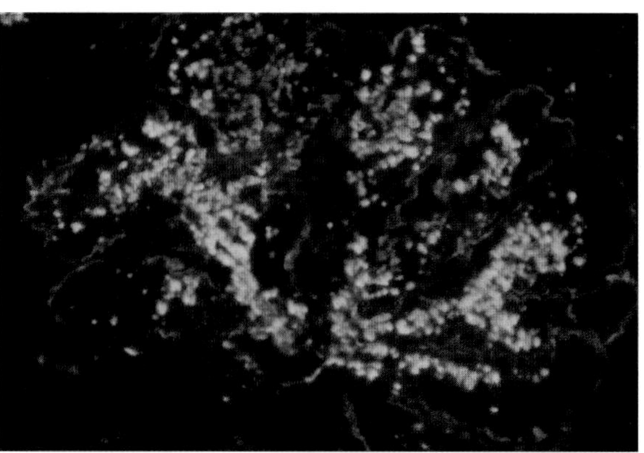

Figure 10-32

MPGN TYPE 2

The strong staining for C3 outlines ring-shaped forms within the mesangium, with weaker staining of the glomerular capillary walls (immunofluorescence micrograph).

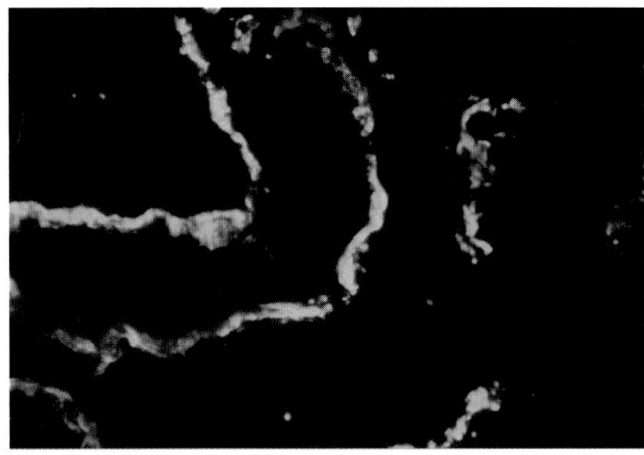

Figure 10-33

MPGN TYPE 2

There are band-like thickenings of the tubular basement membranes with antisera to C3 (immunofluorescence micrograph).

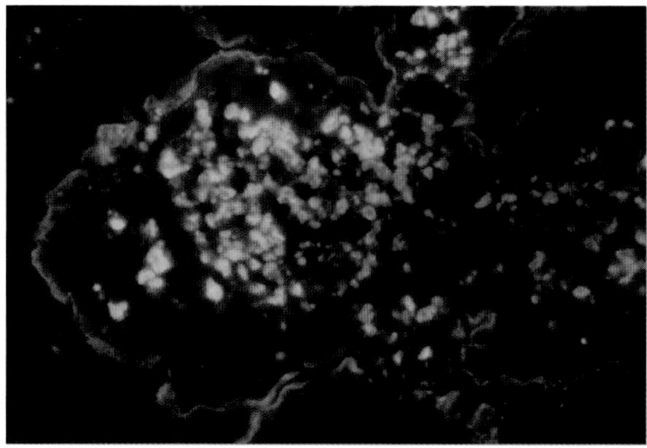

Figure 10-34

MPGN TYPE 2

Detail of the glomerular deposits of C3 within a single glomerular lobule. The mesangial rings produce a coarsely granular staining pattern whereas the glomerular capillary wall deposits appear more delicate and pseudolinear (immunofluorescence micrograph).

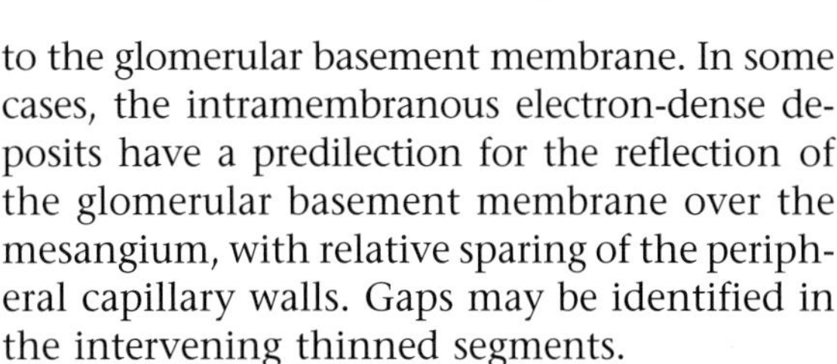

to the glomerular basement membrane. In some cases, the intramembranous electron-dense deposits have a predilection for the reflection of the glomerular basement membrane over the mesangium, with relative sparing of the peripheral capillary walls. Gaps may be identified in the intervening thinned segments.

The mesangium contains electron-dense deposits that tend to form small rounded nodules within the sclerotic mesangial matrix, corresponding to the ring forms seen by immunofluorescence (fig. 10-38). In other cases, the mesangial deposits are more diffusely distributed within the mesangial matrix. Intramembranous dense deposits are also present in Bowman's capsule. In the tubular basement membranes, they may appear intramembranous or appear to fall off and pool in the adjacent interstitium (fig. 10-39). Rarely have deposits been seen in interstitial capillary basement membranes or arteriolar membranes (19).

MPGN Type 3: Pathologic Features. *Light Microscopic and Electron Microscopic Findings.*

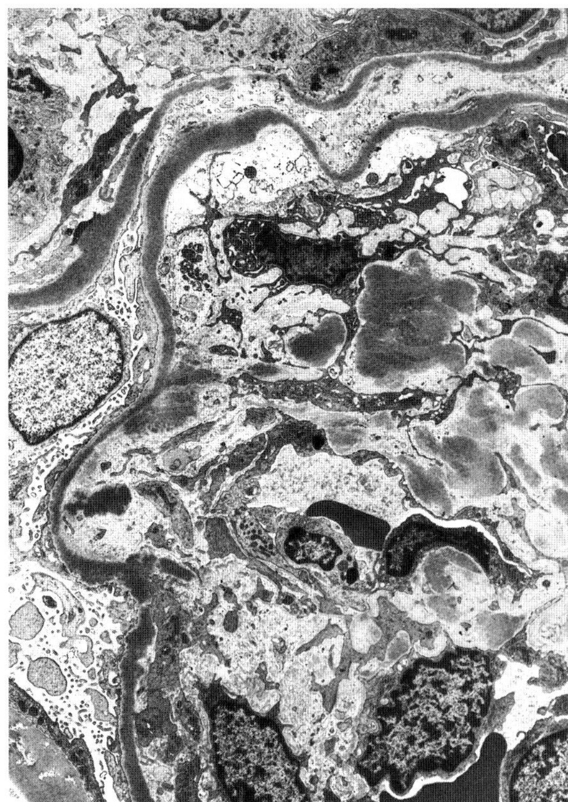

Figure 10-35

MPGN TYPE 2

Same case seen in figures 10-32 through 10-34 reveals distinctive ring-shaped electron-dense deposits within the mesangium and linear band-like electron densities within the lamina densa. The glomerular capillary lumen is severely narrowed (electron micrograph).

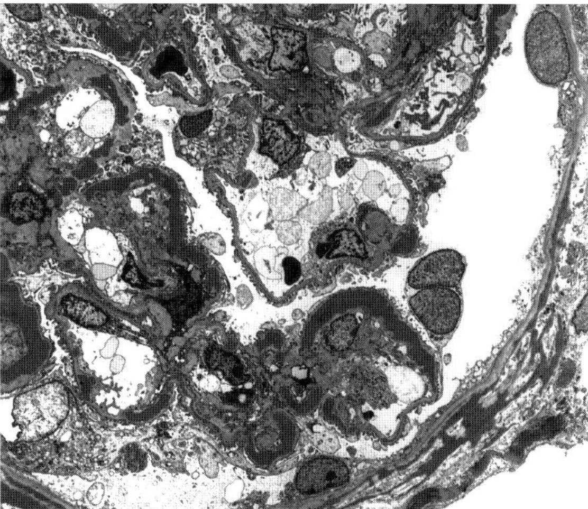

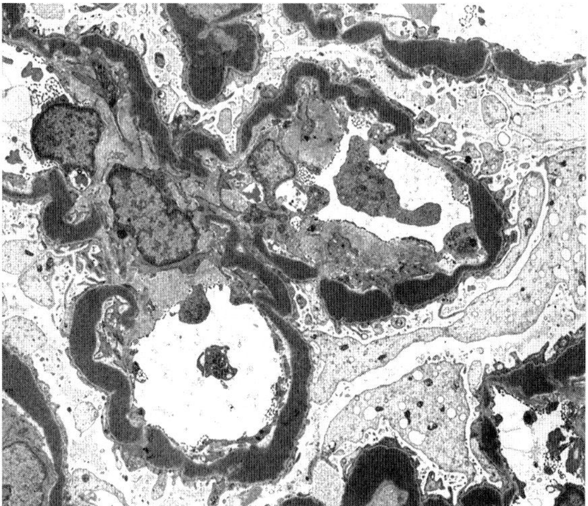

Figure 10-36

MPGN TYPE 2

Top: Low-power view illustrates the segmental, irregular distribution of the ribbon-like thickenings of the glomerular basement membranes by intramembranous, highly electron-dense deposits. There is involvement of both the peripheral capillary walls and the glomerular basement membrane reflection over the mesangium. Deposits are also seen focally involving the outer aspect of Bowman's capsule (electron micrograph).

Bottom: An example with fusiform electron-dense thickening of the lamina densa alternating with thinned segments, producing a "sausage-string" appearance (electron micrograph).

MPGN type 3 occurs in two different subtypes: one defined by Burkholder (5) and the other by Strife and Anders (1,39).

The subtype defined by Burkholder has combined features of MPGN type 1 and membranous glomerulopathy (5). By light microscopy, it is identified by complex thickening of the glomerular capillary walls owing to mesangial interposition, double contours of glomerular basement membranes, and subepithelial spikes (fig. 10-40). With the trichrome stain, fuchsinophilic deposits may be identified in combined mesangial, subendothelial, and subepithelial locations. There are varying degrees of mesangial proliferation and exudation of inflammatory cells, similar to the spectrum seen in type 1 MPGN. By electron microscopy, the Burkholder variant has discrete, granular electron-dense deposits in the mesangium, as well as in the subendothelial and subepithelial regions. The thickening of the glomerular capillary wall is extremely complex, with subendothelial and subepithelial deposits, as well as spike formation along the outer aspect

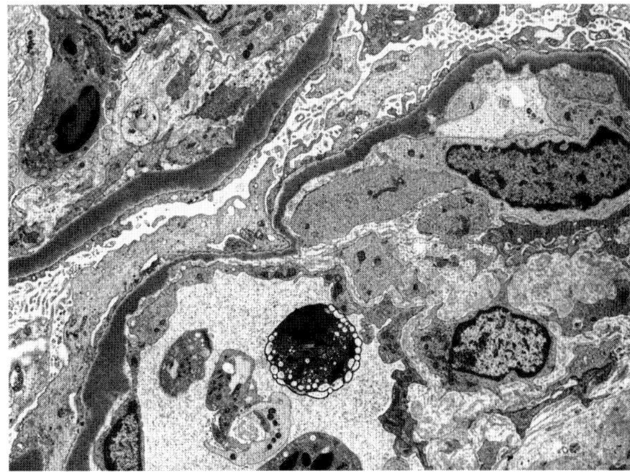

Figure 10-37

MPGN TYPE 2

High-power microscopic view shows the ribbon-like thickening of the lamina densa, with relative sparing of a thin layer of lamina rara interna and externa (electron micrograph).

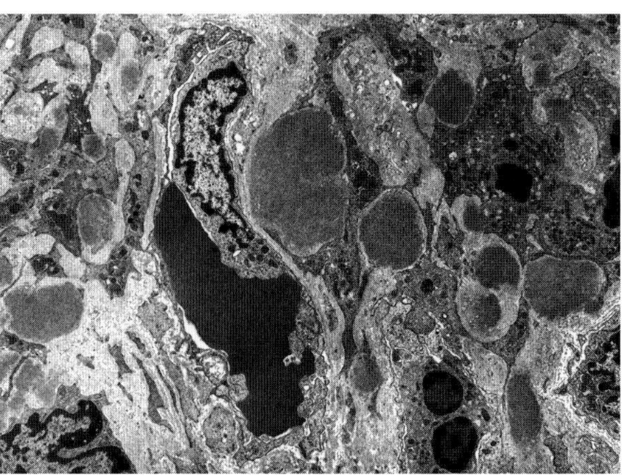

Figure 10-38

MPGN TYPE 2

High-power microscopic view of mesangial ring forms shows them to be composed of rounded aggregates of granular electron-dense material (electron micrograph).

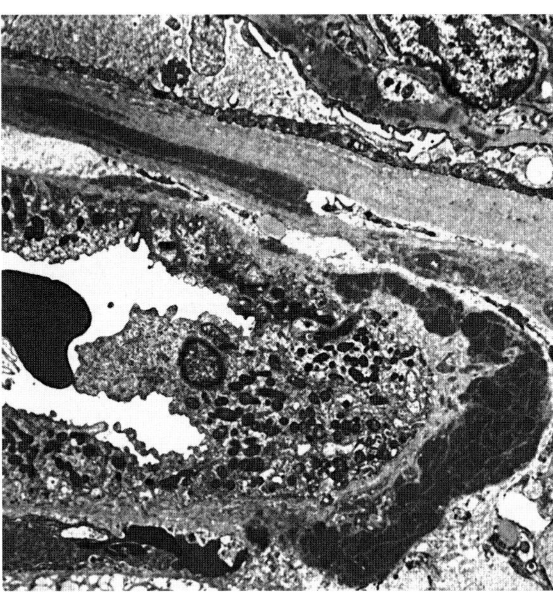

Figure 10-39

MPGN TYPE 2

The tubular basement membrane and Bowman's capsule contain electron-dense deposits that tend to pool along their outer aspect (electron micrograph).

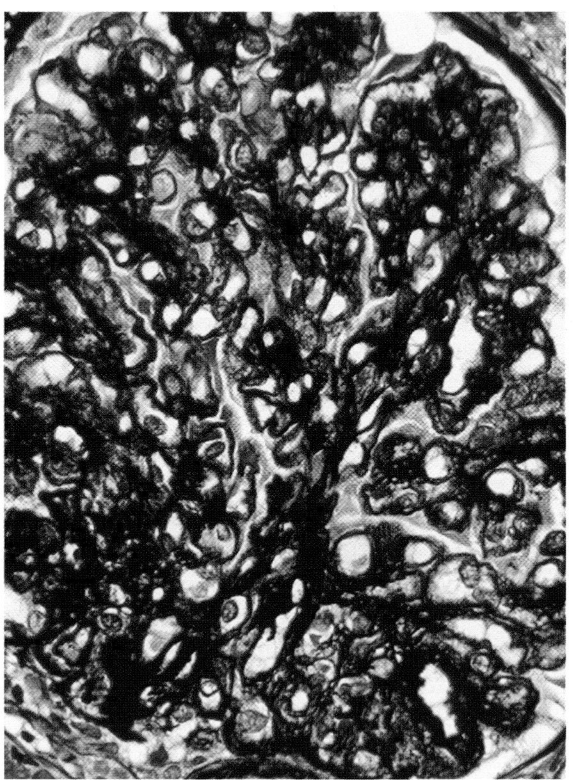

Figure 10-40

MPGN TYPE 3 OF BURKHOLDER

A glomerulus shows the combined features of MPGN type 1 (with mesangial proliferation, mesangial interposition, and double contours) and features of membranous glomerulopathy (with spiking of the glomerular basement membranes) (JMS stain).

and irregular lamellation of basement membrane material along the inner aspect (fig. 10-41).

The second variant, described independently by both Strife and Anders in 1977, was defined using silver impregnation electron microscopic

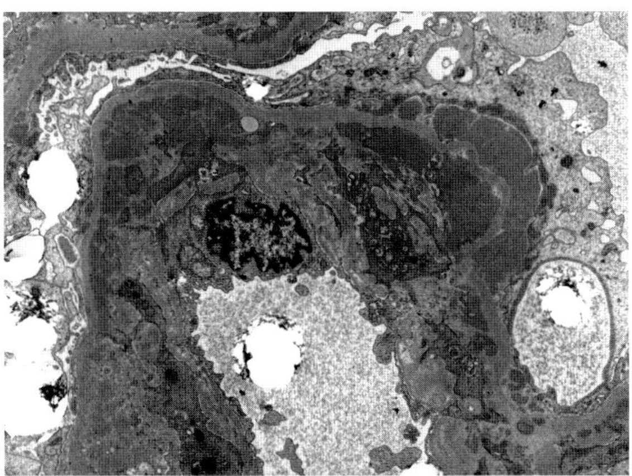

Figure 10-41

MPGN TYPE 3 OF BURKHOLDER

There are subendothelial deposits with circumferential mesangial interposition as well as subepithelial deposits (electron micrograph).

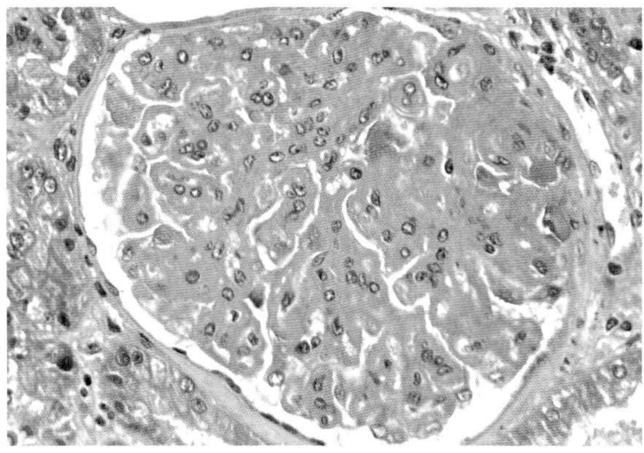

Figure 10-42

MPGN TYPE 3 OF STRIFE AND ANDERS

There is a relatively mild mesangial proliferation but severe thickening of glomerular capillary walls by glassy eosinophilic deposits (H&E stain). (Figs. 10-42 and 10-43 are from the same patient.)

techniques (1,39,41). It is characterized by subendothelial as well as complex intramembranous deposits that impart an irregularly thickened appearance to the glomerular capillary walls. By light microscopy, the intramembranous deposits form irregular, highly eosinophilic, PAS-positive thickenings (fig. 10-42). These intramembranous deposits tend to be JMS negative. With the silver stain, the glomerular basement membranes appear disrupted, frayed, and moth-eaten (fig. 10-43). By electron microscopy, the intramembranous deposits are not concentrated in the lamina densa, as they are in dense deposit disease. Rather, they appear to extend from the subendothelial to the subepithelial aspect, producing breaks and lamellations in the intervening lamina densa (fig. 10-44). The deposits are not as highly electron dense as the intramembranous deposits seen in dense deposit disease. In fact, in many cases the deposits are ill-defined, with a moderate electron density that is difficult to distinguish from that of the surrounding basement membrane material. Thus, in silver-impregnated samples, the lamina densa acquires a characteristic woven, laminated, disrupted appearance (1). In this subtype, it is not uncommon to find adjacent capillaries with more distinct subendothelial or subepithelial deposits. Thus, examination of many capillaries is often required to distinguish this variant from that

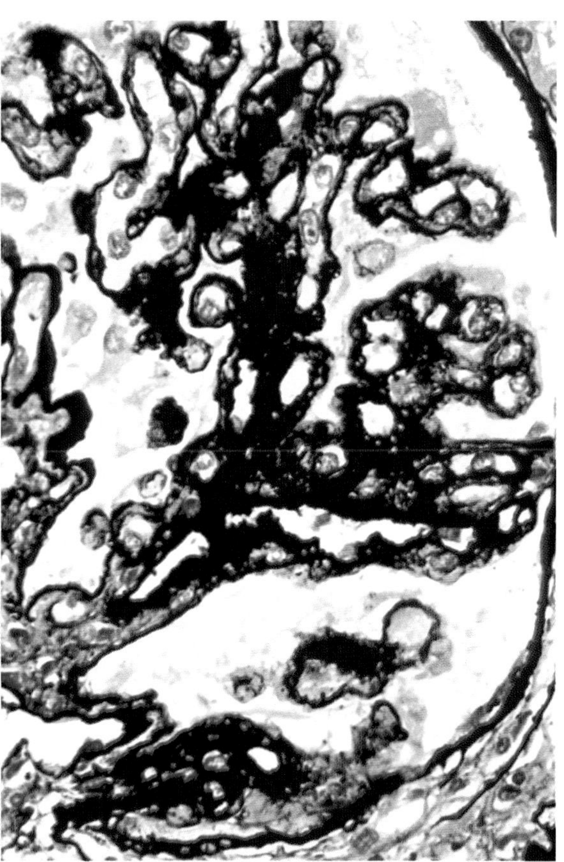

Figure 10-43

MPGN TYPE 3 OF STRIFE AND ANDERS

A motheaten appearance is seen in the glomerular capillary walls with the JMS stain.

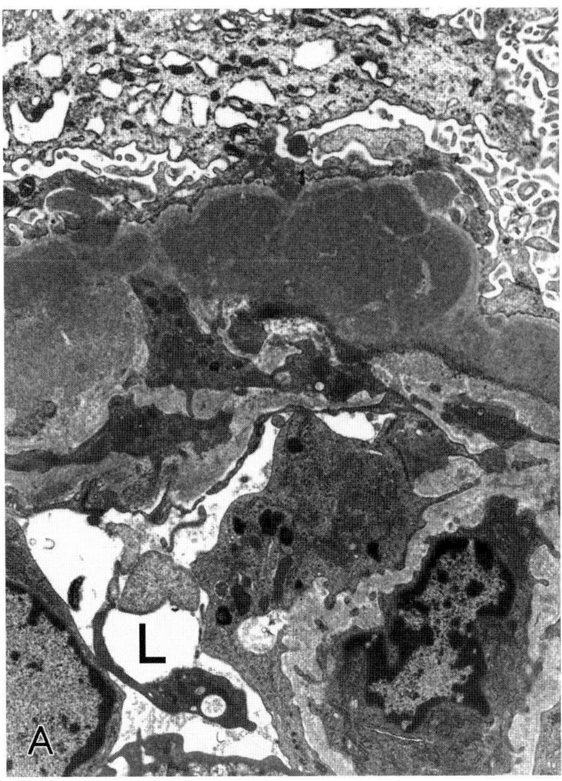

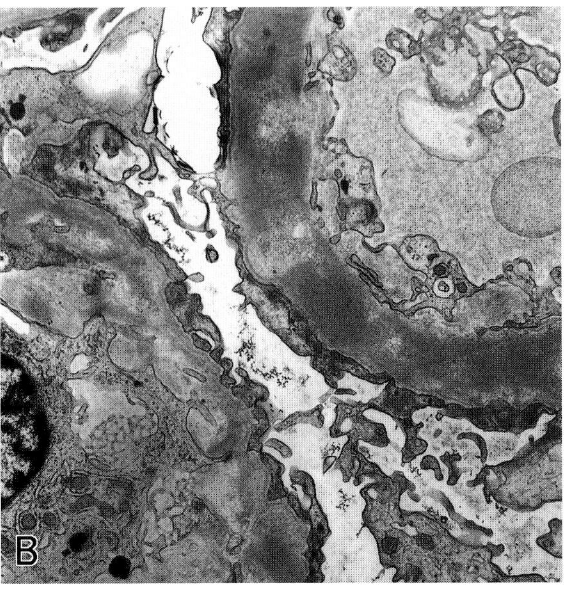

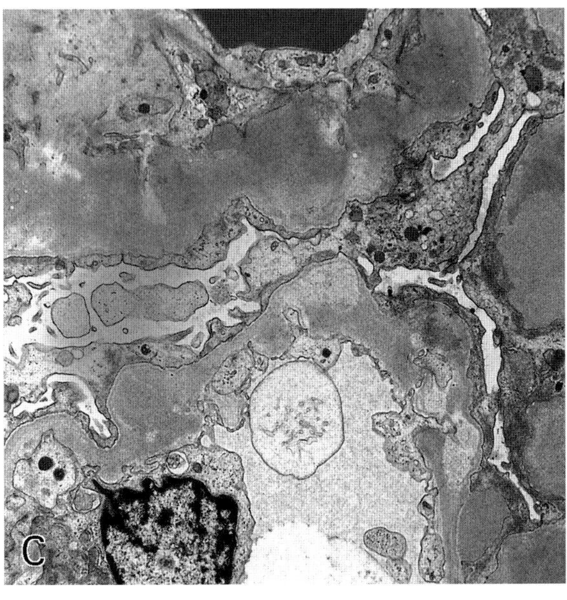

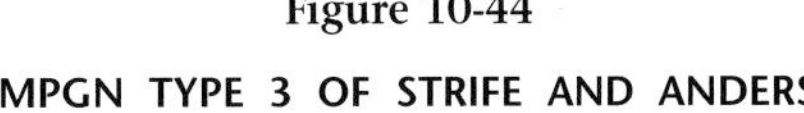

Figure 10-44

MPGN TYPE 3 OF STRIFE AND ANDERS

A: The glomerular capillary walls are thickened by transmembranous electron-dense deposits that extend from the subendothelial to the subepithelial aspect, causing disruptions and fraying of the lamina densa. Beneath the glomerular basement membrane, mesangial interposition can be seen (L=lumen) (electron micrograph).

B: There is irregular thickening of the glomerular capillary walls by complex intramembranous deposits that have variable electron density.

C: The intramembranous deposits appear complex, producing variable and irregular thickening of the glomerular capillary walls. These intramembranous deposits lack the highly electron-dense, uniform appearance of the deposits seen in dense deposit disease.

of Burkholder. Tubular basement membrane deposits are identified in about a third of cases.

Immunofluorescence Findings. By immunofluorescence, both subtypes of MPGN type 3 have similar findings. Approximately half the cases have combined staining for immunoglobulin (predominantly IgG) and C3, with more variable and less intense staining for IgM, IgA, and C1q. The staining for C3 is usually much more intense than the staining for IgG. The other half of cases stain for C3 only. Deposits are seen in the mesangium as well as involving the peripheral capillary walls, although the degree to which each of these glomerular compartments is involved can vary considerably from case to case. The glomerular capillary wall deposits tend to be bulky and coarsely granular (figs. 10-45, 10-46). Focal tubular basement membrane staining for C3, exhibiting a semilinear to granular texture, is present in about a third of cases (fig. 10-47).

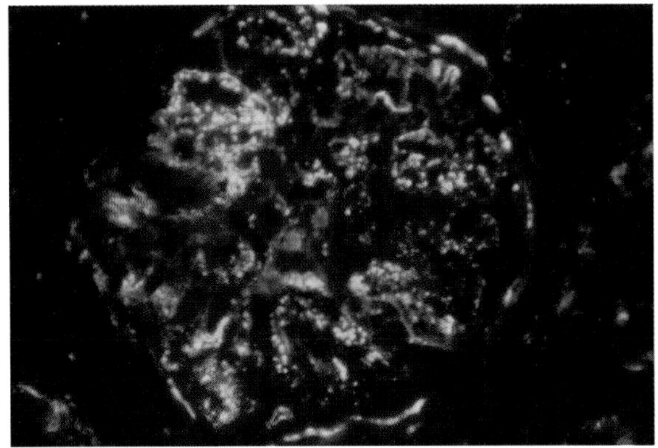

Figure 10-45

MPGN TYPE 3 OF BURKHOLDER

There is strong (3+) staining for C3 outlining mesangial, subendothelial, and subepithelial deposits, as well as Bowman's capsule (immunofluorescence micrograph).

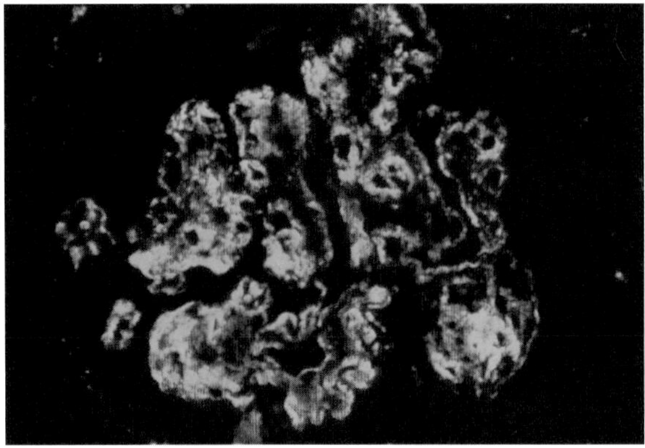

Figure 10-46

MPGN TYPE 3 OF STRIFE AND ANDERS

The intramembranous deposits have a confluent granular to semilinear texture (immunofluorescence micrograph).

Differential Diagnosis. The approach to the membranoproliferative pattern of renal disease requires first the differentiation of primary MPGN from the many secondary forms listed in Table 10-2 (35). A complete clinical history and serologies are essential. By careful analysis of the immunofluorescence and electron microscopic findings, it is possible to distinguish MPGN related to immune complex disease from forms due to paraprotein deposition (monoclonal immunoglobulin, light chain, or heavy chain) or forms lacking immune deposits (such as thrombotic microangiopathy or transplant glomerulopathy).

If the MPGN pattern is associated with immune complexes, underlying autoimmune disease or infection should be considered. The possibilities of systemic lupus erythematosus, hepatitis B or C infection, endocarditis (3), shunt nephritis (2), visceral infections (26), malaria (46), cryoglobulinemia, or the other conditions listed in Table 10-2, must be ruled out by clinical history and serologic evaluation. In this sense, the diagnosis of primary MPGN is a diagnosis of exclusion. IgA nephropathy and Henoch-Schönlein purpura nephritis can also present with a membranoproliferative pattern, but are readily distinguished by their dominant or co-dominant immunostaining for IgA, with positive C3, trace to negative C1, and frequent lambda dominance.

In subacute or chronic thrombotic microangiopathies with a membranoproliferative pattern, no immune deposits are seen (fig. 10-48). Rather, the material found between the double contours of glomerular basement membrane consists of organizing products of coagulation, with predominant immunofluorescence staining for fibrin/fibrinogen (fig. 10-49). By electron microscopy, the thrombotic microangiopathies display subendothelial accumulation of relatively electron-lucent, flocculent material ("fluff") rather than electron-dense deposits (figs. 10-50, 10-51), (20). Membranoproliferative lesions in chronic liver disease, such as due to alcoholic cirrhosis, typically have electron-lucent glomerular deposits

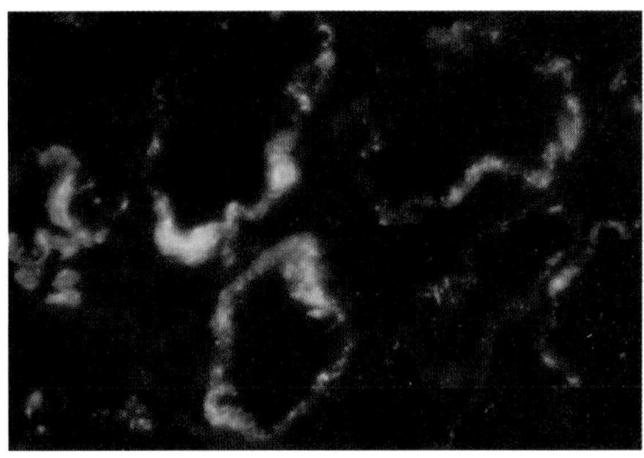

Figure 10-47

MPGN TYPE 3 OF STRIFE AND ANDERS

There are focal tubular basement membrane deposits of C3 (immunofluorescence micrograph).

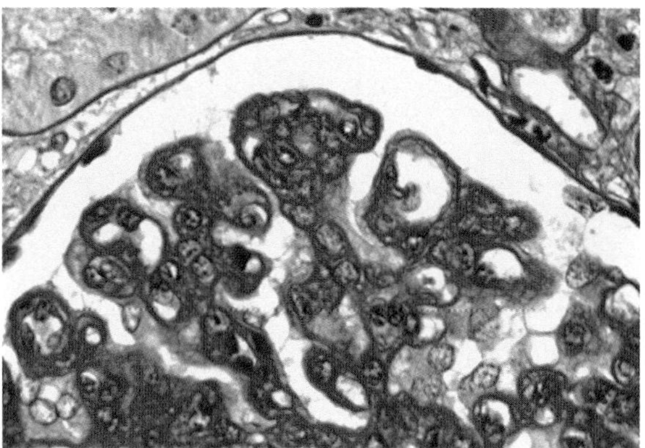

Figure 10-48

MPGN SECONDARY TO SICKLE CELL DISEASE

There are narrow reduplications of the glomerular basement membranes associated with minimal mesangial proliferation (PAS stain).

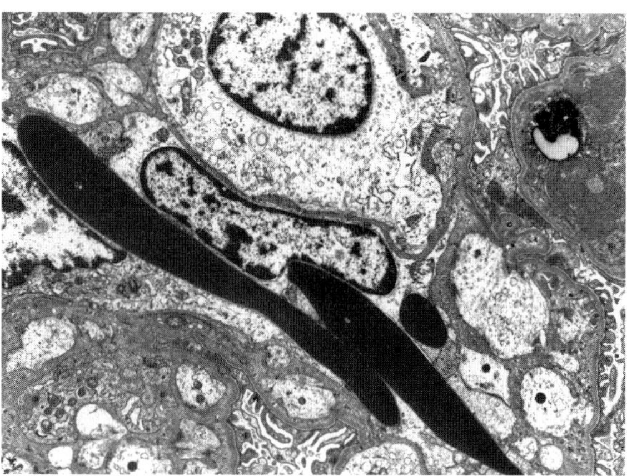

Figure 10-50

MPGN SECONDARY TO SICKLE CELL DISEASE

There is extensive mesangial interposition, with scanty deposits, endothelial swelling, and sickled intraluminal red blood cells (electron micrograph).

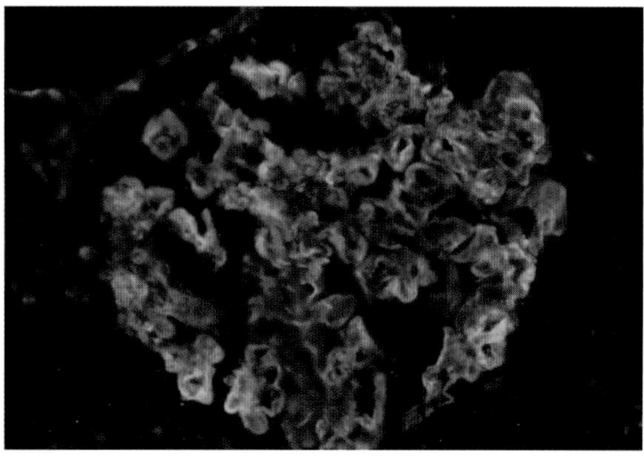

Figure 10-49

MPGN SECONDARY TO SICKLE CELL DISEASE

Immunofluorescence reveals positivity for fibrin/fibrinogen outlining the glomerular lobules (immunofluorescence micrograph).

resembling lipid rather than immune deposits. An exception is the rare form seen in alpha-1-antitrypsin deficiency, in which the deposits are more granular and electron dense (38). In sickle cell disease, some forms of secondary MPGN resemble chronic thrombotic microangiopathies, whereas others have electron-dense deposits (33).

In the dysproteinemias, there may be glomerular deposition of a variety of paraproteins, some of which are monoclonal. For example, in light chain deposition disease, the glomerular deposits consist of a single pathogenic light chain (kappa in 80 percent). Because the light chain deposits do not consist of immune complexes, no associated positivity for complement components is identified. In heavy chain deposition disease, there is staining for a single heavy chain (usually gamma, rarely alpha), without an associated light chain. Because complement can be activated on the truncated, mutated heavy chain, co-deposits of C3 and C1 may be found.

In fibrillary glomerulonephritis, the deposits consist predominantly of polyclonal IgG and complement, with the diagnostic ultrastructural finding of randomly oriented fibrils, 16 to 24 nm in diameter, involving the mesangium and glomerular basement membranes (12). In immunotactoid glomerulopathy, the deposits also usually consist of polyclonal immunoglobulins, forming highly organized deposits with a tubulofibrillar substructure that ranges from 30 to 50 nm in diameter (fig. 10-52).

Once secondary forms of MPGN have been excluded, the three subtypes of primary MPGN must then be differentiated. For this task, a well-prepared silver stain, careful immunofluorescence analysis, and detailed electron microscopic studies are essential.

Etiology and Pathogenesis. The nature of the antigenic stimulus in primary MPGN is unknown. However, the demonstration of circulating immune complexes in over half of

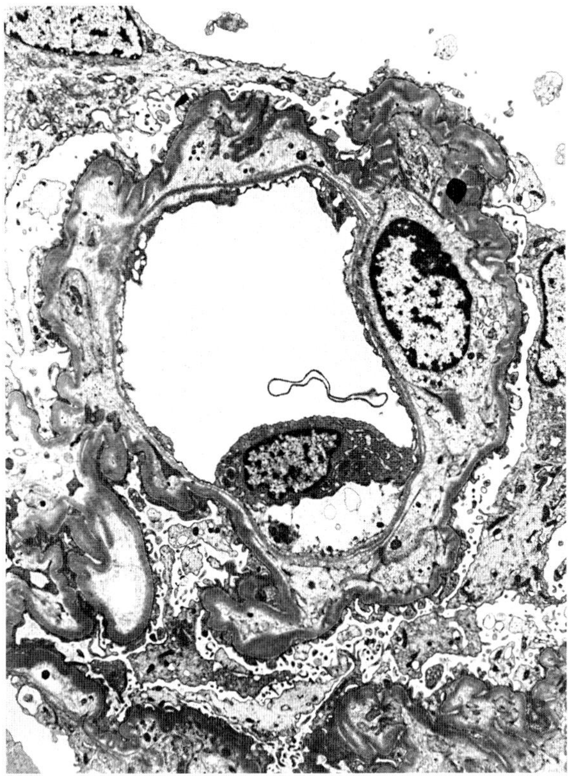

Figure 10-51

MPGN SECONDARY TO SYSTEMIC SCLEROSIS

There is circumferential mesangial interposition and duplication of glomerular basement membranes. Electron-lucent flocculent material is present between the double contours and in the mesangium, without evidence of electron-dense deposits. These features resemble those seen in other forms of chronic thrombotic microangiopathy (electron micrograph).

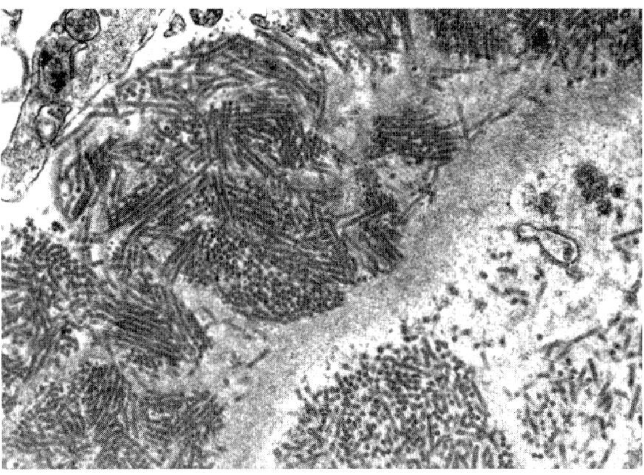

Figure 10-52

MPGN TYPE 3 SECONDARY TO IMMUNOTACTOID GLOMERULONEPHRITIS

The subepithelial and subendothelial deposits are composed of highly organized microtubular structures, 30 nm in diameter, that are stacked into parallel arrays (electron micrograph).

patients with MPGN type 1 and hypocomplementemia in nearly three quarters, strongly supports an immune complex pathogenesis. A process of immune complex deposition in the mesangium and glomerular capillary wall, followed by complement activation, leukocyte chemotaxis, platelet activation, and release of cytokines mitogenic for mesangial cells, is likely central to the mediation of primary MPGN. Experimental models of chronic serum sickness produced by repeated injection of foreign antigen closely mimic MPGN. In models of passive administration of preformed immune complexes, complexes of intermediate size and variable charge (cationic, neutral, or anionic) deposit in the mesangial and subendothelial zones to produce a membranoproliferative pattern of glomerulonephritis (14). Although data are limited, the pathogenesis of MPGN type 3 is probably similar to that of type 1.

The pathogenesis of MPGN type 2 is unknown. The pathomechanism is probably quite different from that for types 1 and 3. In MPGN type 2, no circulating immune complexes have been identified and the glomerular deposits consist of C3 only, without immunoglobulins. These patients have evidence of systemic electron-dense deposits that affect splenic sinusoids and Bruch's membrane of the retina (19). Some also have partial lipodystrophy. Lipid extraction techniques applied to the ultrathin sections used for electron microscopy cause the electron-dense deposits to lose their distinctive appearance, suggesting that they may consist of lipids rich in unsaturated fatty acids, although their chemical composition and origin are unknown. It has been postulated that factor D of the complement system, a serine protease adipsin synthesized by adipocytes which converts factor B of the preconvertase C3bB to the activated form C3bBb, may provide a pathogenetic link between partial lipodystrophy and MPGN type 2.

Treatment and Prognosis. The optimal therapy in children and adults with primary MPGN type 1 has not been defined (6,11,13,29, 42,45). Limited data are available for MPGN types 2 and 3. Most randomized clinical trials are flawed

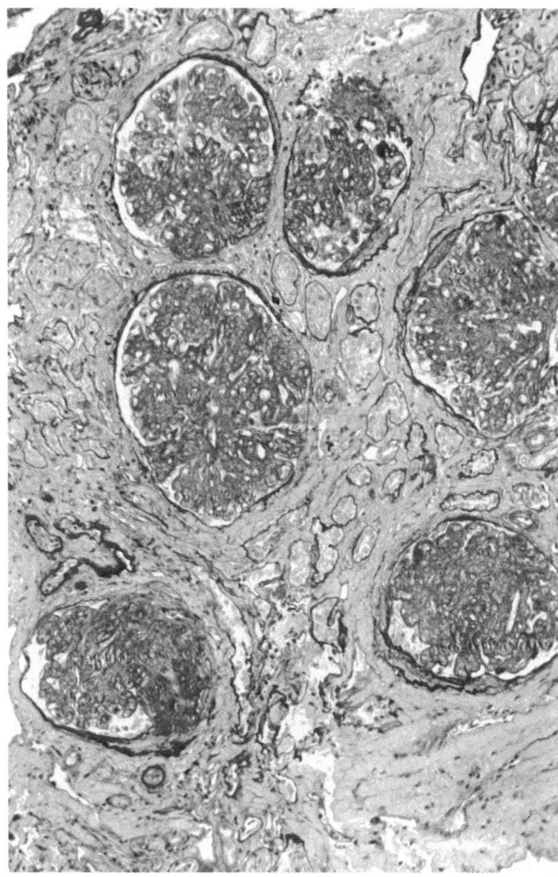

Figure 10-53

MPGN TYPE 1 BEFORE TREATMENT

Biopsy from an 8-year-old child prior to initiation of alternate day steroid therapy. There is exuberant glomerular proliferation and enlargement (PAS stain).

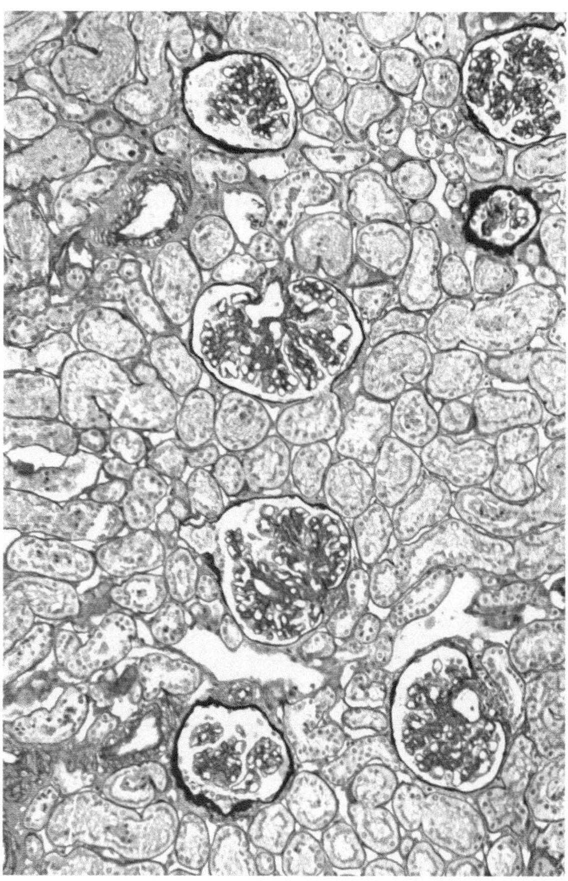

Figure 10-54

MPGN TYPE 1 AFTER TREATMENT

A rebiopsy of the same case 5 years after treatment with alternate day steroids shows striking improvement in the severity of the glomerulonephritis, with regression of the proliferation and restoration of luminal patency (PAS stain).

by short-term follow-up periods of only 1 to 4 years. The interpretation of the findings is hampered by the failure of earlier studies to identify hepatitis C as an associated risk factor.

Most treatment modalities for children with primary MPGN employ long-term low-dose steroid therapy (2 mg/kg every other day for 1 year, tapered gradually to 20 mg every other day for up to 5 to 10 years). Several studies by the International Study of Kidney Disease in Children (ISKDC) have documented stabilization or improvement in renal function and proteinuria with this regimen (42). There is a risk of steroid toxicity, however, including hypertension and growth retardation. Biopsies are repeated routinely by some nephrologists at 5 years from initiation of treatment to monitor histologic improvement to determine the need for continued therapy (figs. 10-53, 10-54).

The role of corticosteroid therapy in adults is less well documented. Most nephrologists offer steroids in a regimen similar to that of children to adults with significant active disease and nephrotic syndrome. Antiplatelet agents (aspirin and dipyridamole) have been utilized alone or in conjunction with steroids in some patients (10). Compared to earlier 10-year renal survival rates of approximately 50 percent for patients with primary MPGN, more recent studies of patients receiving therapy have reported improved rates of 60 to 85 percent for both children and adults (25).

In all types of MPGN, the pathologic features that portend a poor outcome include greater percentage of sclerotic glomeruli, numerous crescents, and more severe tubular atrophy and interstitial fibrosis. Negative clinical prognostic features include severe unremitting nephrotic syndrome, elevated serum creatinine level at biopsy, and hypertension. The outcome appears to be better in patients with asymptomatic hematuria and subnephrotic proteinuria who have more focal and milder membranoproliferative features on biopsy (40).

MPGN type 1 tends to be a slowly progressive disease, with few spontaneous remissions. The 10-year survival rate is approximately 50 percent. Treatment produces a partial or complete clinical remission in a subgroup of patients. Median renal survival time for patients with MPGN type 1 is 9 to 12 years, compared to 5 to 12 years for those with type 2. Patients with MPGN type 2 tend to have a worse prognosis, and a more aggressive course to renal failure. The prognosis of patients with MPGN type 3 closely resembles that of type 1.

For those patients who progress to renal failure and receive a renal transplant, there is a high risk of recurrence of MPGN in the allograft, especially within the first 6 months to 1 year post-transplant. Approximately 30 percent of children with MPGN type 1 who have had transplants develop recurrence, some in several successive allografts. Up to 40 percent of these recurrences lead to graft failure. The rate of recurrence of MPGN type 2 is much higher, approaching 80 to 100 percent, depending on how carefully it is sought and whether immunofluorescence and electron microscopy have been performed. Recurrences tend to be clinically mild and only 10 to 20 percent are responsible for graft failure.

SECONDARY MPGN

The membranoproliferative pattern of glomerular disease (defined as mesangial hypercellularity and nodular mesangial expansion, mesangial interposition and double contouring of the glomerular basement membranes) may be seen in a variety of underlying conditions. These fall into several major subheadings: infections, autoimmune diseases, dysproteinemias, chronic liver diseases, and thrombotic microangiopathies (see Table 10-2). A detailed description of many of these entities can be found in other chapters of this Fascicle. Only those related to cryoglobulinemia, hepatitis C, and hepatitis B are considered in depth here.

MPGN Secondary to Cryoglobulinemia (Cryoglobulinemic Glomerulonephritis)

Definition. Cryoglobulinemic glomerulonephritis is a form of glomerulonephritis, often with membranoproliferative features, that results from glomerular deposition of cryoglobulins. Cryoglobulins are immunoglobulins that have the physical property of reversibly precipitating in the cold. Three main types of cryoglobulins have been identified by Brouet (4): type 1 cryoglobulins consist of a single monoclonal immunoglobulin (usually IgG kappa or IgM kappa); type 2 cryoglobulins are mixed cryoglobulins consisting of a monoclonal immunoglobulin (usually IgM kappa) complexed to a polyclonal immunoglobulin (usually IgG); and type 3 cryoglobulins are mixed cryoglobulins containing two polyclonal components (usually IgG-IgM or IgG-IgG).

Clinical Features. The renal manifestations of cryoglobulinemic glomerulonephritis are hematuria, proteinuria, and renal insufficiency (8,9). The systemic manifestations resemble those of systemic vasculitis, including palpable purpura due to leukocytoclastic vasculitis, arthralgias and arthritis, distal necrosis and skin ulcerations, Raynaud's phenomenon, peripheral neuropathy, and abdominal pain (24,30). Hypocomplementemia is a common feature, including reduced CH50 in 90 percent of cases, reduced C4 in 79 percent, and reduced C3 in 50 percent. Common underlying systemic diseases include infections, autoimmune diseases, and dysproteinemias.

Type 1 cryoglobulins are seen in association with dysproteinemias (such as myeloma, B-cell lymphomas, and Waldenström's macroglobulinemia). Type 2 cryoglobulinemia is the form most frequently associated with glomerulonephritis. In the past, such cases were labeled "mixed essential cryoglobulinemia" because the etiology of the cryoglobulinemia was unknown. In the last decade, many cases of cryoglobulinemic glomerulonephritis associated with type 2 cryoglobulins have been linked

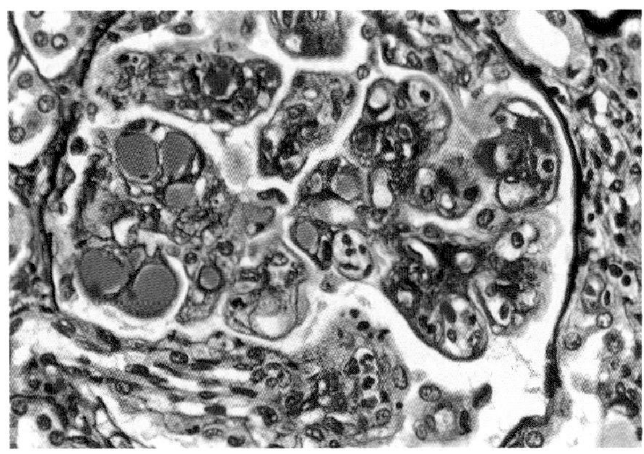

Figure 10-55

MPGN TYPE 1 IN A PATIENT WITH TYPE 2 CRYOGLOBULINEMIA

There are numerous intracapillary "protein thrombi" and double contours (JMS stain).

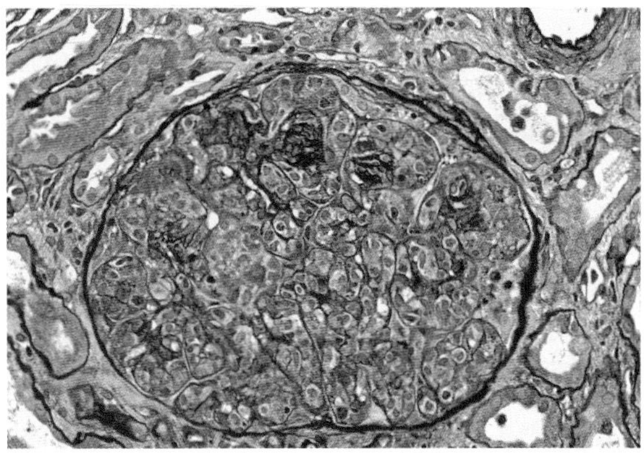

Figure 10-56

MPGN ASSOCIATED WITH TYPE 2 CRYOGLOBULINEMIA

An example with more exudative glomerulonephritis than in figure 10-55 contains abundant infiltrating monocytes (PAS stain).

to chronic hepatitis C infection. Type 2 cryoglobulinemia may also occur in association with dysproteinemias, other infections (such as hepatitis B, Epstein-Barr virus [EBV] infection, bacterial endocarditis) and autoimmune conditions (such as systemic lupus erythematosus, Sjögren's disease, and rheumatoid arthritis). Type 3 cryoglobulins are common in autoimmune and infectious diseases but are less frequently implicated in the development of glomerulonephritis than are the type 2 cryoglobulins.

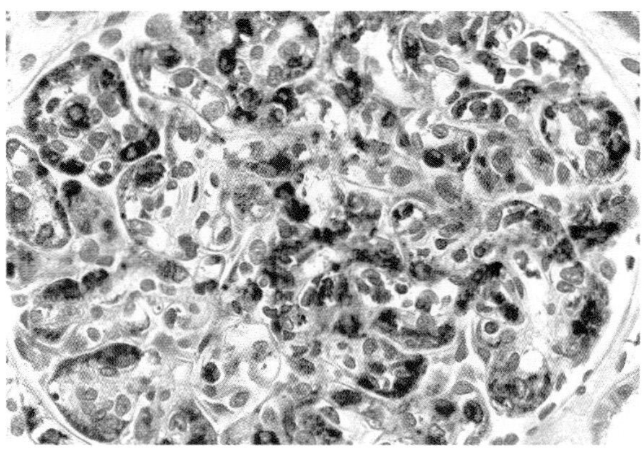

Figure 10-57

MPGN ASSOCIATED WITH TYPE 2 CRYOGLOBULINEMIA

The numerous infiltrating cells of monocyte/macrophage lineage are revealed with an immunostain for CD68 (immunoperoxidase stain).

Light Microscopic Findings. In cryoglobulinemic glomerulonephritis, MPGN type 1 is the most common pattern (fig. 10-55), followed by MPGN type 3. In some examples, there is a diffuse, endocapillary proliferative and exudative glomerulonephritis with few membranoproliferative features (fig. 10-56). Glomerular infiltration by large numbers of monocytes, as well as neutrophils, is common (fig. 10-57) (32). The glomerular deposits of cryoglobulin are found in subendothelial and intraluminal locations, forming intracapillary "protein thrombi," with less conspicuous mesangial deposition (fig. 10-58). There may be prominent phagocytosis of the intraluminal deposits by the infiltrating monocytes, which display large phagosomes that are visible by light and electron microscopy (figs. 10-59–10-61). Fibrinoid necrosis of the glomerular tuft is never seen. Crescents are extremely rare.

In less than one third of cases, vasculitis is identified in the renal biopsy. The arteritis or arteriolitis of cryoglobulinemia often consists of an endarteritis, with inflammation involving the endothelial and intimal layers, but sparing the media (fig. 10-62). The involved vessels frequently contain intimal or intraluminal cryoglobulin deposits with similar properties, as seen by light and fluorescence microscopy, to those in the glomerular capillaries (figs. 10-62, 10-63). In rare cases, a transmural necrotizing arteritis, resembling microscopic polyangiitis or macroscopic polyarteritis, occurs in the kidney.

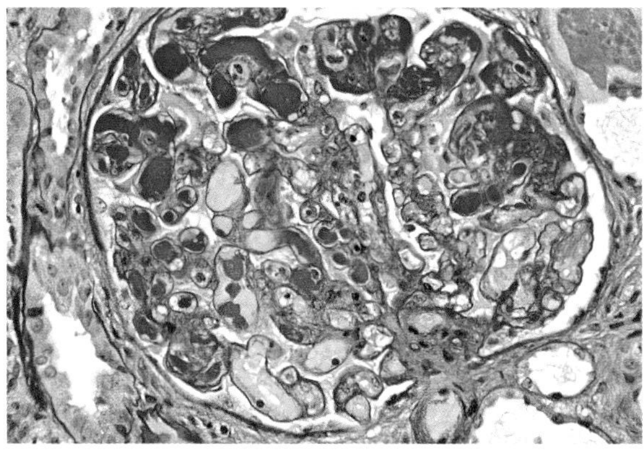

Figure 10-58

MPGN ASSOCIATED WITH TYPE 1 CRYOGLOBULINEMIA FROM A PATIENT WITH CHRONIC LYMPHOCYTIC LEUKEMIA AND A MONOCLONAL IgM KAPPA CRYOGLOBULIN

There is relatively little glomerular hypercellularity but massive intracapillary protein thrombi (PAS stain).

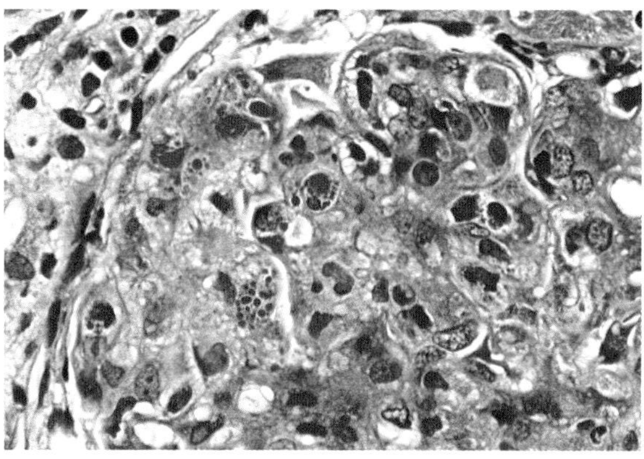

Figure 10-59

MPGN ASSOCIATED WITH TYPE 2 CRYOGLOBULINEMIA

The trichrome stain highlights the red phagosomes within the infiltrating monocytes as well as the intraluminal deposits (electron micrograph).

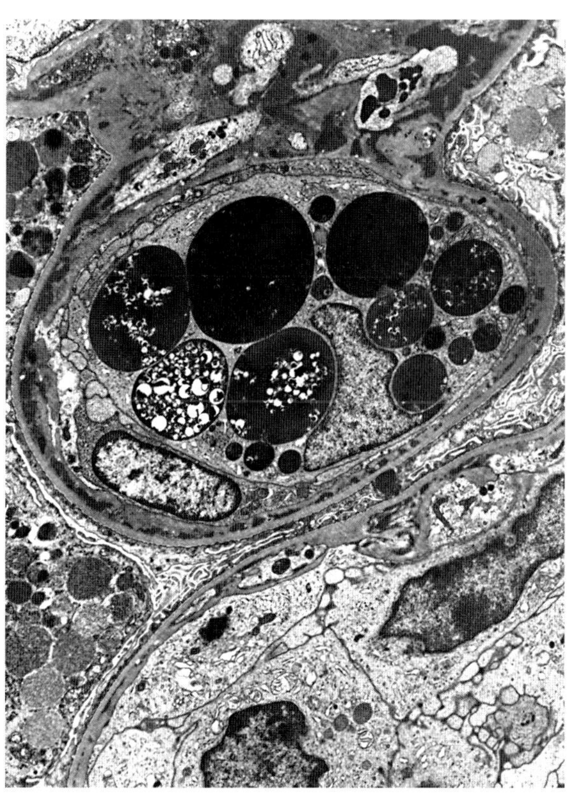

Figure 10-60

MPGN ASSOCIATED WITH TYPE 2 CRYOGLOBULINEMIA

There are mesangial and subendothelial deposits associated with large intraluminal monocytes with prominent phagosomes (electron micrograph).

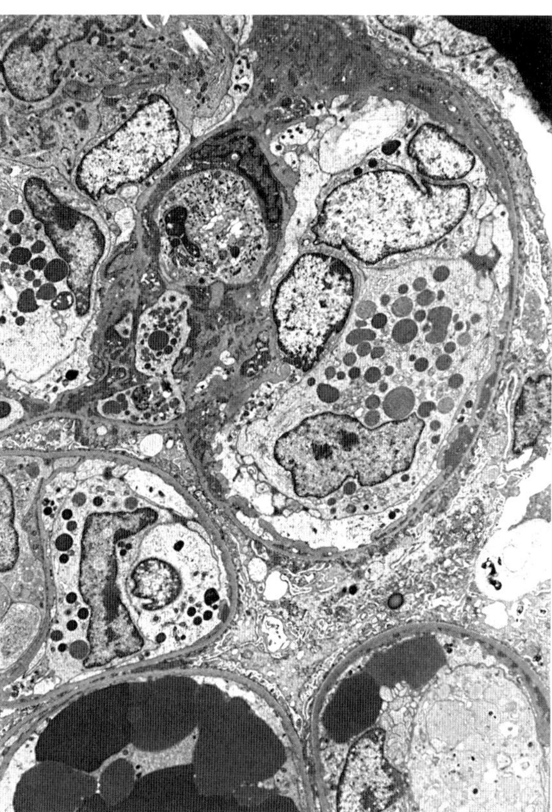

Figure 10-61

MPGN ASSOCIATED WITH TYPE 2 CRYOGLOBULINEMIA

The majority of endocapillary cells are monocytes, as identified by their numerous phagolysosomes (electron micrograph).

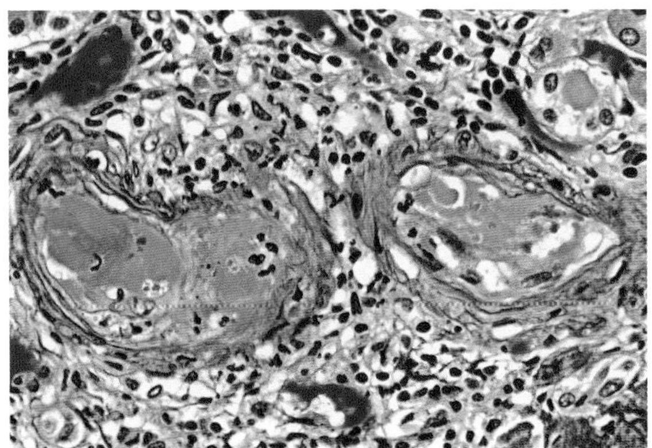

Figure 10-62

CRYOGLOBULINEMIC VASCULITIS

An interlobular artery displays endarteritis with predominantly intimal infiltration by leukocytes and large intimal and intraluminal cryoglobulin deposits (JMS stain).

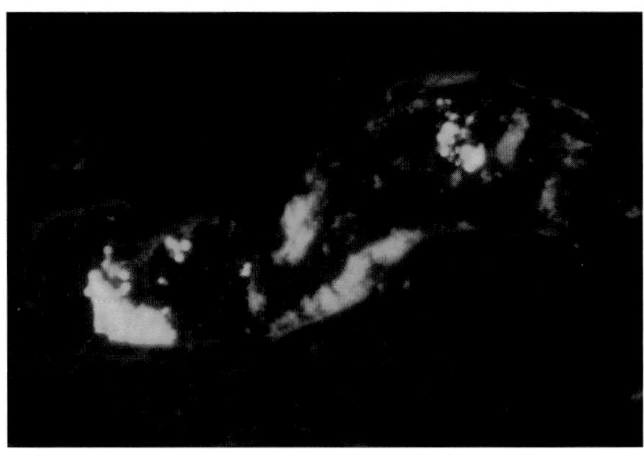

Figure 10-63

CRYOGLOBULINEMIC VASCULITIS

An interlobular artery stains strongly for IgM (as well as IgG, not shown) in the distribution of the intimal cryoglobulin deposits (immunofluorescence micrograph).

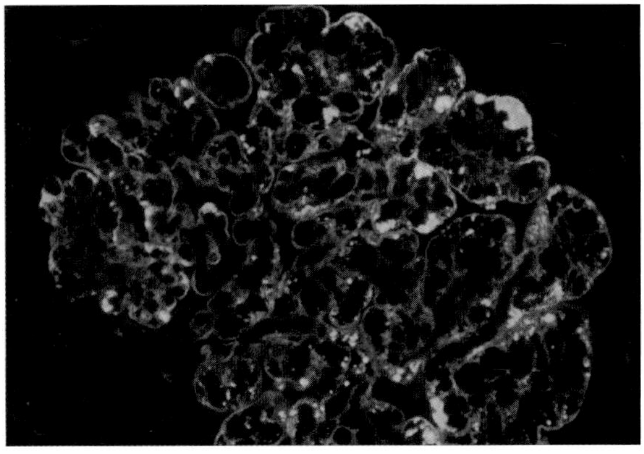

Figure 10-64

MPGN SECONDARY TO TYPE 2 CRYOGLOBULINEMIA AND HEPATITIS C INFECTION

There is intense (2+) positivity for IgM in the distribution of the subendothelial and intracapillary deposits (immunofluorescence micrograph).

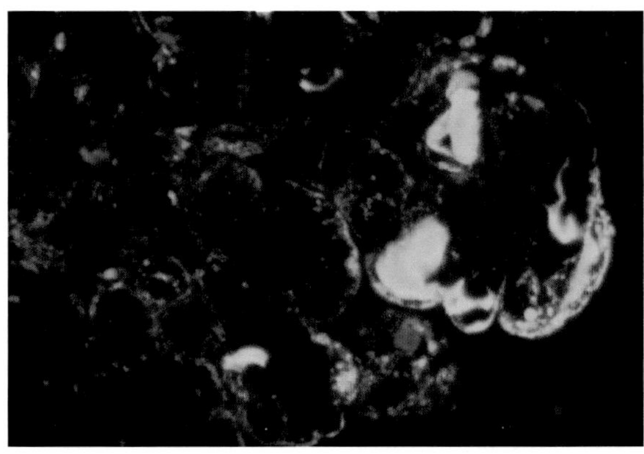

Figure 10-65

MPGN SECONDARY TO TYPE 2 CRYOGLOBULINEMIA AND HEPATITIS C INFECTION

High-power microscopic view shows strong staining for IgM outlining the intracapillary protein thrombi as well as the more delicate subendothelial deposits (immunofluorescence micrograph). (Figs. 10-65 and 10-66 are from the same patient.)

Immunofluorescence Findings. In cryoglobulinemia, the glomerular deposits detected by immunofluorescence reflect the composition of the cryoprecipitate in the serum. For example, in type 1 cryoglobulinemia, they consist of a single monoclonal immunoglobulin component (frequently IgG kappa). In cases associated with Waldenström's macroglobulinemia, they consist of monoclonal IgM (usually IgM kappa). Some patients with type 1 cryoglobulins have evidence of complement activation (C3 or C1q) in the glomerular deposits, whereas others do not.

In the more common type 2 cryoglobulinemia, the deposits usually stain for both IgG and IgM, complement components C3 and C1, as well as kappa and lambda light chains. The staining for IgM and kappa may be most intense, reflecting the presence of a monoclonal IgM-kappa component (figs. 10-64–10-66).

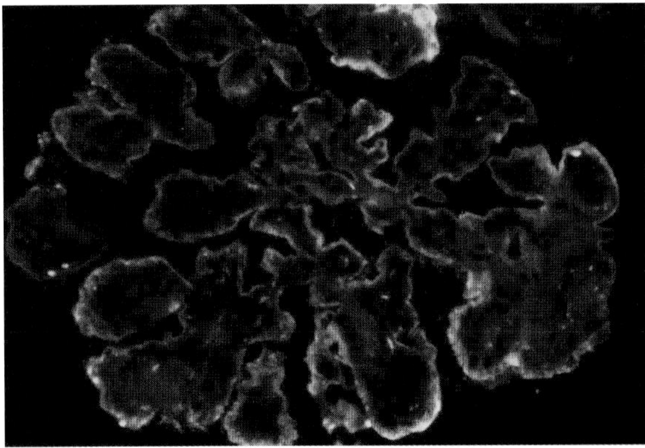

Figure 10-66

MPGN SECONDARY TO TYPE 2 CRYOGLOBULINEMIA AND HEPATITIS C INFECTION

There is weaker (1+) positivity for IgG. The combination of intense staining for IgM and weaker co-deposits of IgG is commonly observed in cases of type 2 cryoglobulinemia composed of monoclonal IgM and polyclonal IgG (immunofluorescence micrograph).

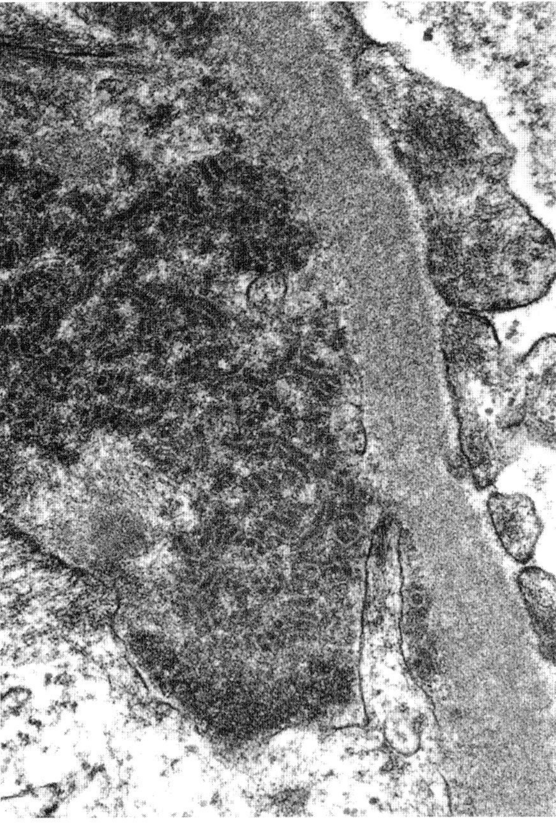

Figure 10-67

MPGN ASSOCIATED WITH TYPE 2 CRYOGLOBULINEMIA

The subendothelial deposits exhibit an organized substructure composed of 30-nm annular-tubular arrays (electron micrograph).

Electron Microscopic Findings. The glomerular capillaries are infiltrated by monocytes, which are recognized by their large phagolysosomes (figs. 10-60, 10-61). The glomerular deposits may be granular or organized. Organized deposits are more common in the forms of cryoglobulinemia that contain a monoclonal component (type 1 or 2). In type 1 cryoglobulinemia, fibrillar deposits may be seen. In type 2, the organized deposits typically exhibit a curvilinear annular-tubular substructure, with a tubular diameter of 20 to 35 nm (fig. 10-67). The areas of organization usually involve some, but not all, of the glomerular electron-dense deposits. Organized deposits are identified in less than half of cases and usually require examination under high-power magnification (more than 20,000X). The patterns of organization in the glomerular deposits resemble those seen on ultrastructural examination of the serum cryoprecipitate.

Treatment and Prognosis. Interferon-alpha is the mainstay of long-term therapy for patients with hepatitis C–associated cryoglobulinemia (22,31). Ribavirin has also been used in recent years (15). A course of aggressive immunosuppressive therapy (pulse methylprednisolone followed by oral steroids and cyclophosphamide) is usually reserved for patients with severe acute vasculitis and multisystem manifestations (16,21). This regimen should be used cautiously in patients with underlying hepatitis C infection, due to the possible reactivation of the virus. Plasmapheresis is occasionally useful. Cryofiltration, which precipitates out the cryoglobulins by cooling the patient's plasma, and then reinfuses the patient's rewarmed plasma, can obviate the need for replacement fluid.

Secondary MPGN Due to Hepatitis C Infection

Definition. Hepatitis C–associated glomerulonephritis is an immune complex–mediated glomerular disease occurring in patients with hepatitis C infection, as determined by hepatitis C viral serologies. Glomerulonephritis occurring in patients with hepatitis C infection may or may not be associated with cryoglobulinemia.

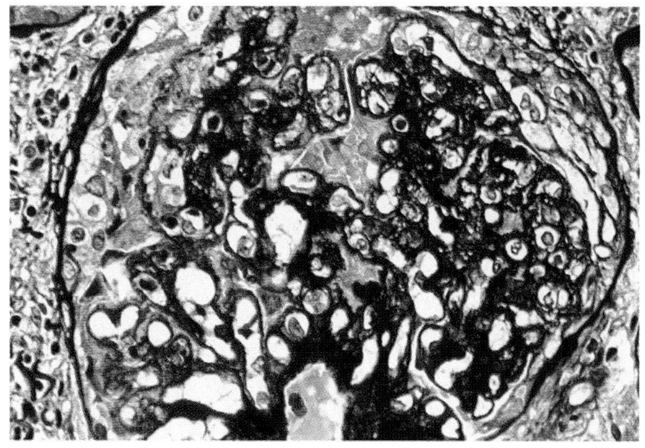

Figure 10-68

MPGN TYPE 3 ASSOCIATED WITH HEPATITIS C INFECTION

There are combined membranous features with glomerular basement membrane spikes and membranoproliferative features with glomerular basement membrane duplication and mesangial interposition. A crescent is also seen (JMS stain).

If cryoglobulinemia is present, the glomerulonephritis is termed *cyroglobulinemic glomerulonephritis*. If there is no evidence of cryoglobulinemia, the most appropriate designation is *hepatitis C–associated glomerulonephritis*.

Clinical Features. Hepatitis C is now recognized as one of the most common causes of secondary MPGN. Approximately one third of patients with hepatitis C–associated glomerular disease lack documented cryoglobulinemia (23). In some patients, the development of glomerulonephritis precedes by months or years the clinical demonstration of cryoglobulinemia. Glomerulonephritis is a relatively late manifestation of hepatitis C infection, occurring at least 10 years and often many decades after infection. For this reason, it is primarily a disease of adults. Over 60 percent of patients have abnormal liver function tests but only about 20 percent have documented advanced chronic hepatitis or cirrhosis of the liver. Hypocomplementemia is present in 50 to 90 percent, with more frequent reductions in C4 than C3. The most common renal presentation is proteinuria (which is nephrotic in about 70 percent of cases) and mild azotemia. Hematuria and nephritic features are present in about 25 percent of patients.

Light Microscopic Findings. The most common form of glomerular disease in patients with hepatitis C infection is MPGN type 1 (over 80 percent), followed by MPGN type 3 (of Burkholder), membranous glomerulopathy, and acute proliferative and exudative glomerulonephritis (fig. 10-68) (34,36). There are recent reports of fibrillary glomerulonephritis and immunotactoid glomerulopathy associated with hepatitis C infection (27).

Immunofluorescence Findings. The glomerular immune deposits usually stain for IgG, IgM, C3, C1, and kappa and lambda light chains, with varying intensity of each. However, some cases may have IgM and complement only, without associated IgG.

Electron Microscopic Findings. Electron-dense deposits are identifiable by electron microscopy in mesangial, subendothelial, and subepithelial locations, depending on the histologic pattern. In some cases, the deposits are surprisingly scanty relative to the degree of glomerular hypercellularity. Organized deposits are more common in those with documented type 2 cryoglobulinemia.

Etiology and Pathogenesis. The presumed pathogenesis involves glomerular deposition of circulating immune complexes in the setting of chronic viral antigenemia. Although viral antigens (including hepatitis C nucleocapsid/core protein C22-3) are concentrated in the circulating cryoglobulins of patients with hepatitis C virus infection, it has been difficult to demonstrate viral antigen in the glomerular immune deposits (23).

Treatment and Prognosis. Antiviral therapy, including interferon-alpha and ribavirin, is the treatment of choice. Immunosuppression is contraindicated because it can promote viral replication. Reduction of the viral burden following interferon therapy has led to significant improvement in proteinuria, although the renal insufficiency appears to be less responsive.

Secondary MPGN Due to Hepatitis B Infection

Definition. *Hepatitis B–associated glomerulonephritis* is defined as a form of immune complex–mediated glomerulonephritis, typically with membranoproliferative features, occurring in a patient with hepatitis B surface antigenemia. If a cryoglobulin is identified, the designation *cryoglobulinemic glomerulonephritis* is preferred.

Clinical Features. Hepatitis B–associated glomerulonephritis is more common in children than adults. Some patients with hepatitis B infection develop acute multisystem vasculitis, including renal vasculitis, within weeks or months of the acute hepatitis. They often manifest an acute serum sickness–like picture with fever, rash, arthralgias, and abdominal pain. The serologic profile includes positive HBsAg (hepatitis B surface antigen), positive HBcAb (hepatitis B core antibody), and negative HBsAb (hepatitis B surface antibody) titers. By contrast, MPGN or membranous glomerulonephritis occurs in the setting of more chronic hepatitis B viral infection and persistent HBsAg antigenemia. Patients typically have positive HBsAg, positive HBeAg (hepatitis B e antigen), and positive HBcAb titers, but are negative for HBsAb and HBeAb (44). Hypocomplementemia is detected in over 50 percent of cases, including both membranoproliferative and membranous forms. The most common presentation of hepatitis B virus–associated MPGN is nephrotic proteinuria, often with associated hematuria and renal insufficiency.

Light Microscopic Findings. A variety of patterns of glomerular disease are associated with hepatitis B infection. These include membranous glomerulopathy, MPGN type 1, MPGN type 3 (of Burkholder), MPGN secondary to cryoglobulinemia, IgA nephropathy, and renal vasculitis. The MPGN pattern by light microscopy may be indistinguishable from that of primary MPGN type 1 or type 3 (see fig. 10-8). In those with associated cryoglobulinemia, exudative features and intraluminal deposits are frequently seen.

Immunofluorescence Findings. Deposits of IgG, IgM, C3, and C1 are most commonly identified. Special studies have revealed hepatitis B antigens (including surface, core, and e antigens) in the subendothelial and subepithelial deposits (44).

Electron Microscopic Findings. Electron-dense deposits may be identified in mesangial, subendothelial, and subepithelial locations. An annular-tubular pattern of the deposit substructure may be seen in cases with associated cryoglobulinemia.

Pathogenesis. The pathogenesis involves the glomerular deposition of immune deposits in response to chronic hepatitis B virus antigenemia. This is one of the rare forms of secondary MPGN in which viral antigens are demonstrated in the glomerular immune deposits.

Treatment and Prognosis. In hepatitis B–associated MPGN, the glomerulonephritis often resolves spontaneously or following interferon therapy. Immunosuppression may be contraindicated due to the increased risk of activation of the hepatitis.

REFERENCES

1. Anders D, Agricola B, Sippel M, Thoenes W. Basement membrane changes in membranoproliferative glomerulonephritis II. Characterization of a third type by silver impregnation of ultra thin sections. Virchows Arch A Pathol Anat Histol 1977;376:1–19.
2. Arze RS, Rashid H, Morley R, Ward MK, Kerr DN. Shunt nephritis: report of two cases and review of the literature. Clin Nephrol 1983;19:48–53.
3. Beaufils M, Gibert C, Morel-Maroger L, et al. Glomerulonephritis in severe bacterial infections with and without endocarditis. Adv Nephrol Necker Hosp 1977;7:217–34.
4. Brouet JC, Clauvel JP, Danon F, Klein M, Seligmann M. Biologic and clinical significance of cryoglobulins. A report of 86 cases. Am J Med 1974;57:775–88.
5. Burkholder PM, Marchand A, Krueger RP. Mixed membranous and proliferative glomerulonephritis. A correlative light, immunofluorescence, and electron microscopic study. Lab Invest 1970;23:459–79.
6. Cameron JS, Turner DR, Heaton J, et al. Idiopathic mesangiocapillary glomerulonephritis. Comparison of types I and II in children and adults and long-term prognosis. Am J Med 1983;74:175–92.
7. D'Agati V. Membranoproliferative glomerulonephritis. In: Greenberg A, Cheung AK, Coffman TM, Falk RJ, Jeannette JC, eds. National Kidney Foundation primer on kidney diseases, 2nd ed. San Diego: Academic Press; 1998:153–60.

8. D'Amico G. Renal involvement in hepatitis C infection: cryoglobulinemic glomerulonephritis. Kidney Int 1998;54:650–71.
9. D'Amico G, Fornasieri A. Cryoglobulinemic glomerulonephritis: a membranoproliferative glomerulonephritis induced by hepatitis C virus. Am J Kidney Dis 1995;25:361–9.
10. Donadio JV Jr, Anderson CF, Mitchell JC 3rd, et al. Membranoproliferative glomerulonephritis. A prospective clinical trial of antiplatelet therapy. N Engl J Med 1984;310:1421–6.
11. Donadio JV Jr, Offord KP. Reassessment of treatment results in membranoproliferative glomerulonephritis, with emphasis on life-table analysis. Am J Kidney Dis 1989;14:445–51.
12. Fogo A, Qureshi N, Horn RG. Morphologic and clinical features of fibrillary glomerulonephritis versus immunotactoid glomerulopathy. Am J Kidney Dis 1993;22:367–77.
13. Ford DM, Briscoe DM, Shanley PF, Lum GM. Childhood membranoproliferative glomerulonephritis type I: limited steroid therapy. Kidney Int 1992;41:1606–12.
14. Gallo GR, Caulin-Glaser T, Lamm ME. Charge of circulating immune complexes as a factor in glomerular basement membrane localization in mice. J Clin Invest 1981;67:1305–13.
15. Garini G, Allegri L, Carnevali L, Catellani W, Manganelli P, Buzio C. Interferon-alpha in combination with ribavirin as initial treatment for hepatitis C virus-associated cryoglobulinemic membranoproliferative glomerulonephritis. Am J Kidney Dis 2001;38:E35.
16. Giannico G, Manno C, Schena FP. Treatment of glomerulonephritides associated with hepatitis C virus infection. Nephrol Dial Transplant 2000;15(Suppl 8):34–8.
17. Habib R, Gubler MC, Loirat C, Maiz HB, Levy M. Dense deposit disease: a variant of membranoproliferative glomerulonephritis. Kidney Int 1975;7:204–15.
18. Habib R, Kleinknecht C, Gubler MC, Levy M. Idiopathic membranoproliferative glomerulonephritis in children. Report of 105 cases. Clin Nephrol 1973;1:194–214.
19. Holley KE, Donadio JV Jr. Membranoproliferative glomerulonephritis. In: Tisher CC, Brenner BM, eds. Renal pathology, with clinical and functional correlations, 2nd ed. Philadelphia: Lippincott; 1994:294–329.
20. Hsu HC, Suzuki Y, Churg J, Grishman E. Ultrastructure of transplant glomerulopathy. Histopathology 1980;4:351–67.
21. Jefferson JA, Johnson RJ. Treatment of hepatitis C-associated glomerular disease. Semin Nephrol 2000;20:286–92.
22. Johnson RJ, Gretch DR, Couser WG, et al. Hepatitis C virus-associated glomerulonephritis. Effect of alpha-interferon therapy. Kidney Int 1994;46:1700–4.
23. Johnson RJ, Gretch DR, Yamabe H, et al. Membranoproliferative glomerulonephritis associated with hepatitis C virus infection. N Engl J Med 1993;328:465–70.
24. Johnson RJ, Willson R, Yamabe H, et al. Renal manifestations of hepatitis C virus infection. Kidney Int 1994;46:1255–63.
25. Levin A. Management of membranoproliferative glomerulonephritis: evidence-based recommendations. Kidney Int 1999;70(Suppl):S41–6.
26. Magil AB. Monocytes and glomerulonephritis associated with remote visceral infection. Clin Nephrol 1984;22:169–75.
27. Markowitz GS, Cheng JT, Colvin RB, Trebbin W, D'Agati VD. Hepatitis C viral infection is associated with fibrillary glomerulonephritis and immunotactoid glomerulopathy. J Am Soc Nephrol 1998;9:2244–52.
28. McCoy RC. Ultrastructural alterations in the kidney of patients with sickle cell disease and the nephrotic syndrome. Lab Invest 1969;21:85–95.
29. McEnery PT, McAdams AJ, West CD. The effect of prednisone in a high-dose, alternate-day regimen on the natural history of idiopathic membranoproliferative glomerulonephritis. Medicine 1985;64:401–24.
30. Mehta S, Levey JM, Bonkovsky HL. Extrahepatic manifestations of infection with hepatitis C virus. Clin Liv Dis 2001;5:979–1008.
31. Misiani R, Bellavita P, Fenili D, et al. Interferon alpha-2a therapy in cryoglobulinemia associated with hepatitis C virus. N Engl J Med 1994;330:751–6.
32. Monga G, Mazzucco G, di Belgiojoso GB, Busnach G. The presence and possible role of monocyte infiltration in human chronic proliferative glomerulonephritides. Light microscopic, immunofluorescence, and histochemical correlations. Am J Pathol 1979;94:271–84.
33. Pardo V, Strauss J, Kramer H, Ozawa T, McIntosh RM. Nephropathy associated with sickle cell anemia: an autologous immune complex nephritis. II. Clinicopathologic study of seven patients. Am J Med 1975;59:650–9.
34. Pouteil-Noble C, Maiza H, Dijoud F, MacGregor B. Glomerular disease associated with hepatitis C virus infection in native kidneys. Nephrol Dial Transplant 2000;(Suppl 8):28–33.
35. Rennke HG. Secondary membranoproliferative glomerulonephritis. Kidney Int 1995;47:643–56.

36. Sabry AA, Sobh MA, Irving WL, et al. A comprehensive study of the association between hepatitis C virus and glomerulopathy. Nephrol Dial Transplant 2002;17:239–45.
37. Sibley RK, Kim Y. Dense intramembranous deposit disease: new pathologic features. Kidney Int 1984;25:660–70.
38. Strife CF, Hug G, Chuck G, McAdams AJ, Davis CA, Kline JJ. Membranoproliferative glomerulonephritis and alpha 1-antitrypsin deficiency in children. Pediatrics 1983;71:88–92.
39. Strife CF, Jackson EC, McAdams AJ. Type III membranoproliferative glomerulonephritis: long-term clinical and morphologic evaluation. Clin Nephrol 1984;21:323–34.
40. Strife CF, McAdams AJ, West CD. Membranoproliferative glomerulonephritis characterized by focal, segmental proliferative lesions. Clin Nephrol 1982;18:9–16.
41. Strife CF, McEnery PT, McAdams AJ, West CD. Membranoproliferative glomerulonephritis with disruption of the glomerular basement membrane. Clin Nephrol 1977;7:65–72.
42. Tarshish P, Bernstein J, Tobin JN, Edelmann CM Jr. Treatment of mesangiocapillary glomerulonephritis with alternate-day prednisone—a report of the International Study of Kidney Disease in Children. Pediatr Nephrol 1992;6:123–30.
43. Varade WS, Forristal J, West CD. Patterns of complement activation in idiopathic membranoproliferative glomerulonephritis types I, II, and III. Am J Kidney Dis 1990;16:196–206.
44. Venkataseshan VS, Lieberman K, Kim DU, et al. Hepatitis-B-associated glomerulonephritis: pathology, pathogenesis, and clinical course. Medicine 1990;69:200–16.
45. West CD. Childhood membranoproliferative glomerulonephritis: an approach to management. Kidney Int 1986;29:1077–93.
46. White RH. Quartan malarial nephrotic syndrome. Nephron 1973;11:147–62.

11 ACUTE POSTINFECTIOUS GLOMERULONEPHRITIS AND OTHER BACTERIAL INFECTIOUS GLOMERULONEPHRITIDES

ACUTE POSTINFECTIOUS GLOMERULONEPHRITIS AND ACUTE DIFFUSE PROLIFERATIVE GLOMERULONEPHRITIS

Definition. Acute postinfectious glomerulonephritis is caused by an acute, usually self-limited, infection. The most common cause is streptococcal infection, in which case the term *acute poststreptococcal glomerulonephritis* is appropriate. During the acute phase, the most frequent histologic pattern of injury is an acute diffuse proliferative glomerulonephritis with conspicuous glomerular capillary neutrophils. Other patterns of proliferative glomerulonephritis are caused by transient infections, and postinfectious acute diffuse proliferative glomerulonephritis evolves through other patterns of injury as it resolves, including mesangioproliferative glomerulonephritis.

Although acute diffuse proliferative glomerulonephritis is most often caused by transient acute bacterial infection, this pattern of injury is not completely specific for this etiology because it also can be caused by more persistent infections with bacteria, viruses, and other pathogens. Glomerulonephritis that accompanies persistent infections often is called "infectious" glomerulonephritis rather than "postinfectious" glomerulonephritis. The first section of this chapter focuses on postinfectious glomerulonephritis and the following sections on other forms of infectious glomerulonephritis caused by bacteria; infectious glomerulonephritis caused by viruses is discussed in other chapters.

Clinical Features. Acute postinfectious glomerulonephritis is most frequent in children but can occur at any age. The peak age of onset is between 5 and 20 years of age (44,47). Recurrences are rare. There is a male predominance of 2 or 3 to 1 (44,47).

Over the past century, this disease has declined in frequency in economically developed countries, but continues to be a major cause of acute nephritis in developing countries, especially in Africa and Asia (16,31,35,55). Although streptococci remain the leading cause of acute postinfectious glomerulonephritis, staphylococci now are a more frequent cause than in the past (31). Predisposing factors for postinfectious and other forms of infectious glomerulonephritis include alcoholism, diabetes, and intravenous drug abuse (31). The frequency of poststreptococcal glomerulonephritis is probably underestimated because some patients with well-developed pathologic lesions have minimal clinical manifestations of nephritis (53). The prognosis is very good in children (greater than 90 percent with complete recovery), but worse in adults (25 percent or more with long-term sequelae) (42,44).

Acute poststreptococcal glomerulonephritis typically becomes clinically apparent 1 to 3 weeks after the onset of pharyngitis and 3 to 6 weeks after the onset of pyoderma (35). The most common clinical and laboratory features of poststreptococcal glomerulonephritis and other forms of acute postinfectious glomerulonephritis are gross or microscopic hematuria, proteinuria (usually greater than 2.5 g/day), and renal insufficiency that may be accompanied by oliguria (44,46). Most patients develop edema and hypertension related to salt and water retention. Hypocomplementemia is frequent. When evaluated during the acute phase, more than 90 percent of patients have decreased complement (C)3 levels and total hemolytic complement (CH) 50, although fewer than 10 percent have decreased C4 levels. C3 typically returns to normal within 2 months. Rising antistreptococcal antibody titers are identified in 80 percent of patients with acute poststreptococcal glomerulonephritis.

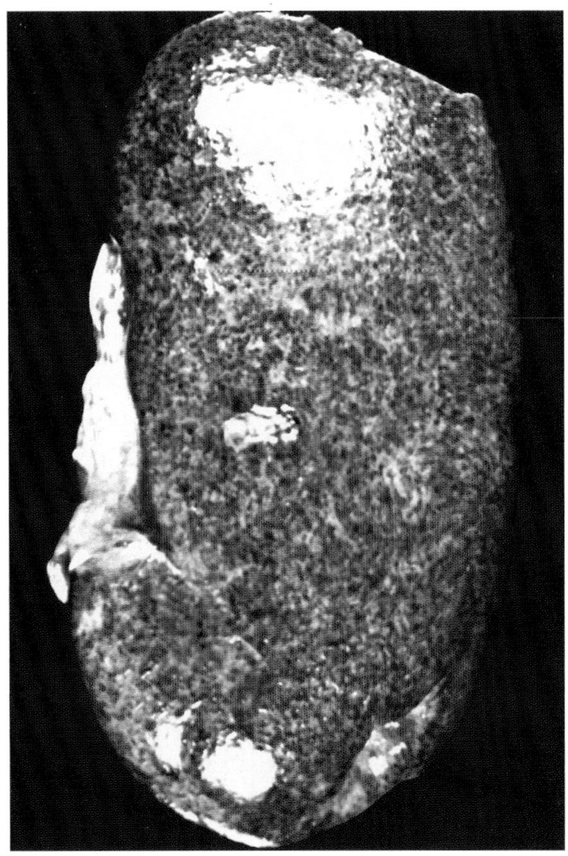

Figure 11-1

POSTINFECTIOUS ACUTE DIFFUSE PROLIFERATIVE GLOMERULONEPHRITIS

Specimen from a child who died of renal failure caused by acute poststreptococcal glomerulonephritis in the 1940s, prior to the availability of dialysis. Note the "flea-bitten" appearance caused by hemorrhage into Bowman's spaces and tubular lumens. (Courtesy of Dr. C. Pirani, New York, NY.)

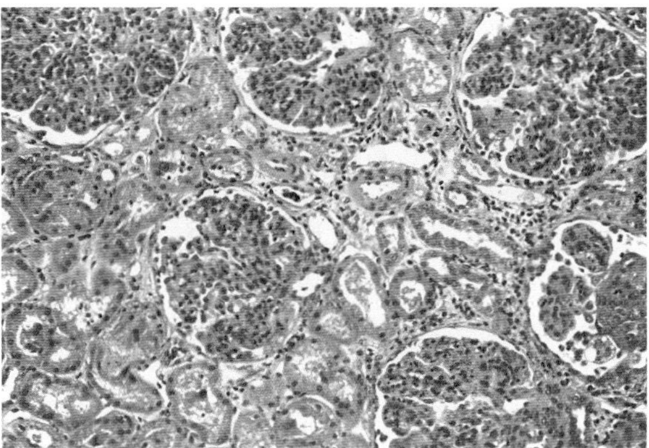

Figure 11-2

POSTINFECTIOUS ACUTE DIFFUSE PROLIFERATIVE GLOMERULONEPHRITIS

There is diffuse, global, marked endocapillary hypercellularity caused by extensive neutrophilic infiltration. There is only slight focal interstitial edema and infiltration of predominantly mononuclear leukocytes (hematoxylin and eosin [H&E] stain).

Evaluation of antistreptolysin O (ASO) titers is more sensitive for documenting streptococcal pharyngitis while analysis of anti-DNase-B is more sensitive for streptococcal pyoderma. Rising titers are more specific than a static elevation. Positive assays for cryoglobulins or C3 nephritic factor do not rule out poststreptococcal glomerulonephritis.

A minority of patients with poststreptococcal glomerulonephritis have crescentic glomerulonephritis, with an unusually aggressive course and poorer outcome (3). In children, poststreptococcal glomerulonephritis is the second most common cause of crescentic glomerulonephritis after lupus nephritis (3,12,55).

A renal biopsy is not required for the management of patients with typical, uncomplicated, self-limited poststreptococcal glomerulonephritis. Atypical clinical features that prompt renal biopsy include absence of antistreptococcal antibodies, absence of hypocomplementemia, more severe or more persistent (more than 6 weeks) renal failure than expected, persistence of hypocomplementemia beyond 2 months, persistence of proteinuria beyond 6 months, or persistence of hematuria beyond 12 months.

Gross Findings. Because typical acute postinfectious glomerulonephritis is not lethal, gross observations are rare. The typical finding is swelling of the kidney and, if there is severe hematuria, a "flea-bitten" appearance characterized by numerous tiny red dots caused by the red blood cells within Bowman's spaces and tubular lumens (fig. 11-1). This is a nonspecific finding that is seen with any type of glomerulonephritis that causes marked hematuria.

Light Microscopic Findings. The most frequent histologic pattern of glomerular injury in acute postinfectious glomerulonephritis, including acute poststreptococcal glomerulonephritis, is acute diffuse proliferative glomerulonephritis (figs. 11-2–11-7). Acute diffuse proliferative glomerulonephritis is characterized by numerous neutrophils ("acute") and endocapillary hypercellularity ("proliferative") affecting all

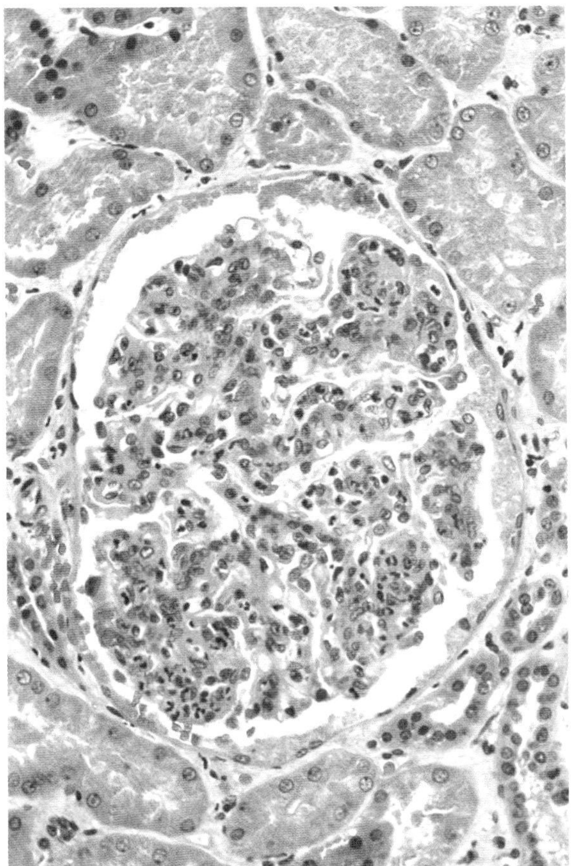

Figure 11-3

POSTINFECTIOUS ACUTE DIFFUSE PROLIFERATIVE GLOMERULONEPHRITIS

Marked global hypercellularity is caused by endocapillary hypercellularity and an influx of leukocytes, including many segmented neutrophils. Many capillary lumens are obscured or occluded. Some of the few capillary walls that can be seen appear thickened (H&E stain).

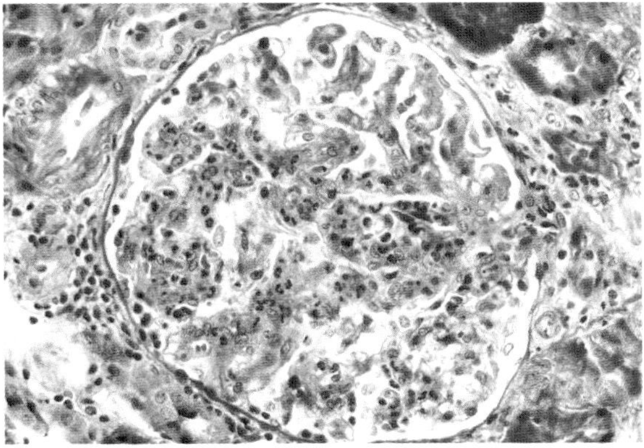

Figure 11-4

POSTINFECTIOUS ACUTE DIFFUSE PROLIFERATIVE GLOMERULONEPHRITIS

This Masson trichrome stain reveals no increase in collagenous mesangial matrix and no replication of glomerular basement membranes, which distinguish this lesion from type 1 membranoproliferative glomerulonephritis. There is slight edema and infiltration by leukocytes in the periglomerular interstitium.

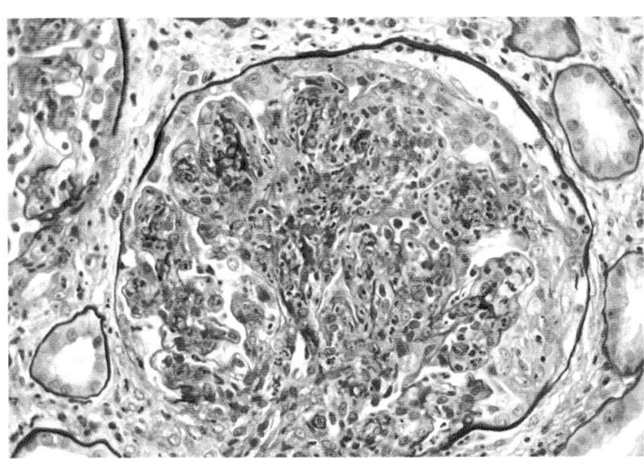

Figure 11-5

POSTINFECTIOUS ACUTE DIFFUSE PROLIFERATIVE GLOMERULONEPHRITIS WITH A CRESCENT

Extracapillary hypercellularity (crescent formation) is seen above and to the right of the tuft. There is intense inflammation of the glomerulus, with numerous neutrophils in capillary lumens and infiltrating the mesangium. There appears to be some lysis of the mesangial matrix, slight focal lysis of glomerular basement membranes, and focal lysis of Bowman's capsule. There is edema and infiltration of neutrophils into the periglomerular interstitium (Jones methenamine sliver [JMS] stain and H&E counterstain).

glomeruli ("diffuse") (15,24,40,44,46,47). This lesion also has been called "exudative" glomerulonephritis because of the numerous neutrophils; however, this is a misnomer because most of the neutrophils are inside capillaries rather than exuded into extravascular sites. Eosinophils may be present in addition to neutrophils (15,24,40). Monocytes, and to a lesser extent lymphocytes, contribute to the endocapillary hypercellularity but are difficult to identify without special immunohistochemical stains (36). Extracapillary hypercellularity (crescent formation) is present in the most severe cases (figs. 11-5, 11-6), however, crescents typically affect less than 50 percent of glomeruli (15,40, 44,46). Segmental necrosis and capillary thrombosis are uncommon (46). With the Masson trichrome stain, large subepithelial immune deposits may be identifiable as fuchsinophilic (red)

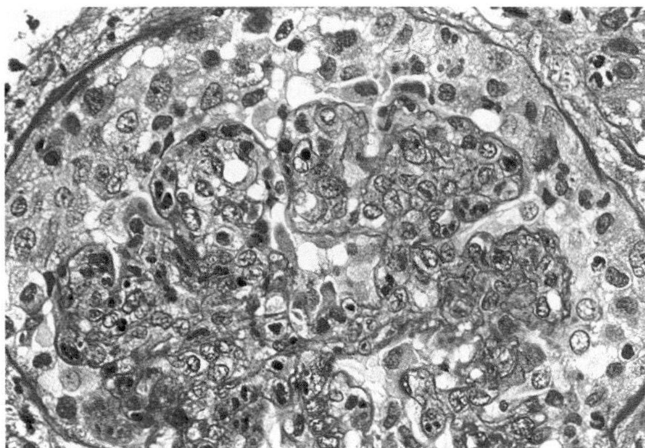

Figure 11-6

POSTINFECTIOUS ACUTE DIFFUSE PROLIFERATIVE GLOMERULONEPHRITIS

The periodic acid–Schiff (PAS) stain demonstrates extensive extracapillary hypercellularity (crescent formation) and extensive endocapillary hypercellularity. The latter is contributed to by the influx of segmented neutrophils as well as by the proliferation of endogenous glomerular cells, including endothelial cells and mesangial cells.

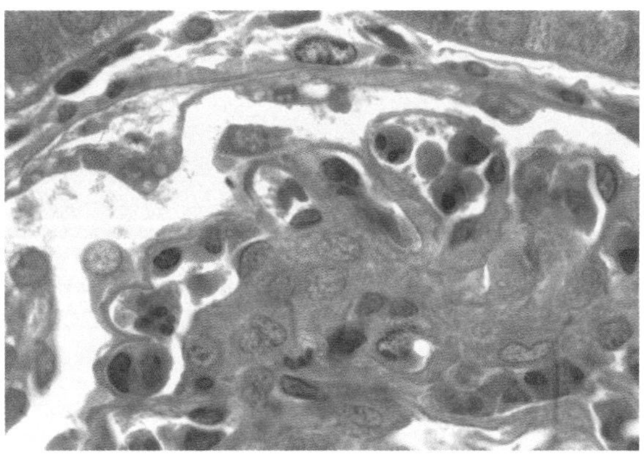

Figure 11-7

POSTINFECTIOUS ACUTE DIFFUSE PROLIFERATIVE GLOMERULONEPHRITIS

High magnification view of a segment showing irregularly thickened capillary walls, increased neutrophils and monocytes in capillary lumens, and endothelial and mesangial hypercellularity. An eosinophil is present in the lower right quadrant (H&E stain).

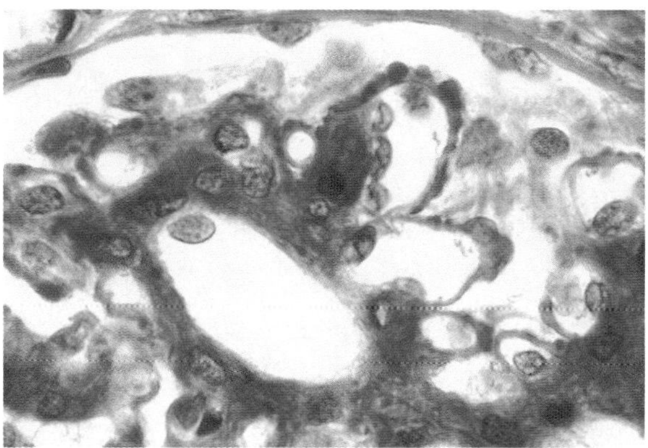

Figure 11-8

POSTINFECTIOUS ACUTE DIFFUSE PROLIFERATIVE GLOMERULONEPHRITIS

High magnification view of a Masson trichrome–stained glomerular segment shows well-defined, subepithelial, fuchsinophilic (red) hump-like deposits sitting on top of the blue glomerular basement membrane.

granules on the outer aspect of capillaries and adjacent to paramesangial basement membranes (fig. 11-8). Intramembranous, subendothelial, and mesangial deposits are more difficult to identify. Staining of sections that are oblique to glomerular basement membranes with the Jones methenamine silver (JMS) stain may reveal small, round, pale (less silver-positive) foci that correspond to intramembranous deposits (49). Glomerular basement membrane replication is rare in acute postinfectious glomerulonephritis (46), which helps to distinguish it from type 1 membranoproliferative glomerulonephritis.

There may be little or no tubulointerstitial changes in the early phase of overt acute postinfectious glomerulonephritis (fig. 11-2). The most frequent finding is slight interstitial edema and mild periglomerular interstitial infiltration by predominantly mononuclear leukocytes (40). If the acute glomerular inflammation is severe, there may be more pronounced interstitial edema and interstitial infiltration by leukocytes, including neutrophils (fig. 11-9). Neutrophilic tubulitis may occur. Tubular lumens often contain red blood cells and occasionally, neutrophils (fig. 11-10).

As the acute inflammation typically resolves between 1 and 2 months after onset, the glomerular lesions progressively lose neutrophils and the endocapillary hypercellularity evolves into pure mesangial hypercellularity, which in turn resolves to leave a normal-appearing glomerulus (24,40,44,46,49). The first change is a loss of neutrophils and an opening of the lumens that have been narrowed or occluded by endocapillary

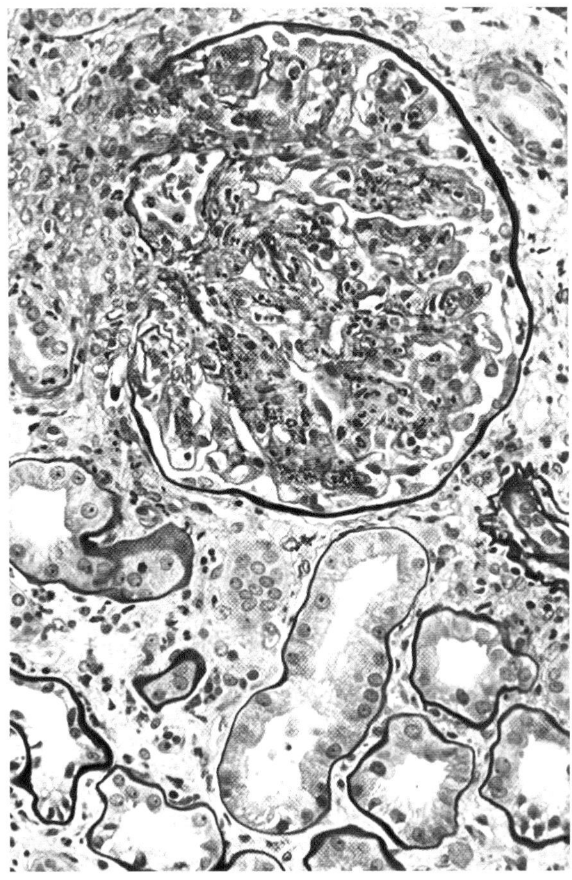

Figure 11-9

POSTINFECTIOUS ACUTE DIFFUSE PROLIFERATIVE GLOMERULONEPHRITIS

There is periglomerular interstitial edema and infiltration by leukocytes, including neutrophils. The distal tubule adjacent to the hilum shows acute tubulitis with neutrophils between epithelial cells (JMS stain).

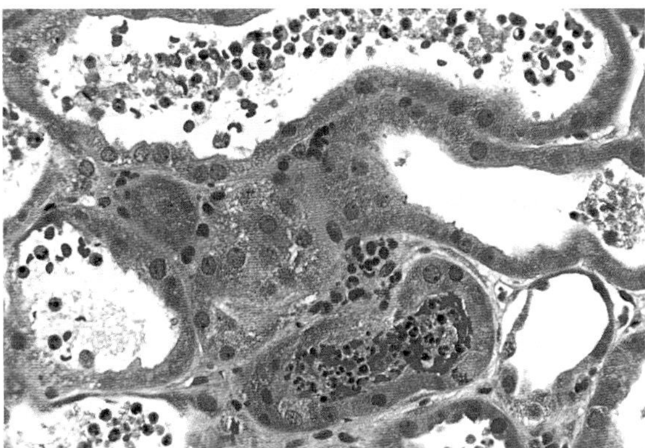

Figure 11-10

ACUTE POSTINFECTIOUS GLOMERULONEPHRITIS

Tubular lumens contain red blood cells and neutrophils that have spilled out of acutely inflamed glomeruli.

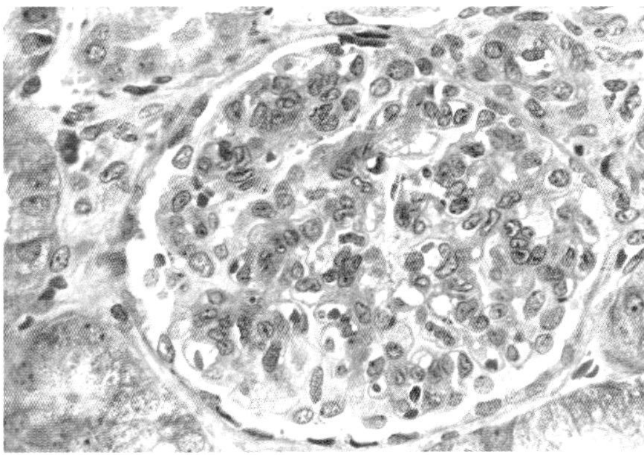

Figure 11-11

RESOLVING POSTINFECTIOUS GLOMERULONEPHRITIS

This specimen was obtained 2 months into the course of a streptococcal pyoderma–induced postinfectious glomerulonephritis that resulted in unusually persistent renal insufficiency (serum creatinine, 2.5 mg/dL), hematuria, and proteinuria. There is diffuse proliferative glomerulonephritis with substantial endocapillary hypercellularity but no neutrophils (see figure 11-17 for immunofluorescence findings) (Masson trichrome stain).

hypercellularity and leukocyte influx (fig. 11-11) (24). During the first 2 weeks after onset, over 75 percent of specimens show marked glomerular neutrophil infiltration, compared to less than 20 percent at 3 to 4 weeks after onset, and none at 6 weeks after onset (46). As the neutrophils disappear, the complex endocapillary hypercellularity simplifies to pure mesangial hypercellularity, with varying degrees of increased mesangial matrix (fig. 11-12) (40). Mild mesangial hypercellularity or matrix expansion may persist for several years. Eventually, in most patients, even the mesangial expansion resolves and the glomerulus recovers its normal histology (8,40). However, the most destructive inflammatory glomerular lesions evolve into focal, usually segmental, sclerotic glomerular lesions that persist (fig. 11-13) (40,49). Active glomerular inflammation that persists longer than 6 months raises the possibility of an infectious glomerulonephritis other than postinfectious glomerulonephritis.

The histologic appearance of postinfectious glomerulonephritis varies in severity among

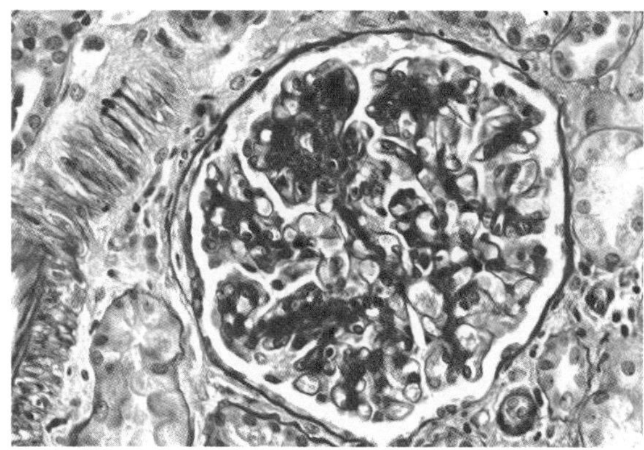

Figure 11-12

RESOLVING POSTINFECTIOUS GLOMERULONEPHRITIS

This specimen is from a patient who had persistent proteinuria (over 2 g/day) and hematuria 4 months after streptococcal pharyngitis and an earlier episode of even more active nephritis. Most glomeruli were normal by light microscopy, but others, such as the one illustrated here, had segmental mesangial hypercellularity (see figure 11-18 for the immunofluorescence results) (PAS stain).

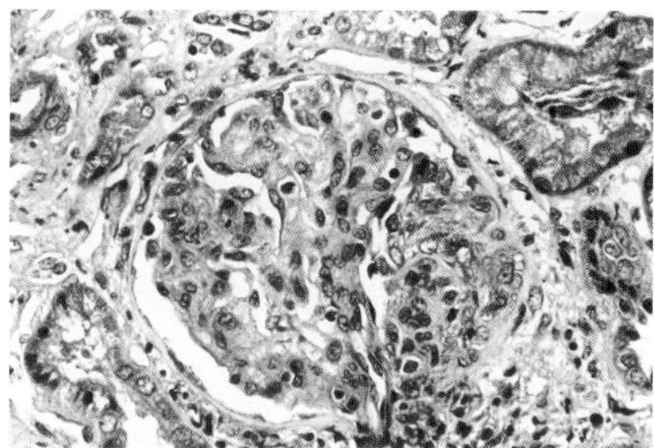

Figure 11-13

POSTINFECTIOUS SCLEROSING GLOMERULONEPHRITIS

Glomerular scarring developed secondary to poststreptococcal glomerulonephritis. There is residual endocapillary hypercellularity with increased matrix material and an adhesion to Bowman's capsule. Adjacent to the glomerulus is interstitial fibrosis, chronic inflammation, and tubular atrophy (Masson trichrome stain).

different patients, and varies over time in an individual patient. All of the pathologic expressions, not just the classic acute presentation, must be recognized to accurately diagnose postinfectious glomerulonephritis.

Immunofluorescence Findings. As is true for the histology, the findings by immunohistology vary in severity and pattern among different patients, and over time in individual patients (44,46,47). In fact, the different glomerular distributions of immune reactants probably are the basis for the variations in the histologic appearance of the glomerular lesions. In the acute phase of postinfectious glomerulonephritis, the most common finding is a coarsely granular capillary wall and mesangial staining for complement alone, or complement and immunoglobulins (figs. 11-14–11-17) (44,46). Rarely in the acute phase, but commonly in the resolving phase, there is mesangial staining without capillary wall staining (fig. 11-18). Staining for C3 and other complement components is more frequent and usually more intense than staining for immunoglobulins (Table 11-1; figs. 11-16, 11-17) (30–32,35,46). Staining for C3 degradation products (such as C3d) and terminal complement components, including the membrane attack complex, often is intense (fig. 11-17C) (36).

There is controversy over how often and when immunoglobulins are seen. Some investigators conclude that immunoglobulin deposition usually occurs early (e.g., during the first 2 weeks) (46), whereas others suggest that it occurs after complement deposition (35). This issue is discussed further in the section on pathogenesis. Immunoglobulin (Ig)G is seen most often and most intensely in acute postinfectious glomerulonephritis whereas IgM is seen most often and most intensely in glomerulonephritis caused by persistent infections (Table 11-1).

Sorger and associates (46,47) have categorized the immunostaining seen with acute postinfectious glomerulonephritis into three patterns: starry sky pattern, garland pattern, and mesangial pattern. The description of these patterns provides a basis for understanding the spectrum of staining patterns seen in acute postinfectious glomerulonephritis, but many specimens have mixed patterns of staining that cannot be placed readily into one category.

The starry sky pattern is characterized by many, relatively discrete granules of staining scattered over the glomerular tuft, thus mimicking the random distribution of stars in the sky (fig. 11-14, right). The ultrastructural basis for this pattern is the occurrence of scattered subepithelial, intramembranous, subendothelial,

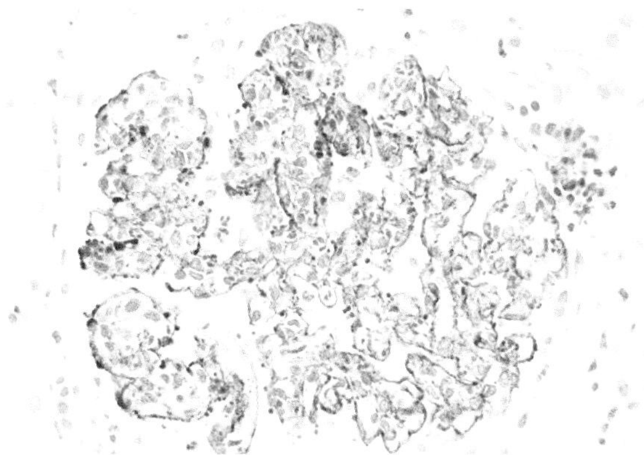

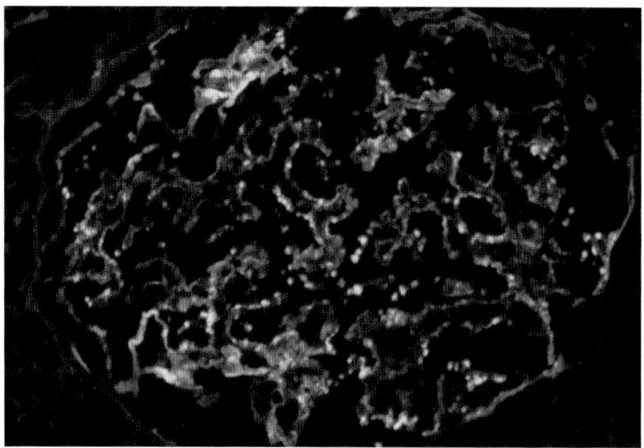

Figure 11-14

COMPLEMENT (C)3 IMMUNOSTAINING IN POSTINFECTIOUS ACUTE DIFFUSE PROLIFERATIVE GLOMERULONEPHRITIS

Immunoenzyme microscopy (left) and immunofluorescence microscopy (right) show coarse granular staining of capillary walls and adjacent to paramesangial basement membranes, and less pronounced staining in the mesangium.

and mesangial immune deposits (46). The absence of a predominance of deposits in any one glomerular location causes the scattered pattern seen by immunohistology.

The garland pattern is characterized by a closely aligned, sometimes confluent, subepithelial granular to band-like staining pattern (fig. 11-16A) (46). The more intense peripheral staining in the glomerular segments produces a peripheral band that resembles a garland around the segments. The ultrastructural basis for the garland pattern is the presence of numerous subepithelial immune deposits, most with a hump configuration but some with broad bases (46). Subendothelial and mesangial deposits are less frequent than in the starry sky pattern. The garland pattern often is more apparent in some glomerular segments than others. In fact, some specimens have quite variable mixtures of starry sky and garland staining patterns in different segments within glomeruli and among different glomeruli.

As indicated by the name, the mesangial pattern is characterized by predominantly or exclusively mesangial staining (fig. 11-18) (46). The staining usually is predominantly or exclusively for complement, with little or no staining for immunoglobulins (32,46). This pattern occurs most often in specimens obtained late after onset, and in many instances probably represents the resolving phase of acute postinfectious glomerulonephritis that at an earlier time had more widespread deposits. Some milder cases, however, never develop glomerular lesions that are more severe than mesangial deposits with mesangial hypercellularity alone. Ultrastructural findings in patients with acute postinfectious glomerulonephritis who have the mesangial staining pattern also suggest that this represents resolving disease because the subepithelial deposits that are present are primarily adjacent to the paramesangial basement membranes and often have low electron density, which are features of resolving subepithelial deposits (46).

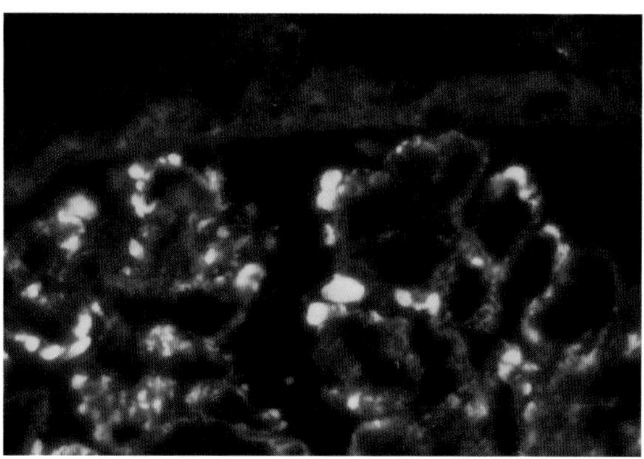

Figure 11-15

C3 IMMUNOSTAINING IN POSTINFECTIOUS ACUTE DIFFUSE PROLIFERATIVE GLOMERULONEPHRITIS

High magnification microscopy shows bright staining for C3 in large subepithelial deposits and low intensity staining of small intramembranous/subendothelial and mesangial deposits.

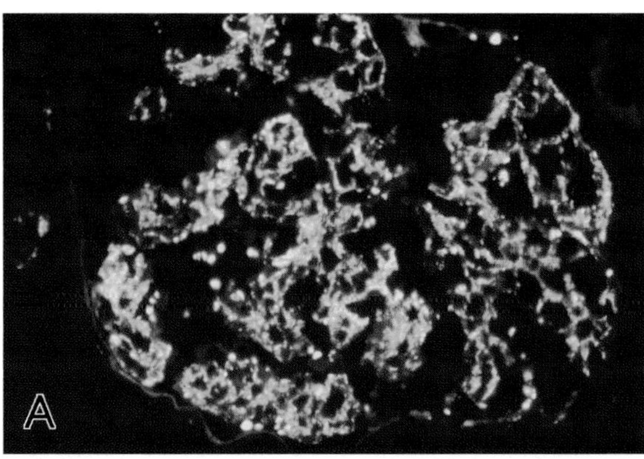

Figure 11-16

POSTINFECTIOUS ACUTE DIFFUSE PROLIFERATIVE GLOMERULONEPHRITIS

There is intense, coarsely granular staining for C3 (A) with only minor staining for IgG (B) or IgM (C).

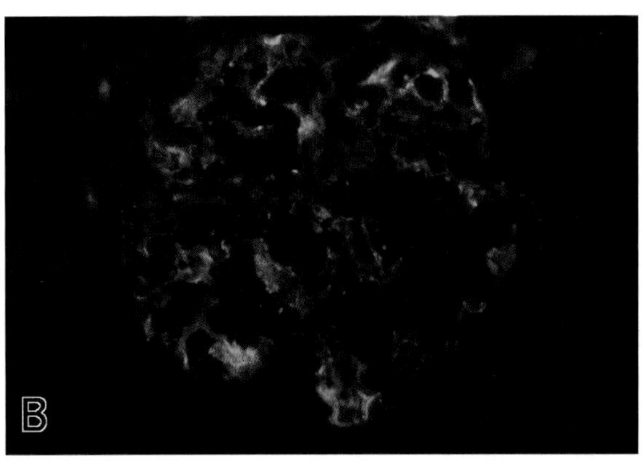

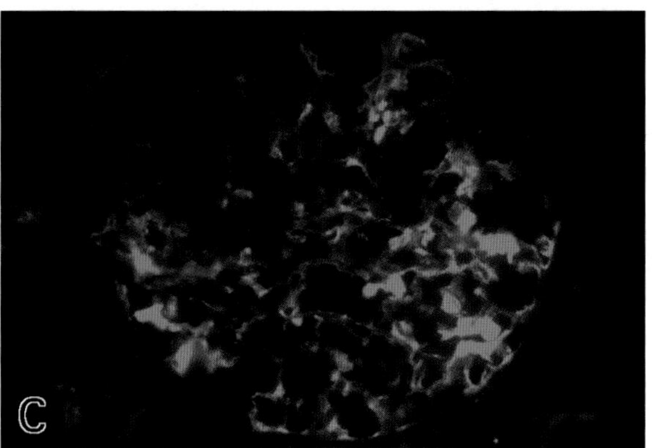

Table 11-1

GLOMERULAR IMMUNE DEPOSITS DETECTED BY IMMUNOFLUORESCENCE MICROSCOPY AND ELECTRON MICROSCOPY[a]

	Acute Postinfectious Glomerulonephritis n = 52	Endocarditis Glomerulonephritis n = 9	Shunt Glomerulonephritis n = 4
Immunofluorescence Microscopy			
IgG	72% / 1.4+[b]	89% / 1.2+	50% / 1.5+
IgM	42% / 0.7+	89% / 1.8+	100% / 2.2+
IgA	47% / 0.7+	78% / 0.8+	50% / 0.5+
C3	100% / 3.0+	89% / 2.3+	100% / 2.1+
C1q	23% / 0.7+	78% / 1.5+	100% / 2.0+
Dense Deposits by Electron Microscopy			
Mesangial	92%	89%	100%
Subendothelial	85%	89%	100%
Subepithelial	86%	33%	50%
M and IgG (not shown)			

[a]Consecutive patients with acute diffuse proliferative glomerulonephritis consistent with postinfectious glomerulonephritis, infectious endocarditis glomerulonephritis, and infectious shunt glomerulonephritis were evaluated at the University of North Carolina Nephropathology Laboratory.

[b]The immunofluorescence microscopy results are expressed as the percent of specimens that were positive and the mean intensity when positive on a scale of 0 to 4+.

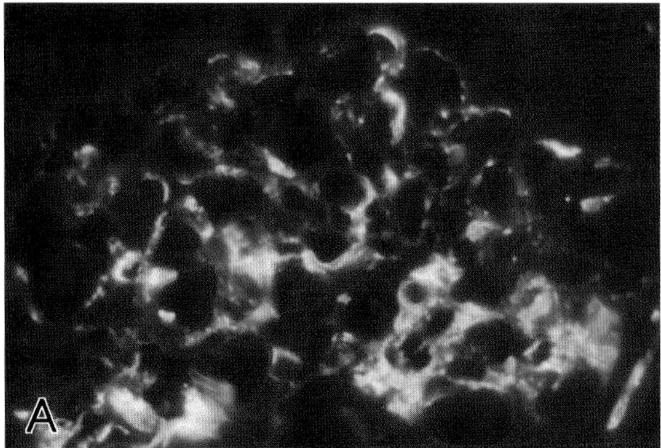

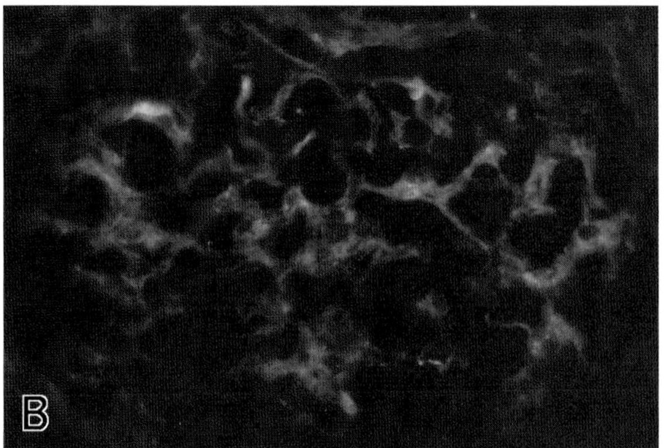

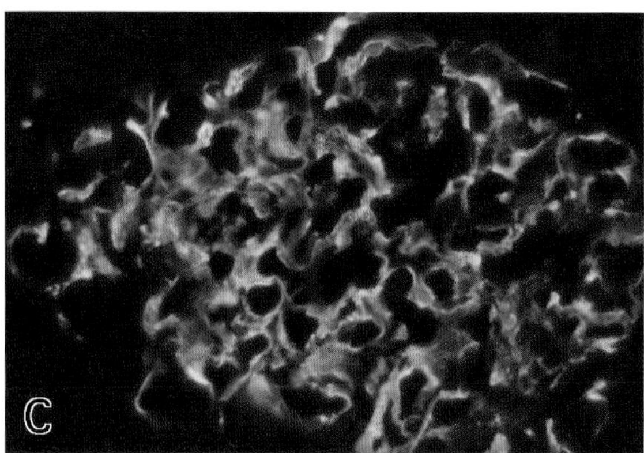

Figure 11-17

RESOLVING POSTINFECTIOUS GLOMERULONEPHRITIS

Immunofluorescence microscopy on same specimen as in figure 11-11 shows segmental capillary wall staining and prominent mesangial staining with anti-C3 (A) but not with a polyspecific antibody that reacts with IgG, IgA, and IgM (B). There is extensive capillary wall and mesangial staining with an antiserum specific for C3d (C).

Electron Microscopic Findings. The most distinctive ultrastructural feature of acute postinfectious glomerulonephritis is the presence of electron-dense deposits, especially the large subepithelial deposits called "humps" (figs. 11-19–11-22). During the acute phase (initial several weeks), most glomeruli have subepithelial, intramembranous, subendothelial (figs. 11-21, 11-22), and mesangial electron-dense deposits (16,24,30,44,46,47,49). The subepithelial deposits (humps) usually are very conspicuous. In general, they are larger, more variable in size and shape, less numerous, and less regularly distributed than the subepithelial electron-dense deposits of membranous glomerulopathy. Unlike membranous glomerulopathy, there are no adjacent projections of basement membrane material ("spikes"). Some specimens have numerous (seven or more per capillary loop), sometimes confluent, subepithelial deposits that correspond to the garland pattern of staining by immunofluorescence microscopy (figs. 11-19, 11-20) (16,46,47). Other specimens have fewer subepithelial deposits and more numerous subendothelial and mesangial deposits (fig. 11-22). This ultrastructural pattern corresponds to the starry sky pattern by immunofluorescence microscopy (16). Mild acute and resolving lesions have predominantly or exclusively

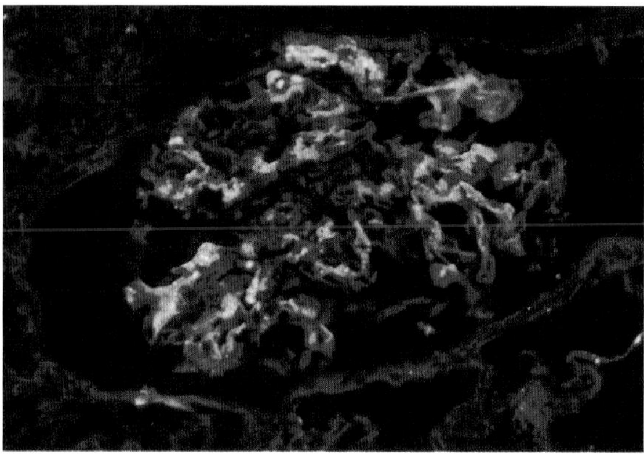

Figure 11-18

RESOLVING POSTINFECTIOUS GLOMERULONEPHRITIS

Same specimen as in figure 11-12 shows predominantly mesangial staining for C3. There was no staining for IgG, IgM, or IgA.

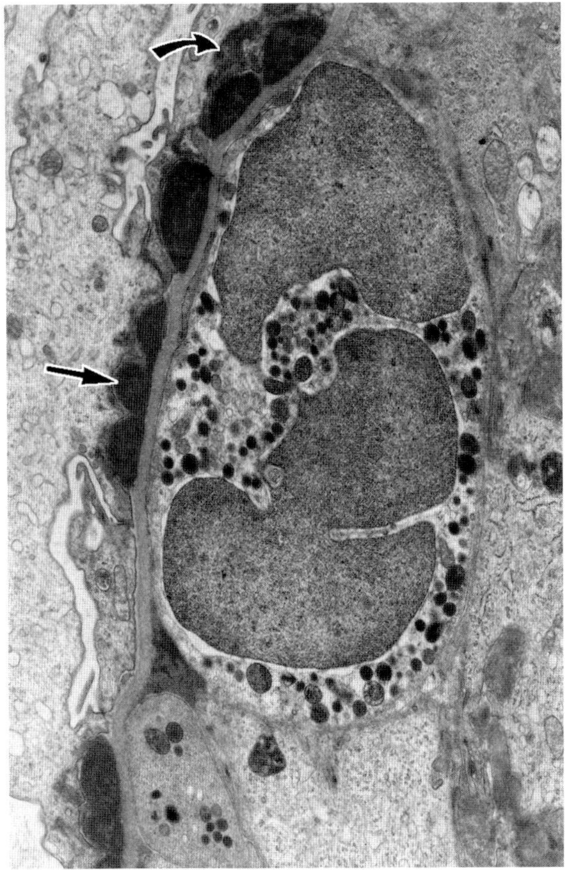

Figure 11-19

ACUTE POSTINFECTIOUS GLOMERULONEPHRITIS

Numerous subepithelial electron-dense deposits (humps; straight arrow) are covered by visceral epithelial cytoplasm. Effaced foot processes and dense condensations of cytoskeleton (curved arrow) are adjacent to the subepithelial deposits. The neutrophil, which contains numerous cytoplasmic granules, is marginated directly against the glomerular basement membrane at a site of endothelial denudation.

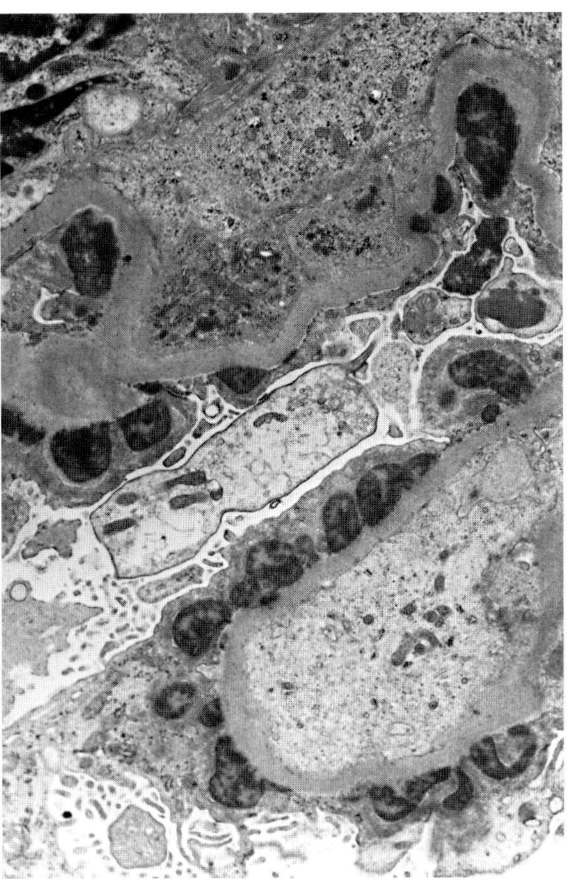

Figure 11-20

ACUTE POSTINFECTIOUS GLOMERULONEPHRITIS

Numerous subepithelial electron-dense deposits have a variegated appearance. There is marked endothelial cell swelling that is occluding the capillary lumens.

mesangial dense deposits that correspond to the mesangial pattern of staining by immunofluorescence microscopy (16). Capillary wall subepithelial deposits tend to resolve first, thus resolving lesions may have subepithelial deposits only in the "notch" region overlying the paramesangial basement membrane.

The largest subepithelial deposits typically have diameters ranging from 1 to 3 μm (49). Initially, they are denser than the lamina densa of the glomerular basement membrane. They are usually homogeneous but may be variegated (fig. 11-20). The deposits, especially in the acute phase, rarely indent the lamina densa or project into the adjacent basement membrane material. There may be thinning or lamination of the glomerular basement membrane beneath the subepithelial deposits or elsewhere in the glomerulus during the acute and resolving phases (fig. 11-23) (30). Gaps may occur in the glomerular basement membrane and often appear to be plugged by invaginations of podocyte cytoplasm. Occasionally, subepithelial, electron-dense deposits are continuous with intramembranous dense deposits (40). The visceral epithelial foot processes overlying subepithelial deposits are effaced, and the epithelial cytoplasm contains condensed cytoskeletal elements, predominantly actin (figs. 11-19, 11-23). Subendothelial deposits usually are small and scattered, and may be overlooked if not sought diligently

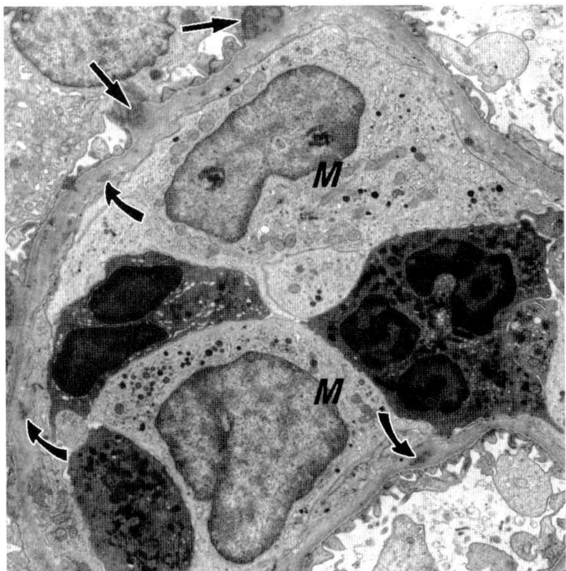

Figure 11-21

ACUTE POSTINFECTIOUS GLOMERULONEPHRITIS

Neutrophils with segmented nuclei and numerous cytoplasmic granules, and monocytes (M) with fewer granules are occluding the capillary lumen. The capillary wall has scattered subepithelial dense deposits (straight arrows) and small subendothelial deposits (curved arrows).

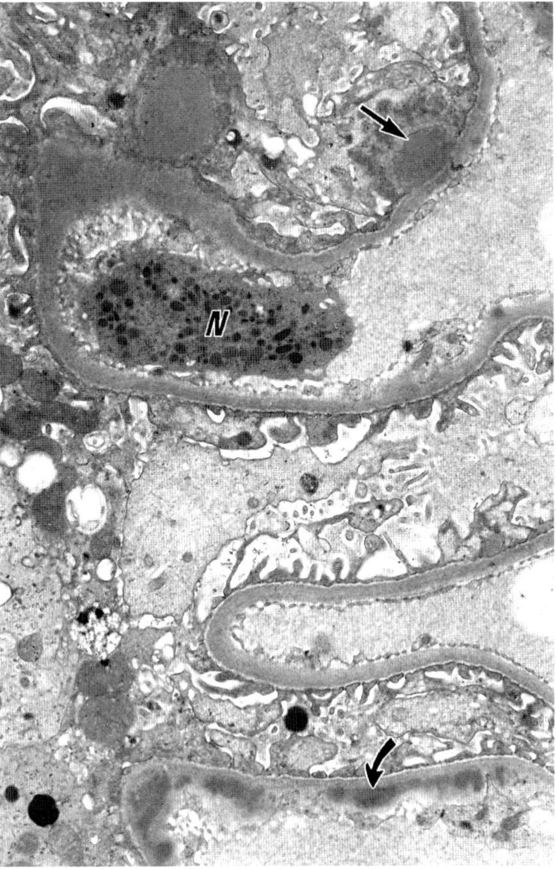

Figure 11-22

ACUTE POSTINFECTIOUS GLOMERULONEPHRITIS

Three capillary loops show scattered subepithelial (straight arrow) and subendothelial (curved arrow) electron-dense deposits. There is a neutrophil in one lumen (N).

(fig. 11-22). In the acute phase, the endothelial cytoplasm often is swollen (fig. 11-20) and may be focally denuded (fig. 11-19) (15). Neutrophils may be marginated on areas of denuded basement membrane (fig. 11-19). Capillary lumens may be narrowed or occluded by endothelial swelling, endothelial proliferation, mesangial proliferation, matrix expansion, and influx of neutrophils and monocytes/macrophages (fig. 11-21) (24). In the most severe lesions, there may be capillary thrombosis.

With resolution of the inflammation, there is a progressive loss of hypercellularity, beginning with loss of neutrophils and ending with resolution of mesangial hypercellularity. The electron-dense subepithelial deposits typically begin to loose their density 4 to 6 weeks after the onset of acute postinfectious glomerulonephritis (fig. 11-24), and eventually disappear completely with resolution of the disease (15,30,49). The number of subepithelial deposits progressively declines over time. Subepithelial deposits in peripheral capillary loops are lost first, leaving subepithelial deposits predominantly external to the paramesangial basement membranes.

As the subepithelial deposits disappear, there is an increase in irregular, variably electron-dense vacuoles in visceral epithelial cells (fig. 11-24), which may be the result of internalization of material from the deposits (30,49). Obliquely cut sections through subepithelial deposits that appear to be completely within the epithelial cytoplasm but at another plane of section are in contact with the glomerular basement membrane may be misinterpreted as intraepithelial vacuoles containing dense material (24).

Although rarely present in the acute phase, in the later phase of acute postinfectious glomerulonephritis there may be projections of glomerular basement membrane material adjacent to fading subepithelial deposits (49). These subepithelial basement membrane irregularities

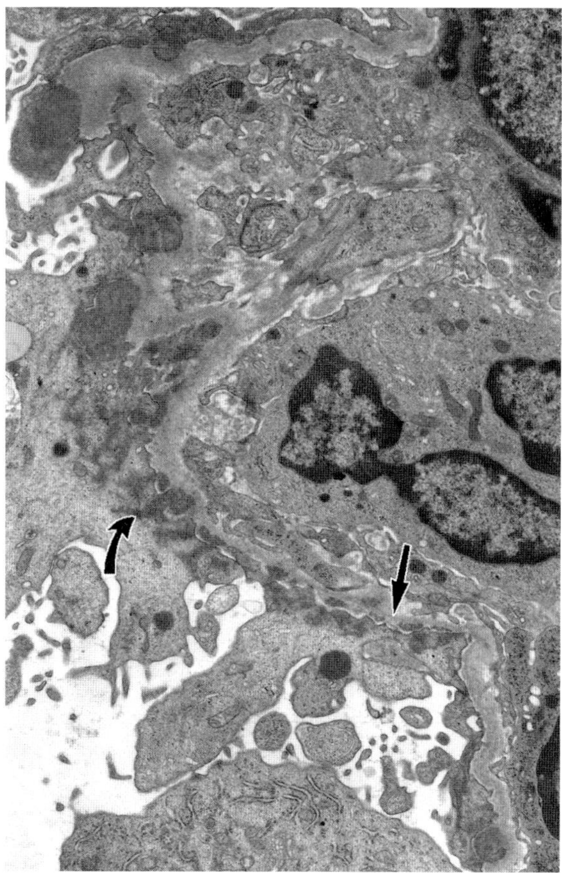

Figure 11-23

ACUTE POSTINFECTIOUS GLOMERULONEPHRITIS

There is a focal area of glomerular basement membrane thinning (straight arrow). Dense cytoskeletal condensations (curved arrow) are seen in the visceral epithelial cytoplasm adjacent to subepithelial dense deposits.

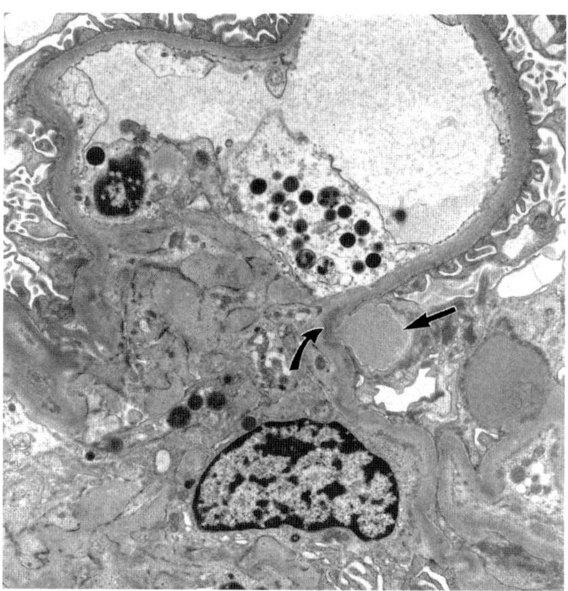

Figure 11-24

RESOLVING POSTINFECTIOUS GLOMERULONEPHRITIS

A subepithelial deposit adjacent to the paramesangial basement membrane is less dense than the lamina densa (straight arrow), suggesting that it is resolving. It is contiguous with residual intramembranous dense material (curved arrow). The capillary lumen at the top is widely patent although the endothelial cell is slightly swollen and contains increased phagosomes.

may persist after the deposits are gone. As acute postinfectious glomerulonephritis evolves, electron-dense and electron-lucent intramembranous deposits become more numerous. Intramembranous deposits are most conspicuous 1 month or more after disease onset (49). In the late phases of resolution, intramembranous deposits are most numerous in the paramesangial portions of glomerular basement membranes (fig. 11-26). Some intramembranous deposits may represent residual material from subepithelial deposits that have been surrounded by the basement membrane material produced by epithelial cells. The findings by electron microscopy suggest that subepithelial deposits disappear by three mechanisms: loss of electron density, internalization into visceral epithelial cells, and incorporation into glomerular basement membranes (49).

The last ultrastructural changes to resolve are focal glomerular basement membrane thickening and wrinkling, especially in the paramesangial basement membrane, and increased mesangial matrix (40). Bowman's capsule also may be slightly thickened. These nonspecific ultrastructural changes may persist for many years.

Differential Diagnosis. The pathologic differential diagnosis of acute postinfectious glomerulonephritis and its spectrum of resolving phenotypes includes most other forms of immune complex glomerulonephritis that can cause diffuse endocapillary hypercellularity, such as types 1 and 2 membranoproliferative glomerulonephritis, lupus glomerulonephritis, and IgA nephropathy. Immunofluorescence microscopy and electron microscopy are most helpful in distinguishing postinfectious glomerulonephritis from these diseases. The light microscopic pattern of injury in lupus nephritis and IgA nephropathy rarely resembles that of typical acute diffuse proliferative postinfectious glomerulonephritis, however, resolving phases of acute postinfectious glomerulonephritis with varying degrees of endocapillary hypercellularity or purely mesangial hypercellularity can be indistinguishable by light microscopy from these entities. IgA nephropathy is distinguished by the dominant or co-dominant immunostaining for IgA, which is rare in acute postinfectious glomerulonephritis with an acute diffuse proliferative glomerulonephritis phenotype, or in the resolving phases of this process. The resolving phases look most like IgA nephropathy by light and electron microscopy, but by immunofluorescence there is staining for complement alone or for predominantly complement with only low level staining for immunoglobulins. There are rare cases of IgA nephropathy developing after *Yersinia enterocolitica* infection, but these look like typical IgA nephropathy rather than acute diffuse proliferative glomerulonephritis (13).

Compared to acute postinfectious glomerulonephritis, lupus nephritis has more frequent and more intense immunostaining for IgG, IgM, IgA, and C1q. Granular staining of the tubular basement membranes is common in lupus nephritis but rare in acute postinfectious glomerulonephritis. By electron microscopy, proliferative lupus glomerulonephritis has more subendothelial dense deposits than postinfectious glomerulonephritis. Endothelial tubuloreticular inclusions are identified in approximately 90 percent of renal biopsy specimens from patients with systemic lupus erythematosus but in less than 5 percent of patients with postinfectious glomerulonephritis.

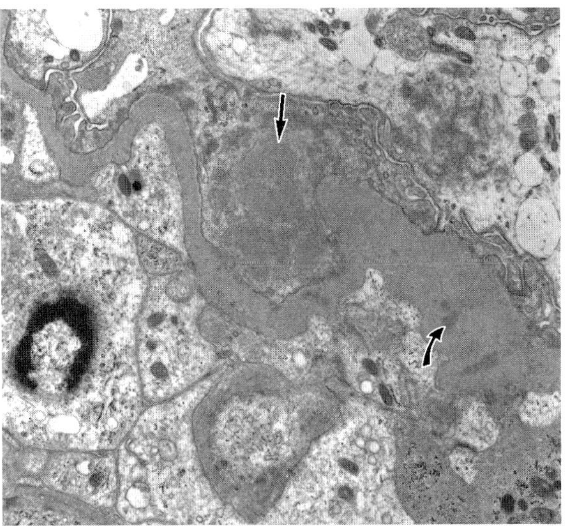

Figure 11-25

RESOLVING POSTINFECTIOUS GLOMERULONEPHRITIS

The epithelial cytoplasm appears to have irregular vacuoles containing relatively low density material that could be internalized immune deposits (straight arrow). Without serial sections, however, obliquely cut subepithelial deposits that touch the glomerular basement membrane at another plane of section cannot be unequivocally ruled out. Small intramembranous deposits also are present (curved arrow).

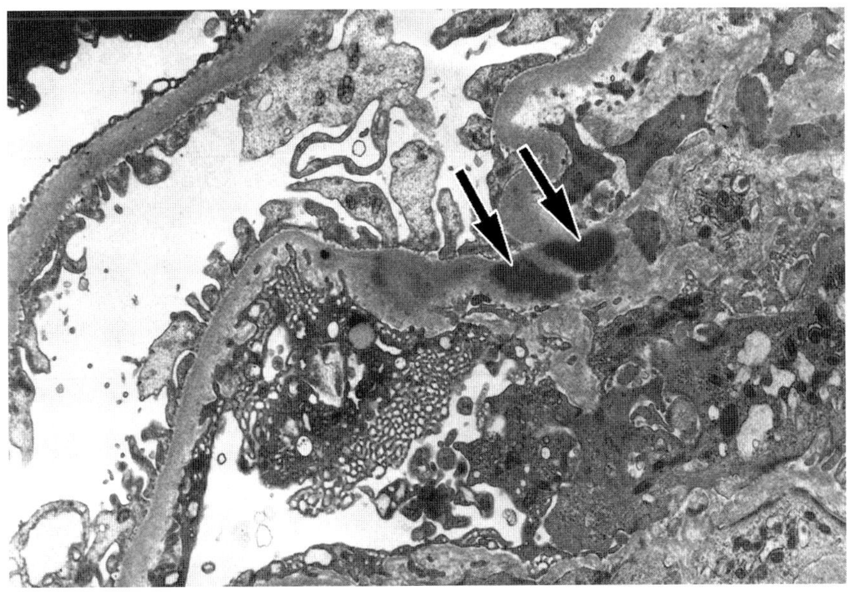

Figure 11-26

RESOLVING POSTINFECTIOUS GLOMERULONEPHRITIS

Electron-dense deposits that appear to be partly intramembranous and partly mesangial are present in the paramesangial region (arrows).

Acute postinfectious glomerulonephritis can occur superimposed on any other form of glomerular disease, such as IgA nephropathy, lupus nephritis, and diabetic glomerulosclerosis. This may prompt biopsy because of a change in the clinical course of a known glomerular disease. For example, if a patient with a clinical or pathologic diagnosis of IgA nephropathy, lupus nephritis, or diabetic glomerulosclerosis experiences a precipitous loss of renal function, a renal biopsy may be performed to determine if the patient has developed an aggressive exacerbation of the known renal disease or has developed an additional disease process. In this setting, unsuspected acute postinfectious glomerulonephritis may be identified superimposed on the chronic disease.

By light microscopy, especially with a hematoxylin and eosin (H&E) stain alone, types 1 and 2 membranoproliferative glomerulonephritis can closely resemble acute postinfectious glomerulonephritis, including the presence of numerous neutrophils. The complement-dominant immunostaining of membranoproliferative glomerulonephritis does not distinguish it from acute postinfectious glomerulonephritis. The distinguishing feature of type 2 membranoproliferative glomerulonephritis (dense deposit disease) is the pathognomonic electron-dense transformation of the glomerular basement membrane and mesangial matrix seen by electron microscopy. Interestingly, type 2 membranoproliferative glomerulonephritis occasionally has subepithelial hump-like deposits similar to those seen in acute postinfectious glomerulonephritis.

Type 1 membranoproliferative glomerulonephritis is distinguished from acute postinfectious glomerulonephritis by extensive replication of glomerular basement membranes, evident by light and electron microscopy, and by the ultrastructural finding of subendothelial dense deposits, subendothelial mesangial interposition, and subendothelial deposition of new basement membrane material. Pathogenetically, type 1 membranoproliferative glomerulonephritis is closely related to acute postinfectious glomerulonephritis. As is discussed in detail later, persistent glomerular injury that is caused by bacterial and other infections often causes type 1 membranoproliferative glomerulonephritis. In fact, some patients with glomerulonephritis that is caused by infection have features that appear to be a mixture of acute diffuse proliferative and type 1 membranoproliferative glomerulonephritis. In addition, infectious glomerulonephritis caused by persistent rather than transient infections can induce glomerulonephritis that is pathologically indistinguishable from acute postinfectious glomerulonephritis, including poststreptococcal glomerulonephritis. The distinction between postinfectious and infectious glomerulonephritis must be made clinically by identifying the character of the nephritogenic infection.

In a consecutive series of 24 patients with pathologic features of acute diffuse proliferative glomerulonephritis and evidence of a preceding infection seen in the University of North Carolina Nephropathology Laboratory, 14 were caused by pharyngitis, 6 by pyoderma, 1 by chronic sinusitis, 1 by osteomyelitis, 1 by a periodontal abscess, and 1 by a lower extremity soft tissue abscess. Three quarters of the patients with pharyngitis or pyoderma had evidence of streptococcal infection. The patients with glomerulonephritis caused by infections at other sites all had staphylococcal infections. The glomerular lesions in the four patients with acute diffuse proliferative glomerulonephritis caused by more persistent infections were indistinguishable from those caused by acute streptococcal pharyngitis or pyoderma. Similar results were reported in a recent series from France which noted that of 44 cases of infection-induced diffuse proliferative glomerulonephritis, 17 were caused by pharyngitis, 11 by pyoderma, 7 by lung infection, 7 by periodontal abscess, and 3 by endocarditis (31).

Patients with cryoglobulinemic glomerulonephritis may have clinical and pathologic features that are difficult to differentiate from acute postinfectious glomerulonephritis. For example, clinically, patients with either disease can have nephritis, hypocomplementemia, type 3 cryoglobulins, and positive rheumatoid factor. Histologically, both often have diffuse global endocapillary hypercellularity with conspicuous neutrophils. Cryoglobulinemic glomerulonephritis is more likely if the specimen has numerous, glomerular capillary, hyaline "thrombi" and extensive glomerular basement membrane replication by light microscopy, or microtubular configurations within the electron-dense deposits by electron microscopy.

In the practice of renal pathology, as many as half of the patients whose renal biopsy specimens have typical features of acute postinfectious glomerulonephritis do not have known evidence of an infectious etiology at the time of biopsy. After the pathologic diagnosis, further evaluation identifies the nephritogenic infection in some of these patients, but no etiology is found in others. In this setting, a morphologic-pathologic diagnosis is appropriate, with a clause or comment indicating that the pattern of injury is consistent with a postinfectious or infectious etiology. There are no universally agreed upon criteria for concluding that a specific example of glomerulonephritis is caused by an infection, however, Montseny and associates (31) have proposed an approach that is reasonable. They consider that a glomerulonephritis is of infectious or postinfectious origin if three of the following five criteria are fulfilled: 1) clinical or laboratory evidence of an infection preceding the onset of glomerulonephritis; 2) close temporal relationship between infection and the first appearance of signs and symptoms of glomerulonephritis; 3) glomerular pathologic findings consistent with an infectious or postinfectious glomerulonephritis; 4) absence of clinical, laboratory, or pathologic evidence of a systemic disease that causes glomerulonephritis; and 5) immunohistologic findings not consistent with IgA nephropathy.

Etiology and Pathogenesis. Acute poststreptococcal glomerulonephritis is most often caused by infection with group A beta-hemolytic streptococci. Staphylococci, the second most common cause, Gram-negative bacteria, and even viruses can cause a pathologically identical glomerulonephritis (31,44). The most frequent site of nephritogenic streptococcal infection is in the nasopharynx in temperate regions and skin in tropical regions. In temperate regions, glomerulonephritis caused by pharyngitis is most frequent in the winter, and glomerulonephritis caused by pyoderma is most frequent in the summer (40). Only a small proportion (less than 0.5 percent) of children, and even fewer adults, who have streptococcal infections develop acute postinfectious glomerulonephritis (1,33). Certain strains are more nephritogenic than others (35).

The immune pathogenesis of postinfectious glomerulonephritis is incompletely understood. Possible mechanisms include glomerular deposition of circulating immune complexes, in situ formation of immune complexes, or in situ localization of cationic bacterial molecules that directly injure glomeruli or activate complement in the absence of immunoglobulins (11, 32,35,36,39,43,54). Combinations of these mechanisms may occur. For example, cationic molecules could first localize and cause injury without the presence of immunoglobulins, and later could be bound by antibody to form immune complexes.

A variety of streptococcal antigens have been identified in the glomeruli of some patients with acute postinfectious glomerulonephritis, including endostreptosin, streptokinase, and streptococcal erythrogenic toxin type B (ETB) (11,30, 35,36,39). After localizing in glomeruli by direct ionic binding to basement membranes and mesangial matrix, ETB may contribute directly to tissue injury by inducing complement activation, leukocyte infiltration, cell proliferation, and apoptosis (11,36,39,51). Cationic staphylococcal proteins may induce the same nephritogenic events (19). Direct activation of complement by bacterial proteins localized in glomeruli would explain the prominent immunostaining for C3, with little or no staining for the immunoglobulins that are seen in most specimens with postinfectious glomerulonephritis. This pathogenic mechanism has not yet been proven.

Treatment and Prognosis. Streptococcal pharyngitis and pyoderma should be treated with antibiotics to eradicate the infection and reduce the risk of secondary complications; however, once poststreptococcal glomerulonephritis develops, treatment with antibiotics has no apparent effect on the outcome of the nephritis. Prophylactic treatment of individuals with streptococcal infection and their contacts with penicillin can reduce the spread of nephritogenic streptococcal infections and the incidence of glomerulonephritis during epidemic outbreaks of poststreptococcal glomerulonephritis (25).

More than 90 percent of children with acute poststreptococcal glomerulonephritis recover completely (17,38,42). Children with crescentic poststreptococcal glomerulonephritis have a lower recovery rate, although this is better than the rate of recovery from other forms of crescentic glomerulonephritis in children (3). Adults with acute poststreptococcal glomerulonephritis have a worse prognosis, with a quarter or more developing persistent renal dysfunction (35,42,44).

There is no specific treatment for uncomplicated acute postinfectious glomerulonephritis other than management of complications from fluid retention, hypertension, or renal failure. Renal insufficiency typically resolves by 6 weeks, hematuria usually resolves within 3 months, proteinuria may persist after the hematuria resolves but usually not longer than 6 months, and hypocomplementemia typically resolves within 2 months. Persistence of any of these abnormalities may prompt a renal biopsy to confirm the diagnosis of postinfectious glomerulonephritis or to detect unusually severe disease. Patients with unusually aggressive postinfectious glomerulonephritis, especially those with numerous crescents, often are treated with high-dose corticosteroids, cytotoxic agents, or both.

Certain pathologic features correlate with the course and outcome of acute postinfectious glomerulonephritis. The presence of crescents, especially if numerous, worsens the prognosis in children and adults (12,44,55). Some investigators have found more crescents in patients with the starry sky pattern (16) while others have found more crescents with the garland pattern (46). The garland pattern of immune deposits correlates with greater proteinuria (over 5 g/day) (16,46), and more persistent proteinuria (47).

INFECTIOUS ENDOCARDITIS GLOMERULONEPHRITIS

Definition. Acute bacterial postinfectious glomerulonephritis follows a short-term acute bacterial infection, most often streptococcal pharyngitis or pyoderma. There are a variety of other settings in which glomerulonephritis is caused by persistent rather than acute bacterial infections, such as endocarditis, osteomyelitis, abscesses, and infected catheters in contact with cardiac chambers, arteries, or veins. Glomerulonephritis that is caused by persistent bacterial infections may be pathologically indistinguishable from acute diffuse proliferative poststreptococcal glomerulonephritis, or may fall anywhere in the spectrum from focal proliferative or necrotizing glomerulonephritis to diffuse proliferative glomerulonephritis to type 1 membranoproliferative glomerulonephritis (5,8,9,31,44).

Infectious endocarditis glomerulonephritis is caused by either acute or subacute bacterial endocarditis (29,34,44). Acute endocarditis usually causes acute diffuse proliferative glomerulonephritis and subacute endocarditis usually causes focal proliferative or necrotizing glomerulonephritis, or type 1 membranoproliferative glomerulonephritis, however, a wide variety of glomerular lesions can be caused by either type of endocarditis (21,29,34,44).

Clinical Features. The clinical manifestations of infectious endocarditis are fever, heart murmurs, anemia, Roth spots, hepatosplenomegaly, and rarely, purpura (21). The renal disease is the presenting feature in 20 percent of patients (29). The rate of glomerulonephritis in patients with infectious endocarditis is poorly determined, with incidences ranging from 2 to 60 percent, but is reduced by early and appropriate antibiotic treatment of the endocarditis (34). Preexisting cardiac valve disease and intravenous drug abuse are major risk factors for endocarditis and endocarditis glomerulonephritis (29,34).

Patients with glomerulonephritis caused by endocarditis have a high frequency of hematuria and proteinuria. Hypocomplementemia, rheumatoid factor, and circulating immune complexes are frequent (34,44). The frequency of hypocomplementemia varies depending on the type of underlying glomerulonephritis. Patients with immune complex–type glomerulonephritis are likely to have hypocomplementemia, whereas patients with no glomerular immune deposits are not (9,29). Hypertension and nephrotic syndrome are rare. The degree of renal failure varies, from none to severe. Mild focal glomerulonephritis usually causes no significant renal insufficiency, diffuse proliferative glomerulonephritis usually causes moderate renal insufficiency, and crescentic glomerulonephritis typically causes severe, rapidly developing renal failure (26,44). Patients with endocarditis who undergo renal biopsy usually have renal insufficiency that has not improved with antibiotic therapy (29).

Gross Findings. The major renal pathologic lesions in patients with infectious endocarditis are renal infarcts caused by valve vegetation emboli, focal or diffuse glomerulonephritis, drug-induced tubulointerstitial nephritis, and drug-induced acute tubular necrosis (21,29,34,44). Renal involvement by secondary amyloidosis is a rare complication of longstanding endocarditis (23). The renal infarcts are most readily identified by gross inspection, however, they are rarely sampled in renal biopsy specimens (29). Approximately 50 percent of patients with infectious endocarditis have renal infarcts identified at the time of postmortem examination (29). These infarcts are caused by embolism of valve vegetations and not by secondary immune-mediated vasculitis.

Light Microscopic Findings. The major findings by light microscopy are features of focal glomerulonephritis, diffuse glomerulonephritis, drug-induced tubulointerstitial nephritis, and drug-induced acute tubular necrosis (5,8,21,29, 34,44). The drug-induced tubulointerstitial nephritis and drug-induced acute tubular necrosis usually are caused by antibiotics, and have the typical pathologic features that are described for these processes elsewhere in this book and are not considered further here.

The glomerular lesions of infectious endocarditis glomerulonephritis are extremely varied and range from typical acute diffuse proliferative glomerulonephritis that is indistinguishable from acute poststreptococcal glomerulonephritis, to immune complex focal or diffuse proliferative glomerulonephritis, to crescentic glomerulonephritis to type 1 membranoproliferative glomerulonephritis, to focal necrotizing glomerulonephritis with no immune deposits, resembling vasculitis-associated pauci-immune necrotizing glomerulonephritis (21, 26,29,34,44). Focal glomerulonephritis is the most common finding (5,44). The older literature emphasizes the frequency of overt immune complex glomerulonephritis (21,27), whereas recent studies have documented the frequent occurrence of the pauci-immune focal glomerulonephritis (29); in a series of 9 renal biopsy specimens and 7 autopsy specimens with infectious endocarditis glomerulonephritis, Majumdar et al. (29) observed focal pauci-immune ("vasculitic") glomerulonephritis in 11, acute diffuse proliferative glomerulonephritis in 3, and type 1 membranoproliferative glomerulonephritis in 2.

Acute diffuse proliferative glomerulonephritis or diffuse proliferative glomerulonephritis caused by infectious endocarditis is pathologically identical to acute postinfectious glomerulonephritis, described in detail earlier in this chapter. In the acute phase, there is marked endocapillary hypercellularity and neutrophil influx (fig. 11-27, left). Crescents may be present but rarely are numerous. With effective treatment of the endocarditis, the glomerular lesions resolve through the same histologic phases as acute postinfectious glomerulonephritis.

Type 1 membranoproliferative glomerulonephritis can be caused by a variety of chronic bacterial and viral infections, including bacterial endocarditis. It is more likely with chronic, subacute endocarditis than acute endocarditis (44). The pathologic changes are no different from idiopathic type 1 membranoproliferative glomerulonephritis, which are described in detail in chapter 10. The major light microscopic findings are diffuse endocapillary hypercellularity, thickened capillary walls, and hypersegmentation (lobulation) (fig. 11-28, left). Special stains reveal prominent glomerular basement membrane replication. Trichrome staining may demonstrate subendothelial fuchsinophilic deposits.

Focal glomerulonephritis was once termed "focal embolic glomerulonephritis" before its pathogenesis was attributed to mechanisms other than embolization (5,21). One of the most compelling observations against an embolic origin is the occurrence of typical focal segmental necrotizing glomerulonephritis in patients with endocarditis limited to the right side of the heart (44). A wide variety of patterns of focal glomerulonephritis are seen in patients with endocarditis, including focal proliferative, focal necrotizing, focal sclerosing, and mixtures of these patterns. Crescents may be present, especially with necrotizing glomerulonephritis (29). Although proliferative and necrotizing glomerular lesions usually are focal and segmental, the same patterns of injury may be diffuse (i.e., affecting more than 50 percent of glomeruli).

The most common focal lesion is focal necrotizing glomerulonephritis, which is characterized by segmental capillary thrombosis and fibrinoid necrosis, sometimes with associated neutrophils (figs. 11-29, 11-30) (5,8,29). Adjacent non-necrotic glomerular segments often are

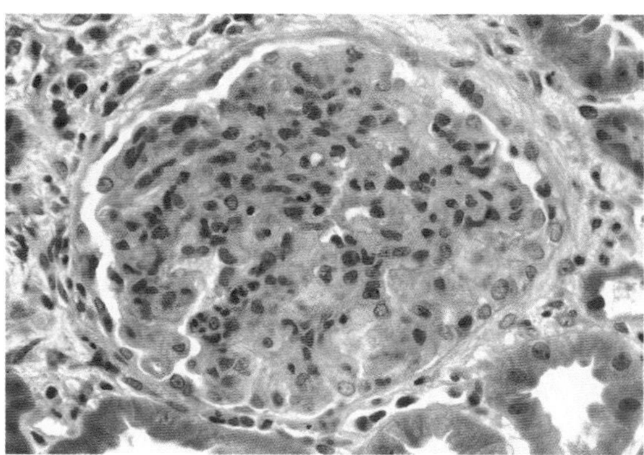
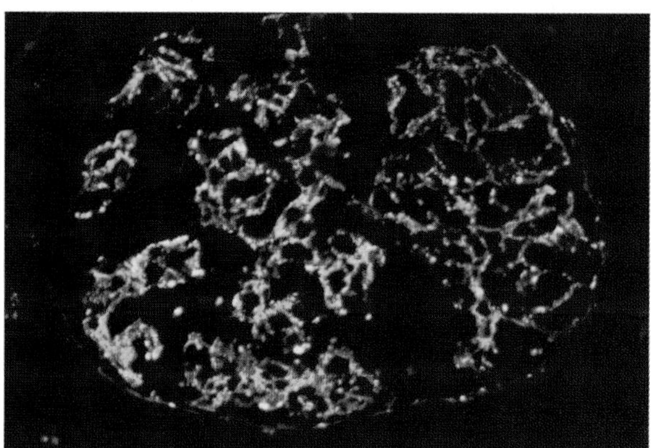

Figure 11-27

INFECTIOUS ENDOCARDITIS GLOMERULONEPHRITIS

This patient with a history of intravenous drug abuse developed endocarditis, purpura, and nephritis.

Left: Light microscopy of a renal biopsy specimen reveals diffuse proliferative glomerulonephritis with segmental influx of neutrophils and segmental capillary wall thickening (H&E stain).

Right: Immunofluorescence microscopy demonstrates coarsely granular capillary wall staining that is intense for C3 and weak for IgG and IgM (not shown).

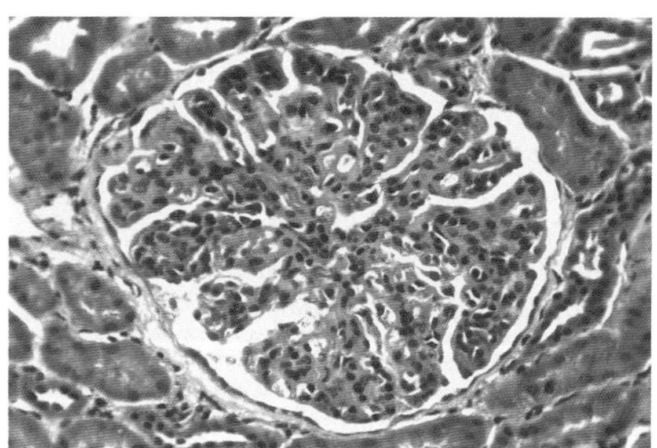
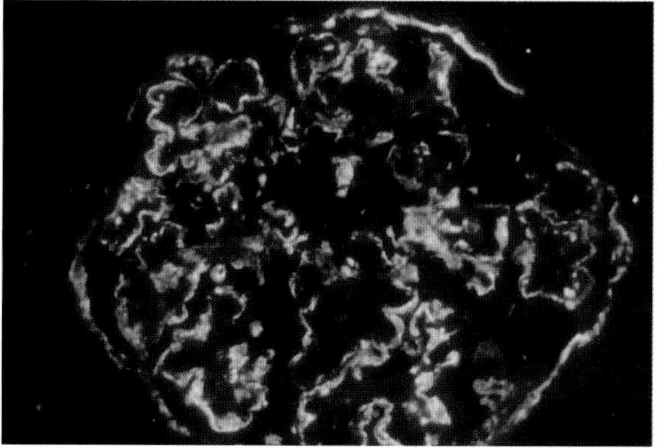

Figure 11-28

INFECTIOUS ENDOCARDITIS GLOMERULONEPHRITIS

The type 1 membranoproliferative glomerulonephritis pattern of endocarditis glomerulonephritis shows hypersegmentation, endocapillary hypercellularity, and capillary wall thickening by light microscopy (H&E stain; left), and band-like or granular capillary wall staining for C3 by immunofluorescence microscopy (right).

histologically unremarkable, however, mixed proliferative and necrotizing lesions also occur. Extensive segmental necrosis often has adjacent crescent formation (fig. 11-30). Necrotizing lesions heal with scarring, and some specimens contain both active focal segmental necrotizing lesions and focal segmental glomerular sclerosis with adhesions to Bowman's capsule.

Proliferative glomerulonephritis caused by endocarditis resembles other types of immune complex glomerulonephritis (figs. 11-27, 11-31). There are varying degrees of segmental to global endocapillary hypercellularity, occasionally with superimposed segmental necrosis. Some specimens with diffuse proliferative glomerulonephritis have focal features consistent with membranoproliferative glomerulonephritis. In fact, the decision to make one or the other of these morphologic diagnoses may be arbitrary in some patients, and does not influence management.

After effective treatment of infectious endocarditis, there is clinical and pathologic

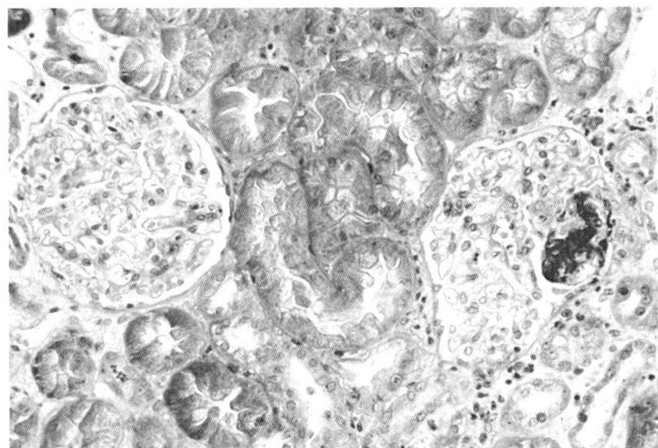

Figure 11-29

FOCAL NECROTIZING INFECTIOUS ENDOCARDITIS GLOMERULONEPHRITIS

There is a single small fuchsinophilic focus of capillary thrombosis and fibrinoid necrosis in one of the two glomeruli. This pattern of injury was once called "focal embolic glomerulonephritis" (Masson trichrome stain).

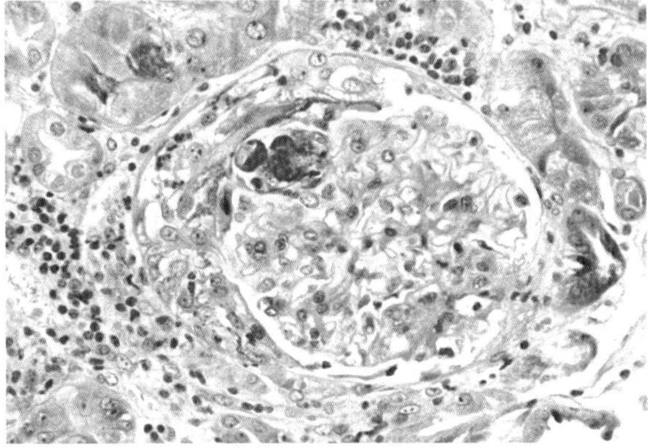

Figure 11-30

FOCAL NECROTIZING INFECTIOUS ENDOCARDITIS GLOMERULONEPHRITIS

This glomerulus has segmental fibrinoid necrosis with an adjacent cellular crescent. The non-necrotic tuft is relatively unremarkable (Masson trichrome stain).

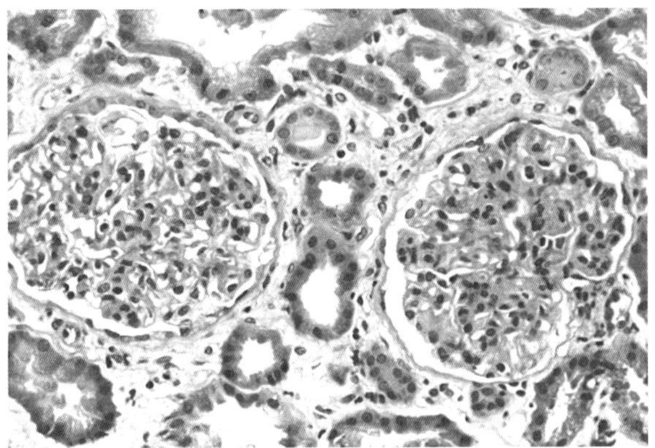

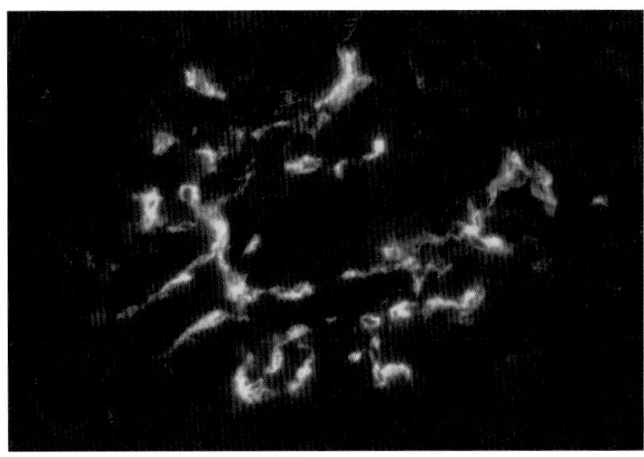

Figure 11-31

MILD PROLIFERATIVE INFECTIOUS ENDOCARDITIS GLOMERULONEPHRITIS

Left: The glomeruli have mild segmental mesangial hypercellularity with minimal endocapillary changes by light microscopy (H&E stain).

Right: By immunofluorescence microscopy, there is staining for mesangial IgM (right) and C3 but not for IgG or IgA (not shown).

resolution of the glomerulonephritis (21). Uncomplicated proliferative glomerulonephritis resolves through a mesangioproliferative stage to normal architecture. Severe inflammatory or necrotizing lesions organize into segmental or global glomerular sclerosis, usually with adhesions to Bowman's capsule.

The extent and character of acute or chronic tubulointerstitial injury should be commensurate with the nature of the glomerular injury. If tubulointerstitial injury is disproportionately severe compared to glomerular disease, the possibility of concurrent tubulointerstitial disease should be considered, especially disease caused by antibiotics or other drugs.

Immunofluorescence Findings. Glomerular staining for immunoglobulins and complement usually is present in proliferative and membranoproliferative infectious endocarditis glomerulonephritis (figs. 11-27, right; 11-28, right; 11-31, right) (21,29,44); necrotizing glomerulonephritis, however, typically has little or no

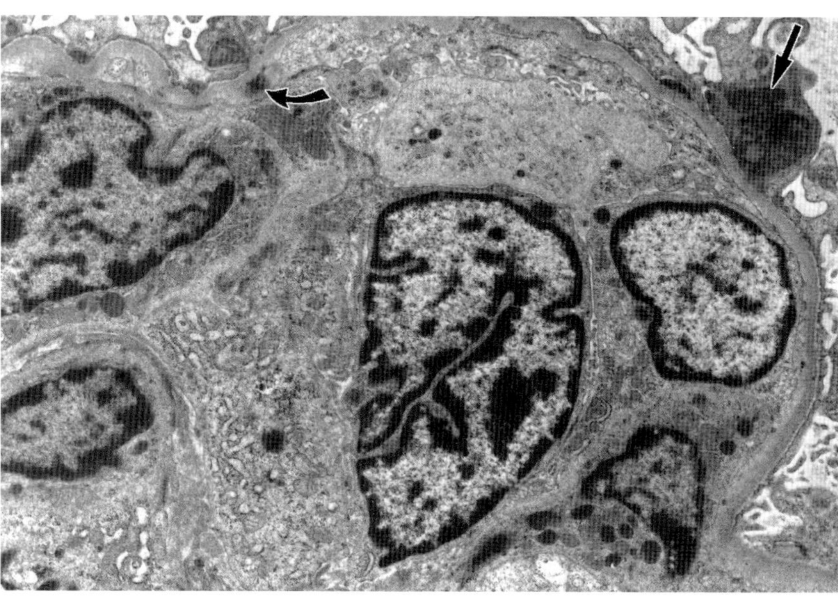

Figure 11-32

INFECTIOUS ENDOCARDITIS GLOMERULONEPHRITIS

The ultrastructural features are identical to those seen with acute postinfectious glomerulonephritis, including hump-like subepithelial electron-dense deposits (straight arrow) and scattered small subendothelial deposits (curved arrow).

staining for immunoglobulins and complement (29). Some specimens of diffuse proliferative glomerulonephritis show no staining for immunoglobulins or complement (9), but this is unusual. Membranoproliferative glomerulonephritis typically has mesangial and extensive capillary wall, band-like or granular staining for complement and immunoglobulins, often with greater staining for IgM than for IgG or IgA (29). IgM-dominant staining is also characteristic of focal or diffuse proliferative glomerulonephritis in patients with endocarditis (see Table 11-1). Large subendothelial immune deposits often appear as bands of capillary wall staining by immunofluorescence microscopy. Otherwise, the capillary wall and mesangial staining is usually granular.

Electron Microscopic Findings. Immune complex–mediated infectious endocarditis glomerulonephritis has varying amounts of subepithelial, intramembranous, subendothelial, and mesangial electron-dense deposits, depending on the phenotype and temporal stage of the glomerular injury (21,29,44). Specimens with acute diffuse proliferative glomerulonephritis by light microscopy are most likely to have conspicuous subepithelial dense deposits (humps) (fig. 11-32); specimens with membranoproliferative glomerulonephritis by light microscopy are most likely to have prominent subendothelial dense deposits (fig. 11-33); and specimens with purely necrotizing glomerulonephritis may have no dense deposits. Nondescript focal or diffuse proliferative glomerulonephritis usually has mesangial and subendothelial dense deposits, occasionally with a few scattered subepithelial deposits. Overall, subepithelial dense deposits occur in about a third of patients with endocarditis glomerulonephritis (fig. 11-33, left).

During the resolution of the glomerulonephritis, after effective treatment of the endocarditis, capillary wall electron-dense deposits are lost, while mesangial dense deposits persist for 6 months or longer (21).

Differential Diagnosis. The glomerular lesions of infectious endocarditis glomerulonephritis have a very broad pathologic differential diagnosis because they are so varied. Each pattern raises somewhat different diagnostic considerations. A finding of acute diffuse proliferative glomerulonephritis raises the possibility of glomerulonephritis secondary to acute bacterial infection at any site. Clinical information is required to determine the source of the infection. Immune complex focal or diffuse proliferative glomerulonephritis raises the possibility of other immune complex glomerulonephritides, such as lupus nephritis. Once again, clinical data helps define the type of immune complex disease. Type 1 membranoproliferative glomerulonephritis caused by infectious endocarditis can be indistinguishable from membranoproliferative glomerulonephritis of other causes. Compared to idiopathic

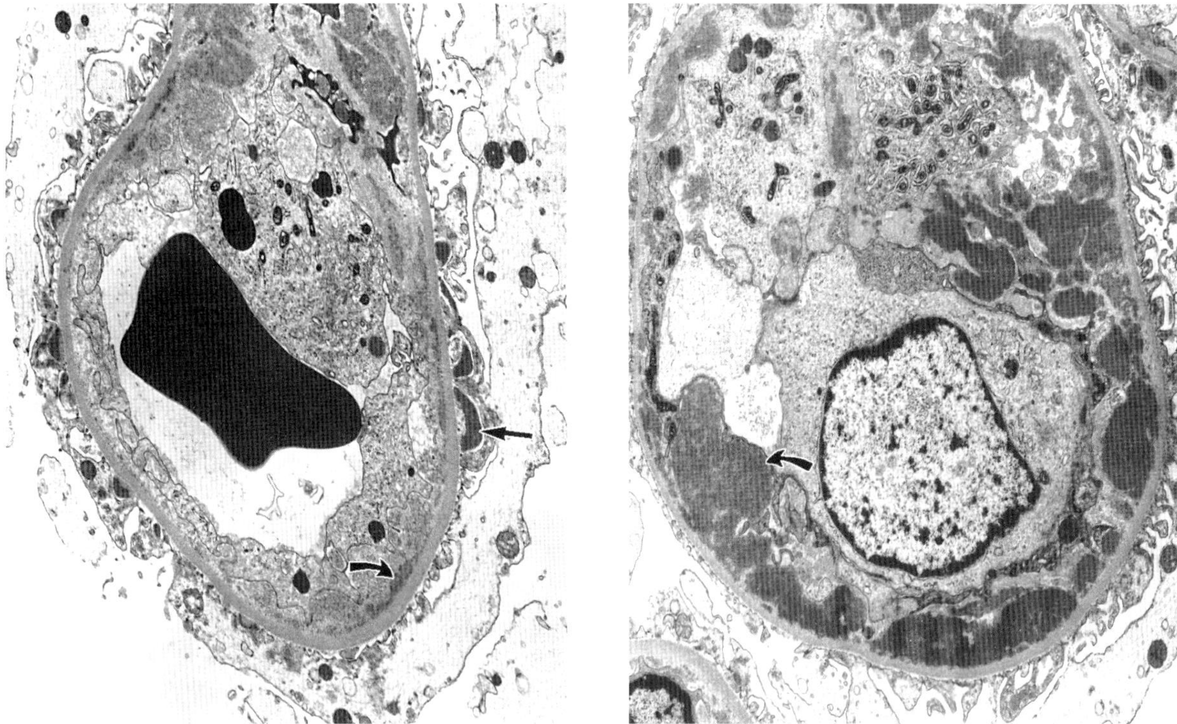

Figure 11-33

INFECTIOUS ENDOCARDITIS GLOMERULONEPHRITIS

This patient with a history of intravenous drug abuse and infectious endocarditis had a membranoproliferative pattern of glomerulonephritis by light microscopy. By electron microscopy, some capillaries have numerous subepithelial dense deposits (straight arrow) and only a few subendothelial dense deposits (curved arrow; left), whereas other capillaries have no subepithelial dense deposits and numerous large subendothelial dense deposits (curved arrow; right).

membranoproliferative glomerulonephritis, endocarditis-induced membranoproliferative glomerulonephritis more often has dominant staining for IgM. The presence of hyaline thrombi by light microscopy or of a microtubular configuration in the dense deposits by electron microscopy should raise the possibility of hepatitis C infection, especially in an intravenous drug abuser. Proliferative or membranoproliferative glomerulonephritis with conspicuous focal segmental necrosis should prompt consideration of the possibility of endocarditis glomerulonephritis (5,21).

Endocarditis-associated focal necrotizing glomerulonephritis with little or no immunostaining for immunoglobulins or complement may be indistinguishable from antineutrophil cytoplasmic antibody (ANCA)-associated pauci-immune necrotizing glomerulonephritis (29). Apparently, an association with infectious endocarditis indicates that the glomerulonephritis will be less aggressive than ANCA-associated pauci-immune glomerulonephritis that is not associated with endocarditis, however, patients with extensive necrosis have a worse prognosis than those with proliferative forms of endocarditis-induced glomerulonephritis (10,29). More data are needed to clarify this issue.

Etiology and Pathogenesis. The introduction of antibiotic therapy altered the epidemiology, etiology, and pathology of infectious endocarditis glomerulonephritis by reducing the frequency of disease caused by streptococci (29, 34,44). *Staphylococcus aureus* currently is the most common cause of infectious endocarditis glomerulonephritis (29). Additional causes include other species of *Staphylococcus* (especially *S. epidermidis*), *Streptococcus, Enterococcus, Proteus, Haemophilus, Neisseria, Pseudomonas coxiella, Cardiobacterium*, and *Actinobacillus*

(28,29,44). Intravenous drug abuse is a major cause of endocarditis and endocarditis glomerulonephritis (31). Approximately 90 percent of patients with infectious endocarditis glomerulonephritis have endocarditis affecting native cardiac valves and 10 percent affecting prosthetic valves (29). Infrequent causes of infectious endocarditis glomerulonephritis are infected permanent pacemakers (6) and implanted central venous devices (52).

The same pathogenic mechanisms that were discussed earlier for postinfectious glomerulonephritis can be proposed for infectious proliferative glomerulonephritis with immune deposits. These include circulating immune complex deposition, in situ immune complex formation, or in situ localization of directly nephritogenic cationic bacterial molecules (19). Persistent circulating immune complexes are the most likely cause of type 1 membranoproliferative glomerulonephritis secondary to endocarditis.

Pauci-immune focal glomerulonephritis may be caused by a cell-mediated rather than an antibody-mediated mechanism (29), however, there is no direct evidence for this. A minority of patients with infectious endocarditis and pauci-immune glomerulonephritis are ANCA positive (29). There is a well-documented low frequency of proteinase 3–specific ANCA (PR3-ANCA) in patients with infectious endocarditis, including patients with glomerulonephritis (10). This at least raises the possibility that ANCA could be involved in the pathogenesis of glomerulonephritis in some patients with endocarditis.

Treatment and Prognosis. Patients with glomerulonephritis caused by any form of persistent infection, including endocarditis, have a worse prognosis than those with postinfectious glomerulonephritis caused by a transient infection (31). The early detection of the glomerulonephritis and the prompt eradication of the nephritogenic infection usually lead to resolution of the nephritis. A brief course of corticosteroid therapy may facilitate recovery from the glomerulonephritis without exacerbating the endocarditis (2,28). For patients with unusually aggressive or recalcitrant disease, treatment includes plasmapheresis, removal of valve vegetations, or valve replacement (2). Prophylactic antibiotic therapy in patients at risk for endocarditis reduces the incidence of endocarditis and resultant glomerulonephritis (34). Patients with necrotizing and crescentic glomerulonephritis have a worse prognosis than those with proliferative or membranoproliferative glomerulonephritis (29).

SHUNT NEPHRITIS

Definition. Shunt nephritis is a glomerulonephritis caused by bacterial infection of cerebrospinal fluid shunts inserted for the treatment of hydrocephalus (4,22,41,50). The etiologic pathogens typically are of low virulence. Shunt nephritis is much more common with ventriculoatrial (VA) shunts than ventriculoperitoneal (VP) shunts, which is one reason why the latter are now favored (22). Patients with portosystemic shunt surgery may develop immune complex glomerulonephritis (45), but this should not be called shunt nephritis.

Clinical Features. Fever is the most common clinical manifestation of shunt infection (4, 22,41,50). Most patients also have anemia and hepatosplenomegaly. Additional clinical features are nausea, vomiting, malaise, and other signs of increased intracranial pressure (4,22). A minority of patients have purpura caused by systemic immune complex small vessel vasculitis (4). Negative blood cultures do not rule out shunt infection (22).

The interval between VA shunt insertion and the diagnosis of glomerulonephritis has a mean of 4 to 5 years and ranges from 1 month to greater than 20 years (4,22). The ubiquitous manifestations of shunt nephritis are hematuria and proteinuria. Nephrotic syndrome occurs in approximately a quarter of patients. Hypertension is uncommon. There are varying degrees of renal insufficiency depending upon the severity of the glomerular injury.

Patients with shunt nephritis have a variety of immunologic abnormalities that support an immune complex pathogenesis for the glomerulonephritis. There is a very high frequency of hypocomplementemia (decreased C3 and C4), cryoglobulins, circulating immune complexes, elevated C-reactive protein, rheumatoid factor, and hypergammaglobulinemia. IgM often is markedly elevated, and to a lesser extent, IgG; this corresponds to a higher frequency and intensity of glomerular staining for IgM than IgG in shunt nephritis (see Table 11-1) (4,44).

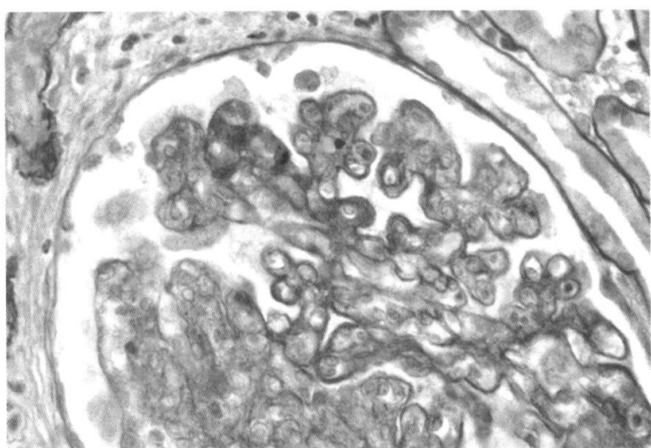

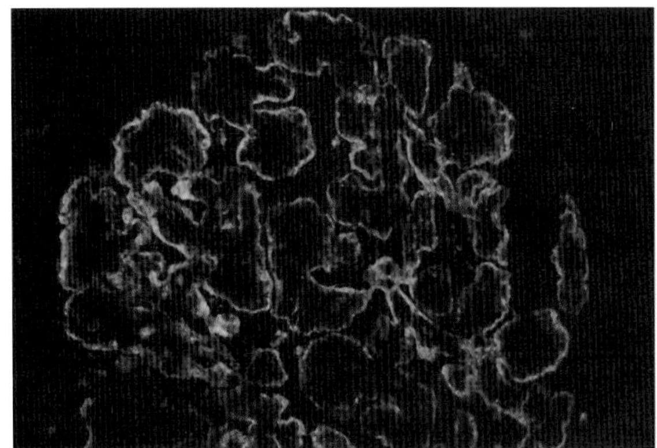

Figure 11-34

SHUNT NEPHRITIS

A 10-year-old with hydrocephalus since birth relieved with a ventriculoatrial (VA) shunt developed membranoproliferative glomerulonephritis.

Left: Light microscopy demonstrates glomerular endocapillary hypercellularity, thick capillary walls, and focal basement membrane replication (PAS stain).

Right: Immunofluorescence microscopy reveals finely granular to confluent peripheral staining of glomerular segments. Staining was most intense for IgM and C3 (not shown).

Light Microscopic Findings. More than half of patients with shunt nephritis have type 1 membranoproliferative glomerulonephritis (mesangiocapillary glomerulonephritis) (fig. 11-34, left) (4,22,44,50). This is characterized by diffuse global endocapillary hypercellularity, capillary wall thickening, and glomerular basement membrane replication. Approximately a third of these patients have focal or diffuse proliferative glomerulonephritis, including a minority of patients with acute diffuse proliferative glomerulonephritis that is indistinguishable from acute postinfectious glomerulonephritis (4). Specimens of proliferative glomerulonephritis often show focal, segmental thickening of capillary walls caused predominantly by subendothelial immune deposits, which occasionally can be identified in trichrome-stained sections as fuchsinophilic deposits. A few patients have exclusively mesangioproliferative glomerulonephritis. Crescent formation occurs in occasional cases but involvement of more than 50 percent of glomeruli is rare.

Immunofluorescence Findings. Immunoglobulins and complement are identified in most specimens of shunt nephritis, and the remaining specimens have complement without detectable immunoglobulin (4,44). An interesting immunohistologic feature of shunt nephritis, which is shared by other forms of glomerulonephritis caused by chronic bacterial infection, is a higher frequency and greater intensity of staining for IgM compared to IgG (Table 11-1; fig. 11-34, right) (4); IgA staining is less frequent and of less intensity when present. Shunt nephritis caused by cerebrospinal fluid shunt infection should not be confused with glomerulonephritis caused by portosystemic vascular shunts, which is an IgA-dominant type 1 membranoproliferative glomerulonephritis (45). Staining for C3 is positive in over 90 percent of specimens; a quarter to a third of specimens are positive for C1q and C4. The distribution and pattern of staining for immunoglobulins and complement correspond to the histologic phenotype of the glomerulonephritis. For example, patients with type 1 membranoproliferative glomerulonephritis as seen by light microscopy, have granular to band-like staining of the capillary wall along with mesangial staining. Patients with acute diffuse proliferative glomerulonephritis may have very coarsely granular capillary wall staining caused by large subepithelial deposits. Patients who have a purely mesangioproliferative glomerulonephritis by light microscopy often have only mesangial staining by immunofluorescence microscopy.

Electron Microscopic Findings. Most specimens have well-defined, immune complex–type electron-dense deposits (44). Mesangial and subendothelial deposits are most frequent, but subepithelial deposits, including humps, are identified in a minority of patients (see Table 11-1). The ultrastructural findings parallel the histologic phenotype of injury. For example, patients with type 1 membranoproliferative glomerulonephritis by light microscopy have subendothelial deposits with associated mesangial interposition and deposition of new basement membrane material (fig. 11-35). Patients with acute diffuse proliferative glomerulonephritis may have subepithelial humps identical to those in acute postinfectious glomerulonephritis. Patients with purely mesangioproliferative glomerulonephritis by light microscopy often have only mesangial deposits by electron microscopy. The endothelial and mesangial hypercellularity, and influx of leukocytes, are variable and again parallel the findings by light microscopy. There usually is focal or diffuse effacement of visceral epithelial foot processes.

Differential Diagnosis. The pathologic differential diagnosis is the same as for other postinfectious and infectious glomerulonephritides discussed earlier in this chapter. The possibility of shunt infection, or infection of some other implanted vascular device, should be part of the differential diagnosis, especially when type 1 membranoproliferative glomerulonephritis with IgM-dominant immune deposits is identified in a biopsy specimen.

Etiology and Pathogenesis. While a VA shunt infections are relatively common, glomerulonephritis develops in less than 2 percent of these patients (4). Shunt infection may be facilitated by the adherence of bacteria to the plastic surface of the shunt where they may be protected from antibiotics and immune defenses (41). Analogous forms of immune complex glomerulonephritis can be caused by other implanted vascular devices, such as indwelling catheters and injection reservoirs (37,52).

The most common cause of shunt nephritis is staphylococcal infection, especially with *Staphylococcus epidermidis* and *S. albus* (4,22,41). Many bacteria other than *Staphylococcus* species cause shunt nephritis, including *Propionibacterium, Corynebacterium, Bacillus, Listeria, Pseudomonas, Acinetobacter*, and others (18,22,41). The presumed pathogenesis involves localization of bacterial antigens and bound antibodies in glomeruli. This is supported by the finding in patients with shunt nephritis of high levels of immune complexes in the circulation (41) and of immunoglobulins, complement, and bacterial antigens in glomeruli (4). Cationic staphylococcal proteins also may localize in glomeruli and cause in situ immunoglobulin binding, complement activation, and inflammation (19).

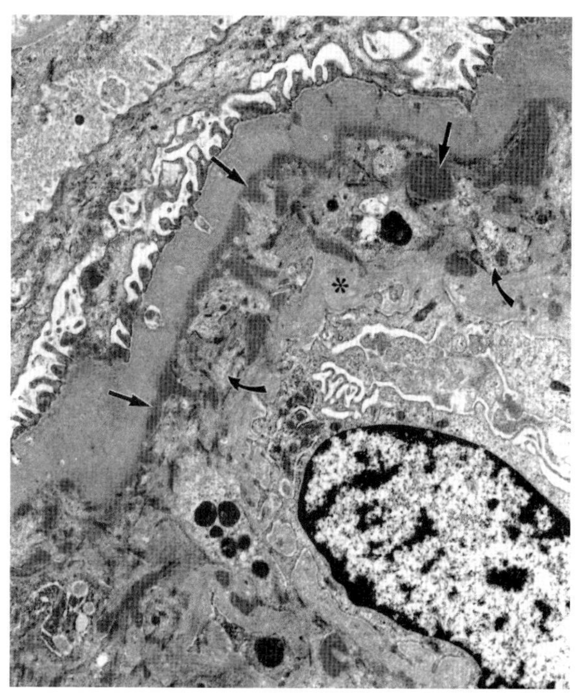

Figure 11-35

SHUNT NEPHRITIS

Features of membranoproliferative glomerulonephritis are present, including subendothelial electron-dense deposits (straight arrows), subendothelial islands of mesangial cytoplasm (curved arrows), and new basement membrane material (asterisk).

Treatment and Prognosis. Shunt nephritis typically resolves after effective treatment of the infection with intravenous antibiotics and removal of the shunt (4,22,41,44). Antibiotic treatment without shunt removal is rarely effective (22). VA shunts that have caused nephritis can be replaced with VP shunts that only rarely cause nephritis (22). If treatment is delayed until irreversible renal damage has occurred, shunt nephritis can progress to end-state renal disease.

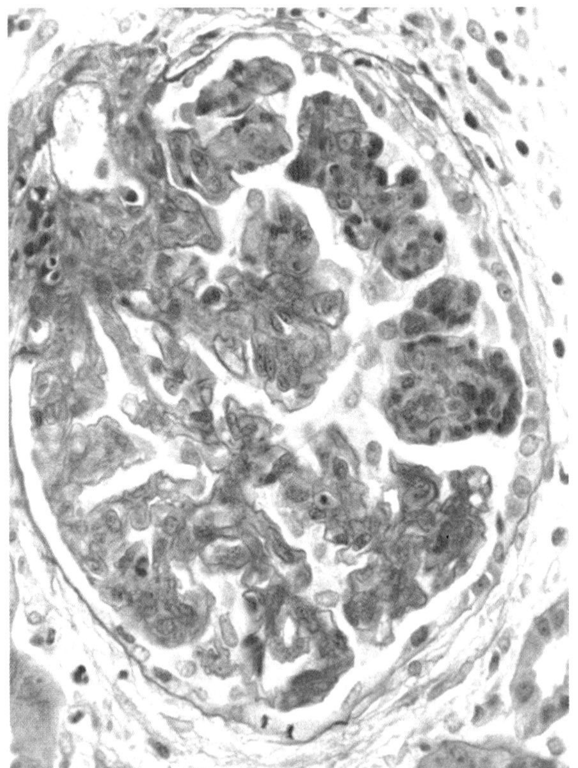

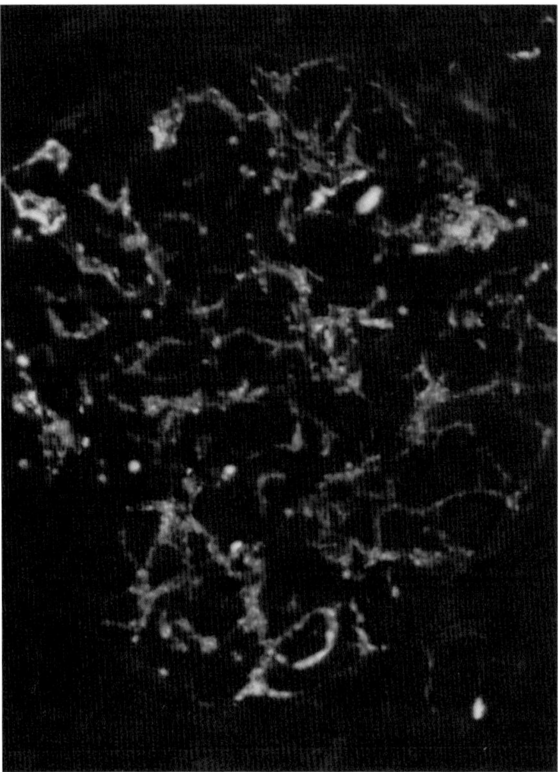

Figure 11-36

ABSCESS GLOMERULONEPHRITIS

Proliferative glomerulonephritis in a patient with a history of staphylococcal periodontal abscesses.

Left: Light microscopy shows segmental endocapillary hypercellularity with influx of neutrophils (PAS stain).

Right: Immunofluorescence microscopy shows coarsely granular capillary wall and mesangial staining for predominantly C3, with slight staining for IgM and IgG (not shown).

Approximately half of patients with shunt nephritis recover completely after appropriate treatment, a quarter have persistent renal abnormalities (especially proteinuria and mild insufficiency), and a quarter develop end-stage renal disease or die of complications related to the glomerulonephritis or infection (4,22).

ABSCESS AND OSTEOMYELITIS GLOMERULONEPHRITIS

Definition. Bacterial abscesses in viscera (e.g., lung and appendix abscesses), soft tissues (e.g., subcutaneous and periodontal abscesses), and bone (osteomyelitis and mastoiditis) can cause infectious glomerulonephritis (7,14,20,31,44, 48). This is not surprising since active bacterial infections in the nasopharynx, skin, and heart valves cause glomerulonephritis.

Clinical Features. The ubiquitous clinical manifestation of the infection is fever (7,31). Other clinical manifestations depend on the site of infection. Purpura caused by systemic small vessel vasculitis that is accompanying the glomerulonephritis may be present (7). The most common features are hematuria and proteinuria. Features of renal insufficiency and hypertension are variable and depend on the severity of the glomerulonephritis. Hypocomplementemia and cryoglobulinemia are common, however, patients usually do not have rheumatoid factor (7).

Light Microscopic Findings. Like other infectious glomerulonephritides, glomerulonephritis caused by abscess and osteomyelitis has a spectrum of histologic phenotypes, including acute diffuse proliferative glomerulonephritis, proliferative glomerulonephritis (fig. 11-36, left), membranoproliferative glomerulonephritis, crescentic glomerulonephritis, and mesangioproliferative glomerulonephritis (7,14,31,44, 48). Some degree of crescent formation is common (7). Renal biopsies that are repeated after clinical recovery may show no pathologic abnormalities, whereas repeat biopsies in patients with persistent or recurrent disease show varying degrees of continued glomerulonephritis or glomerular sclerosis (7).

Immunofluorescence Findings. The predominant finding is substantial glomerular staining for C3 (fig. 11-36, right) (7,44). The degree of staining of the capillary wall versus the mesangium corresponds to the histologic pattern of injury, with some specimens (such as those with membranoproliferative glomerulonephritis) having extensive capillary wall deposits, and others (such as most with mesangioproliferative glomerulonephritis) having exclusively mesangial deposits. There usually is little or no staining for immunoglobulins, differentiating this glomerulonephritis from that seen with endocarditis or shunt glomerulonephritis (7).

Electron Microscopic Findings. Findings by electron microscopy parallel observations by immunofluorescence microscopy and include the spectrum of ultrastructural features that can be produced by all forms of infectious or postinfectious glomerulonephritis.

Differential Diagnosis. The same differential diagnostic considerations that were discussed for other infectious and postinfectious glomerulonephritides should be considered.

Etiology and Pathogenesis. The sites of abscess formation that most often lead to infectious glomerulonephritis are lungs and periodontal tissues (7,31). The most common pathogen is *Staphylococcus aureus* (7,31). Most likely, the same or only slightly modified pathogenic mechanisms cause glomerulonephritis in patients with bacterial abscesses or osteomyelitis as cause glomerulonephritis in patients with bacterial infections in the nasopharynx, skin, and heart valves.

Treatment and Prognosis. Effective antibiotic treatment of the etiologic infection usually results in complete resolution of the glomerulonephritis, whereas delay in institution of therapy or failure to clear the infection may result in persistent or progressive renal failure (7).

REFERENCES

1. Abdel-Rehim M, Degnan B, El-Ghobary A, et al. Serum antibodies to group A streptococcal extracellular and cell-associated antigens in Egyptians with post-streptococcal diseases. FEMS Immunol Med Microbiol 2001;31:21–7.
2. Adam D, Scholz H, Helmerking M. Short-course antibiotic treatment of 4782 culture-proven cases of group A streptococcal tonsillopharyngitis and incidence of poststreptococcal sequelae. J Infect Dis 2000;182:509–16.
3. Anand SK, Trygstad CW, Sharma HM, Northway JD. Extracapillary proliferative glomerulonephritis in children. Pediatrics 1975;56:434–42.
4. Arze RS, Rashid H, Morley R, Ward MK, Kerr DN. Shunt nephritis: report of two cases and review of the literature. Clin Nephrol 1983;19:48–53.
5. Baehr G. Glomerular lesions of subacute bacterial endocarditis. J Exp Med 1912;II:330–47.
6. Barnes E, Frankel A, Brown EA, Woodrow D. Glomerulonephritis associated with permanent pacemaker endocarditis. Am J Nephrol 1995;15:436–8.
7. Beaufils M, Morel-Maroger L, Sraer JD, Kanfer A, Kourilsky O, Richet G. Acute renal failure of glomerular origin during visceral abscesses. N Engl J Med 1976;295:185–9.
8. Bell ET. Glomerular lesions associated with endocarditis. Am J Pathol 1932;8:639–63.
9. Boulton-Jones JM, Sissons JG, Evans DJ, Peters DK. Renal lesions of subacute infective endocarditis. Br Med J 1974;2:11–4.
10. Choi HK, Lamprecht P, Niles JL, Gross WL, Merkel PA. Subacute bacterial endocarditis with positive cytoplasmic antineutrophil cytoplasmic antibodies and anti-proteinase 3 antibodies. Arthritis Rheum 2000;43:226–31.

11. Cu GA, Mezzano S, Bannan JD, Zabriskie JB. Immunohistochemical and serological evidence for the role of streptococcal proteinase in acute post-streptococcal glomerulonephritis. Kidney Int 1998;54:819–26.
12. Cunningham RJ, Gilfoil M, Cavallo T, et al. Rapidly progressive glomerulonephritis in children: a report of thirteen cases and a review of the literature. Pediatr Res 1980;14:128–32.
13. Cusack D, Martin P, Schinittger T, McCafferky M, Keane C, Keogh B. IgA nephropathy in association with Yersinia enterocolitica. Ir J Med Sc 1983;152:311–2.
14. Danovitch GM, Nord EP, Barki Y, Krugliak L. Staphylococcal lung abscess and acute glomerulonephritis. Is J Med Sc 1979;15:840–3.
15. Dodge WF, Spargo BH, Bass PS, Travis LB. The relationship between the clinical and pathologic features of poststreptococcal glomerulonephritis. A study of the early natural history. Medicine 1968;47:227–67.
16. Edelstein CL, Bates WD. Subtypes of acute postinfectious glomerulonephritis: a clinicopathological correlation. Clin Nephrol 1992;38:311–7.
17. el Tayeb SH, Nasr EM, Sattallah AS. Streptococcal impetigo and acute glomerulonephritis in children in Cairo. Br J Dermatol 1978;98:53–62.
18. Frank JA, Friedman HS, Davidson DM, Falletta JM, Kinney TR. Propionibacterium shunt nephritis in two adolescents with medulloblastoma. Cancer 1983;52:330–3.
19. Fujigaki Y, Yousif Y, Morioka T, et al. Glomerular injury induced by cationic 70-kD staphylococcal protein; specific immune response is not involved in early phase in rats. J Pathol 1998;184:436–45.
20. Griffin MD, Bjornsson J, Erickson SB. Diffuse proliferative glomerulonephritis and acute renal failure associated with acute staphylococcal osteomyelitis. J Am Soc Nephrol 1997;8:1633–9.
21. Gutman RA, Striker GE, Gilliland BC, Cutler RE. The immune complex glomerulonephritis of bacterial endocarditis. Medicine 1972;51:1–25.
22. Haffner D, Schindera F, Aschoff A, Matthias S, Waldherr R, Scharer K. The clinical spectrum of shunt nephritis. Nephrol Dial Transplant 1997;12:1143–8.
23. Herbert MA, Milford DV, Silove ED, Raafat F. Secondary amyloidosis from long-standing bacterial endocarditis. Pediatr Nephrol 1995;9:33–5.
24. Herdson PB, Jennings RB, Earle DP. Glomerular fine structure in poststreptococcal acute glomerulonephritis. Arch Pathol 1966;81:117–28.
25. Johnston F, Carapetis J, Patel MS, Wallace T, Spillane P. Evaluating the use of penicillin to control outbreaks of acute poststreptococcal glomerulonephritis. Pediatr Infect Dis J 1999;18:327–32.
26. Kannan S, Mattoo TK. Diffuse crescentic glomerulonephritis in bacterial endocarditis. Pediatr Nephrol 2001;16:423–8.
27. Keslin MH, Messner RP, Williams RC Jr. Glomerulonephritis with subacute bacterial endocarditis. Immunofluorescent studies. Arch Intern Med 1973;132:578–81.
28. Le Moing V, Lacassin F, Delahousse M, et al. Use of corticosteroids in glomerulonephritis related to infective endocarditis: three cases and review. Clin Infect Dis 1999;28:1057–61.
29. Majumdar A, Chowdhary S, Ferreira MA, et al. Renal pathological findings in infective endocarditis. Nephrol Dial Transplant 2000;15:1782–7.
30. Michael AF Jr, Drummond KN, Good RA, Vernier RL. Acute poststreptococcal glomerulonephritis: immune deposit disease. J Clin Invest 1966;45:237–48.
31. Montseny JJ, Meyrier A, Kleinknecht D, Callard P. The current spectrum of infectious glomerulonephritis. Experience with 76 patients and review of the literature. Medicine 1995;74:63–73.
32. Muftuoglu AU, Erbengi T, Harmanci M, Karayel T, Gursoy E, Tahsinoglu M. Acute glomerulonephritis. Immunofluorescent and electron-microscopic observations in sporadic cases. Am J Clin Pathol 1975;63:300–9.
33. Nelson KE, Bisno AL, Waytz P, Brunt J, Moses VK, Haque R. The epidemiology and natural history of streptococcal pyoderma: an endemic disease of the rural southern United States. Am J Epidemiol 1976;103:270–83.
34. Neugarten J, Baldwin DS. Glomerulonephritis in bacterial endocarditis. Am J Med 1984;77:297–304.
35. Nordstrand A, Norgren M, Holm SE. Pathogenic mechanism of acute post-streptococcal glomerulonephritis. Scand J Infect Dis 1999;31:523–37.
36. Parra G, Platt JL, Falk RJ, Rodriguez-Iturbe B, Michael AF. Cell populations and membrane attack complex in glomeruli of patients with poststreptococcal glomerulonephritis: identification using monoclonal antibodies by indirect immunofluorescence. Clin Immunol Immunopathol 1984;33:324–32.
37. Pulik M, Lionnet F, Genet P, Petitdidier C, Vacher B. Immune-complex glomerulonephritis associated with Staphylococcus aureus infection of a totally implantable venous device. Support Care Cancer 1995;3:324–6.
38. Rodriguez-Iturbe B, Gastillo L, Valbuena R, Cuenca L. Acute poststreptococcal glomerulonephritis. A review of recent developments. Paediatrician 1979;8:307–24.

39. Romero M, Mosquera J, Novo E, Fernandez L, Parra G. Erythrogenic toxin type B and its precursor isolated from nephritogenic streptococci induce leukocyte infiltration in normal rat kidneys. Nephrol Dial Transplant 1999;14:1867–74.
40. Roy S 3rd, Pitcock JA, Etteldorf JN. Prognosis of acute poststreptococcal glomerulonephritis in childhood: prospective study and review of the literature. Adv Pediatr 1976;23:35–69.
41. Samtleben W, Bauriedel G, Bosch T, Goetz C, Klare B, Gurland HJ. Renal complications of infected ventriculoatrial shunts. Artif Organs 1993;17:695–701.
42. Sanjad S, Tolaymat A, Whitworth J, Levin S. Acute glomerulonephritis in children: a review of 153 cases. South Med J 1977;70:1202–6.
43. Schafer R, Sheil JM. Superantigens and their role in infectious disease. Adv Pediatr Infect Dis 1995;10:369–90.
44. Silva FG. Acute postinfectious glomerulonephritis and glomerulonephritis complicating persistent bacterial infection. In: Jennette JC, Olson JL, Schwartz MM, Silva FG, eds. Heptinstall's pathology of the kidney, 5th ed. Philadelphia: Lippincott-Raven; 1998:389–453.
45. Soma J, Saito T, Sato H, Ootaka T, Abe K. Membranoproliferative glomerulonephritis induced by portosystemic shunt surgery for noncirrhotic portal hypertension. Clin Nephrol 1997;48:274–81.
46. Sorger K, Gessler M, Hubner FK, et al. Follow-up studies of three subtypes of acute postinfectious glomerulonephritis ascertained by renal biopsy. Clin Nephrol 1987;27:111–24.
47. Sorger K, Gessler U, Hubner FK, et al. Subtypes of acute postinfectious glomerulonephritis. Synopsis of clinical and pathological features. Clin Nephrol 1982;17:114–28.
48. Spector DA, Millan J, Zauber N, Burton J. Glomerulonephritis and Staphylococcal aureus infections. Clin Nephrol 1980;14:256–61.
49. Tornroth T. The fate of subepithelial deposits in acute poststreptococcal glomerulonephritis. Lab Invest 1976;35:461–74.
50. Vella J, Carmody M, Campbell E, Browne O, Doyle G, Donohoe J. Glomerulonephritis after ventriculo-atrial shunt. QJM 1995;88:911–8.
51. Viera NT, Romero MJ, Montero MK, Rincon J, Mosquera JA. Streptococcal erythrogenic toxin B induces apoptosis and proliferation in human leukocytes. Kidney Int 2001;59:950–8.
52. Yared G, Seidner DL, Steiger E, Hall PM, Nally JV. Tunneled right atrial catheter infection presenting as renal failure. JPEN J Parent Enteral Nutr 1999;23:363–5.
53. Yoshizawa N, Suzuki Y, Oshima S, et al. Asymptomatic acute poststreptococcal glomerulonephritis following upper respiratory tract infections caused by group A streptococci. Clin Nephrol 1996;46:96–301.
54. Zelman ME, Lange CF. Immunochemical studies of streptococcal cell membrane antigens immunologically related to glomerular basement membrane. Hybridoma 1995;14:529–36.
55. Zent R, Van Zyl Smit R, Duffield M, Cassidy MJ. Crescentic nephritis at Groote Schuur Hospital, South Africa—not a benign disease. Clin Nephrol 1994;42:22–9.

12 IgA NEPHROPATHY AND HENOCH-SCHÖNLEIN PURPURA

IMMUNOGLOBULIN (Ig)A NEPHROPATHY

Definition. IgA nephropathy is a glomerular disease in which glomerular immunohistologic staining for IgA is more intense or equally intense as staining for IgG and IgM (fig. 12-1). The exception to this definition is the glomerulonephritis seen in patients with systemic lupus erythematosus in which the dominant or co-dominant IgA staining is considered to be lupus glomerulonephritis with extensive IgA deposition rather than IgA nephropathy. Most cases of IgA nephropathy occur as a primary (idiopathic) disease, with no associated systemic diseases. IgA nephropathy, however, may occur as a component of Henoch-Schönlein purpura, or may be associated with, and possibly caused by, a variety of extrarenal diseases, including liver disease, ankylosing spondylitis, psoriasis, Reiter's disease, uveitis, enteritis, inflammatory bowel disease, celiac disease, dermatitis herpetiformis, and human immunodeficiency virus (HIV) infection. The nephritis of Henoch-Schönlein purpura is virtually indistinguishable from primary IgA nephropathy; however, because of its distinctive clinical features and distinctive extrarenal pathologic lesions, Henoch-Schönlein purpura is discussed separately later in this chapter.

Clinical Features. IgA nephropathy is the most common form of primary glomerulonephritis in the world (11,21,23,32,41,60). It accounts for approximately 5 to 10 percent of patients in the United States whose glomerular disease is diagnosed by renal biopsy, 20 percent in Europe, and 40 percent in Asia. Irrespective of geographic location, the frequency of IgA nephropathy varies among ethnic groups, with the highest frequency among Asians and Native Americans, intermediate frequency among Caucasians, and lowest frequency among individuals of African lineage (23,38). One study, however, suggests that IgA nephropathy may be more frequent in African-American children than has previously been thought (54). Familial clustering of IgA nephropathy occurs but is uncommon (53). IgA nephropathy is twice as frequent in men than women. It is usually identified during late childhood or early adulthood, but may be diagnosed at any age (fig. 12-2).

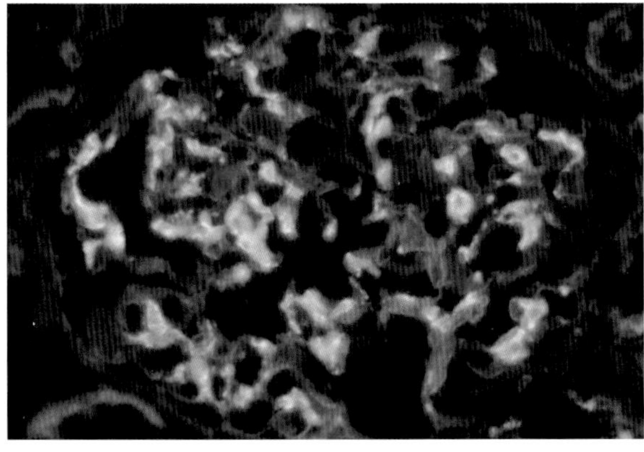

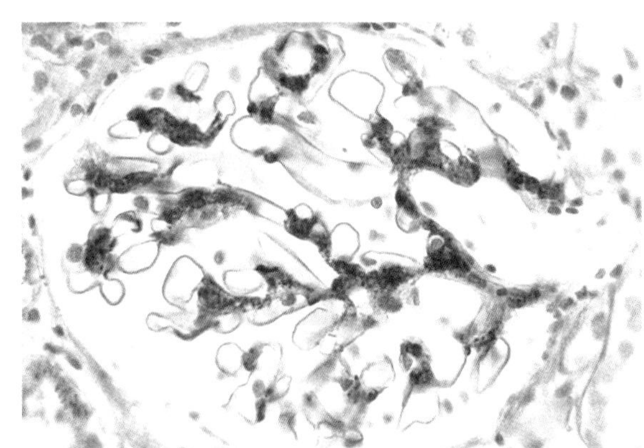

Figure 12-1

IMMUNOGLOBULIN (Ig)A NEPHROPATHY: MESANGIAL DEPOSITS

Immunofluorescence microscopy on frozen tissue (left) and immunoenzyme microscopy on paraffin-embedded tissue (right) demonstrate intense mesangial staining for IgA.

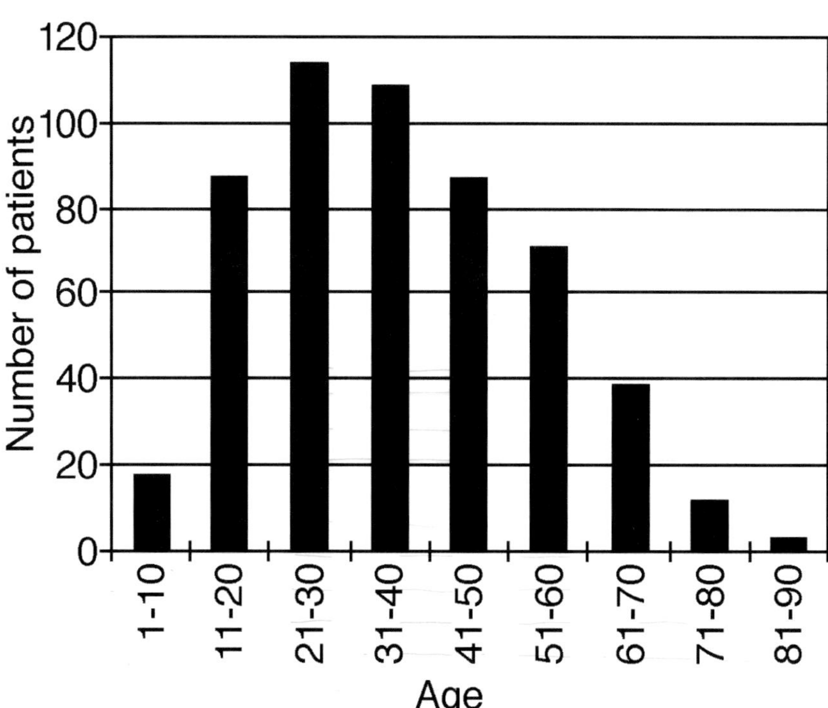

Figure 12-2

AGE DISTRIBUTION OF PATIENTS AT THE TIME OF DIAGNOSIS OF IgA NEPHROPATHY

The chart shows the ages of 544 patients at the time of renal biopsy diagnosis of IgA nephropathy at the University of North Carolina Nephropathology Laboratory. Note the peak in late childhood and early adulthood.

Berger and Hinglais (5) first described IgA nephropathy in 1968. They reported on 25 patients with intense glomerular deposits of IgA and less intense IgG and complement deposits. All the patients had microscopic evidence of hematuria and proteinuria, 50 percent had episodes of gross hematuria, and most had normal renal function. Half of the patients had focal glomerulonephritis with segmental necrosis and sclerosis while the remainder had a variety of other glomerular lesions. The following year, Berger (4) extended his series of what he called "nephropathy with mesangial IgA-IgG deposits" to 55 patients, and reported similar immunohistopathologic findings in patients with Henoch-Schönlein purpura nephritis. Most of these patients had persistent microscopic hematuria, often with bouts of gross hematuria frequently associated with pharyngitis. They usually had proteinuria. Only three patients had renal insufficiency; one eventually required transplantation and had recurrence of IgA nephropathy in the allograft. There was considerable heterogeneity by light microscopy, with 25 patients having focal glomerulonephritis; 20, varying degrees of chronic glomerulonephritis; and 5, no discernible lesions.

Over the years since its discovery, the clinical and pathologic diversity of IgA nephropathy that was noted by Berger has been substantiated (11,21,23,32,60). The clinical presentation of IgA nephropathy spans the gamut of signs and symptoms that can be caused by any glomerular disease. A rough approximation of the proportion of patients with various initial clinical manifestations is: 40 percent with asymptomatic microscopic hematuria, 40 with percent gross hematuria, 10 percent with nephrotic syndrome, and 10 percent with renal failure. Rare patients present with rapidly progressive glomerulonephritis. Serum complement levels are normal and assays for antinuclear antibodies are typically negative. A minority of patients have hypertension at the time of diagnosis but many develop hypertension as the disease progresses. Loin pain (flank pain) is an occasional symptom, especially in patients with gross hematuria.

Gross Findings. The kidneys are rarely available for gross examination during an acute episode of IgA nephropathy because there is almost no acute mortality with the disease. If gross examination could be carried out during active disease when there is extensive hematuria, tiny

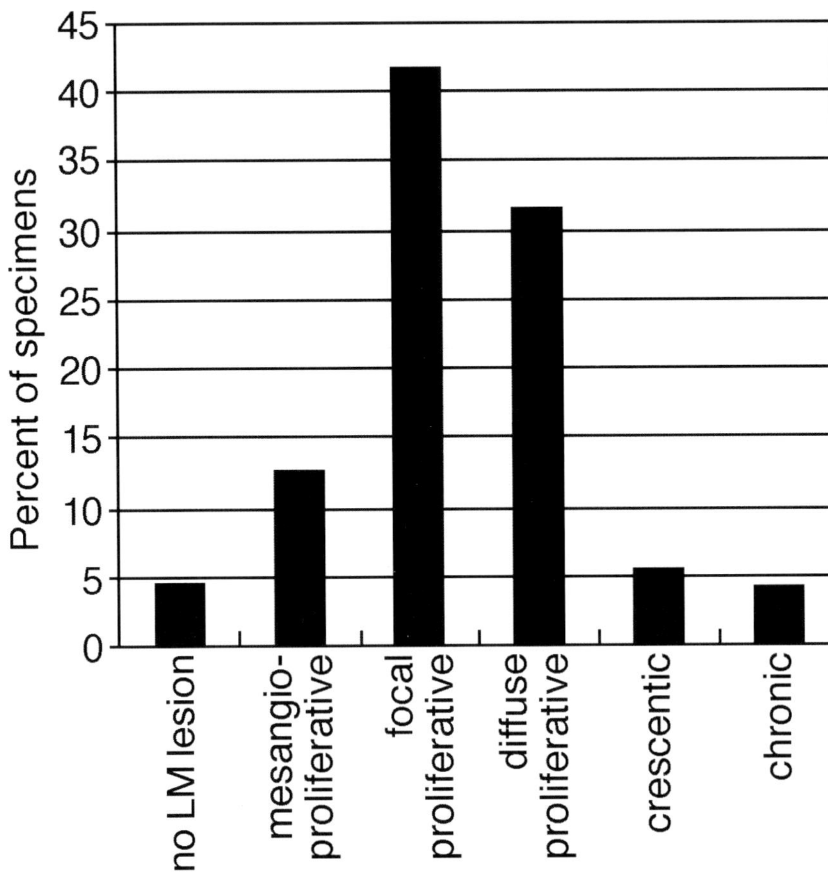

Figure 12-3

FREQUENCY OF DIFFERENT HISTOLOGIC CATEGORIES OF IgA NEPHROPATHY

The chart shows the percentage of 447 renal biopsy specimens that revealed different histologic phenotypes of IgA nephropathy when they were evaluated at the University of North Carolina Nephropathology Laboratory. The relative frequencies vary among different patient cohorts based, in part, on the clinical criteria for biopsy.

red dots would be seen over the capsular and cut kidney surfaces as a result of hemorrhage into Bowman's spaces and the lumens of tubules. This "flea-bitten" appearance is not specific for IgA nephropathy but can be seen with any glomerular disease that causes marked hematuria. With progression of the disease, the cortex gets thinner as a result of glomerular scarring and tubular atrophy. The external surfaces are finely granular and the cut surfaces of the cortex are pale and hard.

Light Microscopic Findings. IgA nephropathy may manifest most of the histologic phenotypes that are caused by immune complex–mediated glomerulonephritis, including no lesion by light microscopy, focal (less than 50 percent glomeruli involved) or diffuse (50 percent or more of glomeruli involved) mesangioproliferative glomerulonephritis, focal or diffuse endocapillary proliferative glomerulonephritis, crescentic glomerulonephritis (uncommon), type 1 membranoproliferative glomerulonephritis (rare), and focal or diffuse sclerosing glomerulonephritis (19,25,37,46,47). The relative frequencies of these different histologic phenotypes depend on the selection criteria used by the referring nephrologists to decide when to biopsy a patient with glomerular hematuria (fig. 12-3). The greater the degree of renal insufficiency or proteinuria required for a decision to biopsy, the higher the proportion of IgA nephropathy specimens that have overt proliferative and sclerosing disease, and the lower the proportion with no light microscopic lesions or only mild mesangial hypercellularity.

A number of different histologic classification systems have been used to categorize the histologic patterns of IgA nephropathy (Table 12-1) (19,25,46,47). An alternative approach is to use the same terminology for IgA nephropathy that is commonly used to categorize lupus nephritis (i.e., the World Health Organization [WHO] system), which precludes the need to learn an additional categorizing system for IgA nephropathy.

Table 12-1

HISTOLOGIC CLASSIFICATION SYSTEMS FOR IgA NEPHROPATHY

Lee IgA Nephropathy System[a]	Haas IgA Nephropathy System[b]	WHO Lupus System
		IIA. No lesion by light microscopy
I. Focal mesangioproliferative	I. Focal mesangioproliferative	IIB. Mesangioproliferative
II. Moderate focal proliferative	III. Focal proliferative	III. Focal proliferative
	II. Focal sclerosing	IIIC. Focal sclerosing
III. Mild diffuse proliferative	IV. Diffuse proliferative	IV. Diffuse proliferative
IV. Moderate diffuse proliferative		
V. Severe diffuse proliferative	V. Chronic sclerosing	VI. Chronic sclerosing

[a]Lee system from reference 46.
[b]Haas system from reference 25.

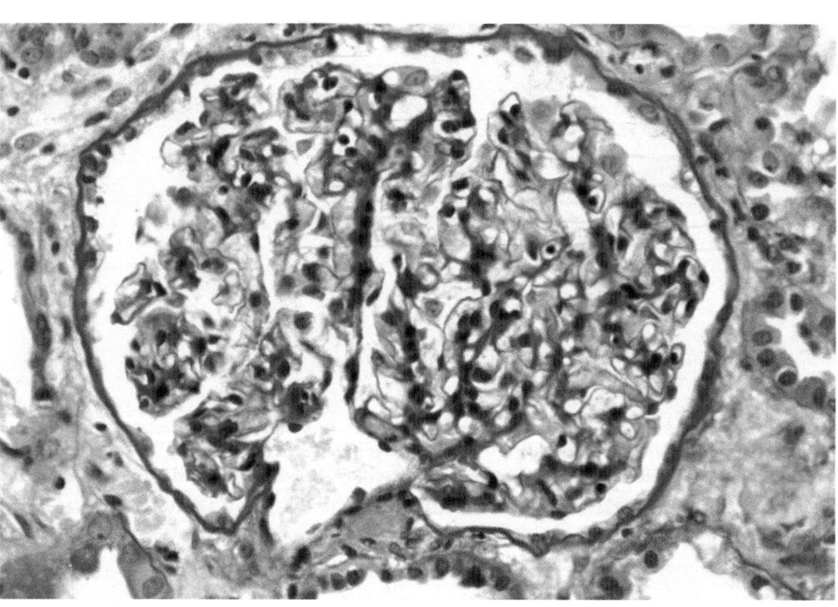

Figure 12-4

IgA NEPHROPATHY WITH NO LESION BY LIGHT MICROSCOPY

The periodic acid–Schiff (PAS) stain demonstrates no discernable glomerular abnormalities, including no increase in mesangial matrix and no mesangial hypercellularity. The normal numbers of mesangial cells and the delicate investment by mesangial matrix are evident when compared with figures 12-6 to 12-8.

Patients with IgA nephropathy who have overt clinical manifestations and typical IgA-dominant mesangial deposits may have no identifiable lesion by light microscopy (fig. 12-4). This is analogous to the mildest expression of lupus nephritis in which the mesangial immune deposits seen by immunofluorescence and electron microscopy are not detected by the light microscope. Even when glomeruli look normal using most staining techniques, a Masson trichrome stain may reveal mesangial fuchsinophilic deposits that correspond to IgA-rich immune deposits (fig. 12-5). These fuchsinophilic deposits can be seen with any histologic phenotype of IgA nephropathy if the immune deposits are large enough and if the trichrome stain is adjusted to differentiate immune deposits. In practice, however, this is not a reliable or sensitive method for identifying mesangial immune deposits. Immunohistology and electron microscopy are the appropriate methods for this purpose.

The most ubiquitous histologic feature of IgA nephropathy is mesangial hypercellularity (figs. 12-6–12-8). A widely accepted definition of mesangial hypercellularity is greater than three cells in one mesangial segment in a 3- to 4-μm section. Mesangial hypercellularity often is accompanied by increased mesangial matrix, which may form a small peripheral nodule of

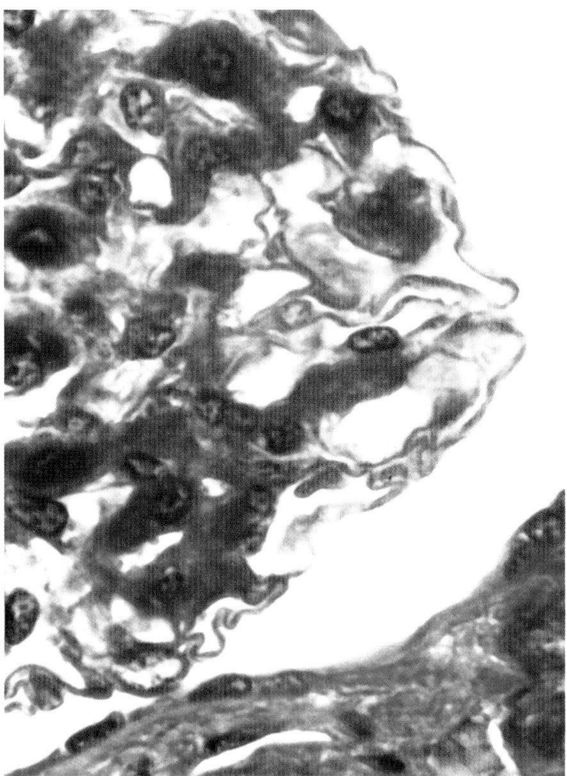

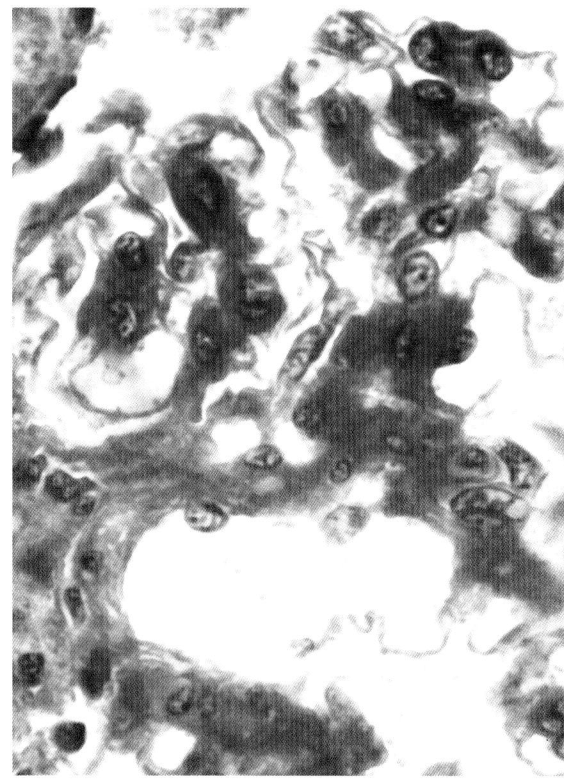

Figure 12-5

IgA NEPHROPATHY WITH FUCHSINOPHILIC MESANGIAL DEPOSITS

This Masson trichrome stain reveals bright red (fuchsinophilic) immune deposits in mesangial regions in the periphery of the tuft (left) and extending into the hilar matrix (right). The deposits do not extend into the juxtaglomerular apparatus (right).

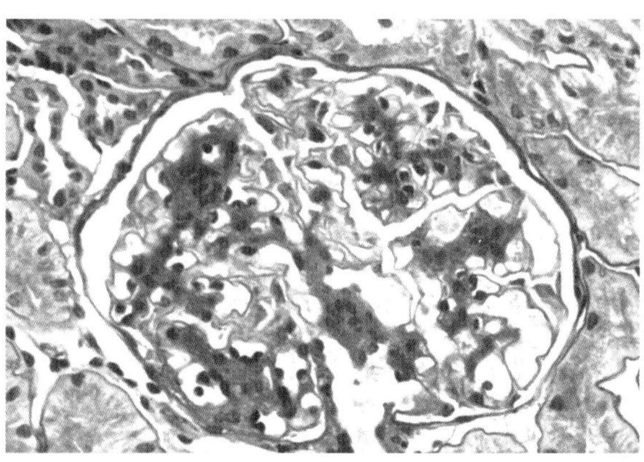

Figure 12-6

IgA NEPHROPATHY WITH MESANGIOPROLIFERATIVE GLOMERULONEPHRITIS

The PAS-stained glomerulus has segmental foci of mesangial hypercellularity and matrix expansion (examples are seen at the 3-o'clock and 10-o'clock positions). These foci have greater than three mesangial cells in a single sector of matrix. The capillary loops are patent and unremarkable.

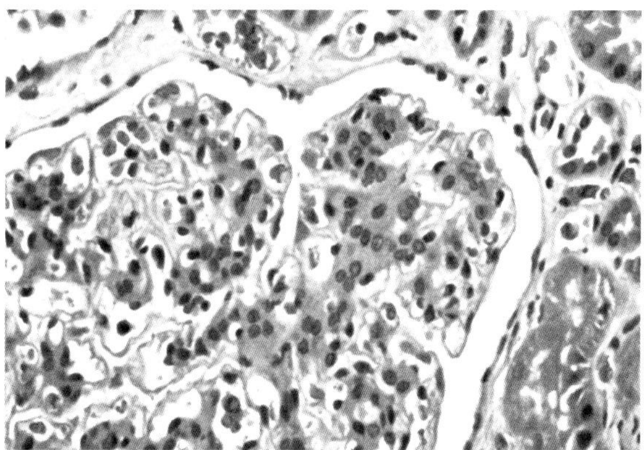

Figure 12-7

IgA NEPHROPATHY WITH MESANGIOPROLIFERATIVE GLOMERULONEPHRITIS

The hematoxylin and eosin (H&E)–stained glomerulus has prominent segmental mesangial hypercellularity, especially in the segment in the upper right. The capillary loops are patent and unremarkable.

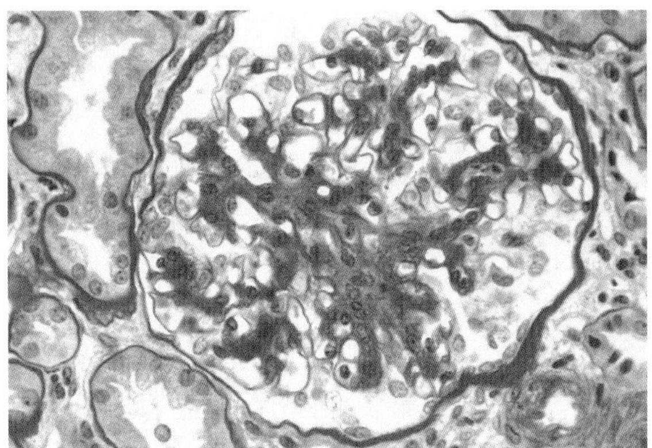

Figure 12-8

IgA NEPHROPATHY WITH MESANGIOPROLIFERATIVE GLOMERULONEPHRITIS

The PAS stain reveals marked segmental mesangial matrix expansion and hypercellularity, especially at the lower right. This may be evolving toward segmental sclerosis, but has not yet caused clear obliteration of glomerular architectural compartments.

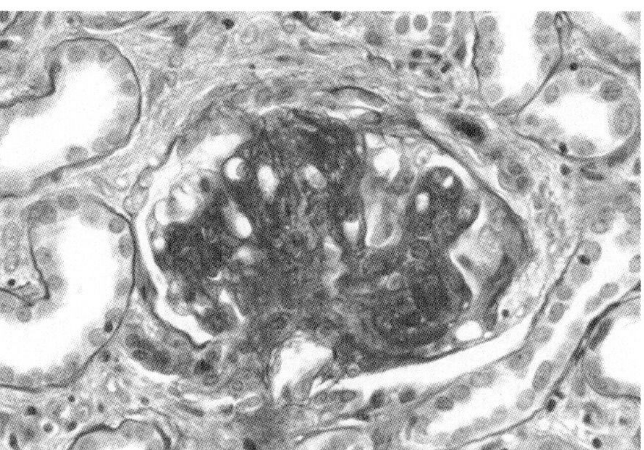

Figure 12-10

IgA NEPHROPATHY WITH GLOBAL GLOMERULAR SCLEROSIS

This glomerulus has progressed to global sclerosis secondary to IgA nephropathy. The lack of glomerular contraction (i.e., as seen with ischemic scarring) and several adhesions to Bowman's capsule indicate postnephritic scarring, but the specific kind of glomerulonephritis that caused the scarring cannot be determined by light microscopy.

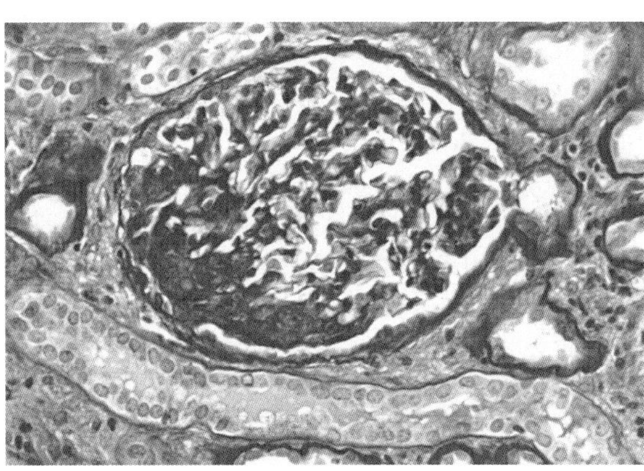

Figure 12-9

IgA NEPHROPATHY WITH FOCAL SCLEROSING GLOMERULONEPHRITIS

This PAS stain demonstrates segmental glomerular scarring with adhesions to Bowman's capsule. By light microscopy alone, this could not be distinguished from focal segmental glomerulosclerosis or other causes of glomerular scarring. The adjacent tubules are atrophied and have thickened basement membranes. There is increased interstitial fibrosis and slight interstitial infiltration by mononuclear leukocytes.

mesangium (fig. 12-6) or produce wider, more irregular expanses of matrix (fig. 12-8). As long as the segments remain distinct and the capillary lumens are patent, the increased collagenous material is referred to as expanded mesangial matrix rather than sclerosis. When the collagenous matrix obliterates capillary lumens or forms adhesions between glomerular segments and Bowman's capsule, it is called glomerular sclerosis, which is either segmental (fig. 12-9) or global (fig. 12-10).

Proliferative glomerulonephritis, which is short for endocapillary proliferative glomerulonephritis, differs from mesangioproliferative glomerulonephritis with respect to the heterogeneity of the cells that are causing the hypercellularity and the extent of obliteration of capillary lumens (figs. 12-11, 12-12). Focal proliferative glomerulonephritis is the most frequent histologic phenotype of IgA nephropathy identified in the University of North Carolina Nephropathology Laboratory (see fig. 12-3) as well as in many published series. For example, in an analysis of 244 IgA nephropathy specimens by Mark Haas (25), focal proliferative glomerulonephritis was found in 45 percent. As noted earlier, the relative frequencies of the different phenotypes vary depending on the biopsy criteria of the referring nephrologists. For example, the proportion of specimens with no lesion by light microscopy or purely mesangioproliferative lesions will be higher if larger numbers of patients with hematuria, normal renal function, and little or no proteinuria are biopsied.

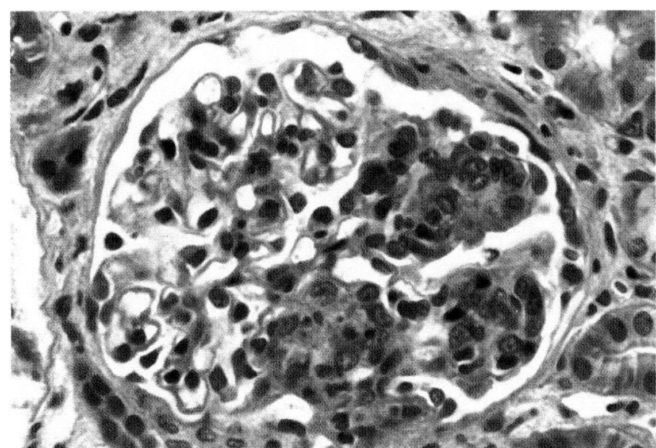

Figure 12-11

IgA NEPHROPATHY WITH PROLIFERATIVE GLOMERULONEPHRITIS

The segmental endocapillary hypercellularity has obscured the capillary lumens. Individual cells could be mesangial cells, endothelial cells, or leukocytes, however, this cannot be determined in this H&E-stained section. There are a few scattered fragments of nuclear debris indicative of karyorrhexis.

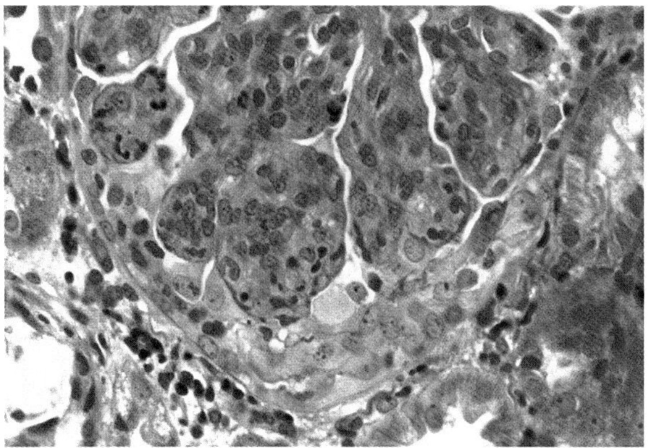

Figure 12-12

IgA NEPHROPATHY WITH PROLIFERATIVE GLOMERULONEPHRITIS

The global endocapillary hypercellularity is accompanied by extracapillary hypercellularity (crescent formation; top of figure). Several polymorphonuclear leukocytes contribute to the endocapillary cellularity. There is slight scattered nuclear pyknosis and karyorrhexis (Masson trichrome stain).

The endocapillary hypercellularity of proliferative glomerulonephritis is a complex mixture of different cell types, including endogenous glomerular cells (mesangial cells and endothelial cells) and infiltrating leukocytes (neutrophils, monocytes, macrophages, and lymphocytes). Without immunohistologic phenotyping, the specific cell types involved in endocapillary hypercellularity cannot be accurately distinguished by light microscopy. Trichrome staining may reveal fuchsinophilic immune deposits in the capillary wall in patients with endocapillary hypercellularity. Rare patients with IgA-dominant mesangial and capillary wall immune deposits detected by immunohistology have a light microscopic pattern of injury consistent with type 1 membranoproliferative (mesangiocapillary) glomerulonephritis (fig. 12-13). These samples have the ultrastructural features of membranoproliferative glomerulonephritis as well as subendothelial dense deposits and mesangial interposition.

Endocapillary hypercellularity in patients with IgA nephropathy may be accompanied by necrosis, which can manifest as scattered pyknotic nuclei and karyorrhectic debris (figs. 12-11, 12-12) or segmental fibrinoid necrosis (fig. 12-14). Focal segmental necrosis is seen in approximately

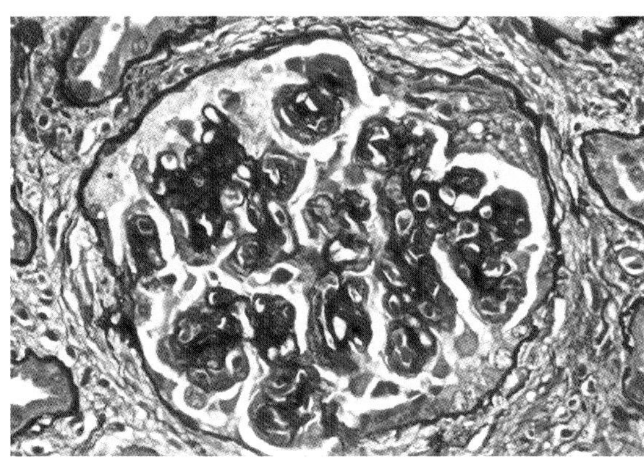

Figure 12-13

IgA NEPHROPATHY WITH MEMBRANOPROLIFERATIVE GLOMERULONEPHRITIS

This glomerulus has accentuated lobulation and segmentally variable glomerular basement membrane thickening and replication. There is a small crescent at the upper right. Immunofluorescence microscopy demonstrated extensive capillary wall and mesangial IgA-dominant staining. Electron microscopy demonstrated numerous subendothelial deposits and focal subendothelial mesangial interposition Jones methenamine silver [JMS] stain).

10 percent of patients and does not predict the presence of Henoch-Schönlein purpura or concurrent antineutrophil cytoplasmic antibody (ANCA) disease (12). Extracapillary hypercellularity (crescent formation) may accompany

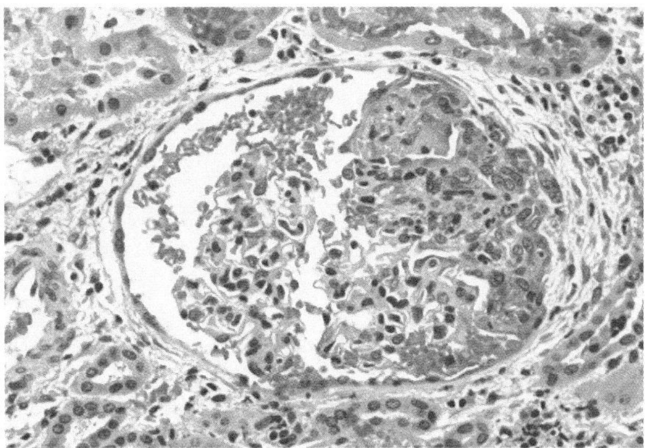

Figure 12-14

IgA NEPHROPATHY WITH PROLIFERATIVE GLOMERULONEPHRITIS AND NECROSIS

There is segmental endocapillary hypercellularity and a focal accumulation of fibrinoid material. This appears to be, in part, fibrinoid necrosis of a glomerular segment and, in part, fibrin spilling into Bowman's space. There is an early epithelial response (JMS stain with H&E counter stain).

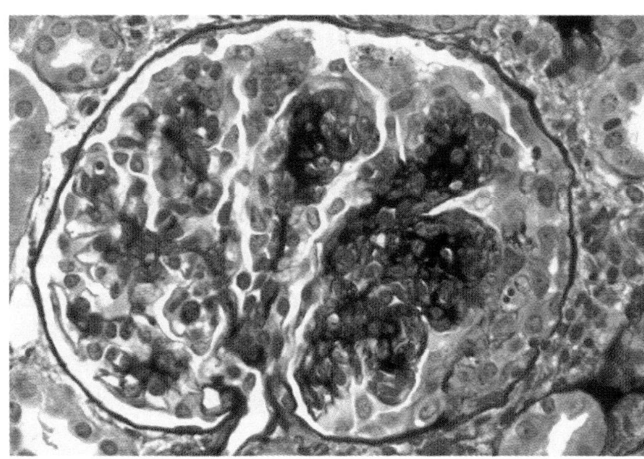

Figure 12-15

IgA NEPHROPATHY WITH PROLIFERATIVE GLOMERULONEPHRITIS AND CRESCENT

On the right, there is endocapillary hypercellularity with overlying extracapillary hypercellularity (crescent formation). The JMS with H&E counter stain helps demarcate the junction between the two.

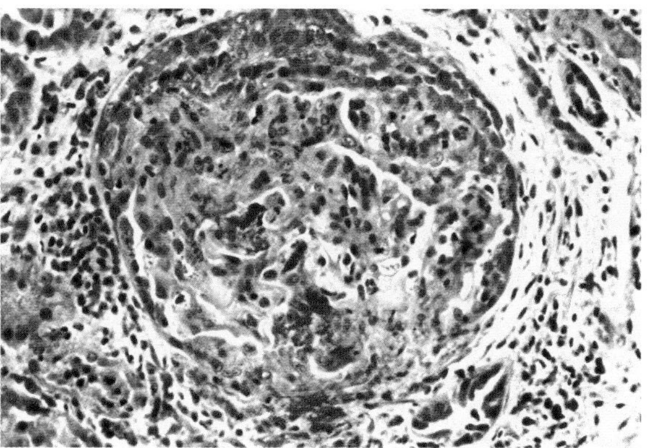

Figure 12-16

IgA NEPHROPATHY WITH PROLIFERATIVE, NECROTIZING AND CRESCENTIC GLOMERULONEPHRITIS ASSOCIATED WITH ANTINEUTROPHIL CYTOPLASMIC ANTIBODIES (ANCA)

This patient had extensive crescent formation and glomerular necrosis even though the IgA-dominant immune deposits were confined to the mesangium. The cellular crescent is at the top and the foci of fuchsinophilic fibrinoid necrosis at the bottom. Serologic testing revealed a high ANCA titer.

endocapillary hypercellularity (figs. 12-12, 12-14, 12-15). Crescents occur in a quarter or less of patients with IgA nephropathy and only 5 percent or less have 50 percent or more of glomeruli with crescents (33). Although crescents and necrosis may be caused by severe IgA nephropathy alone, when they are conspicuous, the possibility of concurrent IgA nephropathy and ANCA disease should be considered (fig. 12-16) (26). The likelihood of concurrent ANCA disease is highest when there are numerous crescents but only mild endocapillary hypercellularity.

The glomerular inflammation of IgA nephropathy can cause glomerular scarring. In some biopsy specimens there is focal segmental glomerular sclerosis without any active glomerular inflammation. Haas (25) observed this in 7 percent of IgA nephropathy specimens. Focal segmental glomerular scarring caused by IgA nephropathy can be impossible to distinguish from focal segmental glomerulosclerosis by light microscopy alone (see fig. 12-9). The finding of typical immune deposits by immunohistology and electron microscopy indicates that the sclerosis is postnephritic scarring. As IgA nephropathy progresses toward end-stage renal disease, more and more glomeruli undergo segmental and global sclerosis (see fig. 12-10). If a specimen contains only globally sclerotic glomeruli, the diagnostic immune deposits of IgA nephropathy may not be detectable by immunohistology.

The tubulointerstitial and extraglomerular vascular injury in IgA nephropathy are commensurate with the glomerular injury. With progressive disease, especially if there is concomitant hypertension, arteriolar and arterial

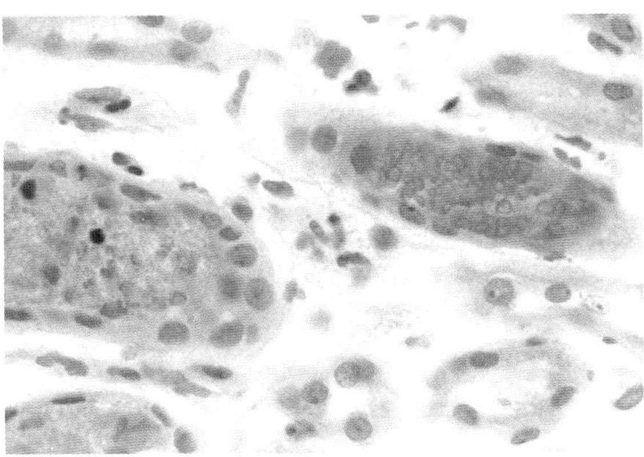

Figure 12-17

DYSMORPHIC ERYTHROCYTES IN TUBULAR LUMENS

Medullary tubular lumens contain erythrocytes with varying degrees of degeneration. This finding documents hematuria of glomerular origin.

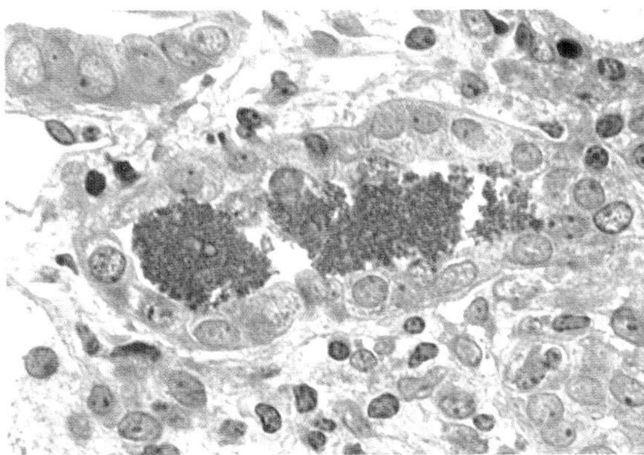

Figure 12-18

GRANULAR HEMOGLOBIN CAST IN TUBULAR LUMEN

A tubular lumen contains granular pigmented material consistent with hemoglobin. This can result from glomerular hematuria. The differential diagnosis includes hemolysis of circulating erythrocytes leading to hemoglobinuria. Hemoglobin casts cannot be distinguished from myoglobin casts by light microscopy alone.

sclerosis develop. The glomerular inflammation does not extend into arterioles in patients with IgA nephropathy. Arteriolitis is rare even in patients with Henoch-Schönlein purpura. The presence of arteriolitis, and especially arteritis, in a patient with the glomerular changes of IgA nephropathy should raise the possibility of Henoch-Schönlein purpura and, to an even greater extent, concurrent ANCA disease.

With mild glomerular injury, the tubulointerstitial tissue may appear completely normal. If there is active hematuria, erythrocytes, erythrocyte casts (fig. 12-17), and pigmented granular casts (fig. 12-18) may be seen within the lumens of tubules. Unaltered erythrocytes alone often spill into tubular lumens during the biopsy procedure and thus are not diagnostic of hematuria. The presence of dysmorphic erythrocytes or pigmented erythrocyte debris in tubular lumens documents hematuria, however. Rarely, tubular obstruction and tubular epithelial injury caused by massive hematuria appear to contribute to an acute loss of renal function in patients with IgA nephropathy (45). Another marker of persistent hematuria is hemosiderin within tubular epithelial cells. This is seen most often in the medulla (fig. 12-19). In a specimen from a patient with IgA nephropathy who has no active hematuria and no glomerular lesion by light microscopy, the presence of tubular epithelial hemosiderin may be the only histologic evidence of glomerular disease.

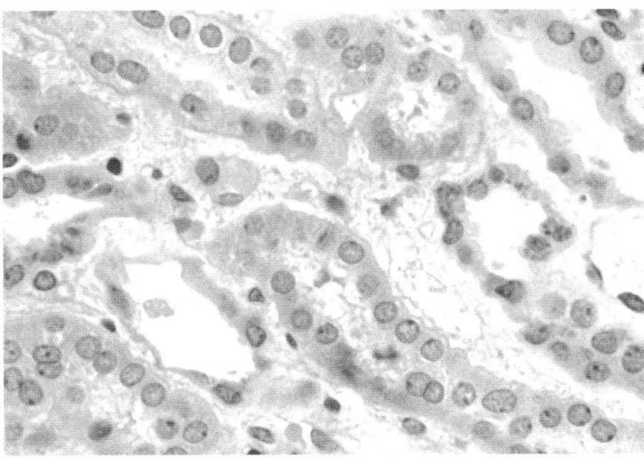

Figure 12-19

TUBULAR EPITHELIAL CELLS WITH HEMOSIDERIN

There is focal accumulation of golden brown hemosiderin pigment within medullary tubular epithelial cells. This supports the presence of persistent renal parenchymal hematuria, especially hematuria of glomerular origin.

With more severe glomerular injury, especially chronic sclerosing injury, there is proportionately more severe tubulointerstitial injury (figs. 12-20, 12-21). This begins as focal interstitial edema and infiltration by mononuclear leukocytes, and progresses to varying degrees of interstitial fibrosis, chronic inflammation, and tubular atrophy. Tubulitis usually is not

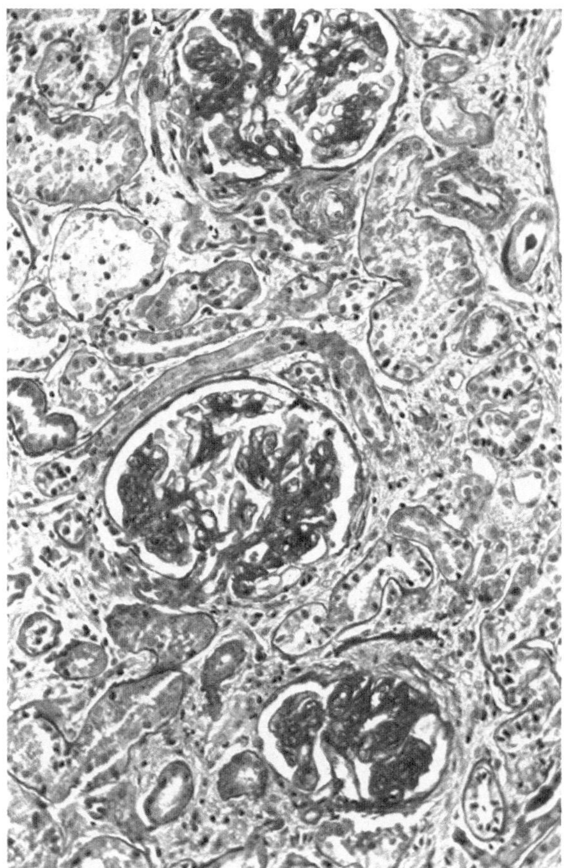

Figure 12-20

IgA NEPHROPATHY WITH MILD TUBULOINTERSTITIAL INJURY

The glomeruli have segmentally variable, proliferative and sclerosing lesions. There is relatively mild interstitial edema and fibrosis with a few interstitial mononuclear leukocytes. There is no significant tubular atrophy.

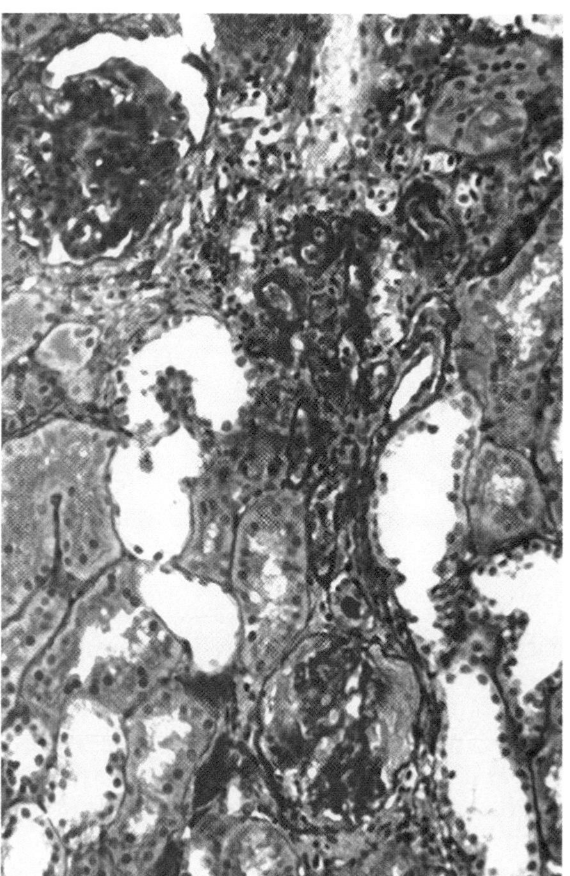

Figure 12-21

IgA NEPHROPATHY WITH CHRONIC TUBULOINTERSTITIAL INJURY

The glomerulus at the top has global endocapillary hypercellularity and the one on the bottom has global sclerosis. Near the center of the figure, there is a swath of severe chronic tubulointerstitial injury, including tubular atrophy, interstitial fibrosis, and interstitial infiltration by mononuclear leukocytes.

conspicuous but may be present, especially with advanced chronic disease.

Immunofluorescence Findings. The sine qua non for IgA nephropathy is immunohistologic detection of dominant or co-dominant staining for IgA in the glomerular mesangium (see fig. 12-1) (34). IgA is essentially always accompanied by C3 (fig. 12-22) and terminal complement components, however, staining for C1q usually is absent or of low intensity. The staining for C3 typically is more granular or particulate than the staining for IgA, although the general distribution of staining is similar. Over 50 percent of specimens have IgG and IgM in the same distribution as the IgA, but by definition IgG and IgM staining are not more intense than the staining for IgA; in most specimens, the staining intensity for IgA is much greater than that for IgG or IgM. Staining for IgA usually is 2+ or stronger (on a scale of 0 to 4+), however, a diagnosis of IgA nephropathy may be appropriate with lower intensity staining if supported by other pathologic and clinical data. A very distinctive feature of IgA nephropathy compared to other immune complex diseases is the high frequency of greater staining for lambda than kappa light chains (34). A few specimens stain for lambda but not kappa (fig. 12-23). Other immune complex–mediated glomerular

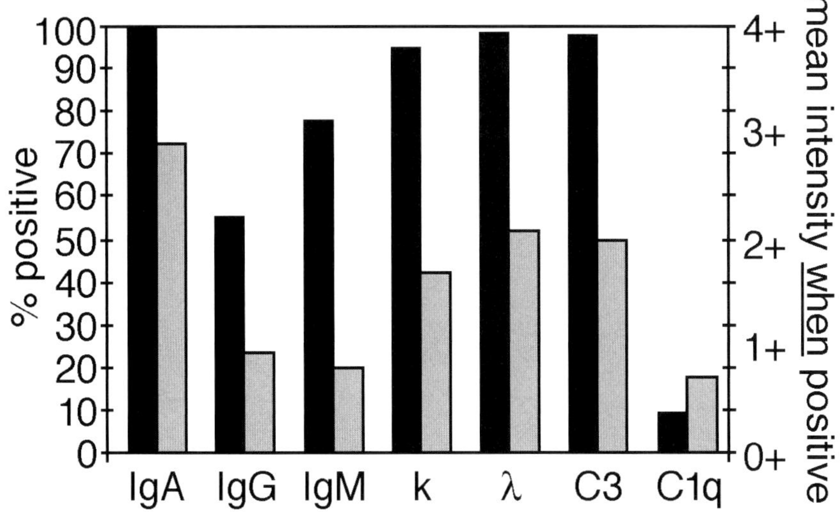

Figure 12-22

IMMUNOGLOBULIN AND COMPLEMENT STAINING IN IgA NEPHROPATHY

The bars on the left show the percentage of 447 IgA nephropathy specimens that stained by direct immunofluorescence for different immunoglobulin and complement molecules. The bars on the right show the mean intensity of staining when positive (i.e., 0 staining was not factored in). The mean intensity of staining for lambda light chains is higher than that for kappa light chains.

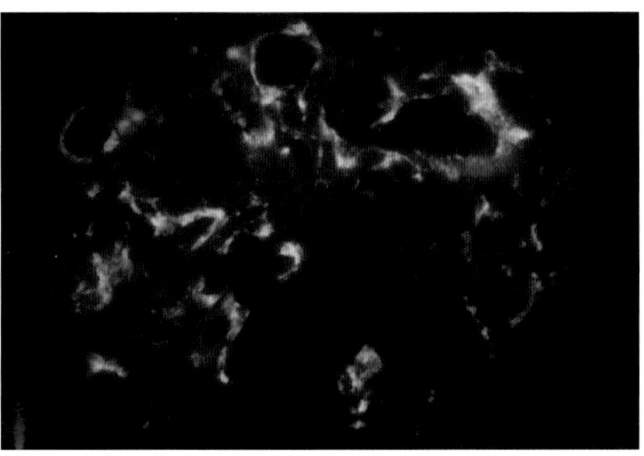

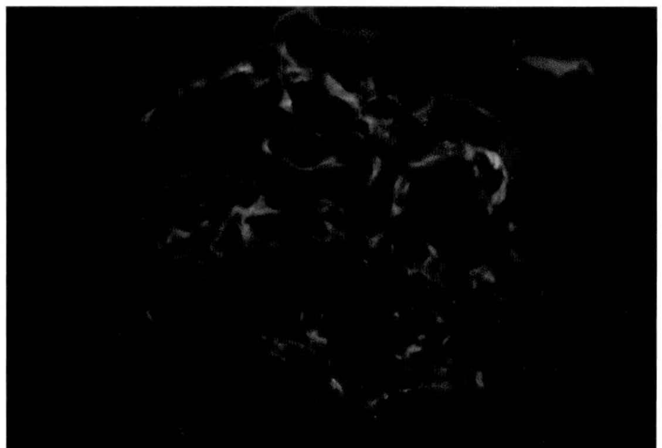

Figure 12-23

IgA NEPHROPATHY WITH LAMBDA LIGHT CHAINS ALONE

The mesangium in this specimen of IgA nephropathy stained intensely for lambda light chains (left) but not for kappa light chains (right). There was also intense staining for IgA and C3 but no staining for IgG or IgM, or C1q. The patient had no evidence of a monoclonal gammopathy.

diseases typically have equal or greater staining for kappa compared to lambda light chains. The greater staining for lambda light chains in IgA nephropathy is a reflection of the fact that IgA molecules have more lambda light chains than do either IgG or IgM molecules, which have a 2 to 1 ratio of kappa to lambda light chains. In fact, patients with IgA nephropathy have an even higher than normal ratio of lambda to kappa light chains in circulating IgA (7).

Examination of the background staining of glomeruli allows delineation of capillary walls from mesangial regions when staining is confined to, or at least predominantly within, the mesangium (figs. 12-1, 12-24). The mesangial staining may be granular or chunky, and sometimes appears as short curvilinear (comma-shaped) or granular bands when the deposits are clustered beneath the paramesangial basement membrane and absent from the central zone of the mesangium. Typically, the mesangial deposits stop abruptly at the juncture of the mesangium with the hilar arterioles (figs. 12-1, 12-25). Extension into the arterioles is rare in IgA nephropathy, and uncommon in Henoch-Schönlein purpura.

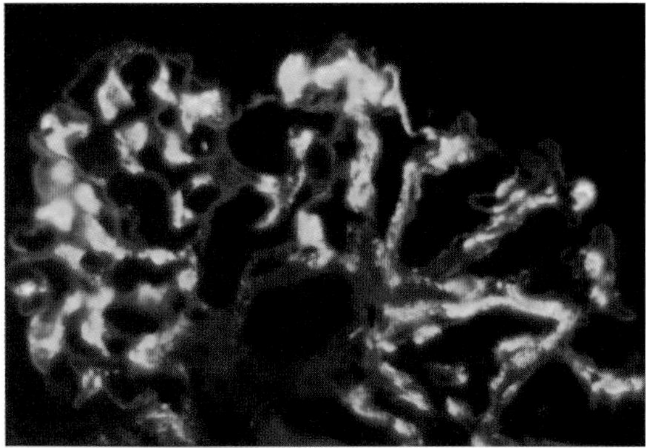

Figure 12-24

IgA NEPHROPATHY WITH MESANGIAL IgA

Direct immunofluorescence microscopy for IgA demonstrates numerous large, bright mesangial deposits but no significant staining in the capillary walls, which can be seen vaguely via the background staining.

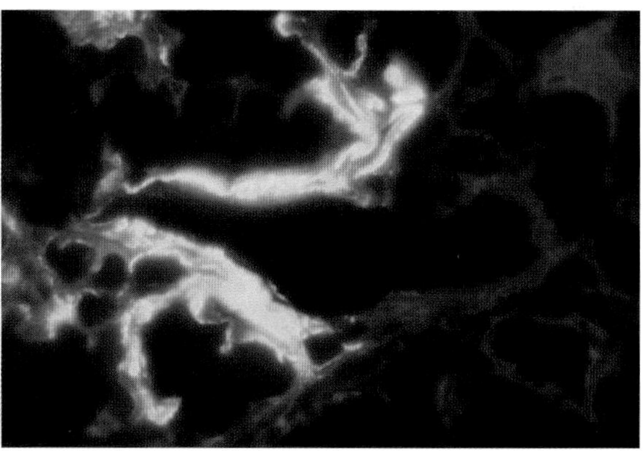

Figure 12-25

IgA NEPHROPATHY WITH MESANGIAL IgA

Direct immunofluorescence microscopy for IgA demonstrates numerous large, bright mesangial deposits that stop abruptly at the junction of the mesangium and the muscularis of the hilar arteriole.

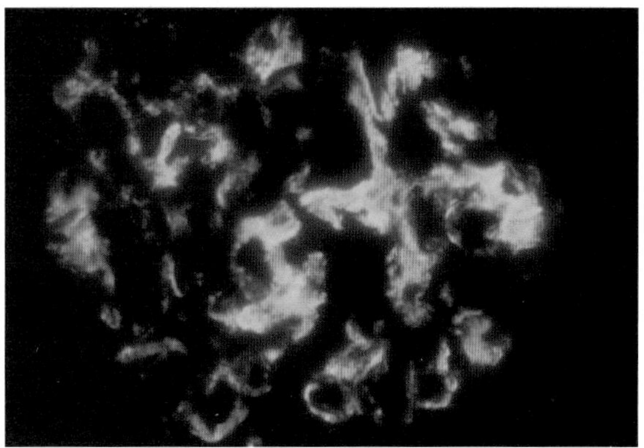

Figure 12-26

IgA NEPHROPATHY WITH MESANGIAL AND CAPILLARY WALL IgA

Direct immunofluorescence microscopy for IgA demonstrates numerous mesangial deposits as well as scattered deposits in a peripheral capillary (the loops at the bottom of the figure).

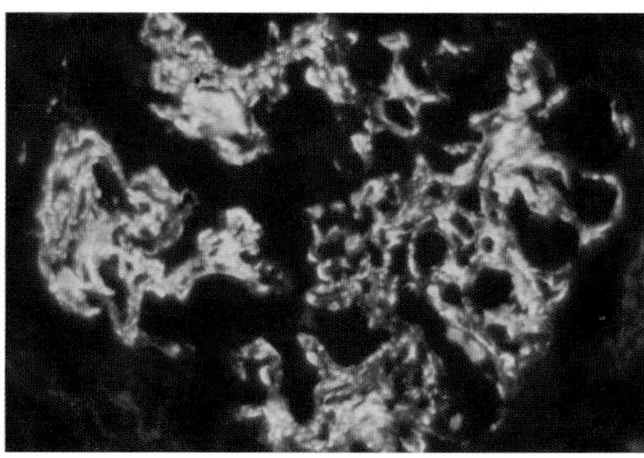

Figure 12-27

IgA NEPHROPATHY WITH EXTENSIVE CAPILLARY WALL DEPOSITS

Direct immunofluorescence microscopy for IgA demonstrates numerous capillary wall deposits in a specimen with a membranoproliferative pattern of glomerular injury as seen by light microscopy. Some of the capillary wall deposits are band-like, suggesting a subendothelial location.

About a quarter of IgA nephropathy specimens have focal segmental capillary wall staining that has the same composition as the mesangial deposits (fig. 12-26). When capillary wall deposits are numerous, the light microscopic pattern of injury consists of endocapillary hypercellularity and possible extracapillary hypercellularity (crescent formation). In rare specimens, the subendothelial capillary wall IgA-dominant deposits are extensive (fig. 12-27) and a type 1 membranoproliferative (mesangiocapillary) glomerulonephritis pattern of injury may be detected by light microscopy (see fig. 12-13).

Another rare finding is IgA nephropathy with mesangial IgA-dominant deposits combined with membranous glomerulopathy with IgG-dominant capillary wall deposits (fig. 12-28) (36,56). Electron microscopy confirms the presence of numerous subepithelial as well as mesangial

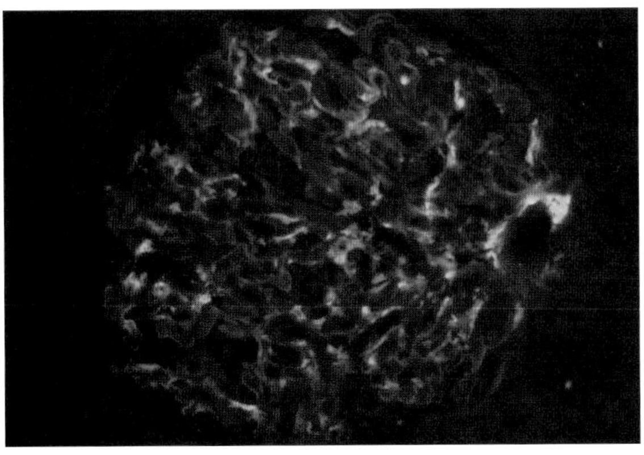

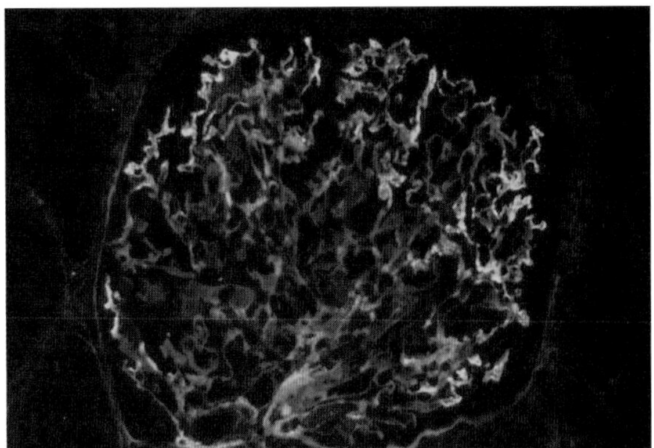

Figure 12-28

COMBINED IgA NEPHROPATHY AND MEMBRANOUS GLOMERULOPATHY

Direct immunofluorescence microscopy for IgA (left) and IgG (right) in the same specimen demonstrates IgA-dominant mesangial deposits indicative of IgA nephropathy (left) as well as IgG-dominant granular capillary wall deposits consistent with membranous glomerulopathy (right) (compare with figure 12-29).

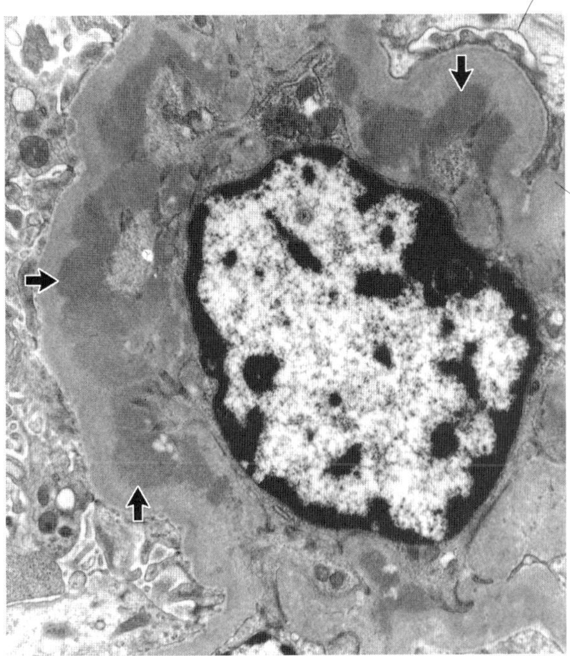

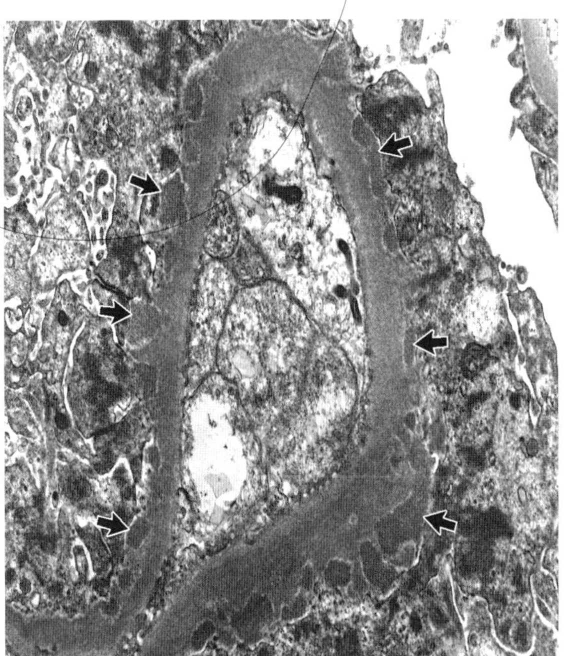

Figure 12-29

COMBINED IgA NEPHROPATHY AND MEMBRANOUS GLOMERULOPATHY

Electron microscopy of the same specimen illustrated in figure 12-28 demonstrates both mesangial electron-dense deposits (arrows) consistent with IgA nephropathy (left) and numerous subepithelial dense deposits (arrows) indicative of membranous glomerulopathy (right).

electron-dense deposits in patients with combined IgA nephropathy and membranous glomerulopathy (fig. 12-29). IgA nephropathy with scattered subepithelial deposits that have the same IgA-dominant composition as the mesangial deposits should not be confused with combined membranous glomerulopathy and IgA nephropathy in which the immunoglobulin composition of the capillary wall deposits is distinctly different from the mesangial immune deposits.

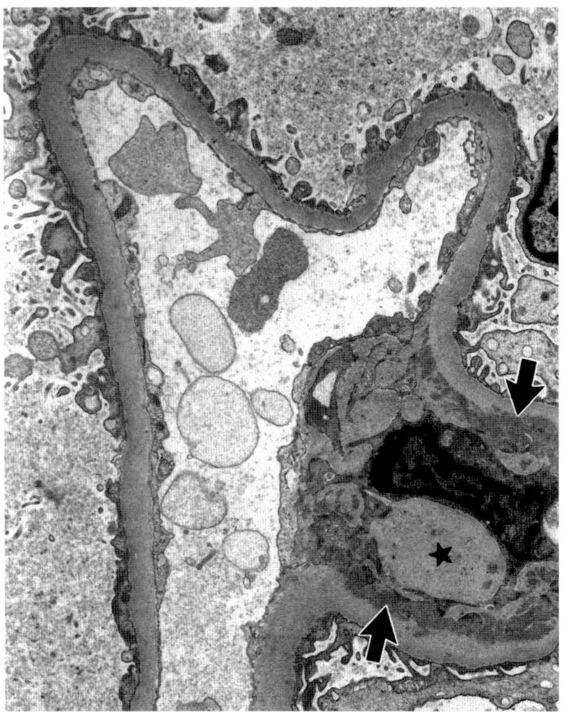

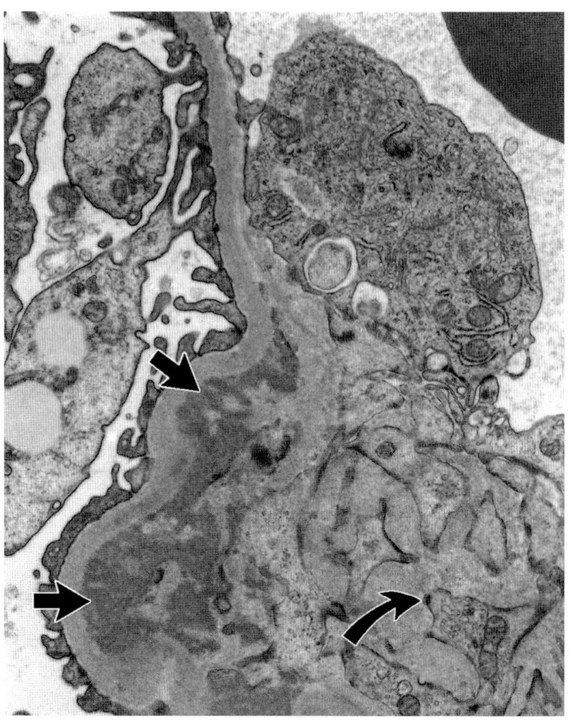

Figure 12-30

IgA NEPHROPATHY WITH MESANGIAL ELECTRON-DENSE DEPOSITS AND MATRIX EXPANSION

The mesangial electron-dense deposits are clustered immediately beneath the paramesangial basement membrane (arrows) (left and right). There is a central zone of mesangial matrix expansion in the left figure (star). In the right figure, there also is mesangial hypercellularity that is evidenced by multiple islands of mesangial cytoplasm with dense plaques (curved arrow) in their surface membranes.

Electron Microscopic Findings. The immune deposits seen by immunohistology appear as electron-dense deposits by electron microscopy (19,44). They are, of course, most numerous in the mesangium, where they are typically concentrated underneath the paramesangial basement membrane (figs. 12-30, 12-31). In this location, the deposits are nevertheless in the mesangium, although they often are called "paramesangial" deposits when in this location. Rare specimens with immunopathologic evidence of IgA nephropathy have no identifiable mesangial dense deposits. An increase in mesangial matrix material, mesangial hypercellularity, or both, often accompanies the mesangial dense deposits (fig. 12-30). Mesangial cells, because of their smooth muscle cell lineage, can be identified ultrastructurally by the presence of dense plaques scattered along the cell surfaces (fig. 12-30, right). The actin filaments of the cytoplasmic contractile apparatus attach to the dense plaques of the membrane to couple the contractile force of the mesangial cells to the mesangial matrix. In specimens with massive immune deposits, the extracellular compartment of the mesangium may be completely filled and expanded by electron-dense immune deposits (fig. 12-31). Especially when there are numerous mesangial deposits, some are in the matrix that lies in direct contact with the capillary lumen via the endothelial pores (fig. 12-32), where they may be more effective at activating inflammatory mediators than the deposits clustered beneath the paramesangial basement membrane.

Capillary wall deposits are seen in a quarter to a third of specimens (25,44). These can be subepithelial, subendothelial, or intramembranous (fig. 12-33). The capillary wall deposits are usually scattered about in some capillary walls but not others. Thus, even when subepithelial deposits are present, they typically are too sparsely distributed to warrant a consideration

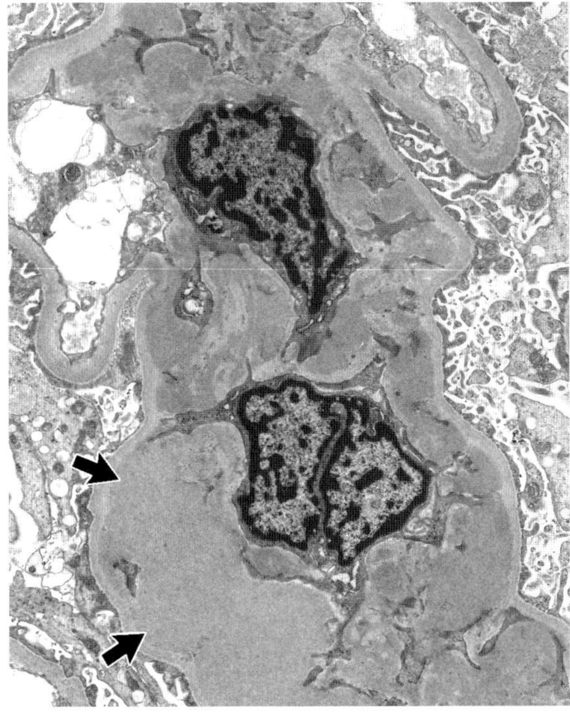

Figure 12-31

IgA NEPHROPATHY WITH MASSIVE MESANGIAL ELECTRON-DENSE DEPOSITS

There is marked expansion of the mesangium by large electron-dense deposits (arrows).

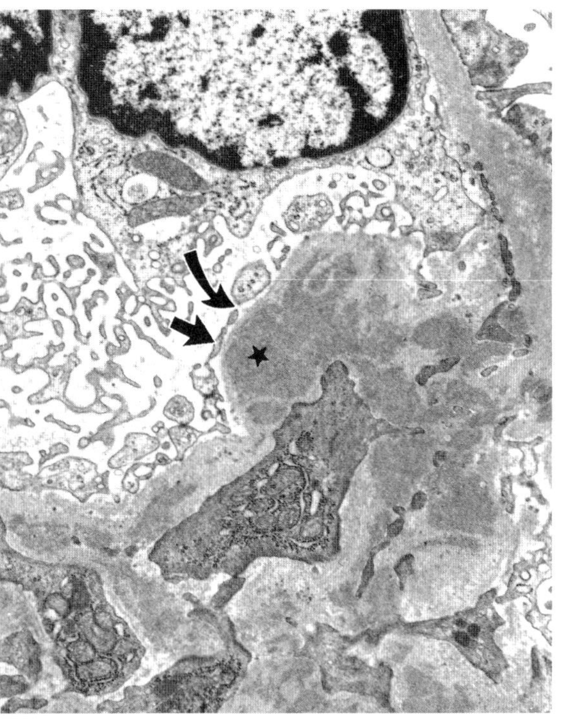

Figure 12-32

IgA NEPHROPATHY WITH MESANGIAL DEPOSITS

The mesangial immune deposits (star) are in apparent direct contact with the plasma through the fenestrations (curved arrow) in the endothelial cell (straight arrow) that covers the luminal surface of the mesangium.

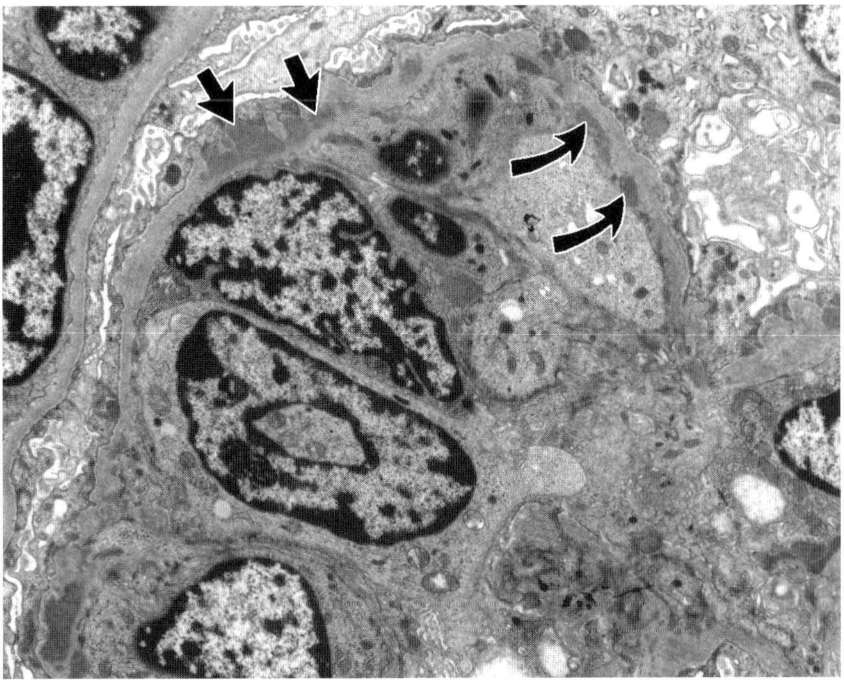

Figure 12-33

IgA NEPHROPATHY WITH CAPILLARY WALL ELECTRON-DENSE DEPOSITS AND ENDOCAPILLARY HYPERCELLULARITY

There are scattered subepithelial (straight arrows) and subendothelial (curved arrows) electron-dense deposits. These are accompanied by endocapillary hypercellularity and obliteration of the capillary lumen.

of membranous glomerulopathy. Capillary wall immune deposits are more frequently identified in specimens that have severe glomerular injury by light microscopy (fig. 12-34). This is

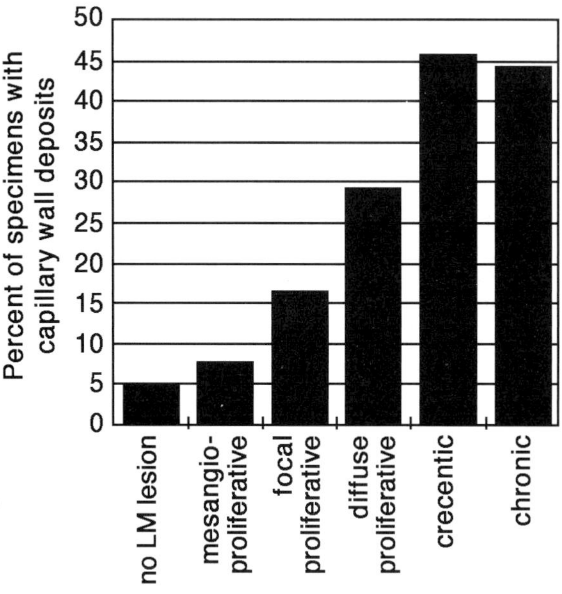

Figure 12-34

CORRELATION OF CAPILLARY WALL DEPOSITS WITH HISTOLOGIC PHENOTYPE OF IgA NEPHROPATHY

The percentage of 447 specimens with capillary wall deposits evaluated at the University of North Carolina Nephropathology Laboratory varies in different histologic categories of IgA nephropathy. There is a higher frequency of capillary wall deposits in specimens with more severe injury.

analogous to lupus nephritis and suggests that capillary wall deposits, especially subendothelial deposits, are more likely to activate inflammatory pathways than mesangial deposits. Studies, however, have failed to show a correlation between capillary wall deposits and a worse long-term prognosis (25). Subendothelial deposits often are accompanied by endocapillary hypercellularity (fig. 12-33) or crescent formation (fig. 12-22), and vice versa. Breaks in glomerular basement membranes often are identified in glomeruli with crescents (fig. 12-35).

Focal areas of glomerular basement membrane thinning are often identified in IgA nephropathy specimens (fig. 12-36) (9,13,21,44). Focal lamination ("basket-weave" pattern) occurs but is less frequent than thinning. Focal effacement of visceral epithelial foot processes is a frequent finding in IgA nephropathy, and usually corresponds in degree to the amount of proteinuria. Foot process effacement, along with visceral epithelial microvillous transformation, is particularly conspicuous in patients who have minimal change-like glomerulopathy superimposed on mild IgA nephropathy (8). These patients present with rapid onset of nephrotic syndrome that is usually steroid responsive.

Differential Diagnosis. The clinical differential diagnosis for patients who ultimately are found to have IgA nephropathy depends on the clinical presentation, which, as was discussed

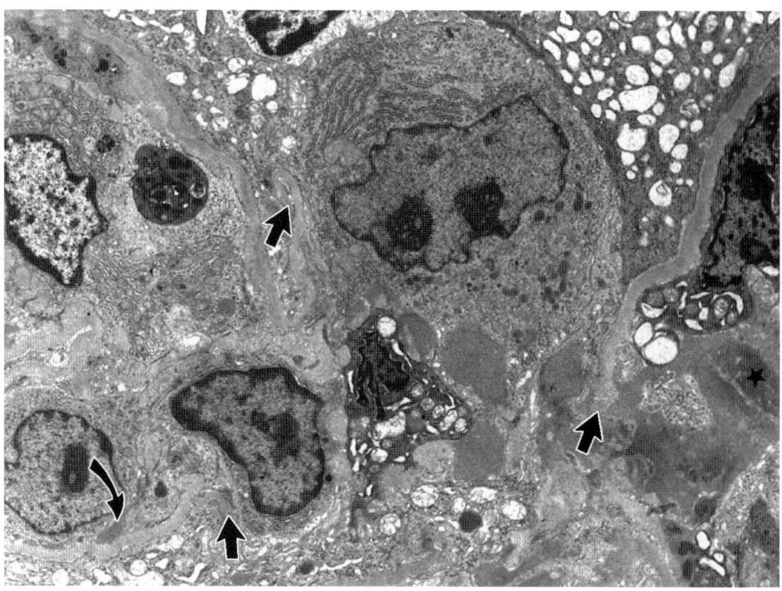

Figure 12-35

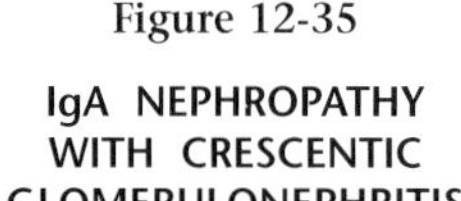

IgA NEPHROPATHY WITH CRESCENTIC GLOMERULONEPHRITIS

The crescent is at the top of the photomicrograph. There are multiple breaks in the glomerular basement membrane (straight arrows), subendothelial deposits (curved arrow), and intraluminal fibrin (star).

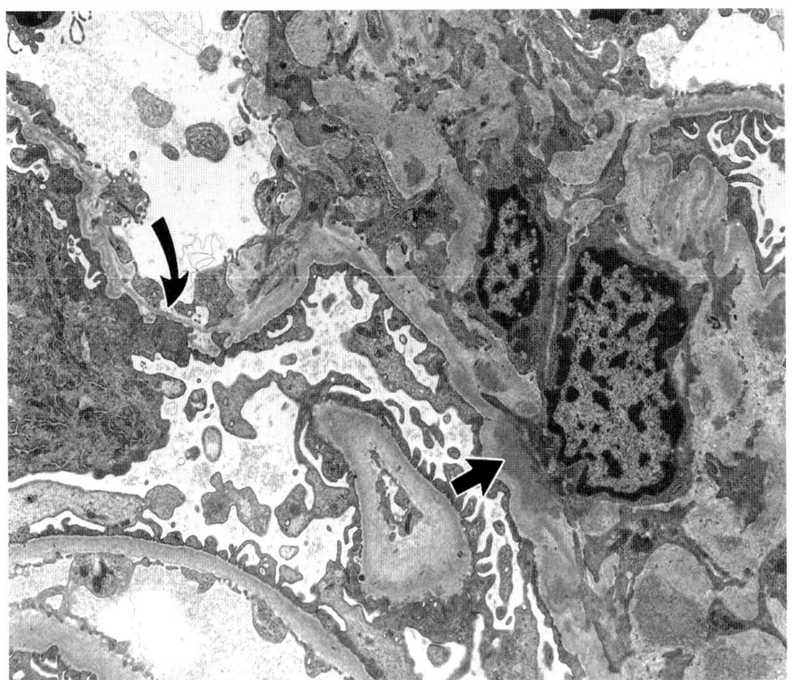

Figure 12-36

IgA NEPHROPATHY WITH FOCAL GLOMERULAR BASEMENT MEMBRANE THINNING

The electron micrograph demonstrates focal thinning of the glomerular basement membrane (curved arrow) and mesangial electron-dense deposits (straight arrow).

in detail earlier, can range from asymptomatic hematuria to nephrotic syndrome to overt nephritis to chronic renal failure. A frequent clinical presentation is with asymptomatic hematuria, normal renal function, and little or no proteinuria. The three most frequent renal biopsy findings in such patients are IgA nephropathy, thin basement membrane nephropathy, and no identifiable pathologic abnormality (fig. 12-37). This latter finding raises the possibility that the hematuria is not of glomerular origin, but does not completely exclude the possibility of an undetectable or unrecognized glomerular lesion. In patients with asymptomatic hematuria and "subnephrotic" proteinuria (less than 3g/day), IgA nephropathy is the most likely diagnosis, but many other glomerular diseases are in the differential diagnosis (fig. 12-37).

The pathologic diagnostic considerations by light microscopy include all other forms of mesangioproliferative and proliferative glomerulonephritis, which includes many types of immune complex glomerulonephritis. This diagnostic problem can be resolved only by immunohistology, which, by definition, differentiates IgA nephropathy from other forms of immune complex glomerulonephritis except for lupus nephritis. Lupus nephritis must be excluded by clinical and serologic data. In a patient with IgA-dominant or IgA-co-dominant glomerular deposits, the pathologic finding of endothelial tubuloreticular inclusions or substantial glomerular staining for C1q should raise the possibility of lupus nephritis. C1q staining is infrequent and weak in IgA nephropathy but is frequent and strong in lupus nephritis (34). In some patients, the light microscopic appearance of IgA nephropathy is indistinguishable from focal segmental glomerulosclerosis (25), however, immunostaining demonstrates that this is in fact a focal sclerosing IgA nephropathy.

Once a pathologic diagnosis of IgA nephropathy is made, additional differential considerations include whether or not it is a component of Henoch-Schönlein purpura or is associated with a number of extrarenal processes, including liver disease, ankylosing spondylitis, psoriasis, Reiter's disease, uveitis, enteritis, inflammatory bowel disease, celiac disease, dermatitis herpetiformis, HIV infection, and neoplastic disease (15,19,23,35). This is determined by carefully correlating clinical and laboratory data. Some secondary forms of IgA nephropathy have little or no clinical manifestations and less severe glomerular inflammation than primary IgA nephropathy, possibly because of less complement activation as evidenced by less immunostaining for complement (15).

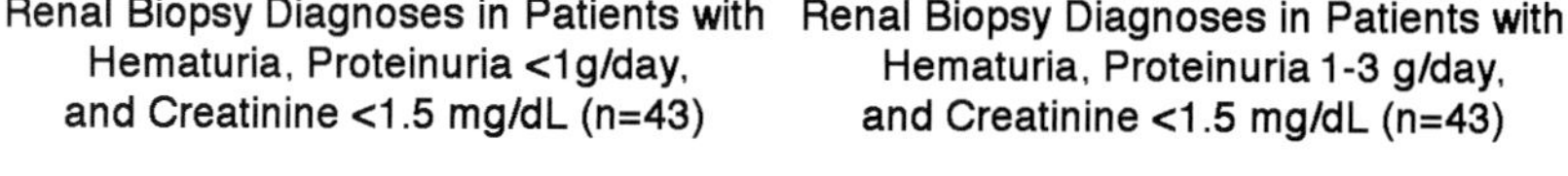

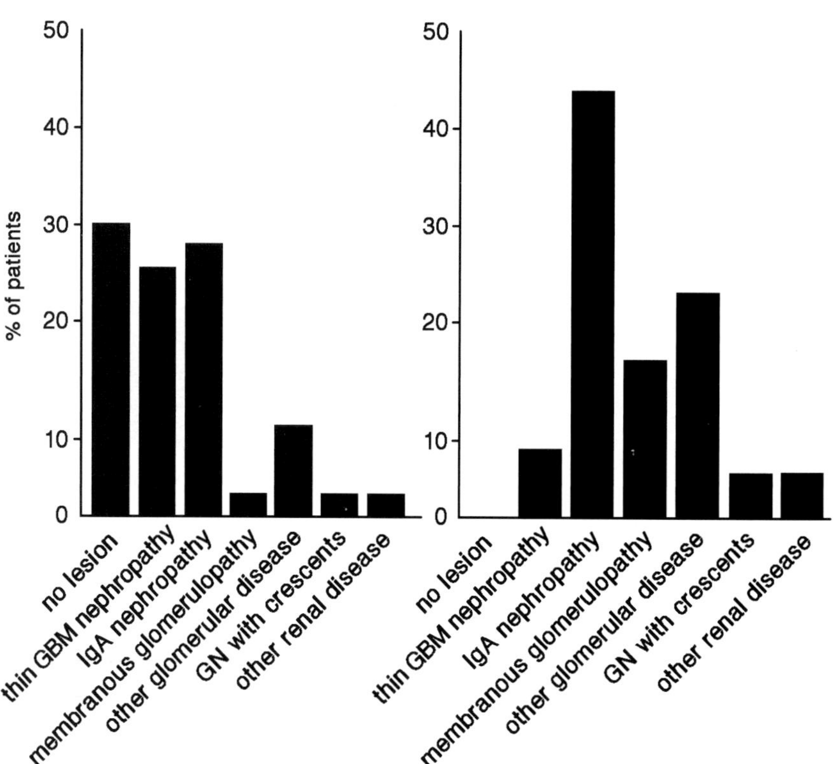

Figure 12-37

FREQUENCY OF IgA NEPHROPATHY WITH DIFFERENT CLINICAL PRESENTATIONS

The two graphs compare the relative frequency of IgA nephropathy in patients with hematuria and normal renal function who undergo renal biopsy and have either less than 1g/day proteinuria (left graph) or 1 to 3 g/day proteinuria (right graph). Thin basement membrane nephropathy is a major differential diagnostic consideration when there is little or no proteinuria, but is less likely with more proteinuria.

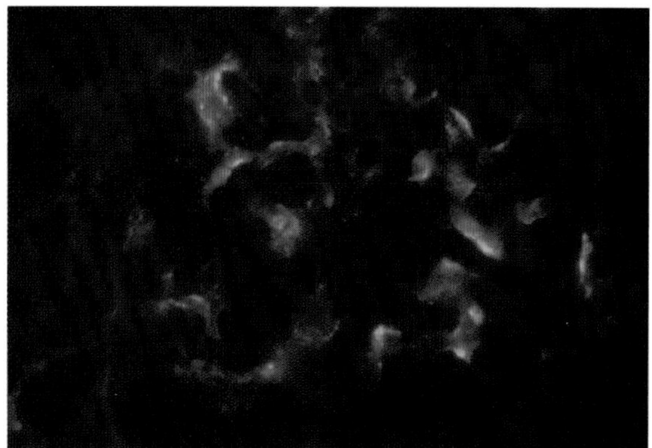

Figure 12-38

LOW-LEVEL MESANGIAL IgA STAINING

This glomerulus has definite but low-level mesangial staining for IgA. This raises the possibility of IgA nephropathy; however, with very low levels of staining, a definitive diagnosis of IgA nephropathy should be made only if clinical data and findings by electron and light microscopy support this diagnosis.

Another diagnostic challenge is deciding when to conclude that low-level immunostaining for IgA (fig. 12-38) is clinically and diagnostically insignificant. This is subjective and difficult. Low-level mesangial IgA staining may be seen in postmortem kidney tissue from patients with no clinical evidence of renal disease, and may be present in the background of renal biopsy specimens that have other obvious well-defined disease processes that explain the renal dysfunction that prompted the biopsy. This is analogous to low-level mesangial IgM or C3 staining that also may be seen as apparently insignificant background staining. The absence of mesangial dense deposits by electron microscopy in a specimen with low-level IgA immunostaining supports the possibility that the IgA is of no pathogenic or clinical significance. Low-level immunostaining for IgA should always be noted in the renal biopsy report, but if further clinical or pathologic evidence of IgA nephropathy is lacking, it is unwise to conclude that the patient has unequivocal IgA nephropathy. Patients with hepatic cirrhosis may develop "hepatic glomerulosclerosis" with or without IgA nephropathy. Hepatic glomerulosclerosis (hepatic glomerulopathy) is characterized by thickened glomerular basement membranes and increased mesangial matrix, sometimes accompanied by mesangial and subendothelial lipid deposits.

Etiology and Pathogenesis. One widely held hypothesis for the pathogenesis of IgA nephropathy proposes that mucosal antigenic exposure results in the generation of nephritogenic IgA antibodies that form immune complexes in the circulation, deposit in glomeruli, and mediate inflammation. If this hypothesis is correct, IgA nephropathy could result from multiple different abnormalities, including: 1) excessive mucosal exposure to antigen; 2) excessive permeability of mucosa to antigen; 3) excessive IgA antibody response to mucosal antigen exposure; 4) reduced clearance of circulating IgA complexes; or 5) enhanced glomerular mesangial deposition or impaired mesangial clearance. These abnormalities could in turn result from abnormalities in the immune system, glomerular structure, or IgA molecular structure. There are observations in some patients with IgA nephropathy that support the presence of one or more of these abnormalities. IgA nephropathy may be a phenotype of injury that is the final common pathway for many different abnormalities.

Circulating and glomerular IgA deposits are predominantly IgA1. Mucosa-derived IgA is predominantly IgA2, whereas IgA derived from other lymphoid sites is predominantly IgA1. Thus, the nephritogenic IgA may be derived from a systemic immune response rather than a mucosal response, however, the antigen still could enter across a mucosal surface. Patients with IgA nephropathy have quantitative and qualitative abnormalities in circulating IgA and IgA-bearing B cells (1,2,19,27,29,39,42,43,49, 59). They have increased circulating IgA, increased IgA-bearing B cells, and increased B-cell secretion of IgA. There is increased circulating heavy IgA that is either multimeric, complexed with other molecules, or both.

Some secondary forms of IgA nephropathy may be caused by the increased entry of IgA complexes into the circulation (e.g., inflammatory bowel disease) or decreased clearance from the circulation (e.g., hepatic cirrhosis). IgA complexes are cleared from the circulation predominantly by the liver. Thus, reduced hepatic clearance may be the basis for the increased incidence of IgA nephropathy in patients with liver disease, especially cirrhosis.

The role of reduced galactosylation of the O-linked glycans of the IgA1 hinge region in the pathogenesis of IgA nephropathy has received a lot of attention over the past few years (1–3,29). This could lead to increased self-aggregation of IgA in the circulation, decreased clearance of abnormal IgA because of lack of receptor engagement, and/or increased affinity of IgA for mesangial matrix. The abnormally galactosylated IgA may also become a target for autoantibody binding that would produce nephritogenic immune complexes (39). The basis for this abnormal galactosylation may be a B-cell–restricted reduction of beta 1,3 galactosyltransferase activity (2). Other genetic abnormalities could contribute to the pathogenesis of IgA nephropathy (31), such as abnormalities in other genes that control immunoglobulin molecules, molecules involved in the IgA trafficking, or molecules involved in IgA-mediated inflammation.

Treatment and Prognosis. IgA nephropathy is a persistent and usually slowly progressive disease (11,21,23,32,41,60). Complete remission is uncommon; 10 to 15 percent of patients reach end-stage renal disease after 10 years, and 25 to 35 percent after 20 years (15,17,19). There is a substantial risk of progression of disease even if the initial clinical and pathologic manifestations are mild (57). The risk of progression is greater if the initial clinical manifestations of renal dysfunction are more severe, such as higher serum creatinine, more proteinuria, and worse hypertension (50). Marked proteinuria usually corresponds to severe disease and poor outcome, except in the rare patients who appear to have concurrent IgA nephropathy and minimal change glomerulopathy (8). The severity of acute and chronic injury seen by light microscopy correlates to a degree with outcome (25,46,50,58), but has not been used extensively to guide therapy. The severity of the chronic changes in all renal compartments, including glomerular sclerosis, interstitial fibrosis, and vascular sclerosis, correlates well with outcome (50,58).

The appropriate treatment strategy for patients with IgA nephropathy is controversial (21,23, 30,60). Many nephrologists advocate minimal nontoxic treatment because of the usually mild initial manifestations and the slowly progressing course in most patients. Angiotensin converting enzyme inhibitors are used in most patients irrespective of the presence of hypertension. This reduces the proteinuria and may stabilize renal function. Fish oil supplements that contain a high concentration of omega 3 fatty acids are a widely used and apparently benign treatment for IgA nephropathy, although the efficacy of this treatment is still debated (21). The studies by Donadio and associates (16,18) suggest that prolonged treatment with fish oil slows renal progression for high-risk patients with IgA nephropathy if treatment is begun prior to the development of advanced disease. Trials with corticosteroids have given inconsistent results, but suggest that such treatment may reduce proteinuria and stabilize glomerular filtration rate (30,60). Corticosteroid treatment is most effective in the rare patients who have minimal change–like glomerulopathy superimposed on mild IgA nephropathy. Unusually aggressive IgA nephropathy with extensive crescent formation warrants immunosuppressive therapy.

A variety of other therapies also have been tried, such as plasmapheresis; administration of cyclosporin, intravenous gamma globulin, anticoagulants, gluten restrictors, phenytoin, or mycophenolate mofetil; and tonsillectomy. The beneficial effects of these therapies have not been proven.

The pathologic recurrence rate of IgA nephropathy in renal allografts is approximately 50 percent, as defined by the presence of IgA deposits in the mesangium; approximately a quarter to a third of these patients lose their graft because of progressive recurrent IgA nephropathy (21,61). There are some data to suggest that a well-matched allograft from a living related donor is at greater risk for recurrent IgA nephropathy than a less well-matched kidney (61). However, evidence of this is controversial and inadequate to preclude living related donor allografts in patients with IgA nephropathy (22).

HENOCH-SCHÖNLEIN PURPURA

Definition. Henoch-Schönlein purpura is small vessel (i.e., capillaries, venules, and arterioles) vasculitis with vessel wall IgA-dominant immune complex deposits (15,51). Involvement of small arteries is rare. The skin, gut, joints, and renal glomeruli are the most frequently involved tissues.

Clinical Features. In 1837, Johann Schönlein (52), a German physician, noticed the association of purpura with arthralgias and arthritis. In 1868, Eduard Henoch (28), a German pediatrician who had been Schönlein's pupil, described the association of purpura with abdominal pain and arthritis, especially in children. Henoch later described the association of purpura not only with abdominal pain and arthritis but also nephritis. This syndrome was initially called Henoch's purpura and later Henoch-Schönlein purpura. Some have advocated using the more chronologically correct term Schönlein-Henoch purpura, however, Henoch was more instrumental in defining the syndrome and thus deserves primacy in the name.

Berger (4) was the first to document that the nephritis of Henoch-Schönlein purpura was immunopathologically identical to IgA nephropathy. Later, Faille-Kuyber (20), a Dutch dermatologist, demonstrated that there were IgA deposits not only in renal glomeruli but also in skin vessels in these patients. This supports the proposition that Henoch-Schönlein purpura is a systemic expression of small vessel vasculitis caused by the vascular localization of IgA-rich immune deposits, whereas IgA nephropathy is the renal-limited expression of this process.

Henoch-Schönlein purpura has a greater predilection for young children than does IgA nephropathy (15). Henoch-Schönlein purpura is most frequent in children, especially children under 10 years of age, although it can begin at any age. As is true for IgA nephropathy, Henoch-Schönlein purpura nephritis is twice as common in males than females, and is uncommon in individuals of African descent (51). The onset of Henoch-Schönlein purpura is usually in the spring and fall. The disease often is initially diagnosed during or immediately following an upper respiratory tract infection. Less frequently, the onset of disease is associated with drug therapy or the development of a neoplasm (51).

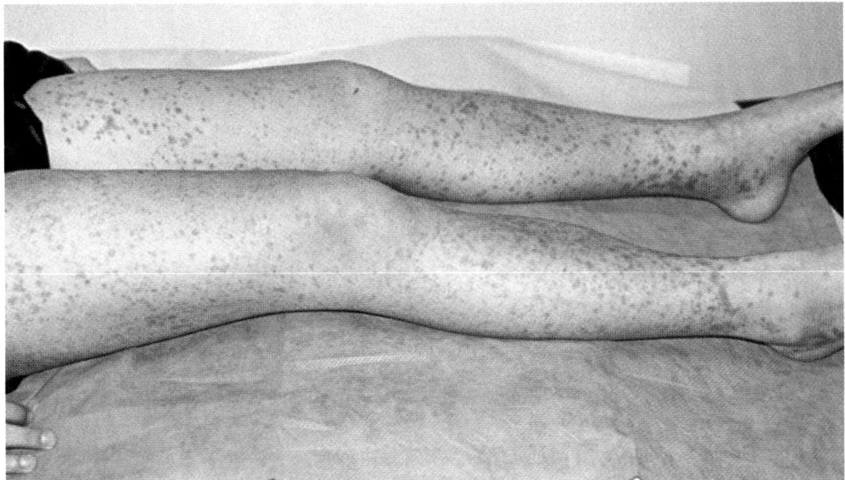

Figure 12-39

HENOCH-SCHÖNLEIN PURPURA

The lower extremities of this patient with Henoch-Schönlein purpura are covered by numerous variably sized and variably shaped purpuric lesions.

Purpura, arthralgias, and colicky abdominal pain are the most frequent manifestations (48). Approximately half of the patients have hematuria and proteinuria but only a minority have reduced renal function. The onset of nephritis is almost always within 3 months of the onset of purpura.

Gross Findings. The gross appearance of the kidney is the same as for IgA nephropathy. The major gross lesion is the cutaneous purpura (fig. 12-39). The purpura are palpable, and usually occur first and sometimes exclusively on the lower extremities and buttocks. Blister or ulcer formation is uncommon.

Light Microscopic Findings. The glomerular pathology is indistinguishable from isolated IgA nephropathy (14,19,48,51,55). Focal proliferative glomerulonephritis is the most frequent light microscopic phenotype, followed in order of decreasing frequency by diffuse proliferative glomerulonephritis, mesangioproliferative glomerulonephritis, and no detectable lesion (48,55). More diffuse lesions are seen during later stages of the disease (55).

As with IgA nephropathy, there are multiple classification systems for the different phenotypes of light microscopic injury observed with Henoch-Schönlein purpura nephritis (19,48,51). There is substantial confusion over which system to use and how to apply a given system (19). The simplest approach is to use the lupus nephritis classification system for not only Henoch-Schönlein purpura nephritis but also IgA nephropathy. This provides histologic categories that approximate those described in other classification systems but avoids the need to learn multiple different numerical class designations for different categories of immune complex glomerulonephritis that all have the same basic variations in histologic pattern of injury, i.e., no lesion by light microscopy (lupus class I), mesangioproliferative glomerulonephritis (class II), focal proliferative glomerulonephritis (class III), diffuse proliferative glomerulonephritis (class IV), focal sclerosing glomerulonephritis (class IIIC), diffuse sclerosing glomerulonephritis (class VI). Focal and diffuse proliferative Henoch-Schönlein purpura nephritis can have varying degrees of focal segmental necrosis and crescent formation (fig. 12-40), however, crescent formation in greater than 50 percent of glomeruli is uncommon. Necrosis and crescents are more frequent in Henoch-Schönlein purpura nephritis specimens than in IgA nephropathy specimens (15,33,51), but this may reflect a tendency to perform renal biopsies more frequently in those patients with more severe nephritis. Approximately 50 percent of patients have some crescent formation (19,38). Rare patients have a type I membranoproliferative (mesangiocapillary) phenotype of injury.

Vasculitis in extraglomerular renal vessels is rare (14,51); when it occurs, it is essentially confined to arterioles. Thus, the presence of any vasculitis in a specimen with IgA nephropathy, especially vasculitis in an artery, should raise the possibility of another concurrent vasculitis, especially ANCA small vessel vasculitis.

The characteristic cutaneous lesion of Henoch-Schönlein purpura is a leukocytoclastic angiitis affecting primarily venules in the upper dermis

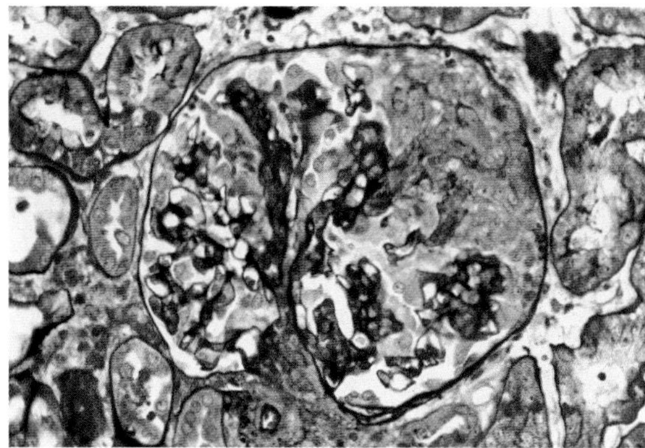

Figure 12-40

HENOCH-SCHÖNLEIN PURPURA GLOMERULONEPHRITIS WITH CRESCENTS AND NECROSIS

The JMS stain with H&E counterstain demonstrates segmental disruption of glomerular basement membranes at the upper right of the tuft, with adjacent crescent formation in Bowman's space.

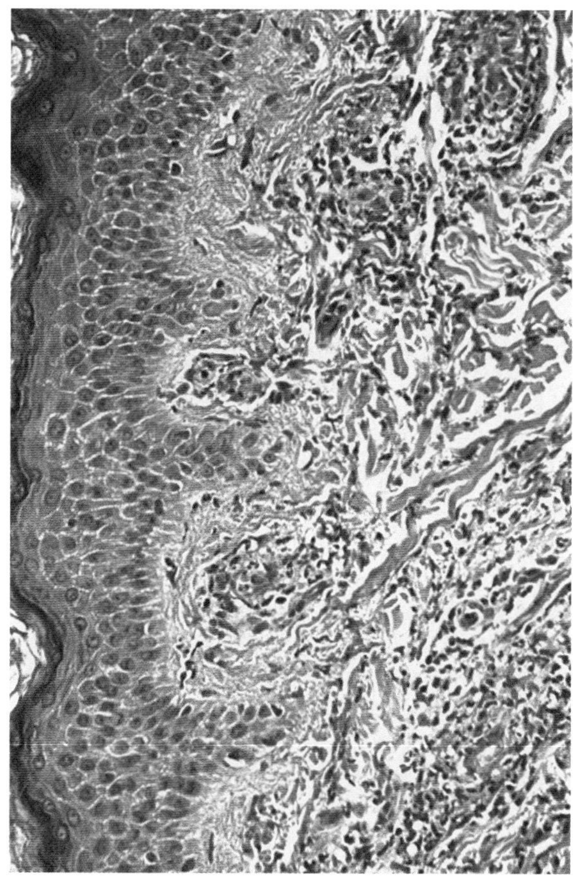

Figure 12-41

DERMAL LEUKOCYTOCLASTIC ANGIITIS CAUSED BY HENOCH-SCHÖNLEIN PURPURA

Many small dermal vessels are infiltrated by and surrounded by leukocytes, including many neutrophils. There is conspicuous leukocytoclasia and slight hemorrhage. By light microscopy alone, the specific cause of this leukocytoclastic angiitis could not be determined.

(fig. 12-41). Similar lesions occur in the gut. On the basis of light microscopy alone, this lesion cannot be confidently distinguished from other types of immune complex small vessel vasculitides, such as cryoglobulinemic vasculitis, or pauci-immune (ANCA) small vessel vasculitides, such as microscopic polyangiitis. Of course, immunohistology can make this distinction.

Immunofluorescence Findings. The glomerular immunohistology is indistinguishable from that of isolated IgA nephropathy (fig. 12-42) (51,55). There is a tendency toward more frequent and more intense staining for fibrin (15, 19), but this depends in part on the nature of the fibrin antibody. There is a higher frequency of capillary wall deposits (15,19), however, this does not allow pathologic differentiation of a specific case of Henoch-Schönlein purpura nephritis from IgA nephropathy. Irregular glomerular staining for fibrin corresponds with foci of fibrinoid necrosis, and fibrin in Bowman's space corresponds with crescent formation.

Focal IgA-dominant immune deposits occur in arterioles and peritubular capillaries in 20 percent or fewer patients (fig. 12-43) (19). C3 staining alone in hilar arterioles is more common but is nonspecific.

In patients with Henoch-Schönlein purpura, IgA-dominant immune deposits can be identified not only in the kidneys, but also in the small vessels of the skin and gut (fig. 12-44) (3,15). This is not of value, however, in differentiating Henoch-Schönlein purpura from IgA nephropathy because many patients with IgA nephropathy who have no evidence of systemic vasculitis nevertheless have IgA in dermal venules.

Electron Microscopic Findings. The electron microscopic findings in Henoch-Schönlein purpura nephritis are not distinguishable from those of isolated IgA nephropathy (19,51,55). In line with the immunohistologic findings, capillary wall electron-dense deposits are seen more frequently than with IgA nephropathy (15,19). Glomerular basement membrane thinning is similar to that in IgA nephropathy.

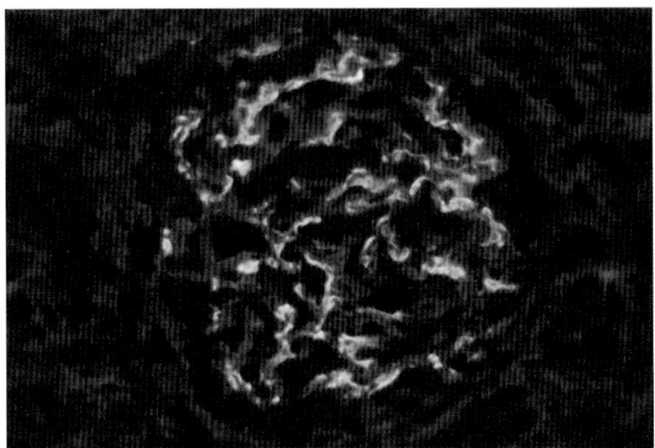

Figure 12-42

HENOCH-SCHÖNLEIN PURPURA NEPHRITIS WITH MESANGIAL IgA

The intense mesangial staining for IgA in a patient with Henoch-Schönlein purpura is indistinguishable from that seen with IgA nephropathy. This patient also had ankylosing spondylitis, which is associated with a higher incidence of IgA nephropathy and Henoch-Schönlein purpura.

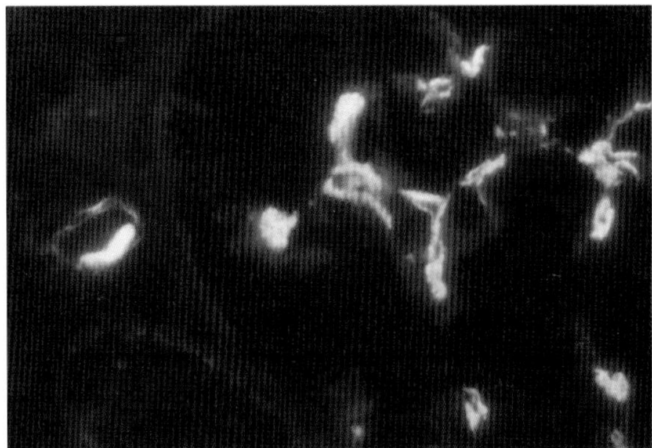

Figure 12-43

HENOCH-SCHÖNLEIN PURPURA WITH GLOMERULAR AND ARTERIOLAR IgA

The arteriole to the left of the glomerulus stains intensely for IgA, similar to that in the mesangium of the glomerulus.

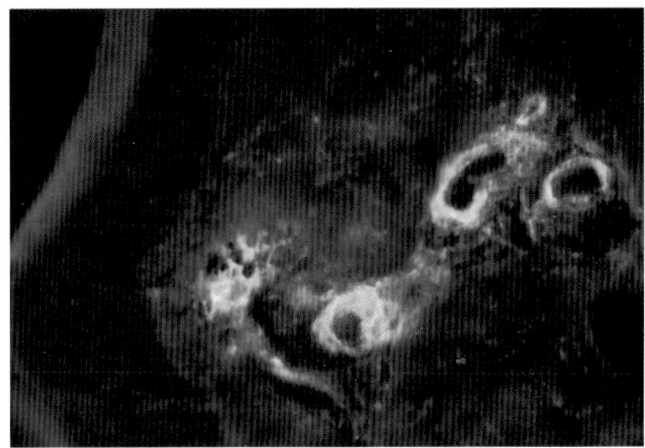

Figure 12-44

HENOCH-SCHÖNLEIN PURPURA WITH DERMAL VASCULAR IgA

The epidermis is to the left and the dermis to the right. There is intense granular staining of the walls of small dermal vessels with an antibody specific for IgA. There was similar staining for C3 but only low intensity staining for IgG and IgM.

Differential Diagnosis. The clinical differential diagnosis in a patient with purpura and glomerulonephritis includes not only Henoch-Schönlein purpura, but also cryoglobulinemic vasculitis, microscopic polyangiitis, Wegener's granulomatosis, Churg-Strauss syndrome, and other forms of small vessel vasculitis. Clinical, serologic, and pathologic findings allow differentiation among these. Cryoglobulinemic vasculitis has circulating cryoglobulins, hypocomplementemia, and usually a type 1 membranoproliferative glomerulonephritis pattern of glomerular injury, with IgG or IgM as the major immunoglobulins in the immune deposits. Microscopic polyangiitis, Wegener's granulomatosis, and Churg-Strauss syndrome usually have circulating ANCA and a pauci-immune necrotizing and crescentic glomerulonephritis, with little or no glomerular staining for immunoglobulin. However, occasional patients with ANCA crescentic glomerulonephritis and small vessel vasculitis have low levels (i.e., a paucity) of IgA immunostaining. This does not warrant a diagnosis of concurrent IgA nephropathy unless the degree of IgA staining and the amount of electron-dense deposits seen by electron microscopy are comparable to that seen with typical IgA nephropathy or Henoch-Schönlein purpura nephritis. In addition, IgA nephropathy or Henoch-Schönlein purpura nephritis that is accompanied by ANCA disease typically has much more endocapillary hypercellularity than ANCA glomerulonephritis alone.

Etiology and Pathogenesis. Patients with Henoch-Schönlein purpura have the same immunologic abnormalities as patients with isolated IgA nephropathy (15,40,51). Henoch-Schönlein purpura patients have larger circulating IgA-containing immune complexes and a greater incidence of increased plasma IgA (15). Patients with nephritis have the same IgA hinge region glycosylation defect as do patients with IgA nephropathy, however, patients who do not have nephritis lack this defect (15). Why systemic small vessel vasculitis develops in patients with Henoch-Schönlein purpura but not IgA nephropathy is not known. This may involve subtle differences in immune complex composition or differences in the cytokine milieu (15).

Treatment and Prognosis. Most patients with Henoch-Schönlein purpura have only one episode of purpura that resolves completely; a few have one or more minor flare-ups. The major long-term complication is persistent and progressive renal disease. Some data indicate that only about 5 percent of patients with Henoch-Schönlein purpura eventually develop end-stage renal disease (10,24), however, other studies suggest that the risk of end-stage disease is as high as 20 percent after 20 years (15, 51). More severe clinical manifestations of nephritis and more severe pathologic lesions, especially the presence of crescents, are predictors of poor outcome (10,24,51).

No specific treatment is given to patients with Henoch-Schönlein purpura when they first develop the disease unless they have severe renal involvement, which is usually treated with corticosteroids and immunosuppressive drugs (6,51). Nonsteroidal anti-inflammatory drugs relieve joint pain.

Approximately a third of patients who receive renal allografts for end-stage renal disease caused by Henoch-Schönlein purpura nephritis develop recurrent IgA nephropathy in the transplant within 5 years (51), although there is no recurrence of the systemic vasculitis. Approximately a third of the patients with recurrence have graft insufficiency attributable to the recurrent disease.

REFERENCES

1. Allen A, Feehally J. IgA glycosylation in IgA nephropathy. Adv Exp Med Biol 1998;435:175–83.
2. Allen A, Harper S, Feehally J. Origin and structure of pathogenic IgA in IgA nephropathy. Biochem Soc Trans 1997;25:486–90.
3. Allen AC, Topham PS, Harper SJ, Feehally J. Leucocyte beta 1,3 galactosyltransferase activity in IgA nephropathy. Nephrol Dial Transplant 1997;12:701–6.
4. Berger J. IgA glomerular deposits in renal disease. Transplant Proc 1969;1:939–44.
5. Berger J, Hinglais N. [Intercapillary deposits of IgA-IgG.] J Urol Nephrol (Paris) 1968;74:694–5.
6. Bergstein J, Leiser J, Andreoli SP. Response of crescentic Henoch-Schoenlein purpura nephritis to corticosteroid and azathioprine therapy. Clin Nephrol 1998;49:9–14.
7. Chui SH, Lam CW, Lewis WH, Lai KN. Light-chain ratio of serum IgA 1 in IgA nephropathy. J Clin Immunol 1991;11:219–23.
8. Clive DM, Galvanek EG, Silva FG. Mesangial immunoglobulin A deposits in minimal change nephrotic syndrome: a report of an older patient and review of the literature. Am J Nephrol 1990;10:31–6.
9. Cosio FG, Falkenhain ME, Sedmak DD. Association of thin glomerular basement membrane with other glomerulopathies. Kidney Int 1994; 46:471–4.
10. Counahan R, Winterborn MH, White RH, et al. Prognosis of Henoch-Schonlein nephritis in children. Br Med J 1977;2:11–4.
11. D'Amico G, Imbasciati E, Barbiano Di Belgioioso G, et al. Idiopathic IgA mesangial nephropathy. Clinical and histological study of 374 patients. Medicine 1985;64:49–60.
12. D'Amico G, Napodano P, Ferrario F, Rastaldi MP, Arrigo G. Idiopathic IgA nephropathy with segmental necrotizing lesions of the capillary wall. Kidney Int 2001;59:682–92.
13. Danilewicz M, Wagrowska-Danilewicz M. Glomerular basement membrane thickness in primary diffuse IgA nephropathy: ultrastructural morphometric analysis. Int Urol Nephrol 1998;30:513–9.
14. Danilewicz M, Wagrowska-Danilewicz M. Morphometric analysis of glomerular and interstitial lesions in idiopathic IgA nephropathy and Schoenlein-Henoch nephritis. Pol J Pathol 1998;49:303–7.

15. Davin JC, Ten Berge IJ, Weening JJ. What is the difference between IgA nephropathy and Henoch-Schoenlein purpura nephritis? Kidney Int 2001;59:823–34.
16. Donadio JV Jr, Bergstralh EJ, Offord KP, Spencer DC, Holley KE. A controlled trial of fish oil in IgA nephropathy. Mayo Nephrology Collaborative Group. N Engl J Med 1994;331:1194–9.
17. Donadio JV Jr, Grande JP. Immunoglobulin A nephropathy: a clinical perspective. J Am Soc Nephrol 1997;8:1324–32.
18. Donadio JV Jr, Grande JP, Bergstralh EJ, Dart RA, Larson TS, Spencer DC. The long-term outcome of patients with IgA nephropathy treated with fish oil in a controlled trial. Mayo Nephrology Collaborative Group. J Am Soc Nephrol 1999;10:1772–7.
19. Emancipator SN. IgA nephropathy and Henoch-Schoenlein syndrome. In: Jennette JC, Olson JL, Schwartz MM, Silva FG, eds. Heptinstall's pathology of the kidney, 5th ed. Philadelphia: Lippincott-Raven; 1998:479–539.
20. Faille-Kuyber EH, Kater L, Kooiker CJ, Dorhout ME. IgA-deposits in cutaneous blood-vessel walls and mesangium in Henoch-Schoenlein syndrome. Lancet 1973;1:892–3.
21. Floege J, Feehally J. IgA nephropathy: recent developments. J Am Soc Nephrol 2000;11:2395–403.
22. Frohnert PP, Donadio JV Jr, Velosa JA, Holley KE, Sterioff S. The fate of renal transplants in patients with IgA nephropathy. Clin Transplant 1997;11:127–33.
23. Galla JH. IgA nephropathy. Kidney Int 1995;47:377–87.
24. Goldstein AR, White RH, Akuse R, Chantler C. Long-term follow-up of childhood Henoch-Schonlein nephritis. Lancet 1992;339:280–2.
25. Haas M. Histologic subclassification of IgA nephropathy: a clinicopathologic study of 244 cases. Am J Kidney Dis 1997;29:829–42.
26. Haas M, Jafri J, Bartosh SM, Karp SL, Adler SG, Meehan SM. ANCA-associated crescentic glomerulonephritis with mesangial IgA deposits. Am J Kidney Dis 2000;36:709–18.
27. Hale GM, McIntosh SL, Hiki Y, Clarkson AR, Woodroffe AJ. Evidence for IgA-specific B cell hyperactivity in patients with IgA nephropathy. Kidney Int 1986;29:718–24.
28. Henoch E. Uber den zusammenhang von purpura und intestinal-stoerungen. Berl Klin Wochenschur 1868;5:517–9.
29. Hiki Y, Kokubo T, Iwase H, et al. Underglycosylation of IgA1 hinge plays a certain role for its glomerular deposition in IgA nephropathy. J Am Soc Nephrol 1999;10:760–9.
30. Hogg RJ, Waldo B. Advances in treatment: immunoglobulin A nephropathy. Semin Nephrol 1996;16:511–6.
31. Hsu SI, Ramirez SB, Winn MP, Bonventre JV, Owen WF. Evidence for genetic factors in the development and progression of IgA nephropathy. Kidney Int 2000;57:1818–35.
32. Ibels LS, Gyory AZ. IgA nephropathy: analysis of the natural history, important factors in the progression of renal disease, and a review of the literature. Medicine 1994;73:79–102.
33. Jennette JC. Crescentic glomerulonephritis. In: Jennette JC, Olson JL, Schwartz MM, Silva FG, eds. Heptinstall's pathology of the kidney, 5th ed. Philadelphia: Lippincott-Raven; 1998:625–56.
34. Jennette JC. The immunohistology of IgA nephropathy. Am J Kidney Dis 1988;12:348–52.
35. Jennette JC, Ferguson AL, Moore MA, Freeman DG. IgA nephropathy associated with seronegative spondyloarthropathies. Arthritis Rheum 1982;25:144–9.
36. Jennette JC, Newman WJ, Diaz-Buxo JA. Overlapping IgA and membranous nephropathy. Am J Clin Pathol 1987;88:74–8.
37. Jennette JC, Wall SD. The clinical and pathologic heterogeneity of IgA nephropathy. Kidney 1983;16:17–23.
38. Jennette JC, Wall SD, Wilkman AS. Low incidence of IgA nephropathy in blacks. Kidney Int 1985;28:944–50.
39. Kokubo T, Hashizume K, Iwase H, et al. Humoral immunity against the proline-rich peptide epitope of the IgA1 hinge region in IgA nephropathy. Nephrol Dial Transplant 2000;15:28–33.
40. Kubota R. [Peripheral blood IgA bearing cells in children with Henoch-Schoenlein purpura nephritis and IgA nephropathy. Relationship between IgA bearing cells and clinico-pathological findings or T alpha 4 cells.] Nippon Jinzo Gakkai Shi 1992;34:1149–59.
41. Lai KN, Wang AY. IgA nephropathy: common nephritis leading to end-stage renal failure. Int J Artif Organs 1994;17:457–60.
42. Launay P, Grossetete B, Arcos-Fajardo M, et al. Fcalpha receptor (CD89) mediates the development of immunoglobulin A (IgA) nephropathy (Berger's disease). Evidence for pathogenic soluble receptor-IgA complexes in patients and CD89 transgenic mice. J Exp Med 2000;191: 1999–2009.
43. Layward L, Allen AC, Hattersley JM, Harper SJ, Feehally J. Elevation of IgA in IgA nephropathy is localized in the serum and not saliva and is restricted to the IgA1 subclass. Nephrol Dial Transplant 1993;8:25–8.

44. Lee HS, Choi Y, Lee JS, Yu BH, Koh HI. Ultrastructural changes in IgA nephropathy in relation to histologic and clinical data. Kidney Int 1989;35:880–6.
45. Lee HS, Pyo HJ, Koh HI. Acute renal failure associated with hematuria in IgA nephropathy. Am J Kidney Dis 1988;12:236–9.
46. Lee SM. Prognostic indicators of progressive renal disease in IgA nephropathy: emergence of a new histologic grading system. Am J Kidney Dis 1997;29:953–8.
47. Lee SM, Rao VM, Franklin WA, et al. IgA nephropathy: morphologic predictors of progressive renal disease. Hum Pathol 1982;13:314–22.
48. Meadow SR, Glasgow EF, White RH, Moncrieff MW, Cameron JS, Ogg CS. Schoenlein-Henoch nephritis. Q J Med 1972;41:241–58.
49. Montenegro V, Monteiro RC. Elevation of serum IgA in spondyloarthropathies and IgA nephropathy and its pathogenic role. Curr Opin Rheumatol 1999;11:265–72.
50. Radford MG Jr, Donadio JV Jr, Bergstralh EJ, Grande JP. Predicting renal outcome in IgA nephropathy. J Am Soc Nephrol 1997;8:199–207.
51. Rai A, Nast C, Adler S. Henoch-Schoenlein purpura nephritis. J Am Soc Nephrol 1999;10:2637–44.
52. Schoenlein JL. Allgemeine und specielle pathologie und therapie, 3rd ed. Herisau, Switzerland: Literatur-Comptoir; 1837:48.
53. Scolari F. Familial IgA nephropathy. J Nephrol 1999;12:213–9.
54. Sehic AM, Gaber LW, Roy S 3rd, Miller PM, Kritchevsky SB, Wyatt RJ. Increased recognition of IgA nephropathy in African-American children. Pediatr Nephrol 1997;11:435–7.
55. Sinniah R, Feng PH, Chen BT. Henoch-Schoenlein syndrome: a clinical and morphological study of renal biopsies. Clin Nephrol 1978;9:219–28.
56. Stokes MB, Alpers CE. Combined membranous nephropathy and IgA nephropathy. Am J Kidney Dis 1998;32:649–56.
57. Szeto CC, Lai FM, To KF, et al. The natural history of immunoglobulin A nephropathy among patients with hematuria and minimal proteinuria. Am J Med 2001;110:434–7.
58. To KF, Choi PC, Szeto CC, et al. Outcome of IgA nephropathy in adults graded by chronic histological lesions. Am J Kidney Dis 2000;35:392–400.
59. van Es LA, van den Wall Bake AW, Stad RK, van den Dobbelsteen ME, Bogers MJ, Daha MR. Enigmas in the pathogenesis of IgA nephropathy. Contrib Nephrol 1995;111:169–75.
60. Waldo FB, Wyatt RJ, Hogg RJ, Andreoli SP, Milliner DS. Current concepts and controversies in IgA nephropathy. Pediatr Nephrol 1998;12:498–504.
61. Wang AY, Lai FM, Yu AW, et al. Recurrent IgA nephropathy in renal transplant allografts. Am J Kidney Dis 2001;38:588–96.

13 SYSTEMIC LUPUS ERYTHEMATOSUS AND OTHER RHEUMATOLOGIC DISEASES

SYSTEMIC LUPUS ERYTHEMATOSUS

Systemic lupus erythematosus (SLE) is a systemic autoimmune disease that affects multiple organs, including skin, joints, kidney, serous membranes, lungs, and central nervous system. The 1982 American Rheumatism Association (ARA) criteria, which were updated in 1997, recognize 11 cardinal features of SLE (24,46). These include: malar rash, discoid rash, photosensitivity, oral ulcers, nondeforming arthritis, serositis, renal disease (defined as persistent proteinuria greater than 500 mg daily or 3+ by dipstick, or cellular casts of any type), neurologic disease, hematologic disorders (including hemolytic anemia, leukopenia, lymphopenia, or thrombocytopenia), positive immune serologic tests (for antiphospholipid antibody, lupus anticoagulant, anti-DNA antibody, anti-Smith antibody, or false-positive VDRL [venereal disease research laboratories]), and a positive antinuclear antibody (ANA) test. The development of any four of these features in concert or sequentially is highly sensitive and specific for SLE. It is estimated that clinical renal disease occurs in approximately 50 percent of SLE patients, especially within the first few years following disease onset (16). Some investigators believe that a much higher percentage would be shown to have morphologic renal involvement if renal biopsies were performed systematically on all patients with SLE.

The term *lupus nephritis* denotes the spectrum of immune complex–mediated renal diseases secondary to SLE. The renal manifestations of SLE are extremely heterogeneous and may affect any or all renal compartments, including glomeruli, tubules, interstitium, and blood vessels (3,8,11,23,33,44). Investigators have attempted to define and quantify the many morphologic lesions of lupus nephritis in a comprehensive, systematic fashion. Three classification systems are in use. Historically, the most widely used and universally accepted is the original World Health Organization (WHO) classification (Table 13-1). This classification scheme was formulated in 1974 in Buffalo, New York, under the auspices of the WHO (32). It recognizes five major classes of lupus nephritis. In 1982, a revised WHO classification was proposed by the International Study of Kidney Disease in Children (ISKDC) (12) and was further revised in 1995 (Table 13-2) (13). It defines six major classes of lupus nephritis and a large number of subclasses, with emphasis on distribution, activity, and chronicity of the lesions. Although it is much more detailed and precise than the original WHO classification, it has not been as widely accepted. Resistance to the use

Table 13-1

ORIGINAL WORLD HEALTH ORGANIZATION CLASSIFICATION OF LUPUS NEPHRITIS (1974)[a]

Class I	Normal glomeruli (by LM, IF, and EM)[b]
Class II	Purely mesangial disease
a.	Normocellular mesangium by LM, but mesangial deposits by IF and/or EM
b.	Mesangial hypercellularity, with mesangial deposits by IF and/or EM
Class III	Focal proliferative glomerulonephritis (<50% glomeruli)
Class IV	Diffuse proliferative glomerulonephritis (≥50% glomeruli)
Class V	Membranous glomerulonephritis

[a]Adapted from references 3 and 32.

[b]LM = light microscopy; IF = immunofluorescence microscopy; EM = electron microscopy.

Table 13-2

MODIFIED WORLD HEALTH ORGANIZATION CLASSIFICATION OF LUPUS NEPHRITIS (1982)[a]

Class I	Normal glomeruli
a.	Nil (by all techniques)
b.	Normal by LM but deposits seen by IF and/or EM[b]
Class II	Purely mesangial alterations (mesangiopathy)
a.	Mesangial widening and/or moderate mesangial alterations
b.	Moderate hypercellularity (++)
Class III	Focal segmental glomerulonephritis (associated with mild or moderate mesangial alterations)
a.	With active necrotizing lesions
b.	With active and sclerosing lesions
c.	With sclerosing lesions
Class IV	Diffuse glomerulonephritis (severe mesangial, endocapillary, or mesangiocapillary proliferation, and/or extensive subendothelial deposits). Mesangial deposits are present invariably and subepithelial deposits often, and may be numerous.
a.	Without segmental lesions
b.	With active necrotizing lesions
c.	With active and sclerosing lesions
d.	With sclerosing lesions
Class V	Membranous glomerulonephritis
a.	Pure membranous glomerulonephritis
b.	Associated with lesions of category II (a or b)
c.	Associated with lesions of category III (a, b, or c)[c]
d.	Associated with lesions of category IV (a, b, c, or d)[c]
Class VI	Advanced sclerosing glomerulonephritis

[a]Adapted from references 12 and 13.

[b]LM = light microscopy; IF = immunofluorescence microscopy; EM = electron microscopy.

[c]Deleted from the 1995 modified WHO classification (ref. 12).

of the revised classification can be explained by its greater complexity due to excessive reliance on subclasses. Moreover, its handling of mixed or overlapping classes of lupus nephritis has remained a source of controversy.

A third classification was proposed in 2004 by a consensus conference organized jointly by the International Society of Nephrology (ISN) and the Renal Pathology Society (RPS) (47). It retains the simplicity of the original WHO classification while incorporating some of the refinements introduced by the revised WHO system (Table 13-3). This new classification is expected to supersede prior classifications.

All three classifications are based entirely on the evaluation of glomerular alterations. Accurate classification requires the careful assessment of the glomerular alterations by light microscopy, followed by the integration of the immunofluorescence and electron microscopic findings. The first step is to determine whether there is glomerular hypercellularity in the mesangial, endocapillary, or extracapillary zones. The distribution of this hypercellularity (focal or diffuse) is assessed. Attention is given to the presence of infiltrating leukocytes, necrotizing lesions, and glomerular basement membrane thickening. These light microscopic findings are then interpreted in the context of the distribution of the glomerular immune deposits in mesangial, subendothelial, and subepithelial locations as detected by light, immunofluorescence, and electron microscopy. Although some deposits are large enough to be identified by light microscopy, immunofluorescence and electron microscopy are the most sensitive techniques for the detection of immune deposits. Ideally, the same pathologist should study the biopsy by the three microscopic modalities to accurately integrate the findings. Because some lesions are focal, a proper classification depends on the adequacy of the glomerular sampling.

Table 13-3

INTERNATIONAL SOCIETY OF NEPHROLOGY (ISN)/RENAL PATHOLOGY SOCIETY (RPS) CLASSIFICATION OF LUPUS NEPHRITIS (2004)[a]

Class I	**Minimal Mesangial Lupus Nephritis** Normal glomeruli by LM, but mesangial immune deposits by IF[b]
Class II	**Mesangial Proliferative Lupus Nephritis** Purely mesangial hypercellularity of any degree and/or mesangial matrix expansion by LM, with mesangial immune deposits. A rare isolated subepithelial or subendothelial deposit may be visible by IF or EM, but not by LM.
Class III	**Focal Lupus Nephritis** Active or inactive focal, segmental, or global endo- or extracapillary glomerulonephritis involving <50% of glomeruli, typically with focal subendothelial immune deposits, with or without mesangial alterations. **III (A)** Active lesions (focal proliferative lupus nephritis) **III (A/C)** Active and chronic lesions (focal proliferative sclerosing lupus nephritis) **III (C)** Chronic inactive lesions with scars (focal sclerosing lupus nephritis) **Indicate the proportion of glomeruli with active and with sclerotic lesions* **Indicate the proportion of glomeruli with fibrinoid necrosis and with cellular crescents* **Indicate and grade (mild, moderate, severe) tubular atrophy, interstitial inflammation and fibrosis, arteriosclerosis or other vascular disease*
Class IV	**Diffuse Lupus Nephritis** Active or inactive diffuse, segmental, or global endo- and/or extracapillary glomerulonephritis involving ≥50% of all glomeruli, typically with diffuse subendothelial immune deposits, with or without mesangial alterations. This class is divided into diffuse segmental (IV-S) when ≥50% of the involved glomeruli have segmental lesions, and diffuse global (IV-G) when ≥50% of the involved glomeruli have global lesions. Segmental is defined as a glomerular lesion that involves less than half of the glomerular tuft. This class includes cases with diffuse wire-loop deposits, but with little or no glomerular proliferation. **IV-S (A) or IV-G (A)** Active lesions (diffuse segmental or global proliferative lupus nephritis) **IV-S (A/C) or IV-G (A/C)** Active and chronic lesions (diffuse segmental or global proliferative and sclerosing lupus nephritis) **IV-S (C) or IV-G (C)** Chronic inactive lesions with scars (diffuse segmental or global sclerosing lupus nephritis) **Indicate the proportion of glomeruli with active and with sclerotic lesions* **Indicate the proportion of glomeruli with fibrinoid necrosis and with cellular crescents* **Indicate and grade (mild, moderate, severe) tubular atrophy, interstitial inflammation and fibrosis, arteriosclerosis or other vascular disease*
Class V	**Membranous Lupus Nephritis** Global or segmental subepithelial immune deposits or their morphologic sequelae by LM and by IF or EM, with or without mesangial alterations **May occur in combination with III or IV, in which case both will be diagnosed* **May show advanced sclerosis*
Class VI	**Advanced Sclerosing Lupus Nephritis** ≥90% of glomeruli globally sclerosed without residual activity

[a]Adapted from reference 47.
[b]LM = light microscopy; IF = immunofluorescence microscopy; EM = electron microscopy.

General Clinical Features

The prevalence of SLE has been estimated at from 4 to 250 cases/100,000 population, and is higher among African Americans and Asian Americans than Caucasian Americans. SLE is about 10 times more common in women of reproductive age than men, with reduced female predominance in childhood and old age.

The clinical signs and symptoms of lupus nephritis are diverse, ranging from asymptomatic microhematuria or proteinuria, to nephrotic syndrome or rapidly progressive renal failure. In most patients with SLE, renal biopsy is not necessary to establish a diagnosis, but is performed to define the quality and severity of the renal lesions as a guide to treatment. However, in some patients, the diagnosis of SLE may be in doubt until a renal biopsy reveals the characteristic morphologic and immunopathologic features. This is particularly true of some patients with class II or class V lupus nephritis, in whom renal manifestations may precede by months or years the development of serologic abnormalities or other systemic features of the disease.

The renal biopsy provides the most accurate means of predicting prognosis and guiding therapy in patients with lupus nephritis. Clinical renal abnormalities are relatively insensitive predictors of the class and activity of the renal lesions seen on renal biopsy (1,3). In fact, an extremely small percentage of patients with severe class IV lupus nephritis may have no detectable renal abnormalities ("silent" diffuse proliferative lupus nephritis) (30). Nonetheless, most centers do not advocate performing a renal biopsy on every newly diagnosed patient with SLE without clinical evidence of renal involvement. Most clinicians believe that renal biopsy should be performed if there is the new appearance of any significant marker of renal disease, such as hematuria, proteinuria, nephrotic syndrome, or elevated serum creatinine. Repeat renal biopsies are commonly performed in patients with documented lupus nephritis to gauge the efficacy of treatment and the need for continued or modified treatment (22). Lupus nephritis has the capacity to reactivate or transform from one class to another spontaneously or following treatment. Therefore, repeat biopsies are frequently required if there is a change in clinical renal findings (such as worsening renal function, proteinuria, or hematuria) that may herald such a transformation.

Glomerular Pathologic Findings by Class (According to 2004 ISN/RPS Classification):

Class I (Minimal Mesangial Lupus Nephritis)

Definition. In the original WHO classification system, class I was defined as a normal renal biopsy from a patient who fulfills the ARA criteria for SLE. There are few examples of class I lupus nephritis so defined because these patients generally have no clinical renal abnormalities and are not referred to a nephrologist for biopsy. In the ISN/RPS classification (Table 13-3), the normal category was eliminated and replaced with the original WHO category IIa, because it was deemed contradictory to classify a normal biopsy as a form of "lupus nephritis" (47). Thus, according to the ISN/RPS classification, class I denotes normal glomeruli by light microscopy, but mesangial immune deposits detected by immunofluorescence and/or electron microscopy.

Clinical Features. Patients with class I lupus nephritis usually have minimal urinary findings of microhematuria or mild subnephrotic proteinuria. Renal function is normal. Despite the very mild clinical renal abnormalities, the systemic manifestations of lupus and lupus serologies may be active.

Light Microscopic Findings. There are no histologic abnormalities. The glomerular tuft is normocellular (fig. 13-1).

Immunofluorescence Findings. There are immune deposits limited to the mesangium (fig. 13-2). The mesangial deposits tend to be small and vary from segmental to global in distribution.

Electron Microscopic Findings. Small electron-dense deposits are present in the mesangium (fig. 13-3). No electron-dense deposits are identified involving the peripheral glomerular capillary walls.

Class II (Mesangial Proliferative Lupus Nephritis)

Definition. Class II designates glomerular disease limited to the mesangium. In the original WHO classification, class II was subdivided into class IIa and IIb according to the absence or presence of mesangial hypercellularity, respectively. In the ISN/RPS classification, the original WHO class IIa has now become class I and the original WHO class IIb has become class II. According to the ISN/RPS schema, class II has been redefined as purely mesangial hypercellularity of any degree and/or mesangial matrix expansion, as detected by light microscopy, with mesangial immune deposits. There may be rare isolated subepithelial or subendothelial deposits detected by immunofluorescence or electron microscopy that are not visible by light microscopy.

Clinical Features. The clinical renal manifestations of class II lupus nephritis are mild. Fewer than 50 percent of patients have mild hematuria or proteinuria, which generally does not exceed 1 g/day. The nephrotic syndrome is virtually never observed. Renal insufficiency is uncommon, although up to 15 percent of patients have mildly reduced creatinine clearance. Despite the relatively mild and inactive glomerulonephritis, serologic tests for SLE are strongly positive in up to 25 percent of cases.

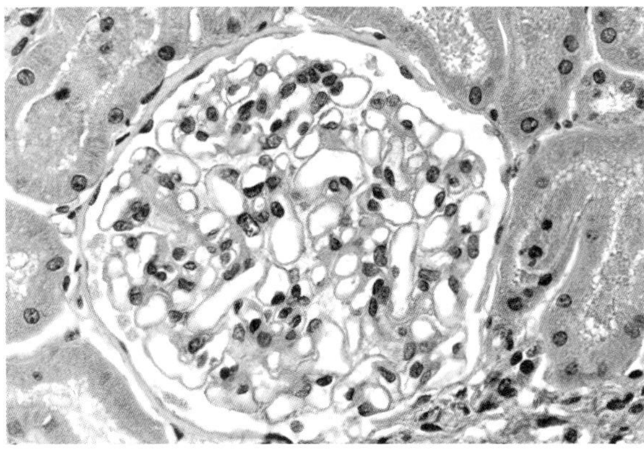

Figure 13-1

LUPUS NEPHRITIS CLASS I

The mesangium is normocellular and the glomerular capillary walls appear normal in thickness (hematoxylin and eosin [H&E] stain).

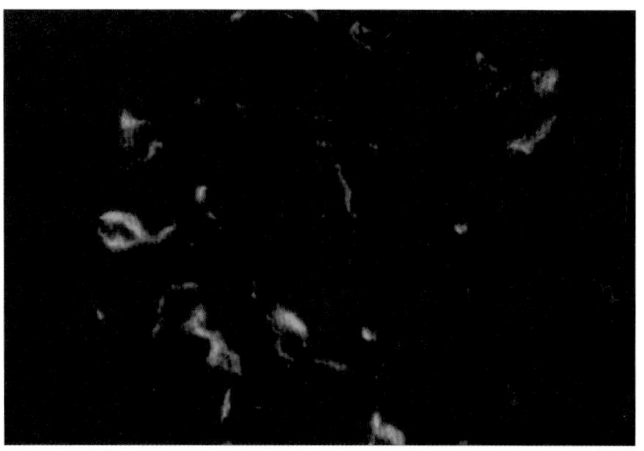

Figure 13-2

LUPUS NEPHRITIS CLASS I

Immunofluorescence micrograph shows small segmental deposits of complement (C)1q confined to the mesangium. Immunoglobulin (Ig)G, IgM, and IgA stained in the same distribution.

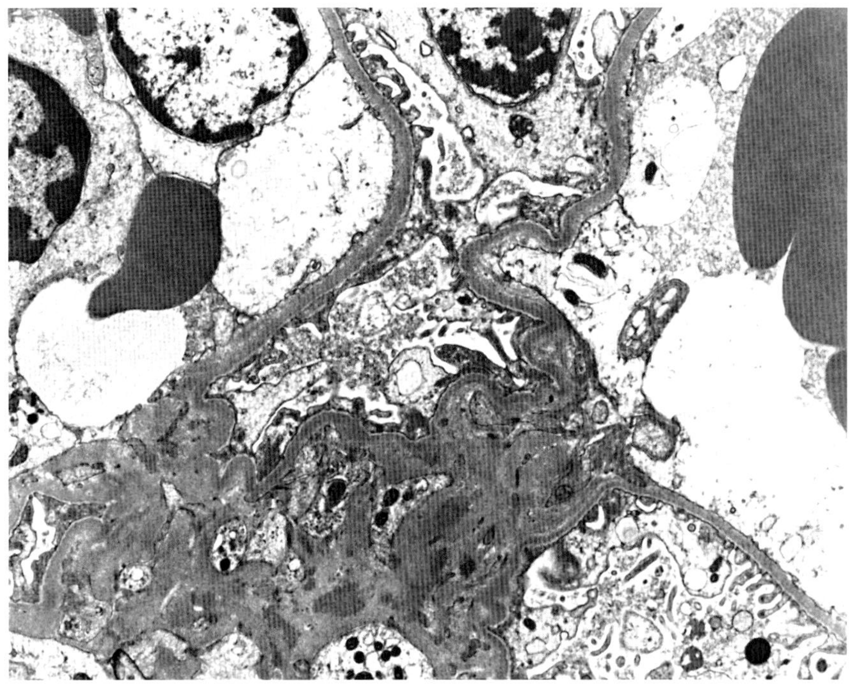

Figure 13-3

LUPUS NEPHRITIS CLASS I

There are small electron-dense deposits in the mesangium. No deposits involve the peripheral glomerular basement membranes, which are normal in thickness. The foot processes are well preserved, correlating with the absence of significant proteinuria.

Light Microscopic Findings. There is mesangial proliferation of any severity (fig. 13-4). Mesangial hypercellularity is defined as greater than three mesangial cells in mesangial areas away from the vascular pole, assessed in 3-µm–thick histologic sections. The mesangial proliferation is usually mild to moderate and does not significantly compromise the glomerular capillary lumen. It may vary in distribution from focal to diffuse and may involve the glomerular tuft segmentally or globally. A variable increase in mesangial matrix may accompany the mesangial hypercellularity. Usually, the mesangial deposits are not large enough to be identified by light microscopy. In some cases, however, large deposits expand the mesangium and impart a glassy, hypereosinophilic appearance to the mesangial matrix.

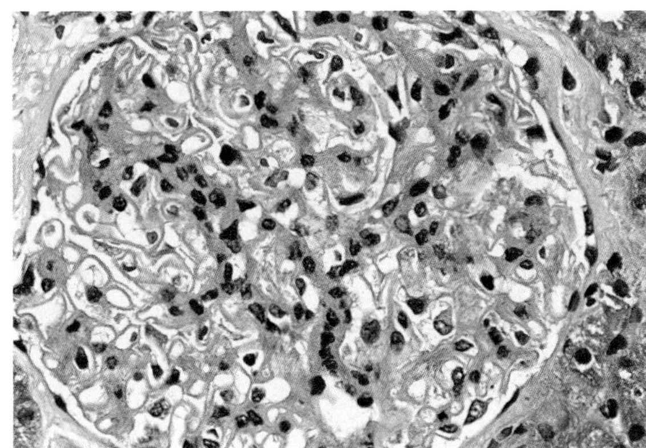

Figure 13-4

LUPUS NEPHRITIS CLASS II

There is mild segmental mesangial hypercellularity, defined as mesangial zones containing more than three mesangial cells (in a 3-µm–thick section). Glomerular capillary lumens are patent and the glomerular basement membranes appear normal in thickness (H&E stain).

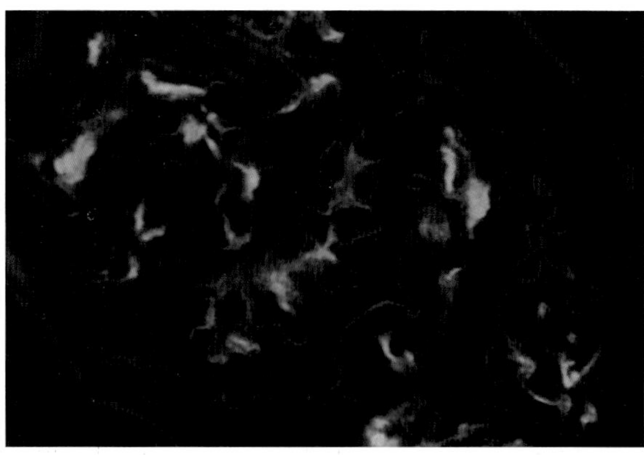

Figure 13-5

LUPUS NEPHRITIS CLASS II

Immunofluorescence micrograph shows global mesangial deposits of IgG. Nonspecific weak linear positivity of the glomerular basement membranes represents background staining. IgM, IgA, C3, and C1q were positive in the mesangial areas.

Cases of lupus nephritis with severe but purely mesangial hypercellularity, without obliteration of the capillary lumens, may pose difficulties in classification. Proper classification requires the careful assessment of the immunofluorescence and electron microscopic findings. If the immune deposits are limited to the mesangium, even cases of severe diffuse mesangial proliferation should be classified as class II. If significant subendothelial deposits are present by immunofluorescence or electron microscopy, or if subendothelial deposits are visible by light microscopy, the case should be classified as focal proliferative if subendothelial deposits are segmentally distributed and diffuse proliferative if globally distributed.

Immunofluorescence Findings. There are granular immune deposits confined to the mesangium (fig. 13-5). The pattern by immunofluorescence outlines the axial framework of the glomerulus, corresponding to the mesangial stalk.

Electron Microscopic Findings. There are electron-dense deposits confined to the mesangial matrix (fig. 13-6). Strictly speaking, pure class II lupus nephritis should have no detectable subendothelial or subepithelial deposits. In practice, however, some cases of purely mesangial proliferative lupus nephritis manifest rare, small subendothelial electron-dense deposits, especially as extensions from the paramesangial region. Such nonconforming cases are problematic and are not adequately addressed by the original WHO classification system. Because the presence of any subendothelial deposits whatsoever in a purely mesangial proliferative glomerulonephritis raises the question of unsampled focal proliferative (class III) lupus nephritis or at least the possibility of imminent transformation to class III or class IV, the presence of subendothelial deposits should be reported. According to the ISN/RPS classification, cases of mesangial proliferative lupus nephritis with rare minute subendothelial or subepithelial deposits (visible only by immunofluorescence or electron microscopy) should be classified as class II (47). However, the presence of any sizeable (visible by light microscopy) or numerous subendothelial deposits in an otherwise mesangial proliferative glomerulonephritis exceeds what is acceptable in pure class II disease and warrants a designation of class III or IV, depending on the distribution and quantity of the deposits.

Differential Diagnosis. Class II lupus nephritis must be distinguished from immunoglobulin (Ig)A nephropathy and other mesangial proliferative glomerulonephritides such as mild membranoproliferative glomerulonephritis or resolving postinfectious glomerulonephritis. The latter two conditions are usually accompanied by hypocomplementemia.

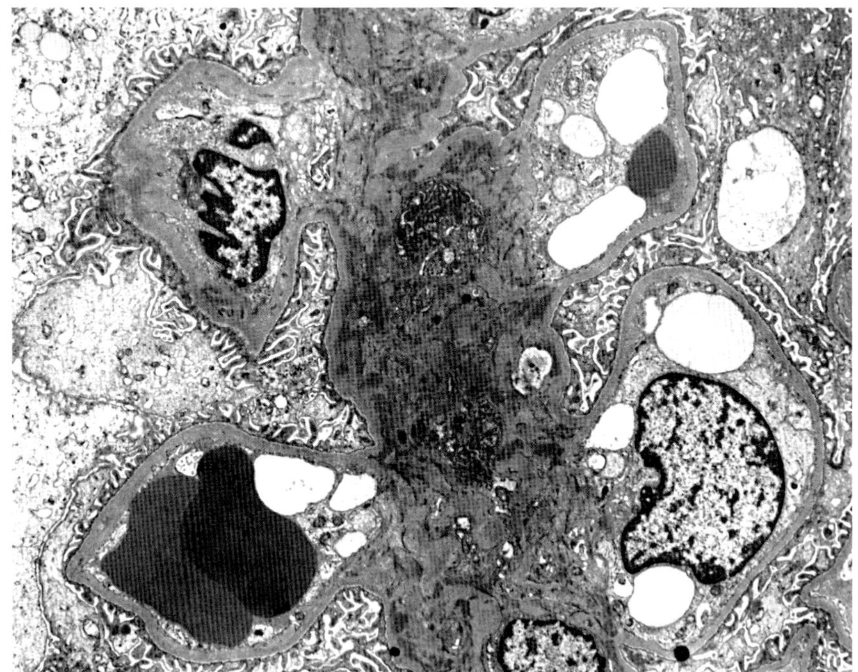

Figure 13-6

LUPUS NEPHRITIS CLASS II

Large electron-dense deposits are confined to the mesangium, or centrilobular region, between adjacent glomerular capillaries. No electron-dense deposits are identified involving the glomerular basement membranes, which appear normal in thickness (electron micrograph).

The most problematic diagnostic consideration in daily practice is the differentiation from IgA nephropathy. Immunofluorescence and electron microscopy are particular helpful in this regard. In IgA nephropathy, the mesangial deposits tend to form in the paramesangial areas, subjacent to the reflection of the glomerular basement membrane. By contrast, they are more uniformly distributed throughout the mesangial matrix in class II lupus nephritis. IgA nephropathy has been defined by immunofluorescence as dominant or co-dominant staining for IgA (usually 2+ or greater) and less than 2+ for C1q, using a scale of 0 to 4+ (25). In IgA nephropathy, where complement is activated through the alternative pathway, C3 is usually positive, with weak or absent C1q. By contrast, over 90 percent of cases of lupus nephritis have C1q staining according to one study (25), with a mean of 3+ intensity. The intensity of IgA immunostaining is greater in IgA nephropathy (mean, 3.2+) than lupus nephritis (mean, 1.8+) (25). Over 90 percent of patients with IgA nephropathy have an intensity of IgA staining greater than that of IgG. By contrast, in 85 percent of lupus nephritis biopsies, IgG more intensely than IgA, and only in 1 percent is IgA more intense. When IgA is present in lupus nephritis, there are virtually always co-deposits of IgG. By contrast, up to 40 percent of patients with IgA nephropathy lack IgG altogether. Lambda light chain dominance is also more common in IgA nephropathy (67 percent) than lupus nephritis (29 percent) (25). Thus, careful assessment of the immunofluorescence features helps differentiate between these two conditions.

Class III (Focal Lupus Nephritis) and Class IV (Diffuse Lupus Nephritis)

Most investigators consider the glomerular lesions of class III and class IV lupus nephritis to be qualitatively similar, differing only in severity and distribution. Therefore, these two related classes are described together.

Definition. Class III lupus nephritis is defined as focal segmental or global endocapillary proliferative glomerulonephritis affecting less than 50 percent of the total glomeruli sampled. Class IV is defined as diffuse segmental or global endocapillary proliferative glomerulonephritis affecting greater than 50 percent of glomeruli. Both class III and class IV manifest subendothelial immune deposits (relatively focal in class III and diffuse in class IV), with or without mesangial alterations. The ISN/RPS classification subdivides lupus nephritis class IV into those cases with diffuse segmental versus diffuse global proliferation (Table 13-3). This subdivision

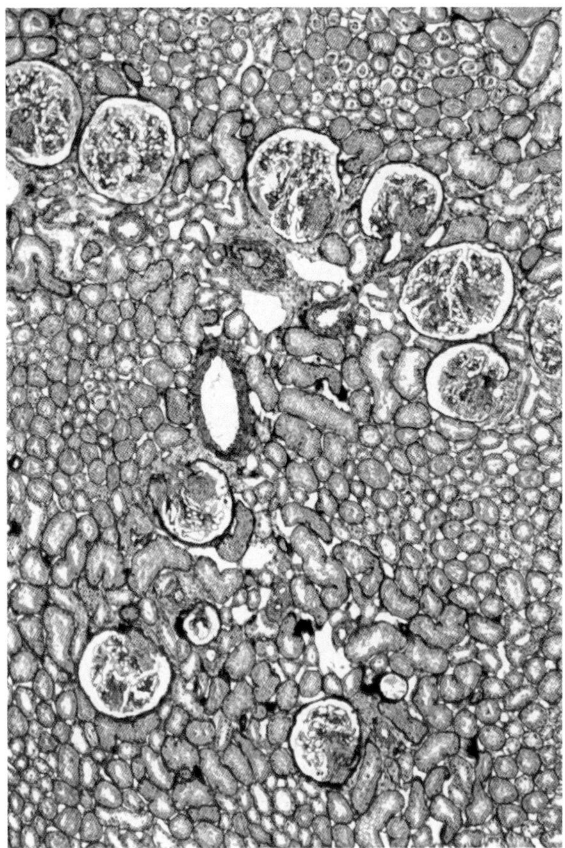

Figure 13-7

LUPUS NEPHRITIS CLASS III

Low-power microscopic view shows focal and segmental endocapillary proliferation accompanied by segmental crescents. The lesions of endocapillary proliferation are discretely segmental, involving a small portion of the tuft. Although most glomeruli in this field are involved, overall the biopsy had focal endocapillary proliferation involving less than 50 percent of the total glomeruli sampled, qualifying as class III lupus nephritis (Jones methenamine silver [JMS] stain).

was proposed to facilitate future studies addressing possible differences in outcome and pathogenesis between these subgroups (27,34). Both class III and class IV nephritis may manifest active (proliferative) and/or inactive (sclerosing) lesions. In determining the percentage of total glomeruli affected by glomerulonephritis, both the proliferative and sclerosing lesions must be taken into account. Although most active glomerular lesions are endocapillary proliferative in nature, both class III and class IV factor in glomerular lesions that are membranoproliferative, extracapillary proliferative, or consist of "wire-loop" deposits without associated proliferation. For these reasons, the ISN/RPS classification prefers the broader terms "focal lupus nephritis" and "diffuse lupus nephritis" over the more restrictive terms "focal proliferative lupus nephritis" and "diffuse proliferative lupus nephritis" used in the original WHO classification.

Clinical Features. Patients with class III lupus nephritis have a variable clinical picture (28). About 50 percent have active urinary sediment and 25 to 50 percent have proteinuria, which may be accompanied by nephrotic syndrome in up to one third. Renal insufficiency, however, is uncommon, affecting only 10 to 25 percent of patients. Hypertension may develop in up to a third. Serologic abnormalities are common and over half of patients manifest anti-DNA antibodies and/or hypocomplementemia.

Patients with class IV lupus nephritis have the most severe and active clinical presentation. Not surprisingly, they comprise the largest group in most biopsy-based series of cases (1,3). Proteinuria is detected in over 95 percent of patients and up to half manifest full nephrotic syndrome. Nearly 75 percent have active urinary sediment. Renal insufficiency, however, is detectable in just over half, using measurements of the glomerular filtration rate (GFR), although serum creatinine levels may be in the normal range. Serologic features of lupus such as positive ANA and anti-DNA antibody, and reduced serum complement levels, are found in 50 to 90 percent of patients.

Light Microscopic Findings. Although endocapillary proliferation affects less than 50 percent of glomeruli in patients with class III and over 50 percent of glomeruli in those with class IV lupus nephritis, the glomerular lesions in the two classes are qualitatively similar. The endocapillary proliferative lesions in class III tend to be relatively segmental (involving only a portion of the glomerular tuft), although some glomeruli may be affected globally (figs. 13-7, 13-8). In class IV, the endocapillary proliferation is typically more diffuse and global (figs. 13-9, 13-10); however, some examples of class IV have a diffuse and segmental distribution (designated class IV-S in the ISN/RPS classification). In both class III and class IV, the endocapillary proliferation usually occurs on a background of mesangial hypercellularity that may be focal or diffuse. Thus, mesangial proliferation and mesangial immune deposits can be considered the substratum upon which the more complex classes (III, IV, and V) are built.

Common light microscopic features seen in class III and class IV lupus nephritis include wire-loop deposits, hyaline thrombi, leukocyte infiltration, necrosis, hematoxylin bodies, cellular crescents, and glomerular scarring, each of which is described below.

In class III and class IV lupus nephritis, subendothelial immune deposits may be large enough to detect by light microscopy, forming wire-loop thickenings of the glomerular capillary walls (figs. 13-11, 13-12). Special stains such as trichrome or Jones methenamine silver (JMS) reveal the deposits to be entirely or largely subendothelial, with preservation of an outer peripheral layer of glomerular basement membrane (fig. 13-13). With the trichrome stain, subendothelial deposits appear orange-red against the blue of the glomerular basement membrane (figs. 13-13, 13-14); with the JMS stain, the deposits appear pink against the black argyrophilic glomerular basement membrane. In some cases, the subendothelial deposits are incorporated into the glomerular capillary wall by a subendothelial layer of neomembrane, producing a double contour. This may be accompanied by mesangial interposition, giving a membranoproliferative appearance.

Some cases of class III or class IV lupus nephritis manifest large intracapillary deposits, forming "hyaline thrombi" (figs. 13-11, 13-12,

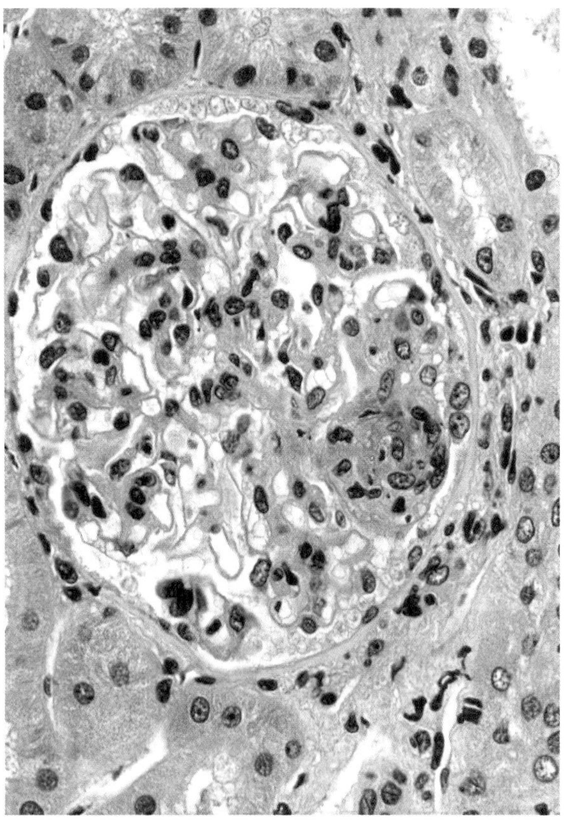

Figure 13-8

LUPUS NEPHRITIS CLASS III

There is segmental endocapillary proliferation with necrotizing features. The involved lobule contains highly eosinophilic material, consistent with the fibrinoid necrosis associated with pyknotic nuclear debris. The adjacent lobules show a background of mild mesangial hypercellularity, with patent capillary lumens (H&E stain).

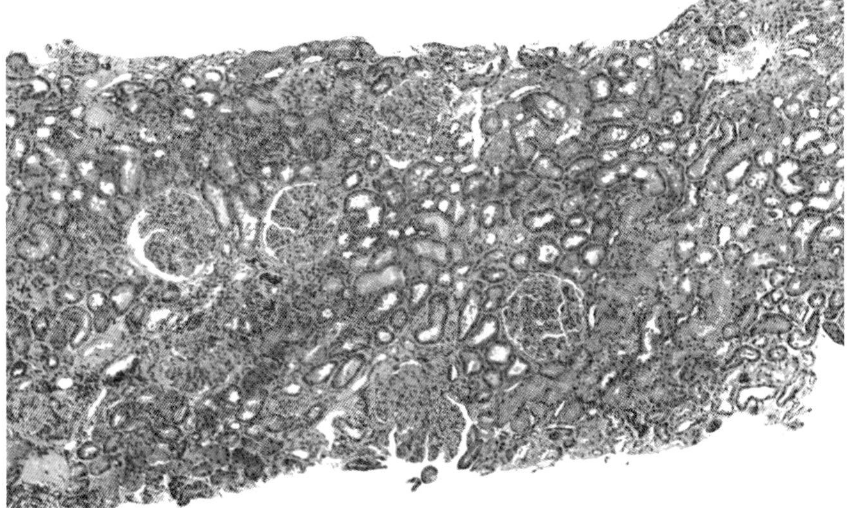

Figure 13-9

LUPUS NEPHRITIS CLASS IV

Low-power microscopic view shows the diffuse and global nature of the glomerular endocapillary proliferation. The glomeruli are involved uniformly, with occlusion of the glomerular capillary lumens by voluminous endocapillary proliferation. The interstitium contains a moderate inflammatory infiltrate (H&E stain).

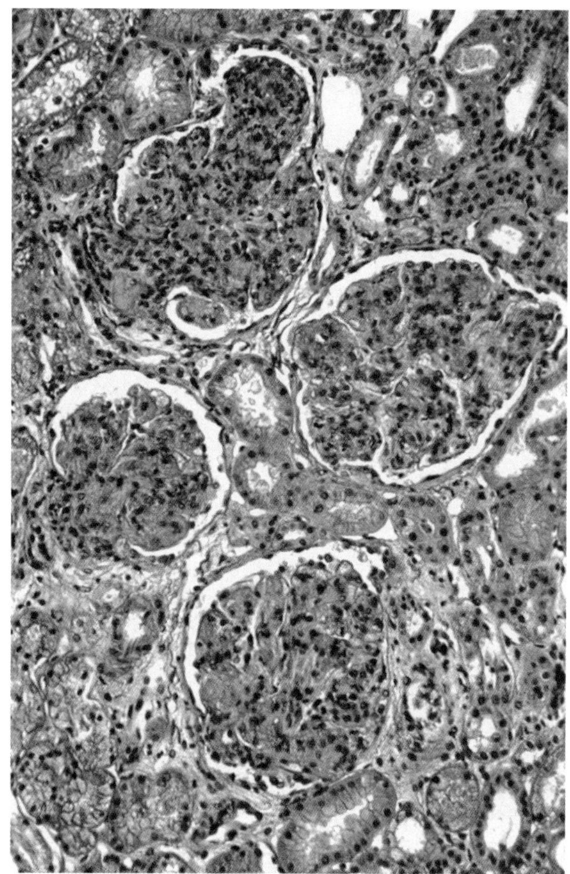

Figure 13-10

LUPUS NEPHRITIS CLASS IV

Glomerular capillary lumens are occluded by diffuse and global endocapillary proliferation. The endocapillary cells include endothelial and mesangial cells, as well as infiltrating mononuclear and polymorphonuclear leukocytes (H&E stain).

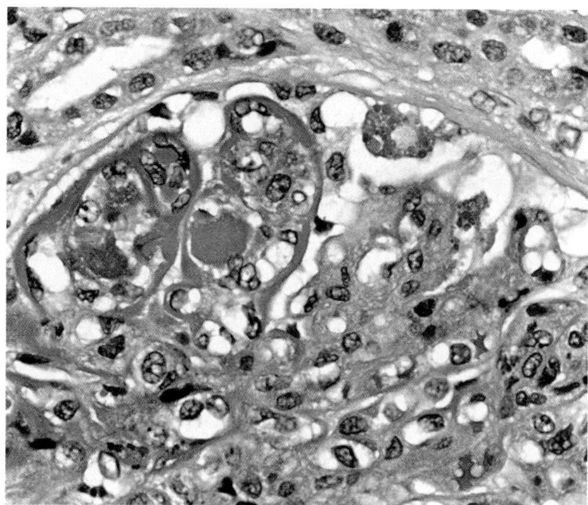

Figure 13-11

LUPUS NEPHRITIS CLASS IV

Several capillaries contain "wire-loop" deposits and "hyaline thrombi." The wire-loop deposits are subendothelial deposits so large that they are visible by light microscopy as glassy, eosinophilic, band-like thickenings of the glomerular capillary walls. The hyaline thrombi are not true fibrin thrombi, but consist of intraluminal immune deposits that form rounded, eosinophilic, intracapillary masses. Other glomerular capillaries show endocapillary proliferation, including infiltrating leukocytes (H&E stain).

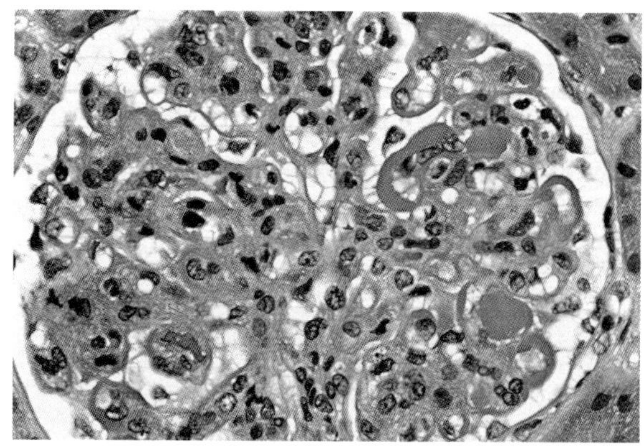

Figure 13-12

LUPUS NEPHRITIS CLASS IV

Several glomerular capillaries in the right portion of the field have wire-loop thickenings of the glomerular capillary walls caused by massive subendothelial immune deposits. Several capillaries also contain eosinophilic intraluminal deposits that form hyaline thrombi (H&E stain).

13-15–13-17). This term is actually a misnomer because these do not represent true fibrin thrombi but massive intracapillary immune deposits with the same composition by immunofluorescence as the neighboring subendothelial immune deposits. The affected capillaries often exhibit less exuberant endocapillary hypercellularity than the adjacent capillaries, suggesting differences in their ability to incite a proliferative response (fig. 13-18).

In most cases of class III and class IV lupus nephritis, the endocapillary hypercellularity results from the proliferation of glomerular endothelial and mesangial cells, as well as by leukocyte infiltration, including infiltration of neutrophils, monocytes, and lymphocytes (fig. 13-19). However, the modified WHO classification (see Table 13-2) recognizes several morphologic

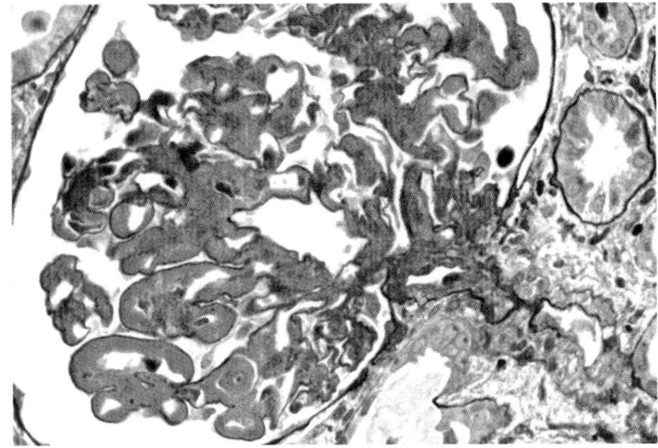

Figure 13-13

LUPUS NEPHRITIS CLASS IV

The trichrome stain delineates global, large subendothelial deposits involving all the glomerular capillaries and corresponding to the wire-loop deposits seen with the H&E stain. The subendothelial deposits are fuchsinophilic (orange-red) with the trichrome stain and contrast with the blue staining of the overlying glomerular basement membranes. Most of the glomeruli in the biopsy had this appearance. Although there is no significant endocapillary proliferation, the diffuse and global distribution of the subendothelial deposits qualifies as class IV lupus nephritis.

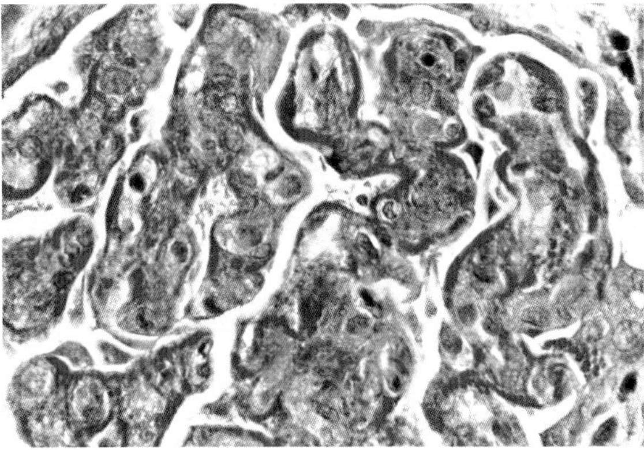

Figure 13-14

LUPUS NEPHRITIS CLASS IV

With the trichrome stain, subendothelial deposits are red against the blue of the glomerular basement membrane. Fuchsinophilic deposits are also identified in the mesangial areas. The glomerular capillary lumens are narrowed by global mild endocapillary proliferation.

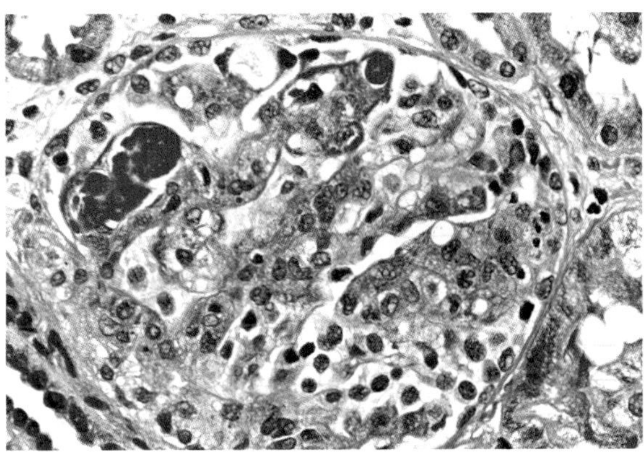

Figure 13-15

LUPUS NEPHRITIS CLASS IV

Hyaline thrombi stain orange-red with the trichrome stain. The intracapillary deposits have a homogeneous glassy texture, unlike true fibrin which is more fibrillar. Smaller subendothelial fuchsinophilic deposits are also present in several capillaries.

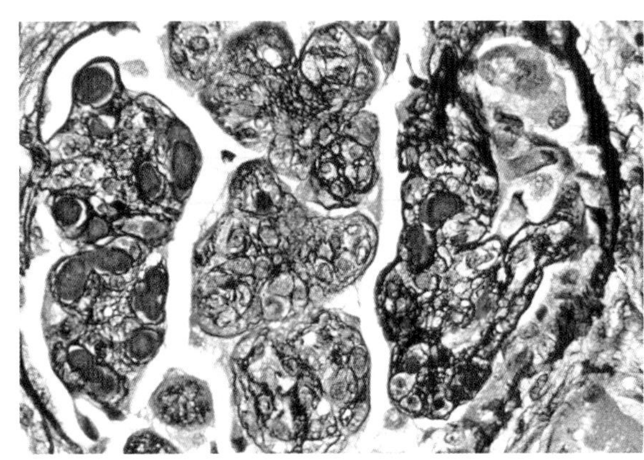

Figure 13-16

LUPUS NEPHRITIS CLASS IV

Hyaline thrombi seen by the JMS stain appear pink against the black outlines of the surrounding glomerular basement membranes. Basement membrane stains help delineate the intracapillary location of the immune deposits.

variants of class IV that lack the typical picture of florid endocapillary proliferation with leukocyte infiltration (12,13). The first is the membranoproliferative variant. In this form, the endocapillary proliferation has a distinctly membranoproliferative aspect, with extensive mesangial interposition and duplication of the glomerular basement membrane, resembling that seen in membranoproliferative glomerulonephritis type 1 (fig. 13-20). The glomerular capillary lumens are typically narrowed by the peripheral mesangial interposition, but without luminal closure. Other variants include severe mesangial proliferation with diffuse subendothelial

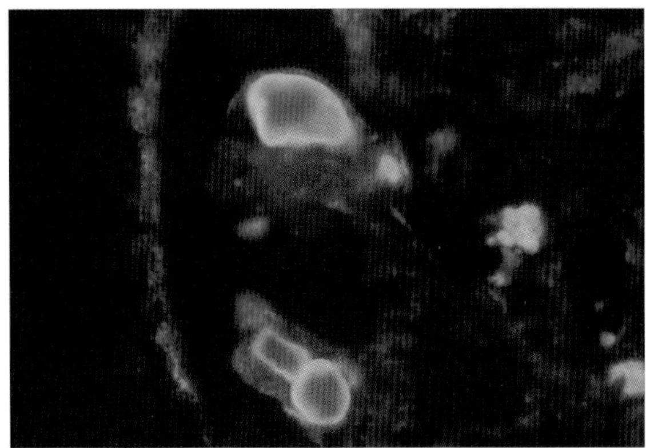

Figure 13-17

LUPUS NEPHRITIS CLASS IV

Immunofluorescence micrograph stained for IgA highlights several intraluminal deposits (hyaline thrombi). Similar staining was observed for IgG, IgM, C3, and C1q. Smaller and more granular deposits are also identified in some glomerular capillary walls and Bowman's capsule.

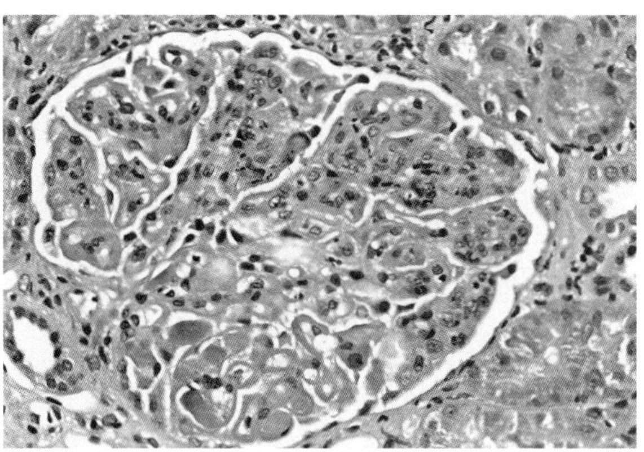

Figure 13-18

LUPUS NEPHRITIS CLASS IV

Glomerular lobules with large subendothelial and intracapillary deposits (towards the bottom of the field) exhibit less endocapillary hypercellularity than adjacent lobules (H&E stain).

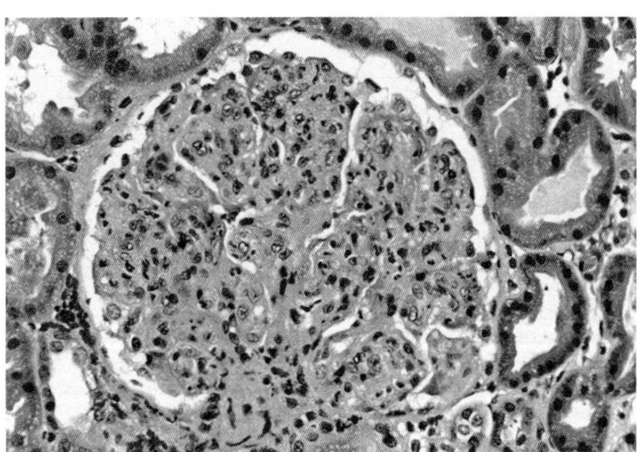

Figure 13-19

LUPUS NEPHRITIS CLASS IV

There is a marked global endocapillary proliferation, including many infiltrating neutrophils. Some of the leukocytes are undergoing apoptosis, producing pyknotic karyorrhectic debris. Small foci of fibrinoid necrosis are visible as smudgy eosinophilic material in several capillaries (H&E stain).

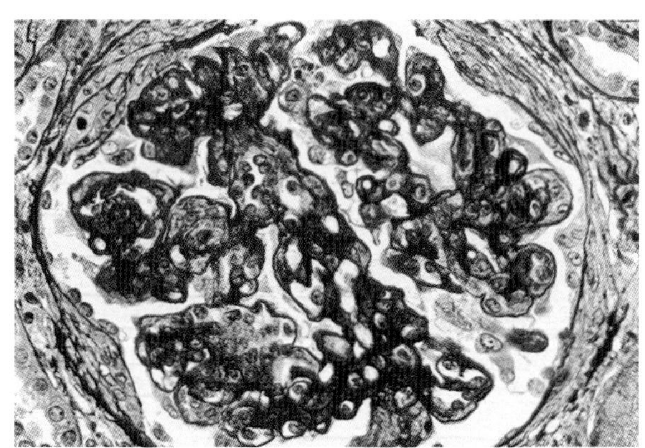

Figure 13-20

LUPUS NEPHRITIS CLASS IV

Membranoproliferative variant with numerous double contours of the glomerular basement membrane. By light microscopy, the findings are indistinguishable from those of idiopathic membranoproliferative glomerulonephritis type 1 (JMS stain).

deposits (fig. 13-21) or extensive subendothelial deposits with minimal glomerular hypercellularity (see fig. 13-12). In all these variants, the sine qua non of class IV disease is diffuse subendothelial deposits, albeit with variable patterns of glomerular proliferation.

Glomerular necrosis is a feature of class III and class IV lupus nephritis and is never observed in pure mesangial proliferative (class II) or membranous (class V) disease. A necrotizing lesion consists of a focus of smudgy fibrinoid obliteration of the glomerular tuft. The necrosis may be accompanied by any or all of the following: deposition of intracapillary fibrin; glomerular basement membrane rupture or gap formation; and apoptosis of infiltrating neutrophils producing pyknotic or karyorrhectic nuclear debris ("nuclear dust") (figs. 13-22, 13-23).

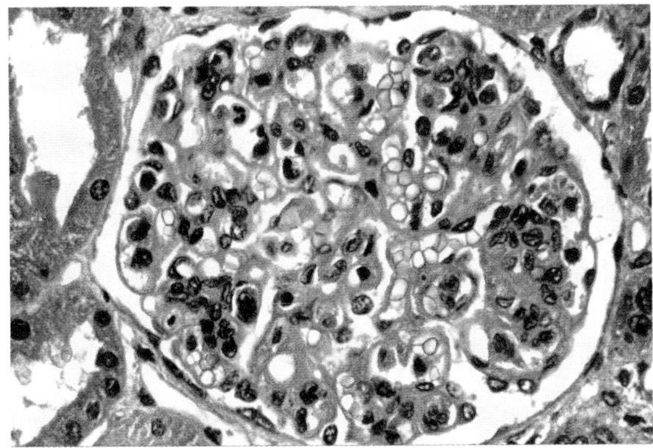

Figure 13-21

LUPUS NEPHRITIS CLASS IV

A variant with mesangial hypercellularity and diffuse subendothelial deposits causes thickening of the glomerular capillary walls, but without overt endocapillary proliferation (H&E stain).

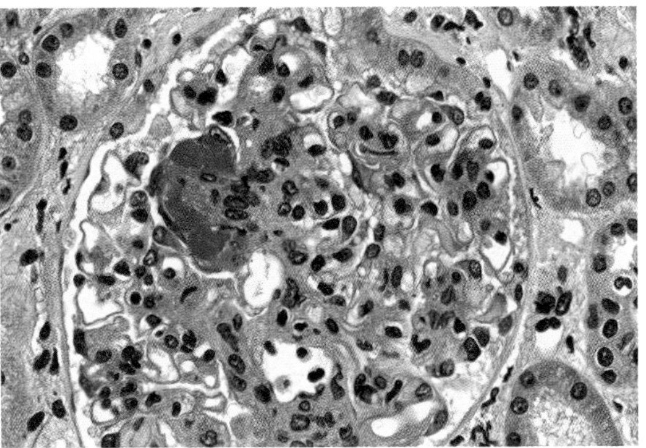

Figure 13-22

LUPUS NEPHRITIS CLASS III

A segmental necrotizing lesion with endocapillary fibrin and pyknosis involves a single glomerular capillary. Adjacent lobules display mild mesangial hypercellularity (H&E stain).

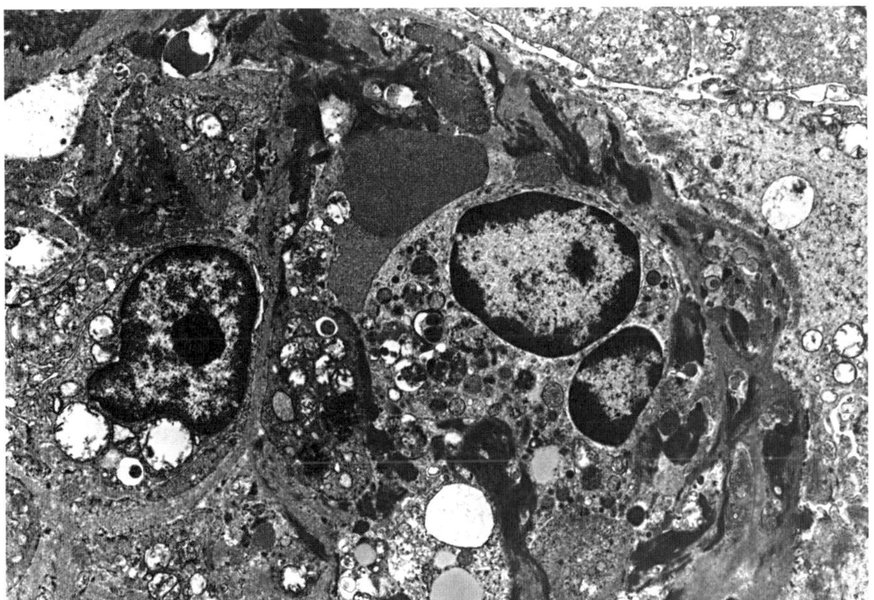

Figure 13-23

LUPUS NEPHRITIS CLASS IV

Electron micrograph shows a necrotizing lesion with infiltrating neutrophils, endothelial necrosis, and intraluminal fibrin. Although both fibrin and immune deposits are electron dense, the fibrin can be differentiated by its fibrillar substructure and tendency to bundle, forming fibrin "tactoids." There is complete foot process effacement of the overlying podocytes.

Necrotizing lesions are typically segmental in distribution, but more than one glomerular lobule may be affected, particularly in diffuse proliferative lupus nephritis.

Hematoxylin bodies are the only truly pathognomonic lesion of lupus nephritis. However, they are extremely uncommon, affecting less than 2 percent of biopsy specimens (44). They consist of smudgy, lilac-staining structures that may be smaller or larger than normal nuclei (figs. 13-24, 13-25). They usually have indistinct borders and merge with the background tissue, with surrounding flecks of hematoxyphilic material. They may be isolated or clustered. Usually they occur in glomeruli with very active proliferative and necrotizing lesions. Hematoxylin bodies are the tissue equivalent of the LE body; they are naked nuclei whose chromatin has been altered following cell death, with extrusion of the nucleus and binding to ambient circulating ANA (14).

Cellular crescents are a feature of active lupus nephritis that may be encountered frequently

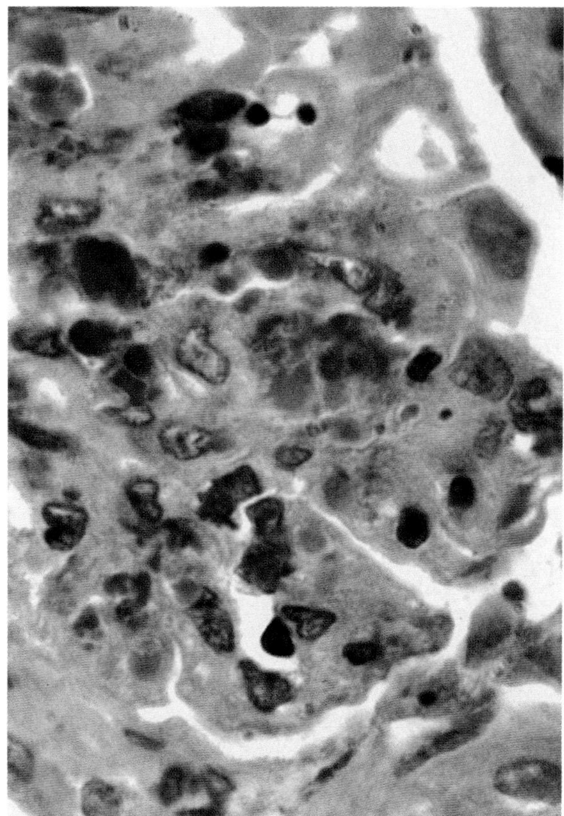

Figure 13-24

LUPUS NEPHRITIS CLASS IV

Hematoxylin bodies appear lilac colored with the H&E stain. They consist of extruded nuclei (probably from infiltrating leukocytes) that have bound to ambient antinuclear antibody, causing swelling and clumping of the nuclear chromatin (H&E stain).

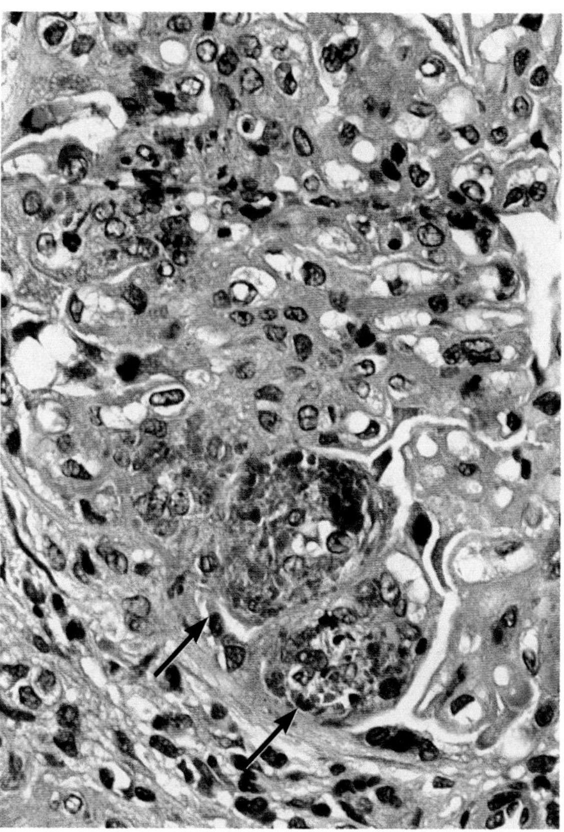

Figure 13-25

LUPUS NEPHRITIS CLASS IV

An example with segmentally distributed hematoxylin bodies, which can be identified as rounded lilac-colored inclusions in several glomerular capillaries (arrows). Other glomerular capillary lumens display endocapillary proliferation (H&E stain).

in both class III and class IV specimens (fig. 13-26). They are common overlying necrotizing lesions but also occur in glomeruli with non-necrotizing endocapillary proliferative lesions. By definition, they never occur in pure mesangial proliferative (class II) disease. Likewise, they are not seen in pure membranous lupus nephritis (modified WHO class Va or Vb).

Glomerular scarring is a feature of chronic glomerular injury in class III and class IV lupus nephritis. In class III, the glomerular scarring is often initially focal and segmental, mirroring the distribution of the proliferative and necrotizing lesions. Associated fibrous crescents may form synechiae to the sclerotic segments. In chronic class IV lupus nephritis, the glomerular scarring is typically more global and diffuse. Of course, glomerular obsolescence is not restricted to class III and class IV, but also can supervene on class V disease. Glomerular sclerosis in lupus nephritis may also occur in the course of aging or as a complication of hypertensive arterionephrosclerosis, and does not necessarily imply scarring in the course of immunologically mediated injury.

Immunofluorescence Findings. In classes III and IV lupus nephritis, the subendothelial immune deposits generally follow the distribution of the endocapillary proliferation. Thus they tend to be relatively focal and segmental in class III and more diffuse and global in class IV lupus nephritis (figs. 13-27–13-29). These subendothelial

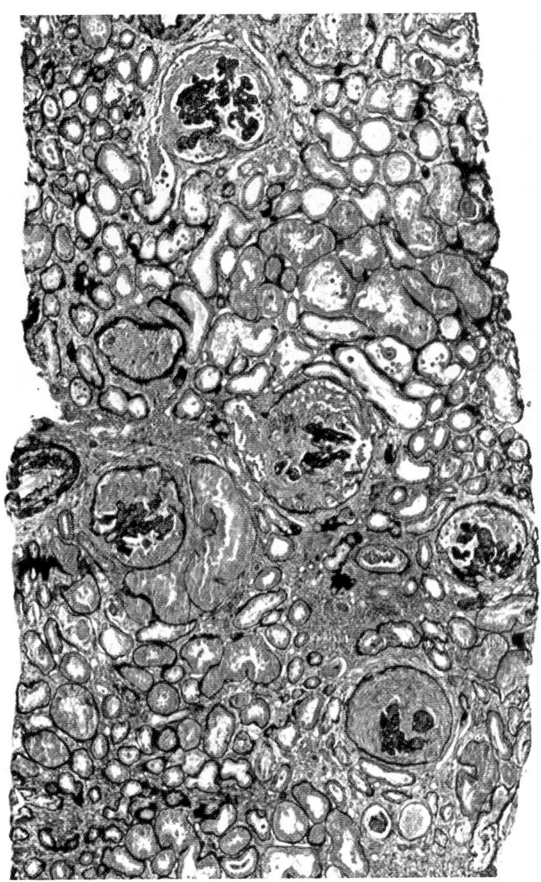

Figure 13-26

LUPUS NEPHRITIS CLASS IV

A severe example with diffuse cellular crescents involving all the glomeruli in this field. The glomerular tufts are compressed by the voluminous circumferential extracapillary proliferation (JMS stain).

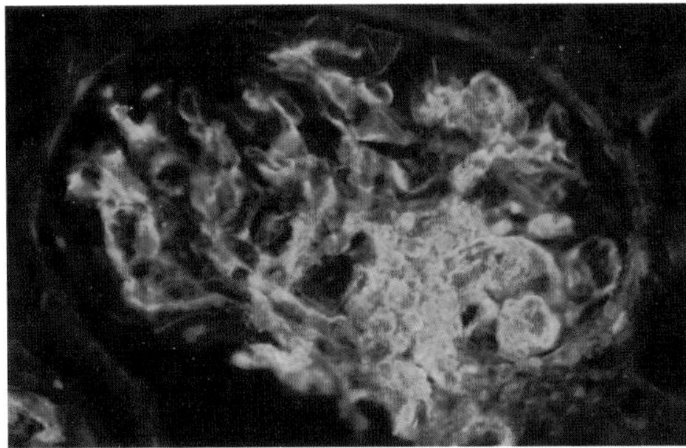

Figure 13-27

LUPUS NEPHRITIS CLASS III

By immunofluorescence, deposits of IgG involve the glomerular capillary walls in a segmental distribution, corresponding to subendothelial deposits. Adjacent lobules contain mesangial deposits.

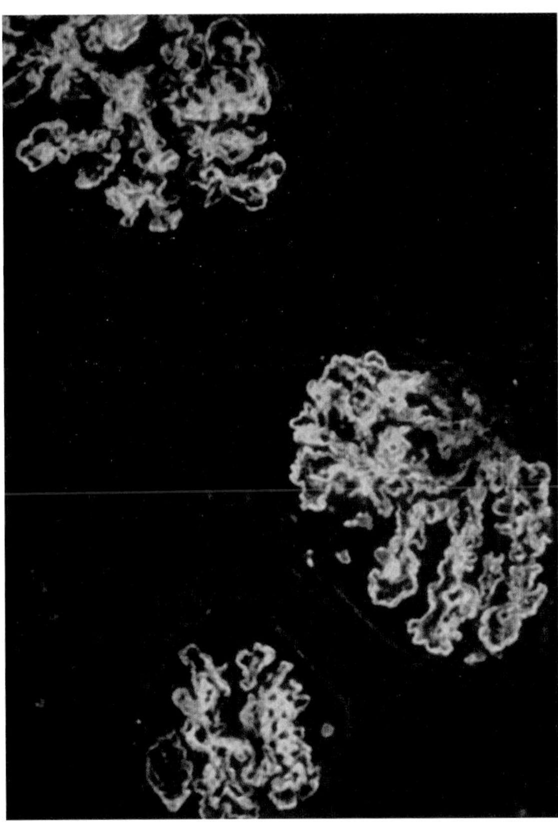

Figure 13-28

LUPUS NEPHRITIS CLASS IV

Immunofluorescence micrograph shows IgG deposited in the mesangium and in the peripheral glomerular capillary walls in a diffuse and global distribution. The glomerular capillary wall deposits appear confluent and semilinear, corresponding to subendothelial immune deposits.

deposits are typically superimposed on generalized mesangial immune deposits. Subendothelial deposits are usually comma-shaped, with a loop pattern, and vary from granular to semilinear (fig. 13-30). Wire-loop–type subendothelial deposits may be massive and ring shaped. They typically have a smooth outer contour corresponding to the delimiting outer glomerular basement membrane (fig. 13-31). Hyaline thrombi form occlusive intracapillary globular deposits (see fig. 13-17). Scattered subepithelial deposits are common in classes III and IV and usually have a more finely granular quality. However, according to the ISN/RPS classification, the presence of regular subepithelial deposits that involve over 50 percent of the glomerular capillary

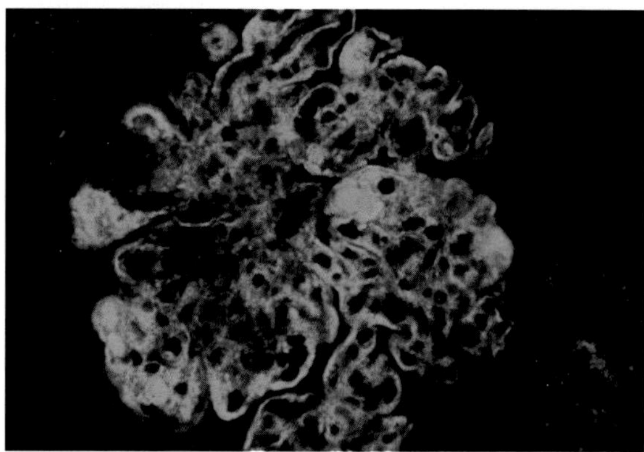

Figure 13-29

LUPUS NEPHRITIS CLASS IV

Immunofluorescence micrograph shows global, large mesangial and subendothelial deposits of IgG. The texture of the subendothelial deposits varies from granular to semilinear. Some of the subendothelial deposits are so massive that they bulge into the glomerular capillary lumens, probably corresponding to hyaline thrombi.

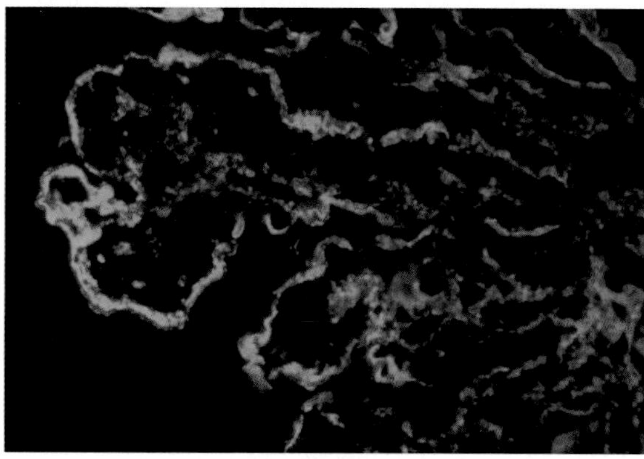

Figure 13-30

LUPUS NEPHRITIS CLASS IV

There are numerous subendothelial and mesangial deposits of IgG as well as a few small subepithelial deposits. In capillaries with both subendothelial and subepithelial deposits, a double layer of immune deposition can be seen. There was similar staining for IgM, IgA, C3, and C1q (immunofluorescence micrograph).

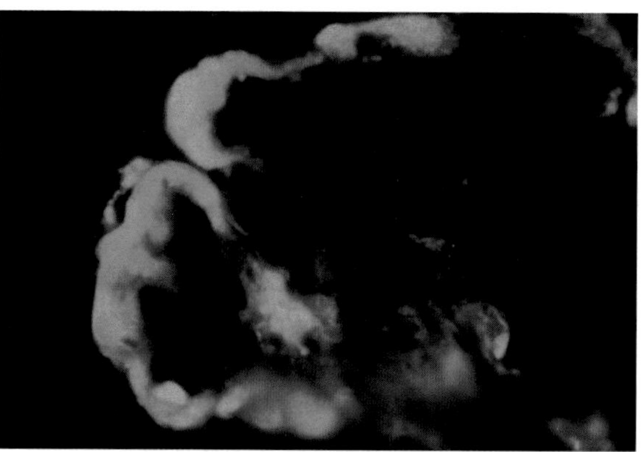

Figure 13-31

LUPUS NEPHRITIS CLASS IV

A wire-loop deposit is seen by immunofluorescence staining for IgG. The deposit is ring-shaped, with a smooth outer contour that conforms to the overlying glomerular basement membrane.

surface area of at least 50 percent of glomeruli exceeds what is acceptable in class III or IV alone and warrants the additional diagnosis of membranous lupus nephritis class V.

Electron Microscopic Findings. Both class III and class IV lupus nephritis usually have mesangial electron-dense deposits. Superimposed on this substratum of mesangial deposits are subendothelial electron-dense deposits that tend to be focal and segmental in class III and more diffuse and global in class IV disease (fig. 13-32). The extent and distribution of the deposits seen by electron microscopy usually parallels that seen by immunofluorescence.

Some cases of class III lupus nephritis have relatively sparse subendothelial deposits relative to the extent and severity of the active necrotizing lesions. Such cases resemble examples of pauci-immune focal segmental necrotizing glomerulonephritis associated with antineutrophil cytoplasmic antibodies (ANCAs) (31).

Differential Diagnosis. Focal proliferative lupus nephritis (class III) must be distinguished from IgA nephropathy, Henoch-Schönlein purpura nephritis, pauci-immune focal segmental necrotizing and crescentic glomerulonephritis, endocarditis-associated glomerulonephritis, and other forms of acute postinfectious glomerulonephritis. Correlation with the pattern of immunofluorescence reactivity, electron microscopic findings, and serologies is required for accurate diagnosis. In general, class III lupus nephritis has baseline mesangial proliferative features in lobules without endocapillary proliferation. This contrasts with pauci-immune focal segmental necrotizing glomerulonephritis, in which uninvolved glomeruli tend to be normocellular.

Diffuse proliferative lupus nephritis (class IV) must be distinguished from severe forms of IgA

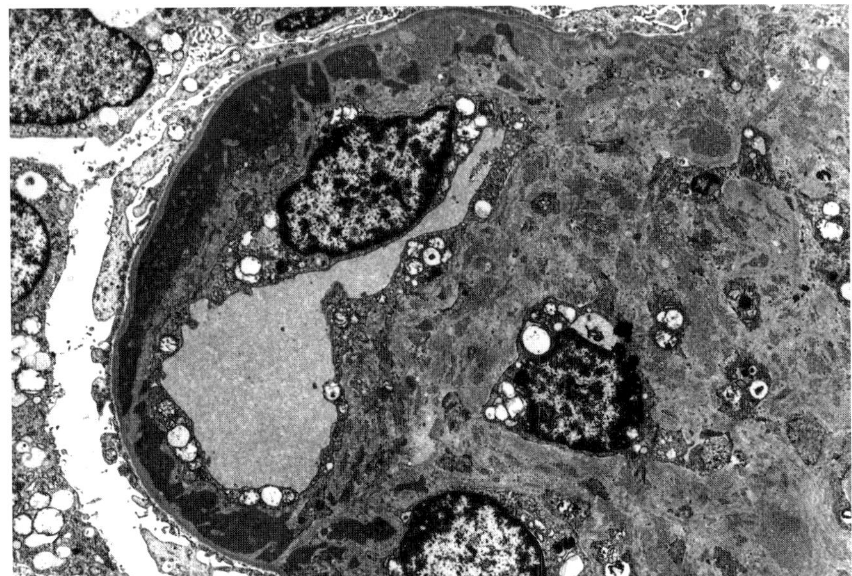

Figure 13-32

LUPUS NEPHRITIS CLASS IV

Electron micrograph shows a large subendothelial electron-dense deposit and smaller mesangial deposits. The subendothelial deposit narrows the capillary lumen and is so large that it would probably be visible by light microscopy as a wire-loop thickening.

nephropathy, membranoproliferative glomerulonephritis, cryoglobulinemic glomerulonephritis, acute postinfectious glomerulonephritis, and pauci-immune crescentic glomerulonephritis. The presence of many endothelial tubuloreticular inclusions and deposits in tubulointerstitial and vascular compartments is a particularly helpful clue to a diagnosis of lupus nephritis.

Class V (Membranous Lupus Nephritis)

Definition. Class V designates membranous lupus nephritis, which is defined by the presence of subepithelial immune deposits or their morphologic sequelae (as seen in the various stages of idiopathic membranous glomerulopathy). According to the INS/RPS classification, a diagnosis of class V is based on the presence of global or segmental continuous granular subepithelial immune deposits. The membranous alterations may be present alone or on a background of mesangial hypercellularity and mesangial immune deposits. Any degree of mesangial hypercellularity may occur in class V. There may be few small subendothelial immune deposits identified by immunofluorescence and/or electron microscopy, but not by light microscopy (47). If visible by light microscopy, subendothelial deposits warrant a combined diagnosis of lupus nephritis classes III and V. Because scattered subepithelial deposits may also be encountered in class III and class IV lupus nephritis, the threshold for an additional diagnosis of membranous lupus nephritis in a proliferative class is membranous involvement of more than 50 percent of the tuft of more than 50 percent of the glomeruli by light microscopy or immunofluorescence.

Clinical Features. In large biopsy series of patients with lupus nephritis, 8 to 22 percent have pure class V (modified WHO class Va or Vb) lupus nephritis. Virtually all patients have proteinuria at presentation, and 60 to 70 percent have the nephrotic syndrome. Hematuria is detectable in about half and hypertension in about one fourth of cases. Renal insufficiency at presentation is uncommon, ranging from 0 to 25 percent of patients. Renal insufficiency and active urine sediment are more common in combined endocapillary proliferative and membranous (modified WHO class Vc or Vd) lupus nephritis than pure membranous forms (modified WHO class Va or Vb).

It has long been recognized that patients with membranous lupus nephritis (class V) differ significantly from those with the proliferative classes III and IV with respect to presenting serologic findings and multisystem disease. Up to one third of patients with class V lupus nephritis present with isolated renal disease before other systemic manifestations of SLE, and approximately one third are ANA negative. Thus the renal biopsy is of particular importance in distinguishing membranous lupus nephritis

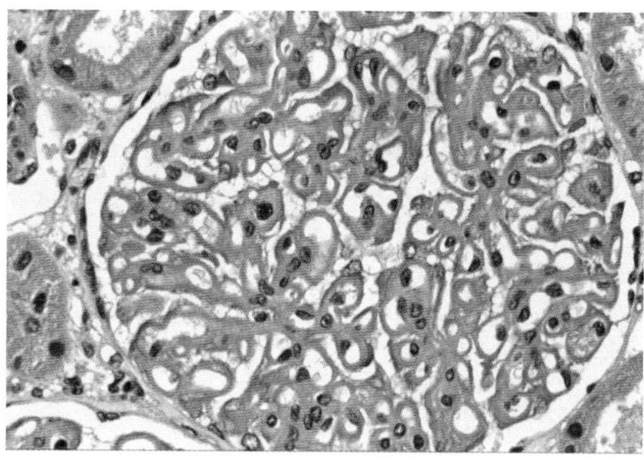

Figure 13-33

LUPUS NEPHRITIS CLASS V (MODIFIED WHO CLASS Va)

The glomerular capillary walls are uniformly thickened, with a rigid aspect. The mesangium is normocellular. By light microscopy, the findings are indistinguishable from those of idiopathic membranous glomerulopathy (H&E stain).

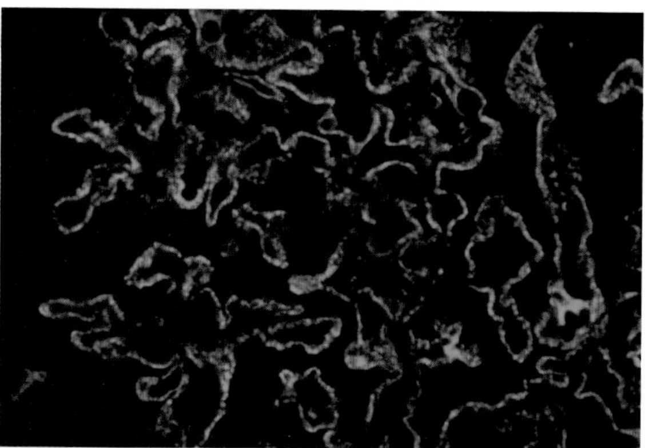

Figure 13-34

LUPUS NEPHRITIS CLASS V (MODIFIED WHO CLASS Va)

Immunofluorescence micrograph shows delicate global subepithelial deposits of IgG, producing a granular pattern, without obvious mesangial deposits.

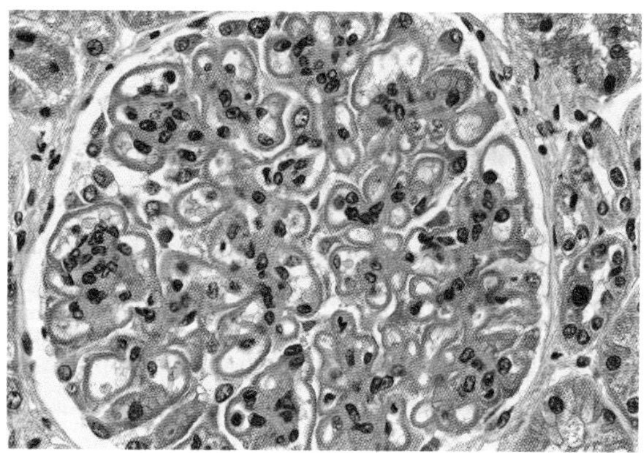

Figure 13-35

LUPUS NEPHRITIS CLASS V (MODIFIED WHO CLASS Vb)

There is moderate global mesangial hypercellularity as well as glomerular capillary wall thickening, with a typical membranous aspect (H&E stain).

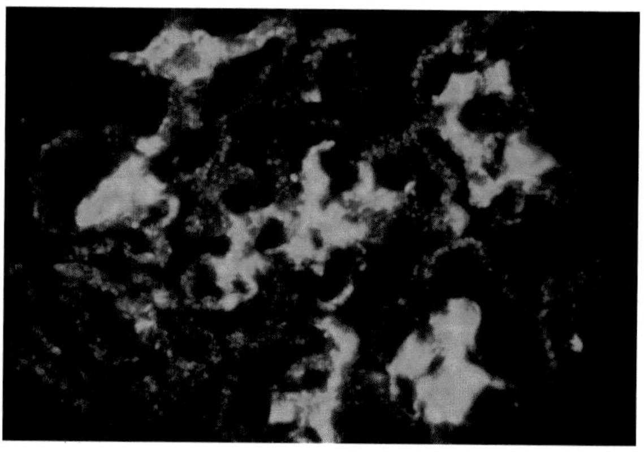

Figure 13-36

LUPUS NEPHRITIS CLASS V (MODIFIED WHO CLASS Vb)

Immunofluorescence micrograph shows heavy deposits of IgG in the mesangium with more delicate global subepithelial deposits. Similar staining was seen for IgA and C3.

from idiopathic membranous glomerulopathy in this population.

Light Microscopic Findings. The modified WHO classification recognizes four subclasses (designated Va through Vd) of membranous class V lupus nephritis (13,40). Class Va consists of cases of pure membranous lupus nephritis without associated mesangial hypercellularity or mesangial immune deposits (figs. 13-33, 13-34). This is a lesion morphologically indistinguishable from idiopathic membranous glomerulopathy. Class Vb denotes a form of class Va plus class II, which may consist of mesangial deposits alone, without mesangial hypercellularity (superadded original WHO class IIa), or mesangial deposits accompanied by mesangial hypercellularity (superadded original WHO class IIb) (figs. 13-35–13-37). The ISN/RPS classification does not subdivide membranous glomerulonephritis into subgroups based on mesangial hypercellularity,

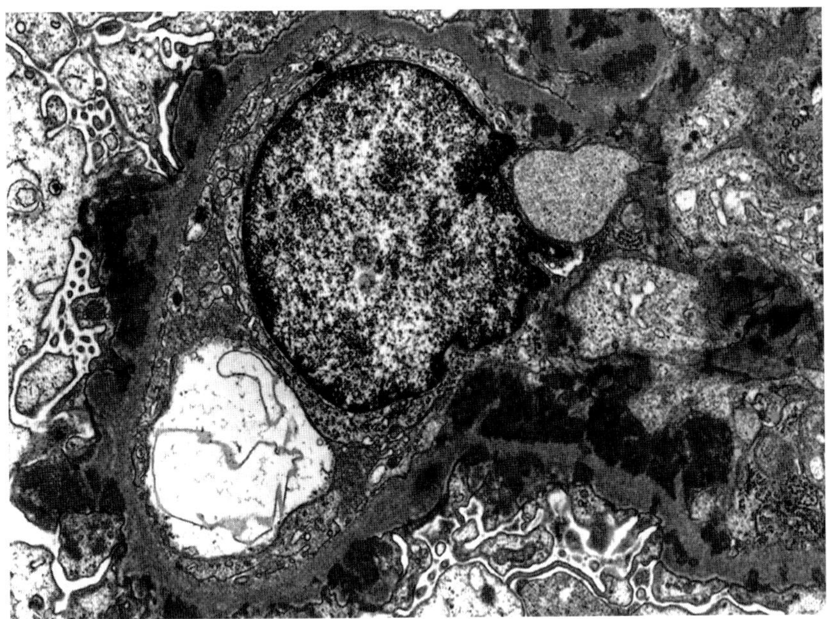

Figure 13-37

LUPUS NEPHRITIS CLASS V (MODIFIED WHO CLASS Vb)

Electron micrograph shows global subepithelial electron-dense deposits as well as mesangial immune deposits. Some of the subepithelial deposits are separated by spike-like projections of glomerular basement membrane. There is extensive foot process effacement.

and any membranous glomerulonephritis is designated simply as class V irrespective of the severity of mesangial hypercellularity or the presence of mesangial immune deposits (47).

In the early stages of class V lupus nephritis, the glomerular capillary walls may appear normal in thickness and texture. However, even at this early stage, the glomerular basement membranes typically display a rigid appearance, with swelling of visceral epithelial cells. If the subepithelial deposits are small, they may not be visible by light microscopy, and are detectable by immunofluorescence and electron microscopy. Well-established membranous features consist of uniform thickening of the glomerular basement membrane, with subepithelial trichrome-red deposits and basement membrane spikes that are best delineated with the JMS stain (fig. 13-38). In later stages, the subepithelial deposits may become incorporated into the glomerular basement membrane by overlying neomembrane formation, producing a vacuolated glomerular basement membrane profile analogous to stage 3 alterations observed in idiopathic membranous glomerulopathy.

The 1982 modified WHO classification also recognized class Vc (combined classes Va and III) and class Vd (combined classes Va and IV) (13). Class Vc denotes focal proliferative glomerulonephritis superimposed on membranous lupus nephritis. Similarly, class Vd denotes diffuse proliferative glomerulonephritis superimposed on membranous lupus nephritis (figs. 13-39, 13-40). A disadvantage of the modified classification was its placement of classes Vc and Vd lesions under the membranous heading. This put undue emphasis on the membranous component by implying that it is the dominant and most clinically relevant lesion, and detracted from the more serious proliferative component. For this reason, classes Vc and Vd were eliminated from the 1995 revised WHO classification (12).

According to the ISN/RPS classification, as in the original WHO classification, the designation, mixed class III and class V, replaces the Vc lesion. Similarly, a designation of mixed class IV and class V replaces the Vd lesion. In the ISN/RPS scheme, the additional designation of class V in the setting of class III or IV requires membranous involvement of at least 50 percent of the glomerular capillary surface area of at least 50 percent of glomeruli, detected by light or immunofluorescence microscopy. This approach is amply supported by clinical-pathologic studies demonstrating that patients with class Vd have an extremely poor prognosis, even worse than those with pure diffuse proliferative class IV disease (40,43).

Patients with lupus nephritis class V are at risk for the development of renal vein thrombosis. Examination of the renal biopsy may provide clues to the occurrence of superimposed renal

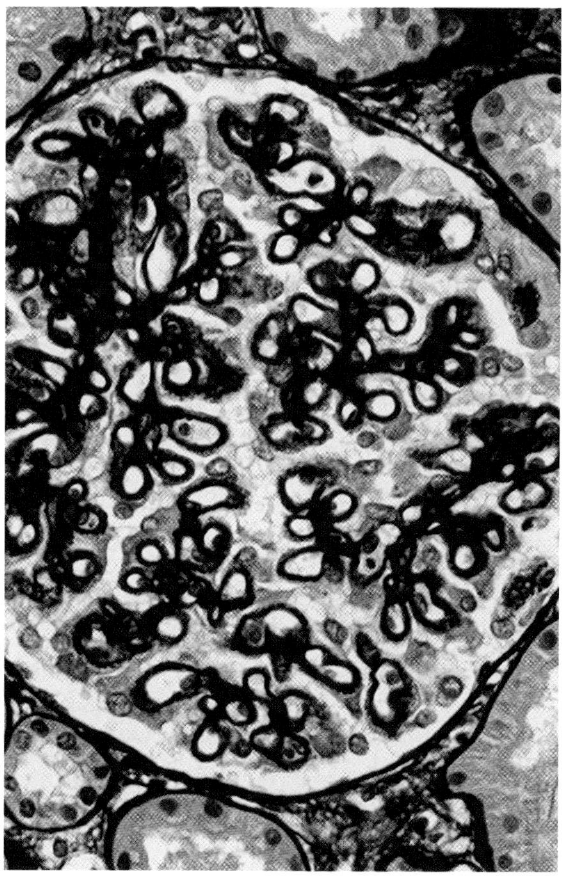

Figure 13-38

LUPUS NEPHRITIS CLASS V (MODIFIED WHO CLASS Vb)

Glomerular basement membrane spikes are best delineated with the JMS stain. Spikes appear as small argyrophilic projections at right angles to the glomerular basement membrane, like the bristles on a comb. There is no endocapillary proliferation. The podocytes appear swollen.

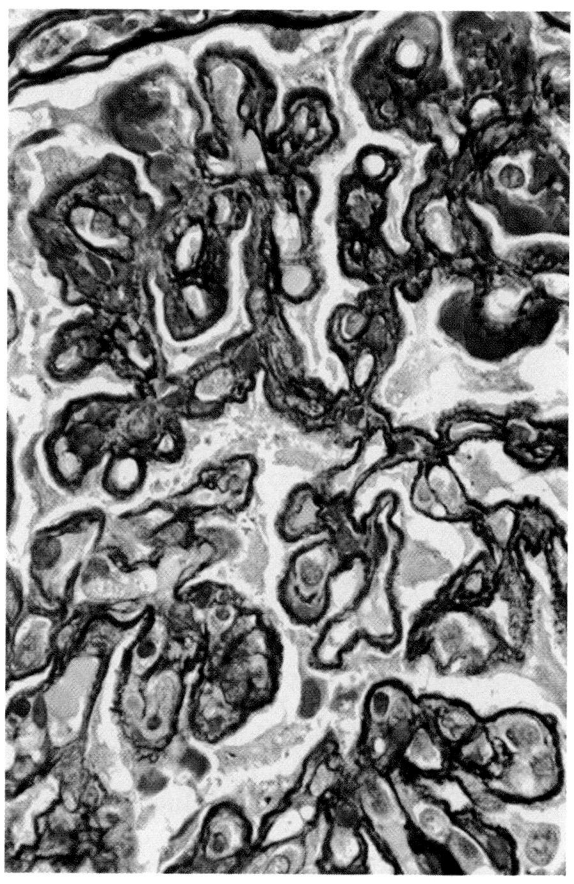

Figure 13-39

LUPUS NEPHRITIS CLASS IV AND V (MODIFIED WHO CLASS Vd)

The glomerular capillary walls demonstrate complex thickening due to combined subendothelial deposits (some of which are incorporated into the capillary wall by neomembrane-producing double contours), as well as subepithelial deposits separated by basement membrane spikes (JMS stain).

vein thrombosis. Suspicious findings include erythrocyte congestion and focal fibrin thrombosis of the glomerular capillaries as well as diffuse interstitial edema (fig. 13-41). In chronic renal vein thrombosis, there may be diffuse tubular atrophy and interstitial fibrosis out of proportion to the degree of glomerular sclerosis.

Immunofluorescence Findings. Granular deposits with a typical membranous (subepithelial) pattern outline the peripheral glomerular capillary walls. In general, subepithelial deposits tend to be more distinctly granular than subendothelial deposits (see fig. 13-34). A background of mesangial immune deposits is commonly observed (fig. 13-36).

Electron Microscopic Findings. Electron-dense subepithelial deposits range from small to large, but involve the majority of capillaries (see fig. 13-37). As the disease progresses, the same ultrastructural stages seen in idiopathic membranous glomerulopathy may evolve. Glomerular basement membrane spikes often separate the subepithelial deposits. In more chronic cases, the deposits become overlaid by neomembrane and later become resorbed and relatively electron lucent. There is extensive foot process effacement in the distribution of the subepithelial deposits. Mesangial electron-dense deposits are commonly observed (fig. 13-37).

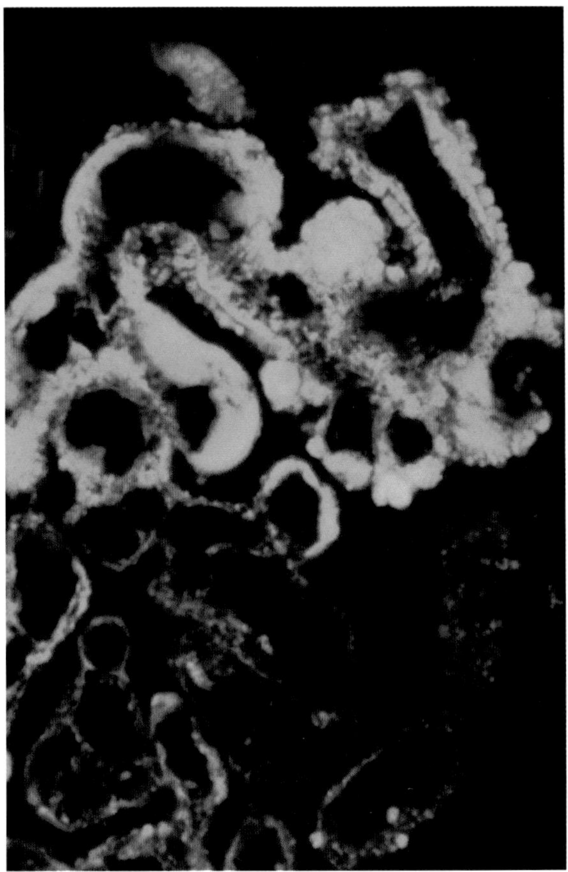

Figure 13-40

LUPUS NEPHRITIS CLASS IV AND V (MODIFIED WHO CLASS Vd)

By immunofluorescence, deposits of IgG are seen in combined subendothelial and subepithelial locations.

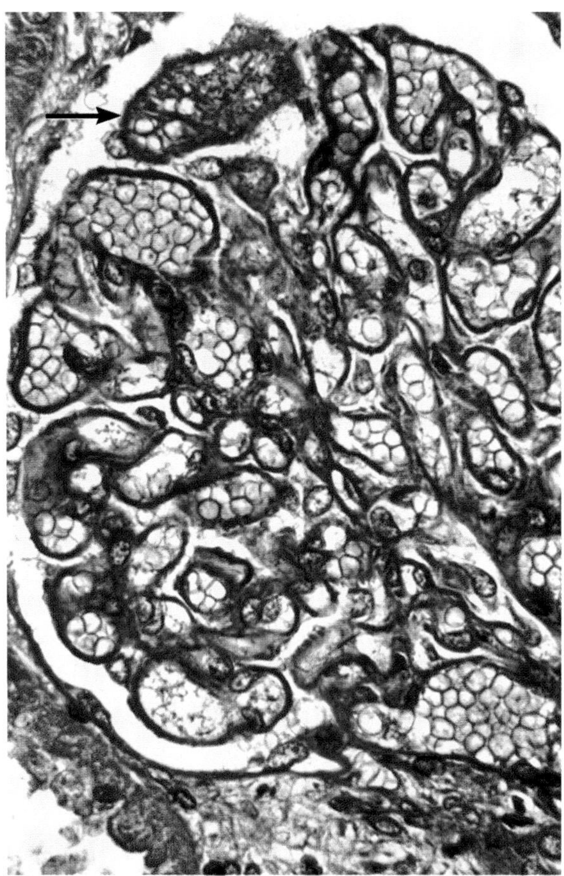

Figure 13-41

LUPUS NEPHRITIS CLASS V WITH SUPERIMPOSED ACUTE RENAL VEIN THROMBOSIS

There is congestion of the glomerular capillaries, indicating a hemodynamic disturbance. Fibrin strands are seen as red thread-like inclusions in one glomerular capillary lumen (arrow) (Masson trichrome stain).

Sparse small subendothelial electron-dense deposits also may be found, but are not accompanied by endocapillary proliferation.

Differential Diagnosis. Membranous lupus nephritis class V must be distinguished from idiopathic membranous glomerulopathy (15,26) and other secondary forms, such as related to hepatitis B or C infection. Because membranous lupus nephritis may present early in the course of SLE, before the appearance of systemic features or positive lupus serologies, differentiation from idiopathic membranous glomerulopathy is particularly important. The presence of mesangial hypercellularity, mesangial immune deposits, "full house" immunoglobulin staining (positive for IgA, IgG, and IgM), strong C1q-staining, sparse subendothelial deposits, tubulointerstitial deposits, arterial deposits, tubuloreticular inclusions, and tissue ANA, individually or in combination, is a helpful clue to a diagnosis of membranous lupus nephritis (26). Of these, tubulointerstitial deposits and subendothelial deposits are the most sensitive features to distinguish membranous lupus nephritis from idiopathic membranous glomerulopathy (26). Secondary membranous glomerulopathy due to hepatitis B or C infection also commonly manifests mesangial hypercellularity, mesangial immune deposits, and hypocomplementemia; however, extraglomerular deposits and endothelial tubuloreticular inclusions are rarely encountered in these forms.

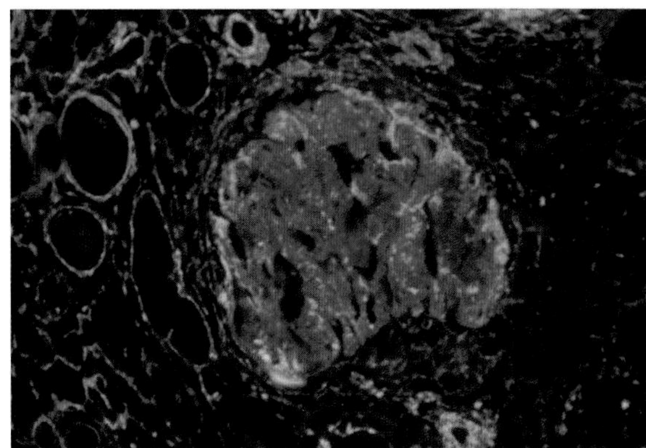

Figure 13-42

LUPUS NEPHRITIS CLASS VI

Sclerotic glomeruli contain residual IgG deposits, seen by immunofluorescence. There are also tubulointerstitial immune deposits.

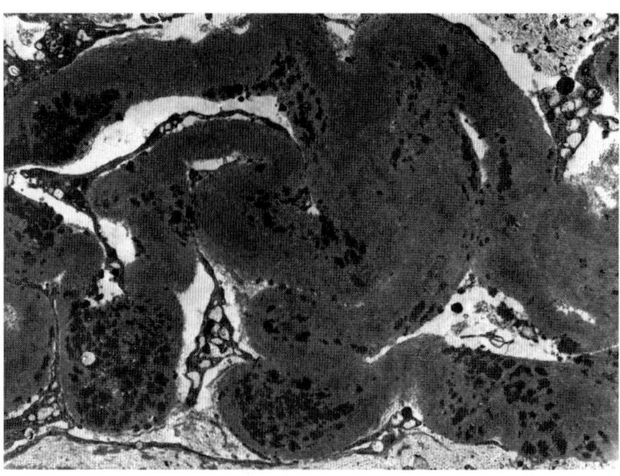

Figure 13-43

LUPUS NEPHRITIS CLASS VI

By electron microscopy, residual electron-dense deposits are still visible in thickened and wrinkled glomerular basement membranes of the obsolescent glomeruli.

Class VI (Advanced Sclerosing Lupus Nephritis)

Definition. The modified WHO classification introduced a sixth class in which the findings are those of extremely chronic advanced glomerulonephritis with widespread glomerular scarring affecting most glomeruli (12,13). The ISN/RPS schema defines class VI more precisely as advanced sclerosing lupus nephritis with global glomerular sclerosis affecting more than 90 percent of glomeruli without residual activity (47).

Most examples of class VI lupus nephritis undoubtedly represent advanced class IV disease. Class V, however, may also progress to end-stage renal disease and manifest this pattern late in the course of disease.

Clinical Features. Patients with class VI lupus nephritis are typically in advanced renal failure, with subnephrotic but variable proteinuria and inactive urinary sediment. Hypertension is common. Lupus serologies are often inactive, leading to a designation of "burnt out" lupus nephritis.

Light Microscopic Findings. There is extensive global glomerular sclerosis involving over 90 percent of glomeruli, without significant ongoing activity. Some glomeruli may be segmentally sclerotic. Glomeruli with less advanced sclerosis may display residual hypercellularity or thickening of the glomerular basement membranes. Vestiges of old crescents may be discernible with the periodic acid–Schiff (PAS) stain as subcapsular fibrous proliferations with disruptions of Bowman's capsule. Severe tubular atrophy, interstitial fibrosis, inflammation, and arteriosclerosis usually accompany the glomerular sclerosis. In some cases, the process is so end-stage that a diagnosis of chronic lupus nephritis is difficult on morphologic grounds.

Immunofluorescence Findings. There are usually some residual immune deposits in the few nonsclerotic glomeruli, as well as in the obsolescent glomeruli (fig. 13-42). Granular deposits may also be detected in the tubulointerstitial compartment or vessel walls.

Electron Microscopic Findings. Despite the advanced glomerular scarring, small electron-dense granular deposits may still be detectable in the sclerosing tuft, as well as in the tubulointerstitial and vascular compartments (fig. 13-43).

Differential Diagnosis. Advanced lupus nephritis can be difficult to distinguish from other chronic glomerular diseases in which there has been progression to severe glomerulosclerosis. This is because the characteristic features of lupus nephritis become less and less obvious as the disease progresses to end-stage. Knowledge that the patient has a history of SLE, review of prior renal biopsies taken during the more active phase of the disease, identification of immune deposits in extraglomerular sites by immunofluorescence and electron microscopy, and positive tissue ANA are all helpful for diagnosing class VI lupus nephritis.

Tubulointerstitial Lesions

Definition. Tubulointerstitial disease may be encountered in all classes of lupus nephritis (35). It is most common in class IV, but also occurs frequently in class III disease. It occurs less commonly in class V and with lowest frequency in class II. The lesions that affect the tubulointerstitial compartment vary from acute to chronic.

Light Microscopic Findings. Acute tubulointerstitial lesions include interstitial inflammation and edema (fig. 13-44). The interstitial infiltrate consists predominantly of mononuclear inflammatory cells, including lymphocytes, monocytes, and plasma cells. Neutrophils and eosinophils are rarely identified. These leukocytic infiltrates vary from sparse to dense and are sometimes associated with lymphocytic infiltration of the tubules (tubulitis). Casts of erythrocytes, neutrophils, and shed tubular epithelial cells are readily identified in active class III or IV lupus nephritis. Intratubular oval fat bodies, consisting of lipid-laden desquamated tubular epithelial cells, may be found in cases of longstanding severe nephrotic syndrome, particularly in the setting of class V disease. Chronic tubulointerstitial disease usually accompanies the chronic sclerosing phase of glomerular disease. These chronic features include tubular atrophy, interstitial fibrosis, and inflammation.

There is no correlation between the severity of the interstitial inflammation and the prevalence of tubulointerstitial immune deposits (35). Indeed, in some biopsies that show severe interstitial inflammation, no tubulointerstitial immune deposits are detected. There is a general correlation, however, between the severity of the tubulointerstitial damage and the degree of renal functional impairment. In most cases of severe tubulointerstitial disease in lupus nephritis, the tubular atrophy, interstitial fibrosis, and inflammation accompany severe glomerular lesions; however, there are rare reports of severe tubulointerstitial disease in the setting of minimal or no glomerular disease.

Immunofluorescence and Electron Microscopic Findings. Tubulointerstitial immune deposits are detected by immunofluorescence and electron microscopy in approximately 50 percent of patients with lupus nephritis (35). They occur most frequently in diffuse proliferative lupus nephritis, but they may also occur in focal proliferative, membranous, and mesangial proliferative forms. Deposits can be found in tubular basement membranes (particularly at the interstitial interface), interstitial capillary basement membranes, and interstitial collagen (fig. 13-45). By immunofluorescence, these deposits have a granular to semilinear aspect that tends to outline the profiles of the tubular basement membranes and interstitial capillary walls (figs. 13-46, 13-47).

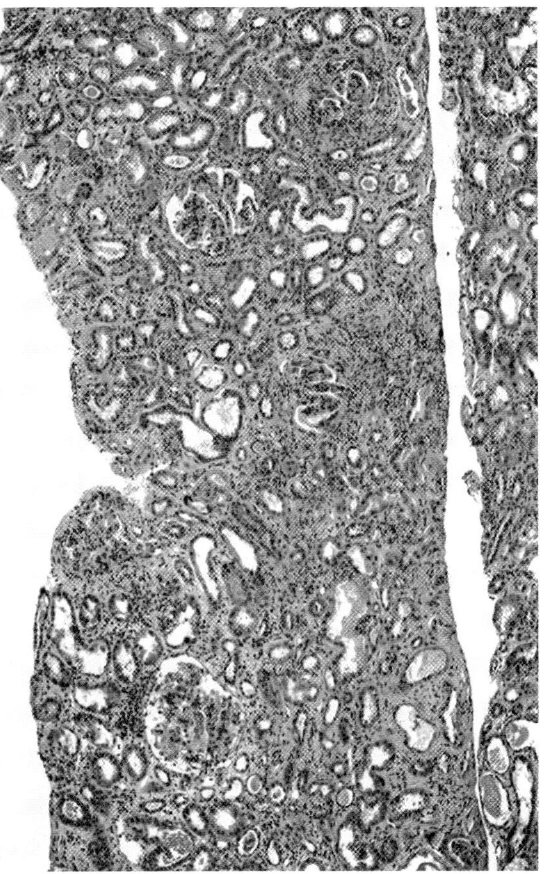

Figure 13-44

LUPUS NEPHRITIS CLASS IV

The cortical interstitium is diffusely expanded by severe interstitial inflammation and edema. The glomeruli display diffuse and global endocapillary proliferation with focal crescents (H&E stain).

Vascular Lesions

Vascular disease is common in lupus nephritis and may assume several morphologically distinct forms (2). Although vascular lesions

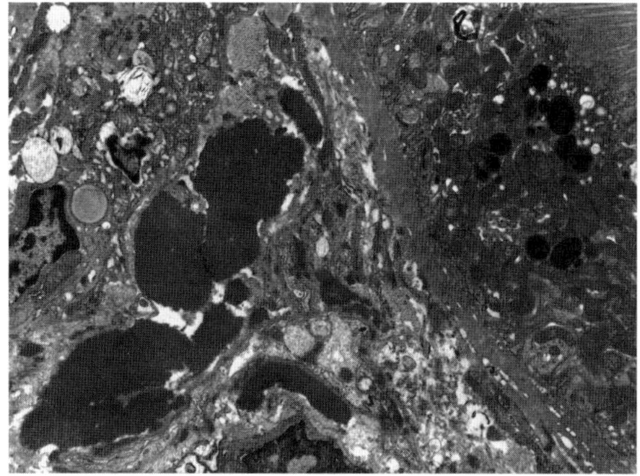

Figure 13-45

LUPUS NEPHRITIS CLASS IV

There are large interstitial electron-dense deposits. A portion of a tubule with tubular basement membrane is seen at the right (electron micrograph).

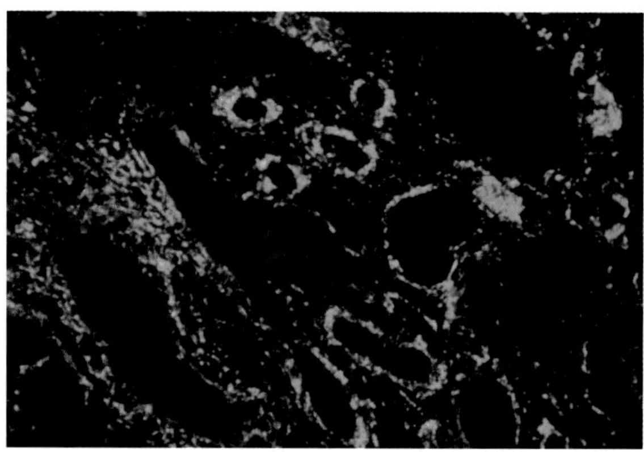

Figure 13-46

LUPUS NEPHRITIS CLASS IV

Abundant deposition of C1q is seen in interstitial connective tissue and tubular basement membranes. There was weaker positivity for IgG and C3 in the same distribution (immunofluorescence micrograph).

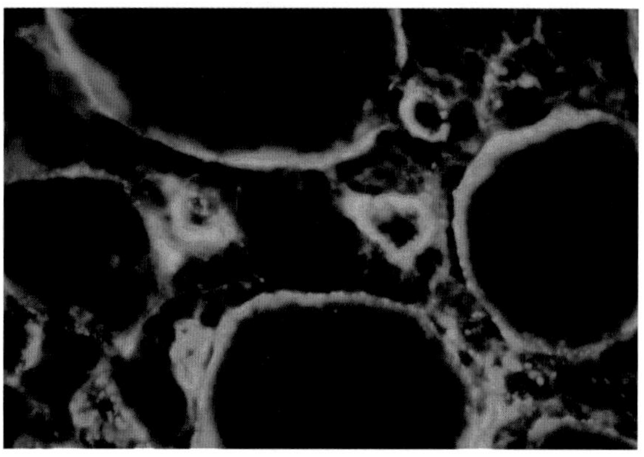

Figure 13-47

LUPUS NEPHRITIS CLASS IV

There is extensive deposition of IgG in the tubular basement membranes and the walls of interstitial capillaries (outlining smaller rounded structures between individual tubules) (immunofluorescence micrograph).

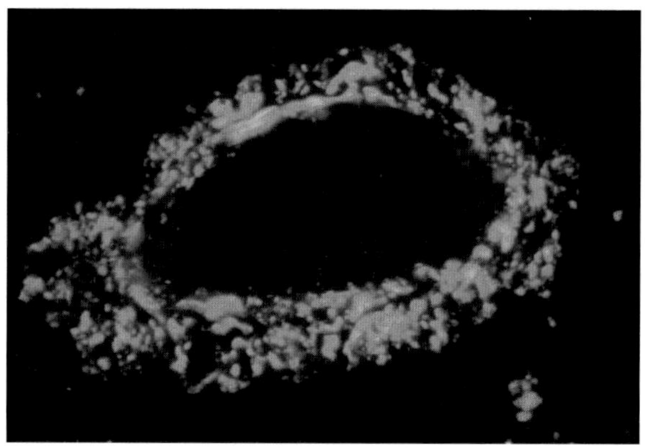

Figure 13-48

LUPUS NEPHRITIS CLASS IV

Abundant granular deposits of IgG are present in the wall of a small artery, involving both the media and intima (immunofluorescence micrograph).

contribute to disease severity and may influence prognosis, they are not factored into the WHO classification or the activity and chronicity indices (9).

Arteriosclerosis and *arteriolosclerosis* are the most common and nonspecific vascular lesions. They may occur in chronic lupus nephritis of all classes, with or without associated hypertension. *Uncomplicated vascular immune deposits* are a common and highly specific feature of lupus nephritis. They are most common in classes III and IV lupus nephritis, but may be found in classes II and V as well. They affect predominantly small arteries and arterioles, and to a lesser extent veins. By immunofluorescence and electron microscopy, granular immune deposits are detectable in the extracellular matrix of the media or the intimal basement membrane (fig. 13-48). The presence of immunoglobulins, as well as complement components C3 and C1q, distinguishes these vascular immune deposits from the nonspecific vascular staining for C3 commonly

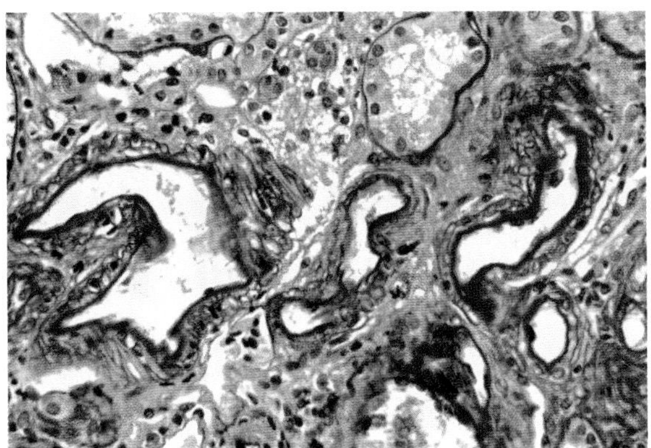

Figure 13-49

LUPUS NEPHRITIS CLASS IV WITH VASCULAR IMMUNE DEPOSITS

Vascular immune deposits cause slight thickening of the arterial subendothelial basement membranes, but without luminal narrowing. There is no inflammation of the vessel wall (periodic acid–Schiff [PAS] stain).

observed in ordinary arteriosclerosis and arteriolosclerosis. Usually, these vascular deposits produce no obvious light microscopic changes. Rarely, thickening of the vascular basement membranes is identified, but without significant compromise of the lumen (fig. 13-49). They have no effect on clinical course or prognosis.

Lupus vasculopathy is a term that refers to a noninflammatory necrotizing vascular lesion that primarily affects arterioles, most frequently in severe class IV lupus nephritis (10). The vascular wall is obscured by smudgy, eosinophilic fibrinoid material that typically expands the intima and may occlude the lumen (fig. 13-50). There is frequent necrosis of medial myocytes and endothelial cells, but without inflammation of the vessel wall. Thus, this is a vasculopathy rather than a true inflammatory vasculitis. By immunofluorescence and using the Lendrum stain for fibrin, both immunoglobulins and fibrin-related antigens are detectable in the intima and media, indicating injury from combined immune deposition and intravascular coagulation (figs. 13-51, 13-52). By electron microscopy, there is endothelial necrosis. The vessel wall and lumen contain granular electron-dense material suggestive of insuded plasma proteins and immune deposits with focal fibrillar fibrin. Patients with this lesion have a poor prognosis, with frequent associated hypertension and a rapid course to renal failure (2,9).

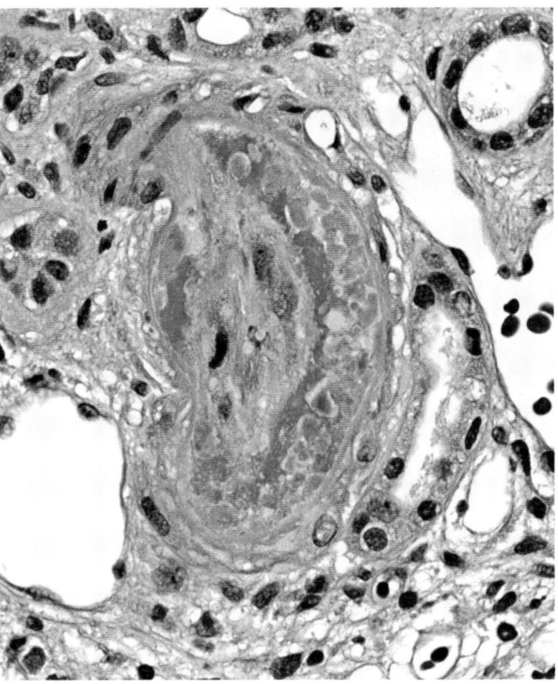

Figure 13-50

LUPUS NEPHRITIS CLASS IV WITH LUPUS VASCULOPATHY

The lumen of this arteriole is occluded by eosinophilic material that consists of fibrin (darkly eosinophilic material internal to the swollen endothelium) and immune deposits (paler and more smudgy, homogeneous eosinophilic material between the fibrin and the media). There is no evidence of inflammatory infiltration of the vessel wall. Thus, this lesion is best termed a "vasculopathy," and not a form of vasculitis (H&E stain).

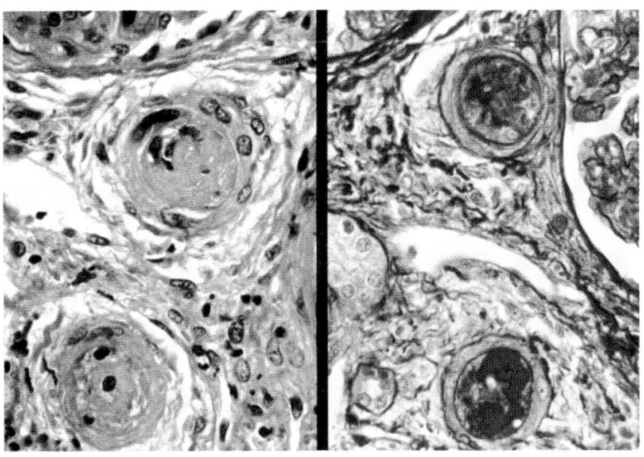

Figure 13-51

LUPUS NEPHRITIS CLASS IV WITH LUPUS VASCULOPATHY

Several preglomerular arterioles are occluded by smudgy eosinophilic material (left) that stains for fibrin (H&E), appearing orange with the Lendrum stain (right).

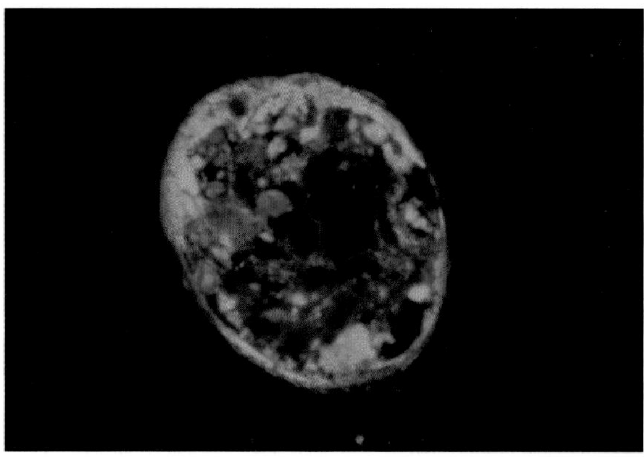

Figure 13-52

LUPUS NEPHRITIS CLASS IV WITH LUPUS VASCULOPATHY

The intimal and intraluminal deposits in this small artery stain for IgG by immunofluorescence. Staining for fibrin/fibrinogen was also seen admixed with the immune deposits.

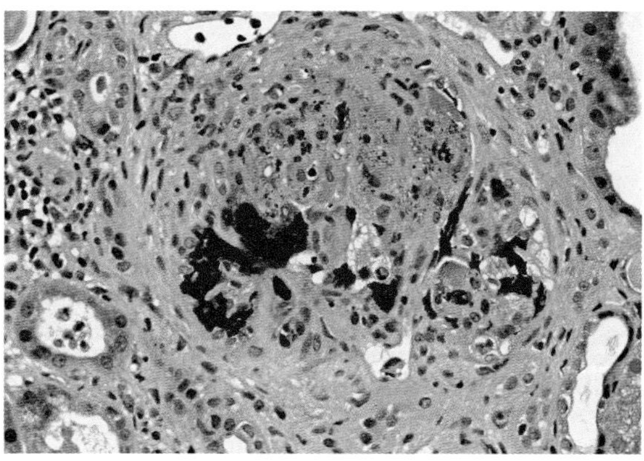

Figure 13-53

THROMBOTIC MICROANGIOPATHY IN LUPUS NEPHRITIS

Renal biopsy from a patient with thrombotic thrombocytopenic purpura-like syndrome shows a glomerulus with fibrin thrombi, endothelial necrosis, and entrapped schistocytes. Some of these patients have an autoantibody to the von Willebrand factor cleaving protease (H&E stain).

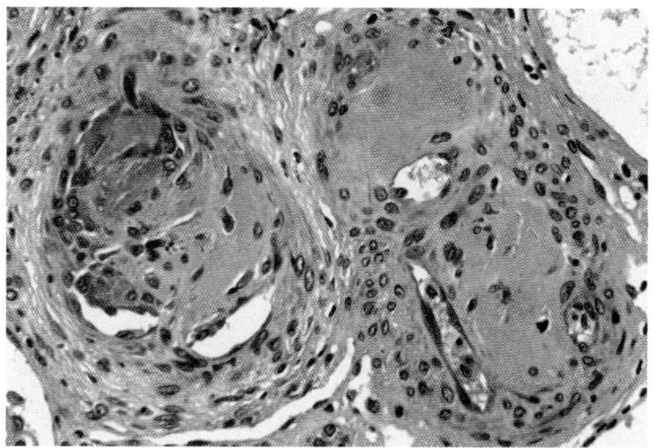

Figure 13-54

LUPUS ANTICOAGULANT SYNDROME

Several interlobular arteries contain organizing thrombi with recanalization. This patient with SLE had prolongation of the activated partial thromboplastin time (APTT) and an anticardiolipin antibody was demonstrated by enzyme-linked immunosorbent assay (ELISA). Although the presence of anticardiolipin antibody prolongs coagulation tests in vitro (hence the name lupus "anticoagulant"), it has procoagulant effects in vivo, leading to glomerular and renal vascular thrombosis (H&E stain).

Thrombotic microangiopathy may affect small arteries, arterioles, and glomerular capillaries. It occurs in several distinct clinical settings including lupus anticoagulant (antiphospholipid antibody) syndrome, hemolytic uremic syndrome, thrombotic thrombocytopenic purpura (associated with autoantibody to the von Willebrand factor cleaving protease), and systemic sclerosis (mixed connective tissue disease) (2, 17–19). Thrombotic microangiopathy may supervene on any class of lupus nephritis. It should be suspected whenever there is intravascular coagulation that cannot be explained by the activity of the glomerular disease. Light microscopic features include fibrin thrombosis of glomerular capillaries and small arteries or arterioles, mesangiolysis, mucoid intimal edema, and entrapment of fragmented erythrocytes in the thrombi (fig. 13-53). Vascular thrombi may become organized and recanalized (fig. 13-54). There is secondary ischemic glomerulosclerosis and tubulointerstitial scarring. Unlike lupus vasculopathy, these thrombotic lesions predominantly contain fibrin-related antigens, detected by immunofluorescence, without associated immune deposits.

True necrotizing vasculitis is rarely identified in patients with lupus nephritis (2,9). It may be renal limited or associated with systemic vasculitis. It resembles microscopic polyangiitis with fibrinoid necrosis and inflammatory infiltration of the vessel wall (fig. 13-55). No vascular immune deposits are detectable by immunofluorescence or electron microscopy. This lesion may occur in any class of lupus nephritis, regardless of the activity of the glomerular disease. It carries an extremely poor prognosis and

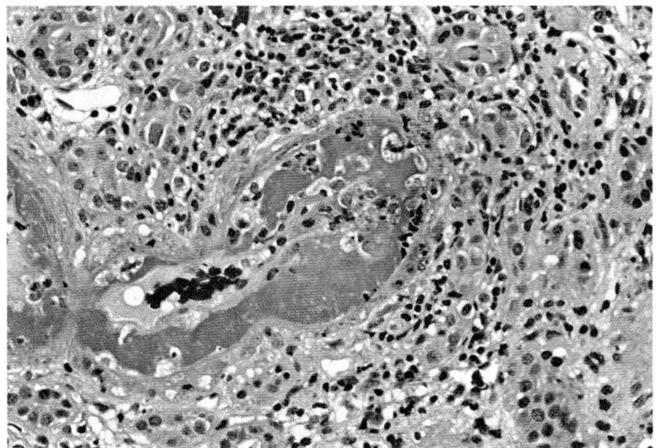

Figure 13-55

LUPUS NEPHRITIS WITH NECROTIZING ARTERITIS

There are transmural inflammation and fibrinoid necrosis in an interlobular artery. These changes represent a true inflammatory vasculitis and are indistinguishable from the vasculitis seen in antineutrophil cytoplasmic antibody (ANCA)-associated microscopic polyangiitis (H&E stain).

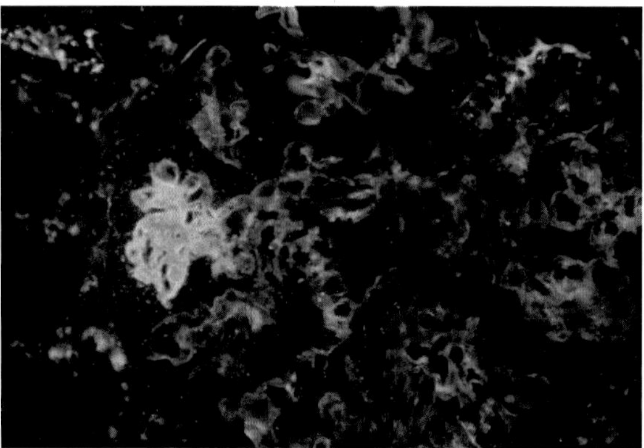

Figure 13-56

LUPUS NEPHRITIS CLASS IV

Strong smudgy immunofluorescence positivity for fibrinogen is seen in the distribution of a segmental necrotizing lesion to the left. The adjacent glomerular lobules have a weaker and more generalized positivity for fibrin, corresponding to areas of non-necrotizing endocapillary proliferation.

must be treated aggressively with an immunosuppressive regimen like that used for ANCA-associated microscopic polyangiitis.

General Immunofluorescence Features in Lupus Nephritis

Lupus nephritis is one of the few diseases in which immune deposits can be detected in any or all of the renal compartments, including glomeruli, tubules, interstitium, and blood vessels. IgG is found almost universally (16). Codeposits of IgM and IgA are present in most specimens. When all three immunoglobulin isotypes are found, the designation "full house" staining is often used. The corresponding presence of both light chains indicates the polyclonal nature of the immunoglobulin deposits. IgG is usually dominant in intensity. Although IgA may be co-dominant with IgG, it is rarely, if ever, more intense than IgG (25). C3 is present in over 90 percent of specimens and C1q in over 80 percent. Intense staining for C1q may be observed. Although not routinely studied, C4, properdin, and membrane attack complex (C5b-9) have also been reported in the glomerular immune deposits. The presence of early complement components C1q and C4, as well as properdin, attests to the activation of complement by both the classic and alternative pathways. Fibrin/fibrinogen is commonly detected in the distribution of the necrotizing lesions and crescents (figs. 13-56, 13-57). More delicate and weaker reactivity for fibrinogen may be detected more diffusely in the distribution of non-necrotizing endocapillary proliferative lesions.

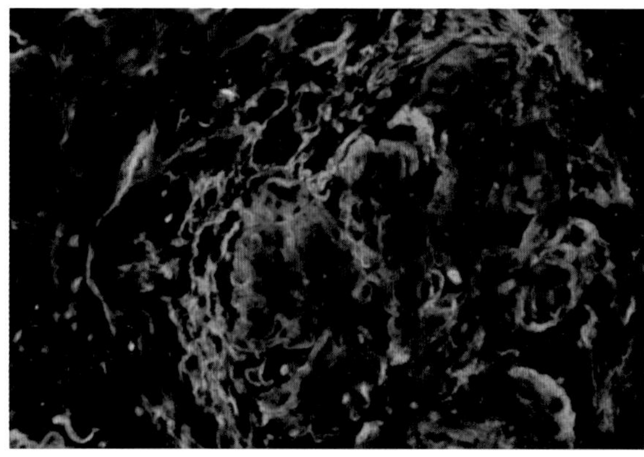

Figure 13-57

LUPUS NEPHRITIS CLASS IV

Staining for fibrin is present in the distribution of crescents, outlining the urinary space. There is also weaker positivity for fibrin in the underlying tuft, corresponding to areas of endocapillary proliferation (immunofluorescence micrograph).

Tissue ANA refers to the commonly observed phenomenon of nuclear staining of renal tubular or glomerular cells with fluoresceinated

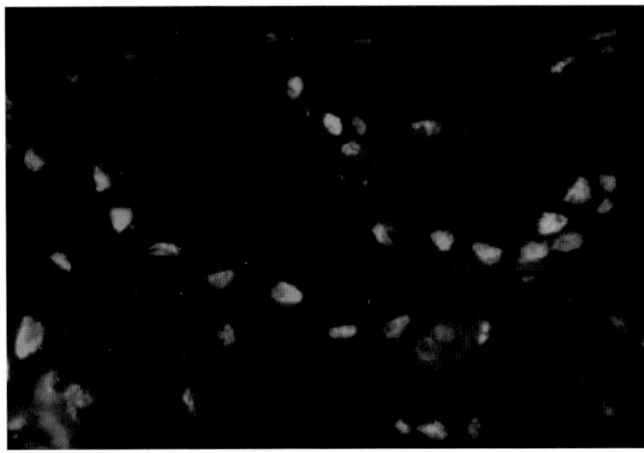

Figure 13-58

LUPUS NEPHRITIS WITH TISSUE ANTINUCLEAR ANTIBODY (ANA)

Tubular nuclei stain for IgG by direct immunofluorescence. This phenomenon, known as "tissue ANA," occurs when cryostat sections expose nuclei in the renal tissue to ambient ANA in the patient's own serum. The ANA, which is usually of IgG class, binds to the exposed nuclei and is revealed when the sections are stained with fluoresceinated-rabbit antihuman IgG.

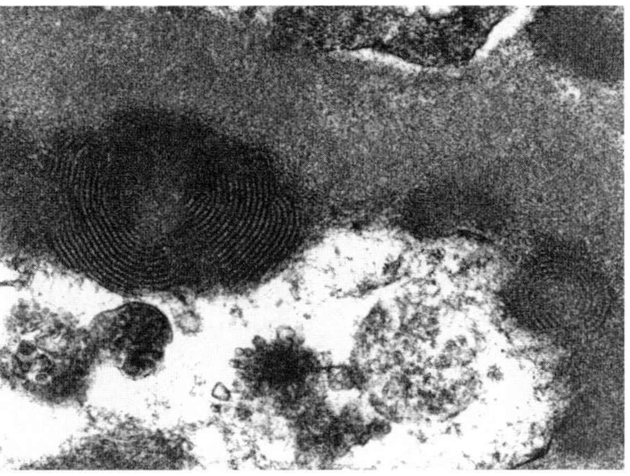

Figure 13-59

LUPUS NEPHRITIS CLASS IV

The subendothelial region contains deposits with a fingerprint substructure, forming curvilinear parallel bands approximately 10 to 15 nm in diameter. Delicate cross-hatching is visible between the parallel bands. Fingerprint substructure is common in the deposits of lupus nephritis and probably corresponds to the presence of type 3 (mixed) cryoglobulins. Usually, the substructure is identified in only a minority of glomerular electron-dense deposits, the remainder of which have the usual granular texture (electron micrograph).

antisera to IgG in routine immunofluorescence preparations (fig. 13-58). This is interpreted as an in vitro artifact of cryostat sectioning, allowing ambient ANA in the patient's serum to bind to nuclei exposed in the course of tissue sectioning. The patient's own IgG with ANA activity is then revealed with secondary fluoresceinated rabbit antihuman IgG.

General Electron Microscopy Features in Lupus Nephritis

The distribution of immune deposits seen by electron microscopy corresponds to that observed by immunofluorescence (37). Mesangial electron-dense deposits are typically observed in all classes of lupus nephritis (with the exception of the original WHO class I). Thus, they may be considered the common substratum upon which the other classes are built. Class III and class IV lupus nephritis display subendothelial as well as mesangial deposits. The distribution of the subendothelial deposits is more focal and segmental in class III and more diffuse and global in class IV, corresponding to the general distribution of the endocapillary proliferative lesions. While scattered subepithelial deposits may also be detected in class III and class IV, regular subepithelial deposits are a distinguishing feature of class V.

In most cases, the texture of the glomerular electron-dense deposits is granular. However, in a small percentage of cases, the deposits are organized into curvilinear microtubular or fibrillar structures composed of bands ranging from 10 to 15 nm in diameter (fig. 13-59). The substructure is known as "fingerprinting." Usually only a portion of an otherwise granular deposit exhibits an organized substructure. Fingerprint substructure is more common in lupus patients with circulating type 3 cryoglobulins.

A common ultrastructural finding in lupus nephritis is the presence of *endothelial tubuloreticular inclusions* (TRIs). These 24-nm interanastomosing tubular structures are commonly encountered in the dilated cisternae of the endoplasmic reticulum of renal endothelial cells (fig. 13-60). They are readily identified in all classes of lupus nephritis, regardless of disease activity. However, these structures are not specific for lupus nephritis. TRIs are also common in renal biopsies from patients infected with the human immunodeficiency virus (HIV)-1. They are also observed in other renal conditions lacking

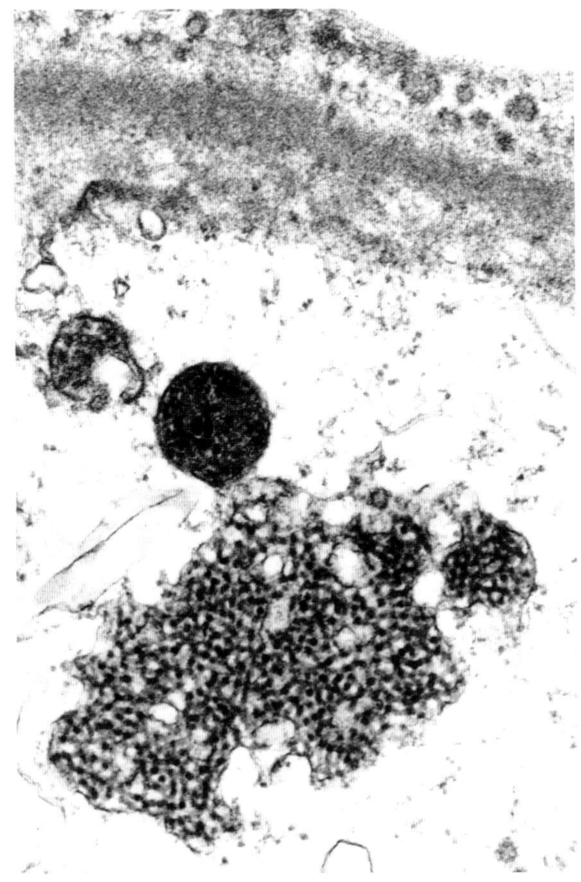

Figure 13-60

LUPUS NEPHRITIS CLASS IV

A large tubuloreticular inclusion is present in this glomerular capillary endothelial cell. These structures are known as "interferon footprints" because they can be induced in normal endothelial cells or leukocytes on exposure to interferon. They consist of 24-nm interanastomosing tubular structures located within dilated cisternae of endoplasmic reticulum (electron micrograph).

known viral associations. Because they appear to be induced by exposure to interferon, TRIs have been termed "interferon footprints."

Activity and Chronicity Indices

The attempt to quantify the degree of activity and chronicity of the lesions of lupus nephritis is based on the intuitive assumption that active lesions are more amenable to therapy and chronic lesions represent largely irreversible damage. Thus, assessment of disease activity and chronicity is a helpful guide to prognosis and treatment. Activity indices were first formulated by Pirani and Morel-Maroger (33). They were later refined and popularized by Austin and Balow (6,7) as the NIH (National Institutes of Health) activity and chronicity indices (Table 13-4). Hill et al. (21) have proposed a more comprehensive index that incorporates immunofluorescence findings and quantitation of glomerular and tubular macrophage infiltration. The persistence of active lesions in biopsies repeated after a course of aggressive immunosuppressive therapy indicates resistant disease with a greater likelihood of progression to renal failure (22).

Table 13-4

ACTIVITY AND CHRONICITY INDICES[a]

Index of Activity (0-24)	
Endocapillary hypercellularity	(0-3+)
Leukocyte infiltration	(0-3+)
Subendothelial hyaline deposits	(0-3+)
Fibrinoid necrosis/karyorrhexis	(0-3+) x 2
Cellular crescents	(0-3+) x 2
Interstitial inflammation	(0-3+)
Index of Chronicity (0-12)	
Glomerular sclerosis	(0-3+)
Fibrous crescents	(0-3+)
Tubular atrophy	(0-3+)
Interstitial fibrosis	(0-3+)

[a]Adapted from references 6 and 7.

According to the NIH schema, the activity index is calculated by summing the score for each of six histologic features, which are graded individually on a scale of 0 to 3+. These include glomerular endocapillary proliferation, glomerular leukocyte infiltration, glomerular subendothelial hyaline deposits, glomerular fibrinoid necrosis or karyorrhexis, cellular crescents, and interstitial inflammation. A score of 0 = absent, 1+ = less than 25 percent of glomeruli affected, 2+ = 25 to 50 percent of glomeruli affected, 3+ = greater than 50 percent of glomeruli affected. The scores for glomerular necrosis and cellular crescents are accorded double weight due to their more ominous importance. Interstitial inflammation is graded as 1+, mild; 2+, moderate; 3+, severe. The sum of these values gives a total possible activity score of 0 to 24. Similarly, chronicity is graded on a scale of 0 to 12 by summing each of four features of chronicity: glomerular sclerosis, fibrous crescents, tubular atrophy, and interstitial fibrosis.

The NIH group initially found that an activity index of greater than 12 and a chronicity of greater than 4 were predictors of poor outcome (6,7). Subsequent studies have failed to confirm these data. Schwartz and co-workers (41,42) have noted problems in interobserver and intraobserver reproducibility. While there does not appear to be a precise cut-off for activity and chronicity that predicts outcome, there is general agreement that higher chronicity portends a worse prognosis. Morever, these indices are of particular value when biopsies are repeated in individual patients to monitor disease evolution and response to treatment. Despite these limitations, it is standard practice for renal biopsy reports of patients with lupus nephritis to include an activity and chronicity index. The ISN/RPS classification specifies that the proportion of glomeruli with active and sclerosing lesions, and particularly with fibrinoid necrosis or cellular crescents, should be indicated in each biopsy report. It also encourages, but does not mandate, the use of the NIH (or other) system for systematic quantitation of activity and chronicity.

Pathogenesis

SLE is a chronic immune complex disease of unknown etiology. The development of autoimmunity involves loss of self tolerance due to inadequate control or elimination of self-reactive lymphocyte clones (20). A role of dysregulated apoptosis and ineffective removal of nuclear debris has also been proposed (45). There is likely to be a complex genetic basis that is modulated by hormonal and environmental influences. The importance of genetic factors is exemplified by the familial association of the disease, the high concordance of disease in monozygotic twins, human leukocyte antigen (HLA) associations (such as DR2, DR3, and B8), inherited complement deficiencies (such as C2 and C4), and the existence of numerous genetic murine models. The importance of hormonal factors is illustrated by the strong female preponderance in humans, and by the ability to attenuate the disease in murine models by hormonal manipulation.

The pathogenesis of lupus nephritis is incompletely understood. In recent years, emphasis has shifted away from the concept of deposition of preformed immune complexes to embrace the role of local immune deposition at the level of the glomerulus. Factors that may influence immune complex formation include the class and subclass of immunoglobulin, the electric charge of the immunoglobulin, autoantibody specificity and cross reactivity with glomerular constituents, and binding of autoantigens to glomerular constituents through charge interactions (20). For example, in murine models, there is evidence that nucleosomes consisting of DNA bound to histone have affinity for glomerular basement membrane components such as collagen, fibronectin, and laminin. Histones in particular are highly cationic and may interact with negative charge sites in the glomerular basement membrane. Once planted in the glomerular basement membrane, these autoantigens are then free to interact with circulating autoantibodies. There is also new evidence that anti-DNA antibodies exhibit a broad range of cross-reactivities to normal glomerular constituents, such as heparan sulfate proteoglycans, laminin, and type IV collagen, leading to in situ immune complex formation (20).

The glomerular deposition of immune complexes leads to local complement activation, release of chemotactins, influx of leukocytes, and release of inflammatory and fibrogenic cytokines that promote proliferation of indigenous glomerular cells and progressive glomerular sclerosis.

Therapy and Prognosis

The features of the renal biopsy remain the most valuable objective criteria on which to base therapeutic decisions in patients with lupus nephritis (4). Patients with mesangial lesions (ISN/RPS class I or II) require no treatment for their renal disease, and therapy should be directed to their extrarenal disease manifestations. For those with class III lupus nephritis, very mild and focal disease lacking substantial subendothelial deposits or necrotizing features can usually be managed with steroids alone. Class III patients with very active or severe glomerulonephritis are usually treated with vigorous therapy comparable to that recommended for active diffuse proliferative lupus nephritis class IV. Most investigators agree that low-dose steroids are inadequate to treat active diffuse proliferative disease. Most regimens use steroids in combination with cyclophosphamide. A particularly popular regimen is intravenous cyclophosphamide administered monthly with oral steroids, followed by follow-up doses every third month. Treatment of membranous lupus nephritis (class V) is controversial. Patients at high risk for progression, such as those with severe nephrotic syndrome or renal insufficiency, are usually offered a 4- to 6-month trial of aggressive immunosuppressive therapy to achieve remission of the nephrotic syndrome. It is advisable to discontinue therapy after 6 months if there is no response due to the increasing risk of morbidity from prolonged immunosuppressive therapy.

The prognosis of patients with lupus nephritis varies with the class, activity, and chronicity of the disease as well as the development of transformations from one class to another (5,29,38,39). Overall 5-year renal survival rates for those with class II lupus nephritis is over 90 percent, but drops to 85 to 90 percent for those with class III, 60 to 90 percent for class IV, and 70 to 90 percent for class V. Factors that predict poor survival for patients with class IV disease include black race, higher serum creatinine levels, and lower hematocrit (5). A combination of cellular crescents and interstitial fibrosis was found by the NIH group to portend a worse prognosis (5). In the membranous group (class V), long-term outcome is worse in the subgroup with persistent nephrotic syndrome (36). Outcome is also worse in those patients with class V membranous lupus nephritis who transform to a mixed proliferative and membranous form.

Lupus nephritis is not a static entity but has the capacity to transform over time, either spontaneously or following treatment. Transformations occur in 15 to 40 percent of patients undergoing repeat biopsy (16). Virtually all possible directions of transformation have been reported, including mesangial to diffuse, focal to diffuse, focal to membranous, diffuse to membranous, diffuse to mesangial, membranous to diffuse, and membranous to combined membranous and proliferative. Not surprisingly, one of the most common transformations is focal to diffuse proliferative, which many consider movement along a disease continuum. Transformation from class IV to class V following therapy is also common. The transformation from class IV to class II following treatment is considered a sign of effective therapy.

MIXED CONNECTIVE TISSUE DISEASE

Definition. Mixed connective tissue disease was first defined by Sharp and colleagues in 1972 (54) as an overlap syndrome with mixed features of SLE, systemic sclerosis (scleroderma), and polymyositis.

Clinical Features. The serologic features include a high titer of ANA and antibody to extractable nuclear antigen (ENA) that is ribonuclease sensitive. In recent years, the concept of mixed connective tissue disease has been supplanted by the concept of *undifferentiated autoimmune rheumatic and connective tissue disorder* (50). Many of these patients eventually convert to a clinical picture of SLE, systemic sclerosis, or rheumatoid arthritis (56). The clinical features include arthritis, Raynaud's phenomenon, sclerodactyly, alopecia, rash, restrictive lung disease, and lymphadenopathy. Central nervous system and renal manifestations are uncommon.

Light Microscopic Findings. Renal involvement may take the form of immune complex–mediated disease resembling lupus nephritis, thrombotic microangiopathy resembling renal systemic sclerosis, or a combination of both (48, 49,51–53,55). Membranous glomerulonephritis is one of the most common lesions, accounting for 35 to 40 percent of renal biopsy diagnoses. Other diagnoses include mesangial proliferative glomerulonephritis (7 to 35 percent), focal or diffuse proliferative glomerulonephritis (7 to 10 percent), and scleroderma vascular disease (22 percent). The immune complex–mediated glomerular diseases resemble the lesions described for classes II, III, IV, and V lupus nephritis. The renal vascular lesions of scleroderma renal disease range from fibrinoid necrosis of arterioles and mucoid edema of interlobular arteries to more chronic onion-skin type intimal fibroplasia of small and medium-sized arteries (fig. 13-61).

Immunofluorescence Findings. The same patterns of immune staining described for the various classes of lupus nephritis are encountered. Patients with exclusively scleroderma renal disease often have tissue ANA but typically lack parenchymal immune deposits. Their renal biopsies may display vascular staining for

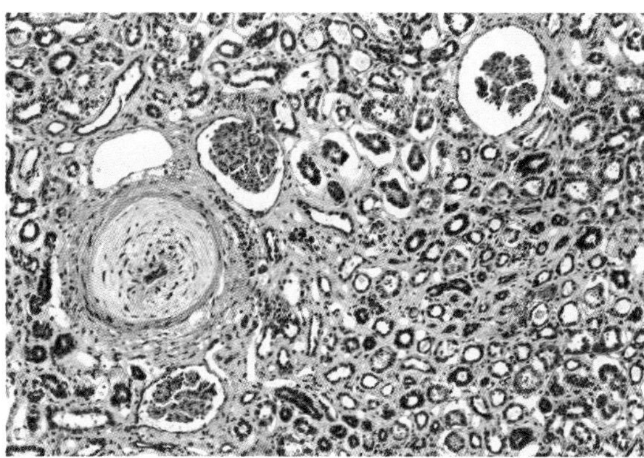

Figure 13-61

MIXED CONNECTIVE TISSUE DISEASE WITH FEATURES OF SCLERODERMA

A patient with mixed connective tissue disease and predominant manifestations of scleroderma developed acute renal failure and severe hypertension. Renal biopsy shows features of subacute thrombotic microangiopathy with marked narrowing of interlobular arteries by concentric mucoid intimal edema. The adjacent glomeruli display ischemic retraction of the tuft with wrinkling of glomerular basement membranes. There is diffuse interstitial fibrosis and tubular atrophy. Immunofluorescence revealed fibrin in the vessel walls, but no evidence of any immune deposits typical of lupus nephritis (H&E stain).

fibrin/fibrinogen, IgM, and C3, identical to that observed in other forms of thrombotic microangiopathy.

Electron Microscopic Findings. The ultrastructural findings are indistinguishable from those observed in the various classes of lupus nephritis or scleroderma renal disease.

Differential Diagnosis. The differential diagnosis includes all the entities listed for the different classes of lupus nephritis above. In patients with purely scleroderma renal disease, the differential diagnosis includes other causes of thrombotic microangiopathy, such as lupus anticoagulant syndrome, malignant hypertension, hemolytic uremic syndrome, and thrombotic thrombocytopenic purpura.

Treatment and Prognosis. For patients with lupus nephritis, immunosuppressive therapy is directed to the class of nephritis identified by renal biopsy, and prognosis will vary accordingly. In the situation of scleroderma renal disease, the mainstay of therapy is angiotensin converting enzyme inhibitors or angiotensin receptor blockade.

SJÖGREN'S SYNDROME

Definition. In 1933, the Swedish ophthalmologist Henrik Sjögren (68) first described a sicca complex of xerostomia and xerophthalmia caused by chronic inflammation of the exocrine salivary and lacrimal glands. The syndrome may occur as a primary process or a secondary condition associated with a spectrum of autoimmune diseases (67).

Clinical Features. Approximately 40 percent of cases of Sjögren's syndrome are primary (without other disease associations). It has been estimated that up to 50 percent of patients with Sjögren's syndrome have rheumatoid arthritis, about 5 percent have systemic sclerosis, and another 5 percent have SLE. Association with Epstein-Barr viral infection has been described in some of the apparently primary forms (60). Serologic manifestations include hypergammaglobulinemia, rheumatoid factor, mixed cryoglobulinemia, ANA, anti-Ro/SSA, and anti-La/SSB. Hypocomplementemia is rare unless the syndrome occurs in association with SLE.

The clinical renal manifestations are diverse and vary with the type of renal pathologic lesion, including tubulointerstitial, glomerular, and vascular. Those with tubulointerstitial nephritis may present with distal renal tubular acidosis, impaired renal concentrating ability, hypercalciuria, osteomalacia, Fanconi's syndrome, and renal insufficiency. Those with glomerulonephritis present with a spectrum of active urine sediment, proteinuria, and renal insufficiency similar to that seen with lupus nephritis. Patients with vascular lesions usually present with renal insufficiency and hypertension.

Light Microscopic Findings. The most common pathologic lesion is tubulointerstitial nephritis (57,64–66,69), which usually has the appearance of a chronic, but active, process with patchy dense cellular infiltrates of lymphocytes, monocytes, and fewer plasma cells (fig. 13-62). Eosinophils and neutrophils are not generally identified. Granulomas are not seen. Varying degrees of tubulitis, tubular atrophy, and interstitial fibrosis are usually present. Nephrocalcinosis may lead to intratubular and interstitial calcifications. Glomeruli are relatively spared, except for the development of pericapsular fibrosis.

A small percentage of patients with Sjögren's syndrome develop immune complex–mediated glomerulonephritis (59,61,63). All the glomerular patterns that have been described in SLE, including mesangial proliferative, focal proliferative, diffuse proliferative, and membranous, have been reported. Some membranoproliferative forms have been linked to the presence of associated cryoglobulinemia.

A rare manifestation of Sjögren's syndrome is the development of necrotizing vasculitis in the kidney, as well as in extrarenal sites (62). This complication is more common in patients with antibodies to Ro/SSA.

Immunofluorescence Findings. Some patients with tubulointerstitial nephritis have tubular basement membrane deposits of IgG and C3. Others lack evidence of tubulointerstitial immune deposits. Patients with lupus-like glomerulonephritis have glomerular immune deposits identical to those seen in the various classes of lupus nephritis.

Electron Microscopic Findings. In patients with tubulointerstitial nephritis, electron-dense deposits are identified in the tubular basement membrane and interstitium in less than half. In those with glomerulonephritis, glomerular electron-dense deposits are found in the same distribution expected for the corresponding class of lupus nephritis.

Differential Diagnosis. The differential diagnosis of the tubulointerstitial nephritis primarily includes drug-induced (allergic) and infectious (pyelonephritic) forms. The absence of granulomas is helpful to exclude sarcoidosis.

Etiology and Pathogenesis. The etiology of the renal involvement in Sjögren's disease is unknown. Cell-mediated immune response to Epstein-Barr virus (EBV) infection has been proposed for some forms of tubulointerstitial nephritis based on the identification of the EBV viral genome in tubular cells (58). It is likely that the immune complex–mediated forms of glomerulonephritis are due to autoantibody production, as occurs in lupus nephritis.

Treatment and Prognosis. Immunosuppressive therapy is tailored to the type of glomerulonephritis as for the different classes of lupus nephritis. Patients with interstitial nephritis often respond to high-dose steroids. Patients with necrotizing vasculitis are treated with steroids and cyclophosphamide in a similar regimen as used for microscopic polyangiitis.

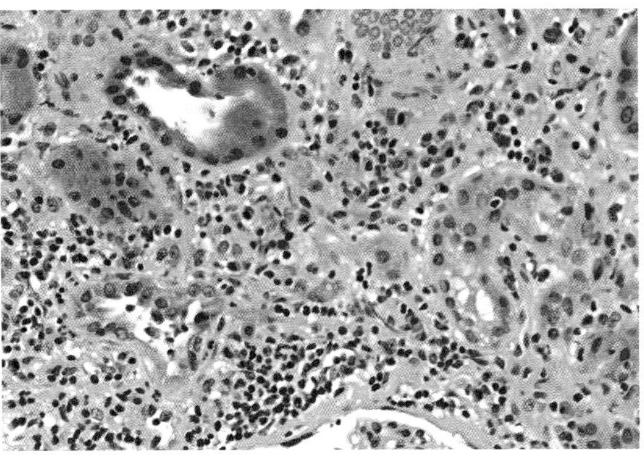

Figure 13-62

SJÖGREN'S SYNDROME WITH TUBULOINTERSTITIAL NEPHRITIS

The interstitium is expanded by edema, fibrosis, and dense inflammatory infiltrates of mononuclear leukocytes and plasma cells. There is focal mild tubulitis (inflammatory infiltration of the tubular epithelium) (H&E stain).

RHEUMATOID ARTHRITIS

Rheumatoid arthritis is an autoimmune inflammatory disease of the joints that may be accompanied by extra-articular manifestations, including rheumatoid nodules and systemic vasculitis. The 1987 revised American College of Rheumatology (ACR) criteria for diagnosis of RA include the following seven criteria: morning stiffness in and around the joints, arthritis of three or more joint areas, arthritis of hand joints, symmetric arthritis, rheumatoid nodules, serum rheumatoid factor, and radiographic changes such as erosions or bony decalcification adjacent to involved joints. Extra-articular disease includes mononeuritis multiplex, pericarditis, pulmonary nodules, pulmonary interstitial fibrosis, episcleritis, and systemic vasculitis. Compared to other autoimmune diseases, the incidence of primary renal disease complicating rheumatoid arthritis is low.

Renal disease in patients with rheumatoid arthritis falls into three major categories: amyloidosis, complications of drug therapy, and renal disease directly related to rheumatoid arthritis itself or overlapping with other autoimmune diseases. Each of these is described individually.

Amyloidosis

Clinical Features. The prevalence of amyloidosis in autopsy series of patients with rheumatoid arthritis is approximately 15 percent (71).

In general, it is more common in patients with a history of longstanding rheumatoid arthritis exceeding 10 to 15 years. Clinical features include proteinuria, often accompanied by the nephrotic syndrome, and variable renal insufficiency.

Light Microscopic Findings. Amyloidosis may affect the glomeruli, tubular basement membranes, interstitium, or blood vessels, in any combination (80). It is indistinguishable morphologically from amyloidosis occurring in other settings. The renal amyloid deposits are glassy and eosinophilic, weakly PAS positive, trichrome gray, and nonargyrophilic. A definitive diagnosis requires the demonstration of Congo red positivity with apple-green birefringence under polarized light. Rotation of the polarizer 45 degrees gives dichroism, producing a yellow to green transformation of the birefringence.

Immunofluorescence Findings. Because the amyloid is of the secondary (AA) type, it is strongly reactive for serum amyloid A (SAA) protein detectable by immunohistochemistry or immunofluorescence when performed on formalin-fixed or frozen sections of renal tissue (fig. 13-63). Unlike AL amyloid, there is no dominant staining for either light chain by immunofluorescence. Routine immunofluorescence staining is usually negative for all immunoglobulins and complement components; however, some cases exhibit weak uniform staining with antisera to immunoglobulins, complement, and albumin due to nonspecific trapping of plasma proteins in the distribution of the amyloid deposits.

Electron Microscopic Findings. Electron microscopy reveals deposits of randomly oriented fibrils ranging from 8 to 12 nm in diameter.

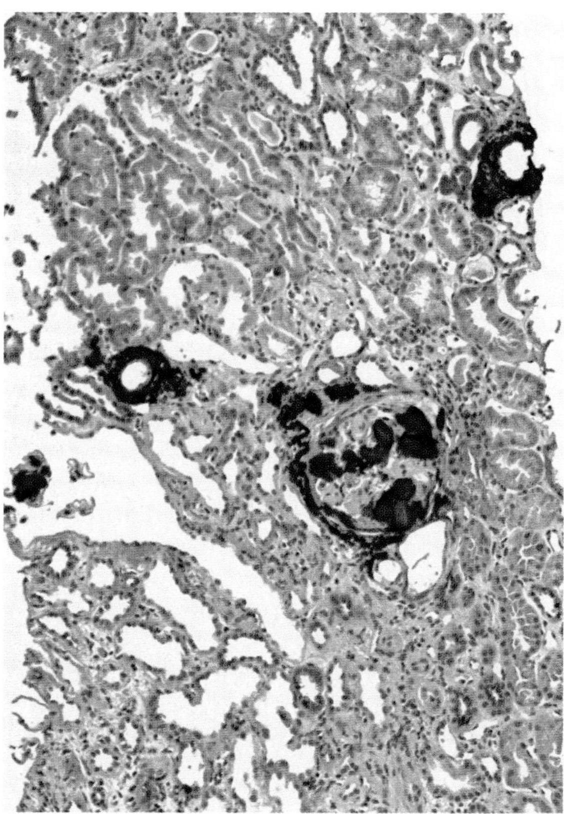

Figure 13-63

RHEUMATOID ARTHRITIS WITH SECONDARY AMYLOIDOSIS

This patient with a history of rheumatoid arthritis for 18 years developed nephrotic syndrome and progressive renal failure. Renal biopsy revealed abundant amyloid deposits in the glomeruli and vessel walls. Immunostain for serum amyloid A (SAA) protein is strongly positive in the distribution of the amyloid deposits, indicating a secondary (AA) amyloidosis (SAA immunoperoxidase stain).

Treatment-Related Renal Disease

Analgesic Nephropathy. The incidence of analgesic nephropathy complicating rheumatoid arthritis has diminished in the modern era due to the less frequent use of combination analgesic compounds and the withdrawal of phenacetin from the market. Features of analgesic nephropathy include papillary necrosis and chronic interstitial nephritis (79).

Nonsteroidal Anti-inflammatory Drugs (NSAID). The use of NSAIDs in patients with rheumatoid arthritis has been associated with the development of episodes of reversible acute renal failure due to the inhibition of cyclo-oxygenase and reduced renal synthesis of vasodilatory prostaglandins. Patients are particularly at risk for acute renal failure if they have intrinsic renal disease or underlying conditions that jeopardize renal perfusion, such as volume depletion, congestive heart failure, or ascites. Other manifestations include acute interstitial nephritis, minimal change disease, or a combination of acute interstitial nephritis and minimal change disease. Patients usually present after many months of NSAID use with an acute onset of nephrotic syndrome, pyuria, and renal insufficiency. These are usually reversible with drug withdrawal and recovery may be hastened by steroid therapy.

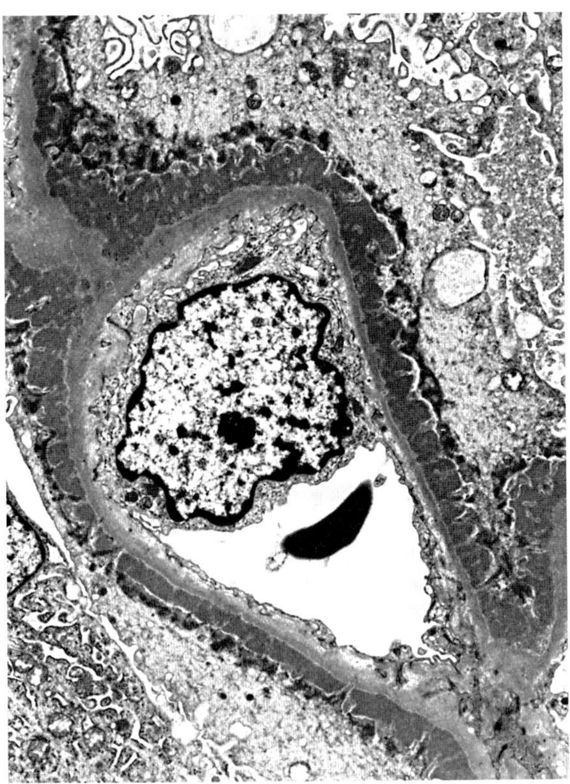

Figure 13-64

RHEUMATOID ARTHRITIS WITH GOLD-INDUCED MEMBRANOUS GLOMERULOPATHY

By electron microscopy, there are abundant subepithelial electron-dense deposits with focal intervening spikes, consistent with stage 2 membranous glomerulopathy. The findings in this form of drug-induced membranous glomerulopathy resemble those of idiopathic membranous glomerulopathy. A few minute mesangial electron-dense deposits are present at the right, however, there is no mesangial proliferation or endothelial tubuloreticular inclusions. Nephrotic syndrome is readily reversible following discontinuation of gold therapy.

Cyclosporine. Treatment with cyclosporine is associated with various forms of nephrotoxicity, like those described in transplant recipients (78). These include acute nephrotoxicity due to vasoconstriction, which has no morphologic correlate and is readily reversible; isometric vacuolization of the proximal tubules (toxic tubulopathy); interstitial fibrosis (stripe-like or diffuse); hyaline arteriolopathy; and thrombotic microangiopathy.

Gold and Penicillamine. Patients treated with gold salts or penicillamine may develop membranous glomerulopathy (72–75). Proteinuria develops as a complication of treatment with these agents in 1 to 10 percent of patients. There is no good correlation between the total cumulative dose and the likelihood of developing this complication. Resolution of the proteinuria is achieved in the majority of patients within 1 year of drug discontinuation. The glomerular lesion is indistinguishable from that of idiopathic membranous glomerulopathy (fig. 13-64). A characteristic feature of gold-induced membranous glomerulopathy, however, is the identification of gold inclusions forming electron-dense filamentous strands within lysosomes of proximal tubular epithelial cells, and more rarely, glomerular epithelial cells and mesangial cells (see chapter 7, fig. 7-55). A rare complication of penicillamine therapy is the development of a focal segmental necrotizing and crescentic glomerulonephritis, sometimes associated with renal vasculitis and pulmonary hemorrhage (70). This condition appears to represent a pauci-immune form of focal crescentic glomerulonephritis.

Antitumor Necrosis Factor (TNF)-Alpha. Treatment of rheumatoid arthritis patients with antitumor necrosis factor–alpha agents may lead to autoantibody formation and de novo renal disease. The inciting agents include etanercept, adalimumab, and infliximab. Complications of therapy include the development of proliferative or membranous lupus nephritis (with new onset anti-DNA antibodies and hypocomplementemia), pauci-immune necrotizing and crescentic glomerulonephritis (with new onset antineutrophil cytoplasmic antibody), and renal vasculitis (81).

Other Renal Diseases Related to Rheumatoid Arthritis

The existence of other renal diseases in patients with rheumatoid arthritis, independent of drug effect or amyloidosis, appears to be exceedingly rare. Most common are reports of a mild mesangial proliferative glomerulonephritis (77) or membranous glomerulopathy (76).

Patients with the mesangial lesion may present with isolated hematuria, isolated proteinuria, or combined hematuria and proteinuria. Mild mesangial hypercellularity and increased mesangial matrix are present. By immunofluorescence, IgM is most commonly identified, with more variable weak positivity for C3, IgA,

C1q, and IgG. Small paramesangial electron-dense deposits have been described.

Patients with membranous glomerulopathy usually present with severe proteinuria, sometimes accompanied by the nephrotic syndrome. The duration of rheumatoid arthritis prior to the onset of renal disease varies from 3 to 22 years. Some patients have exclusively subepithelial deposits of IgG and C3. Rarely are co-deposits of IgM or IgA observed. A few patients have mesangial deposits as well.

There are rare reports of pauci-immune focal segmental necrotizing and crescentic glomerulonephritis in patients with rheumatoid arthritis not exposed to penicillamine. Some of these patients have positive ANCA. Rheumatoid vasculitis involving the major renal artery or its branches has been reported in a few cases. Thrombotic microangiopathy secondary to antiphospholipid antibody has also been described.

REFERENCES

Systemic Lupus Erythematosus

1. Appel GB, Cohen DJ, Pirani CL, Meltzer JI, Estes DR. Long-term follow-up of patients with lupus nephritis. A study based on the classification of the World Health Organization. Am J Med 1987;83:877–85.
2. Appel GB, Pirani CL, D'Agati VD. Renal vascular complications of systemic lupus erythematosus. J Am Soc Nephrol 1994;4:499–515.
3. Appel GB, Silva FG, Pirani CL, Meltzer JI, Estes D. Renal involvement in systemic lupus erythematosus (SLE): a study of 56 patients emphasizing histologic classification. Medicine (Baltimore) 1978:57:371–410.
4. Appel GB, Valeri A. The course and treatment of lupus nephritis. Annu Rev Med 1994;45:525–37.
5. Austin HA 3rd, Boumpas DT, Vaughan EM, Balow JE. Predicting renal outcomes in severe lupus nephritis: contributions of clinical and histologic data. Kidney Int 1994;45:544–50.
6. Austin HA 3rd, Muenz LR, Joyce KM, Antonovych TT, Balow JE. Diffuse proliferative lupus nephritis: identification of specific pathologic features affecting renal outcome. Kidney Int 1984;25:689–95.
7. Austin HA 3rd, Muenz LR, Joyce KM, et al. Prognostic factors in lupus nephritis. Contribution of renal histological data. Am J Med 1983;75: 382–91.
8. Baldwin DS, Gluck MC, Lowenstein J, Gallo GR. Lupus nephritis. Clinical course as related to morphologic forms and their transitions. Am J Med 1977;62:12–30.
9. Banfi G, Bertani T, Boeri V, et al. Renal vascular lesions as a marker of poor prognosis in patients with lupus nephritis. Gruppo Italiano per lo Studio della Nefrite Lupica (GISNEL). Am J Kidney Dis 1991;18:240–8.
10. Bhathena DB, Sobel BJ, Migdal SD. Noninflammatory renal microangiopathy of systemic lupus erythematosus ('lupus vasculitis'). Am J Nephrol 1981;1:144–59.
11. Cameron JS, Turner DR, Ogg CS, et al. Systemic lupus with nephritis: a long-term study. Q J Med 1979;48:1–24.
12. Churg J, Bernstein J, Glassock RJ. Renal disease: classification and atlas of glomerular diseases, 2nd ed. New York: Igaku-Shoin; 1995.
13. Churg, J, Sobin LH. Renal disease: classification and atlas of glomerular disease, 1st ed. Tokyo: Igaku-Shoin; 1982.
14. Cohen AH, Zamboni L. Ultrastructural appearance and morphogenesis of renal glomerular hematoxylin bodies. Am J Pathol 1977;89:105–18.
15. Comparison of idiopathic and systemic lupus erythematosus-associated membranous glomerulonephropathy in children. The Southwest Pediatric Nephrology Study Group. Am J Kidney Dis 1986;7:115–24.
16. D'Agati V. Renal disease in systemic lupus erythematosus, mixed connective tissue disease, Sjogren's syndrome, and rheumatoid arthritis. In: Jennette JC, Olson JL, Schwartz MM, Silva, FG, eds. Heptinstall's pathology of the kidney, 5th ed. Philadelphia: Lipincott Raven; 1998:541–624.
17. D'Agati V, Kunis C, Williams G, Appel GB. Anticardiolipin antibody and renal disease: a report of three cases. J Am Soc Nephrol 1990;1:777–84.
18. Daugas E, Nochy D, Huong du LT, et al. Antiphospholipid syndrome nephropathy in systemic lupus erythematosus. J Am Soc Nephrol 2002;13:42–52.
19. Farrugia E, Torres VE, Gastineau D, Michet CJ, Holley KE. Lupus anticoagulant in systemic lupus erythematosus: a clinical and renal pathological study. Am J Kidney Dis 1992;20:463–71.
20. Foster MH, Cizman B, Madaio MP. Nephritogenic autoantibodies in systemic lupus erythematosus: immunochemical properties, mechanisms of immune deposition, and genetic origins. Lab Invest 1993;69:494–507.

21. Hill GS, Delahousse M, Nochy D, et al. A new index for evaluation of renal biopsies in lupus nephritis. Kidney Int 2000;58:1160–73.
22. Hill GS, Delahousse M, Nochy D, et al. Predictive power of the second renal biopsy in lupus nephritis: significance of macrophages. Kidney Int 2001;59:304–16.
23. Hill GS, Hinglais N, Tron F, Bach JF. Systemic lupus erythematosus. Morphologic correlations with immunologic and clinical data at the time of biopsy. Am J Med 1978;64:61–79.
24. Hochberg MC. Updating the American College of Rheumatology revised criteria for the classification of systemic lupus erythematosus. Arthritis Rheum 1997;40:1725.
25. Jennette JC. The immunohistology of IgA nephropathy. Am J Kidney Dis 1988;12:348–52.
26. Jennette JC, Iskandar SS, Dalldorf FG. Pathologic differentiation between lupus and nonlupus membranous glomerulopathy. Kidney Int 1983;24:377–85.
27. Korbet SM, Lewis EJ, Schwartz MM, Reichlin M, Evans J, Rohde RD. Factors predictive of outcome in severe lupus nephritis. Lupus Nephritis Collaborative Study Group. Am J Kidney Dis 2000;35:904–14.
28. Magil AB, Ballon HS, Rae A. Focal proliferative lupus nephritis. A clinicopathologic study using the W.H.O. classification. Am J Med 1982;72: 620–30.
29. Magil AB, Puterman ML, Ballon HS, et al. Prognostic factors in diffuse proliferative lupus glomerulonephritis. Kidney Int 1988;34:511–7.
30. Mahajan SK, Ordonez NG, Feitelson PJ, Lim VS, Spargo BH, Katz A. Lupus nephropathy without clinical renal involvement. Medicine (Baltimore) 1977;56:493–501.
31. Marshall S, Dressler R, D'Agati V. Membranous lupus nephritis with antineutrophil cytoplasmic antibody-associated segmental necrotizing and crescentic glomerulonephritis. Am J Kidney Dis 1997;29:119–24.
32. McCluskey RT. Lupus nephritis. In: Sommers SC, ed. Kidney pathology decennial 1966-1975. East Norwalk, CT: Appleton-Century-Crofts; 1975:435.
33. Morel-Maroger L, Mery JP, Droz D, et al. The course of lupus nephritis: contribution of serial renal biopsies. In: Hamburger J, Crosnier J, Maxwell MH, eds. Advances in nephrology. Chicago: Year Book Medical; 1976:79.
34. Najafi CC, Korbet SM, Lewis EJ, Schwartz MM, Reichlin M, Evans J. Significance of histologic patterns of glomerular injury upon long-term prognosis in severe lupus glomerulonephritis. Kidney Int 2001;59:2156–63.
35. Park MH, D'Agati V, Appel GB, Pirani CL. Tubulointerstitial disease in lupus nephritis: relationship to immune deposits, interstitial inflammation, glomerular changes, renal function, and prognosis. Nephron 1986;44:309–19.
36. Pasquali S, Banfi G, Zucchelli, A, Moroni G, Ponticelli C, Zuchelli P. Lupus membranous nephropathy: long-term outcome. Clin Nephrol 1993;39:175–82.
37. Pirani CL, Olesnicky L. Role of electron microscopy in the classification of lupus nephritis. Am J Kidney Dis 1982;2(1 Suppl 1):150–63.
38. Schwartz MM, Bernstein J, Hill GS, Holley K, Philips EA. Predictive value of renal pathology in diffuse proliferative lupus glomerulonephritis. Lupus Nephritis Collaborative Study Group. Kidney Int 1989;36:891–6.
39. Schwartz MM, Kawala KS, Corwin HL, Lewis EJ. The prognosis of segmental glomerulonephritis in systemic lupus erythematosus. Kidney Int 1987;32:274–9.
40. Schwartz MM, Kawala K, Roberts JL, Humes C, Lewis EJ. Clinical and pathological features of membranous glomerulonephritis of systemic lupus erythematosus. Am J Nephrol 1984;4:301–11.
41. Schwartz MM, Lan SP, Bernstein J, Hill GS, Holley K, Lewis EJ. Irreproducibility of the activity and chronicity indices limits their utility in the management of lupus nephritis. Lupus Nephritis Collaborative Study Group. Am J Kidney Dis 1993;21:374–7.
42. Schwartz MM, Lan SP, Bernstein J, Hill GS, Holley K, Lewis EJ. Role of pathology indices in the management of severe lupus glomerulonephritis. Lupus Nephritis Collaborative Study Group. Kidney Int 1992;42:743–8.
43. Schwartz MM, Lan SP, Bonsib SM, Gephardt GN, Sharma HM. Clinical outcome of three discrete histologic patterns of injury in severe lupus glomerulonephritis. Am J Kidney Dis 1989;13:273–83.
44. Silva FG. The nephropathies of systemic lupus erythematosus. In: Rosen S, ed. Pathology of glomerular disease. New York: Churchill Livingstone; 1983:79–124.
45. Stuart L, Hughes J. Apoptosis and autoimmunity. Nephrol Dial Transplant 2002;17:697–700.
46. Tan EM, Cohen AS, Fries JF, et al. The 1982 revised criteria for the classification of systemic lupus erythematosus. Arthritis Rheum 1982;25: 1271–7.
47. Weening JJ, D'Agati VD, Schwartz MM, et al. The classification of glomerulonephritis in systemic lupus erythematosus revisited. Kidney Int 2004; 65:521–30.

Mixed Connective Tissue Disease

48. Bennett RM. Mixed connective tissue disease. In: Grishman R, Churg J, Needle MA, Venkataseshan VS eds, The kidney in collagen vascular diseases. New York: Raven Press; 1993:167–77.
49. Bennett RM, Spargo BH. Immune complex nephropathy in mixed connective tissue disease. Am J Med 1977;63:534–41.
50. Black C, Isenberg DA. Mixed connective tissue disease—goodbye to all that. Br J Rheumatol 1992;31:695–700.

51. Cohen AH. Renal pathology forum. Am J Nephrol 1985;5:305–11.
52. Kitridou RC, Akmal M, Turkel SB, Ehresmann GR, Quismorio FP Jr, Massry SG. Renal involvement in mixed connective tissue disease: a longitudinal clinicopathologic study. Semin Arthritis Rheum 1986;16:135–45.
53. Kobayashi S, Nagase M, Kimura M, Ohyama K, Ikeya M, Honda N. Renal involvement in mixed connective tissue disease. Report of 5 cases. Am J Nephrol 1985;5:282–9.
54. Sharp GC, Irvin WS, Tan EM, Gould RG, Holman HR. Mixed connective tissue disease—an apparently distinct rheumatic disease syndrome associated with a specific antibody to an extractable nuclear antigen (ENA). Am J Med 1972;52:148–59.
55. Singsen BH, Swanson VL, Bernstein BH, Heuser ET, Hanson V, Landing BH. A histologic evaluation of mixed connective tissue disease in childhood. Am J Med 1980;68:710–7.
56. Van den Hoogen FH, Spronk PE, Boerbooms AM, et al. Long-term follow-up of 46 patients with anti-(U1)snRNP antibodies. Br J Rheumatol 1994;33:1117–20.

Sjögren's Syndrome

57. Andrassy K, Gebest J, Tan E, Thoednes W, Ritz E. Interstitial nephritis in a patient with atypical Sjogren's syndrome. Klin Wochenschr 1980; 58:563–7.
58. Becker JL, Miller F, Nuovo GJ, Josepovitz C, Schubach WH, Nord EP. Epstein-Barr virus infection of renal proximal tubule cells: possible role in chronic interstitial nephritis. J Clin Invest 1999;104:1673–81.
59. Font J, Cervera R, Lopez-Soto A, Darnell A, Ingelmo M. Mixed membranous and proliferative glomerulonephritis in primary Sjogren's syndrome. Br J Rheumatol 1989;28:548–50.
60. Fox RI, Pearson G, Vaughan JH. Detection of Epstein-Barr virus-associated antigens and DNA in salivary gland biopsies from patients with Sjogren's syndrome. J Immunol 1986;137:3162–8.
61. Khan MA, Akhtar M, Taher SM. Membranoproliferative glomerulonephritis in a patient with primary Sjogren's syndrome. Am J Nephrol 1988;8:235–9.
62. Molina R, Provost TT, Alexander EL. Two types of inflammatory vascular disease in Sjogren's syndrome. Differential association with seroreactivity to rheumatoid factor and antibodies to Ro (SS-A) and with hypocomplementemia. Arthritis Rheum 1985;28:1251–8.
63. Moutsopoulos HM, Balow JE, Lawley TJ, Stahl NI, Antonovych TT, Chused TM. Immune complex glomerulonephritis in sicca syndrome. Am J Med 1978;64:955–60.
64. Pasternack A, Linder E. Renal tubular acidosis: an immunopathological study on four patients. Clin Exp Immunol 1970;7:115–23.
65. Pavlidis NA, Karsh J, Moutsopoulos HM. The clinical picture of primary Sjogren's syndrome: a retrospective study. J Rheumatol 1982;9:685–90.
66. Rayadurg J, Koch AE. Renal insufficiency from interstitial nephritis in primary Sjogren's syndrome. J Rheumatol 1990;17:1714–8.
67. Reveille JD, Wilson RW, Provost TT, Bias WB, Arnett FC. Primary Sjogren's syndrome and other autoimmune diseases in families. Prevalence and immunogenetic studies in six kindreds. Ann Intern Med 1984;101:748–56.
68. Sjogren H. Zur Kenntnis der Keratoconjuctivitis Sicca (Kratitis folliforms bei hypojunktion der tramemdrusen). Acta Ophthalmol Copenh 1933;11:1–151.
69. Tu WH, Shearn MA, Lee JC, Hopper J Jr. Interstitial nephritis in Sjogren's syndrome. Ann Intern Med 1968;69:1163–70.

Rheumatoid Arthritis

70. Almirall J, Alcorta I, Botey A, Revert L. Penicillamine-induced rapidly progressive glomerulonephritis in a patient with rheumatoid arthritis. Am J Nephrol 1993;13:286–8.
71. Boers M. Renal disorders in rheumatoid arthritis. Semin Arthritis Rheum 1990;20:57–68.
72. Hall CL. Gold nephropathy. Nephron 1988;50: 265–72.
73. Hall CL. The natural course of gold and penicillamine nephropathy: a long-term study of 54 patients. Adv Exp Med Biol 1989;252:247–56.
74. Hall CL, Fothergill NJ, Blackwell MM, Harrison PR, MacKenzie JC, MacIver AG. The natural course of gold nephropathy: long term study of 21 patients. Br Med J 1987;295:745–8.
75. Hall CL, Jawad S, Harrison PR, et al. Natural course of penicillamine nephropathy: a long term study of 33 patients. Br Med J 1988;296:1083–6.
76. Honkanen E, Tornroth T, Pettersson E, Skrifvars B. Membranous glomerulonephritis in rheumatoid arthritis not related to gold or D-penicillamine therapy: a report of four cases and review of the literature. Clin Nephrol 1987;27:87–93.
77. Korpela M, Mustonen J, Pasternack A, Helin H. Mesangial glomerulopathy in rheumatoid arthritis patients. Clinical follow-up and relation to antirheumatic therapy. Nephron 1991;59:46–50.
78. Ludwin D, Alexopoulou I. Cyclosporin A nephropathy in patients with rheumatoid arthritis. Br J Rheumatol 1993;32(Suppl 1):60–4.
79. Nanra RS. Renal papillary necrosis in rheumatoid arthritis. Med J Aust 1975;1:194–7.
80. Pollak VE, Pirani CL, Steck IE, Kark RM. The kidney in rheumatoid arthritis: studies by renal biopsy. Arthritis Rheum 1962;5:1–9.
81. Stokes MB, Foster K, Markowitz GS, et al. Development of glomerulonephritis during anti-TNF-alpha therapy for rheumatoid arthritis. Nephrol Dial Transplant 2005;20:1400–6.

14 ANTIGLOMERULAR BASEMENT MEMBRANE GLOMERULONEPHRITIS AND GOODPASTURE'S SYNDROME

ANTIGLOMERULAR BASEMENT MEMBRANE DISEASES

Definition. Antiglomerular basement membrane (anti-GBM) disease is vascular injury mediated by anti-GBM antibodies. Included in this category are *anti-GBM glomerulonephritis, anti-GBM pulmonary capillaritis,* and *Goodpasture's syndrome.* The term Goodpasture's syndrome has been used in the past as a generic term for the concurrence of pulmonary hemorrhage and glomerulonephritis, the so-called pulmonary-renal vasculitic syndrome. Current usage, however, restricts Goodpasture's syndrome to pulmonary-renal vasculitic syndrome that is caused by anti-GBM antibodies.

Clinical Features. Glomerulonephritis is the most common expression of anti-GBM disease (10,47). Most patients already have severe renal failure at the time of presentation (Table 14-1). In fact, pathologically and clinically, anti-GBM glomerulonephritis is the most destructive form of glomerulonephritis (Table 14-2) (20,24). Proteinuria is usually between 1 and 2 g/day, but some patients have nephrotic range proteinuria. Anti-GBM disease has an unusual bimodal age distribution, with one peak in adolescence and young adults, and another peak after the sixth decade of life (fig. 14-1). There is a male predominance among the younger patients and a female predominance among the older patients. Anti-GBM disease is much less frequent in blacks compared to whites (Table 14-1). Rare patients have an initially mild nephritis (31), but this often transforms into rapidly progressive nephritis within days to weeks if not treated with immunosuppressive therapy. Anti-GBM pulmonary disease most often manifests as hemoptysis and dyspnea, which may be mild or life threatening.

Approximately 50 percent of patients initially present with anti-GBM glomerulonephritis alone, less than 5 percent have anti-GBM pulmonary capillaritis alone, and 45 percent have Goodpasture's syndrome with pulmonary and renal disease; accurate incidences, however, are difficult to obtain because percentages vary among different cohorts of patients (46,47,57). Patients who initially have clinical evidence of glomerulonephritis alone or pulmonary capillaritis

Table 14-1

CLINICAL FEATURES OF PATIENTS WITH ANTIGLOMERULAR BASEMENT MEMBRANE (ANTI-GBM) CRESCENTIC GLOMERULONEPHRITIS COMPARED TO THOSE WITH PAUCI-IMMUNE OR IMMUNE COMPLEX CRESCENTIC GLOMERULONEPHRITIS[a]

	Mean Age (range)	Male:Female	Black:White[b]	Creatine (mg/dL) (range)	Proteinuria (g/24 hrs) (range)
Anti-GBM Crescentic Glomerulonephritis	52±21 (14-84) n=92	1:1 45:47 n=92	1:9 7:63 n=70	9.7±7.2 (0.8-50.0) n=86	1.67±3.35 (0.20-16.20) n=68
Pauci-immune Crescentic Glomerulonephritis	56±20 (2-92) n=377	1:0.9 202:177 n=379	1:3.7 65:239 n=304	6.5±4.0 (0.8-22.1) n=338	1.94±2.95 (0.11-18.00) n=331
Immune Complex Crescentic Glomerulonephritis	33±17 (4-77) n=154	1:1.6 61:95 n=156	1:0.9 67:62 n=129	4.9±3.8 (0.8-21.7) n=145	4.39±4.77 (0.30-22.00) n=136

[a]From reference 21.

[b]Approximate black:white ratio in the referral population is 1:3.

Table 14-2

EXTENT OF CRESCENT FORMATION IN VARIOUS FORMS OF GLOMERULAR DISEASES[a]

Type of Glomerular Disease	N[b]	% With Any Crescents	% With >50% Crescents	Average % Glomerular Crescents[c]	Glomerular Necrosis (0-4+)	Glomerular Hyper-cellularity[d] (0-4+)
Anti-GBM Glomerulonephritis[e]	105	97.1%	84.8%	77%	1.7+	0.8+
ANCA Glomerulonephritis	181	89.5%	50.3%	49%	1.2+	0.8+
Lupus Glomerulonephritis (III and IV)	784	56.5%	12.9%	31%	1.7+	2.2+
H-S Purpura Glomerulonephritis	31	61.3%	9.7%	27%	0.4+	1.5+
IgA Nephropathy	853	32.5%	4.0%	21%	0.1+	1.4+
Postinfectious Glomerulonephritis	120	33.3%	3.3%	19%	0.3+	2.7+
Type 1 Membranoproliferative Glomerulonephritis	307	23.8%	4.6%	25%	0.2+	2.8+
Type 2 Membranoproliferative Glomerulonephritis	16	43.8%	18.8%	48%	0.2+	1.8+
Fibrillary Glomerulonephritis	101	22.8%	5.0%	26%	0+	0.6+
Monoclonal Immunoglobulin Deposition Disease	54	5.6%	0%	13%	0	0.3+
Thrombotic Microangiopathy	251	5.6%	0.9%	26%	0.4+	0.3+
Diabetic Glomerulosclerosis	648	3.2%	0.3%	20%	0+	0.3+
Idiopathic Membranous Glomerulopathy	1,092	3.2%	0.1%	15%	0	0.1+

[a]In general, those diseases that most often have crescents also have the largest percentage of glomeruli involved by crescents. From reference 21.

[b]Number of cases.

[c]Average percent of glomeruli with crescents when crescents were present.

[d]Endocapillary (not extracapillary) hypercellularity.

[e]Anti-GBM = antiglomerular basement membrane; ANCA = antineutrophil cytoplasmic autoantibody; H-S = Henoch-Schönlein.

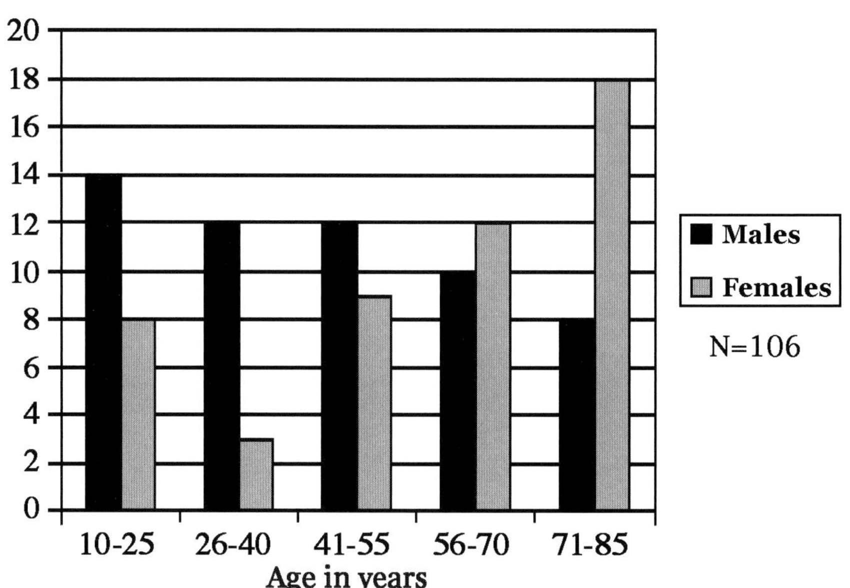

Figure 14-1

AGE DISTRIBUTION OF ANTIGLOMERULAR BASEMENT MEMBRANE (ANTI-GBM) GLOMERULONEPHRITIS

Age at onset of anti-GBM glomerulonephritis shows a peak incidence in males during the second decade of life and two peaks in females, one early and one late. (Based on 106 consecutive patients diagnosed with anti-GBM glomerulonephritis at the Nephropathology Laboratory at the University of North Carolina at Chapel Hill.)

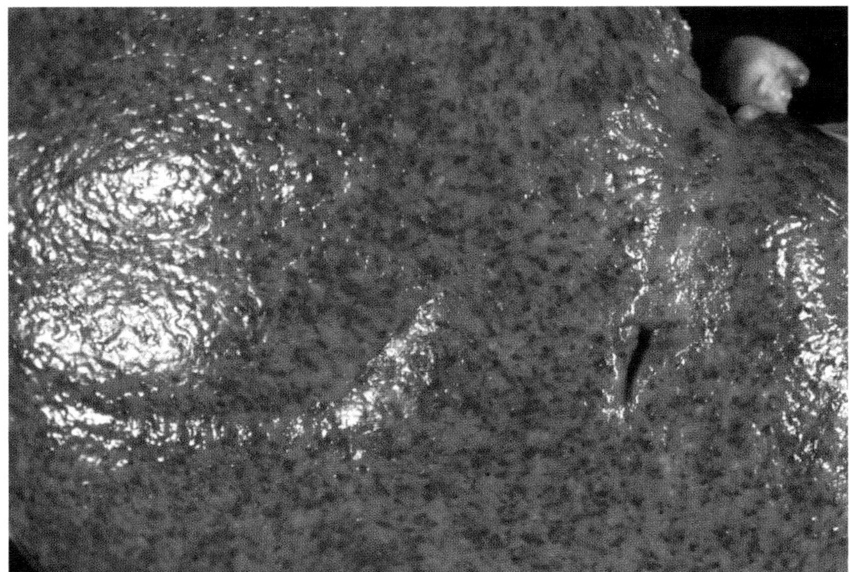

Figure 14-2

"FLEA-BITTEN" KIDNEY

This kidney from a patient with anti-GBM pulmonary-renal vasculitic syndrome (Goodpasture's syndrome) has numerous small red dots on the surface. These are caused by spillage of blood into Bowman's spaces and tubular lumens as a result of extensive inflammatory rupture of glomerular capillaries.

alone may eventually develop pulmonary-renal syndrome (Goodpasture's syndrome). Young men with anti-GBM disease have the highest frequency of pulmonary involvement, and older females have the lowest (47).

Ernest Goodpasture (16) reported in 1919 the association of pulmonary hemorrhage with severe glomerulonephritis in an 18-year-old male with a flu-like illness. Later, the term Goodpasture's syndrome was applied to any patients with concurrent pulmonary hemorrhage and glomerulonephritis (49). In the 1960s, when immunofluorescence microscopy was applied to the evaluation of renal biopsy specimens, a subset of patients with pulmonary-renal vasculitic syndrome who had linear localization of immunoglobulin (Ig)G along the glomerular and pulmonary capillary basement membranes was discovered (49,54). This linear staining was proven to be the result of deposition of pathogenic anti-GBM antibodies (34). Immunohistologic evaluation of renal and pulmonary tissue from patients with pulmonary-renal vasculitic syndrome, as well as serologic testing, demonstrated that only a minority of patients had anti-GBM disease (40); the most common cause of pulmonary-renal vasculitic syndrome is small vessel vasculitis associated with antineutrophil cytoplasmic autoantibodies (ANCAs), such as microscopic polyangiitis, Wegener's granulomatosis, and Churg-Strauss syndrome (40). Thus, an approach to nomenclature is required that separates anti-GBM antibody–mediated pulmonary-renal vasculitic syndrome from pulmonary-renal vasculitic syndrome of other causes. This led to the convention of restricting the term Goodpasture's syndrome to pulmonary-renal vasculitic syndrome caused by anti-GBM antibodies (37).

Gross Findings. When severe anti-GBM glomerulonephritis is present, the external surface of the kidney has numerous small red dots that correspond to blood in Bowman's spaces and the lumens of tubules (fig. 14-2). Similar red dots are seen on the cut surfaces of the kidney, along with coiled red profiles that correspond to blood within the lumens of convoluted tubules. This "flea-bitten" appearance is not specific for anti-GBM glomerulonephritis because it is seen with any form of severe glomerulonephritis that causes marked hematuria. The external and cut surfaces of lungs with anti-GBM capillaritis have focal or diffuse dark red discoloration caused by intra-alveolar hemorrhage (fig. 14-3).

Light Microscopic Findings. Almost all cases of anti-GBM glomerulonephritis have crescent formation at the time of biopsy, with more than 80 percent of specimens having crescents in greater than 50 percent of glomeruli (Table 14-2; fig. 14-4) (24). Most renal pathologists reserve the diagnostic term *crescentic glomerulonephritis* for glomerulonephritis with 50 percent or more of glomeruli with crescents, but include the percent of glomeruli affected in the diagnostic line if it is less than 50 percent. For example, using

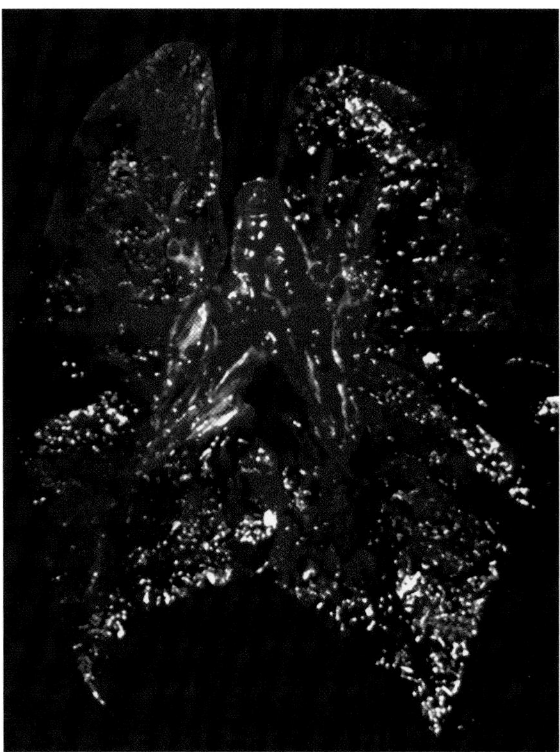

Figure 14-3

PULMONARY HEMORRHAGE

These lungs, from the same patient as in figure 14-2 with anti-GBM pulmonary-renal vasculitic syndrome (Goodpasture's syndrome), have massive pulmonary hemorrhage filling most of the alveolar air spaces and spilling into the bronchi and trachea. The patient died of hemorrhagic asphyxiation.

this approach, anti-GBM glomerulonephritis with 75 percent crescents would be called "crescentic anti-GBM glomerulonephritis" whereas anti-GBM glomerulonephritis with 35 percent crescents would be called "anti-GBM glomerulonephritis with 35 percent crescents."

The earliest identifiable acute glomerular lesion of anti-GBM glomerulonephritis is focal segmental fibrinoid necrosis (fig. 14-5) (20,38,55). This usually is accompanied by a mild accumulation of leukocytes, predominantly neutrophils, at the sites of necrosis. Occasional specimens have moderate numbers of glomerular neutrophils (fig. 14-6), and rare specimens have intense neutrophilic infiltration (fig. 14-7).

Special stains are useful for demarcating glomerular necrosis and crescent formation. Stains that highlight the basement membranes, such as the periodic acid–Schiff (PAS) (fig. 14-5, right), Masson trichrome (fig. 14-6), and Jones methenamine silver (JMS) (figs. 14-8,14-9), are useful for identifying breaks in the GBM and Bowman's capsule that occur at sites of necrosis, and also are useful for identifying the junction between glomerular tufts and cellular crescents, which often is difficult to discern on hematoxylin and eosin (H&E)–stained sections (figs. 14-5, left; 14-7). Trichrome stains distinguish between fibrinoid necrosis, which stains red (fuchsinophilic) (fig. 14-10, left), and sclerosis, which stains blue or green, depending on the staining method used (fig. 14-10, right). This is useful because necrosis and sclerosis both are acidophilic with H&E staining, and have different implications about the activity and chronicity of the glomerular injury.

Injured capillaries often have perforated or fragmented basement membranes which correspond to areas of rupture that have allowed plasma constituents and necrotic debris to spill into Bowman's space (fig. 14-9). Plasma coagulation factors contact thrombogenic stimuli, including tissue factor, resulting in capillary thrombosis and the formation of extravascular fibrin in the areas of necrosis, i.e., fibrinoid necrosis. After rupture of glomerular capillaries, fibrin also forms within Bowman's space and contributes to the induction of cellular crescent formation (fig. 14-11). Fully formed crescents may be very cellular and completely surround the tuft (fig. 14-12).

Glomeruli and glomerular segments that are not affected by necrotizing lesions often appear remarkably normal, with no hypercellularity and no thickening of capillary walls (figs. 14-8;14-10, left). When present, glomerular leukocyte infiltration or other features of endocapillary hypercellularity usually are associated with sites of necrosis or sclerosis. Occasional specimens have prominent capillary neutrophils. Rare examples of anti-GBM glomerulonephritis have more widespread endocapillary hypercellularity.

The lack of substantial glomerular endocapillary hypercellularity or capillary wall thickening, even when there is extensive extracapillary hypercellularity (crescent formation), is similar to pauci-immune ANCA glomerulonephritis but different from immune complex glomerulonephritis. Immune complex glomerulonephritis typically has well-established endocapillary

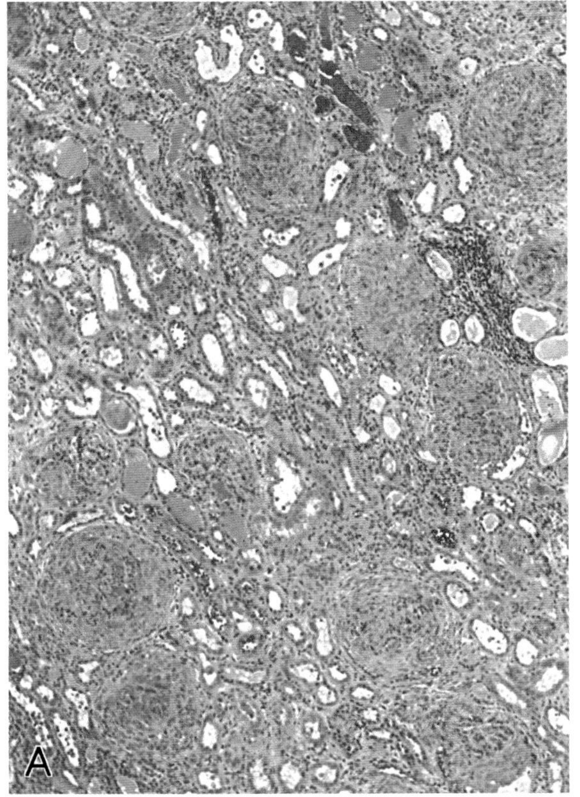

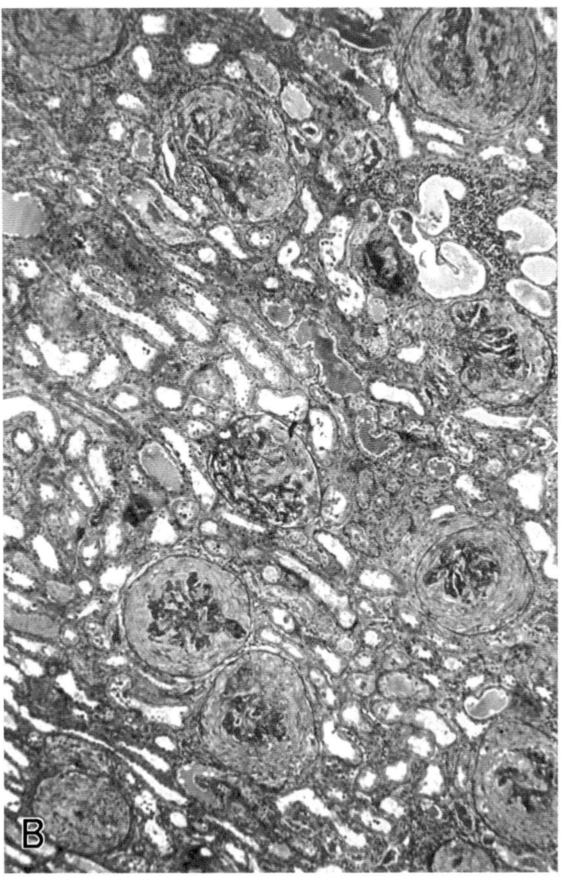

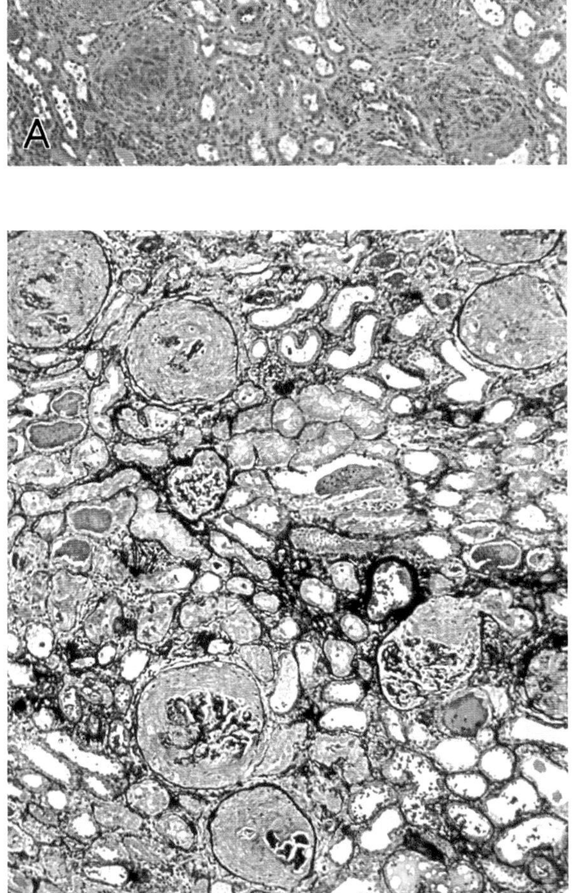

Figure 14-4

CRESCENTIC ANTI-GBM GLOMERULONEPHRITIS

Low-power magnification demonstrates crescentic anti-GBM glomerulonephritis with 100 percent crescents. The large cellular crescents can be demarcated from the injured glomerular tufts better in the sections stained with periodic acid–Schiff (PAS) (B) and Jones methenamine silver (JMS) (C) than in the hematoxylin and eosin (H&E)-stained section (A). There is focal interstitial edema and slight infiltration by predominantly mononuclear leukocytes. Tubules have focal epithelial simplification and some contain red blood cell casts or hemoglobin pigmented casts.

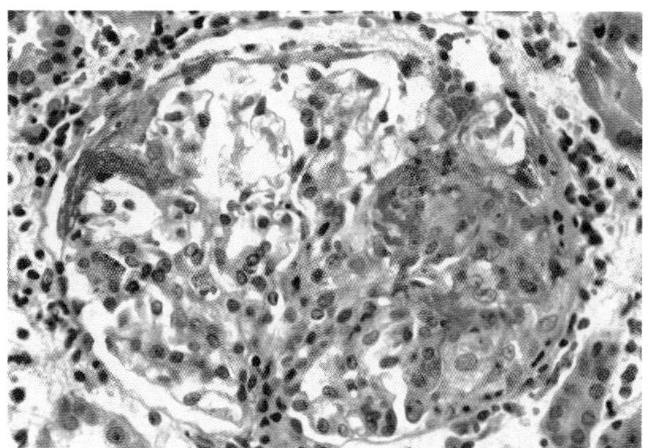
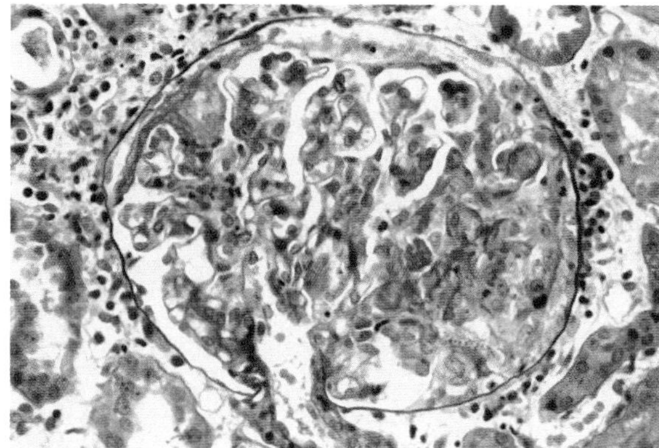

Figure 14-5

ANTI-GBM GLOMERULONEPHRITIS WITH SEGMENTAL NECROSIS AND SMALL CRESCENT

The right side of the glomerulus in both panels shows segmental fibrinoid necrosis and a small crescent. With the H&E stain (left) it is difficult to distinguish between intracapillary and extracapillary cells. A section adjacent to the one illustrated on the left is stained with PAS, which allows better demarcation of segmental necrosis. The intact GBM can be seen on the left but has been destroyed on the right. Note the edema and leukocyte infiltration in the periglomerular interstitium.

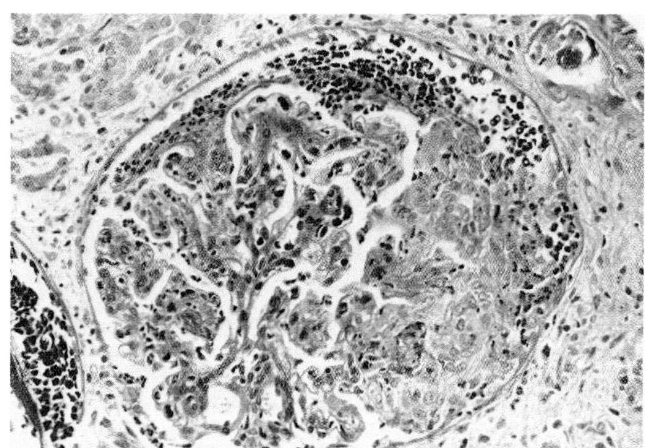
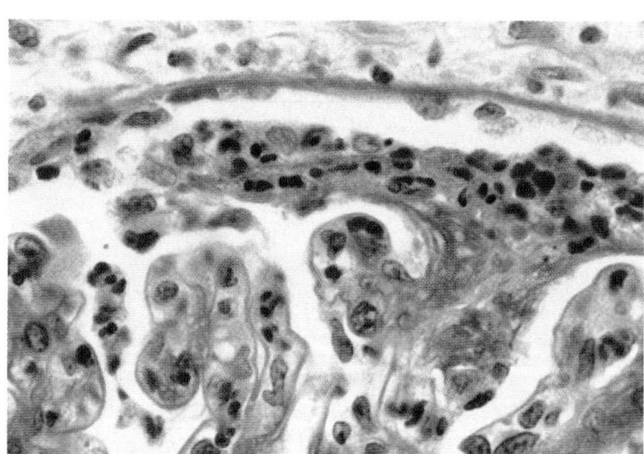

Figure 14-6

ANTI-GBM GLOMERULONEPHRITIS WITH NEUTROPHILS

Left: The low-power magnification shows a cellular crescent to the right and hemorrhage into Bowman's space at the top.
Right: Higher magnification of the same tuft reveals numerous neutrophils in glomerular capillaries, some of which have gnawed their way into Bowman's space.

hypercellularity, often accompanied by capillary wall thickening when it is severe enough to cause crescent formation.

Fully formed cellular crescents range from small segmental structures (see fig. 14-5) to large circumferential crescents (fig. 14-12). The fibrinoid material between the cells of the crescents stains dark blue with the phosphotungstic acid-hematoxylin (PTAH) stain (fig. 14-11). The cellular components of crescents are predominantly mixtures of epithelial cells and macrophages. Monocytes or macrophages can enter Bowman's space either through glomerular capillaries or through breaks in Bowman's capsule, which often occur in anti-GBM glomerulonephritis (fig. 14-13). Epithelial cells usually predominate when Bowman's capsule remains intact, whereas macrophages often predominate when there is disruption of Bowman's capsule (14). In general, there is greater disruption of Bowman's capsule and greater numbers of macrophages in crescents with anti-GBM glomerulonephritis and ANCA glomerulonephritis than with immune complex glomerulonephritis (14,36).

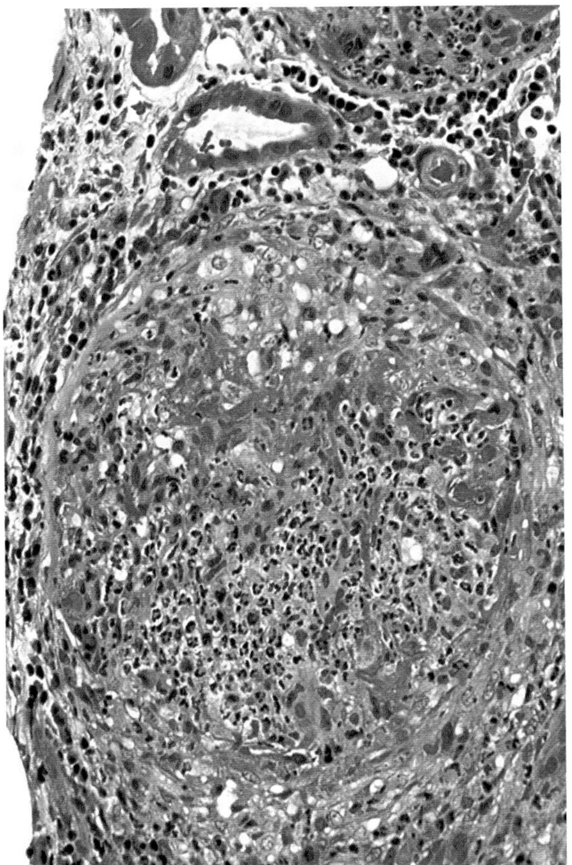

Figure 14-7

ANTI-GBM GLOMERULONEPHRITIS WITH NUMEROUS NEUTROPHILS

The H&E-stained glomerulus has crescent formation to the top, and fibrinoid necrosis and extensive infiltration by neutrophils (especially on the bottom).

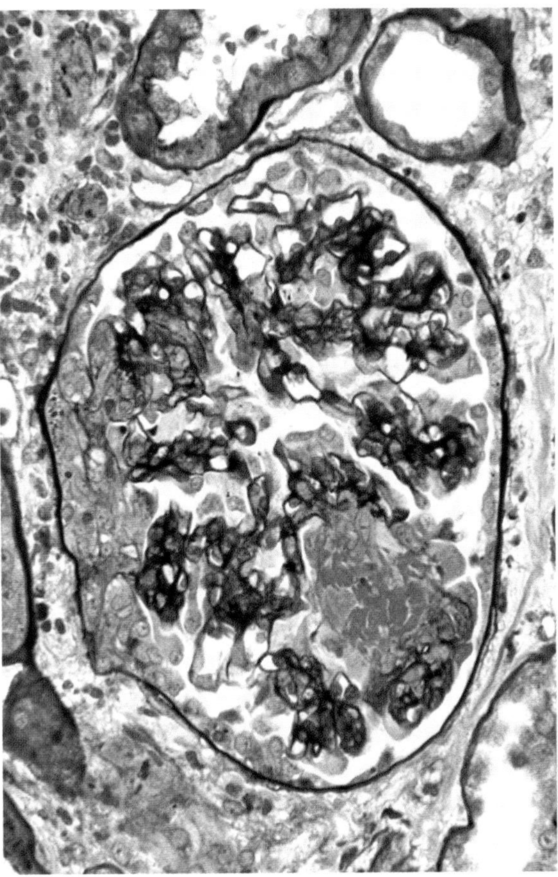

Figure 14-8

ANTI-GBM GLOMERULONEPHRITIS WITH SEGMENTAL NECROSIS AND SMALL CRESCENT

This Jones methenamine silver (JMS) stain with an H&E counterstain clearly delineates a focus of segmental fibrinoid necrosis in the lower right segment. Note the lysis of the GBM cells and mesangial matrix. There is a small cellular crescent at the left.

Periglomerular interstitial inflammation is enhanced in response to disruption of Bowman's capsule. This periglomerular inflammation can have a granulomatous appearance, including the presence of multinucleated giant cells (fig. 14-14). Periglomerular granulomatous inflammation is a nonspecific response to severe glomerular injury and can be seen not only with anti-GBM glomerulonephritis but also with pauci-immune ANCA glomerulonephritis, including both renal-limited ANCA glomerulonephritis and ANCA glomerulonephritis occurring as a component of Wegener's granulomatosis, microscopic polyangiitis, or Churg-Strauss syndrome (3,20).

With chronic evolution of the glomerular injury, there is progressive scarring of cellular crescents, advancing to fibrocellular crescents and finally fibrotic crescents. Tubularization is a less frequent expression of crescent organization that can be seen in cellular or fibrocellular crescents (fig. 14-15). In advanced chronic disease, the demarcation between fibrotic crescents and fibrotic glomerular tufts that have been destroyed by necrotizing injury can be difficult to discern (fig. 14-16). Special stains may help by revealing residual GBMs if there are any. The initial cause of advanced chronic glomerular injury can be difficult to establish in a specimen that has glomerular scarring but

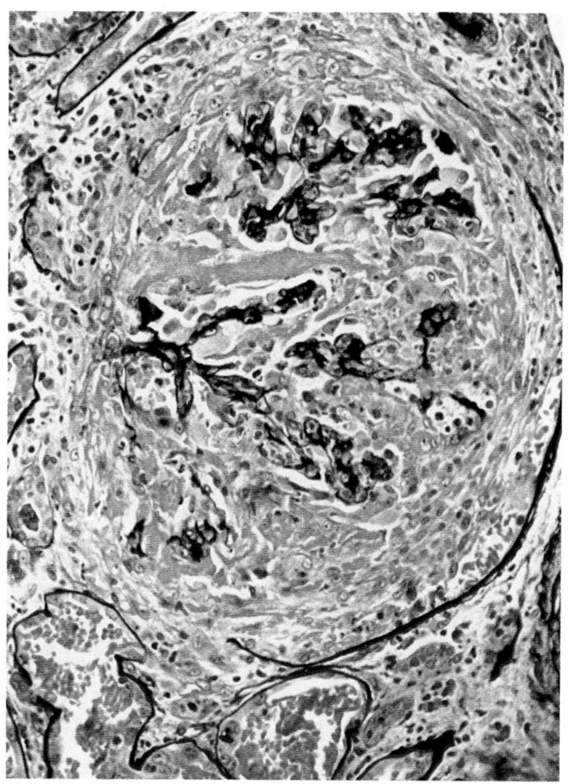

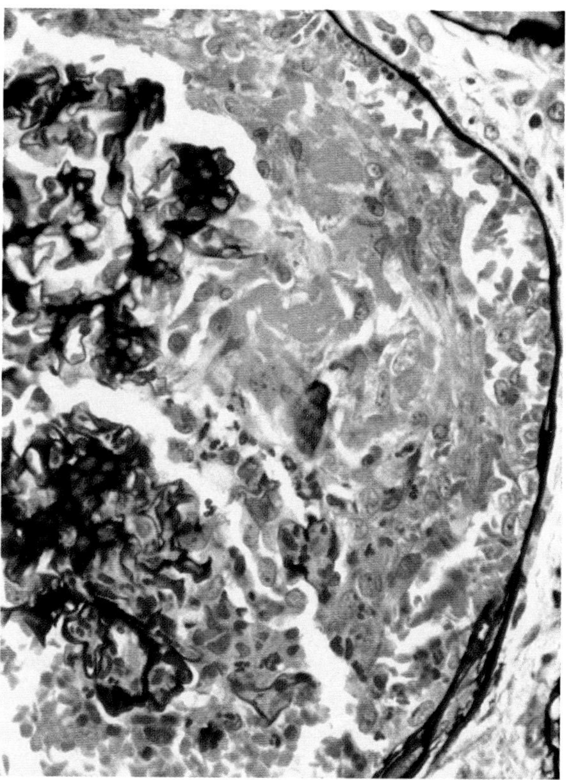

Figure 14-9

ANTI-GBM GLOMERULONEPHRITIS WITH CRESCENT FORMATION

Left: The JMS stain demonstrates extensive lysis of Bowman's capsule as well as segmental lysis of the glomerular tuft. Bowman's space is completely filled by a young crescent with an admixture of fibrin and cells. There is continuity between the exudate in Bowman's space and the periglomerular inflammation, which includes edema and infiltration by predominantly mononuclear leukocytes. Tubular lumens contain numerous erythrocytes, indicative of marked hematuria.

Right: The higher magnification demonstrates extensive spillage of blood constituents (plasma and cells) into Bowman's space where numerous fibrin tactoids are admixed with a few leukocytes and large epithelial/epithelioid cells.

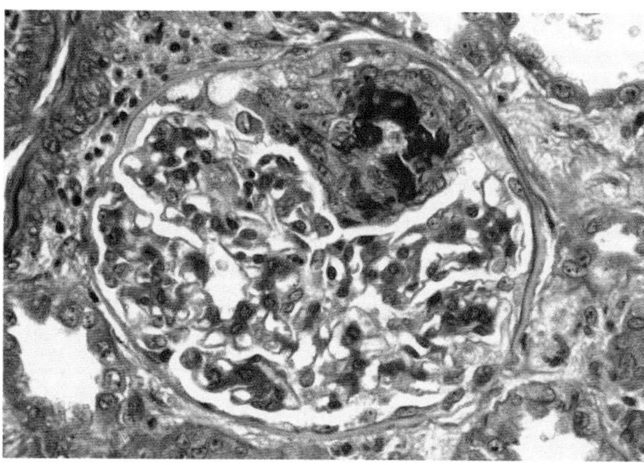

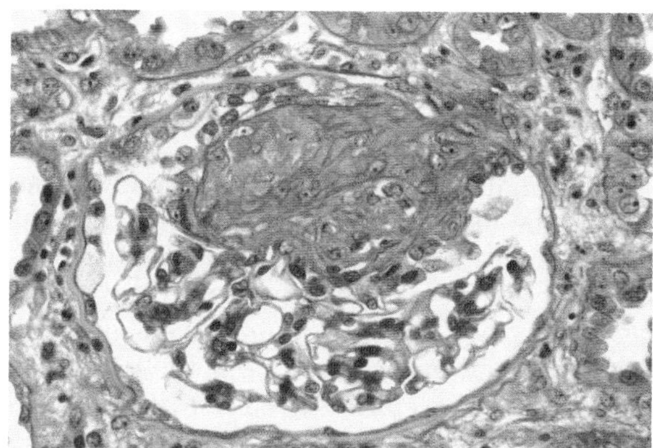

Figure 14-10

ANTI-GBM GLOMERULONEPHRITIS WITH SEGMENTAL NECROSIS AND SEGMENTAL SCLEROSIS

The Masson trichrome stain is useful for distinguishing between foci of fibrinoid necrosis, which stain red (left), and sclerosis, which stain blue (right). Both necrosis and sclerosis stain red with an H&E stain. The uninvolved segments are unremarkable.

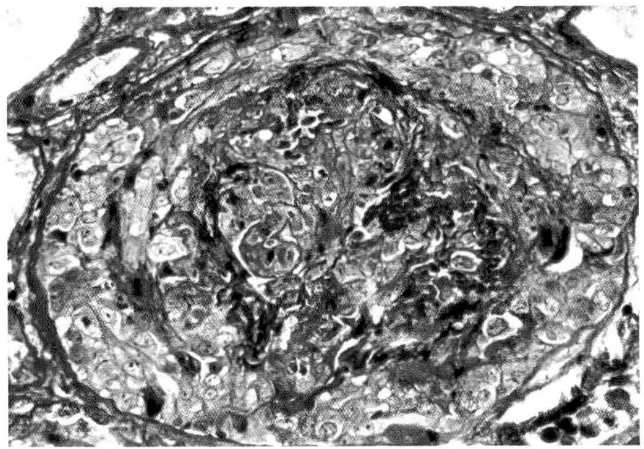

Figure 14-11

ANTI-GBM GLOMERULONEPHRITIS WITH CELLULAR CRESCENT

Fibrin stains dark blue with the phosphotungstic acid-hemotoxylin (PTAH) stain at sites of glomerular fibrinoid necrosis and between some cells within the large circumferential crescent.

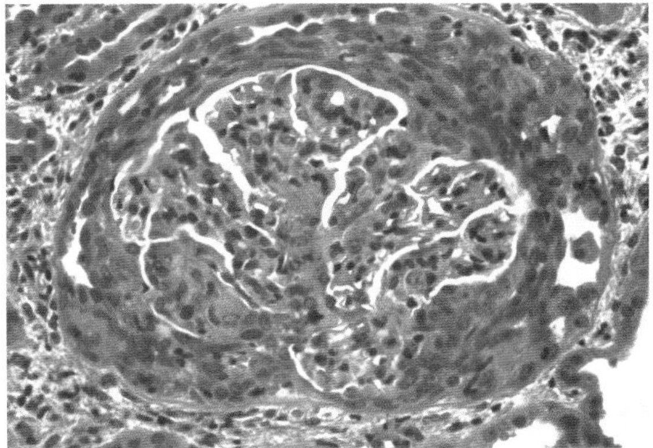

Figure 14-12

ANTI-GBM GLOMERULONEPHRITIS WITH CELLULAR CRESCENT

Bowman's space is completely filled with a large cellular crescent. The glomerular tuft has slight hypercellularity, however, this is difficult to delineate with the H&E stain. There is edema and leukocyte infiltration in the periclomerular interstitum.

no active inflammation or necrosis. Extensive disruption of glomerular basement membranes or Bowman's capsule, which is seen best with the PAS or JMS stain, supports the conclusion that the glomerular scarring is secondary to earlier necrotizing inflammation rather than a less lytic processes, such as ischemia.

The amount of tubulointerstitial injury that accompanies anti-GBM glomerulonephritis usually is commensurate with the amount of glomerular injury and the duration of the disease. In the active phase of acute glomerular injury, tubular lumens in the cortex and medulla contain red blood cell casts or pigmented casts derived from the breakdown of red blood cell casts (fig. 14-17). Varying degrees of interstitial edema, interstitial leukocyte infiltration, tubulitis, and tubular epithelial simplification often accompany acute anti-GBM glomerulonephritis (figs. 14-4–14-19). IgG localized along tubular basement membranes may correlate with more severe tubulointerstitial inflammation (2). This staining typically is restricted to distal tubules that express the alpha 3 chain of type IV collagen. The interstitial infiltrates are most pronounced adjacent to inflamed glomeruli, however, the infiltration may be confluent throughout the cortex if the glomerulonephritis is extensive and diffuse. The infiltrating leukocytes are predominantly mononuclear; however, especially during acute disease, there are varying numbers of admixed neutrophils and eosinophils. As mentioned earlier, periglomerular infiltrates may have a granulomatous appearance, with multinucleated giant cells (fig. 14-14). This periglomerular granulomatous reaction can be caused by anti-GBM glomerulonephritis alone and thus

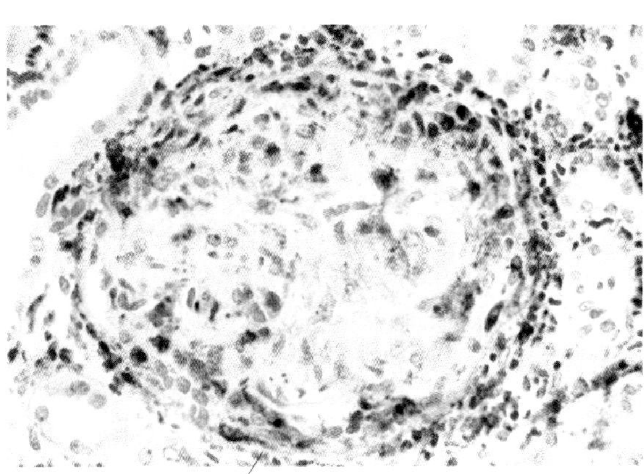

Figure 14-13

ANTI-GBM GLOMERULONEPHRITIS WITH MACROPHAGES IN A CELLULAR CRESCENT

This immunoenzyme microscopy preparation using an antibody specific for monocytes and macrophages (anti-CD68) demonstrates numerous macrophages in a circumferential cellular crescent. Note also the macrophages in the periglomerular interstitium.

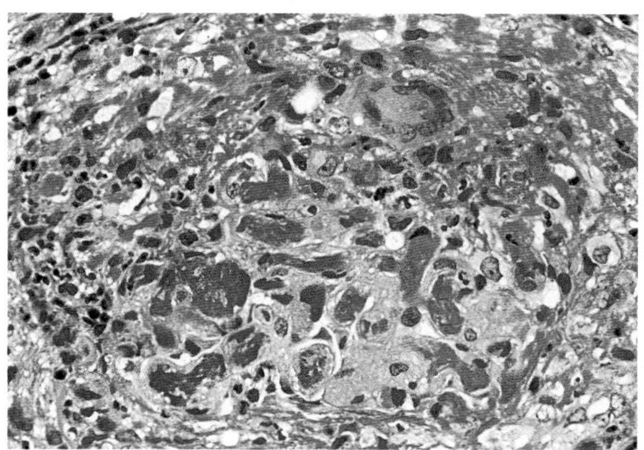

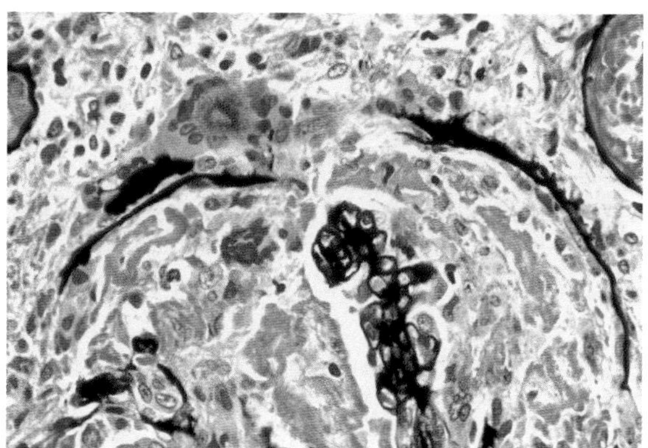

Figure 14-14

ANTI-GBM GLOMERULONEPHRITIS WITH MULTINUCLEATED GIANT CELLS ASSOCIATED WITH DISRUPTION OF BOWMAN'S CAPSULE

Left: The borders between the inflamed glomerulus, crescent, and periglomerular interstitium are difficult to discern in this H&E-stained section. At the top of the panel is a multinucleated giant cell, apparently near where Bowman's capsule should be.

Right: The JMS stain demonstrates extensive disruption of Bowman's capsule. At the site of rupture at the top, there is a multinucleated giant cell in the periglomerular interstitium.

does not require concurrent ANCA disease such as Wegener's granulomatosis (3). Focal acute tubular epithelial simplification (fig. 14-19), which resembles the epithelial injury of ischemic acute renal failure, is most apparent in patients with severe crescentic anti-GBM glomerulonephritis with marked renal failure.

As the glomerulonephritis evolves from an acute to mostly chronic phase, the interstitial edema and tubular epithelial simplification are replaced by interstitial fibrosis and tubular atrophy (fig. 14-16). Acute tubular epithelial simplification and chronic tubular atrophy both have flattened epithelial cells. The former is distinguished by a normal tubular diameter, normal basement membrane thickness, and adjacent interstitial edema (fig. 14-19), whereas the latter is characterized by a reduced tubular diameter, thickened wrinkled basement membranes, and adjacent fibrosis (fig. 14-16).

There is no conclusive evidence that anti-GBM disease alone causes inflammation in vessels other than glomerular capillaries and pulmonary capillaries. Before ANCA vasculitis was recognized, there were case reports of patients with anti-GBM disease who had arteritis. In retrospect, these patients probably had concurrent anti-GBM and ANCA disease. Approximately a quarter to a third of patients with anti-GBM disease patients have ANCAs (8,9,19,52). Patients with both diseases are at risk for developing any of the many renal and systemic expressions of vasculitis that are associated with ANCAs, including arteritis and medullary angiitis in the kidney (20). Thus, identification of arteritis or medullary angiitis in a specimen with anti-GBM glomerulonephritis should prompt serologic testing for ANCAs if it has not already been done. In fact, ANCA testing should be done in any patient with anti-GBM disease because of the high frequency of ANCAs in patients with this disease and the implications for long-term management. Compared to patients who have anti-GBM alone, patients with both anti-GBM and ANCA are older, have somewhat less severe disease, and a better prognosis for response to treatment (Table 14-3) (9,56).

Immunofluorescence Findings. The pathologic sine qua non of anti-GBM glomerulonephritis is linear immunostaining of the GBM for immunoglobulins (figs. 14-20, 14-21) (20,37,44, 47). This is usually accompanied by overt glomerulonephritis, as seen by light microscopy, however, anti-GBM antibodies can be localized in capillaries in specimens that have no identifiable glomerular injury by light microscopy (46). Distal tubular basement membranes may have linear staining as well (fig. 14-20) (2,33), which may contribute to tubulointerstitial injury (2). The results of glomerular and tubular

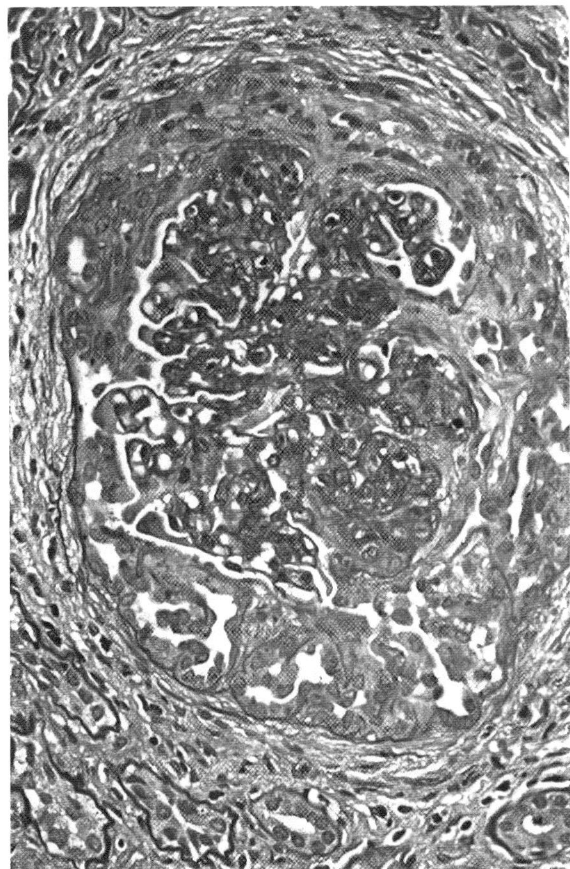

Figure 14-15

ANTI-GBM GLOMERULONEPHRITIS WITH TUBULARIZATION OF A CRESCENT

Epithelial cells within the crescent, especially on the right side, have taken on the appearance of tubules, with lumens and poorly defined basement membranes.

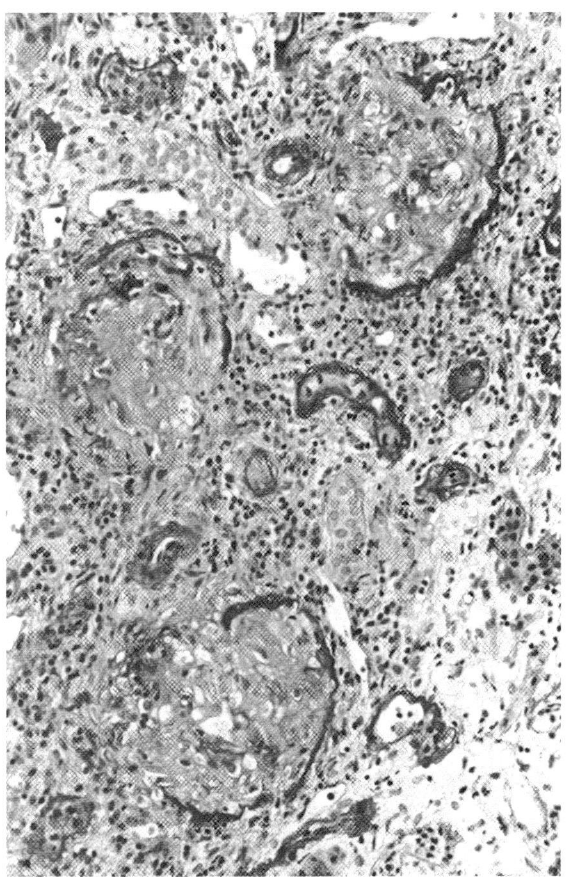

Figure 14-16

CHRONIC ANTI-GBM GLOMERULONEPHRITIS WITH EXTENSIVE GLOMERULAR SCARRING

One year earlier, a renal biopsy revealed severe crescentic anti-GBM glomerulonephritis in this patient. With aggressive immunosuppressive treatment, renal function improved. At the time of the repeat biopsy, proteinuria and renal failure were increasing. Now there is extensive glomerular sclerosis. The demarcation between sclerotic glomeruli and fibrotic crescents is not clear. The extensive disruption of Bowman's capsule and the loss of identifiable GBM cells are consistent with earlier severe necrotizing injury. There are extensive chronic tubulointerstitial changes, including tubular atrophy, interstitial fibrosis, and interstitial infiltration by chronic inflammatory cells.

staining almost always are predominantly positive for IgG, although lesser staining for IgM and IgA often are identified (Table 14-4). Staining is most intense for IgG subclasses IgG1 and IgG4 (50). Rare cases of IgA-dominant anti-GBM glomerulonephritis have been reported (fig. 14-22) (7). The mesangium does not stain for IgG because there is no alpha 3 chain in the collagen of the mesangial matrix. Granular or discontinuous linear GBM staining for C3 and other complement components is usually, but not always, identified (fig. 14-23).

Slight nonspecific linear staining of GBMs for IgG is a frequent finding in many specimens, especially from older patients and from autopsy specimens. The linear staining of anti-GBM disease typically is clearly more intense than this background staining for IgG. On a scale of 0 to 4+, nonspecific background staining usually is trace to 1+ whereas true positive anti-GBM staining usually is 3+ to 4+ (Table 14-4). Intermediate to low-intensity linear staining for IgG should not be considered diagnostic for anti-GBM disease without serologic confirmation of circulating anti-GBM antibodies.

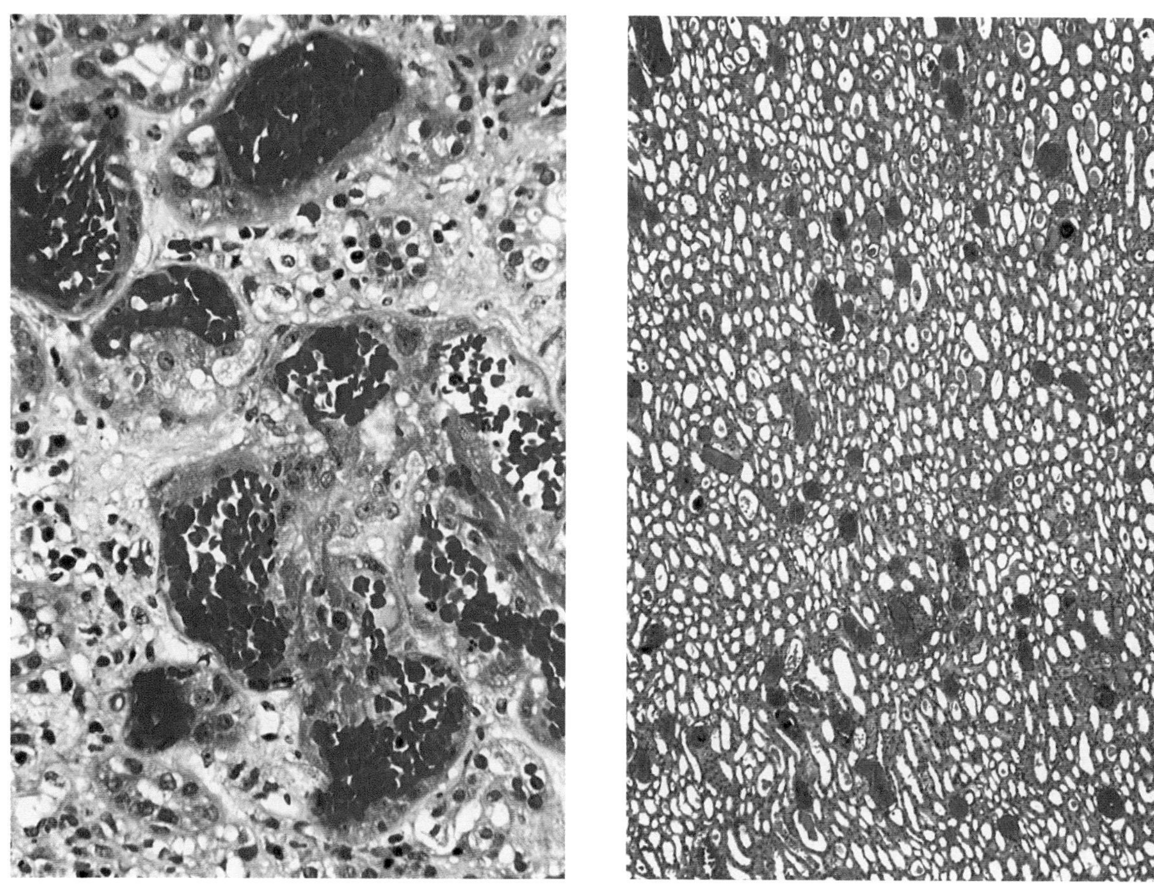

Figure 14-17

ANTI-GBM GLOMERULONEPHRITIS

The numerous red blood cell casts in the cortex (left) and medulla (right) are caused by disruption of glomerular capillaries by anti-GBM disease.

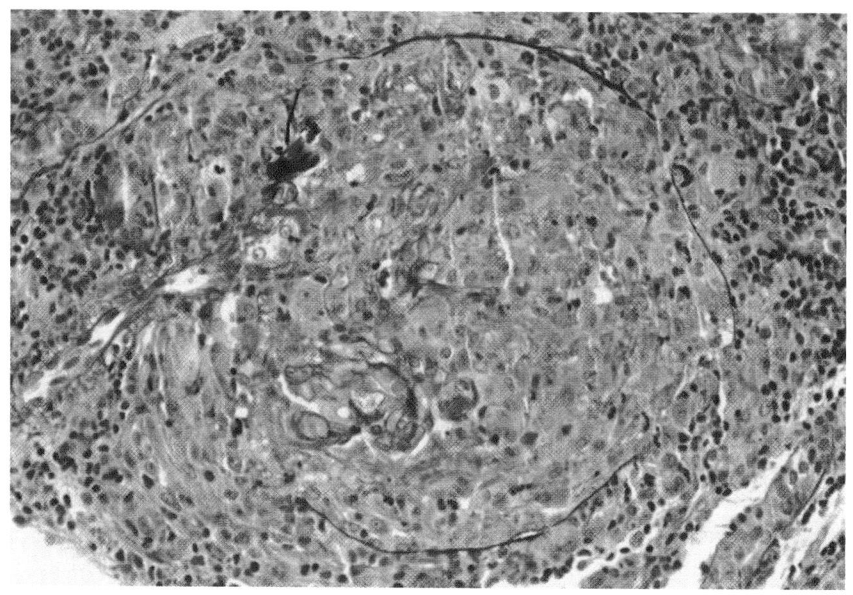

Figure 14-18

ANTI-GBM GLOMERULONEPHRITIS WITH SEVERE GLOMERULAR AND TUBULOINTERSTITIAL INFLAMMATION

This PAS stain reveals intense tubulointerstitial inflammation adjacent to a glomerulus, with extensive lysis of Bowman's capsule and the glomerular tuft. There is extensive interstitial infiltration by mononuclear leukocytes, and some tubules have leukocytes on the epithelial side of the tubular basement membrane (tubulitis).

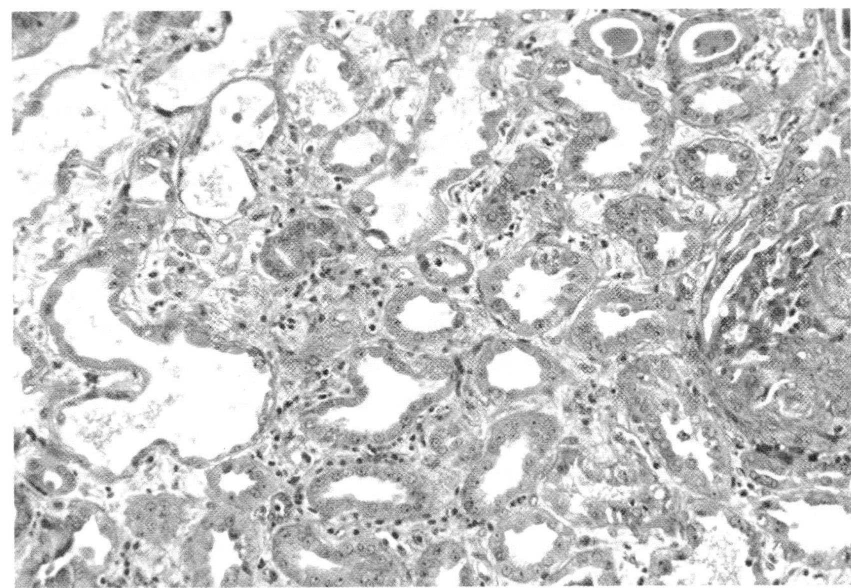

Figure 14-19

ANTI-GBM GLOMERULONEPHRITIS WITH ACUTE TUBULAR EPITHELIAL SIMPLIFICATION

There is focally variable flattening of epithelial cells in a pattern that resembles the epithelial changes of ischemic acute renal failure in the tubules in the upper left corner. There also is interstitial edema and slight infiltration by leukocytes.

Table 14-3

COMPARISON OF CLINICAL AND PATHOLOGIC FEATURES IN PATIENTS WITH ANTIGLOMERULAR BASEMENT MEMBRANE (ANTI-GBM) DISEASE BUT WITHOUT ANTINEUTROPHIL CYTOPLASMIC AUTOANTIBODIES (ANCA) WITH THOSE WHO HAVE BOTH ANTI-GBM AND ANCA DISEASES AT THE TIME OF BIOPSY[a]

	Anti-GBM Positive and ANCA Negative	Anti-GBM Positive and ANCA Positive	P
Number of cases	28	25	
Age	41±21	68±13	*0.0001*
Creatinine at biopsy (mg/dL)	10.0±9.1	9.6±5.3	*0.73*
Anti-GBM titer	579.7	350.5	*0.041*
ANCA titer	<20	72.3±25.0	*<0.0001*
% crescents per specimen	84±21	67±32	*0.027*
Patients with >50% crescents	93%	62%	*0.003*
Glomerular necrosis (0-4+)	2.1+	2.1+	*0.93*
Glomerular sclerosis (0-4+)	1.1+	1.2+	*0.56*

[a]Note that patients with both anti-GBM and ANCA are older and have less extensive crescent formation at the time of diagnosis. Data derived from reference 21.

Table 14-4

IMMUNOFLUORESCENCE MICROSCOPY FINDINGS IN 58 PATIENTS WITH ANTIGLOMERULAR BASEMENT MEMBRANE (ANTI-GBM) GLOMERULONEPHRITIS EVALUATED AT THE UNC NEPHROPATHOLOGY DEPARTMENT[a]

	IgG	IgA	IgM	Kappa	Lambda	C3	C1q
% of specimens positive	100%	39%	55%	100%	100%	96%	10%
Mean intensity when positive (0.5+ to 4+)	3.4+	0.9+	0.8+	2.9+	2.5+	1.6+	0.7+

[a]Positive staining was scored from 0.5+ (trace staining) to 4+ (maximum staining). (Table 14-4 from Jennette JC. Crescentic glomerulonephritis. In: Jennette JC, Olson JL, Schwartz MM, Silva FG, eds. Heptinstall's pathology of the kidney, 5th ed. Philadelphia: Lippincott-Raven; 1998:625–56.); UNC = University of North Carolina.

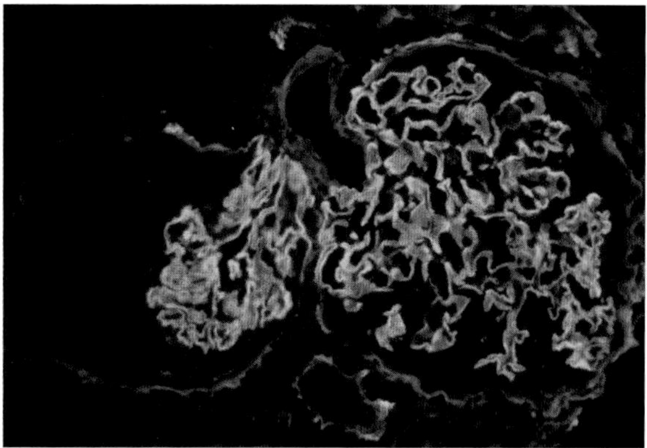

Figure 14-20

LINEAR GBM STAINING FOR IMMUNOGLOBULIN (Ig)G IN ANTI-GBM GLOMERULONEPHRITIS

Two glomeruli have intense linear staining of the GBM with anti-IgG. There is also focal linear staining of tubular basement membranes (e.g., center bottom). The glomerulus on the left has a large negative area within Bowman's space caused by displacement of the tuft by a large crescent.

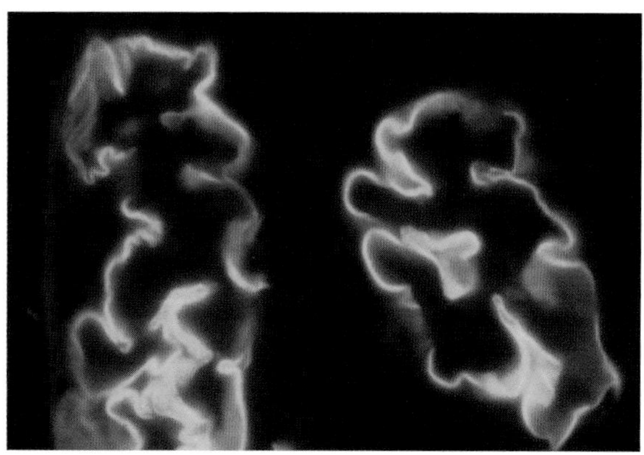

Figure 14-21

LINEAR GBM STAINING FOR IgG IN ANTI-GBM GLOMERULONEPHRITIS

High-power magnification of GBM staining with anti-IgG. There are several breaks in the GBM.

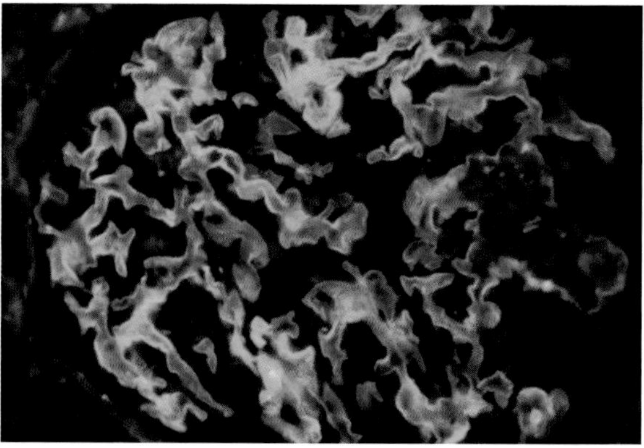

Figure 14-22

LINEAR GBM STAINING FOR IgA IN ANTI-GBM GLOMERULONEPHRITIS

This patient developed end-stage renal disease secondary to Goodpasture's syndrome. She received a renal allograft and 1 year later developed crescentic glomerulonephritis in the transplant. As shown here, the transplant biopsy revealed linear localization of IgA along the GBMs. There was granular staining for C3 but not for IgG or IgM.

The linear staining for immunoglobulins is diffuse and global. However, there may be variability of staining among different glomerular segments and among different glomeruli because of destruction of the GBM by necrosis. In a glomerulus with segmental necrosis, the necrotic segments have no linear staining for immunoglobulins but the intact segments do; glomeruli with extensive necrosis have only a few scattered profiles of residual GBM that have linear staining for IgG (fig. 14-24); and in a glomerulus with total global necrosis, there is no linear GBM staining. A specimen that has only globally necrotic glomeruli with no intact GBMs to examine can cause a misdiagnosis of pauci-immune crescentic glomerulonephritis, that is, crescentic glomerulonephritis with an absence or paucity of immunoglobulin staining. When using immunofluorescence microscopy to examine a specimen with crescentic glomerulonephritis, always use the background fluorescence to identify intact GBM that does not stain for immunoglobulins before making a diagnosis of pauci-immune crescentic glomerulonephritis.

Rare specimens have glomerular anti-GBM localization combined with another type of immune complex localization. The most common combined deposits are subepithelial immune complex deposits indicative of membranous glomerulopathy (23,29,32,39,43). At first glance and at low-power magnification, this may look like anti-GBM glomerulonephritis alone (fig. 14-25, left) or membranous glomerulopathy alone. At higher magnification, however, and with more careful examination, an inner linear and an outer granular staining pattern can be discerned (fig. 14-25, right). The membranous glomerulopathy component is confirmed by electron microscopic demonstration of numerous

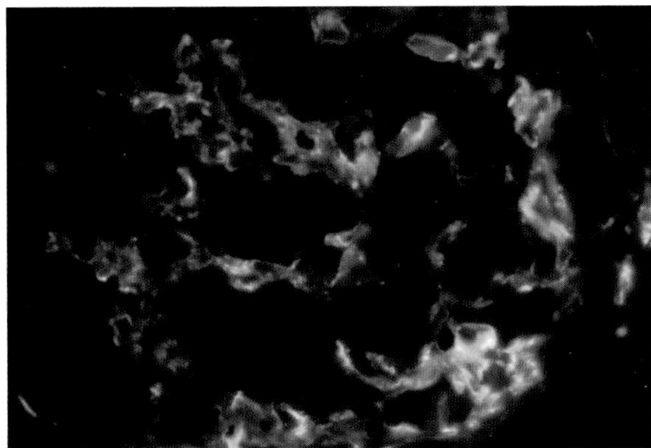

Figure 14-23

GRANULAR C3 STAINING IN ANTI-GBM GLOMERULONEPHRITIS

Unlike the linear staining for IgG, staining for C3 usually is granular, as in this figure. Less commonly, there is a component of discontinuous linear staining for C3.

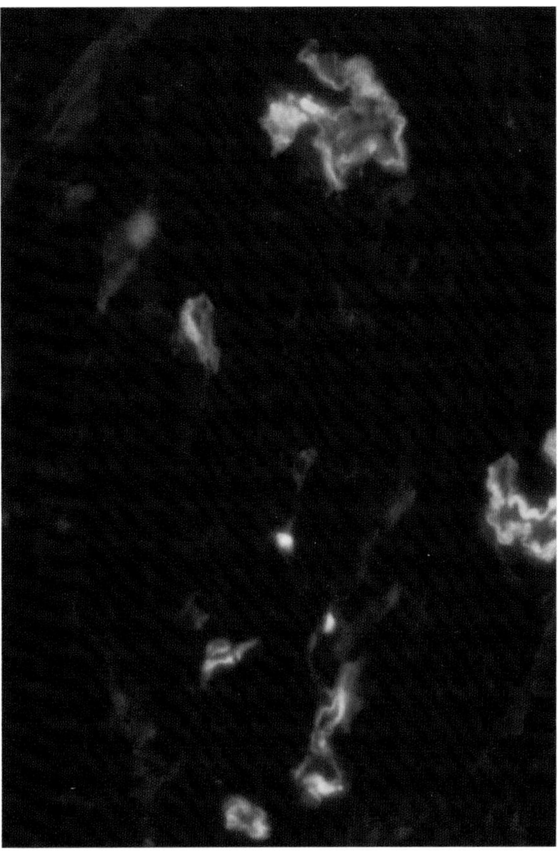

Figure 14-24

FRAGMENTED LINEAR GBM STAINING FOR IgG IN ANTI-GBM GLOMERULONEPHRITIS

There is linear staining of only a few GBM residual fragments in this patient with extensive glomerular necrosis. The light microscopic findings resembled those seen in figure 14-15.

subepithelial electron-dense deposits (fig. 14-26). This combined localization may be present in an initial biopsy or may appear in a second biopsy in a patient who earlier had localization of a single type of immunoglobulin.

Immunostaining for fibrin highlights areas of glomerular necrosis and crescent formation (figs. 14-27,14-28). In Bowman's space, fibrin staining precedes crescent formation. Once crescents form, fibrin staining is most intense in the cellular phase and is progressively lost as the crescents become fibrocellular and then fibrotic. Fibrin staining spills into the periglomerular interstitium at sites of disruption of Bowman's capsule.

Patients with pulmonary involvement have linear localization of IgG and granular localization of C3 along alveolar capillary basement membranes (fig. 14-29, left). In an analogous fashion to the fibrin in Bowman's space after anti-GBM–induced glomerular capillary disruption, alveolar air spaces contain fibrin that can be detected by immunohistology (fig. 14-29, right). In a patient with Goodpasture's syndrome, the diagnostic linear pattern of staining for IgG often is much easier to conclusively recognize in renal biopsy specimens than pulmonary specimens.

Serologic confirmation of anti-GBM disease should always be sought; however, a negative result does not rule out anti-GBM disease in a patient with compelling pathologic evidence. Current immunochemical assays, usually designed as immunoenzyme assays, use purified fragments of type IV collagen or the alpha 3 chain of type IV collagen (27). If true positives are defined as crescentic glomerulonephritis with 3+ or greater linear staining for IgG, the sensitivity of the anti-GBM assay is approximately 80 to 90 percent. On the other hand, if a positive result in an assay for antibodies to type IV collagen is considered to be the gold standard of a true positive, there are a few patients who have pathologic evidence of anti-GBM disease who are negative in such an assay for anti-type IV collagen. These patients may have antibodies to GBM constituents other than

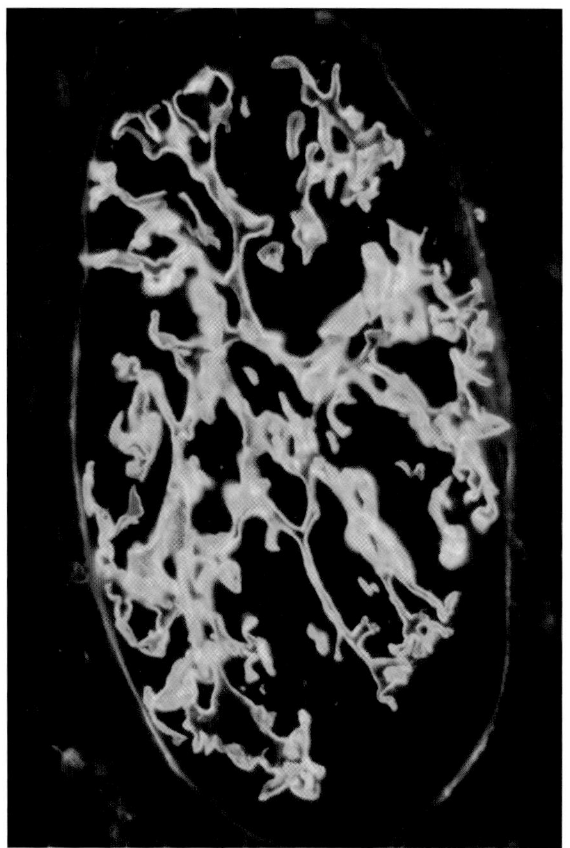

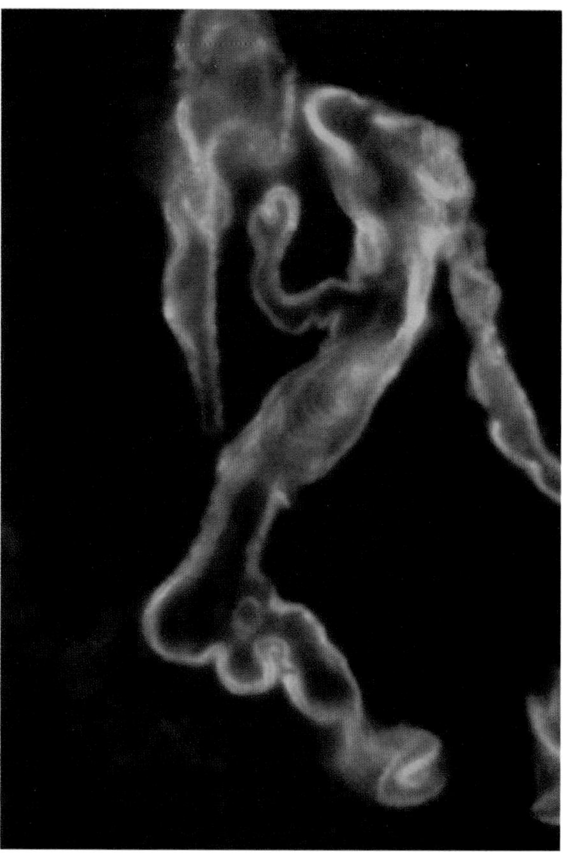

Figure 14-25

CONCURRENT ANTI-GBM GLOMERULONEPHRITIS AND MEMBRANOUS GLOMERULOPATHY

At low-power magnification (left), there seems to be linear staining of GBMs with anti-IgG, however, at high-power magnification (right), an inner linear and an outer granular layer of staining can be discerned in some locations.

Figure 14-26

CONCURRENT ANTI-GBM GLOMERULONEPHRITIS AND MEMBRANOUS GLOMERULOPATHY

Electron microscopy of the same specimen illustrated in figure 14-25 demonstrates numerous subepithelial electron-dense deposits (arrows).

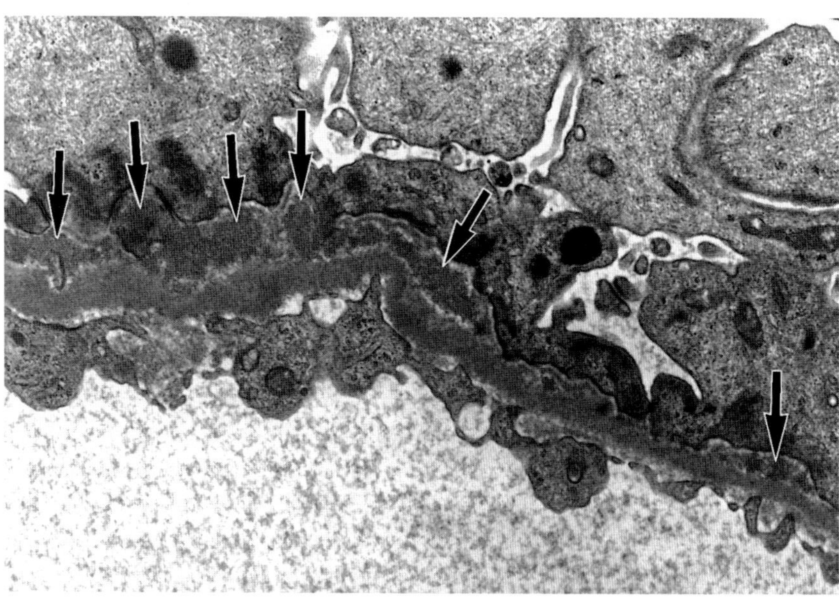

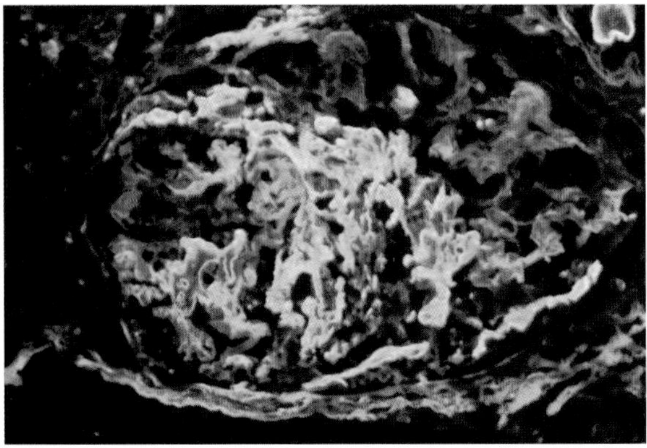

Figure 14-27

FIBRIN STAINING IN FIBRINOID NECROSIS OF ANTI-GBM GLOMERULONEPHRITIS

There is irregular staining for fibrin in areas of segmental fibrinoid necrosis.

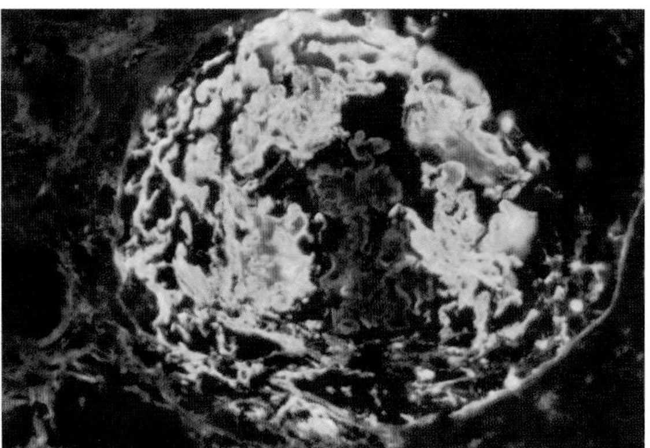

Figure 14-28

FIBRIN STAINING IN A CRESCENT OF ANTI-GBM GLOMERULONEPHRITIS

There is irregular staining for fibrin in a crescent that surrounds a compressed glomerular tuft.

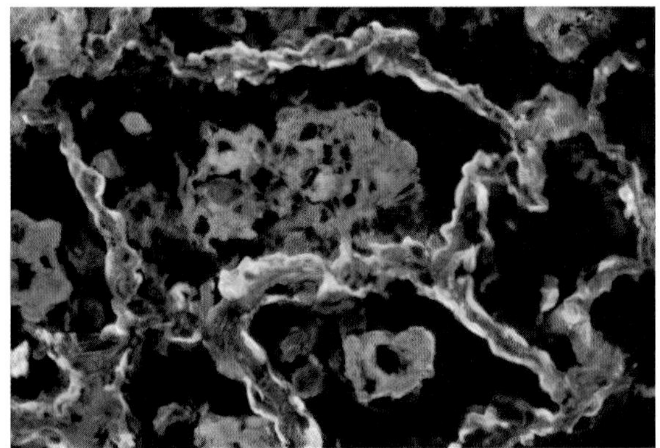

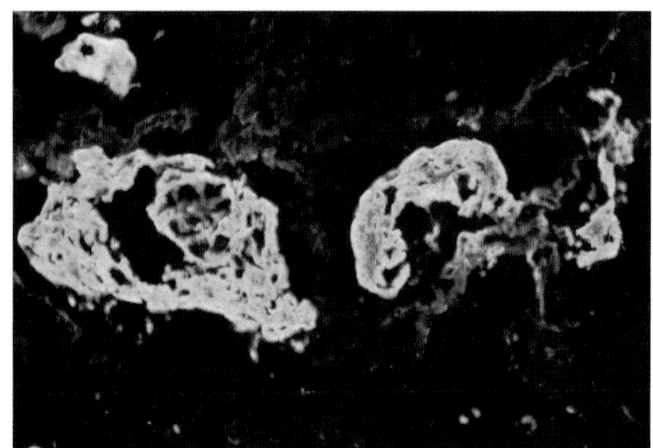

Figure 14-29

GOODPASTURE'S SYNDROME

There is linear staining for IgG along alveolar capillary basement membranes caused by the binding of anti-GBM antibodies (left) and irregular staining for fibrin within the alveolar air spaces caused by hemorrhage (right).

the alpha 3 chain of type IV collagen, for example, antibodies to entactin (48).

Electron Microscopic Findings. Examination of anti-GBM glomerulonephritis by electron microscopy does not reveal specific diagnostic features, but does provide characteristic findings to support the diagnosis (10,20,44,55). The most useful ultrastructural finding is the absence of immune complex–type electron-dense deposits (figs. 14-30, 14-31). This ultrastructural finding in a patient with crescentic glomerulonephritis detected by light microscopy is consistent with anti-GBM glomerulonephritis but is by no means diagnostic because pauci-immune crescentic glomerulonephritis (ANCA crescentic glomerulonephritis), which is much more common than anti-GBM glomerulonephritis, also usually has no immune complex–type electron-dense deposits (20,22). The presence of immune complex–type electron-dense deposits does not completely rule out anti-GBM disease because there are rare examples of concurrent immune complex and anti-GBM glomerulonephritis, especially concurrent membranous glomerulopathy and anti-GBM glomerulonephritis (fig. 14-26) (23,29,32,39,43).

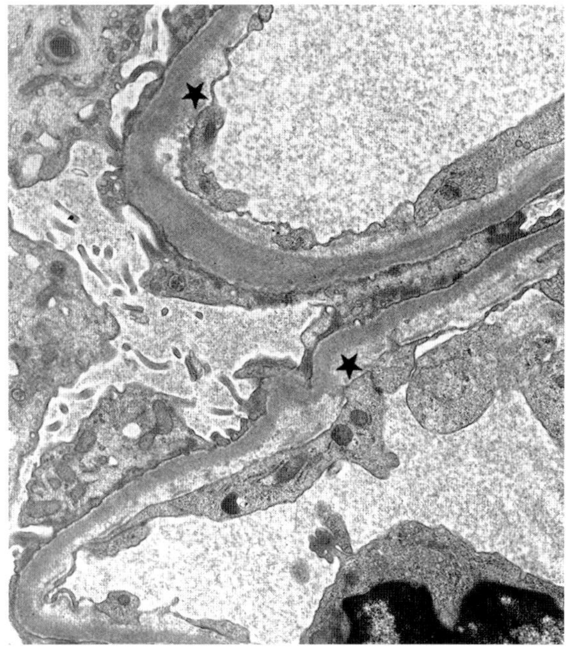

Figure 14-30

SUBENDOTHELIAL LUCENT EXPANSION IN ANTI-GBM GLOMERULONEPHRITIS

The slight irregular lucent expansion of the subendothelial zone (stars) is a common but nonspecific ultrastructural feature of anti-GBM glomerulonephritis. This presumably represents injury caused by the localization of anti-GBM autoantibodies along the adjacent GBM.

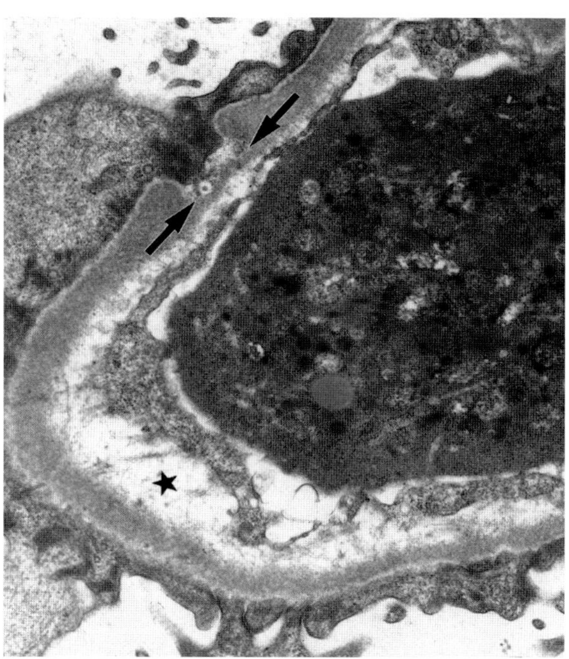

Figure 14-31

PARTIAL GBM BREAK IN ANTI-GBM GLOMERULONEPHRITIS

The arrows delineate an area of partial lysis of the GBM. There is an activated neutrophil in the underlying capillary lumen. Note the lucent expansion of the subendothelial zone (star).

A frequent but nonspecific ultrastructural feature of anti-GBM glomerulonephritis is slight lucent expansion of the subendothelial zone (lamina rara interna) (figs. 14-30, 14-31). In common with other forms of crescentic glomerulonephritis, anti-GBM glomerulonephritis has focal disruption of the GBMs that can be identified by electron microscopy. By transmission electron microscopy, breaks are documented by finding segments of GBM that come to an end (figs. 14-31, 14-32). Normally, the GBM is endless because it is continuous with Bowman's capsule at the hilum, extends uninterrupted around all the capillary loops and paramesangial regions, and eventually merges with the basement membrane of the proximal tubule.

Neutrophils and monocytes may be identified within capillary lumens, especially along stretches of GBM that are denuded of endothelial cytoplasm. At sites of segmental necrosis, electron-dense fibrin is found in capillary thrombi, zones of fibrinoid necrosis, and the interstices between the cells comprising crescents (figs. 14-32, 14-33). The ultrastructural appearance of fibrin varies from amorphous electron-dense material to angular or curvilinear fibrillary tactoids. Care must be taken not to confuse electron-dense fibrin deposits with electron-dense immune complex deposits. This is more of a problem with the amorphous fibrin deposits than the fibrillary fibrin tactoids. If immune complex–type deposits are suspected, the most intact areas of the tuft contain sites of typical mesangial, subendothelial, or subepithelial deposits. If the electron-dense material is confined to areas of severe injury, especially necrosis, this is not adequate evidence of immune complex disease.

Most cells within cellular crescents have the ultrastructural features of epithelial cells or macrophages. The cells in cellular crescents often are surrounded by fibrin tactoids (fig. 14-33). Neutrophils are seen occasionally. At sites of rupture of Bowman's capsule, there is continuity between the crescent and the periglomerular

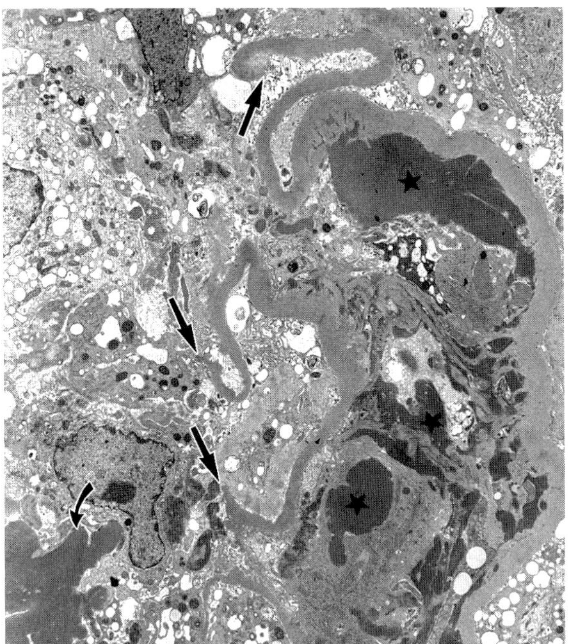

Figure 14-32

GBM BREAKS AND NECROSIS IN ANTI-GBM GLOMERULONEPHRITIS

The GBM terminations (straight arrows) indicate breaks. The capillary lumen contains fibrin thrombi (stars) and there is loss of glomerular cells due to necrosis. This would appear as an area of fibrinoid necrosis by light microscopy. Note also the fibrin in Bowman's space (curved arrow).

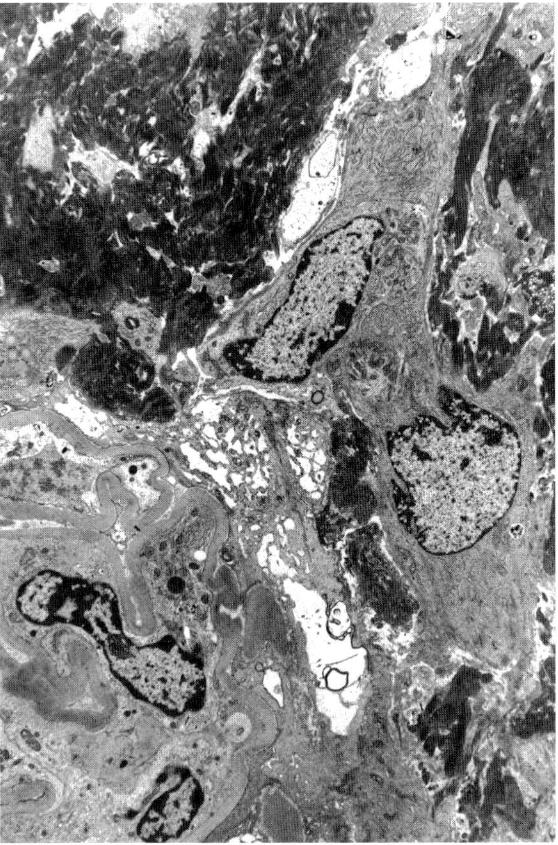

Figure 14-33

CRESCENT IN ANTI-GBM GLOMERULONEPHRITIS

An injured portion of the glomerular tuft is in the lower left quadrant of the electron micrograph. The remainder of the image shows a crescent with electron-dense fibrin tactoids mixed with cells with the ultrastructural features of epithelial cells.

inflammation. As crescents age, they are composed of progressively greater numbers of fibroblasts surrounded by collagen.

Differential Diagnosis. The light microscopic pathologic differential diagnosis of anti-GBM glomerulonephritis includes all other forms of glomerulonephritis with crescent formation. In general, anti-GBM glomerulonephritis has more necrosis and crescent formation and less endocapillary hypercellularity and capillary wall thickening than immune complex glomerulonephritis that is severe enough to cause crescent formation. Thus, a crescentic glomerulonephritis with marked endocapillary hypercellularity and capillary wall thickening is most likely some form of immune complex disease. Pauci-immune crescentic glomerulonephritis, which usually is ANCA-associated glomerulonephritis, is indistinguishable from anti-GBM glomerulonephritis by light microscopy because it also has a propensity for marked segmental to global necrosis and extensive crescent formation, without endocapillary hypercellularity or thick capillary walls.

Of course, detection by immunohistology of linear localization of immunoglobulins, almost always predominantly IgG, along the GBM is the most definitive pathologic evidence for anti-GBM glomerulonephritis. Probably the most difficult distinction is between anti-GBM glomerulonephritis and pauci-immune crescentic glomerulonephritis that has slight nonspecific linear accentuation of IgG staining. This is seen in many specimens, especially from older patients. Each pathologist must develop an internal standard for the expected background staining for IgG in specimens from the laboratory providing the preparations. Staining for albumin is a useful means of establishing the relative level of nonspecific background staining in a specimen. This varies from specimen to specimen and from lab to lab. Confidence in a diagnosis of anti-GBM glomerulonephritis is directly proportional to the intensity of IgG staining above the expected background. An accompanying typical staining pattern for C3 supports the diagnosis.

The differential diagnosis for linear GBM staining of immunoglobulins includes diabetic glomerulosclerosis and monoclonal immunoglobulin deposition disease. Both of these usually have different clinical presentations and different patterns of glomerular injury. Neither is characterized by fibrinoid necrosis or substantial crescent formation, and both produce predominantly mesangial matrix expansion (often nodular) rather than glomerular inflammation. Patients with diabetic glomerulosclerosis should have clinical evidence of diabetes, and patients with monoclonal immunoglobulin deposition disease often have clinical evidence of a monoclonal gammopathy. Patients with monoclonal immunoglobulin deposition disease also have monoclonal immunoglobulin chains causing the linear staining, which are evident if antibodies to immunoglobulin light chains are used for renal biopsy evaluation. For example, a patient with gamma heavy chain deposition disease will have linear GBM staining with an anti-IgG antibody but will have negative staining for kappa and lambda light chains.

Keep in mind that patients with anti-GBM glomerulonephritis can have concurrent ANCA or immune complex disease. Thus, an ANCA-positive patient with pulmonary-renal vasculitic syndrome or rapidly progressive glomerulonephritis could have concurrent anti-GBM glomerulonephritis (8,9,19,52). Likewise, a patient with unequivocal glomerular immune complex deposits, especially in a membranous glomerulopathy pattern, could have concurrent anti-GBM glomerulonephritis (23,29,32,39,43).

Etiology and Pathogenesis. Lerner, Glassock, and Dixon (34) reported in 1967 that the serum and kidneys from patients with glomerulonephritis and linear IgG staining contained antibodies specific for antigens in the GBM. In addition, they demonstrated that these antibodies caused glomerulonephritis when they were injected into monkeys. This confirmed the pathogenicity of anti-GBM antibodies, which already had been demonstrated in sheep and goats that had been immunized with GBM antigens (15,41,53). The pathogenicity of anti-GBM antibodies also is demonstrated in patients with Alport's syndrome who develop anti-GBM glomerulonephritis in transplanted kidneys, although this occurs only in a minority of patients (30,42,51). Patients with Alport's syndrome do not express the anti-GBM target antigen in their own GBMs and thus may develop an immune response to the normally expressed GBM antigens in renal allografts, which can result in the induction of anti-GBM glomerulonephritis in the transplant.

The major epitope for anti-GBM antibodies resides in the noncollagenous domain of the type IV collagen molecule and is in the alpha 3 chain (17,24,26). The specificity of anti-GBM antibodies is the same in patients with Goodpasture's syndrome and anti-GBM glomerulonephritis alone (27). An additive pathogenic factor, such as injurious agents in cigarette smoke or other hydrocarbons, or respiratory tract infection (e.g., influenza) may be required for the development of pulmonary capillary injury (5,13,26). The initial impetus for the immunogenesis of the anti-GBM response is unknown. Injury to the GBM with release or modification of collagen epitopes, has been postulated, for example by hydrocarbons, such as fumes from glue (6), or fragmentation, such as disruption by lithotripsy (59).

Susceptibility to developing anti-GBM disease is influenced by the human leukocyte antigen (HLA) DR and DQ genotypes (18,59). This raises the possibility that the capacity or character of major histocompatibility complex (MHC) antigen presentation is important for GBM immunogenicity or for leukocyte pathogenicity.

T lymphocytes and macrophages are involved in the mediation of vascular injury in anti-GBM disease (4,24). This could be as secondary mediators without specific antigen recognition by the T lymphocytes, or as a component of the primary immune injury with T-lymphocyte activation by specific recognition of GBM antigens. Support for a major role for T lymphocytes in anti-GBM disease comes from experimental models of glomerulonephritis induced in rats by injection of GBM antigens in adjuvant (45). In this model, blockade of T-lymphocyte function markedly ameliorated anti-GBM glomerulonephritis.

Treatment and Prognosis. Anti-GBM glomerulonephritis, whether it occurs alone or as a component of Goodpasture's syndrome, usually is an aggressive disease that warrants rapid institution of vigorous immunosuppressive therapy (10,11,25,35). Standard treatment includes high-dose corticosteroids (e.g., intravenous or oral methylprednisolone followed by oral prednisone), cytotoxic drugs (e.g., cyclophosphamide), and plasmapheresis.

The severity of the renal injury and the serum creatinine level at the time treatment is initiated influence the prognosis (25,35). Of 71 patients with anti-GBM glomerulonephritis who received plasma exchange, prednisolone, and cyclophosphamide, those with an initial creatinine level of less than 5.7 mg/dL had 100 percent patient and 95 percent renal survival rates at 1 year, those with creatinine levels over 5.7 mg/dL and not requiring dialysis initially had patient and renal survival rates of 83 and 82 percent at 1 year, and those who required dialysis at presentation had patient and renal survival rates of 65 and 8 percent at 1 year (35). Thus, making a diagnosis of anti-GBM glomerulonephritis rapidly and beginning therapy immediately is extremely important for optimum outcome.

Patients with anti-GBM glomerulonephritis have a worse prognosis than those with ANCA glomerulonephritis or immune complex glomerulonephritis (11). A positive ANCA in a patient with anti-GBM disease correlates with a better prognosis (9). This may be because patients with anti-GBM and ANCA diseases have less severe findings at the time of initial biopsy than patients with anti-GBM glomerulonephritis alone (see Table 14-3) (56).

Once the initial episode of acute injury enters remission, recurrences of active disease are uncommon, but may occur even many years later (12,28,58). Anti-GBM glomerulonephritis can recur in renal allografts (1) but this is uncommon if transplantation is delayed until anti-GBM antibodies are undetectable in the serum (10).

REFERENCES

1. Almkuist RD, Buckalew VM Jr, Hirszel P, Maher JF, James PM, Wilson CB. Recurrence of anti-glomerular basement membrane antibody mediated glomerulonephritis in an isograft. Clin Immunol Immunopathol 1981;18:54–60.
2. Andres G, Brentjens J, Kohli R, et al. Histology of human tubulo-interstitial nephritis associated with antibodies to renal basement membranes. Kidney Int 1978;13:480–91.
3. Bajema IM, Hagen EC, Ferrario F, et al. Renal granulomas in systemic vasculitis. EC/BCR Project for ANCA-Assay Standardization. Clin Nephrol 1997;48:16–21.
4. Bolton WK, Innes DJ Jr., Sturgill BC, Kaiser DL. T-cells and macrophages in rapidly progressive glomerulonephritis: clinicopathologic correlations. Kidney Int 1987;32:869–76.
5. Bombassei GJ, Kaplan AA. The association between hydrocarbon exposure and anti-glomerular basement membrane antibody-mediated disease (Goodpasture's syndrome). Am J Ind Med 1992;21:141–53.
6. Bonzel KE, Muller-Wiefel DE, Ruder H, Wingen AM, Waldherr R, Weber M. Anti-glomerular basement membrane antibody-mediated glomerulonephritis due to glue sniffing. Eur J Ped 1987;146:296–300.
7. Border WA, Baehler RW, Bhathena D, Glassock RJ. IgA antibasement membrane nephritis with pulmonary hemorrhage. Ann Intern Med 1979; 91:21–5.
8. Bosch X, Mirapeix E, Font J, et al. Anti-myeloperoxidase autoantibodies in patients with necrotizing glomerular and alveolar capillaritis. Am J Kidney Dis 1992;20:231–9.
9. Bosch X, Mirapeix E, Font J, et al. Prognostic implication of anti-neutrophil cytoplasmic autoantibodies with myeloperoxidase specificity in anti-glomerular basement membrane disease. Clin Nephrol 1991;36:107–13.
10. Briggs WA, Johnson JP, Teichman S, Yeager HC, Wilson CB. Antiglomerular basement membrane antibody-mediated glomerulonephritis and Goodpasture's syndrome. Medicine 1979;58: 348–61.

11. Couser WG. Rapidly progressive glomerulonephritis: classification, pathogenetic mechanisms, and therapy. Am J Kidney Dis 1988;11:449–64.
12. Dahlberg PJ, Kurtz SB, Donadio JV, et al. Recurrent Goodpasture's syndrome. Mayo Clin Proc 1978;53:533–7.
13. Donaghy M, Rees AJ. Cigarette smoking and lung hemorrhage in glomerulonephritis caused by autoantibodies to glomerular basement membrane. Lancet 1983;2:1390–3.
14. Ferrario F, Tadros MT, Napodano P, Sinico RA, Fellin G, D'Amico G. Critical re-evaluation of 41 cases of "idiopathic" crescentic glomerulonephritis. Clin Nephrol 1994;41:1–9.
15. Germuth FG Jr, Choi IJ, Taylor JJ, Rodriguez E. Antibasement membrane disease. I. The glomerular lesions of Goodpasture's disease and experimental disease in sheep. Johns Hopkins Med J 1972;131:367–84.
16. Goodpasture EW. The significance of certain pulmonary lesions in relation to the etiology of influenza. Am J Med Sci 1919;158:863–70.
17. Hellmark T, Johansson C, Wieslander J. Characterization of anti-GBM antibodies involved in Goodpasture's syndrome. Kidney Int 1994;46:823–9.
18. Huey B, McCormick K, Capper J, et al. Association of HLA-DR and HLA-DQ types with anti-GBM nephritis by sequence-specific oligonucleotide probe hybridization. Kidney Int 1993;44:307–12.
19. Jayne DR, Marshall PD, Jones SJ, Lockwood CM. Autoantibodies to GBM and neutrophil cytoplasm in rapidly progressive glomerulonephritis. Kidney Int 1990;37:965–70.
20. Jennette JC. Crescentic glomerulonephritis. In: Jennette JC, Olson JL, Schwartz MM, Silva FG, eds. Heptinstall's pathology of the kidney, 5th ed. Philadelphia: Lippincott-Raven; 1998:625–56.
21. Jennette JC. Rapidly progressive crescentic glomerulonephritis. Kidney Int 2003;63:1164–77.
22. Jennette JC, Falk RJ. The pathology of vasculitis involving the kidney. Am J Kidney Dis 1994;24:130–41.
23. Jennette JC, Lamanna RW, Burnette JP, Wilkman AS, Iskander SS. Concurrent antiglomerular basement membrane antibody and immune complex mediated glomerulonephritis. Am J Clin Pathol 1982;78:381–6.
24. Johnson JP, Moore J Jr, Austin HA 3rd, Balow JE, Antonovych TT, Wilson CB. Therapy of anti-glomerular basement membrane antibody disease: analysis of prognostic significance of clinical, pathologic and treatment factors. Medicine 1985;64:219–27.
25. Jones DA, Jennette JC, Falk RJ. Goodpastures's syndrome revisited. A new perspective on glomerulonephritis and alveolar hemorrhage. N C Med J 1990;51:411–5.
26. Kalluri R, Sun MJ, Hudson BG, Neilson EG. The Goodpasture autoantigen. Structural delineation of two immunologically privileged epitopes on alpha3(IV) chain of type IV collagen. J Biol Chem 1996;271:9062–8.
27. Kalluri R, Wilson CB, Weber M, et al. Identification of the alpha 3 chain of type IV collagen as the common autoantigen in antibasement membrane disease and Goodpasture syndrome. J Am Soc Nephrol 1995;6:1178–85.
28. Klasa RJ, Abboud RT, Ballon HS, Grossman L. Goodpasture's syndrome: recurrence after a five-year remission. Case report and review of the literature. Am J Med 1988;84:751–5.
29. Klassen J, Elwood C, Grossberg AL, et al. Evolution of membranous nephropathy into anti-glomerular-basement-membrane glomerulonephritis. N Engl J Med 1974;290:1340–4.
30. Kleppel MM, Fan WW, Cheong HI, Kashtan CE, Michael AF. Immunochemical studies of the Alport antigen. Kidney Int 1992;41:1629–37.
31. Knoll G, Rabin E, Burns BF. Antiglomerular basement membrane antibody-mediated nephritis with normal pulmonary and renal function. A case report and review of the literature. Am J Nephrol 1993;13:494–6.
32. Kurki P, Helve T, von Bonsdorff M, et al. Transformation of membranous glomerulonephritis into crescentic glomerulonephritis with glomerular basement membrane antibodies. Serial determinations of anti-GBM before the transformation. Nephron 1984;38:134–7.
33. Lehman DH, Wilson CB, Dixon FJ. Extraglomerular immunoglobulin deposits in human nephritis. Am J Med 1975;58:765–7.
34. Lerner RA, Glassock RJ, Dixon FJ. The role of anti-glomerular basement membrane antibody in the pathogenesis of human glomerulonephritis. J Exp Med 1967;126:989–1004.
35. Levy JB, Turner AN, Rees AJ, Pusey CD. Long-term outcome of anti-glomerular basement membrane antibody disease treated with plasma exchange and immunosuppression. Ann Intern Med 2001;134:1033–42.
36. Magil AB, Wadsworth LD. Monocyte involvement in glomerular crescents: a histochemical and ultrastructural study. Lab Invest 1982;47:160–6.
37. Martinez JS, Kohler PF. Variant "Goodpasture's syndrome"? The need for immunologic criteria in rapidly progressive glomerulonephritis and hemorrhagic pneumonitis. Ann Intern Med 1971;75:67–76.

38. McPhaul JJ Jr, Mullins JD. Glomerulonephritis mediated by antibody to glomerular basement membrane. Immunological, clinical, and histopathological characteristics. J Clin Invest 1976;57:351–61.
39. Moorthy AV, Zimmerman SW, Burkholder PM, Harrington AR. Association of crescentic glomerulonephritis with membranous glomerulonephropathy: a report of three cases. Clin Nephrol 1976;6:319–25.
40. Niles JL, Bottinger EP, Saurina GR, et al. The syndrome of lung hemorrhage and nephritis is usually an ANCA-associated condition. Arch Intern Med 1996;56:440–5.
41. Ohnuki T. Crescentic glomerulonephritis induced in the goat by immunization with homologous or heterologous glomerular basement membrane antigen. Acta Pathol Jpn 1975;25: 319–31.
42. Oliver TB, Gouldesbrough DR, Swainson CP. Acute crescentic glomerulonephritis associated with antiglomerular basement membrane antibody in Alport's syndrome after second transplantation. Nephrol Dial Transplant 1991;6:893–5.
43. Pettersson E, Tornroth T, Miettinen A. Simultaneous anti-glomerular basement membrane and membranous glomerulonephritis: case report and literature review. Clin Immunol Immunopathol 1984;31:171–80.
44. Poskitt TR. Immunologic and electron microscopic studies in Goodpasture's syndrome. Am J Med 1970;49:250–7.
45. Reynolds J, Tam FW, Chandraker A, et al. CD28-B7 blockade prevents the development of experimental autoimmune glomerulonephritis. J Clin Invest 2000;105:643–51.
46. Saraf P, Berger HW, Thung SN. Goodpasture's syndrome with no overt renal disease. Mt Sinai J Med 1978;45:451–4.
47. Savage CO, Pusey CD, Bowman C, Rees AJ, Lockwood CM. Antiglomerular basement membrane antibody mediated disease in the British Isles 1980-4. Br Med J (Clin Res Ed) 1986;292: 301–4.
48. Saxena R, Bygren P, Arvastson B, Wieslander J. Circulating autoantibodies as serological markers in the differential diagnosis of pulmonary renal syndrome. J Intern Med 1995;238:143–52.
49. Scheer RL, Grossman MA. Immune aspects of glomerulonephritis associated with pulmonary hemorrhage. Ann Intern Med 1964;60:1009–21.
50. Segelmark M, Butkowski R, Wieslander J. Antigen restriction and IgG subclasses among anti-GBM autoantibodies. Nephrol Dial Transplant 1990;5:991–6.
51. Shah B, First MR, Mendoza NC, Clyne DH, Alexander JW, Weiss MA. Alport's syndrome: risk of glomerulonephritis induced by anti-glomerular-basement-membrane antibody after renal transplantation. Nephron 1988;50:34–8.
52. Short AK, Esnault VL, Lockwood CM. Anti-neutrophil cytoplasm antibodies and anti-glomerular basement membrane antibodies: two coexisting distinct autoreactivities detectable in patients with rapidly progressive glomerulonephritis. Am J Kidney Dis 1995;26:439–45.
53. Steblay RW. Glomerulonephritis induced in sheep by injections of heterologous glomerular basement membrane and Freund's complete adjuvant. J Exp Med 1962;116:253–72.
54. Sturgill BC, Westervelt FB. Immunofluorescence studies in a case of Goodpasture's syndrome. JAMA 1965;194:914–16.
55. Teague CA, Doak PB, Simpson IJ, Rainer SP, Herdson PB. Goodpasture's syndrome: an analysis of 29 cases. Kidney Int 1978;13:492–504.
56. Wilkman AS, Hogan SL, Falk RJ, Jennette JC. Clinicopathologic features of concurrent ANCA and anti-GBM glomerulonephritis. Clin Exp Immunol 2000;120(Suppl 1):58.
57. Wilson CB, Dixon FJ. Anti-glomerular basement membrane antibody-induced glomerulonephritis. Kidney Int 1973;3:74–89.
58. Wu MJ, Moorthy AV, Beirne GJ. Relapse in anti-glomerular basement membrane antibody mediated crescentic glomerulonephritis. Clin Nephrol 1980;13:97–102.
59. Xenocostas A, Jothy S, Collins B, Loertscher R, Levy M. Anti-glomerular basement membrane glomerulonephritis after extracorporeal shock wave lithotripsy. Am J Kidney Dis 1999;33:128–32.

15 ANTINEUTROPHIL CYTOPLASMIC AUTOANTIBODY–ASSOCIATED PAUCI-IMMUNE GLOMERULONEPHRITIS AND VASCULITIS, AND OTHER VASCULITIDES

The kidneys are highly vascularized organs and thus are susceptible to involvement by many forms of vasculitis. Every type of vasculitis listed in Table 15-1, as well as others, can affect the kidneys (29,30). Figure 15-1 demonstrates that different types of vasculitis have different distributions of renal vascular involvement. The small vessel vasculitides are the most frequent in the kidneys, most often manifesting as glomerulonephritis. These include microscopic polyangiitis, Wegener's granulomatosis, Churg-Strauss syndrome, Henoch-Schönlein purpura, and cryoglobulinemic vasculitis (31,32). Henoch-Schönlein purpura and cryoglobulinemic vasculitis are reviewed in detail in other chapters and are mentioned here primarily in discussions of differential diagnosis. Because of their importance as causes of renal disease, pauci-immune small vessel vasculitis (antineutrophil cytoplasmic autoantibody [ANCA] small vessel vasculitis) and its renal-limited variant, pauci-immune crescentic glomerulonephritis, are emphasized.

Table 15-1

CATEGORIES OF VASCULITIS THAT ARE NOT KNOWN TO BE CAUSED BY DIRECT INVASION OF VESSEL WALLS BY INFECTIOUS PATHOGENS[a]

Large Vessel Vasculitis (Chronic Granulomatous Arteritis)
Giant cell arteritis
Takayasu's arteritis
Medium-Sized Vessel Vasculitis (Necrotizing Arteritis)
Kawasaki's disease
Polyarteritis nodosa
Small Vessel Vasculitis (Necrotizing Polyangiitis)
Henoch-Schönlein purpura[b]
Cryoglobulinemic vasculitis[b]
Infection-induced immune complex vasculitis (e.g., secondary to hepatitis B or C)[b]
Lupus vasculitis[b]
Rheumatoid vasculitis[b]
Serum sickness vasculitis[b]
Goodpasture's syndrome[b]
Wegener's granulomatosis[c]
Microscopic polyangiitis[c]
Churg-Strauss syndrome[c]

[a]All of these vasculitides can affect the kidney, however, the small vessel vasculitides have the greatest predilection for renal involvement.

[b]Immune complex–mediated vasculitis.

[c]Antineutrophil cytoplasmic autoantibody (ANCA)-associated vasculitis.

PAUCI-IMMUNE CRESCENTIC GLOMERULONEPHRITIS, MICROSCOPIC POLYANGIITIS, WEGENER'S GRANULOMATOSIS, AND CHURG-STRAUSS SYNDROME

Definition. *Pauci-immune crescentic glomerulonephritis* is characterized by crescent formation and an absence or paucity of glomerular immunoglobulins or complement. It is one of the three major immunopathologic categories of crescentic glomerulonephritis (fig. 15-2). The other two categories are *immune complex crescentic glomerulonephritis* and *antiglomerular basement membrane (anti-GBM) antibody crescentic glomerulonephritis.* An alternative designation for pauci-immune crescentic glomerulonephritis is *ANCA-associated crescentic glomerulonephritis* (or *ANCA crescentic glomerulonephritis*) because approximately 80 percent of patients with this form of glomerulonephritis have ANCAs in the circulation (12,19,22,26,34,43,45). Yet another term for pauci-immune crescentic glomerulonephritis is *renal-limited vasculitis* because the glomerular lesion is identical to the glomerular injury that occurs as a component of pauci-immune small vessel vasculitis. In fact, pauci-immune crescentic glomerulonephritis is accompanied by systemic pauci-immune small vessel vasculitis in about 75 percent of patients. Pauci-immune small vessel vasculitis includes microscopic polyangiitis, Wegener's granulomatosis, and Churg-Strauss syndrome.

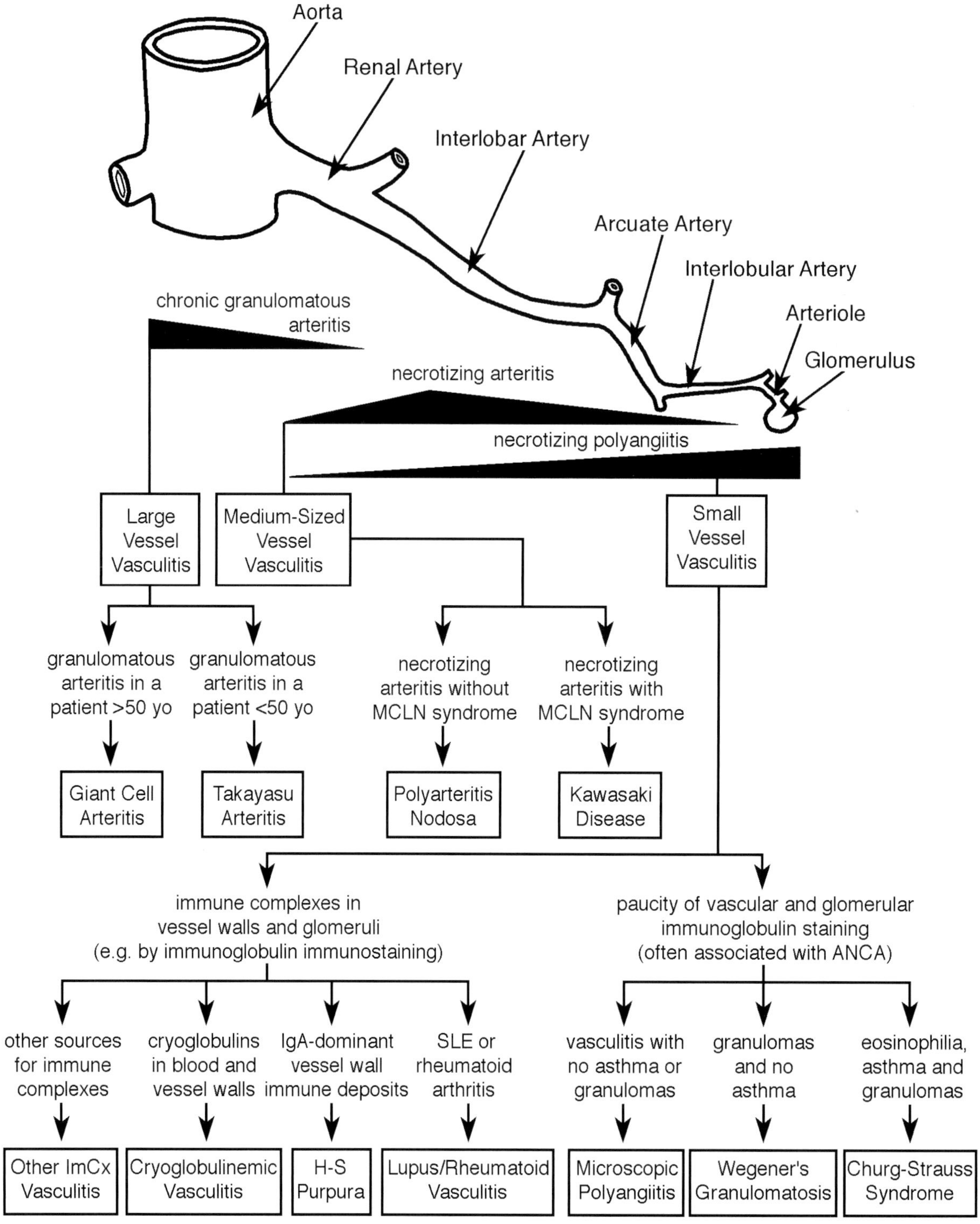

Figure 15-1

VASCULITIS IN THE KIDNEY

Diagram depicting the major distributions of vessel involvement in the kidney by various types of systemic vasculitis. When there is symptomatic involvement of the kidneys, large vessel vasculitis usually causes renovascular hypertension, medium-sized vessel vasculitis causes infarcts and hemorrhage, and small vessel vasculitis causes glomerulonephritis.

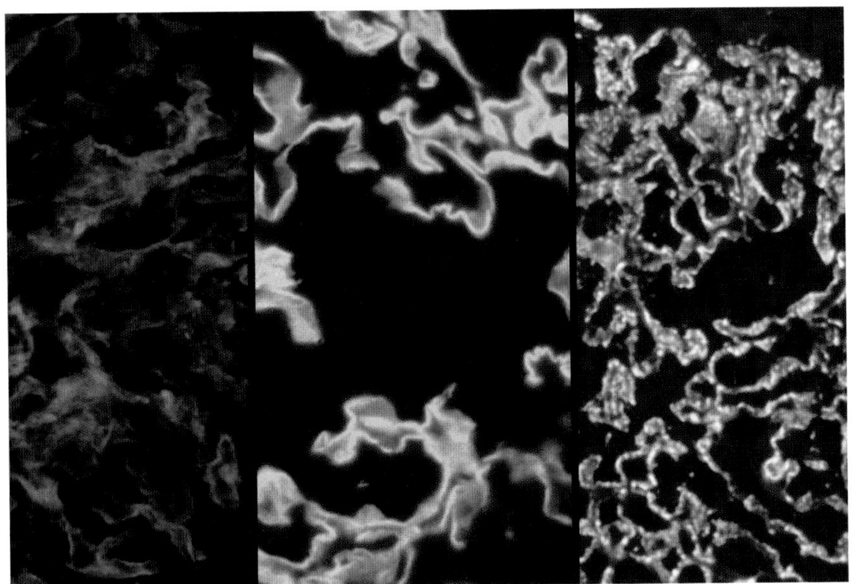

Figure 15-2

IMMUNOPATHOLOGIC CATEGORIES OF CRESCENTIC GLOMERULONEPHRITIS

The three major patterns of glomerular immunoglobulin staining seen by immunofluorescence microscopy in crescentic glomerulonephritis are little or no staining indicative of pauci-immune crescentic glomerulonephritis (left), granular staining indicative of immune complex crescentic glomerulonephritis (center), and linear glomerular basement membrane (GBM) staining indicative of anti-GBM crescentic glomerulonephritis (right) (fluorescein-labeled anti-IgG).

Microscopic polyangiitis is a necrotizing vasculitis with few or no immune deposits that affects small vessels (capillaries, venules, or arterioles) (15,32,33,42,44). Crescentic glomerulonephritis is frequent. Necrotizing arteritis involving small and medium-sized arteries may or may not be present. An alternative term for this form of vasculitis is *microscopic polyarteritis,* however, this is a less desirable designation because many patients have no evidence of arteritis. For example, a patient with microscopic polyangiitis could have dermal venulitis (purpura), pulmonary capillaritis, and crescentic glomerulonephritis but no evidence of arteritis. Although once subsumed in the category of polyarteritis nodosa, current knowledge justifies separating microscopic polyangiitis from polyarteritis nodosa.

Patients with *Wegener's granulomatosis* and *Churg-Strauss syndrome* have a systemic pauci-immune small vessel vasculitis that is indistinguishable from microscopic polyangiitis, however, each syndrome has its own distinguishing diagnostic features (Table 15-2) (1,7,14,16,32). Wegener's granulomatosis is distinguished by the presence of necrotizing granulomatous inflammation, which most often affects the upper or lower respiratory tract, although any organ can be affected (14,32). Churg-Strauss syndrome is differentiated from microscopic polyangiitis and Wegener's granulomatosis by the presence of asthma and blood eosinophilia (13,32).

Microscopic polyangiitis, Wegener's granulomatosis, and Churg-Strauss syndrome are all variants of pauci-immune small vessel vasculitis. Since most patients with pauci-immune small vessel vasculitis are ANCA positive, pauci-immune small vessel vasculitis is almost synonymous with ANCA-associated small vessel vasculitis. In fact, the evidence that ANCAs are directly involved in the pathogenesis is so strong that *ANCA small vessel vasculitis* also is an acceptable term.

Clinical Features. Patients with pauci-immune crescentic glomerulonephritis, whether or not it is accompanied by systemic small vessel vasculitis, usually present with rapidly progressive renal failure and clinical features of glomerulonephritis, such as dysmorphic erythrocyturia, erythrocyte cylindruria, and proteinuria of greater than 2 g/day (11,24,28,31, 42,44). Less commonly, patients present with more indolent acute disease, or chronic disease. Most patients have a prodrome of fever and flu-like symptoms. Patients with pauci-immune crescentic glomerulonephritis alone (renal-limited vasculitis) have no evidence of systemic vasculitis. Minor arthralgias and myalgias often are components of the prodromal inflammatory symptoms and should not be taken as evidence of vasculitis.

Pauci-immune crescentic glomerulonephritis, with or without systemic vasculitis, is the

Table 15-2

NAMES AND DEFINITIONS OF VASCULITIS ADOPTED BY THE CHAPEL HILL CONSENSUS CONFERENCE ON THE NOMENCLATURE OF SYSTEMIC VASCULITIS[a]

Large Vessel Vasculitis (Chronic Granulomatous Arteritis)[b]	
Giant cell arteritis	Granulomatous arteritis of the aorta and its major branches, with a predilection for the extracranial branches of the carotid artery. Often involves the temporal artery. Usually occurs in patients older than 50 and often is associated with polymyalgia rheumatica.
Takayasu's arteritis	Granulomatous inflammation of the aorta and its major branches. Usually occurs in patients younger than 50.
Medium-Sized Vessel Vasculitis (Necrotizing Arteritis)[b]	
Polyarteritis nodosa	Necrotizing inflammation of medium-sized or small arteries without glomerulonephritis or vasculitis in arterioles, capillaries, or venules.
Kawasaki's disease	Arteritis involving large, medium-sized, and small arteries, and associated with mucocutaneous lymph node syndrome. Coronary arteries are often involved. Aorta and veins may be involved. Usually occurs in children.
Small Vessel Vasculitis (Necrotizing Polyangiitis)[b]	
Wegener's granulomatosis[c,d]	Granulomatous inflammation involving the respiratory tract, and necrotizing vasculitis affecting small to medium-sized vessels, e.g., capillaries, venules, arterioles, and arteries. Necrotizing glomerulonephritis is common.
Churg-Strauss syndrome[c,d]	Eosinophil-rich and granulomatous inflammation involving the respiratory tract and necrotizing vasculitis affecting small to medium-sized vessels, and associated with asthma and blood eosinophilia.
Microscopic polyangiitis[c,d]	Necrotizing vasculitis, with few or no immune deposits, affecting small vessels, i.e., capillaries, venules, or arterioles. Necrotizing arteritis involving small and medium-sized arteries may be present. Necrotizing glomerulonephritis is very common. Pulmonary capillaritis often occurs.
Henoch-Schönlein purpura[d]	Vasculitis with IgA-dominant immune deposits affecting small vessels, i.e., capillaries, venules, or arterioles. Typically involves skin, gut, and glomeruli, and is associated with arthralgias or arthritis.
Essential cryoglobulinemic vasculitis[d]	Vasculitis with cryoglobulin immune deposits affecting small vessels, i.e., capillaries, venules, or arterioles, and associated with cryoglobulins in serum. Skin and glomeruli are often involved.
Cutaneous leukocytoclastic angiitis	Isolated cutaneous leukocytoclastic angiitis without systemic vasculitis or glomerulonephritis.

[a]Modified from reference 32.

[b]Large vessel refers to the aorta and the largest arterial branches directed toward major body regions (e.g., to the extremities and the head and neck); medium-sized vessel refers to the main visceral arteries (e.g., renal, hepatic, coronary, and mesenteric arteries); and small artery refers to the distal arterial radicals that connect with arterioles (e.g., renal arcuate and interlobular arteries). Some small and large vessel vasculitides may involve medium-sized arteries; but large and medium-sized vessel vasculitides do not involve vessels smaller than arteries.

[c]Strongly associated with antineutrophil cytoplasmic autoantibodies (ANCAs).

[d]May be accompanied by glomerulonephritis and can manifest as nephritis or pulmonary-renal vasculitic syndrome.

most common form of crescentic glomerulonephritis (Table 15-3). Although it may occur at any age, it is most frequent in older patients (Table 15-4).

When pauci-immune crescentic glomerulonephritis occurs as a component of microscopic polyangiitis, Wegener's granulomatosis, or Churg-Strauss syndrome, the nephritic features can be accompanied by a wide variety of manifestations of vasculitis, involving a broad range of vessels in many different tissues (31). Any organ in the body can be affected. Table 15-5 shows the relative frequency of organ involvement by the different clinicopathologic categories of pauci-immune small vessel vasculitis. Involvement of dermal venules and

Table 15-3

FREQUENCY OF IMMUNOPATHOLOGIC CATEGORIES OF CRESCENTIC GLOMERULONEPHRITIS IN OVER 3,000 CONSECUTIVE NATIVE KIDNEY BIOPSIES EVALUATED BY IMMUNOFLUORESCENCE MICROSCOPY IN THE UNIVERSITY OF NORTH CAROLINA NEPHROPATHOLOGY LABORATORY[a]

Immunohistology	Any Crescents (n = 540)	>50% Crescents (n = 193)	Arteritis in Biopsy (n = 37)
Pauci-immune (<2+ Ig)	51% (227/540)	61% (118/193)[b]	84% (31/37)
Immune Complex (>2+ Ig)	44% (238/540)	29% (56/193)	14% (5/37)[c]
Anti-GBM	5% (25/540)[d]	11% (21/193)	3% (1/37)[e]

[a]Table 3 from Jennette JC, Falk RJ. The pathology of vasculitis involving the kidney. Am J Kidney Dis 1994;24:130–41.

[b]70 of 77 patients tested for ANCA were positive (91%) (44 P-ANCA and 26 C-ANCA). P = perinuclear; C = cytoplasmic; ANCA = antineutrophil cytoplasmic autoantibody; GBM = glomerular basement membrane.

[c]Four patients had lupus and 1 poststreptococcal glomerulonephritis.

[d]3 of 19 patients tested for ANCA were positive (16%) (2 P-ANCA and 1 C-ANCA).

[e]This patient also had a P-ANCA (MPO-ANCA). MPO = myeloperoxidase.

Table 15-4

RELATIVE FREQUENCY OF IMMUNOPATHOLOGIC CATEGORIES OF CRESCENTIC GLOMERULONEPHRITIS WITH RESPECT TO AGE IN PATIENTS WHOSE RENAL BIOPSIES WERE EVALUATED IN THE UNIVERSITY OF NORTH CAROLINA NEPHROPATHOLOGY LABORATORY[a]

Age	10-19	20-39	40-64	≥65
Number	20	42	61	65
Anti-GBM CGN	15%	24%	2%	11%
Immune Complex CGN	50%	48%	30%	8%
Pauci-immune CGN[b,c]	35%	28%	69%	82%

[a]Crescentic glomerulonephritis (CGN) is defined as greater than 50% of glomeruli with crescents. GBM = glomerular basement membrane.

[b]Approximately 90% associated with antineutrophil cytoplasmic autoantibody (ANCA).

[c]Note the high frequency of pauci-immune (usually ANCA-associated) disease in the elderly.

Table 15-5

COMPARISON OF APPROXIMATE FREQUENCY OF MANIFESTATIONS OF MICROSCOPIC POLYANGIITIS TO SEVERAL OTHER FORMS OF SMALL VESSEL VASCULITIS[a]

Manifestations	Microscopic Polyangiitis	Wegener's Granulomatosis	Churg-Strauss Syndrome	Henoch-Schönlein Purpura	Cryoglob-ulinemic Vasculitis
Renal	90%	80%	45%	50%	55%
Cutaneous	40%	40%	60%	90%	90%
Pulmonary	50%	90%	70%	<5%	<5%
Ear, nose, and throat	35%	90%	50%	<5%	<5%
Musculoskeletal	60%	60%	50%	75%	70%
Neurologic	30%	50%	70%	10%	40%
Gastrointestinal	50%	50%	50%	60%	30%

[a]Table 4 from Jennette JC, Falk RJ. Small vessel vasculitis. N Engl J Med 1997;337:1512–23.

capillaries causes purpura and petechiae. Pulmonary capillaritis causes pulmonary hemorrhage and hemoptysis. When this is accompanied by glomerulonephritis, the *pulmonary-renal vasculitic syndrome* occurs. In fact, ANCA small vessel vasculitis is the most common cause of pulmonary-renal vasculitic syndrome (40). Involvement of dermal and subcutaneous arteries causes tender erythematous nodules, infarcts, and ulceration. Involvement of epineural arteries causes peripheral neuropathy that usually manifests as mononeuritis multiplex. Abdominal pain can be caused by ischemia in the gut, liver, pancreas, kidneys, or other abdominal organs. Visceral ischemia also can result in infarcts and elevation in circulating tissue enzymes, thus mimicking (causing) pancreatitis, hepatitis, enteritis, myositis, and other inflammatory diseases. Eye, ear, nose, or throat involvement can occur with any variant of pauci-immune small vessel vasculitis, however, it is most common with Wegener's granulomatosis. Manifestations include necrotizing sinusitis or rhinitis, otitis media, ocular inflammation (conjunctivitis, scleritis, uveitis, keratitis, proptosis, or orbital pseudotumor), and subglottic stenosis.

Patients with Wegener's granulomatosis have clinical evidence of granulomatous inflammation: 1) pulmonary nodules or cavities in the absence of evidence of infection, or 2) destructive bone or cartilage lesions in the upper respiratory tract, which may result in destruction of the nasal septum and saddle nose deformity.

The initial clinical manifestation of Churg-Strauss syndrome is asthma or severe allergic rhinitis, which may precede the development of vasculitis by decades (7,17,18). Eosinophilic inflammation of tissues, such as eosinophilic pneumonia and eosinophilic enteritis, also may precede the vasculitis. The vasculitic phase of Churg-Strauss syndrome usually begins in the fourth or fifth decade of life.

Although glomerulonephritis is a very frequent component of pauci-immune small vessel vasculitis, each category includes a minority of patients with no apparent renal involvement (Table 15-5) (28). Patients with Churg-Strauss syndrome have the lowest frequency of renal involvement and it tends to be less severe when present.

ANCA serology is useful for diagnosing and following patients with pauci-immune crescentic glomerulonephritis and small vessel vasculitis (19,22,26,34,46). ANCAs have specificity for proteins in the primary granules of neutrophils and the peroxidase-positive lysosomes of monocytes. In patients with glomerulonephritis and vasculitis, the two major antigen specificities are for proteinase 3 (PR3-ANCA) and myeloperoxidase (MPO-ANCA). The best assays for detecting MPO-ANCA and PR3-ANCA use purified MPO and PR3, respectively, as substrates (for example in an enzyme-linked immunosorbent assay [ELISA]). A slightly more sensitive but less specific assay uses alcohol-fixed normal human neutrophils as a substrate for an indirect immunofluorescence assay (IIFA). With this assay, PR3-ANCA usually causes cytoplasmic staining of the substrate neutrophils (C-ANCA) and MPO-ANCA causes perinuclear staining (P-ANCA) because the MPO is artifactually redistributed to the nucleus during substrate preparation (fig. 15-3).

Table 15-6 gives the approximate frequency of ANCAs in the different categories of pauci-immune small vessel vasculitis; figure 15-4 depicts the relationship of ANCA specificity to the clinicopathologic categories of crescentic glomerulonephritis and small vessel vasculitis. Each clinicopathologic variant can be associated with PR3-ANCA (C-ANCA) or MPO-ANCA (P-ANCA), and a minority of patients with each category of injury are ANCA negative. Therefore, the absence of positive ANCA serology does not rule out a diagnosis of pauci-immune small vessel vasculitis, and the specificity of the ANCA antigen does not indicate a specific clinicopathologic category of pauci-immune small vessel vasculitis. Nevertheless, ANCA serology is very helpful in the diagnosis of pauci-immune small vessel vasculitis.

Table 15-7 details the predictive value of ANCA results for diagnosing pauci-immune crescentic glomerulonephritis, with or without systemic vasculitis, in patients with different manifestations of renal disease (34). Based on the relative prevalence of pauci-immune crescentic glomerulonephritis versus immune complex or anti-GBM crescentic glomerulonephritis, the pretest likelihood of the former is approximately 50 percent in patients with clinical evidence of rapidly progressive glomerulonephritis. In this setting, a positive ANCA test provides strong

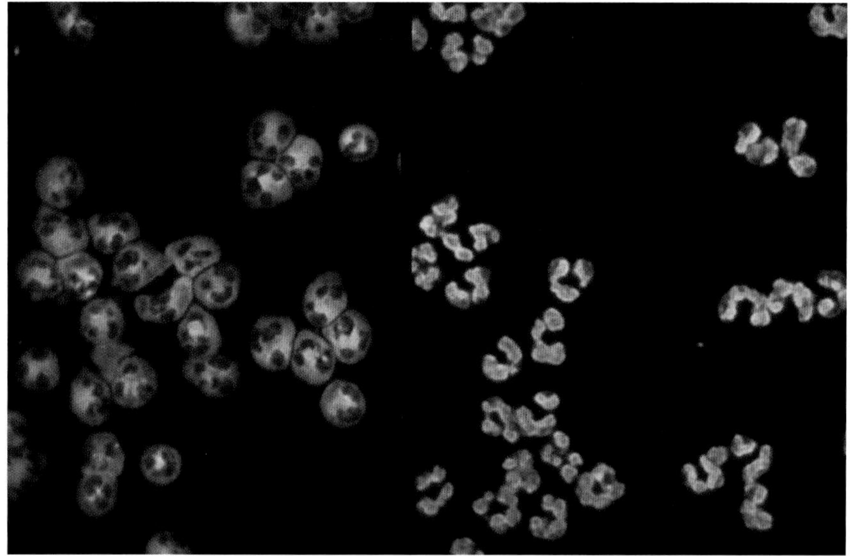

Figure 15-3

ANTINEUTROPHIL CYTOPLASMIC AUTOANTIBODY (ANCA) PATTERNS

Positive indirect immunofluorescence microscopy assay results for ANCA produce either a cytoplasmic staining pattern (C-ANCA) (left) or a perinuclear pattern (P-ANCA) (right).

Table 15-6

APPROXIMATE FREQUENCY OF ANTINEUTROPHIL CYTOPLASMIC AUTOANTIBODY (ANCA) WITH SPECIFICITY FOR PROTEINASE 3 (PR3-ANCA) OR MYELOPEROXIDASE (MPO-ANCA) IN PATIENTS WITH ACTIVE UNTREATED RENAL-LIMITED PAUCI-IMMUNE CRESCENTIC GLOMERULONEPHRITIS, MICROSCOPIC POLYANGIITIS, WEGENER'S GRANULOMATOSIS, AND CHURG-STRAUSS SYNDROME

	Renal-Limited Pauci-Immune Crescentic Glomerulonephritis	Microscopic Polyangiitis	Wegener's Granulomatosis	Churg-Strauss Syndrome
PR3-ANCA	20%	40%	75%	10%
MPO-ANCA	60%	50%	20%	60%
Negative	20%	10%	5%	30%

Table 15-7

PREDICTIVE VALUE FOR PAUCI-IMMUNE CRESCENTIC GLOMERULONEPHRITIS OF COMBINED IMMUNOFLUORESCENCE ASSAY AND ENZYME IMMUNOASSAY ANTINEUTROPHIL CYTOPLASMIC AUTOANTIBODY (ANCA) TESTING[a]

Adult With	Prevalence (Pre-test Likelihood)	PPV[b] (Post-test Likelihood	NPV (Post-test Unlikelihood)
RPGN[b]	47%	95%	85%
Hematuria, proteinuria, creatinine >3 mg/dL	21%	84%	95%
Hematuria, proteinuria, creatinine 1.5-3.0 mg/dL	7%	60%	99%
Hematuria, proteinuria, creatinine <1.5 mg/dL	2%	29%	100%

[a]Data derived from an analysis of 2,315 patients, with ANCA assay sensitivity 81% and specificity 96%, cited in reference ___.
[b]PPV = positive predictive value; NPV = negative predictive value; RPGN = rapidly progressive glomerulonephritis.

support for a diagnosis of pauci-immune crescentic glomerulonephritis (with or without systemic small vessel vasculitis) but a negative ANCA test does not rule out the possibility of ANCA-negative pauci-immune crescentic glomerulonephritis. When there is only weak clinical evidence of pauci-immune crescentic glomerulonephritis, such as hematuria and proteinuria with little

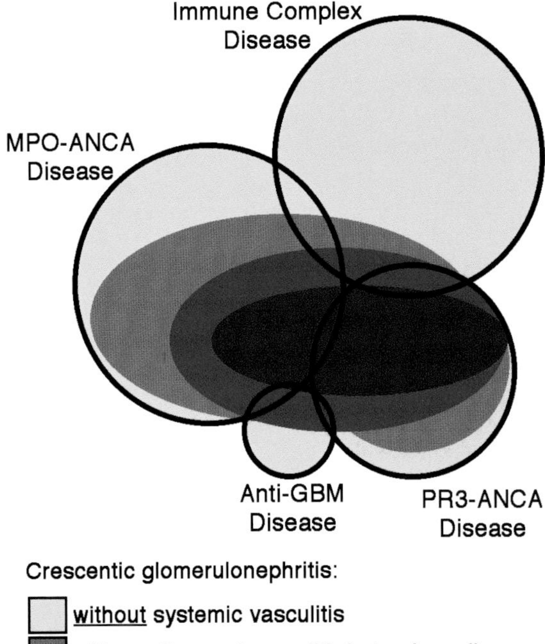

Figure 15-4

RELATIONSHIPS BETWEEN SMALL VESSEL VASCULITIS AND CRESCENTIC GLOMERULONEPHRITIS

The diagram depicts the immunopathologic categories of crescentic glomerulonephritis (circles) and their relationship to different forms of systemic vasculitis (colored areas). Only a small proportion of cases of crescentic immune complex glomerulonephritis are accompanied by systemic vasculitis (e.g., cryoglobulinemic vasculitis, lupus vasculitis), whereas most cases of ANCA-associated glomerulonephritis are a component of systemic small vessel vasculitis (e.g., microscopic polyangiitis, Wegener's granulomatosis). Most cases of renal-limited ANCA glomerulonephritis are associated with MPO-ANCA, whereas most Wegener's granulomatosis are associated with PR3-ANCA.

or no renal insufficiency, a positive ANCA result has only poor positive predictive value, however, a negative result has very high negative predictive value. In addition, even though a positive result in this setting is not diagnostic for pauci-immune crescentic glomerulonephritis, it increases the likelihood to a level that warrants more careful and expeditious evaluation because ANCA-associated pauci-immune crescentic glomerulonephritis usually is a very aggressive disease that should be treated promptly with high-dose immunosuppressive drugs.

Although a positive ANCA serology is most frequent in patients with pauci-immune crescentic glomerulonephritis, it is important to recognize that approximately a quarter of patients with anti-GBM crescentic glomerulonephritis and a quarter of patients with immune complex crescentic glomerulonephritis are also ANCA positive (19,20,23,45). A positive ANCA result in patients with these glomerulonephritides increases the risk of systemic small vessel vasculitis. In patients with immune complex disease, such as membranous glomerulopathy or immunoglobulin (Ig)A nephropathy, a positive ANCA result increases the likelihood that crescents are present, which suggests a synergistic role for ANCA in the pathogenesis of glomerulonephritis (29,35,36).

Gross Findings. Severe necrotizing and crescentic glomerulonephritis causes numerous tiny red dots on the external surface of the kidneys, the "flea-bitten" appearance (fig. 15-5) (28). This appearance is not specific for pauci-immune crescentic glomerulonephritis (ANCA crescentic glomerulonephritis) because it can be seen with any severe glomerulonephritis that causes massive hemorrhage into the urinary space. The red dots result from blood within Bowman's spaces and the lumens of tubules. Dark red vermiform or corkscrew patterns, caused by blood within the lumens of convoluted tubules, are seen as well in the parenchyma.

When renal arteries are involved by pauci-immune small vessel vasculitis (microscopic polyangiitis, Wegener's granulomatosis, and Churg-Strauss syndrome), the interlobular arteries are involved most often; the arcuate arteries occasionally; and the interlobar and main renal arteries rarely. Thus, grossly identifiable pseudoaneurysms and infarcts are seen infrequently. This is in contradistinction to kidneys that are involved by polyarteritis nodosa or Kawasaki's disease, which frequently have grossly identifiable pseudoaneurysms and infarcts caused by involvement of interlobar and arcuate arteries.

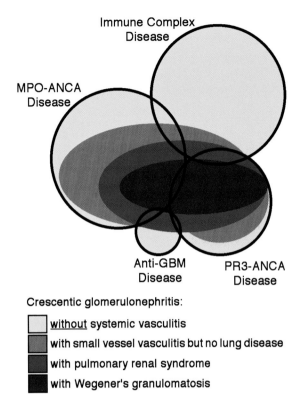

Light Microscopic Findings. Glomerulonephritis is the most common renal lesion in renal-limited as well as systemic ANCA-associated pauci-immune vascular inflammation (28,30). The initial glomerular histologic lesion is segmental fibrinoid necrosis with focal lysis of the glomerular basement membranes and mesangial

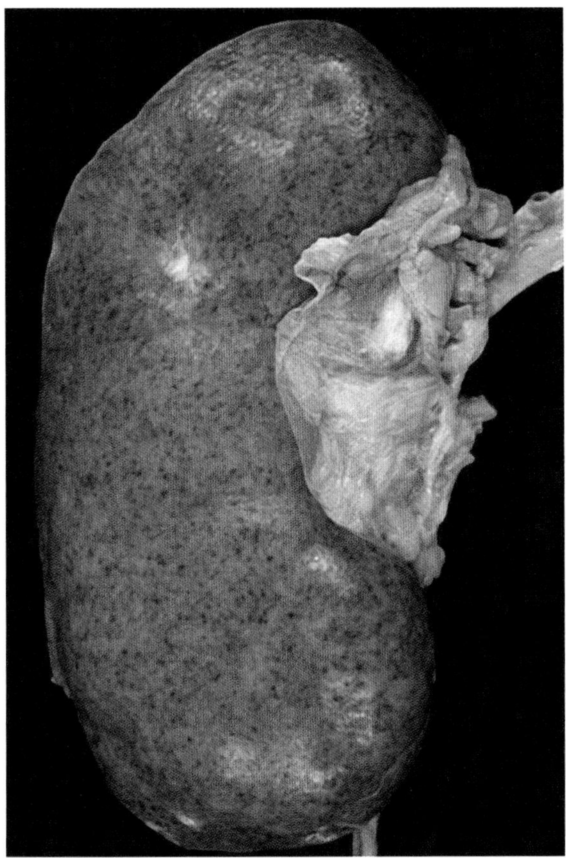

Figure 15-5

"FLEA-BITTEN" KIDNEY

Kidney from a patient who died with C-ANCA crescentic glomerulonephritis has numerous tiny red dots on the surface corresponding to red blood cells that have spilled out of a ruptured glomeruli into Bowman's spaces and tubular lumens.

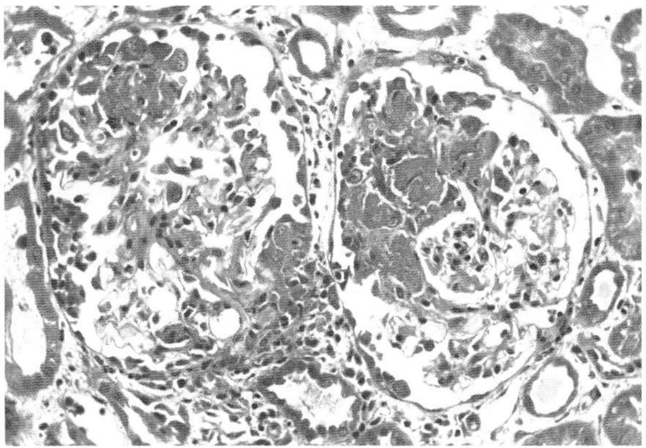

Figure 15-6

FOCAL NECROTIZING ANCA GLOMERULONEPHRITIS

Two glomeruli show deeply acidophilic, segmental fibrinoid necrosis. There is a slight cellular reaction in Bowman's space, but no definite crescent formation.

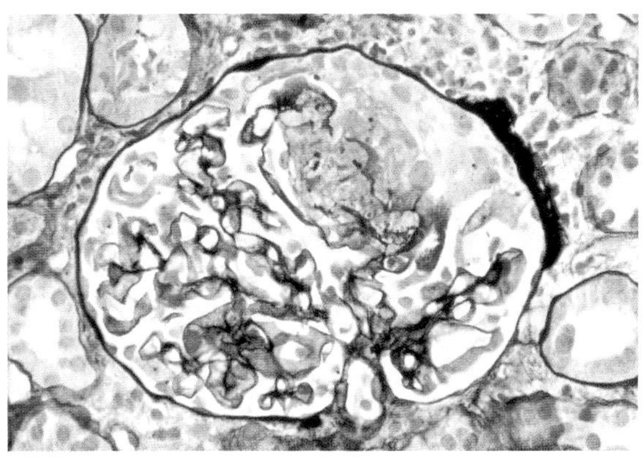

Figure 15-7

FOCAL NECROTIZING ANCA GLOMERULONEPHRITIS

A glomerulus stained with the Jones methenamine silver (JMS) stain shows segmental necrosis demarcated by the lysis of glomerular basement membranes. The non-necrotic segments are histologically unremarkable.

matrix (figs. 15-6, 15-7). Neutrophils, some undergoing leukocytoclasia, often are adjacent to or within areas of early necrosis. Later lesions have a predominance of mononuclear leukocytes, including macrophages. In glomeruli with segmental necrosis, non-necrotic segments often are histologically unremarkable, with no hypercellularity or thickening of capillary walls. Occasionally, there is an increase in marginated neutrophils within otherwise normal-appearing glomeruli. This is in contrast to immune complex glomerulonephritis with segmental necrosis, which typically has endocapillary hypercellularity and capillary wall thickening in segments adjacent to necrosis, and in glomeruli with no necrosis (28). The necrosis of proliferative immune complex glomerulonephritis tends to have more karyorrhexis whereas the necrosis of pauci-immune glomerulonephritis has more fibrinoid material.

Severe segmental or global necrotizing inflammation often causes disruption of Bowman's capsule (figs. 15-8, 15-9). This results in marked periglomerular inflammation that often has a granulomatous appearance and may contain multinucleated giant cells (fig. 15-9). Periglomerular inflammation is difficult to distinguish

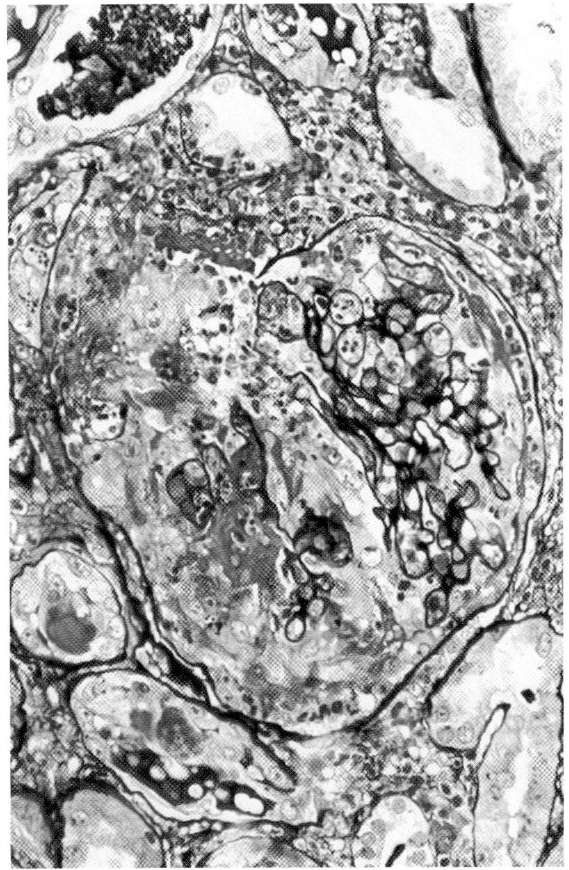

Figure 15-8

NECROTIZING ANCA GLOMERULONEPHRITIS WITH RUPTURE OF BOWMAN'S CAPSULE

In addition to segmental necrosis of the glomerular tuft, the necrotizing process has destroyed a portion of Bowman's capsule. There is intense inflammation in the adjacent interstitium and tubules. Numerous neutrophils are involved in the glomerular and tubulointerstitial inflammation.

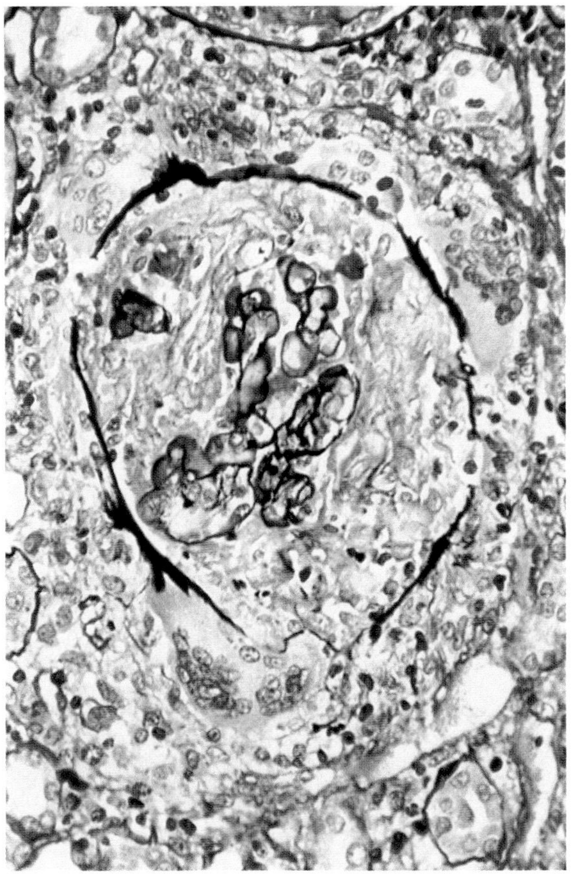

Figure 15-9

GRANULOMATOUS REACTION TO ANCA GLOMERULONEPHRITIS

This glomerulus with ANCA-associated pauci-immune glomerulonephritis has extensive fibrinoid necrosis of the tuft as well as focal lysis of Bowman's capsule, which has resulted in periglomerular granulomatous inflammation with large multinucleated giant cells. Periglomerular granulomatous inflammation is not specific for Wegener's granulomatosis but can occur with any severe necrotizing glomerulonephritis, including microscopic polyangiitis, Churg-Strauss syndrome, renal-limited ANCA glomerulonephritis, and anti-GBM glomerulonephritis.

from interstitial granulomatous inflammation when there is extensive lysis of the glomerular tuft and Bowman's capsule. Serial sections through foci of apparent interstitial necrotizing granulomatous inflammation may reveal residual fragments of glomerular tuft segments or of Bowman's capsule, which identify the lesion as periglomerular rather than interstitial (fig. 15-10). This is an important distinction, because periglomerular granulomatous inflammation is nonspecific and can be seen with renal-limited pauci-immune glomerulonephritis, any form of pauci-immune small vessel vasculitis, and necrotizing anti-GBM glomerulonephritis (4). True renal interstitial granulomatous inflammation that is not adjacent to glomeruli is rare, and is more specific evidence of Wegener's granulomatosis or Churg-Strauss syndrome (fig. 15-11) (1). The interstitial necrotizing granulomatous inflammation of Wegener's granulomatosis and Churg-Strauss syndrome is identified most often in the respiratory tract or skin.

Approximately 90 percent of patients with pauci-immune necrotizing glomerulonephritis have crescents in some glomeruli, with 50 percent glomerular involvement on average (27).

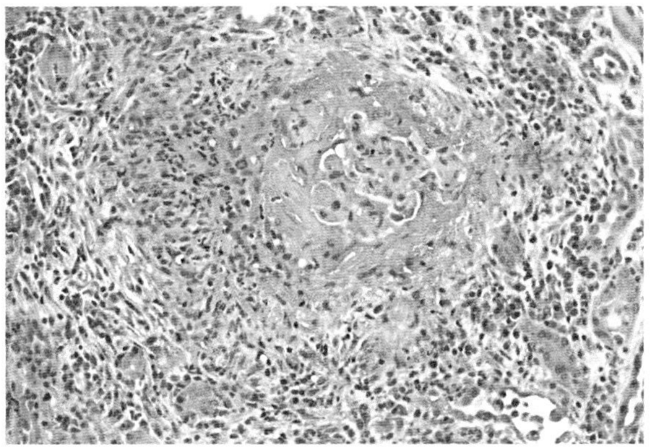

Figure 15-10

PERIGLOMERULAR INFLAMMATION

A glomerulus with severe pauci-immune necrotizing glomerulonephritis and virtually complete destruction of Bowman's capsule is surrounded by intense interstitial inflammation, including numerous macrophages. An off-center plane of section through this lesion that did not include the residual glomerular tuft could be misinterpreted as an interstitial granuloma.

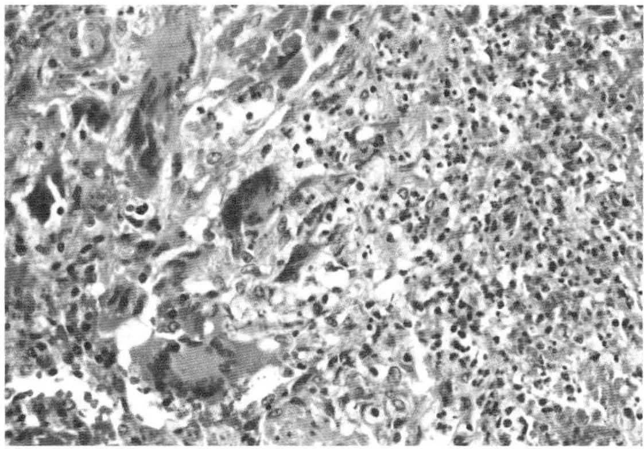

Figure 15-11

NECROTIZING GRANULOMATOUS INTERSTITIAL INFLAMMATION

If not centered on a glomerulus, this pattern of injury is consistent with Wegener's granulomatosis or Churg-Strauss syndrome. Note the admixture of multinucleated giant cells, neutrophils, and pyknotic and karyorrhectic nuclear debris.

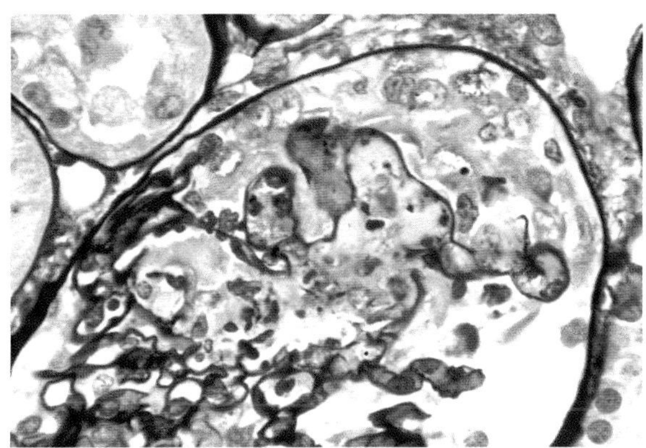

Figure 15-12

ANCA GLOMERULONEPHRITIS WITH SEGMENTAL NECROSIS

A glomerular segment has focal lysis of basement membranes and mesangial matrix documented by glomerular basement membrane terminations and JMS-negative mesangial zones. The spillage of plasma into Bowman's space has resulted in fibrin formation and an early cellular response that leads to crescent formation.

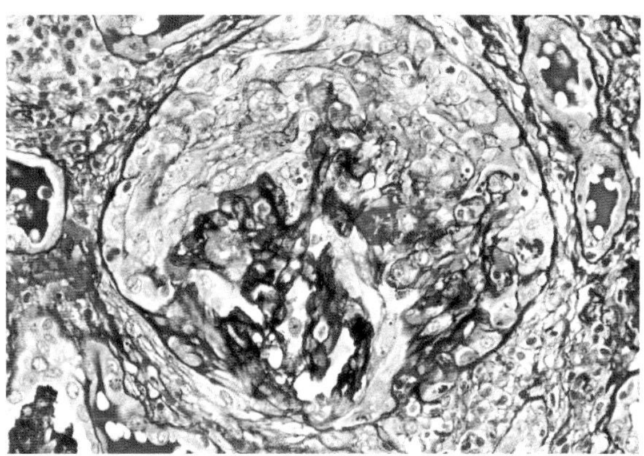

Figure 15-13

CRESCENTIC ANCA GLOMERULONEPHRITIS

A large circumferential cellular crescent surrounds a glomerulus that has lost many peripheral capillary loops and continues to have segmental fibrinoid necrosis.

Glomeruli with early necrotizing lesions may have segmental rupture of capillaries, with spillage of plasma constituents into Bowman's space and resultant fibrin formation, but little or no true crescent formation (fig. 15-12). Eventually, large cellular crescents typically form (fig. 15-13), consisting of a mixture of macrophages and epithelial cells (figs. 15-14, 15-15). Epithelial cells in advanced cellular crescents may align with collagenous matrix to produce "tubularization" of crescents (fig. 15-16). Severe glomerular necrosis with extensive disruption of the glomerular tuft and Bowman's capsule can make the demarcation between tuft and crescent, and between crescent and interstitium, difficult (fig. 15-10). Special stains that highlight basement membrane, such as the periodic acid–Schiff (PAS)

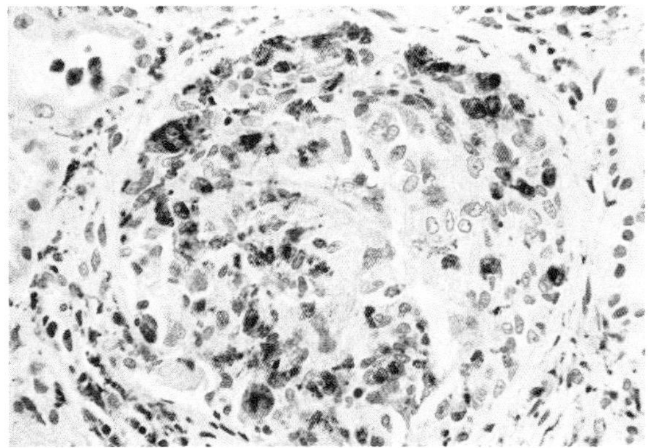

Figure 15-14

MACROPHAGES IN PAUCI-IMMUNE CRESCENTIC ANCA GLOMERULONEPHRITIS

Numerous CD68-positive macrophages are seen within a large cellular crescent and the adjacent periglomerular interstitium.

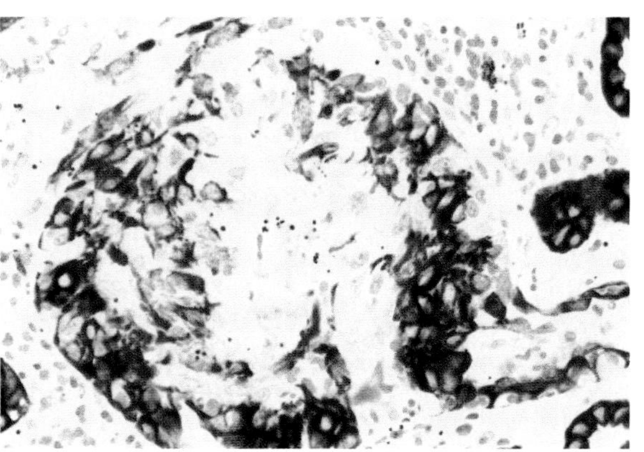

Figure 15-15

EPITHELIAL CELLS IN PAUCI-IMMUNE CRESCENTIC ANCA GLOMERULONEPHRITIS

Cytokeratin-positive (CAM 5.2-positive) epithelial cells are numerous within a cellular crescent and are continuous with cytokeratin-positive epithelial cells in the proximal tubule.

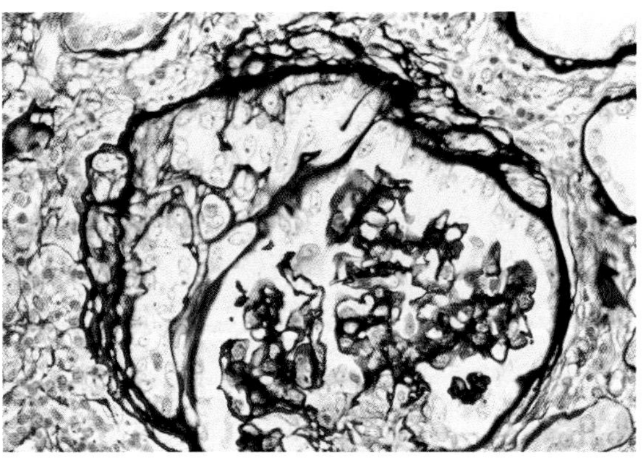

Figure 15-16

CRESCENTIC ANCA GLOMERULONEPHRITIS WITH TUBULARIZATION

Within the crescent, epithelial cells have aligned with basement membrane–like material to form tubular structures.

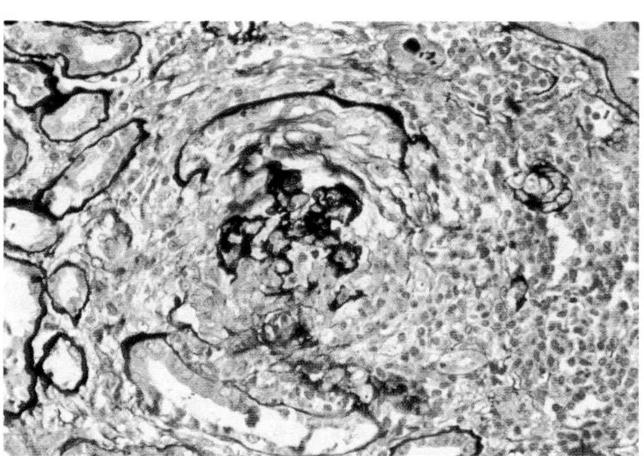

Figure 15-17

ADVANCED CRESCENTIC ANCA GLOMERULONEPHRITIS

There has been so much destruction of the glomerular tuft and Bowman's capsule that this glomerulus would be difficult to see with a hematoxylin and eosin (H&E) stain alone. The JMS stain with a H&E counterstain, however, clearly demarcates the badly injured glomerulus.

or Jones methenamine silver (JMS) stain, are helpful because they demarcate residual fragments of glomerular basement membranes and Bowman's capsule (fig. 15-17).

The necrotizing and crescentic glomerular injury evolves into segmental (fig. 15-18) or global (fig. 15-19) glomerular sclerosis, with adhesions to Bowman's capsule. Again, special stains can indicate earlier necrotizing injury by showing fragmentation of glomerular basement membranes and tufts within the collagenous glomerular scars as opposed to shriveled but continuous basement membranes in glomeruli that have become globally sclerotic secondary to nonnecrotizing glomerular injury. Trichrome stains are useful for differentiating between areas of active necrosis versus sclerosis (fig. 15-20). As in other forms of glomerulonephritis, cellular crescents evolve into fibrocellular and then fibrotic crescents. Glomerular lesions of different ages

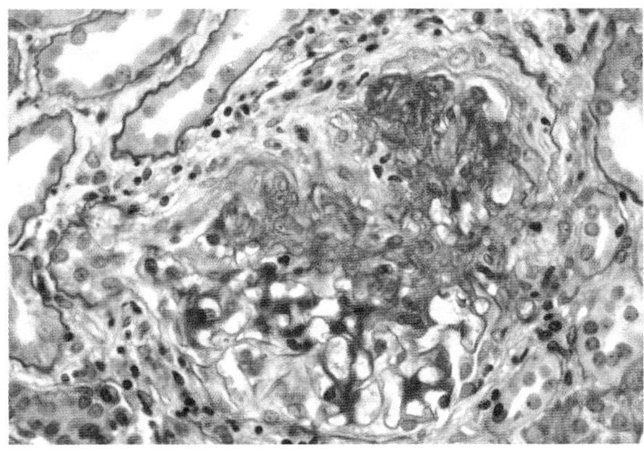

Figure 15-18

SEGMENTAL SCLEROSING ANCA GLOMERULONEPHRITIS

The segmental glomerular scarring is somewhat nonspecific. The extensive disruption of Bowman's capsule and distortion of the residual glomerular basement membranes, however, are consistent with earlier inflammatory injury rather than chronic ischemic injury or a primary sclerosing glomerulopathy such as focal segmental glomerulosclerosis (periodic acid–Schiff [PAS] stain).

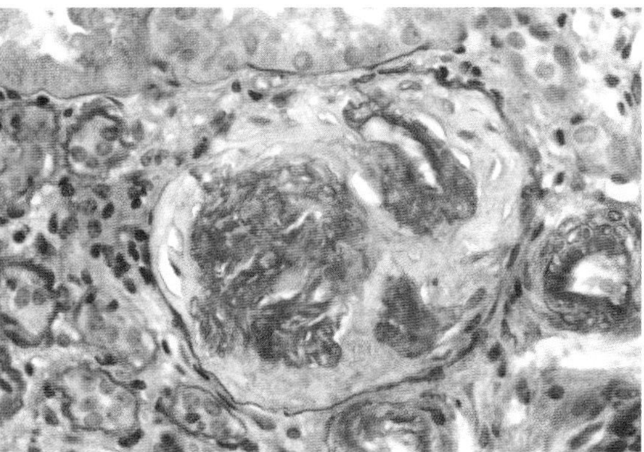

Figure 15-19

GLOBAL SCLEROSING ANCA GLOMERULONEPHRITIS

The PAS stain reveals that the glomerular tuft was torn into fragments before the glomerulus scarred. This is suggestive of earlier destructive necrotizing injury. The disruption of Bowman's capsule also supports this possibility but is a less specific indication.

may occur, which reflects the persistent or recurring nature of pauci-immune necrotizing glomerulonephritis.

Arteriolitis, arteritis, or medullary angiitis is identified in 10 to 20 percent of renal biopsy specimens from patients with pauci-immune small vessel vasculitis (ANCA small vessel vasculitis) (22,27,30,44). The most frequently involved renal arteries are the interlobular arteries, although any artery may be affected. Acute lesions at all vascular sites are characterized by segmental fibrinoid necrosis and infiltrating neutrophils, sometimes with admixed eosinophils or mononuclear leukocytes (fig. 15-21). Leukocytoclasia is frequent in acute lesions. Within a few days, the vasculitic lesions evolve to a predominance of mononuclear leukocytes, usually including conspicuous macrophages (fig. 15-22). The vascular necrosis and inflammation eventually result in irregular vascular and perivascular scarring (fig. 15-23).

The acute arterial lesions are characterized by transmural fibrinoid necrosis with associated leukocyte infiltration. Trichrome stains highlight the fuchsinophilic fibrinoid necrosis (figs. 15-24, 15-25). Rarely, apparently early arterial lesions have partial-thickness intimal inflammation (intimal arteritis) and fibrinoid insudation,

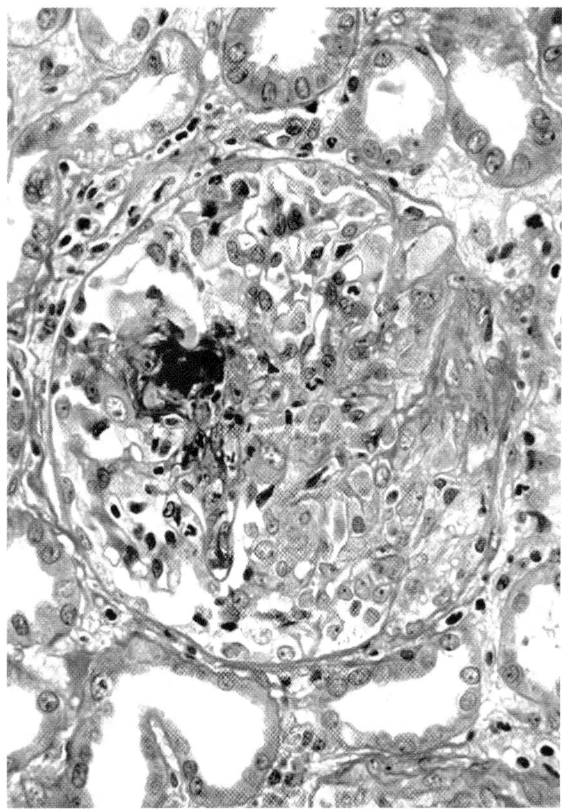

Figure 15-20

CRESCENTIC ANCA GLOMERULONEPHRITIS

The trichrome stain is useful for demonstrating areas of fibrinoid necrosis (red) and sclerosis (blue) in this glomerulus.

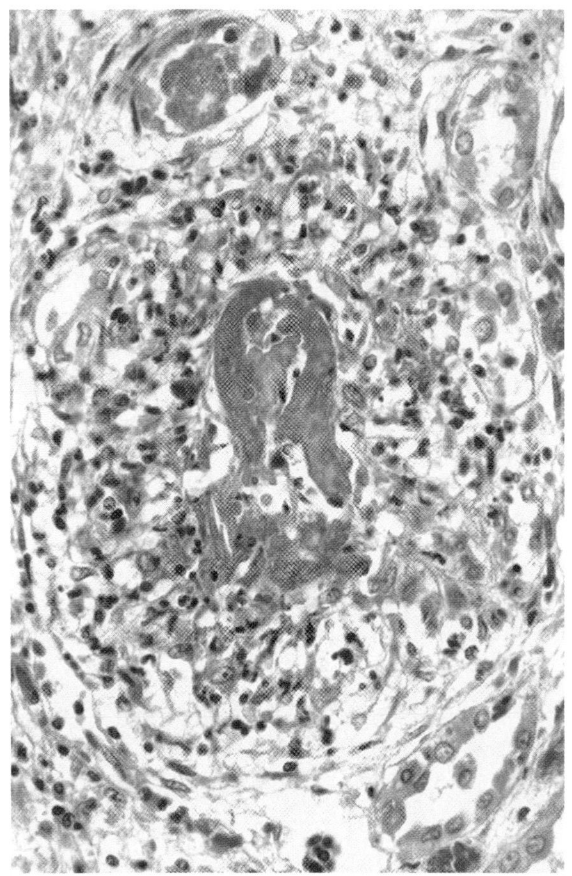

Figure 15-21

ANCA SMALL VESSEL VASCULITIS

Acute necrotizing arteritis completely effaces a small interlobular artery. The muscularis is replaced by fibrinoid material. At this early stage, neutrophils predominate in the associated inflammation.

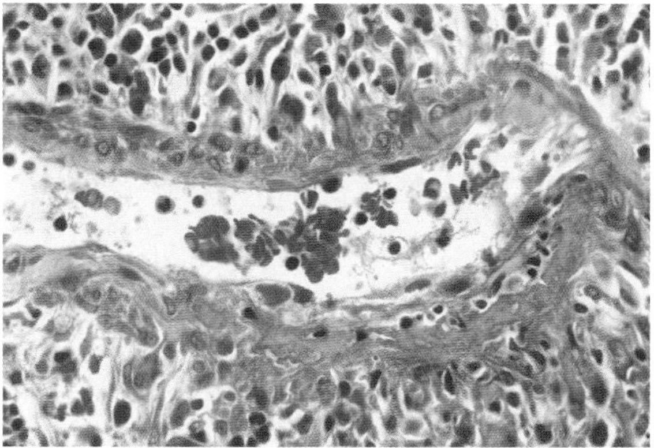

Figure 15-22

ANCA SMALL VESSEL VASCULITIS

This interlobular artery has segmental fibrinoid necrosis with intramural and perivascular infiltration by predominantly mononuclear leukocytes, including macrophages. This pattern of injury can occur not only with microscopic polyangiitis but also with Wegener's granulomatosis and Churg-Strauss syndrome.

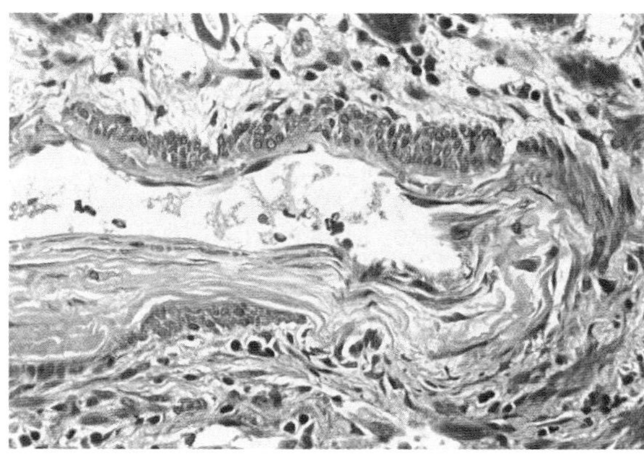

Figure 15-23

ANCA SMALL VESSEL VASCULITIS

This interlobular artery from a patient with microscopic polyangiitis has chronic sclerotic changes secondary to earlier segmental necrotizing arteritis. The focal disruption of the muscularis and, to a lesser extent, the asymmetry of the intimal fibrosis support the inflammatory origin of the scarring. Because of the recurrent and episodic character of ANCA small vessel vasculitis, lesions with different degrees of activity and chronicity may be present in the same specimen.

without disruption of the muscularis. The fibrinoid necrosis can erode completely through the vessel wall into the perivascular tissue, producing a pseudoaneurysm. Thrombosis of the lumen adjacent to an area of inflammation and necrosis may occur. Perivascular inflammation surrounding a site of arteritis is common. The perivascular inflammation often extends along the artery beyond the site of transmural injury; thus, at some planes of section, only the perivascular inflammation is observed. When this is observed, step sectioning may reveal the diagnostic mural involvement. PAS and JMS stains are useful for evaluating the extent of injury in vessel walls because they demarcate areas of matrix dissolution (fig. 15-26).

Leukocytoclastic angiitis affecting the medullary vasa recta is another pattern of renal vascular involvement by pauci-immune small vessel vasculitis (fig. 15-27) (30,49). This distinctive lesion has not been reported in other types of vasculitis. The characteristic features are focal

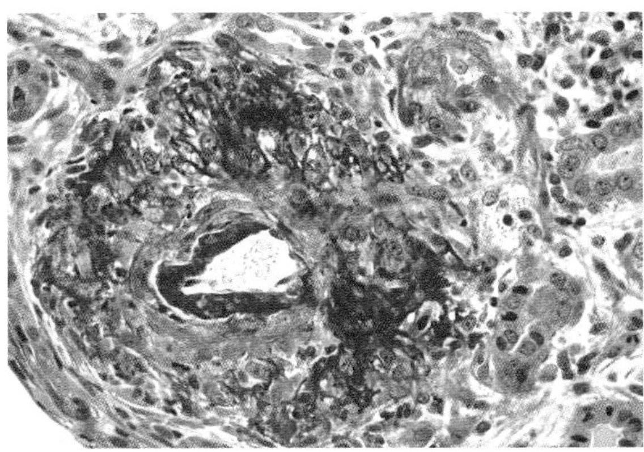

Figure 15-24

ANCA SMALL VESSEL VASCULITIS

An interlobular artery has mural thrombosis and fibroid necrosis, as well as perivascular fibrinoid necrosis and inflammation.

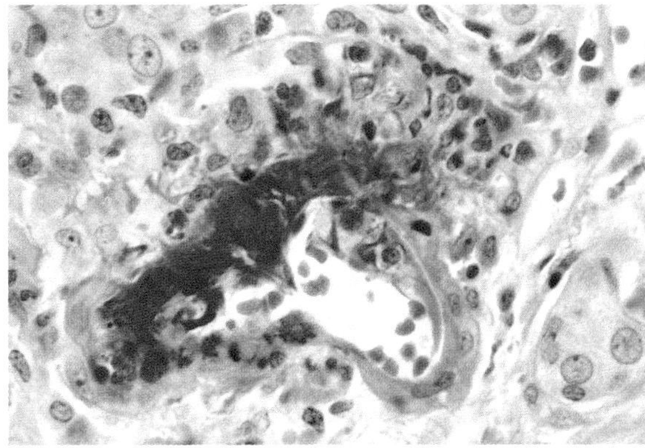

Figure 15-25

ANCA SMALL VESSEL VASCULITIS WITH ANTIGLOMERULAR BASEMENT MEMBRANE (ANTI-GBM) DISEASE

This patient had positive serology for both ANCAs and anti-GBM antibodies. In addition to the necrotizing arteritis shown affecting an interlobular artery, the patient had severe crescentic glomerulonephritis with linear immunoglobulin (Ig)G staining. The necrotizing arteritis is most likely related to the ANCAs rather than the anti-GBM antibodies.

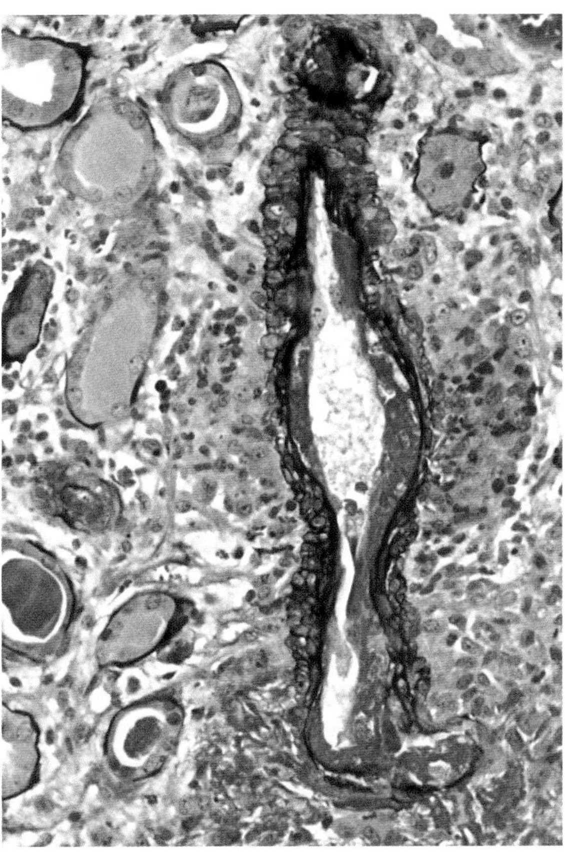

Figure 15-26

ANCA SMALL VESSEL VASCULITIS

This JMS stain with H&E counterstain demonstrates segmental destruction of the muscularis and a small focus of transmural erosion of the artery wall.

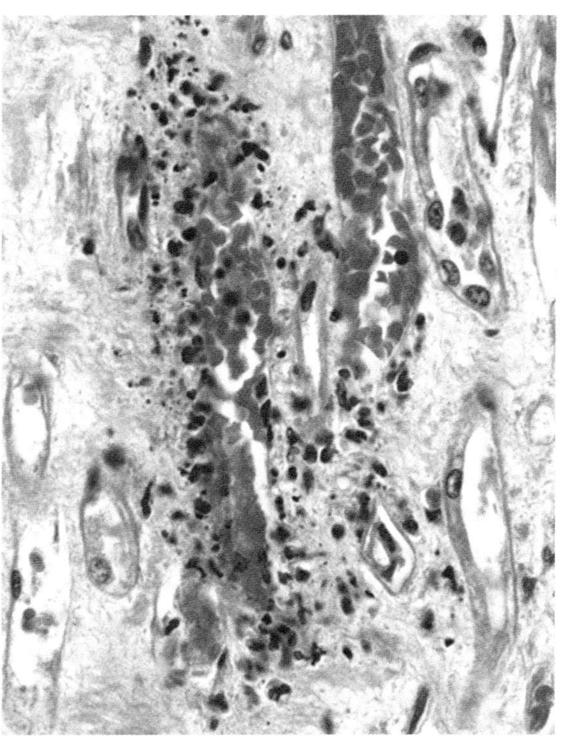

Figure 15-27

MEDULLARY ANGIITIS

Leukocytoclastic angiitis affects the vasa recta in the renal medulla of a patient with Wegener's granulomatosis. This should not be mistaken for acute pyelonephritis.

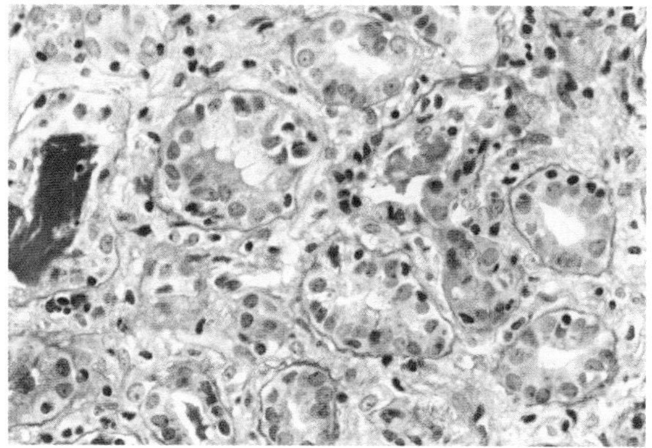

Figure 15-28

TUBULOINTERSTITIAL INFLAMMATION ASSOCIATED WITH ANCA GLOMERULONEPHRITIS

Tubulointerstitial inflammation, including conspicuous tubulitis, is a frequent finding in renal tissue from patients with ANCA glomerulonephritis. The tubulitis usually consists mostly of mononuclear leukocytes, as in this figure, however, neutrophils may be predominant (see figure 15-8).

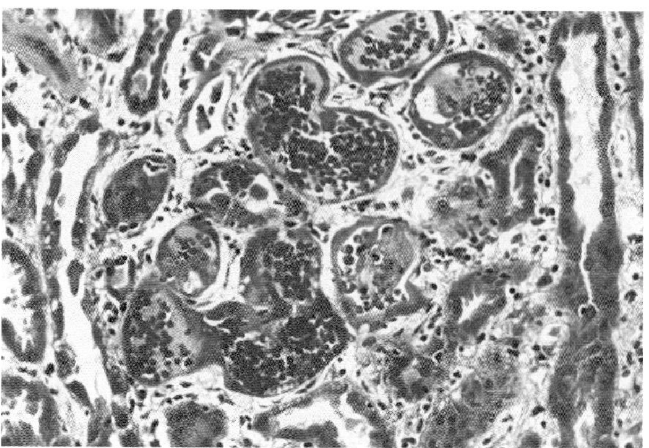

Figure 15-29

TUBULAR EPITHELIAL SIMPLIFICATION ASSOCIATED WITH ANCA GLOMERULONEPHRITIS

The proximal tubular epithelial cells in the center of this figure have irregularly flattened epithelium, indicative of acute injury. Note also the marked hematuria, interstitial edema, and slight tubulitis.

medullary leukocytoclasia and hemorrhage. The involved peritubular vessels are often difficult to identify because of their thin walls and the intensity of the inflammation. However, interstitial hemorrhage associated with interstitial leukocytoclasia is the marker of medullary angiitis. Medullary angiitis may be accompanied by tubulitis and leukocytes within tubular lumens, which should not be confused with pyelonephritis. Severe medullary angiitis may cause papillary necrosis (49).

Cortical tubulointerstitial inflammation accompanies the glomerular inflammation and may be very pronounced (figs. 15-8–15-10,15-17,15-28). In fact, the intensity of the tubulointerstitial inflammation, especially the tubulitis, usually is greater in pauci-immune necrotizing and crescentic glomerulonephritis than in comparably severe immune complex glomerulonephritis. Perhaps this is secondary to the extensive rupture of glomerular capillaries and Bowman's capsule, with the spillage of inflammatory mediators into tubular lumens and the interstitium. Infarcts are rarely identified in renal biopsies from patients with pauci-immune small vessel vasculitis, even when arteritis is present in the specimen. As with other forms of severe glomerulonephritis, there may be simplification of proximal tubular epithelial cells that resembles the changes of ischemic acute renal failure (fig. 15-29).

In addition to renal parenchymal disease, Wegener's granulomatosis and Churg-Strauss syndrome may affect perirenal and urogenital tissues. For example, a rare cause of ureteral obstruction is vasculitic or granulomatous inflammation secondary to Wegener's granulomatosis or Churg-Strauss syndrome.

Figure 15-30 depicts the frequency of different light microscopic patterns in biopsy specimens from ANCA-positive patients with pauci-immune renal disease evaluated at the University of North Carolina. This is similar to the observations made by the European Vasculitis Study Group (22). The highest proportion of patients, almost half, have diffuse necrotizing and crescentic glomerulonephritis (i.e., crescents in more than 50 percent of glomeruli). About a quarter of the patients have necrosis and crescents in less than 50 percent of glomeruli. At the time of biopsy, only 3 percent of patients had focal segmental necrosis without crescent formation. If serial sections are examined, almost all foci of glomerular necrosis have adjacent extracapillary hypercellularity (21). Two patients who were ANCA positive and had clinical evidence of renal disease had tubulointerstitial inflammation but no glomerular lesion identified in the biopsy specimens, and two patients had no lesion at all. These patients may have had focal ANCA glomerulonephritis that was not sampled in the biopsy specimen.

Immunofluorescence Findings. By definition, pauci-immune crescentic glomerulonephritis has a paucity or absence of glomerular staining for immunoglobulins and complement (20,27,47). Pauci-immune refers only to the intensity of staining and does not imply that an immune process does not mediate the injury. As shown in figure 15-31, the likelihood of a positive ANCA serology result is inversely proportional to the intensity of the glomerular staining for immunoglobulins (20). Although most cases of ANCA-associated glomerulonephritis have less than 2+ staining for immunoglobulins, it is important to recognize that patients with overt glomerular immune complex deposits may be ANCA positive, especially if there is glomerular crescent formation and necrosis (20). Therefore, even though a positive ANCA test is most likely in a patient with pauci-immune necrotizing or crescentic glomerulonephritis, patients with overt immune complex glomerulonephritis with crescents and necrosis also may be ANCA positive, especially if the pattern of immune complex localization does not result in substantial necrosis or crescent formation. For example, a patient with exclusively mesangial immune deposits or typical subepithelial immune deposits consistent with membranous glomerulopathy who has substantial necrosis and crescents is more likely to be ANCA positive than a patient with no necrosis or crescents (35,36). The presence of ANCA may act synergistically with the immune complexes to cause more severe injury than would be caused by the immune complex disease alone (29,50).

Approximately a quarter to a third of patients with anti-GBM glomerulonephritis are ANCA positive (23,27). The glomerular injury in these ANCA-positive patients is not pauci-immune because the staining for immunoglobulins is linear along the basement membranes. These patients are at risk for renal and extrarenal vasculitis that does not occur in patients with anti-GBM disease who are ANCA negative (see fig. 15-25).

As in any from of glomerulonephritis, there is nonspecific, irregular localization of immunoglobulins, complement, and other plasma proteins in areas of glomerular necrosis and sclerosis

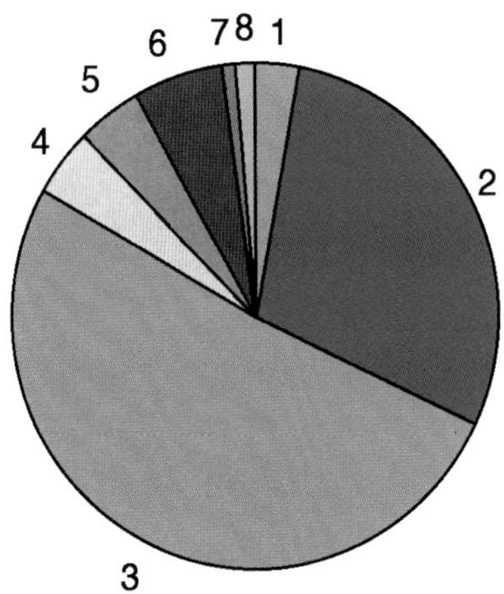

1. Focal necrotizing glomerulonephritis (3%)
2. Focal necrotizing and crescentic glomerulonephritis (27%)
3. Diffuse necrotizing and crescentic glomerulonephritis (48%)
4. Diffuse crescentic glomerulonephritis without necrosis (4%)
5. Focal sclerosing glomerulonephritis (4%)
6. Diffuse sclerosing glomerulonephritis (12%)
7. Tubulointerstitial nephritis alone (1%)
8. No lesion identified (1%)

Figure 15-30

PAUCI-IMMUNE ANCA RENAL DISEASE

This graph depicts the relative frequency of different light microscopic patterns of renal injury in over 200 renal biopsy specimens from ANCA-positive patients with pauci-immune renal disease evaluated in the University of North Carolina Nephropathology Laboratory. Three quarters of the patients had focal or diffuse necrotizing and crescentic glomerulonephritis. A minority had apparently early focal necrotizing glomerulonephritis without crescents, or late focal or diffuse sclerotic disease.

caused by pauci-immune crescentic glomerulonephritis (fig. 15-32). Therefore, when determining whether or not to diagnose pauci-immune glomerulonephritis, the intensity of immunoglobulin staining should be assessed in the most intact glomerular tufts or glomerular segments, where there often is no staining in pauci-immune crescentic glomerulonephritis. A minority of ANCA-positive patients, however, have well-defined but low intensity staining for IgG, IgA, IgM, or multiple immunoglobulins. When IgA staining is dominant, a consideration of IgA

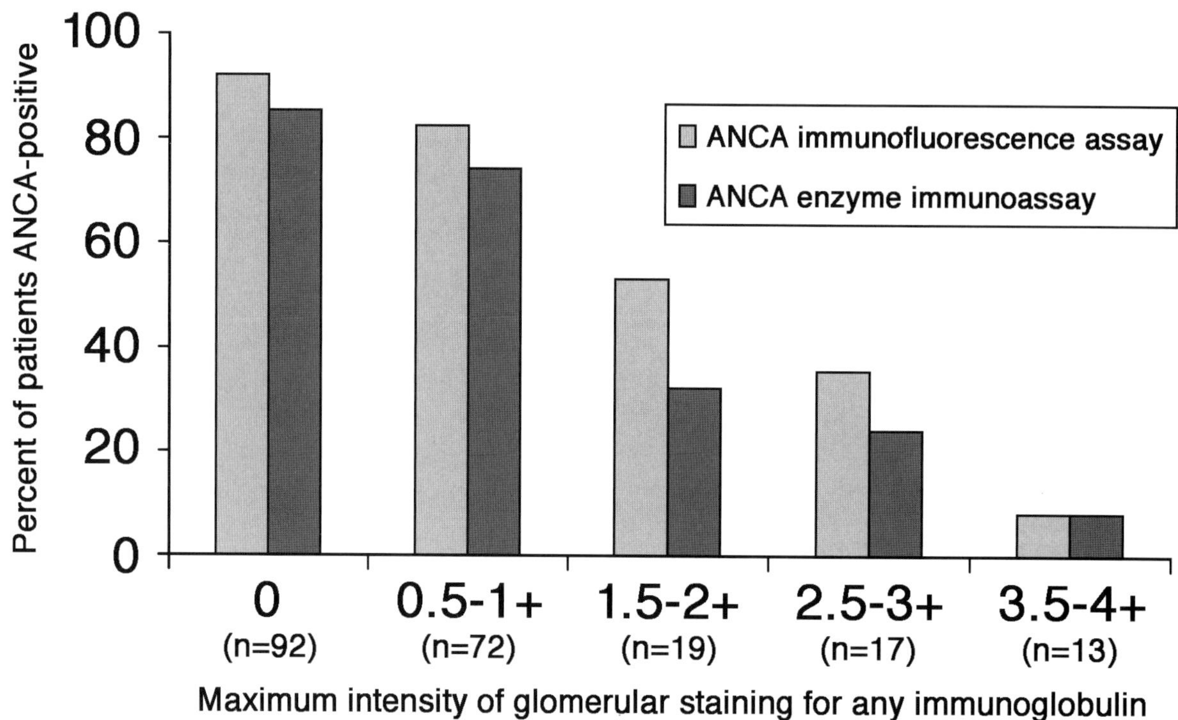

Figure 15-31

LIKELIHOOD OF ANCA RELATIVE TO IMMUNOGLOBULIN STAINING

The data in this chart are from 213 patients with glomerulonephritis with crescent formation. Patients with anti-GBM disease and systemic lupus erythematosus were excluded. Pauci-immune crescentic glomerulonephritis (i.e., with less than 2+ staining for immunoglobulins) has the highest association with ANCA (over 80 percent). A minority of patients with crescentic glomerulonephritis who have well-defined staining for immunoglobulins also are ANCA positive. In these patients, ANCA may play a synergistic pathogenic role along with the immune complexes. (Fig. 6 from Harris AA, Falk RJ, Jennette JC. Crescentic glomerulonephritis with a paucity of glomerular immunoglobulin localization. Am J Kidney Dis 1998;32:179–84.)

nephropathy is appropriate, including IgA nephropathy complicated by superimposed ANCA-induced injury. In the setting of severe necrotizing and crescentic glomerulonephritis, however, slight IgA staining does not warrant a diagnosis other than pauci-immune glomerulonephritis.

Active crescents and foci of glomerular fibrinoid necrosis usually stain for fibrin (figs. 15-32, 15-33). Immunohistochemistry also reveals neutrophil granule proteins, such as MPO, PR3, elastase, and lactoferrin, in foci of necrosis (3). Fibrin staining persists in early fibrocellular crescents but usually is negative in fibrotic crescents. Foci of extraglomerular vasculitis and fibrinoid necrosis also stain for fibrin (fig. 15-34), as well as for plasma constituents, especially complement components and IgM. Because glomerular and arterial lesions are focal, diagnostic foci of pauci-immune glomerular or arterial necrosis may be identified in the tissue by immunofluorescence microscopy but not in the tissue by light microscopy.

Electron Microscopic Findings. The earliest vascular abnormalities in pauci-immune glomerulonephritis or vasculitis are focal endothelial injury and subendothelial accumulation of fibrin (8,10,30). The characteristic, although not specific, ultrastructural feature of overt pauci-immune crescentic glomerulonephritis is focal segmental glomerular necrosis with disruption of basement membranes and Bowman's capsule, and associated localization of electron-dense fibrin tactoids (fig. 15-35) (8). Within and adjacent to sites of glomerular necrosis, capillary thrombi with intraluminal fibrin tactoids and platelets are frequent. Breaks

Figure 15-32

PAUCI-IMMUNE NECROTIZING GLOMERULONEPHRITIS

Direct immunofluorescence microscopy demonstrates slight focal segmental staining for IgG (A) and complement (C) 3 (B), and more extensive irregular staining for fibrin that corresponds to segmental fibrinoid necrosis (C).

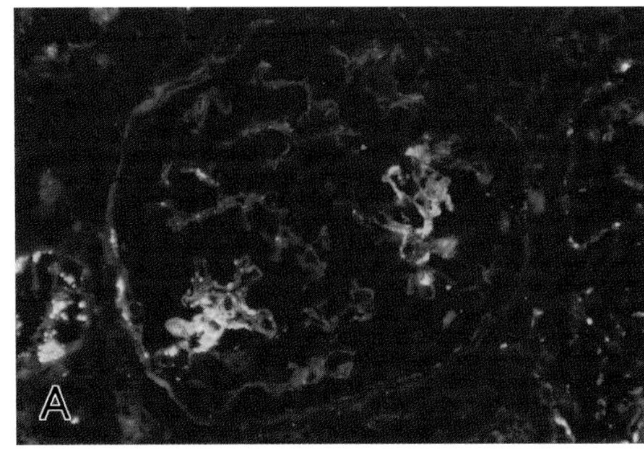

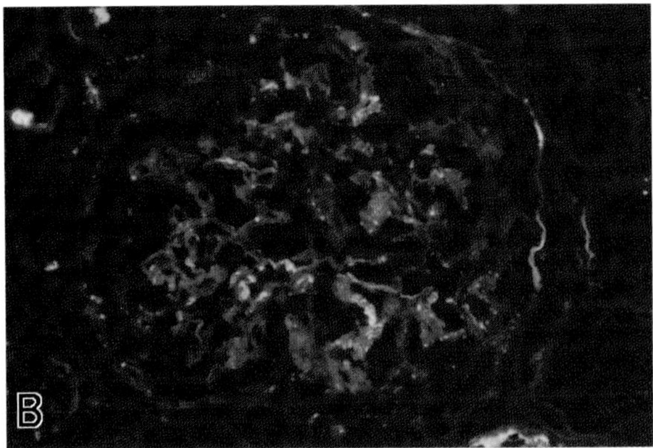

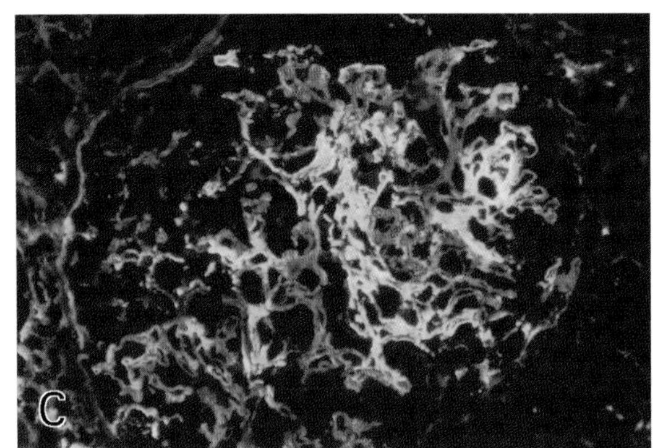

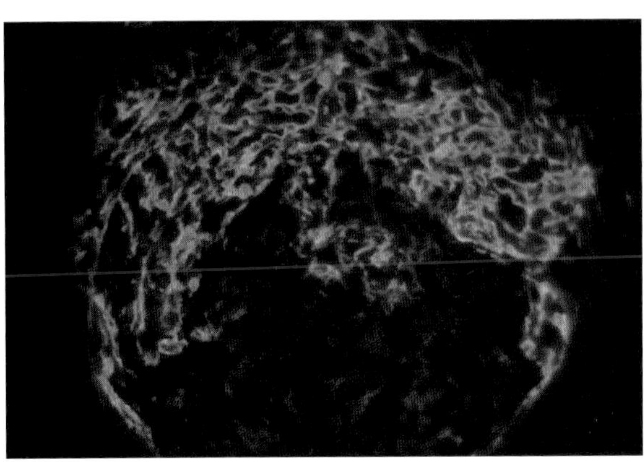

Figure 15-33

FIBRIN IN CRESCENTIC ANCA GLOMERULONEPHRITIS

Direct immunofluorescence microscopy demonstrates fibrin staining in a large crescent from a patient with microscopic polyangiitis and crescentic glomerulonephritis. There also is segmental staining of the glomerular tuft that corresponds to a focus of fibrinoid necrosis.

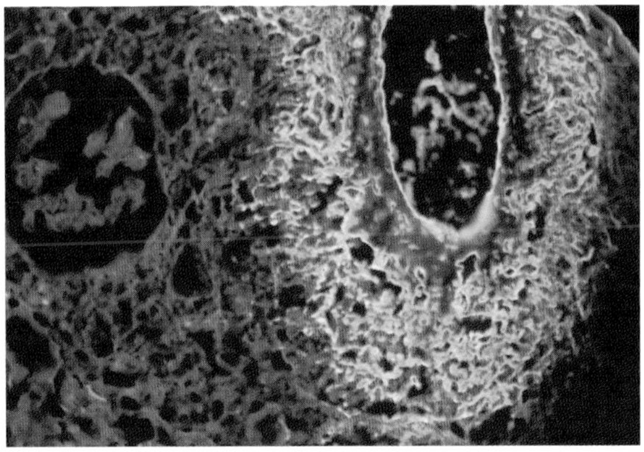

Figure 15-34

FIBRIN IN ANCA ARTERITIS

Direct immunofluorescence microscopy demonstrates fibrin staining in a necrotic interlobular artery from a patient with microscopic polyangiitis. The fibrinoid necrosis extends through the artery wall into the perivascular interstitium. An adjacent glomerulus is negative for fibrin.

in glomerular capillaries and Bowman's capsule are identified by transmission electron microscopy as terminations in glomerular basement membranes and Bowman's capsule. Normally, these structures are endless, because the glomerular basement membranes form an uninterrupted

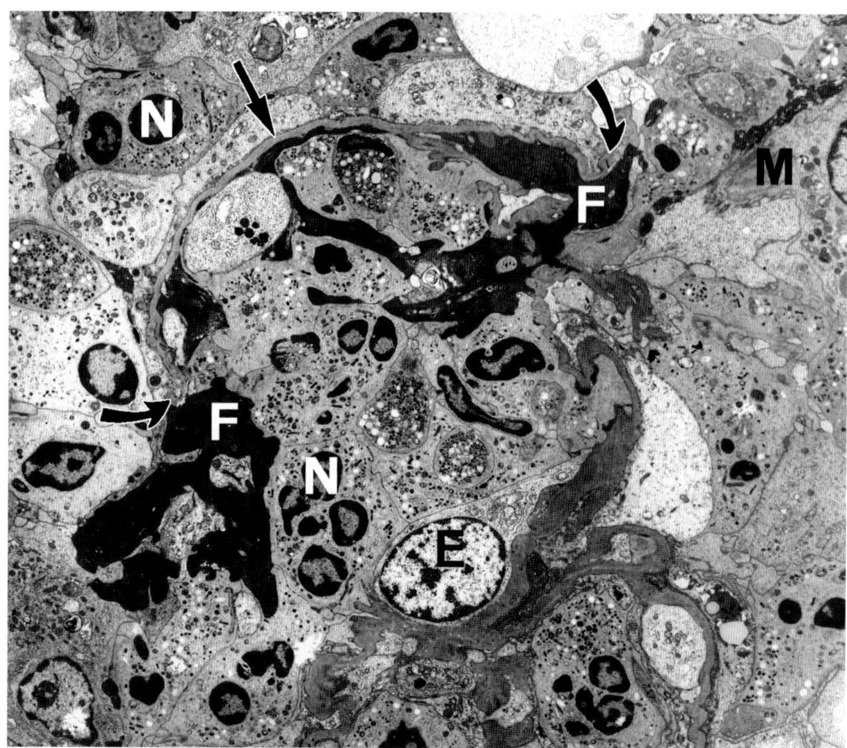

Figure 15-35

PAUCI-IMMUNE NECROTIZING AND CRESCENTIC GLOMERULONEPHRITIS

This electron micrograph of an acute necrotizing lesion shows a single glomerular capillary filling the center of the field. A portion of the peripheral capillary glomerular basement membrane is intact (straight arrow) but as it is traced left or right it terminates at break points (curved arrows). Fibrin (F) extends from the capillary into the adjacent cellular crescent through the breaks in the basement membrane. There are numerous neutrophils (N) in the capillary and the crescent. There is no lumen adjacent to the endothelial cell (E) because it is occluded by fibrin and neutrophils. The crescent also contains macrophages (M).

layer surrounding capillary walls and mesangial regions, then splay out at the hilum to become Bowman's capsule, and eventually merge with the basement membrane of the proximal tubule. Thus, any ends identified by electron microscopy indicate pathologic breaks.

Within and adjacent to acute necrotizing glomerular lesions, often there are neutrophils electron-dense deposits that may have a pattern characteristic of a particular variant of immune complex glomerulonephritis, such as membranous glomerulopathy or membranoproliferative glomerulonephritis.

Electron-dense fibrin tactoids should not be misinterpreted as immune complex–type dense deposits. Fibrin tactoids are more irregular and sometimes have angular edges (fig. 15-35). Chronically injured glomeruli often have nonspecific focal accumulations of entrapped proteinaceous material that may be relatively electron dense (fig. 15-36). This may be confused with immune complex deposits. If the dense material is only at sites of chronic consolidation and not in the most intact segments, it probably is not immune complexes.

The ultrastructural features of necrotizing vasculitis elsewhere in the body are similar to those of necrotizing glomerulonephritis (8). The earliest finding is endothelial injury and subendothelial fibrin formation. In arteries, fibrin accumulates first in the intima and then throughout the media if the necrosis becomes transmural (fig. 15-37). Neutrophils are conspicuous in early arteritis (fig. 15-37), whereas mononuclear leukocytes predominate later.

Differential Diagnosis. Pauci-immune crescentic glomerulonephritis is histologically indistinguishable from anti-GBM glomerulonephritis. Both are characterized by varying degrees of glomerular fibrinoid necrosis and crescent formation, often with disruption of Bowman's capsule. Periglomerular inflammation is common in both, including the presence of multinucleated giant cells. The presence of vasculitis in vessels other than glomerular capillaries is strong evidence for pauci-immune crescentic glomerulonephritis and small vessel vasculitis rather than, or in addition to, anti-GBM disease. Of course, immunofluorescence microscopy readily distinguishes between anti-GBM glomerulonephritis, with intense linear staining of immunoglobulins, and pauci-immune crescentic glomerulonephritis, with little or no staining.

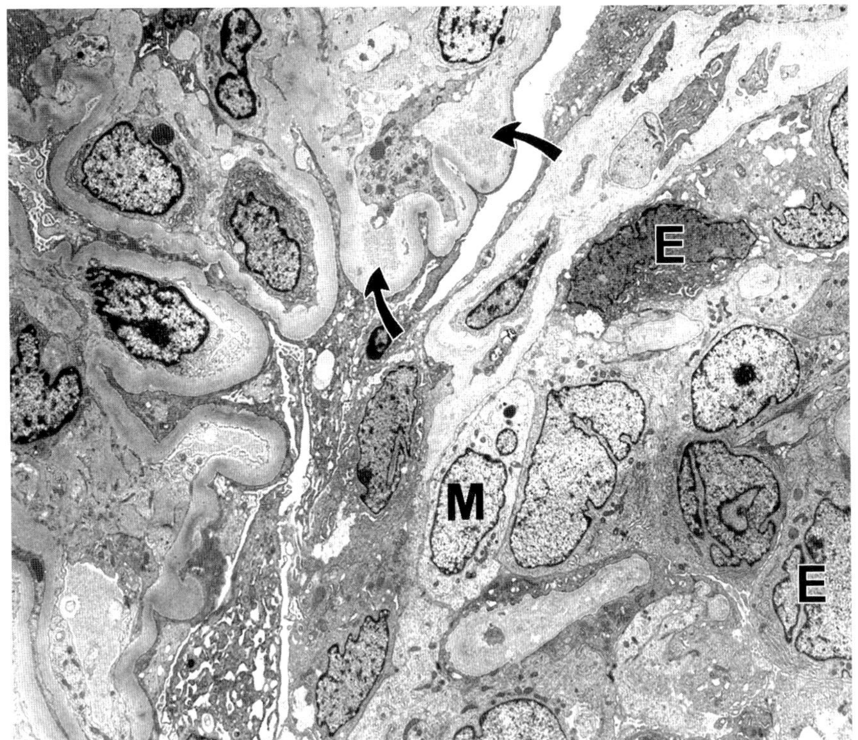

Figure 15-36

PAUCI-IMMUNE CRESCENTIC GLOMERULONEPHRITIS

Compared to the early crescent in figure 15-35, this cellular crescent (lower right) is more mature. It is composed of large mononuclear cells with the ultrastructural features of epithelial cells (E) or macrophages (M). The glomerulus (upper left) shows early chronic changes, including thickening and wrinkling of glomerular basement membranes, increased mesangial matrix material, and accumulation of slightly electron-dense material consistent with protein insudation (curved arrows).

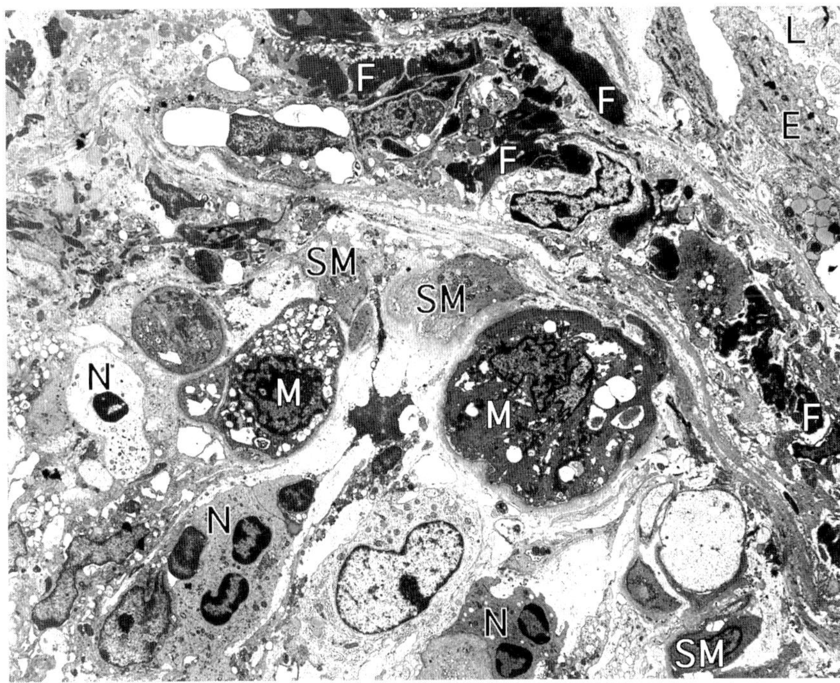

Figure 15-37

MICROSCOPIC POLYANGIITIS

This interlobular artery has extensive necrotizing inflammatory injury. The lumen (L) is at the upper right. The endothelial cell (E) is swollen. There is fibrinoid necrosis with accumulations of electron-dense fibrin (F) in the vessel wall. There is marked disruption of the muscularis, with macrophages (M) and neutrophils (N) infiltrating among residual smooth muscle cells (SM).

Pauci-immune crescentic glomerulonephritis usually can be distinguished from immune complex crescentic glomerulonephritis because the latter typically has hypercellularity and thickening of capillary walls in non-necrotic, nonsclerotic glomerular segments, whereas pauci-immune-crescentic glomerulonephritis often has normal glomerular histology in non-necrotic, nonsclerotic segments, or at most a few marginated neutrophils. The presence of well-defined immune complex staining, detected by immunofluorescence microscopy, rules out pauci-immune crescentic glomerulonephritis. If immune complex glomerulonephritis has more extensive necrosis and crescent formation than would be expected from the type of immune complex localization, the possibility of concurrent pauci-immune crescentic glomerulonephritis should be considered. For example, if the specimen shows a membranous glomerulopathy or IgA nephropathy immunophenotype but has severe necrosis and numerous crescents, ANCA serology should be obtained. If positive, clinical management should be oriented toward pauci-immune crescentic glomerulonephritis rather than typical immune complex glomerulonephritis.

Drug-induced pauci-immune crescentic glomerulonephritis must be distinguished from drug-induced lupus nephritis. A number of drugs, including propylthiouracil and hydralazine, are known to induce circulating ANCAs, which may be accompanied by pauci-immune crescentic glomerulonephritis and vasculitis (9,37,48). Patients with drug-induced ANCAs may also have drug-induced antinuclear antibodies (ANA) and thus also fit the definition of having drug-induced lupus nephritis. The pathology of the glomerulonephritis in patients with drug-induced ANCAs, however, typically is pauci-immune rather than lupus-like. In the absence of ANCAs, patients with drug-induced lupus usually do not have severe glomerulonephritis.

Pauci-immune small vessel vasculitis (ANCA small vessel vasculitis) must be differentiated from other small vessel vasculitides and from the medium-sized vessel vasculitides (polyarteritis nodosa and Kawasaki's disease) (31). Figure 15-1 and Table 15-2 provide approaches for resolving this diagnostic difficulty. Immune complex small vessel vasculitides, such as Henoch-Schönlein purpura and cryoglobulinemic vasculitis, can be distinguished from pauci-immune small vessel vasculitis by identifying immune complex deposits by immunohistology or electron microscopy. In the kidney, the glomerular component of an immune complex small vessel vasculitis typically is some form of proliferative glomerulonephritis, which is only rarely accompanied by inflammation in renal vessels other than the glomeruli. For example, the most common glomerular lesion of Henoch-Schönlein purpura is focal proliferative glomerulonephritis, and the most common glomerular lesion of cryoglobulinemic vasculitis is type 1 membranoproliferative glomerulonephritis. This proliferative glomerular injury differs from the necrotizing pattern of injury seen with pauci-immune small vessel vasculitis.

Pauci-immune small vessel vasculitis can cause necrotizing arteritis that is histologically indistinguishable from the necrotizing arteritis of polyarteritis nodosa and is similar to the arteritis of Kawasaki's disease. These categories of vasculitis are ruled out if capillaries or venules are affected, such as glomerular capillaries, pulmonary capillaries, or dermal venules (32). Arteritis in the kidney should be considered a component of Kawasaki's disease if the patient, usually a child, has the mucocutaneous lymph node syndrome.

Noninflammatory conditions that can mimic systemic small vessel vasculitis include atheroembolization and thrombotic microangiopathy. Atheroembolization is readily distinguished histologically by the presence of cholesterol clefts in vessels. Thrombotic microangiopathy also is histologically distinct, however, care must be taken not to confuse the fibrinoid necrosis of vasculitis with the fibrinoid necrosis of a thrombotic microangiopathy, and vice versa. The fibrinoid necrosis of vasculitis is accompanied by more leukocytes and more extensive destruction of vessel walls.

Etiology and Pathogenesis. The close association of pauci-immune crescentic glomerulonephritis and small vessel vasculitis with ANCAs raises the possibility that ANCAs are involved in the pathogenesis of ANCA-associated vascular inflammation (29,31,50). Drug-induced ANCA disease is the most compelling clinical evidence for the pathogenic potential of ANCAs. A number of drugs are known to induce circulating ANCAs and associated pauci-immune crescentic glomerulonephritis and vasculitis, including propylthiouracil and hydralazine, (9,37,43,45,48). The close temporal association between the induction of ANCAs by drug treatment and the onset of pauci-immune crescentic glomerulonephritis suggests a pathogenic relationship. In addition, ANCA serology becomes negative after discontinuation of the drug, and the glomerulonephritis remits.

ANCAs appear to act synergistically with other inflammatory stimuli to cause neutrophils

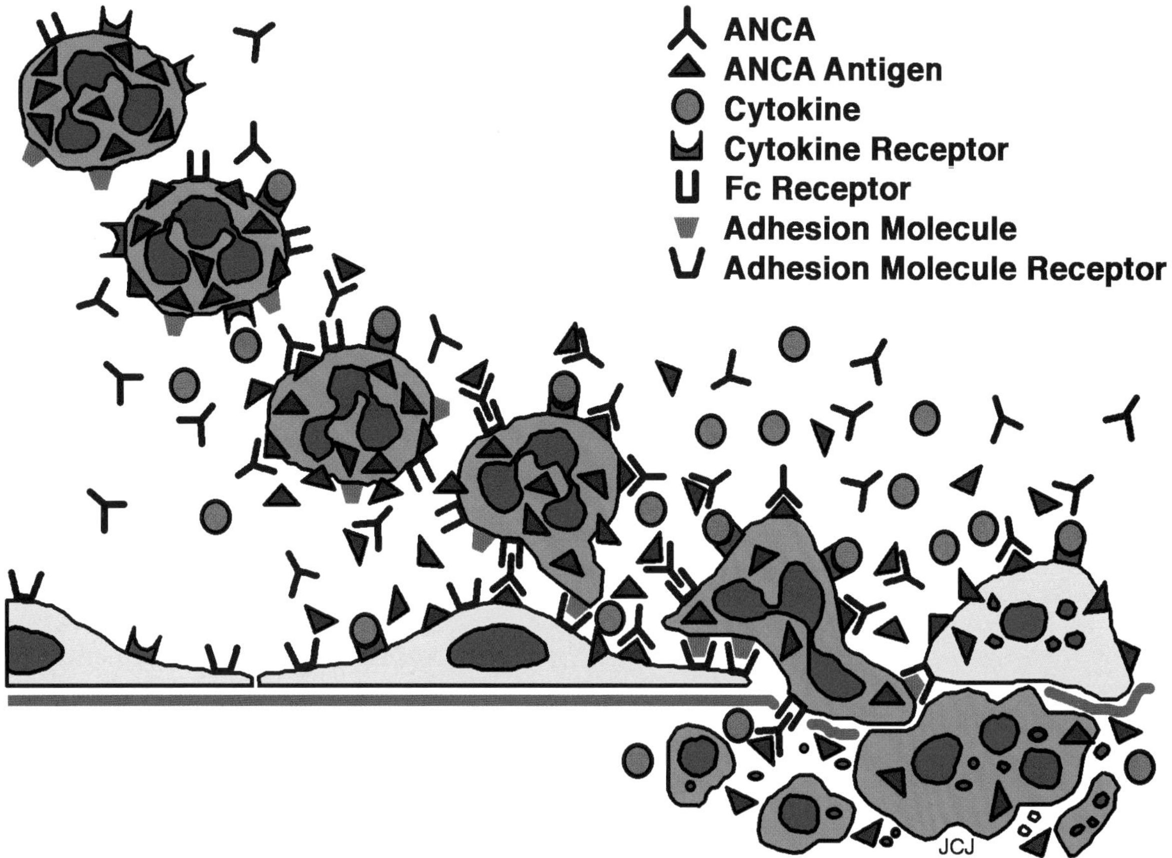

Figure 15-38

PATHOGENESIS OF ANCA VASCULITIS

Figure depicting the hypothetical participation of ANCA in the pathogenesis of vasculitis. Beginning in the upper left corner, proinflammatory stimuli, for example, interactions with cytokines, cause neutrophils (and monocytes, not shown) to express ANCA antigens at the surface. Neutrophils are activated by direct binding of ANCA to the antigens on the surface, and also by Fc receptor engagement by complexes between ANCA and ANCA antigens in the microenvironment around neutrophils and on vessel walls. Activated neutrophils adhere to vessel walls, especially the walls of small vessels, where the neutrophils are in intimate contact with the endothelium. Toxic oxygen metabolites and lytic enzymes cause necrotizing injury to vessel walls and adjacent tissue. (Fig. 1 from reference 29.)

and monocytes to attack vessel walls and cause necrotizing inflammation (fig. 15-38) (29,50). Substantial in vitro evidence and mounting experimental animal data support this hypothesis.

The target antigens for ANCA, such as MPO and PR3, are in granules within the cytoplasm of neutrophils and monocytes. These proteins must be expressed at the surface before they can interact with ANCA. In vitro studies have shown that mild stimulation of neutrophils, for example, with proinflammatory cytokines, causes MPO and PR3 to be expressed at the surface where they can interact with ANCA IgG (29). The interaction of ANCA IgG with cytokine-primed neutrophils results in a respiratory burst, with generation of toxic oxygen metabolites, and degranulation, with release of lytic and toxic enzymes. In vitro, ANCA-activated neutrophils cause apoptosis and necrosis of cultured endothelial cells. If this sequence of in vitro events occurs in vivo, it would cause vasculitis.

The most convincing animal model of ANCA-induced glomerulonephritis and small vessel vasculitis uses MPO gene knock-out mice as a source of pathogenic anti-MPO antibodies (MPO-ANCA) (50). MPO knock-out mice develop high titers of anti-MPO when they are immunized with purified mouse MPO. Passive transfer of anti-MPO IgG into recipient mice, including immune deficient mice that have no antibodies of their own, results in the development of pauci-immune necrotizing and crescentic glomerulonephritis, systemic arteritis, and hemorrhagic capillaritis that closely resemble human ANCA glomerulonephritis and vasculitis (50).

Treatment and Prognosis. Patients with all variants of pauci-immune renal vasculitis are treated similarly with high-dose corticosteroids and immunosuppressive agents when there is active major organ involvement, such as rapidly progressive glomerulonephritis (2,13,15,18, 25,38,41). Treatment can be divided into remission induction, remission maintenance, and relapse treatment (2). Although initial remission is induced in approximately 80 percent of patients, there is a high recurrence rate that requires maintenance of immunosuppressive therapy and retreatment regimens. With appropriate therapy, the 5-year renal and patient survival rates are 60 to 80 percent.

Rapid diagnosis and initiation of treatment are critically important for optimum patient outcome. The serum creatinine level at the time of diagnosis and institution of treatment is the best predictor of outcome (38). The renal biopsy finding that seems to be the best predictor of outcome is the percentage of normal glomeruli (5). Although the ultimate clinical outcomes are similar, patients with C-ANCA (PR3-ANCA) glomerulonephritis have more rapid initial deterioration of renal function than patients with P-ANCA (MPO-ANCA) (12).

Renal transplantation is appropriate in patients with end-stage renal disease secondary to pauci-immune crescentic glomerulonephritis or small vessel vasculitis. The recurrence rate after transplantation is approximately 15 to 20 percent, and does not vary with the initial variant of pauci-immune renal vasculitis, type of antirejection therapy, or persistent ANCA positivity (39). There is no evidence that transplantation should be deferred because of a persistently positive ANCA level in a patient with clinical signs of active disease.

KAWASAKI'S DISEASE

Definition. Kawasaki's disease is a febrile illness of childhood that is defined by the presence of the mucocutaneous lymph node syndrome (53,57,58a,60,61). The mucocutaneous lymph node syndrome is characterized by mucosal changes in the mouth and on the lips, including erythema of the oropharynx and dryness, redness, or fissuring of the lips; cutaneous changes, including erythema, indurative edema, and desquamation; and nonsuppurative lymphadenopathy. Some patients with Kawasaki's disease develop necrotizing vasculitis (51,52,54, 55,58,62,65,67). The arteritis involves large, medium-sized, and small arteries, and is associated with the mucocutaneous lymph node syndrome. Coronary arteries are most often involved. Renal arteries are involved in a quarter to half of patients with fatal Kawasaki's disease.

Clinical Features. Kawasaki's disease usually occurs in young children, with a peak incidence at 1 year of age. Most cases occur sporadically but there are well-documented epidemics that raise the possibility of an infectious etiology. The characteristic presentation of patients with Kawasaki's disease is with the mucocutaneous lymph node syndrome. The most life-threatening complication of Kawasaki's disease is myocardial infarction caused by arteritis of the coronary arteries. In fact, Kawasaki's disease is the most common cause of myocardial infarction in children. Virtually all fatal cases had coronary artery involvement. Renal involvement is rarely clinically significant.

Gross Findings. The major gross feature of Kawasaki's disease arteritis is nodule formation along major arterial branches caused by the formation of inflammatory pseudoaneurysms. Arteries usually are involved between their take-off from the aorta and their penetration into the parenchyma of an organ. For example, the coronary arteries usually are involved within the first few centimeters of their origin from the aorta. In the kidneys, the disease has a strong predilection for the interlobar arteries (65). Even when there is widespread involvement of the lobar arteries, the arcuate and interlobular arteries usually are spared. Renal infarction and hemorrhage are rare. The external surface of the kidneys may be normal even when there is extensive involvement of the interlobar arteries. The renal arterial pseudoaneurysms are seen best by careful examination of the hilum or of the cut surface of the renal sinus.

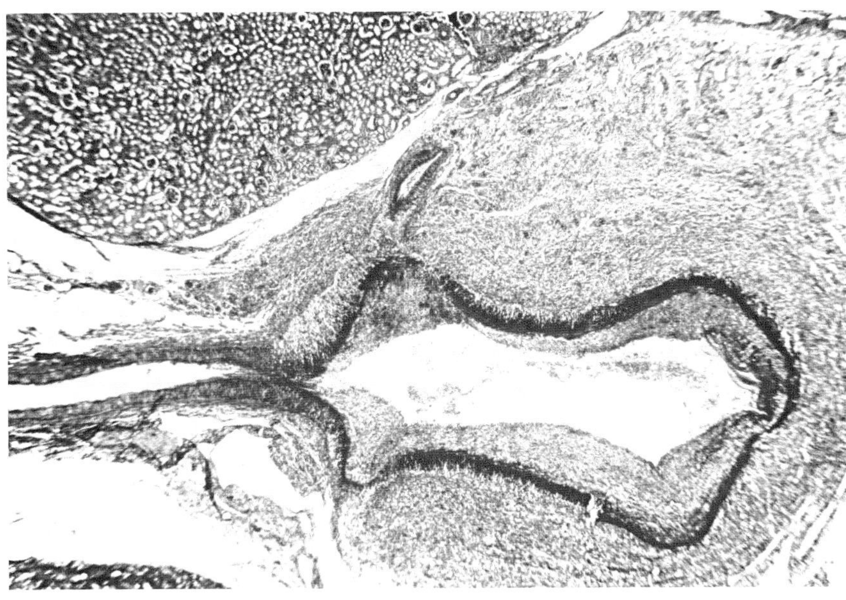

Figure 15-39

KAWASAKI'S DISEASE ARTERITIS

A pseudoaneurysm is seen in an interlobar artery of a young child with Kawasaki's disease. Compare the uninvolved arterial segment on the left to the segment showing extensive fibrinoid necrosis with marked perivascular inflammation in the renal sinus tissue.

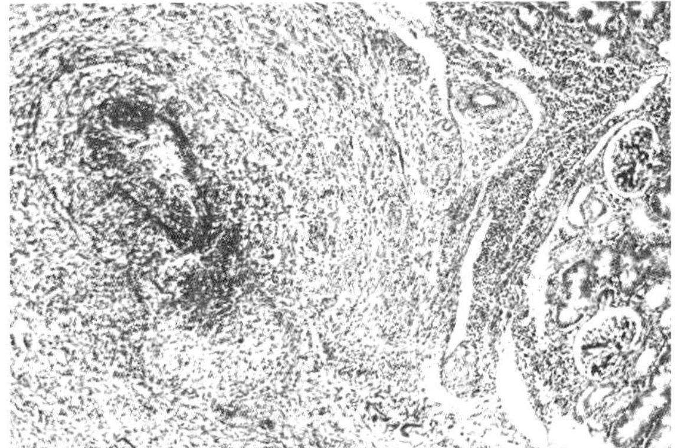

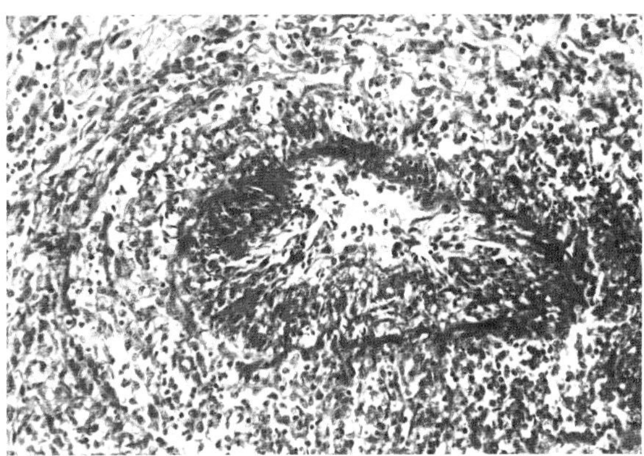

Figure 15-40

KAWASAKI'S DISEASE ARTERITIS

Left: Low-power magnification shows circumferential necrotizing inflammation of an interlobar artery, with perivascular inflammation in the renal sinus but not in the adjacent column of Bertin.

Right: Higher magnification shows the predominance of mononuclear leukocytes and the relatively modest amounts of fibrinoid material.

Light Microscopic Findings. Kawasaki's disease causes a necrotizing arteritis that is characterized by transmural infiltration of predominantly mononuclear leukocytes, accompanied by edema and fibrinoid necrosis (51,52,54,55,58,62, 65,67). Destruction of the vessel wall with erosion of the inflammatory process into the perivascular tissue causes the formation of pseudoaneurysms (fig. 15-39). In Kawasaki's disease arteritis, the edema is more pronounced and the fibrinoid necrosis less pronounced than in the arteritis of polyarteritis nodosa or the ANCA small vessel vasculitides, such as microscopic polyangiitis (figs. 15-40–15-42) (65). All layers of the arteries are affected, although the earliest lesions appear to begin in the intima. In active Kawasaki's disease, there is very conspicuous infiltration of macrophages (fig. 15-43) (59). Marked intimal thickening caused by edema and leukocyte infiltration can narrow lumens and cause ischemia during the acute phase of the disease (figs. 15-40, 15-41). Intimal fibrosis can cause ischemia during the chronic phase. Mild glomerular hypercellularity may occur, in part caused by

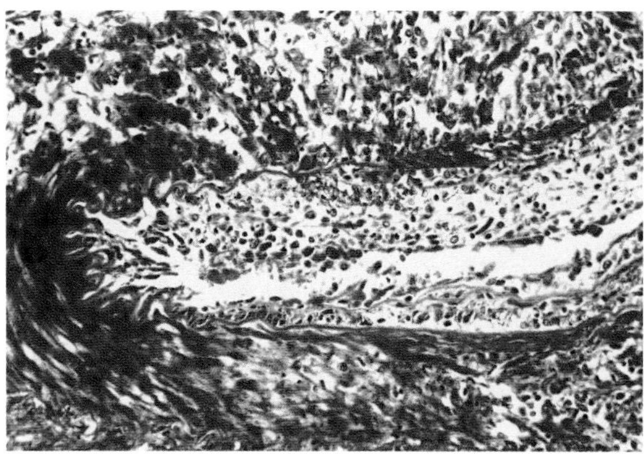

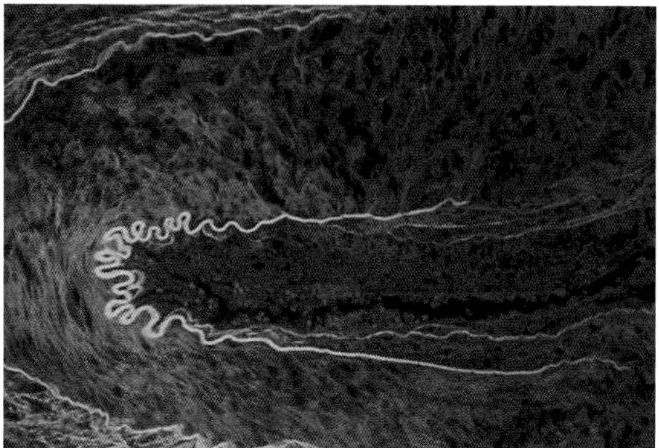

Figure 15-41

KAWASAKI'S DISEASE ARTERITIS

Left: This trichrome-stained section has a relatively intact muscularis in the lower left corner and a markedly edematous muscularis in the upper right portion of the interlobar artery.

Right: This adjacent section stained with H&E and viewed by fluorescence microscopy shows the internal and external elastica as brightly fluorescent lines. The internal elastica is fragmented and disrupted in the area of severe inflammation.

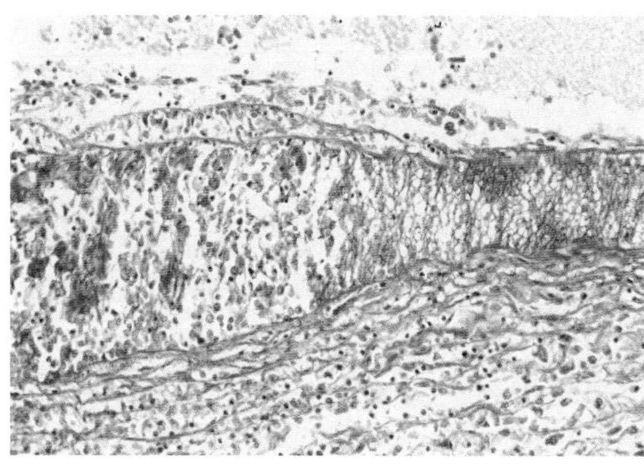

Figure 15-42

KAWASAKI'S DISEASE ARTERITIS

PAS-stained section of an interlobar artery with the lumen at the top of the figure. The muscularis to the right is relatively normal whereas the muscularis to the left has an infiltration of mononuclear leukocytes, severe edema, and focal lysis of smooth muscle cells. The transmural inflammation also involves the intima and adventitia.

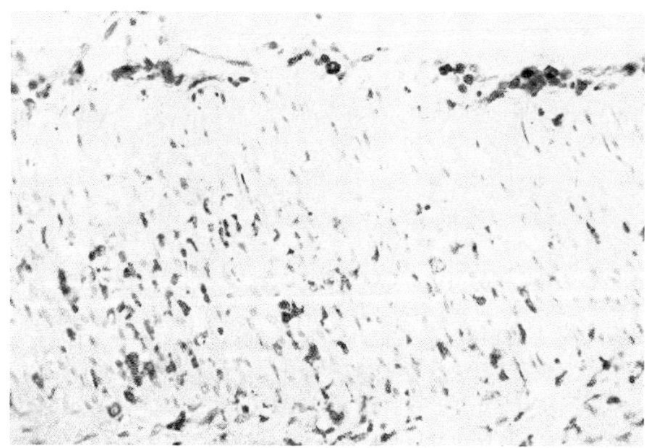

Figure 15-43

KAWASAKI'S DISEASE ARTERITIS

Immunohistochemistry using anti-CD68 antibody demonstrates numerous monocytes and macrophages in the intima and muscularis of a renal lobar artery in a patient with Kawasaki's disease arteritis.

increased glomerular macrophages, but overt glomerulonephritis is not a significant feature.

Immunofluorescence Findings. Immunofluorescence microscopy reveals no immune complex–type deposits. Areas of necrosis and severe edema demonstrate nonspecific entrapment of plasma proteins. There is fibrin staining at sites of fibrinoid material.

Electron Microscopic Findings. No specific ultrastructural features have been reported.

Differential Diagnosis. Kawasaki's disease arteritis must be distinguished from other forms of necrotizing arteritis. Before it was recognized as a distinct entity, Kawasaki's disease was often called infantile polyarteritis nodosa (61). This is not an appropriate designation because it implies that Kawasaki's disease arteritis is merely polyarteritis nodosa occurring in an infant. This is clearly not the case because of the distinctive epidemiology, clinical characteristics, treatment response, and pathologic features of Kawasaki's disease.

Pathologically, the necrotizing arteritis of Kawasaki's disease differs from the necrotizing arteritis of polyarteritis nodosa and the ANCA-associated small vessel vasculitides. In the acute phase, Kawasaki's disease arteritis shows more mural edema, more infiltrating monocytes and macrophages, and less fibrinoid necrosis than these other arteritides, which have more infiltrating neutrophils and more fibrinoid necrosis.

Etiology and Pathogenesis. Antiendothelial cell antibodies (AECAs) are incriminated in the pathogenesis of Kawasaki's disease arteritis (63, 68). The evidence for this is relatively weak, however. The cytotoxic AECAs of Kawasaki's disease are specific for antigens that are expressed only after endothelial cells have been stimulated, for example, by interleukin (IL)-1, tumor necrotic factor (TNF), or interferon. Patients with Kawasaki's disease have increased levels of circulating cytokines, which may activate both endothelial cells and circulating leukocytes. Thus, an interplay between endothelial cells (activated by cytokines, AECAs, or both) and activated leukocytes, especially monocytes and macrophages, could be the basis for the vascular inflammation.

Treatment and Prognosis. The distinction between Kawasaki's disease and other forms of arteritis is more than just a classification exercise because the appropriate treatment for patients with Kawasaki's disease is dramatically different from that for other forms of necrotizing arteritis. The accepted and effective treatment for patients with Kawasaki's disease is aspirin and high-dose intravenous immunoglobulin (IVIG) (56,64,66). If administered early in the course, IVIG markedly reduces the incidence and severity of coronary arteritis, and presumably arteritis elsewhere. The IVIG treatment dampens circulating cytokine levels and may provide anti-idiotypic antibodies to neutralize AECAs.

POLYARTERITIS NODOSA

Definition. Polyarteritis nodosa is necrotizing inflammation of arteries without inflammation in vessels other than arteries (69c,69f,70, 72,73,75,76). Therefore, by this definition, the presence of glomerulonephritis, pulmonary capillaritis, or dermal venulitis rules out polyarteritis nodosa and indicates some form of small vessel vasculitis. Essentially, polyarteritis nodosa is a necrotizing arteritis whereas the small vessel vasculitides are polyangiitides that affect not only arteries but other vessels as well (69e). This definition of polyarteritis nodosa is different from definitions used in the past that subsumed some forms of small vessel vasculitis under the diagnosis. For about the first 50 years after "periarteritis nodosa" was first recognized in the 1800s (71), any patient with gross or microscopic evidence of arteritis was given a diagnosis of "periarteritis nodosa" or the revised term, "polyarteritis nodosa" (31). Over the past half century, however, a succession of distinct variants of vasculitis have been removed from the polyarteritis nodosa category, including Wegener's granulomatosis, Churg-Strauss syndrome, microscopic polyangiitis, and Kawasaki's disease. What remains is a less common category of vasculitis with a more definable natural history, prognosis, and treatment response. This change in definition must be kept in mind when reviewing the literature about the clinical and pathologic features of polyarteritis nodosa because older literature describes features of patients who have a mixture of polyarteritis nodosa, microscopic polyangiitis, and possibly other vasculitides.

Clinical Features. Polyarteritis nodosa usually occurs in adults, but may occur at any age. Kawasaki's disease must be ruled out in any child before a diagnosis of polyarteritis nodosa is considered. Most patients have nonspecific constitutional signs and symptoms of inflammation, such as fever, malaise, arthralgias, myalgias, and anorexia (69c,70,72). Manifestations of tissue injury caused by the arteritis are extremely varied and include tender cutaneous nodules, skin ulceration, peripheral gangrene, livedo reticularis, localized muscle pain, peripheral neuropathy, bowel pain or bleeding, hypertension, testicular pain, myocardial infarction, and elevated tissue enzymes. Visceral arterial aneurysms or thrombotic occlusions may be revealed by imaging studies. The most common initial symptoms are fever, abdominal pain, muscle pain, and peripheral neuropathy, especially mononeuritis multiplex. Renal involvement is frequent and may manifest as hematuria, mild proteinuria, renal insufficiency,

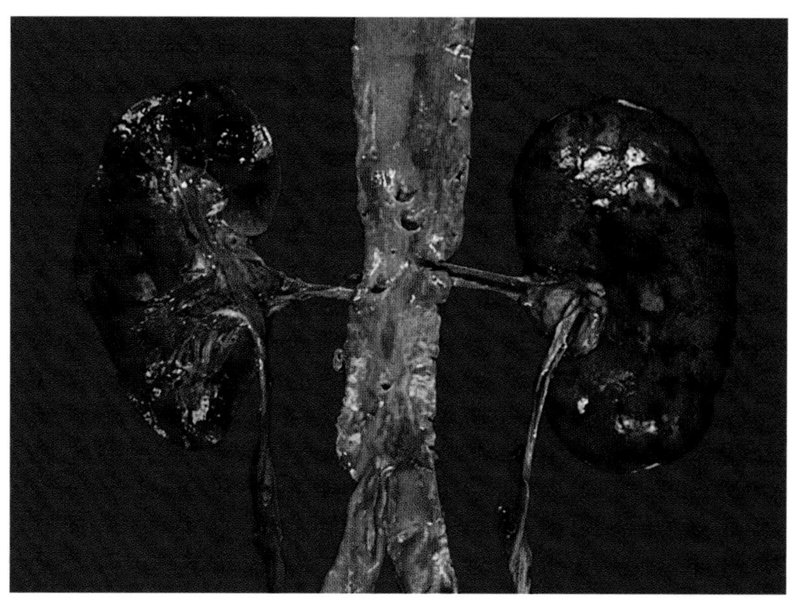

Figure 15-44

POLYARTERITIS NODOSA

The cut surface of the left kidney and the external surface of the right kidney show multiple infarcts with irregular pale centers and hemorrhagic borders. Multiple pseudoaneurysms are seen, especially in the upper pole. The location of these pseudoaneurysms suggests an origin from the interlobar or arcuate arteries.

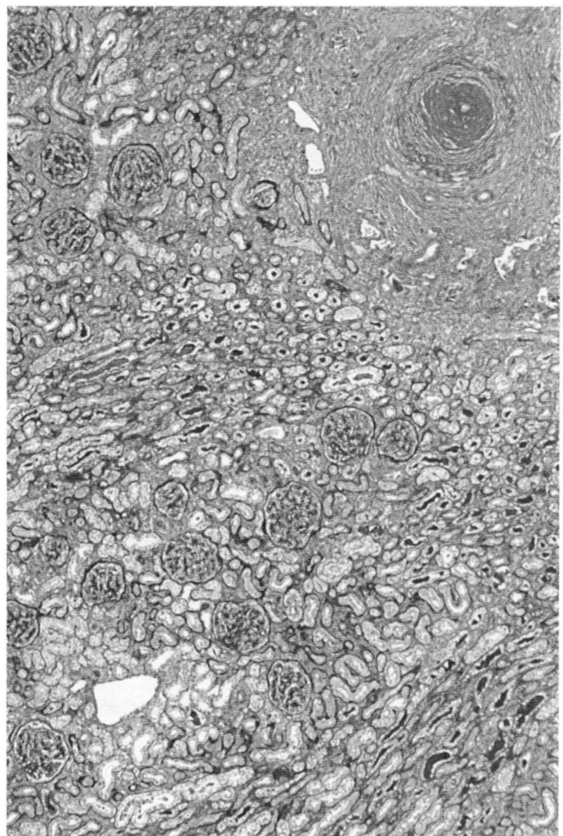

Figure 15-45

POLYARTERITIS NODOSA

Low-power magnification photomicrograph of a PAS-stained section shows arteritis affecting an arcuate artery, but no evidence of glomerulonephritis.

and hypertension as a result of renal infarction and hemorrhage (69,69d). Renovascular hypertension is the most frequent clinically significant renal dysfunction. Rupture of renal pseudoaneurysms can cause fatal retroperitoneal or intraperitoneal hemorrhage (74).

Gross Findings. The presence of pale nodular lesions along the course of major visceral arteries is the classic gross feature, and prompted the designation "nodosa" (69,71). The lesions are most common at branch points. These nodules are the result of expanding pseudoaneurysms and the surrounding inflammation. The leukocytes in the perivascular infiltrates impart the pale color. Cross sections of the pseudoaneurysms often reveal partial or complete occlusion by thrombus. In the kidney, pseudoaneurysms are seen most often at the corticomedullary junction and in the renal sinus because the most frequently involved arteries are the arcuate and interlobar arteries. Thrombosis in pseudoaneurysms and at other sites of arteritis causes infarcts that may be grossly apparent (fig. 15-44). On mucosal and skin surfaces, infarction causes ulcers.

Light Microscopic Findings. The acute lesion of polyarteritis nodosa is segmental transmural fibrinoid necrosis (figs. 15-45–15-48) (69,73,75, 76). The inflammatory infiltrates that accompany the necrosis, and presumably cause it, initially contain numerous neutrophils (fig. 15-46). By the time they are examined histologically,

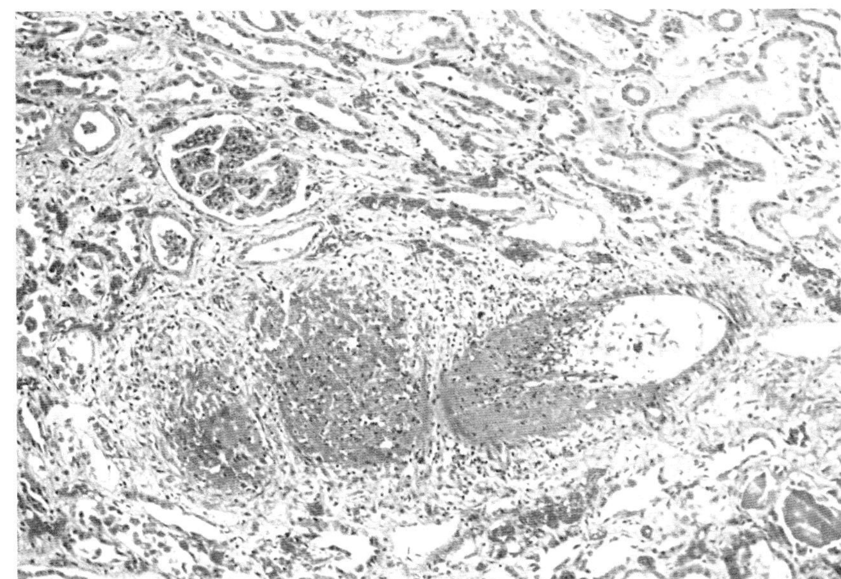

Figure 15-46

POLYARTERITIS NODOSA

Segmental necrotizing inflammation affects an interlobular artery. Note the unremarkable glomerulus. If this same pattern of arteritis was accompanied by necrotizing or crescentic glomerulonephritis, it would be consistent with microscopic polyangiitis, Wegener's granulomatosis, or Churg-Strauss syndrome.

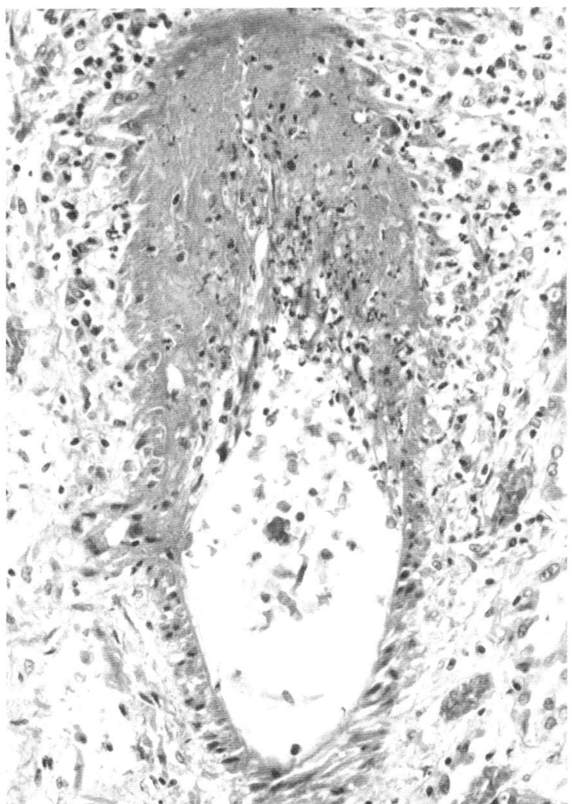

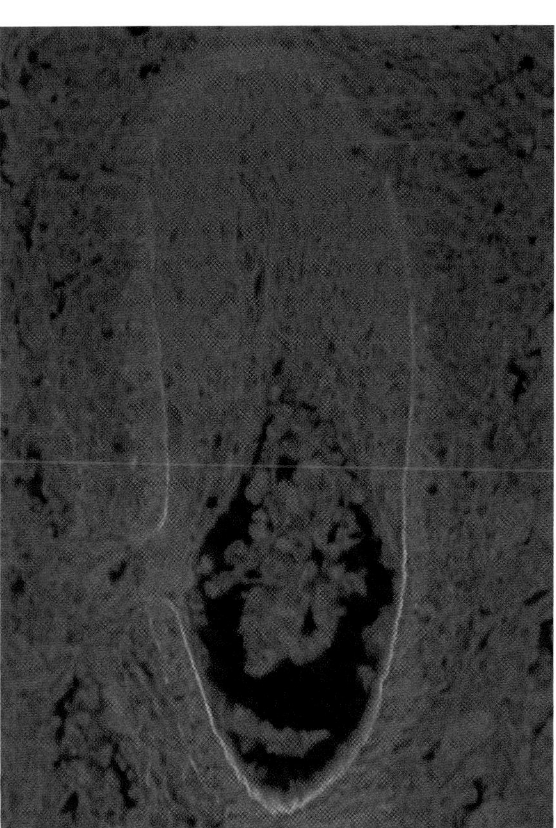

Figure 15-47

POLYARTERITIS NODOSA

Left: Higher magnification of the same artery as in figure 15-46 shows a relatively intact vessel wall at the bottom and severe transmural fibrinoid necrosis at the top. At this early stage, neutrophils are conspicuous.

Right: The same field viewed by fluorescence microscopy. The H&E staining causes fluorescence of the internal elastica under ultraviolet (UV) illumination, which allows identification of segmental rupture on the bottom.

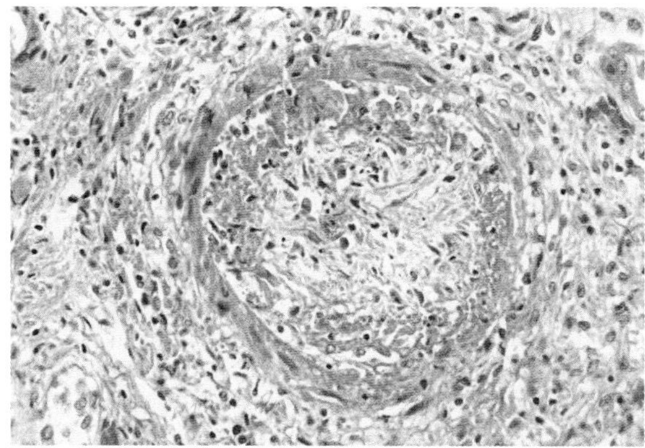

Figure 15-48

POLYARTERITIS NODOSA

Early organizing phase of arteritis, with residual fibrinoid material and nuclear debris in the background and loose connective tissue filling the lumen. The necrosis of the muscularis on the right indicates that the thrombosis is secondary to vasculitis.

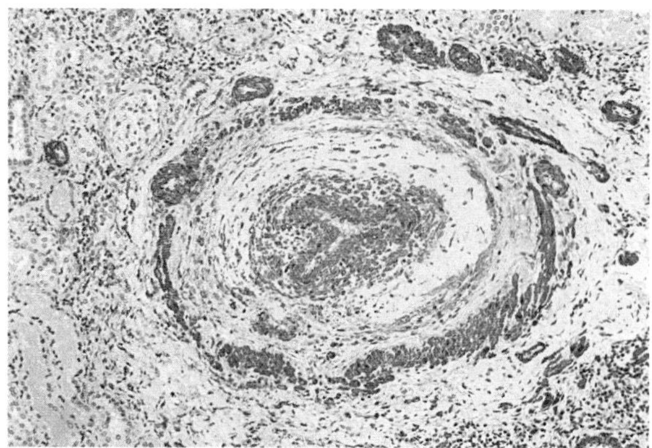

Figure 15-50

POLYARTERITIS NODOSA

Chronic "healed" phase immunostained for smooth muscle actin shows extensive loss and disorganization of smooth muscle cells in the muscularis.

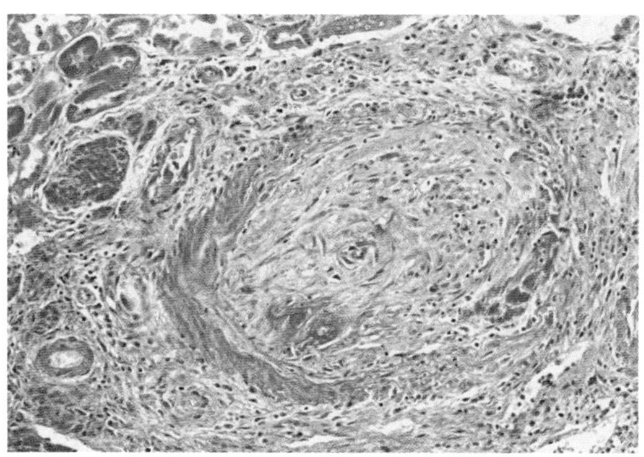

Figure 15-49

POLYARTERITIS NODOSA

Arcuate artery with advanced organization of necrotizing arteritis. The lumen is filled with granulation tissue. The destruction of the muscularis on the right indicates earlier vascular necrosis rather than thrombosis alone.

however, they often have a predominance of mononuclear leukocytes (fig. 15-48). The acute necrotizing lesions evolve through varying stages of organization that eventually lead to arterial scarring (figs. 15-49–15-51). If there is no residual active vasculitis, this arterial scarring may be misinterpreted as hypertensive arteriosclerosis. Focal disruption of the muscularis and internal elastic lamina is a useful histologic marker of earlier arteritis (figs. 15-49–15-51). Trichrome staining (fig. 15-51, left) and immunostaining for smooth muscle actin (fig. 15-50) are useful for identifying injury to the muscularis. Silver staining (fig. 15-51, right) and fluorescence of eosin-stained sections (fig. 15-47, right) are useful for detecting disruption of the elastica.

Any caliber artery, from the main renal artery to the smallest radicals of the interlobular arteries, can be involved by polyarteritis nodosa, however, the presence of glomerulonephritis shifts the diagnosis away from polyarteritis nodosa and into the small vessel vasculitis category (69e,69f,76). An exception to this is reactive inflammation of glomeruli immediately adjacent to areas of intense arteritis or infarction. Similarly, arterial inflammation and necrosis in zones of infarction should not be taken as definitive evidence of arteritis.

Immunofluorescence Findings. Idiopathic polyarteritis nodosa typically has no arterial staining for immunoglobulins or complement except for nonspecific entrapment at sites of inflammation and necrosis (fig. 15-52). Foci of fibrinoid necrosis and thrombosis stain for fibrin. The rare examples of hepatitis-induced vasculitis that have a polyarteritis nodosa pattern may have granular immunoglobulin and complement staining of the vessel wall. Most patients with hepatitis-induced vasculitis, however, have a small vessel vasculitis with involvement not

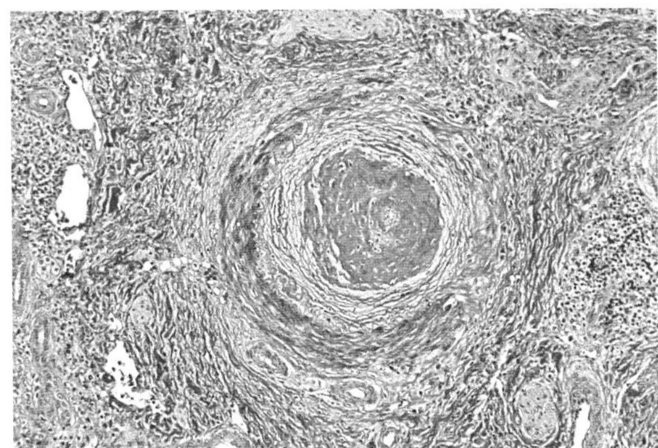

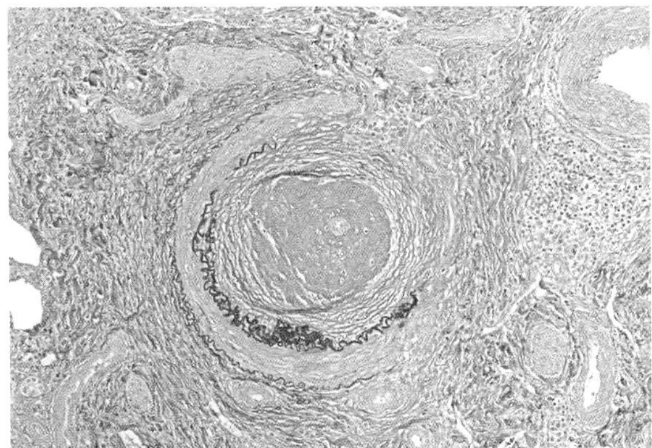

Figure 15-51

POLYARTERITIS NODOSA

Artery with extensive intimal fibrosis, which almost obliterates the lumen, but no active necrosis or inflammation.

Left: The trichrome stain shows that the muscularis has been replaced by fibrosis in a portion of the artery wall at the right.

Right: The JMS stain reveals destruction of the internal and external elastica in a portion of the artery wall at the right, which is indicative of earlier necrotizing injury.

only of arteries but also glomerular capillaries and other small vessels, such as dermal venules.

Electron Microscopic Findings. The ultrastructural features of polyarteritis nodosa do not differ from those of other forms of necrotizing arteritis. These are described earlier in this chapter with pauci-immune small vessel vasculitis.

Differential Diagnosis. Polyarteritis nodosa must be differentiated from other vasculitides that cause necrotizing arteritis, such as Kawasaki's disease, microscopic polyangiitis, Wegener's granulomatosis, and Churg-Strauss syndrome (69e, 69f). Figure 15-1 and Table 15-2 provide approaches for resolving this diagnostic dilemma. Kawasaki's disease should be suspected in any child under 5 years old who has necrotizing arteritis. The presence of mucocutaneous lymph node syndrome distinguishes Kawasaki's disease from polyarteritis nodosa. In addition, pathologically, Kawasaki's disease arteritis has more edema and less fibrinoid necrosis than polyarteritis nodosa.

In a patient with necrotizing arteritis, the concurrence of vasculitis in capillaries or venules indicates some form of small vessel vasculitis, such as microscopic polyangiitis, Wegener's granulomatosis, or Churg-Strauss syndrome, rather than polyarteritis nodosa. Respiratory tract involvement is rare in patients with polyarteritis nodosa but frequent in ANCA small vessel vasculitis.

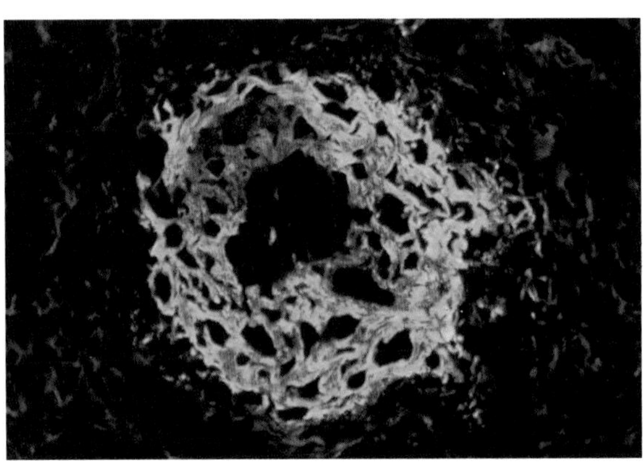

Figure 15-52

POLYARTERITIS NODOSA

Direct immunofluorescence microscopy uses antifibrin antiserum to demarcate extensive fibrin in the wall of an artery with fibrinoid necrosis.

The differential diagnosis for chronic arterial inflammation and scarring includes not only the chronic sclerotic phases of necrotizing arteritides, but also indolent sclerosing vasculitides such as Takayasu's arteritis and giant cell arteritis, and chronic vasculopathies such as arteriosclerosis and fibromuscular dysplasia. This can be a difficult differential to resolve on the basis of histology alone, and the integration of clinical information may be required.

Etiology and Pathogenesis. The etiology of polyarteritis nodosa is unknown. A small proportion of patients with necrotizing arteritis have associated viral (e.g., hepatitis B or C) or bacterial (e.g., streptococcal) infections that may be causing the vasculitis through immune complex localization in artery walls. This accounts for only a minority of patients with the clinicopathologic features of polyarteritis nodosa. Most patients have no evidence of immune complex disease. When microscopic polyangiitis is carefully separated form polyarteritis nodosa, the frequency of ANCAs is low and thus not incriminated in the pathogenesis (69b,69c,70).

Treatment and Prognosis. Patients with polyarteritis nodosa are treated with high-dose corticosteroids, usually in combination with cytotoxic drugs (69a,69c). These patients often require less immunosuppression than those with ANCA small vessel vasculitides, such as microscopic polyangiitis, because recurrences are fewer after induction of remission. The absence of pulmonary involvement and glomerulonephritis in patients with polyarteritis nodosa also improves the prognosis compared to patients with ANCA small vessel vasculitis who frequently have severe pulmonary and renal disease.

TAKAYASU'S ARTERITIS

Definition. Takayasu's arteritis is chronic granulomatous inflammation of the aorta and its major branches that usually occurs in patients younger than 50 years old (77,78a). This disease also has been called *pulseless disease* and *aortic arch disease* because of the ischemic effects caused by sclerotic narrowing of the aortic arch and the major arteries to the extremities.

Clinical Features. Takayasu's arteritis is most common in Asia but occurs throughout the world. The disease has a 9 to 1 female predominance and usually is identified during the second or third decade of life. The clinical course of the disease is marked by recurrent phases of exacerbation and quiescence over months to years (78,81,82). Takayasu's arteritis causes ischemic signs and symptoms that affect the head or extremities, such as reduced pulses, bruits, or claudication (77,78). Imaging of the aorta or its major arterial branches shows focal narrowing of lumens. Renovascular hypertension occurs in approximately half of patients as a result of narrowing of the renal arteries or the abdominal aorta (79).

Gross Findings. Affected arteries have irregular narrowing caused by varying degrees of intimal thickening and fibrotic constriction of the media and adventitia (78,81). Focal post-stenotic dilation adds to the irregularity of the vessel walls. Rare complications include dissecting aneurysms and vessel wall rupture.

Light Microscopic Findings. The arterial and aortic inflammation of Takayasu's arteritis is characterized by transmural inflammation with a predominance of mononuclear leukocytes, sometimes accompanied by multinucleated giant cells (78,81). Plasma cells and eosinophils may be admixed. In early lesions, the most conspicuous inflammation may be in the media, but all layers of the vessel wall eventually are affected (fig. 15-53). Patchy disruption of the medial elastica of the aorta and the elastic lamina of arteries accompanies the inflammation and results in irregular scarring in the media. As Takayasu's arteritis progresses, the amount of intimal and medial fibrosis increases and the leukocyte infiltration diminishes.

In the kidney, the intimal thickening may cause narrowing of the lumen of major renal arteries (fig. 15-54), which can secondarily cause renal ischemia and renovascular hypertension. There are a few reports of various types of glomerular injury in patients with Takayasu's arteritis (80), however, this is so uncommon that it probably is a coincidental, pathogenetically unrelated disease.

Differential Diagnosis. Based on histology alone, the active inflammatory phase of Takayasu's arteritis cannot be distinguished with confidence from the active phase of giant cell arteritis. The best clinical discriminator is the age of the patient (78a). Unless the clinical presentation and vascular distribution are absolutely classic for either Takayasu's arteritis or giant cell arteritis, chronic granulomatous arteritis in a patient younger than 50 years old should be considered Takayasu's arteritis and in a patient older than 50, giant cell arteritis. The chronic sclerotic phase of Takayasu's arteritis is difficult to distinguish from severe arteriosclerosis by histologic examination alone; however, knowledge of the patient's age and clinical course can provide support for a diagnosis of Takayasu's arteritis.

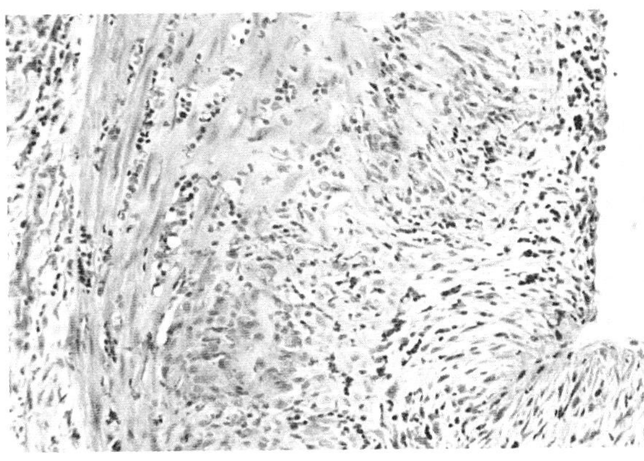

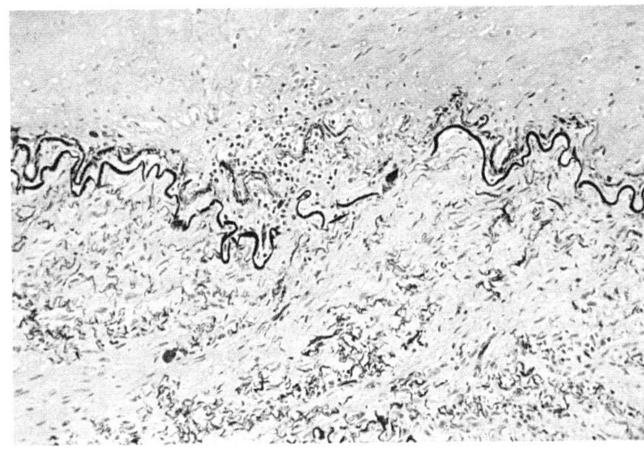

Figure 15-53

TAKAYASU'S ARTERITIS

Top: H&E-stained section shows transmural inflammation of a main renal artery, with infiltrates of mononuclear leukocytes, including macrophages. The intima is thickened and the muscularis has patchy infiltrates. The demarcation between intima and muscularis is obscured by the inflammation.

Bottom: The JMS stain demonstrates fragmentation of the internal elastica caused by the inflammation. The intima above and the media below are extensively infiltrated by mononuclear leukocytes, including macrophages.

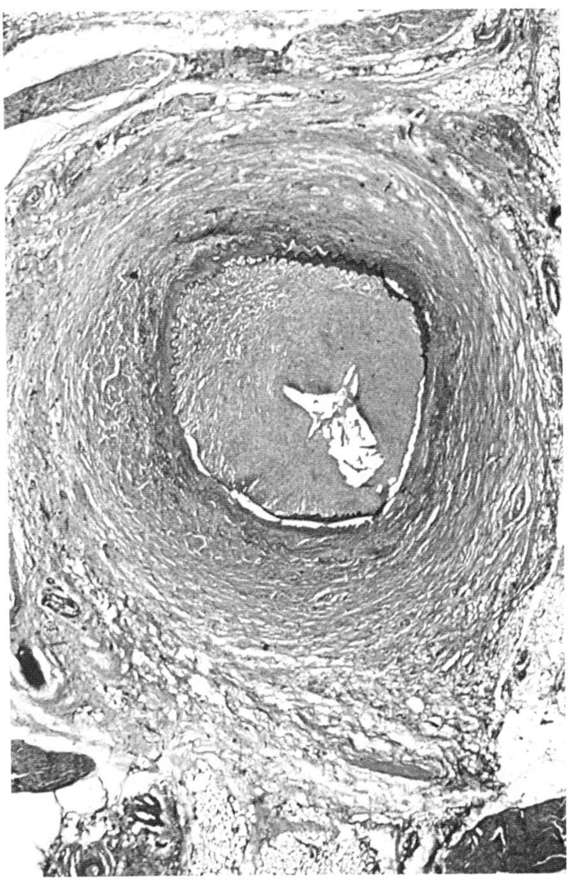

Figure 15-54

TAKAYASU'S ARTERITIS

Advanced chronic injury of a main renal artery caused by Takayasu's arteritis shows extensive intimal and medial fibrosis, and marked narrowing of the lumen. (Fig. 11-2 from Churg J, Bernstein J, Risdon RA, Sobin LH. Renal disease: classification and atlas. New York: Igaku-Shoin; 1987:139.)

Especially when considering the renal arteries, fibromuscular dysplasia is a differential consideration, however, the inflammation or irregular scarring of Takayasu's arteritis is distinct from the less destructive increase in abnormal muscle cells or fibrous tissue seen with renal artery dysplasia.

Etiology and Pathogenesis. The etiology and pathogenesis of Takayasu's arteritis are unknown. The histologic pattern of injury raises the possibility of involvement of a cell mediated immune response, however, no specific pathogenic immune or autoimmune mechanism has been elucidated.

Treatment and Prognosis. Active phases of Takayasu's arteritis are treated with corticosteroids, sometimes augmented with cytotoxic drugs (78,81,82). Sclerotic occlusive vascular disease may require surgical revascularization procedures (79).

GIANT CELL ARTERITIS

Definition. Giant cell arteritis is granulomatous arteritis of the aorta and its major branches, with a predilection for the extracranial branches of the carotid artery (83–86,88). It frequently involves the temporal artery, usually occurs in patients older than 50 years of age, and often is

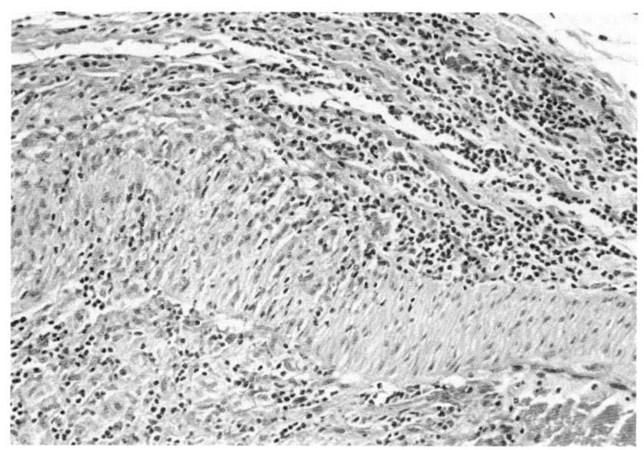

Figure 15-55

GIANT CELL ARTERITIS

The portion of the renal artery wall on the right is relatively intact but the wall on the left has extensive transmural inflammation, including marked intimal and adventitial infiltration by mononuclear leukocytes.

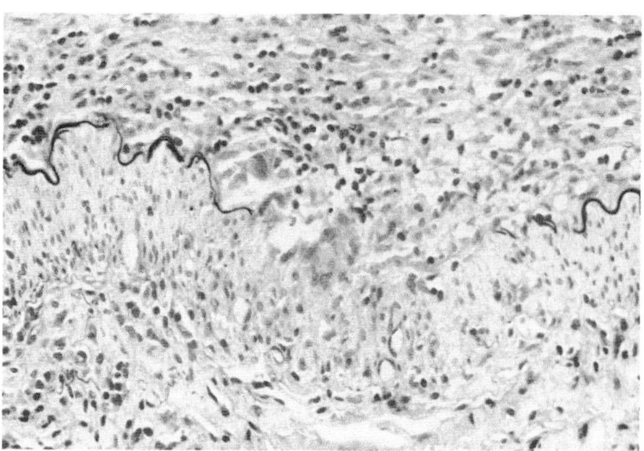

Figure 15-56

GIANT CELL ARTERITIS

The JMS stain demonstrates focal disruption of the internal elastica in a renal artery affected by giant cell arteritis. There are several giant cells near the fragmented elastica. The thickened and inflamed intima is above the elastica.

associated with polymyalgia rheumatica. The term *temporal arteritis* has been used as a synonym for giant cell arteritis, however, this is a less desirable term because all patients with giant cell arteritis do not have temporal artery involvement and all patients with arteritis involving the temporal artery do not have giant cell arteritis (86,89). Temporal artery arteritis can be a component of polyarteritis nodosa, microscopic polyangiitis, and Wegener's granulomatosis.

Clinical Features. Giant cell arteritis is most frequent in northern Europeans and populations of northern European extraction elsewhere in the world. The disease rarely occurs in patients younger than 50 years old (85). Polymyalgia rheumatica occurs in 50 to 75 percent of patients. Most patients present with a combination of nonspecific constitutional symptoms (fever, night sweats, malaise, anorexia, and fatigue) and symptoms caused by ischemia from arterial narrowing (84,85,88). When giant cell arteritis affects the extracranial branches of the carotid artery, common clinical features include headache, temporal artery tenderness or loss of pulse, scalp tenderness, nodularity in the distribution of the temporal artery, tongue or jaw claudication, or loss of vision or other ischemic ocular manifestations. Involvement of arteries supplying the extremities is second in frequency to head and neck disease, and causes reduced pulses and claudication. Clinically significant renal involvement is rare, although a few patients have renovascular hypertension or mild hematuria and proteinuria (87). At least some of the published reports of "giant cell arteritis with glomerulonephritis" probably are misdiagnosed Wegener's granulomatosis.

Gross Findings. Involved arteries have segmentally thickened walls and narrowed lumens. The gross appearance is less irregular than that of Takayasu's arteritis.

Light Microscopic Findings. There is chronic granulomatous inflammation that may be most conspicuous in the media but extends to involve all layers of the artery, including the adventitia (83). The inflammatory infiltrate consists predominantly of mononuclear leukocytes, including macrophages, monocytes, and lymphocytes (figs. 15-55–15-57). At sites of active inflammation, multinucleated giant cells are often identified. Infiltrates occasionally contain scattered eosinophils. The internal, and to a lesser extent the external, elastic lamina are frequently disrupted (figs. 15-56, 15-57). Multinucleated giant cells may be concentrated around the fragmented elastica (fig. 15-56). Intimal thickening is frequent and causes narrowing of the lumen (fig. 15-57). Involvement of the main renal artery or multiple lobar arteries may cause ischemic atrophy of the renal parenchyma (fig. 15-58). Adventitial inflammation may be conspicuous, even in apparently early disease.

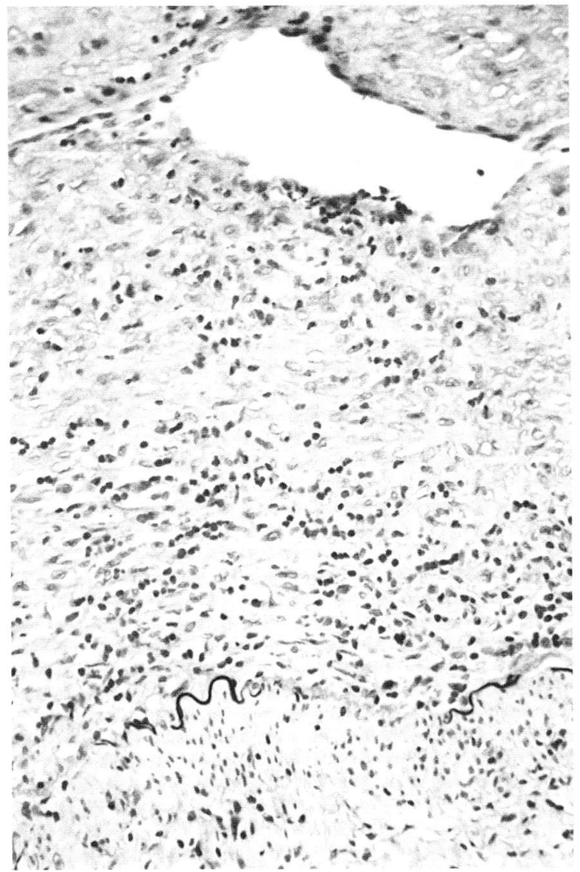

Figure 15-57

GIANT CELL ARTERITIS

There is marked narrowing of the lumen of this main renal artery by extensive intimal thickening. The internal elastica is fragmented (JMS stain).

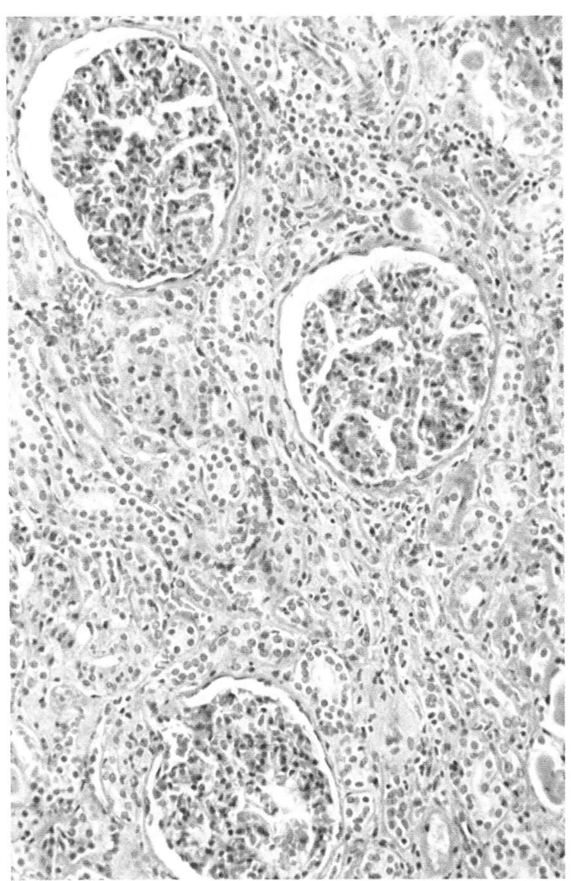

Figure 15-58

ISCHEMIC RENAL ATROPHY SECONDARY TO GIANT CELL ARTERITIS

There is marked atrophy of cortical tubules secondary to renal artery stenosis that was caused by giant cell arteritis. The glomeruli are spared.

Advanced chronic disease has vascular scarring with only slight nonspecific inflammation.

The frequency of renal artery involvement by giant cell arteritis is not well characterized. Renal artery involvement is seen in patients who die with active giant cell arteritis even when there was no clinical evidence of renal dysfunction. There are isolated reports of glomerular injury in patients with giant cell arteritis (87), but at least some of these reports are attributable to small vessel vasculitis, such as Wegener's granulomatosis, that has affected both temporal arteries and glomeruli.

Differential Diagnosis. The major pathologic differential diagnostic consideration is Takayasu's arteritis. Giant cell arteritis and Takayasu's arteritis cannot be reliably distinguished on the basis of histology alone. Clinical and demographic data, especially patient age, must be factored in to reach the most appropriate diagnosis (86).

The chronic sclerotic phase of the necrotizing arteritides, such as polyarteritis nodosa, microscopic polyangiitis, and Wegener's granulomatosis, must be distinguished from giant cell arteritis. It is important to realize that these vasculitides can affect the temporal artery. This distinction is difficult in the chronic phase of the disease, but in the active inflammatory phase, the extensive fibrinoid necrosis of polyarteritis nodosa and the ANCA vasculitides distinguishes them from giant cell arteritis. Small foci of fibrinoid material may occur in the lesions of giant cell arteritis, but large zones of necrosis should raise suspicion of other variants of necrotizing arteritis.

Etiology and Pathogenesis. The etiology of giant cell arteritis is unknown. One hypothesis proposes that a major element of the pathogenesis involves T cells coming from the vasa vasorum of the adventitia (90). Cytokines released by these cells could activate the macrophages that cause the major injury to the artery walls.

Treatment and Prognosis. Corticosteroids are the mainstay of therapy for patients with giant cell arteritis (83,88). The disease usually enters sustained remission within 1 year and corticosteroids can be stopped. Occasional flares can be controlled with corticosteroids.

REFERENCES

Pauci-Immune Crescentic Glomerulonephritis, Microscopic Polyangiitis, Wegener's Granulomatosis, and Churg-Strauss Syndrome

1. Aasarod K, Bostad L, Hammerstrom J, Jorstad S, Iversen BM. Renal histopathology and clinical course in 94 patients with Wegener's granulomatosis. Nephrol Dial Transplant 2001;16:953–60.
2. Bacon PA. Therapy of vasculitis. J Rheumatol 1994;21:788–90.
3. Bajema IM, Hagen EC, de Heer E, van der Woude FJ, Bruijn JA. Colocalization of ANCA-antigens and fibrinoid necrosis in ANCA-associated vasculitis. Kidney Int 2001;60:2025–30.
4. Bajema IM, Hagen EC, Ferrario F, et al. Renal granulomas in systemic vasculitis. EC/BCR Project for ANCA-Assay Standardization. Clin Nephrol 1997;48:16–21.
5. Bajema IM, Hagen EC, Hermans J, et al. Kidney biopsy as a predictor for renal outcome in ANCA-associated necrotizing glomerulonephritis. Kidney Int 1999;56:1751–8.
6. Bajema IM, Hagen EC, van der Woude FJ, Bruijn JA. Wegener's granulomatosis: a meta-analysis of 349 literary case reports. J Lab Clin Med 1997;129:17–22.
7. Churg J, Strauss L. Allergic granulomatosis, allergic angiitis and periarteritis nodosa. Am J Pathol 1951;27:277–301.
8. D'Agati V, Chander P, Nash M, Mancilla-Jimenez R. Idiopathic microscopic polyarteritis nodosa: ultrastructural observations on the renal vascular and glomerular lesions. Am J Kidney Dis 1986;7:95–110.
9. Dolman KM, Gans RO, Vervaat TJ, et al. Vasculitis and antineutrophil cytoplasmic autoantibodies associated with propylthiouracil therapy. Lancet 1993;342:651–2.
10. Donald KJ, Edwards RL, McEvoy JD. An ultrastructural study of the pathogenesis of tissue injury in limited Wegener's granulomatosis. Pathology 1976;8:161–9
11. Falk RJ, Hogan S, Carey TS, Jennette JC. Clinical course of anti-neutrophil cytoplasmic autoantibody-associated glomerulonephritis and systemic vasculitis. The Glomerular Disease Collaborative Network. Ann Intern Med 1990;113: 656–63.
12. Franssen CF, Stegeman CA, Kallenberg CG, et al. Antiproteinase 3- and antimyeloperoxidase-associated vasculitis. Kidney Int 2000;57:2195–206.
13. Gayraud M, Guillevin L, le Toumelin P, Cohen P, Lhote F, Casassus P, Jarrousse B. Long-term followup of polyarteritis nodosa, microscopic polyangiitis, and Churg-Strauss syndrome: analysis of four prospective trials including 278 patients. Arthritis Rheum 2001;44:666–75.
14. Godman GC, Churg J. Wegener's granulomatosis. Pathology and review of the literature. Arch Pathol 1954;58:533–53.
15. Guillevin L, Durand-Gasselin B, Cevallos R, et al. Microscopic polyangiitis: clinical and laboratory findings in eighty-five patients. Arthritis Rheum 1999;42:421–30.
16. Guillevin L, Lhote F. Treatment of polyarteritis nodosa and microscopic polyangiitis. Arthritis Rheum 1998;41:2100–5.
17. Guillevin L, Lhote F, Amouroux J, Gherardi R, Callard P, Casassus P. Antineutrophil cytoplasmic antibodies, abnormal angiograms and pathological findings in polyarteritis nodosa and Churg-Strauss syndrome: indications for the classification of vasculitides of the Polyarteritis Nodosa Group. Br J Rheumatol 1996;35:958–64.
18. Guillevin L, Lhote F, Gherardi R. Polyarteritis nodosa, microscopic polyangiitis, and Churg-Strauss syndrome: clinical aspects, neurologic manifestations, and treatment. Neurol Clin 1997;15:865–86.

19. Hagen EC, Daha MR, Hermans J, et al. Diagnostic value of standardized assays for anti-neutrophil cytoplasmic antibodies in idiopathic systemic vasculitis. EC/BCR Project for ANCA Assay Standardization. Kidney Int 1998;53:743–53.
20. Harris AA, Falk RJ, Jennette JC. Crescentic glomerulonephritis with a paucity of glomerular immunoglobulin localization. Am J Kidney Dis 1998;32:179–84.
21. Hauer HA, Bajema IM, de Heer E, Hermans J, Hagen EC, Bruijn JA. Distribution of renal lesions in idiopathic systemic vasculitis: a three-dimensional analysis of 87 glomeruli. Am J Kidney Dis 2000;36:257–65.
22. Hauer HA, Bajema IM, van Houwelingen HC, et al. Renal histology in ANCA-associated vasculitis: differences between diagnostic and serologic groups. Kidney Int 2002;61:80–9
23. Hellmark T, Niles JL, Collins AB, McCluskey RT, Brunmark C. Comparison of anti-GBM antibodies in sera with or without ANCA. J Am Soc Nephrol 1997;8:376–85.
24. Hoffman GS, Kerr GS, Leavitt RY, et al. Wegener granulomatosis: an analysis of 158 patients. Ann Intern Med 1992;116:488–98.
25. Hogan SL, Nachman PH, Wilkman AS, Jennette JC, Falk RJ. Prognostic markers in patients with antineutrophil cytoplasmic autoantibody-associated microscopic polyangiitis and glomerulonephritis. J Am Soc Nephrol 1996;7:23–32.
26. Hoorntje SJ, Franssen CF, Gans RO, et al. Differences between anti-myeloperoxidase- and anti-proteinase 3-associated renal disease. Kidney Int 1995;47:193–9.
27. Jennette JC. Rapidly progressive crescentic glomerulonephritis. Kidney Int 2003;63:1164–77.
28. Jennette JC. Renal Involvement in systemic vasculitis. In: Jennette JC, Olson JL, Schwartz MM, Silva FG, eds. Heptinstall's pathology of the kidney, 5th ed. Philadelphia: Lippincott-Raven; 1998:1059–96.
29. Jennette JC, Falk RJ. Pathogenesis of the vascular and glomerular damage in ANCA-positive vasculitis. Nephrol Dial Transplant 1998;13 (Suppl 1):16–20.
30. Jennette JC, Falk RJ. The pathology of vasculitis involving the kidney. Am J Kidney Dis 1994;24:130–41.
31. Jennette JC, Falk RJ. Small-vessel vasculitis. N Engl J Med 1997;337:1512–23.
32. Jennette JC, Falk RJ, Andrassy K, et al. Nomenclature of systemic vasculitides. Proposal of an international consensus conference. Arthritis Rheum 1994;37:187–92.
33. Jennette JC, Thomas DB, Falk RJ. Microscopic polyangiitis (microscopic polyarteritis). Semin Diagn Pathol 2001;18:3–13.
33a. Landing BH, Larson EJ. Are infantile periarteritis nodosa with coronary artery involvement and fatal mucocutaneous lymph node syndrome the same? Comparison of 20 patients from North America with patients from Hawaii and Japan. Pediatrics 1977;59:651–62.
34. Lim LC, Taylor JG 3rd, Schmitz JL, et al. Diagnostic usefulness of antineutrophil cytoplasmic autoantibody serology: comparative evaluation of commercial indirect fluorescent antibody kits and enzyme immunoassay kits. Am J Clin Pathol 1999;111:363–9.
35. Marshall S, Dressler R, D'Agati V. Membranous lupus nephritis with antineutrophil cytoplasmic antibody-associated segmental necrotizing and crescentic glomerulonephritis. Am J Kidney Dis 1997;29:119–24.
36. Mathieson PW, Peat DS, Short A, Watts RA. Coexistent membranous nephropathy and ANCA-positive crescentic glomerulonephritis in association with penicillamine. Nephrol Dial Transplant 1996;11:863–6.
37. Morita S, Ueda Y, Eguchi K. Anti-thyroid drug-induced ANCA-associated vasculitis: a case report and review of the literature. Endocr J 2000;47:467–70.
38. Nachman PH, Hogan SL, Jennette JC, Falk RJ. Treatment response and relapse in antineutrophil cytoplasmic autoantibody-associated microscopic polyangiitis and glomerulonephritis. J Am Soc Nephrol 1996;7:33–9.
39. Nachman PH, Segelmark M, Westman K, et al. Recurrent ANCA-associated small vessel vasculitis after transplantation: a pooled analysis. Kidney Int 1999;56:1544–50
40. Niles JL, Bottinger EP, Saurina GR, et al. The syndrome of lung hemorrhage and nephritis is usually an ANCA- associated condition. Arch Intern Med 1996;156:440–5.
41. Pettersson EE, Sundelin B, Heigl Z. Incidence and outcome of pauci-immune necrotizing and crescentic glomerulonephritis in adults. Clin Nephrol 1995;43:141–9.
42. Pusey CD. Microscopic polyangiitis. Clin Exp Immunol 2000;120(Supp l):32.
43. Savage CO. ANCA-associated renal vasculitis. Kidney Int 2001;60:1614–27.
44. Savage CO, Winearls CG, Evans DJ, Rees AJ, Lockwood CM. Microscopic polyarteritis: presentation, pathology and prognosis. Q J Med 1985;56:467–83.
45. Savige J, Davies D, Falk RJ, Jennette JC, Wiik A. Antineutrophil cytoplasmic antibodies (ANCA) and associated diseases: a review of the clinical and laboratory features. Kidney Int 2000;57:846–62.

46. Savige J, Gillis D, Davies D, et al. International Consensus Statement on Testing and Reporting of Antineutrophil Cytoplasmic Antibodies (ANCA). Am J Clin Pathol 1999;111:507–13.
47. Stilmant MM, Bolton WK, Sturgill BC, Schmitt GW, Couser WG. Crescentic glomerulonephritis without immune deposits: clinicopathologic features. Kidney Int 1979;15:184–95.
48. Vogt BA, Kim Y, Jennette JC, Falk RJ, Burke BA, Sinaiko A. Antineutrophil cytoplasmic autoantibody-positive crescentic glomerulonephritis as a complication of treatment with propylthiouracil in children. J Pediatr 1994;124:986–8.
49. Watanabe T, Nagafuchi Y, Yoshikawa Y, Toyoshima H. Renal papillary necrosis associated with Wegener's granulomatosis. Hum Pathol 1983;14:551–7.
50. Xiao H, Heeringa P, Hu P, et al. Antineutrophil cytoplasmic autoantibodies specific for myeloperoxidase cause glomerulonephritis and vasculitis in mice. J Clin Invest 2002;110:955–63.

Kawasaki's Disease

51. Amano S, Hazama F, Hamashima Y. Pathology of Kawasaki disease: I. Pathology and morphogenesis of the vascular changes. Jpn Cir J 1979;43:633–43.
52. Amano S, Hazama F, Hamashima Y. Pathology of Kawasaki disease: II. Distribution and incidence of the vascular lesions. Jpn Cir J 1979; 43:741–8.
53. Bell DM, Brink EW, Nitzkin JL, et al. Kawasaki syndrome: description of two outbreaks in the United States. N Engl J Med 1981;304:1568–75.
54. Fujiwara H, Hamashima Y. Pathology of the heart in Kawasaki disease. Pediatrics 1978;61:100–7.
55. Fujiwara T, Fujiwara H, Nakano H. Pathological features of coronary arteries in children with Kawasaki disease in which coronary arterial aneurysm was absent at autopsy. Quantitative analysis. Circulation 1988;78:345–50.
56. Furusho K, Kamiya T, Nakano H, et al. High-dose intravenous gammaglobulin for Kawasaki disease. Lancet 1984;2:1055–8.
57. Gribetz D, Landing B, Larson EJ. Kawasaki disease: mucocutaneous lymph node syndrome (MCLS). In: Churg A, Churg J, eds. Systemic vasculitides. New York: Igaku-Shoin; 1991:257–72.
58. Hirose S, Hamashima Y. Morphological observations on the vasculitis in the mucocutaneous lymph node syndrome. A skin biopsy study of 27 patients. Eur J Pediatr 1978;129:17–27.
58a. Jennette JC, Falk RJ, Andrassy K, et al. Nomenclature of systemic vasculitides. Proposal of an international consensus conference. Arthritis Rheum 1994;37:187–92.
59. Jennette JC, Sciarrotta J, Takahashi K, Naoe S. Predominance of monocytes and macrophages in the inflammatory infiltrates of acute Kawasaki disease arteritis. Ped Research 2002;53:94A.
60. Kawasaki T, Kosaki F, Okawa S, Shigematsu L, Yanagawa H. A new infantile acute febrile mucocutaneous lymph node syndrome (MLNS). Pediatrics 1974;54:271–6.
61. Landing BH, Larson EJ. Are infantile periarteritis nodosa with coronary artery involvement and fatal mucocutaneous lymph node syndrome the same? Comparison of 20 patients from North America with patients from Hawaii and Japan. Pediatrics 1977;59:651–62.
62. Landing BH, Larson EJ. Pathological features of Kawasaki disease (mucocutaneous lymph node syndrome). Am J Cardiovasc Pathol 1987;1:218–29.
63. Leung DY, Collins T, Lapierre LA, Geha RS, Pober JS. Immunoglobulin M antibodies present in the acute phase of Kawasaki syndrome lyse cultured vascular endothelial cells stimulated by gamma interferon. J Clin Invest 1986;77:1428–35.
64. Nagashima M, Matsushima M, Matsuoka H, Ogawa A, Okumura N. High-dose gammaglobulin therapy for Kawasaki disease. J Pedriatr 1987;110:710–2.
65. Naoe S, Takahashi K, Masuda H, Tanaka N. Kawasaki disease. With particular emphasis on arterial lesions. Acta Pathol Jpn 1991;41:785–97.
66. Newburger JW, Takahashi M, Burns JC, et al. The treatment of Kawasaki syndrome with intravenous gamma globulin. N Engl J Med 1986;315:341–7.
67. Tanaka N, Naoe S, Kawasaki T. Pathological study on autopsy cases of mucocutaneous lymph node syndrome. J Jap Red Cross Cent Hosp 1971;2:85–94.
68. Tizard EJ, Baguley E, Hughes GR, Dillon MJ. Antiendothelial cell antibodies detected by a cellular based ELISA in Kawasaki disease. Arch Dis Child 1991;66:189–92.

Polyarteritis Nodosa

69. Davson J, Ball J, Platt R. The kidney in periarteritis nodosa. Q J Med 1948;17:175–202.
69a. Guillevin L, Lhote F. Treatment of polyarteritis nodosa and microscopic polyangiitis. Arthritis Rheum 1998;41:2100–5.
69b. Guillevin L, Lhote F, Amouroux J, Gherardi R, Callard P, Casassus P. Antineutrophil cytoplasmic antibodies, abnormal angiograms and pathological findings in polyarteritis nodosa and Churg-Strauss syndrome: indications for the classification of vasculitides of the Polyarteritis Nodosa Group. Br J Rheumatol 1996;35:958–64.

69c. Guillevin L, Lhote F, Gherardi R. Polyarteritis nodosa, microscopic polyangiitis, and Churg-Strauss syndrome: clinical aspects, neurologic manifestations, and treatment. Neurol Clin 1997;15:865–86.
69d. Jennette JC. Renal Involvement in systemic vasculitis. In: Jennette JC, Olson JL, Schwartz MM, Silva FG, eds. Heptinstall's pathology of the kidney, 5th ed. Philadelphia: Lippincott-Raven; 1998:1059–96.
69e. Jennette JC, Falk RJ. Small-vessel vasculitis. N Engl J Med 1997;337:1512–23.
69f. Jennette JC, Falk RJ, Andrassy K, et al. Nomenclature of systemic vasculitides. Proposal of an international consensus conference. Arthritis Rheum 1994;37:187–92.
70. Kirkland GS, Savige J, Wilson D, Heale W, Sinclair RA, Hope RN. Classical polyarteritis nodosa and microscopic polyarteritis with medium vessel involvement—a comparison of the clinical and laboratory features. Clin Nephrol 1997;47:176–80.
71. Kussmaul A, Maier R. Ueber eine bisher nicht beschreibene eigenthumliche Arterienerkrankung (Periarteritis nodosa), die mit Morbus Brightii und rapid fortschreitender allgemeiner Muskellahmung einhergeht. Dtsch Arch Klin Med 1866;1:484–518.
72. Lhote F, Guillevin L. Polyarteritis nodosa, microscopic polyangiitis, and Churg-Strauss syndrome. Clinical aspects and treatment. Rheum Dis Clin North Am 1995;21:911–47.
73. Rose GA, Spencer H. Polyarteritis nodosa. Q J Med 1957;26:43–81.
74. Smith DL, Wernick R. Spontaneous rupture of a renal artery aneurysm in polyarteritis nodosa: critical review of the literature and report of a case. Am J Med 1989;87:464–7.
75. Zeek PM. Periarteritis nodosa: a critical review. Am J Clin Pathol 1952;22:777–90.
76. Zeek PM, Smith CC, Weeter JC. Studies on periarteritis nodosa. III. The differentiation between the vascular lesions of periarteritis nodosa and of hypersensitivity. Am J Pathol 1948;24:889–917.

Takayasu's Arteritis

77. Arend WP, Michel BA, Bloch DA, et al. The American College of Rheumatology 1990 criteria for the classification of Takayasu arteritis. Arthritis Rheum 1990;33:1129–34.
78. Churg J. Large vessel vasculitis. Clin Exp Immunol 1993;93(Suppl 1):11–2.
78a. Jennette JC, Falk RJ, Andrassy K, et al. Nomenclature of systemic vasculitides. Proposal of an international consensus conference. Arthritis Rheum 1994;37:187–92.
79. Lagneau P, Michel JB. Renovascular hypertension and Takayasu's disease. J Urol 1985;134:876–9.
80. Lai KN, Chan KW, Ho CP. Glomerulonephritis associated with Takayasu's arteritis: report of three cases and review of literature. Am J Kidney Dis 1986;7:197–204.
81. Lie JT. Takayasu arteritis. In: Churg A, Churg J, eds. Systemic vasculitides. New York: Igaku-Shoin; 1991:159–79.
82. Lupi-Herrera E, Sanchez-Torres G, Marcushamer J, Mispireta J, Horwitz S, Vela JE. Takayasu's arteritis. Clinical study of 107 cases. Am Heart J 1977;93:94–103.

Giant Cell Arteritis

83. Churg J. Large vessel vasculitis. Clin Exp Immunol 1993;93(Suppl 1):11–2.
84. Hamilton CR Jr, Shelley WM, Tumulty PA. Giant cell arteritis: including temporal arteritis and polymyalgia rheumatica. Medicine 1971;50:1–27.
85. Hunder GG, Bloch DA, Michel BA, et al. The American College of Rheumatology 1990 criteria for the classification of giant cell arteritis. Arthritis Rheum 1990;33:1122–8.
86. Jennette JC, Falk RJ, Andrassy K, et al. Nomenclature of systemic vasculitides. Proposal of an international consensus conference. Arthritis Rheum 1994;37:187–92.
87. Klein RG, Hunder GG, Stanson AW, Sheps SG. Larger artery involvement in giant cell (temporal) arteritis. Ann Intern Med 1975;83:806–12.
88. Lupi-Herrera E, Sanchez-Torres G, Marcushamer J, Mispireta J, Horwitz S, Vela JE. Takayasu's arteritis. Clinical study of 107 cases. Am Heart J 1977;93:94–103.
89. Sonnenblick M, Nesher G, Rosin A. Nonclassical organ involvement in temporal arteritis. Sem Arthritis Rheum 1989;19:183–90.
90. Weyand CM, Goronzy JJ. Pathogenic principles in giant cell arteritis. Int J Cardiol 2000;75 (Suppl 1):S9–15.

16 HYPERTENSIVE NEPHROSCLEROSIS, RENAL ARTERY STENOSIS, AND ATHEROEMBOLIZATION

HYPERTENSIVE NEPHROSCLEROSIS

Definition. Hypertensive nephrosclerosis is renal injury caused by chronic mild to moderate hypertension. Such low-level hypertension often is called "benign" hypertension. Thus, a synonym for hypertensive nephrosclerosis is *benign hypertensive nephrosclerosis*, or *benign nephrosclerosis*. The qualifying term benign in these designations, however, is a misnomer because the process is clearly not benign or it would not be contributing to renal injury, as well as injury to other organs, especially the heart and brain. Thus, the term hypertensive nephrosclerosis is a more appropriate designation for renal injury caused by chronic hypertension. This is distinct from malignant hypertensive nephropathy, which is discussed in detail in the next section and is acute renal injury caused by very severe (malignant) hypertension.

All of the pathologic changes of hypertensive nephrosclerosis also are associated with advanced aging in individuals with no evidence of longstanding hypertension (1,20,27,28,39,48). More than 50 percent of individuals over 60 years of age who have no history of hypertension have some degree of renal arteriolar hyalinosis, focal global glomerular sclerosis, or arterial intimal fibrosis.

Arterionephrosclerosis is a generic term that encompasses the vascular and parenchymal changes of both hypertensive nephrosclerosis and age-related arterionephrosclerosis. The term arterionephrosclerosis includes vascular and parenchymal lesions that are accompanied by arterial sclerosis (arteriosclerosis), arteriolar sclerosis (arteriolosclerosis), or both. The term *arteriolonephrosclerosis* implies that the parenchymal injury is caused exclusively by arteriolar rather than arterial sclerosis, which is rarely if ever the case. Hypertensive nephrosclerosis and age-related arterionephrosclerosis are distinct from atheroembolization or chronic renal ischemia caused by renal artery stenosis, which is discussed later in this chapter.

Clinical Features. Patients with hypertension are those who are in "the upper part of a distribution curve of blood pressure readings obtained from a large population" (39). One commonly used cut-off is a diastolic blood pressure over 90 mm Hg or a systolic blood pressure over 140 mm Hg (12). Hypertension affects 20 to 40 percent of the population in Western society (48). Evidence of a link between renal disease and hypertension began with Bright's observation in the early 1800s of an association between small granular atrophic kidneys and left ventricular hypertrophy (5). Approximately 15 percent of patients with "benign" hypertension develop renal dysfunction (17). Chronic hypertension is estimated to be the cause of a third to a quarter of end-stage renal disease in patients in the United States and Europe. This may be an overestimate because the diagnosis of end-stage renal disease secondary to hypertension often is made without pathologic confirmation and because hypertension often supervenes in other chronic renal diseases (13,35). Hypertensive nephrosclerosis is four times more common in blacks than whites, and occurs at an earlier age and progresses more rapidly in blacks (13,27). Hypertensive nephrosclerosis is the leading cause of end-stage renal disease in blacks (13).

Clinical findings that support a diagnosis of hypertensive nephrosclerosis include a history of hypertension that preceded the development of renal dysfunction, a family history of hypertension, and left ventricular hypertrophy. Substantial proteinuria does not rule out a diagnosis of hypertensive nephrosclerosis. In patients with renal biopsy evidence of hypertensive nephrosclerosis and no other disease, proteinuria of more than 1.5 g/day is found in 40 percent and more than 3.0 g/day in 22 percent (17). Nevertheless, substantial proteinuria, especially, overt nephrotic syndrome, should suggest the possibility of some form of glomerular

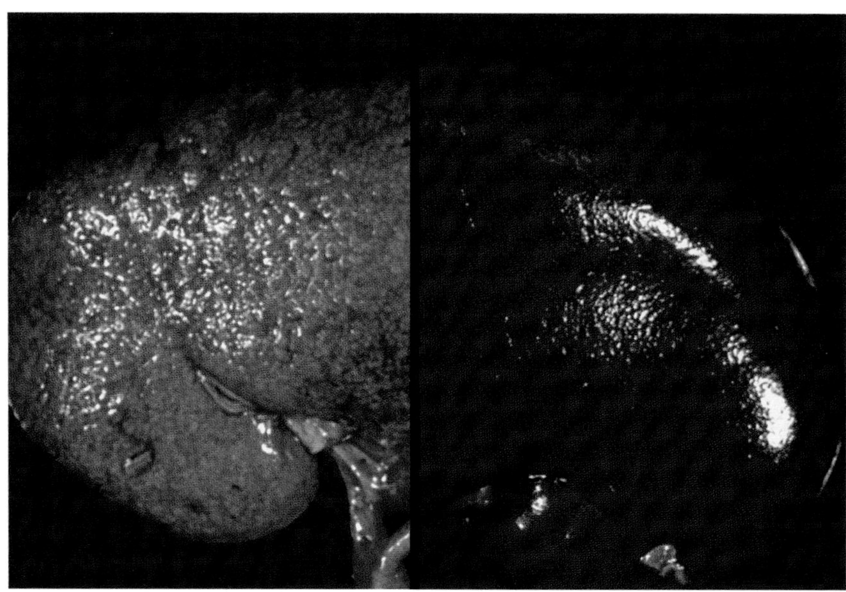

Figure 16-1

HYPERTENSIVE NEPHROSCLEROSIS AND NORMAL KIDNEY

The external surface of a kidney with hypertensive nephrosclerosis (left) is granular and pale compared to the smooth darker surface of a normal kidney (right).

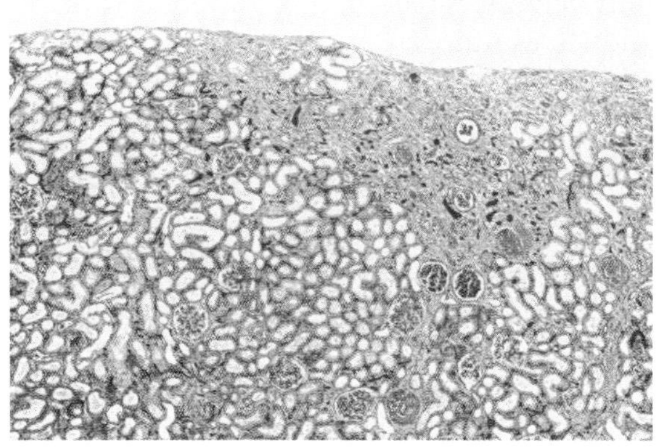

Figure 16-2

FOCAL CORTICAL ATROPHY OF HYPERTENSIVE NEPHROSCLEROSIS

There is a wedge-shaped zone of ischemic atrophy with its base at the capsular surface. The atrophic area has several globally sclerotic glomeruli surrounded by interstitial fibrosis and atrophic tubules.

disease other than, or in addition to, hypertensive nephrosclerosis, including focal segmental glomerulosclerosis that is concurrent with, if not secondary to, hypertensive nephrosclerosis (26).

Gross Findings. Advanced hypertensive nephrosclerosis causes reduced renal size as a result of ischemic renal atrophy. The external surface of the kidney is pale and diffusely finely granular (fig. 16-1) (19,28). There may be scattered irregular depressions, usually 5 to 10 mm in greatest dimension. The fine granularity is caused by depressed areas of chronic ischemic atrophy alternating with residual raised areas of nonatrophic, often hypertrophied, parenchyma (fig. 16-2) (39). Rarely, large hypertrophied glomeruli are seen at the surface as small protruding domes. Larger zones of ischemic atrophy cause larger surface depressions.

The cut surfaces of the kidneys reveal thinning of the cortex caused by chronic ischemic atrophy (fig. 16-3). The cortex is firm as a result of interstitial fibrosis. Arcuate and interlobar arteries usually have thickened pale walls with a "pipe stem" appearance. The medulla should be relatively intact. Substantial chronic erosion of the medulla raises the possibility of chronic pyelonephritis, which can be mistaken clinically for hypertensive nephrosclerosis if a patient presents late in the course of the disease with hypertension and chronic renal failure, and a poor history of urinary tract infections.

Well-defined cortical scars, consistent with earlier infarction or focal cortical necrosis, are not expected with uncomplicated hypertensive nephrosclerosis or age-related arterionephrosclerosis. These lesions should raise the possibility of concurrent episodes of malignant hypertension, atheroembolization, or other causes of acute severe arterial narrowing or occlusion of arteries.

Light Microscopic Findings. The glomeruli, arterioles, arteries, and tubulointerstitial tissue all are affected by hypertensive nephrosclerosis

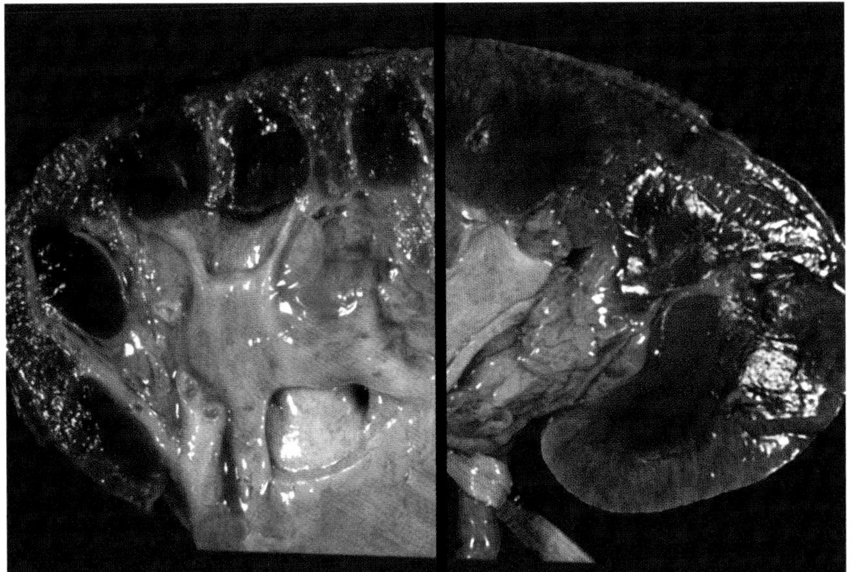

Figure 16-3

HYPERTENSIVE NEPHROSCLEROSIS AND NORMAL KIDNEY

The cut surface of a kidney with hypertensive nephrosclerosis (left) has marked atrophic thinning of the cortex compared to the cortex of the normal kidney (right).

(4,28). The most characteristic changes are focal global glomerular sclerosis, arteriolar hyalinosis and sclerosis, and arterial fibrotic intimal thickening (19,38,39,46). The arteriolar and arterial changes are found in organs in addition to the kidneys in patients with hypertension, however, they are most pronounced in the kidneys (27).

The most frequent and probably earliest changes are in the afferent arterioles (13,27). The severity of arteriolar lesions correlates with the degree of elevation of diastolic blood pressure (38). The most common arteriolar lesion of hypertensive nephrosclerosis and age-related vasculopathy is hyalinosis (figs. 16-4–16-6). Hyaline simply means glassy, which is the histologic appearance of the material that accumulates in vessel walls. This is distinct from the more textured or flat appearance of collagen in areas of fibrosis and sclerosis. The distribution of hyalinosis is dictated by the structure of the internal elastic membrane of arteries and arterioles. Hyalinosis occurs predominantly in small vessels, especially arterioles, that have little or no elastin in their internal elastic membranes (basal laminae) (39).

The hyaline material of arteriolar hyalinosis is eosinophilic, very periodic acid–Schiff (PAS)-positive (fig. 16-5), Jones methenamine silver (JMS) negative, and fuchsinophilic (fig. 16-6) with trichrome staining. The hilar arterioles normally have one or two layers of smooth muscle cells in the media and an incomplete or absent

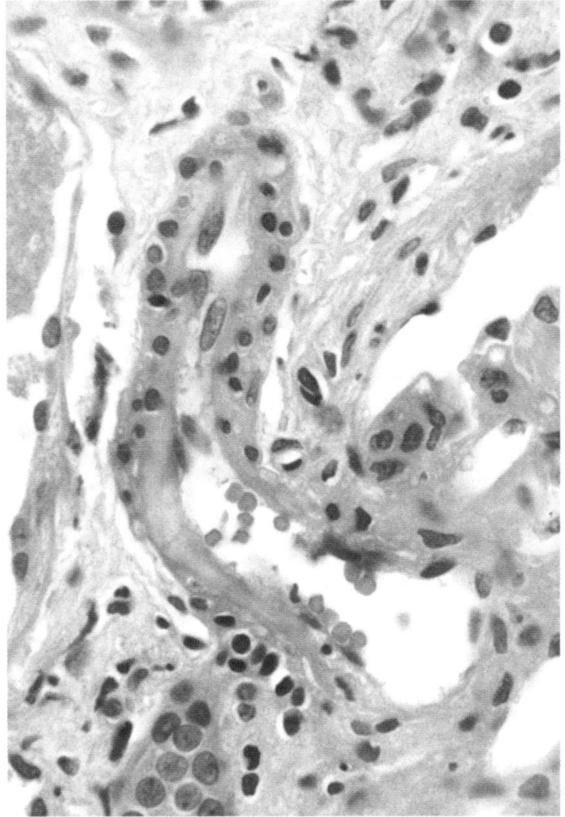

Figure 16-4

ARTERIOLAR HYALINOSIS

Hematoxylin and eosin (H&E)-stained section shows focal hyalinosis of an afferent arteriole. The muscularis has atrophied at the site of hyalinosis.

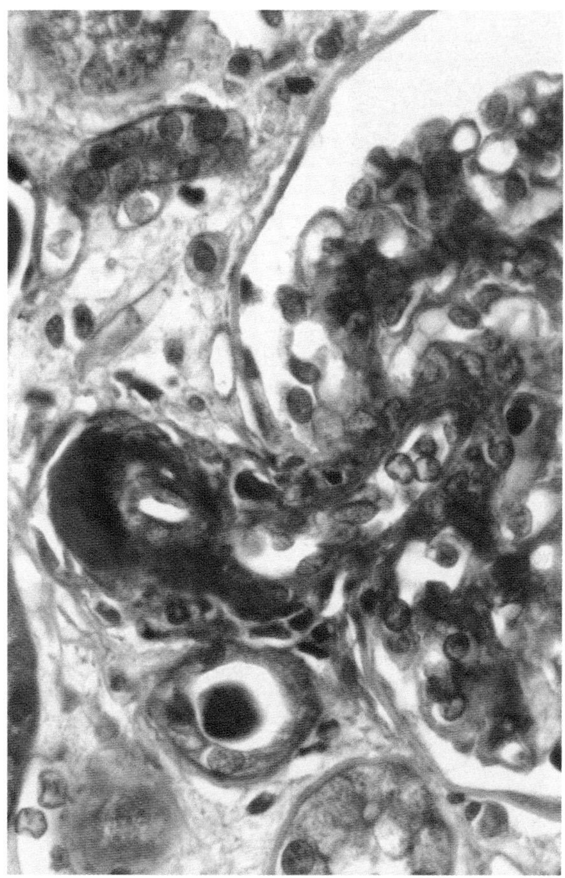

Figure 16-5

ARTERIOLAR HYALINOSIS

Masson trichrome–stained section shows fuchsinophilic hyaline material in the wall of an afferent arteriole.

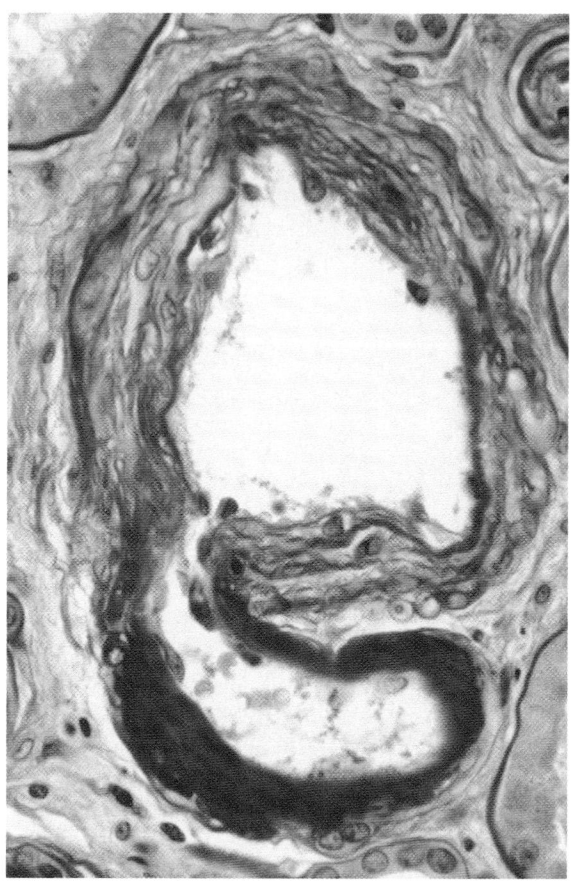

Figure 16-6

ARTERIOLAR HYALINOSIS

Periodic acid–Schiff (PAS)-stained section shows extensive hyalinosis in an arteriole at its origin from an interlobular artery. There has been extensive atrophy of the muscularis of the arteriole. The interlobular artery has medial sclerosis.

internal elastic or collagenous lamina immediately beneath the endothelial cells (12,19). The earliest accumulations of hyaline material occur between the endothelial cells and muscularis, on either side or spanning the internal lamina (39). In cross-section, the earliest hyaline deposits usually are focal rather than circumferential (12,38). Longitudinal sections show segmental involvement of arterioles, which becomes more continuous nearer the glomerulus. With extensive hyalinosis, there may be a broad circumferential band of hyaline material separating the endothelium from the muscularis. There often is atrophy of the smooth muscle cells in the muscularis at sites of hyalinosis (figs. 16-4–16-6). Very severe hyalinosis may be accompanied by complete loss of the arteriolar muscularis.

In addition to or instead of hyalinosis, arterioles may have varying degrees of sclerosis, with accumulation of collagen (fig. 16-7) (12). Arteriolar sclerosis typically has a more textured, less intensely acidophilic appearance than hyalinosis. Foci of sclerosis are blue/green and arteriolar hyalinosis is red with trichrome staining (fig. 16-5). Sclerosis is less PAS positive than hyalinosis.

Arterioles with advanced hypertensive injury may become elongated and tortuous, resulting in more cross-sectional profiles in tissue sections (38). Arteriolar thickening and possibly elongation can be caused, at least in part, by hyperplasia of smooth muscle cells in the muscularis (figs. 16-8,16-9) (27). Hyperplasia of the arteriolar muscularis is much less frequent than

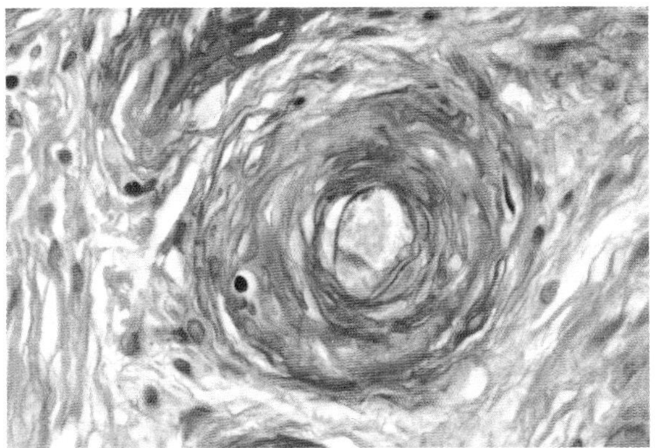

Figure 16-7

ARTERIOLAR SCLEROSIS

The muscularis of this arteriole is largely replaced by fibrosis. The collagenous matrix is textured and thus not consistent with hyalinosis (i.e., not glassy).

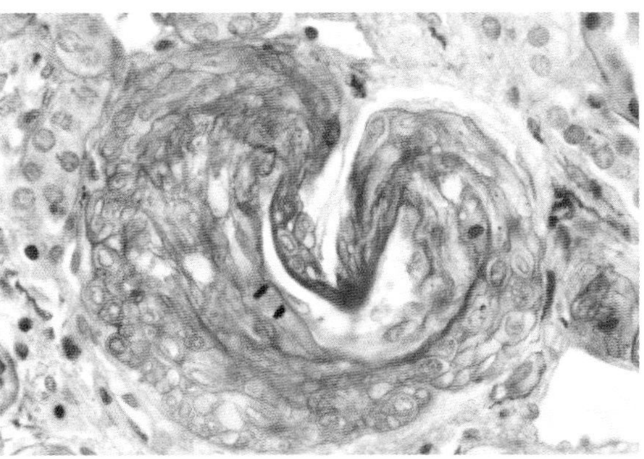

Figure 16-8

ARTERIOLAR SMOOTH MUSCLE HYPERPLASIA

Focal thickening of the muscularis of this arteriole is caused by hyperplasia of smooth muscle cells, including one in the process of mitosis (PAS stain).

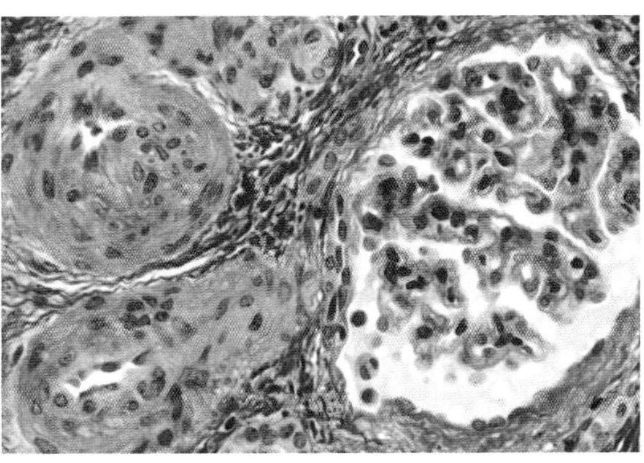

Figure 16-9

ARTERIOLAR SMOOTH MUSCLE HYPERPLASIA

Two arteriolar cross sections (which may be of the same tortuous afferent arteriole) show medial smooth muscle hyperplasia and slight focal medial sclerosis. The adjacent glomerulus has ischemic wrinkling of glomerular basement membranes (Masson trichrome stain).

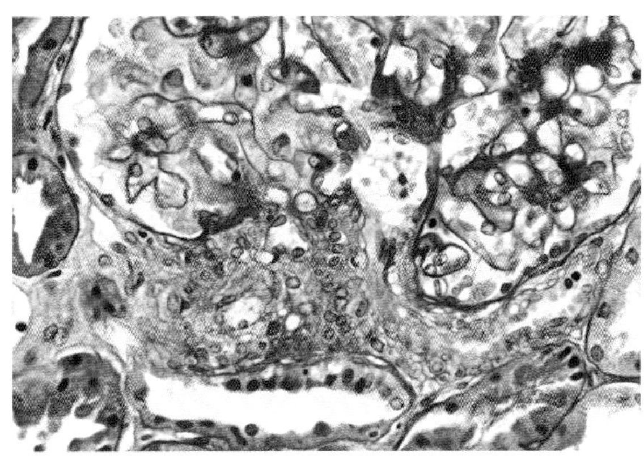

Figure 16-10

JUXTAGLOMERULAR CELL HYPERPLASIA

There is an increase in the number of cells between the macula densa of the distal tubule and the hilus of the glomerulus (PAS stain). Note the reverse polarity of the nuclei in the macula densa, with the nuclei in an apical rather than basal position.

arteriolar hyalinosis or sclerosis. Hyperplasia of the modified smooth muscle cells of the juxtaglomerular apparatus may occur, presumably related to renin hypersecretion (fig. 16-10) (38). Juxtaglomerular cell hyperplasia is most common and most conspicuous in conditions that are causing renovascular hypertension, such as unilateral renal artery stenosis.

The characteristic arterial lesions of hypertensive nephrosclerosis and age-related arteriosclerosis are proliferative and fibrotic intimal thickening, and replication of the internal elastic lamina (figs. 16-11–16-13). The arcuate and interlobar arteries are affected most often, although the lesions may extend into the interlobular arteries (39). Endothelial cells sit on the internal elastic lamina in completely normal interlobular and arcuate arteries. With chronic hypertension or advanced age, the intima is expanded by myofibroblasts, fibroblasts, and progressive accumulation of collagenous matrix (fig. 16-12). This is accompanied by deposition

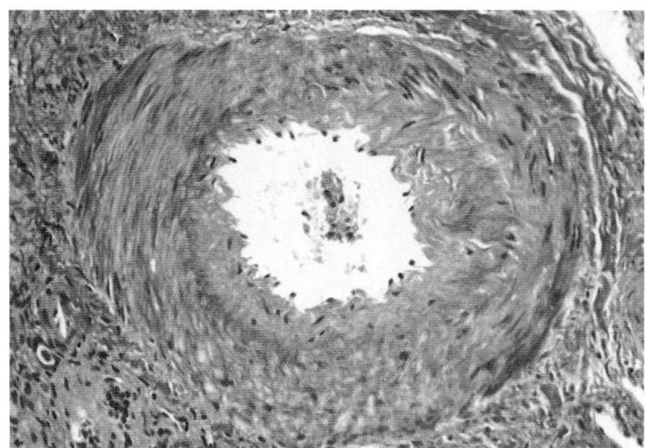

Figure 16-11

ARTERIAL INTIMAL FIBROSIS (ARTERIOSCLEROSIS)

The intima of this arcuate artery is thickened by increased deposition of collagenous matrix that stains blue with the Masson trichrome stain. The internal elastica is a single, slightly fuchsinophilic (red), wavy band at the junction with the media and is seen best in the upper portion of the artery wall.

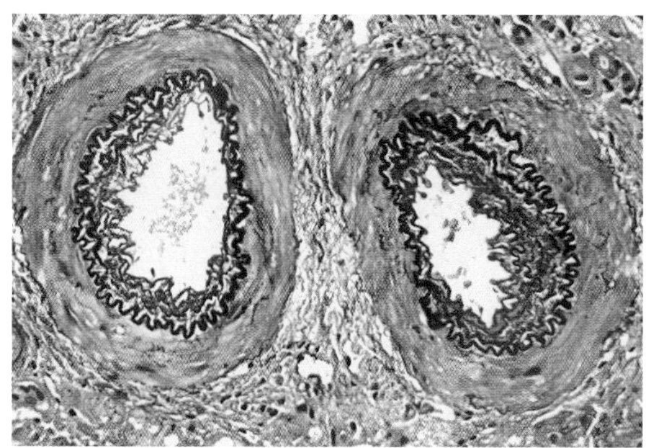

Figure 16-13

ARTERIAL INTIMAL FIBROSIS (ARTERIOSCLEROSIS)

A Verhoeff van Gieson elastic stain highlights the multiple layers of dense collagen in the fibrotic intima of these two arteries. The true internal elastica is the outermost, darker staining, wavy lamina in each vessel.

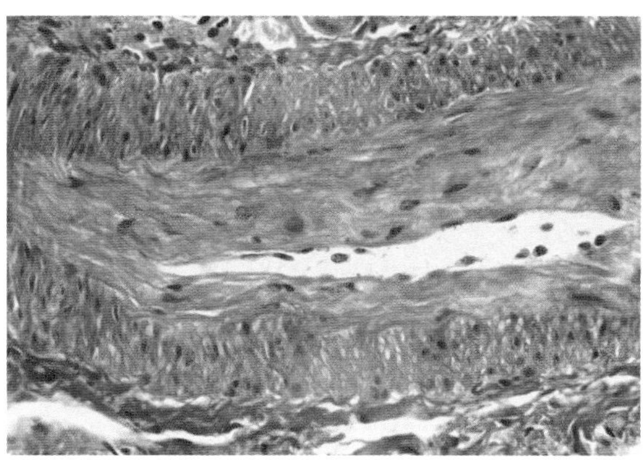

Figure 16-12

ARTERIAL INTIMAL FIBROSIS (ARTERIOSCLEROSIS)

The intima of this longitudinally sectioned arcuate artery is thickened by infiltration, proliferation of fibroblasts, and increased deposition of collagenous matrix that stains blue with the Masson trichrome stain. The lumen is markedly narrowed.

of multiple concentric collagenous laminae that can be seen best with elastic stains (fig. 16-13). Although the increased laminations have the tinctorial properties of elastic fibers (e.g., positive staining with the Verhoeff van Gieson elastic stain), they are composed primarily of collagen rather than elastin (39). Thus, the terms intimal elastosis and intimal fibroelastosis are misleading. In cross-section, the fibrotic intimal thickening may be asymmetric or circumferential, and causes narrowing of the lumen. Complete occlusion is rare unless there is secondary thrombosis, which is exceptional in uncomplicated hypertensive nephrosclerosis.

In hypertensive nephrosclerosis, arterial intimal fibrosis may occur in the absence of discernible changes in the muscularis, however, changes in the muscularis are almost always accompanied by intimal fibrosis. Trichrome staining is useful for assessing changes in the media. The most common medial changes are focal fibrosis and atrophy, which are most pronounced adjacent to intimal fibrosis (fig. 16-14). Medial fibrosis causes replacement of medial smooth muscle cells by collagen. Atrophy causes thinning of the media. Overt medial hyperplasia is much less frequent than medial fibrosis and atrophy.

The classic glomerular lesion of hypertensive nephrosclerosis and age-related arterionephrosclerosis is an acellular wrinkled mass of glomerular basement membranes contracted to the hilar side of Bowman's space and surrounded by collagen that fills Bowman's space (25). In patients with hypertension, focal global glomerular sclerosis usually is accompanied by arteriolar hyalinosis or sclerosis. A few patients have glomerular sclerosis with no arteriolar hyalinosis or sclerosis (25).

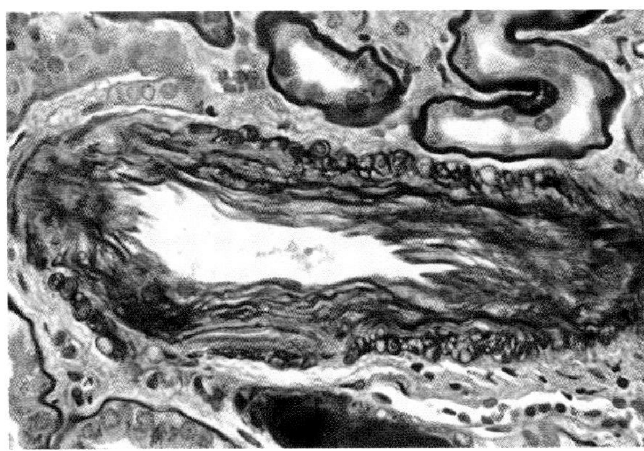

Figure 16-14

ARTERIAL INTIMAL FIBROSIS AND MEDIAL ATROPHY (ARTERIOSCLEROSIS)

This interlobular artery has focally variable intimal fibrosis and focal atrophy of the muscularis. There is complete loss of the muscle cells in the upper left of the vessel wall (Jones methenamine silver [JMS] stain with H&E counterstain).

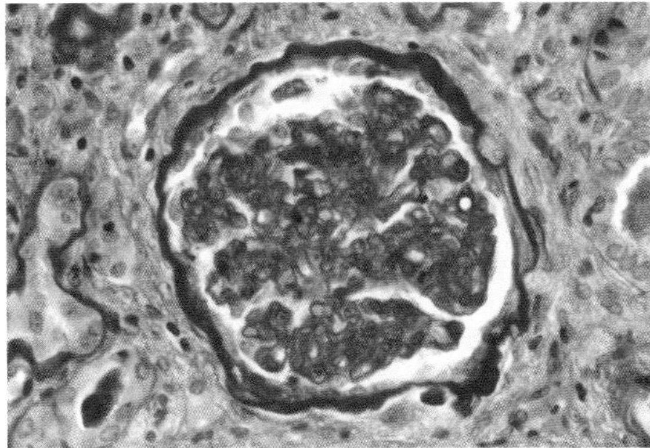

Figure 16-15

EARLY GLOMERULAR CHANGES OF HYPERTENSIVE NEPHROSCLEROSIS

There is global wrinkling and thickening of the glomerular basement membranes, and slight segmental basement membrane replication. Bowman's capsule is thickened. There is interstitial fibrosis, chronic inflammation, and tubular atrophy (PAS stain).

The earliest glomerular changes of hypertensive nephrosclerosis or age-related arterionephrosclerosis are wrinkling and thickening, and sometimes replication, of glomerular basement membranes (figs. 16-9, 16-15) (25). This may be accompanied by mild mesangial matrix expansion. The wrinkling usually is relatively global, but more segmental changes may occur. As the glomerular sclerosis progresses, the structure of the glomerulus may become more simplified, with fewer identifiable capillary loops; visceral epithelial cells become more cuboidal and eventually disappear (25).

In parallel with glomerular tuft sclerosis, there is thickening, wrinkling, and replication of Bowman's capsule (figs. 16-15, 16-16). In addition, collagen accumulates in Bowman's space. This typically begins adjacent to the hilum, but eventually completely fills Bowman's space (figs. 16-16, 16-17) (25). Glomerular basement membranes are more PAS and JMS positive than the collagen that accumulates in Bowman's space. Thus, PAS and JMS stains are useful for documenting this pattern of ischemic glomerular sclerosis (figs. 16-16, 16-17). As glomerular sclerosis becomes advanced, Bowman's capsule may undergo partial or complete dissolution (fig. 16-17). Eventually, the entire globally sclerotic glomerulus disappears, sometimes leaving residual fragments of Bowman's capsule.

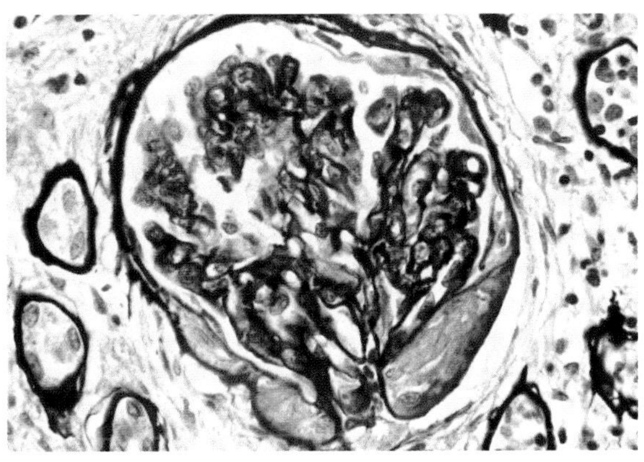

Figure 16-16

EARLY GLOMERULAR CHANGES OF HYPERTENSIVE NEPHROSCLEROSIS

There is global wrinkling and thickening of glomerular basement membranes, and slight segmental basement membrane replication. There is early accumulation of collagen within the perihilar portion of Bowman's space. Bowman's capsule is thickened. Interstitial fibrosis, chronic inflammation, and tubular atrophy are seen (JMS stain with H&E counterstain).

The globally sclerotic glomeruli of hypertensive nephrosclerosis and age-related arterionephrosclerosis are most numerous in the outer cortex, and frequently are clustered at the surface in roughly wedge-shaped zones of chronic ischemic parenchymal atrophy (figs. 16-2, 16-18).

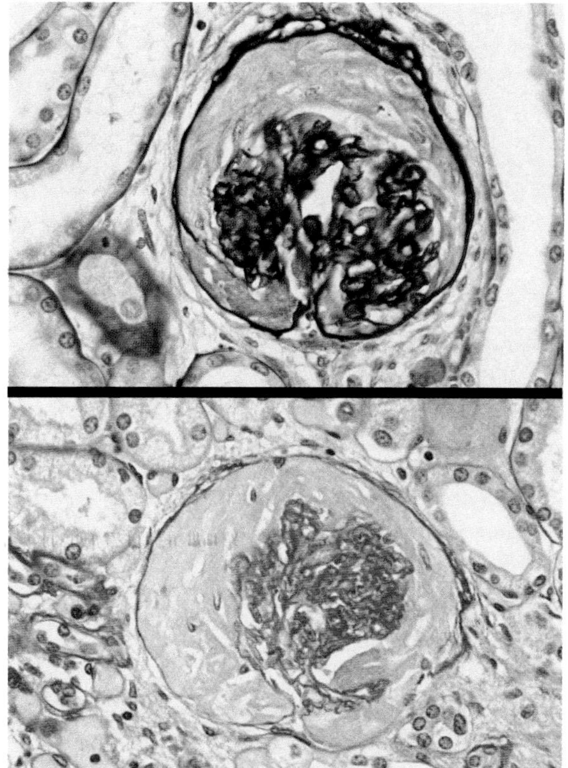

Figure 16-17

LATE GLOMERULAR CHANGES OF HYPERTENSIVE NEPHROSCLEROSIS

The shrunken glomerulus has global wrinkling and thickening of basement membranes, and loss of most cells. Bowman's space is completely filled with collagen that stains less intensely than the glomerular basement membranes. Bowman's capsule is thickened (top; JMS stain with H&E counterstain), and has focal areas of resorption (bottom; PAS stain).

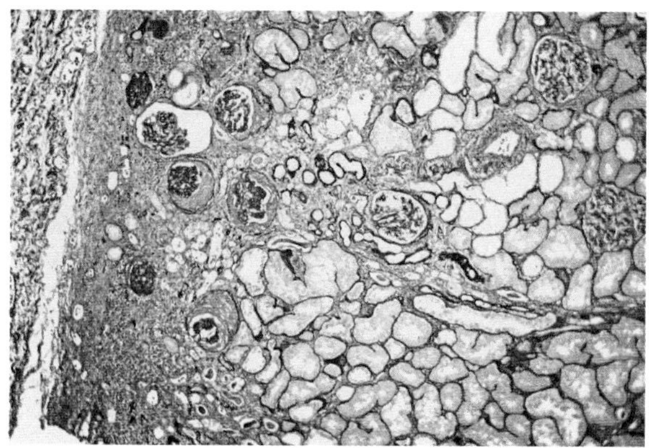

Figure 16-18

HYPERTENSIVE NEPHROSCLEROSIS

There is a peripheral zone of chronic ischemic atrophy, with glomeruli at varying stages of ischemic sclerosis, from glomeruli with wrinkled basement membranes, to those with shriveled tufts surrounded by collagen in Bowman's space, to naked masses of shriveled basement membranes that have lost Bowman's capsule. The sclerotic glomeruli are within a zone of marked interstitial fibrosis, chronic inflammation, and tubular atrophy. The deeper nonatrophic tubules have very little intervening interstitium (JMS stain with H&E counterstain).

This distribution may be difficult to discern in small biopsy specimens but in larger specimens these atrophic zones can be seen alternating with nonatrophic or hypertrophied adjacent parenchyma. Tubular atrophy, interstitial fibrosis, and chronic inflammation surround the globally sclerotic glomeruli (figs. 16-15–16-18). As hypertensive nephrosclerosis progresses, more and more glomeruli are involved until the process evolves into end-stage renal disease with minimal residual intact nephrons.

In advanced arterionephrosclerosis, some glomeruli have a pattern of segmental scarring that is consistent with focal segmental glomerulosclerosis (fig. 16-19) (13). Patients with this pattern of injury often have substantial proteinuria. One interpretation of these findings is that they represent the development of focal segmental glomerulosclerosis secondary to nephron overwork caused by the progressive loss of nephrons to the arterionephrosclerosis. Arterionephrosclerosis with superimposed secondary focal segmental glomerulosclerosis must be differentiated from primary focal segmental glomerulosclerosis with secondary hypertensive changes in the renal parenchyma. This can be difficult and sometimes impossible. Factors that help are the relative severity of the focal segmental glomerulosclerosis versus hypertensive changes, and the history of the time of onset of hypertension versus proteinuria. For example, a patient with changes of both hypertensive nephrosclerosis and focal segmental glomerulosclerosis who initially presented with substantial proteinuria and little or no hypertension several years prior to biopsy but at the time of biopsy has severe hypertension, probably has primary focal segmental glomerulosclerosis with secondary hypertensive nephrosclerosis.

Immunofluorescence Findings. Most sclerotic glomeruli and renal vessels in patients with hypertensive nephrosclerosis or age-

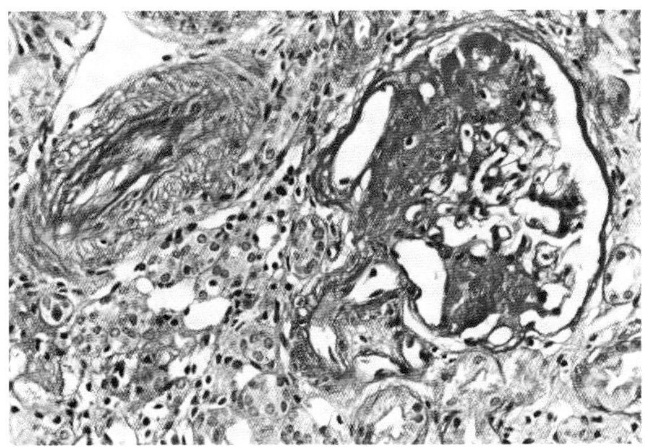

Figure 16-19

FOCAL SEGMENTAL GLOMERULOSCLEROSIS IN HYPERTENSIVE NEPHROSCLEROSIS

This specimen was from a patient who developed nephrotic-range proteinuria after many years of hypertension and slowly progressive renal insufficiency. The photomicrograph shows one of the approximately 20 percent of glomeruli that had segmental, predominantly perihilar sclerosis, often with hyalinosis. The interlobular artery on the left has prominent fibrotic intimal thickening. There is interstitial fibrosis, chronic inflammation, and tubular atrophy. Elsewhere in the biopsy were typical features of hypertensive nephrosclerosis, including clusters of globally sclerotic glomeruli (PAS stain).

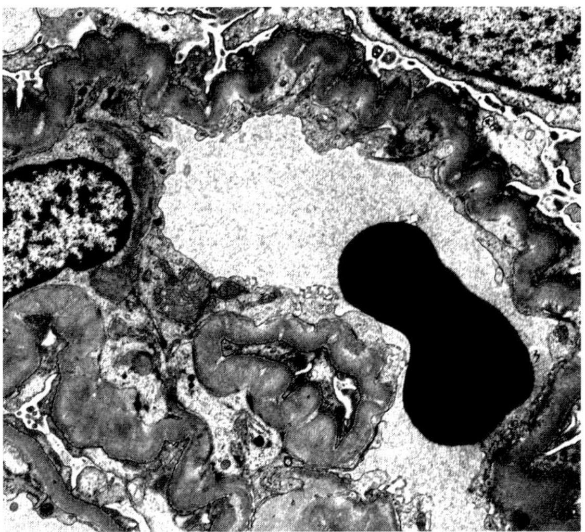

Figure 16-20

GLOMERULAR BASEMENT MEMBRANE WRINKLING IN HYPERTENSIVE NEPHROSCLEROSIS

Electron micrograph demonstrates marked wrinkling and slight thickening of the capillary wall and paramesangial glomerular basement membrane. There is effacement of visceral epithelial cell foot processes.

related arteriosclerosis do not stain significantly for immunoglobulins or complement (28,30). Foci of arteriolar or glomerular hyalinosis may stain irregularly for complement and immunoglobulins, especially IgM. This is similar to the entrapment of complement and immunoglobulins that is observed with any form of glomerular sclerosis.

Electron Microscopic Findings. Glomeruli in hypertensive nephrosclerosis and age-related arterionephrosclerosis have thickened and wrinkled glomerular basement membranes, and increased mesangial matrix material (fig. 16-20) (11,28). There may be smudgy areas of increased density within the mesangial matrix and thickened basement membranes, but typical immune complex–type electron-dense deposits should be absent. If present, the possibility of a sclerotic glomerulonephritis with secondary hypertensive changes should be considered. The thickened basement membranes and mesangial matrix may contain scattered lipid debris in the form of small spheres or droplets, or curvilinear laminated membrane-like fragments. Focal or diffuse visceral epithelial foot process effacement is common, especially in patients with proteinuria. As the sclerosis progresses there is progressive simplification, and ultimately loss, of glomerular cells.

The material that has a hyaline (glassy) appearance by light microscopy appears homogeneous or finely granular, and moderately electron dense by electron microscopy (figs. 16-21, 16-22) (1,11,39,46). In arterioles, it accumulates first between the endothelial cell and the underlying basal lamina (1,39). Larger hyaline lesions extend through the basal lamina and infiltrate into the interstitial spaces between the smooth muscle cells. With extensive arteriolar hyalinosis, there is a continuous band of moderately electron-dense material that separates the endothelial cells from a peripheral ring of smooth muscle cells that often are atrophic (fig. 16-22). The homogeneous hyaline material may contain electron-dense, curvilinear fibrin tactoids or fibrils of banded collagen. Extensive accumulation of collagen indicates arteriolar sclerosis whereas numerous fibrin tactoids indicate arteriolar fibrinoid necrosis rather than hyalinosis.

Swelling of endothelial cells and hypertrophy or proliferation of smooth muscle cells may be seen in arterioles with hyalinosis (fig. 16-21)

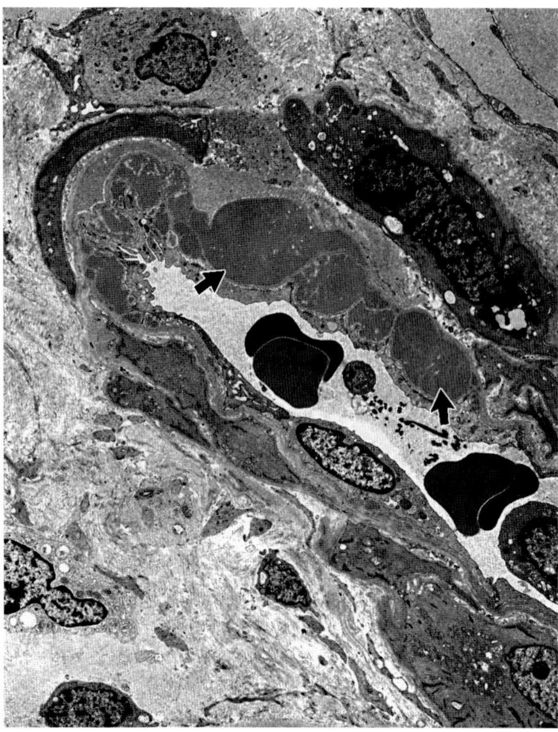

Figure 16-21

EARLY ARTERIOLAR HYALINOSIS

Electron micrograph shows irregular accumulation of finely granular to amorphous, moderately electron-dense material (arrows) that corresponds to early hyalinosis by light microscopy. Most of the hyaline material is between the swollen endothelial cell and the surrounding smooth muscle cells.

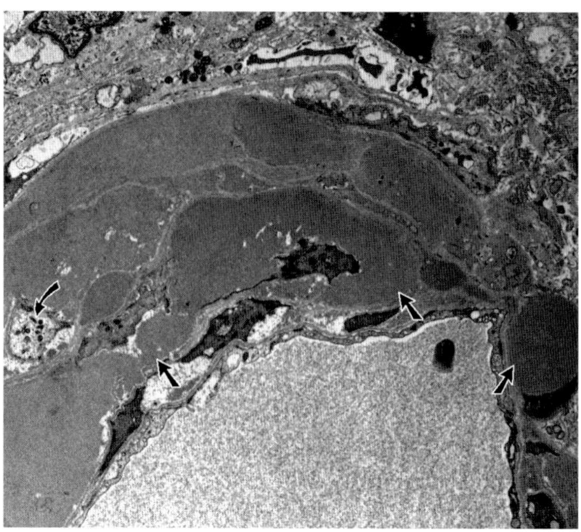

Figure 16-22

LATE ARTERIOLAR HYALINOSIS

The wall of this arteriole is almost completely replaced by amorphous to finely granular, moderately electron-dense material (straight arrows) that corresponds to advanced hyalinosis by light microscopy. A few atrophic smooth muscle cells remain (curved arrow). The adjacent interstitium is fibrotic, with increased collagen fibers.

(1). Even in the absence of hyalinosis, there may be smooth muscle hyperplasia, sclerosis with increased collagenous matrix, or both in the arterioles (fig. 16-23).

The thickened intima of arteries contains varying numbers of myofibroblasts and fibroblasts, with intervening amorphous or fibrillary collagenous matrix (11,46). Cytoplasmic myofilaments and surface membrane-dense attachment plaques characterize the smooth muscle cells and myofibroblasts.

As arterial sclerosis progresses, more and more interstitial collagen accumulates and there is progressive atrophy of the cellular elements. With advanced arterial sclerosis, most of the artery wall becomes acellular collagenous matrix.

Differential Diagnosis. Chronic renal disease secondary to hypertensive nephrosclerosis must be distinguished from other forms of chronic renal disease, such as chronic ischemic nephropathy secondary to renal artery stenosis, chronic thrombotic microangiopathy, chronic glomerulonephritis, and chronic tubulointerstitial nephritis (including chronic pyelonephritis). This may be difficult, especially in a small biopsy specimen.

As is discussed in detail later in this chapter, chronic ischemic nephropathy secondary to renal artery stenosis is characterized by a distinctive pattern of proximal tubular atrophy that results in very small tubules with inapparent lumens and mild to moderate interstitial fibrosis. This reduction in tubular volume brings the glomeruli closer together. Thus, chronic ischemic nephropathy secondary to renal artery stenosis has crowded glomeruli surrounded by tiny tubules, whereas hypertensive nephrosclerosis has zones of globally sclerotic glomeruli and atrophic tubules surrounded by marked interstitial fibrosis and chronic inflammation.

Chronic renal injury secondary to a thrombotic microangiopathy can be difficult to distinguish from hypertensive nephrosclerosis. There often are indistinguishable sclerotic

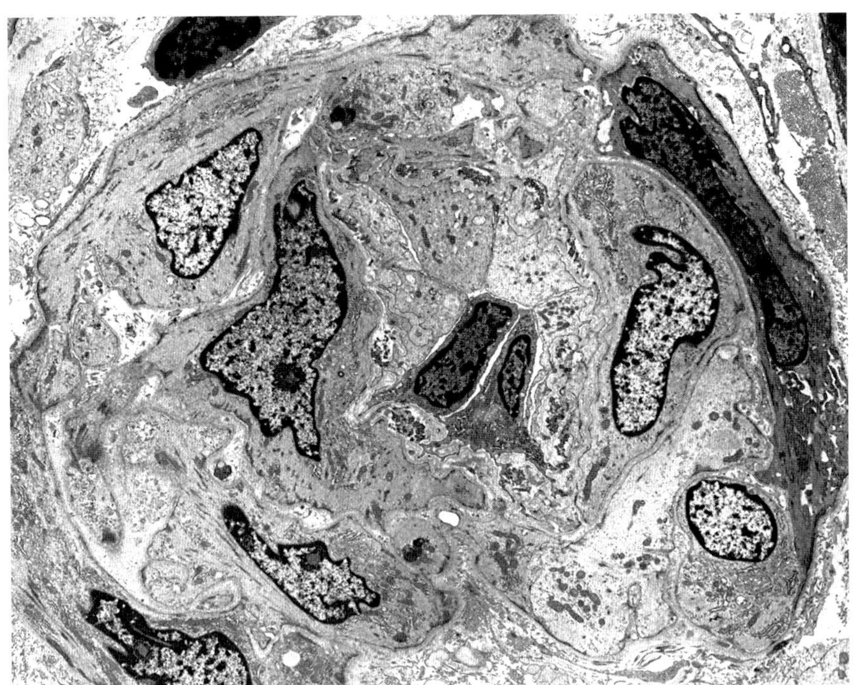

Figure 16-23

ARTERIOLAR SMOOTH MUSCLE HYPERPLASIA

An increased number of slightly disordered smooth muscle cells is seen in the muscularis of an arteriole. There is only a slight increase in interstitial collagenous matrix in the muscularis.

changes in arteries and arterioles, as well as indistinguishable chronic tubular atrophy, interstitial fibrosis, and chronic inflammation. The pattern of glomerular scarring is the most useful differentiating feature. The glomerular sclerosis of hypertensive nephrosclerosis is characterized by a contracted, wrinkled mass of glomerular basement membranes in one corner of Bowman's space, with the rest filled by amorphous collagen. Glomerular scarring secondary to thrombotic microangiopathy results in a sclerotic tuft that is not as contracted and has replication of glomerular basement membranes (see fig. 16-28). Cortical scars consistent with earlier focal cortical necrosis also support a diagnosis of chronic injury secondary to thrombotic microangiopathy rather than hypertensive nephrosclerosis.

Patients with chronic glomerulonephritis often have concurrent features of hypertensive nephrosclerosis, if the hypertension developed secondary to the glomerulonephritis. Therefore, the presence or absence of pathologic changes of hypertensive nephrosclerosis does not rule out chronic glomerulonephritis. The most definitive evidence of chronic glomerulonephritis is the demonstration by immunohistology or electron microscopy of an identifiable feature of a specific form of glomerulonephritis, for example, immune complex–type deposits or deposits of dense deposit disease. The pattern of glomerular sclerosis also may indicate scarring secondary to inflammation rather than chronic ischemia.

All forms of chronic renal disease show some degree of interstitial fibrosis and chronic inflammation, however, a specific pathologic diagnosis of chronic tubulointerstitial nephritis is appropriate only if the tubulointerstitial injury is a primary process and not merely a secondary consequence of vascular or glomerular disease. Support for this conclusion is provided when the severity of tubulointerstitial injury is much worse than the glomerular or vascular disease. For example, a renal biopsy specimen with 20 nonsclerotic glomeruli and mild to moderate vascular sclerosis, but severe diffuse interstitial fibrosis, chronic inflammation, and tubular atrophy is more consistent with chronic tubulointerstitial nephritis than with hypertensive nephrosclerosis or chronic glomerulonephritis.

Etiology and Pathogenesis. For over 100 years, there has been controversy over the nature of the relationship between hypertension and arteriosclerosis (18–20). Two possibilities are: 1) arteriosclerosis is a primary disease that causes hypertension and nephrosclerosis; 2) hypertension is a primary disease that causes arteriosclerosis and nephrosclerosis. The work of

Goldblatt (14) demonstrated that vascular narrowing can cause hypertension and that hypertension can cause vascular sclerosis. However, identical vascular lesions to those apparently caused by hypertension also occur in patients with no hypertension. This raises the possibility that these vascular changes can be caused by processes other than hypertension. In fact, hypertension and vascular sclerosis form a classic vicious cycle because hypertension causes renal vascular sclerosis and renal vascular sclerosis causes hypertension. In most patients, the evidence suggests that the hypertension is primary and the renal vascular sclerosis is secondary. The possibility remains, however, that some patients have a primary propensity for renal vascular sclerosis that secondarily causes hypertension (13).

Renal transplantation studies suggest that there is some process in the kidneys that contributes to the development of "essential" hypertension (hypertension of unknown etiology). Transplantation of normal kidneys into patients with end-stage hypertensive nephrosclerosis results not only in amelioration of the hypertension but also reversal of hypertensive injury in the heart and retinal vessels (6).

Factors in addition to hypertension may contribute to the pathologic lesions of hypertensive nephrosclerosis and age-related arterionephrosclerosis. There is evidence that tobacco smoking (2,3) and hyperlipidemia (9), alone or in combination with hypertension, can cause renal vascular and glomerular sclerosis.

The pathogenesis of the glomerular and vascular lesions of arterionephrosclerosis involves not only increased deposition of collagen and other matrix components, but also, in certain lesions, intramural insudation of plasma proteins and migration and proliferation of cells, especially smooth muscle cells and their progeny. The hyaline of arteriolar hyalinosis is derived, at least in part, from plasma constituents that have leaked across endothelial cells into the intima and muscularis. The plasma proteins accumulate there in association with matrix molecules (11,19). As a result, arterioles with hyalinosis contain increased amounts of water, sodium, calcium, glycosaminoglycans, and collagen (19).

Persistent endothelial injury and insudation of plasma constituents into the intima probably initiate the intimal thickening in arteries. This stimulates smooth muscle cell migration from the muscularis through fenestrations in the elastica and into the intima where they transform into myofibroblasts and fibroblasts (19). These cells produce collagen, which may form dense bands that have the staining properties of elastin.

Glomerular sclerosis involves the production of both type IV and type III collagen by glomerular cells (31). Normally, the glomerulus contains type IV but not type III collagen. Type IV collagen is a major component of Bowman's capsule, glomerular basement membranes, and mesangial matrix. Type III collagen is abundant in the renal interstitium. As glomerular sclerosis progresses, there is an increasing proportion of type III collagen, especially in the collagen that fills Bowman's space (31).

Treatment and Prognosis. Pharmacologic control of blood pressure is the primary therapeutic strategy for preventing the development and slowing the progression of hypertensive nephrosclerosis. The therapeutic goal is to prescribe a combination of lifestyle modifications (e.g., salt restriction, weight loss, exercise) plus the lowest dose of drug(s) that normalizes the blood pressure (12). The target blood pressure is less than 140/90 mm Hg if there is no proteinuria and lower than 125/75 if there is 1 g/day or more proteinuria or significant renal insufficiency. Drug monotherapy usually is not adequate to control blood pressure in patients with hypertensive nephrosclerosis: on average, four drugs are required. Angiotensin converting enzyme inhibitors, and probably angiotensin receptor antagonists, are especially useful in patients with hypertensive nephrosclerosis because they appear to slow the progression of renal failure, possibly because the renal renin-angiotensin system plays an important role in the pathogenesis of sclerotic changes in vessels and glomeruli (12). In addition, angiotensin converting enzyme inhibitors and angiotensin receptor antagonists reduce proteinuria if it is present. Once patients reach end-stage renal disease with hypertensive nephrosclerosis, renal transplantation usually is the optimum form of therapy, and has the added benefit of ameliorating the hypertension (6).

MALIGNANT HYPERTENSIVE NEPHROPATHY

Definition. Malignant hypertension is severe hypertension that causes acute tissue injury in multiple organs. There are many different clinical definitions of malignant hypertension. Generally acceptable criteria are a diastolic blood pressure greater than 130 mm Hg (usually with systolic blood pressure greater than 210 mm Hg), retinal vascular changes, papilledema, and renal functional impairment. Malignant hypertension usually arises in patients with underlying chronic renal disease (39). About half the patients with malignant hypertensive nephropathy have a history of hypertensive nephrosclerosis. Most others have evidence of chronic renal injury of some other cause, such as from chronic pyelonephritis (30). Rarely, malignant hypertensive nephropathy arises de novo in apparently healthy individuals, most often young black men.

Malignant hypertensive nephropathy is a form of thrombotic microangiopathy and thus must be distinguished from other categories of thrombotic microangiopathy, such as hemolytic uremic syndrome, thrombotic thrombocytopenic purpura, systemic sclerosis renal crisis, antiphospholipid antibody syndrome, and acute postpartum renal failure. This differentiation requires knowledge of clinical and laboratory data because of shared pathologic features among all of the thrombotic microangiopathies.

Clinical Features. The clinical manifestations of malignant hypertension include severe headache, blurred vision, nystagmus, neurological symptoms, extensor plantar reflexes, papilledema with hemorrhages and exudates, congestive heart failure, and acute renal failure (12). As with other types of thrombotic microangiopathy, microangiopathic hemolytic anemia and thrombocytopenia may occur, but rarely as the primary vasculopathic process in patients with malignant hypertension. If there is conspicuous microangiopathic hemolytic anemia and thrombocytopenia in a patient with malignant hypertension, the clinical diagnosis usually is hemolytic uremic syndrome with secondary malignant hypertension rather than malignant hypertension with secondary microangiopathic hemolytic anemia.

Gross Findings. Malignant hypertensive nephropathy often is superimposed on chronic hypertensive nephrosclerosis, thus, the pathologic features of the latter may dominate the gross appearance. The acute gross features of malignant hypertensive nephropathy include renal swelling and scattered, irregular red specks or splotches caused by hemorrhage from foci of arteriolar and glomerular fibrinoid necrosis (fig. 16-24) (28,39,46). These red specks are much less frequent than the red dots of the "flea-bitten" kidney of severe acute or crescentic glomerulonephritis.

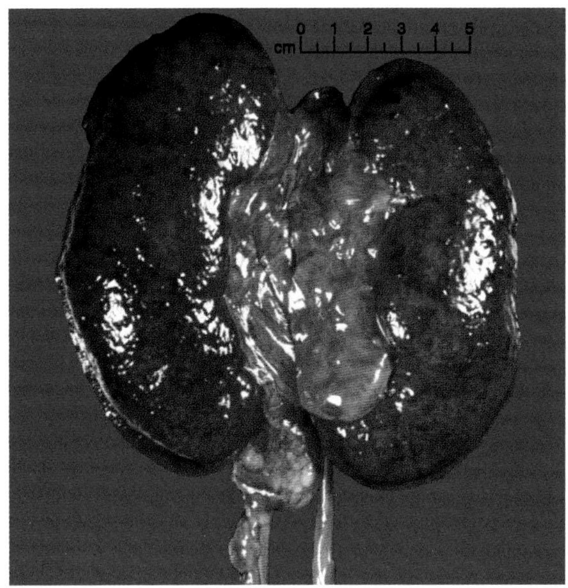

Figure 16-24

MALIGNANT HYPERTENSIVE NEPHROPATHY

The kidneys are swollen and have scattered hemorrhages, for example, on the upper pole of the kidney on the right.

Severe malignant hypertensive nephropathy may lead to grossly visible infarcts if arcuate or large interlobular arteries are occluded by extensive intimal expansion or thrombosis; or to focal cortical necrosis if there is extensive localized occlusion of the microvasculature, including interlobular arteries, arterioles, and glomerular capillaries. Infarcts and foci of cortical necrosis are very pale and slightly swollen, with narrow hemorrhagic margins during the acute phase, and later become depressed as they undergo fibrosis. On the cut surfaces of the kidney, infarcts are more triangular, with the base oriented toward the capsular surface, whereas foci of cortical necrosis are broader,

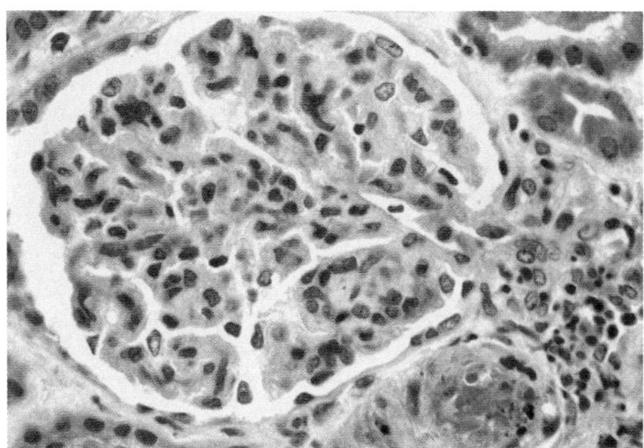

Figure 16-25

MALIGNANT HYPERTENSIVE NEPHROPATHY

The glomerulus is consolidated without being hypercellular. It is relatively "bloodless" because of the lack of erythrocytes in the capillary lumens. The lumens are obscured by swollen endothelial cells and expanded subendothelial zones. The arteriole in the right lower corner has thrombosis in the lumen and fibrinoid necrosis in the wall. Endothelial cells and most smooth muscle cells are replaced by fibrinoid material that contains some karyorrhectic debris and erythrocyte fragments (H&E stain).

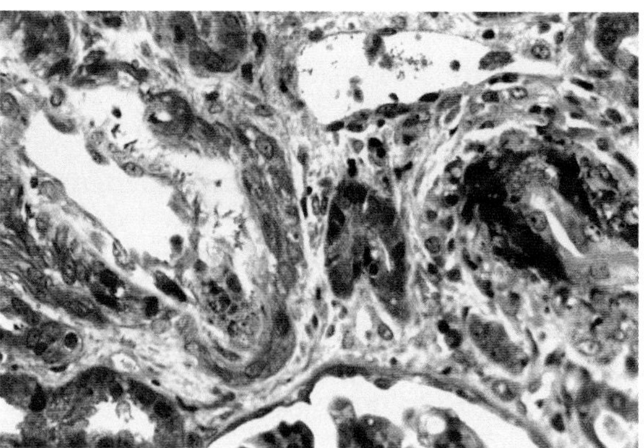

Figure 16-26

MALIGNANT HYPERTENSIVE NEPHROPATHY

The arteriole on the right has ragged, red fibrinoid material beneath swollen endothelial cells that extends between adjacent smooth muscle cells. There is little or no leukocytic infiltration, which distinguishes this from necrotizing vasculitis. The interlobular artery on the left has edematous intimal thickening and narrowing of the lumen (Masson trichrome stain).

more rectangular, and usually do not extend into the medulla.

Light Microscopic Findings. The characteristic lesions are edematous (mucoid, myxoid) intimal thickening in arteries, fibrinoid necrosis in arterioles and glomeruli, and glomerular consolidation (28,39).

The most characteristic although not diagnostically specific arteriolar lesion is fibrinoid necrosis (figs. 16-25, 16-26) (28,39). This affects afferent rather than efferent arterioles. Arteriolar fibrinoid necrosis may extend contiguously into the hilar regions of glomeruli (fig. 16-27). At any site, the fibrinoid necrosis of malignant hypertensive nephropathy and other thrombotic microangiopathies is characterized by effacement of architecture by deeply acidophilic material with irregular margins. This material has the same tinctorial properties as the fibrin in thrombi: it is fuchsinophilic with the trichrome stain (fig. 16-26) and stains dark blue with the phosphotungstic acid–hematoxylin (PTAH) stain. The fibrinoid material may contain erythrocyte fragments and a small amount of scattered nuclear debris (fig. 16-25). The lumens of vessels with fibrinoid necrosis may contain thrombi (fig. 16-25). In these areas, the endothelium often is necrotic or denuded. There is little or no vascular or glomerular infiltration of leukocytes associated with the fibrinoid necrosis of malignant hypertensive nephropathy and other thrombotic microangiopathies. This differs from the fibrinoid necrosis of necrotizing vasculitis (such as polyarteritis nodosa and microscopic polyangiitis) which is accompanied by substantial leukocyte infiltration.

In addition to segmental fibrinoid necrosis, glomeruli often have global, or less frequently, segmental consolidation caused by subendothelial expansion, endothelial swelling, and capillary thrombosis (figs. 16-25, 16-27). This results in "bloodless" glomeruli with obscured or occluded capillary lumens. High-power light microscopic examination sometimes allows documentation of the subendothelial expansion, but this is seen best by electron microscopy. Glomerular capillaries may have thrombosis superimposed on the endothelial injury. Occasional glomeruli have segmental or global capillary congestion, with numerous erythrocytes stuffed into dilated capillary lumens. This probably results from downstream capillary occlusion.

Infarction of individual glomeruli is the mildest expression of focal cortical necrosis (39). Glomerular infarction usually is a component

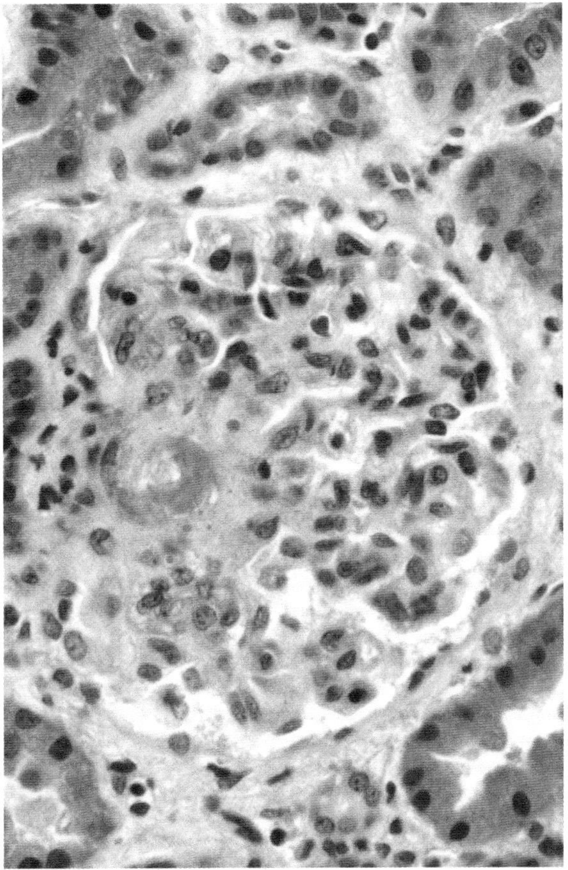

Figure 16-27

MALIGNANT HYPERTENSIVE NEPHROPATHY

The glomerulus is consolidated without being hypercellular. The capillary lumens are obscured by swollen endothelial cells and expanded subendothelial zones. The more deeply acidophilic material of the hilum is thrombosis and fibrinoid necrosis.

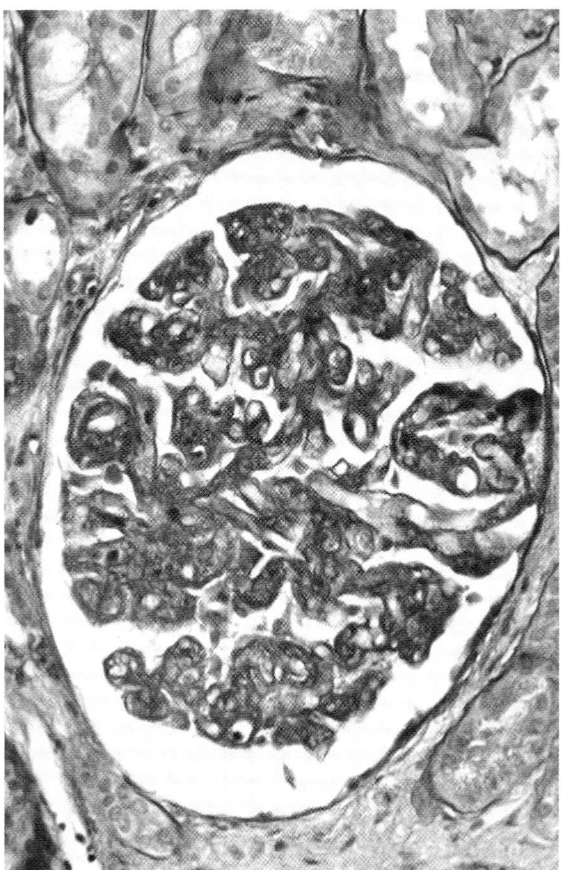

Figure 16-28

CHRONIC GLOMERULAR CHANGES AFTER MALIGNANT HYPERTENSION

Extensive remodeling of the glomerular basement membranes and mesangial matrix follows earlier injury from malignant hypertensive nephropathy. Glomerular basement membranes are replicated or trabeculated (PAS stain).

of focal cortical necrosis that is caused by extensive microvascular injury and the resultant severe ischemia.

The late phase of glomerular injury is characterized by thickening and replication of the basement membrane as a result of mesangial interposition into the expanded subendothelial zone (fig. 16-28). By light microscopy, this can be confused with membranous glomerulopathy or membranoproliferative glomerulonephritis, however, immunohistology and electron microscopy clarify this differential diagnosis.

Edematous or mucoid intimal thickening is the most common alteration in renal arteries with malignant hypertensive nephropathy and other types of thrombotic microangiopathy (figs. 16-26, 16-29–16-31). This is most frequent in interlobular and arcuate arteries, but may affect the interlobar arteries and arterioles (39). The interstitial substance in the earliest edematous lesions stains weakly. The thickened intima may have overlying thrombosis (fig. 16-30). The interstitial substance in older "mucoid" lesions stains more basophilic because of the accumulation of young collagen and other proteins and proteoglycans (fig. 16-31). This eventually evolves into intimal fibrosis, with numerous coarse bands of collagen that stain intensely with the PAS and Verhoeff van Gieson elastic stain. This imparts a laminated ("onion-skin")

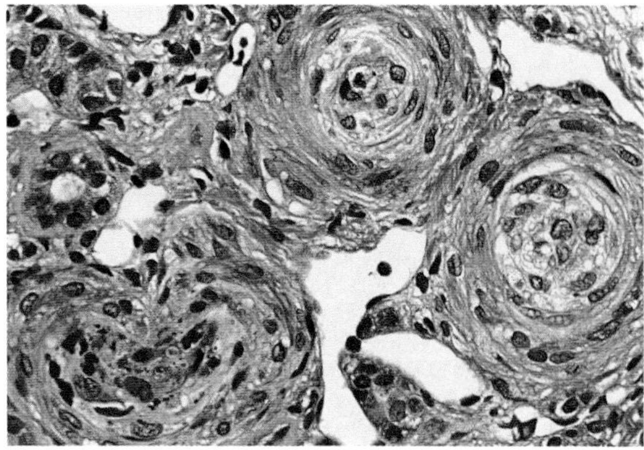

Figure 16-29

MALIGNANT HYPERTENSIVE NEPHROPATHY

The interlobular cross sections demonstrate obliteration of lumens by edematous thickening of the intima. There are schistocytes in the thickened intima of the artery on the far left (Masson trichrome stain).

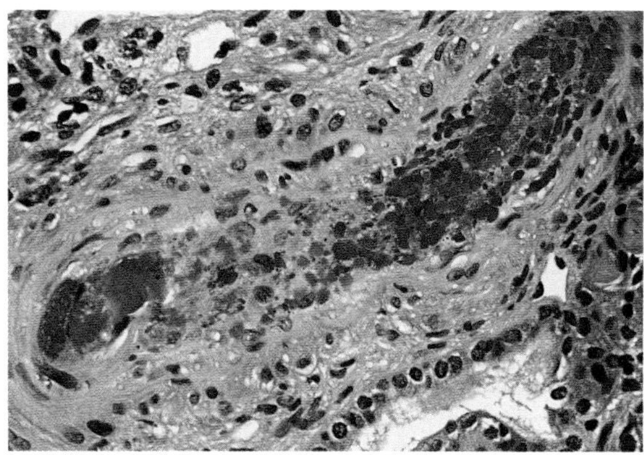

Figure 16-30

MALIGNANT HYPERTENSIVE NEPHROPATHY

Thrombosis in an interlobular artery that has edematous intimal expansion (H&E).

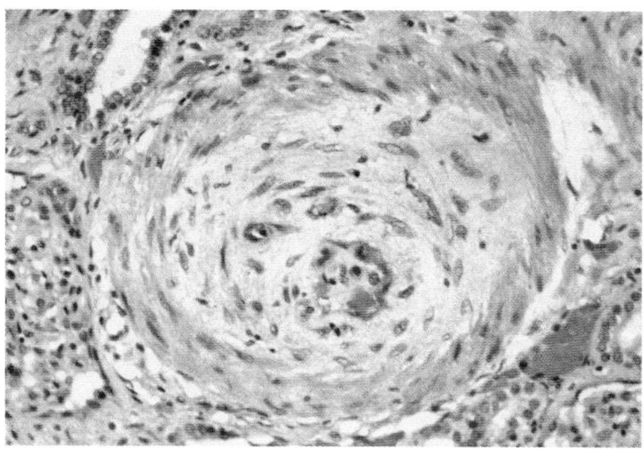

Figure 16-31

MALIGNANT HYPERTENSIVE NEPHROPATHY

There is marked edematous thickening of the intima of an arcuate artery with resultant severe narrowing of the lumen. The intima has a slightly basophilic hue that prompts the designations "mucinous" or "myxoid" intimal expansion (H&E stain).

appearance to the thickened intima and resembles the sclerotic changes that are caused by chronic hypertension (fig. 16-32). This is sometimes called replication of the internal elastica (or elastosis), however, it is not a true replication because the additional laminations are made of collagen and not elastin (39).

Malignant hypertension often is superimposed on chronic hypertensive nephrosclerosis. This results in a combination of features of chronic hypertensive nephrosclerosis and malignant hypertensive nephropathy. For example, the edematous intimal expansion may occur internal to fibrotic intimal thickening (fig. 16-33).

Immunofluorescence Findings. Immunohistology demonstrates various plasma proteins at sites of arteriolar and glomerular fibrinoid necrosis and thrombosis, including fibrin, fibrinogen, complement components, immunoglobulins (especially IgM), and albumin (fig. 16-34) (30,39,46). There is less intense and consistent staining of the acutely thickened intima in arteries. Intimal staining for immunoglobulins and complement diminishes as the lesion progresses from the edematous early phase to the fibrotic late phase.

Electron Microscopic Findings. The most frequent glomerular ultrastructural abnormality is electron-lucent expansion of the subendothelial zone (fig. 16-35). This may be continuous with similarly lucent areas in the mesangium (mesangiolysis). The subendothelial expansion is thought to be the result of insudation of plasma proteins beneath the endothelial cells and into the mesangium, possibly as a result of increased plasma pressure, endothelial injury, or both (19). Conceptually, this is analogous to the insudation of plasma proteins into arteriolar walls that manifests as fibrinoid necrosis, and the insudation of plasma into the intima of arteries that manifests as edematous intimal expansion. Over time, there is extension of

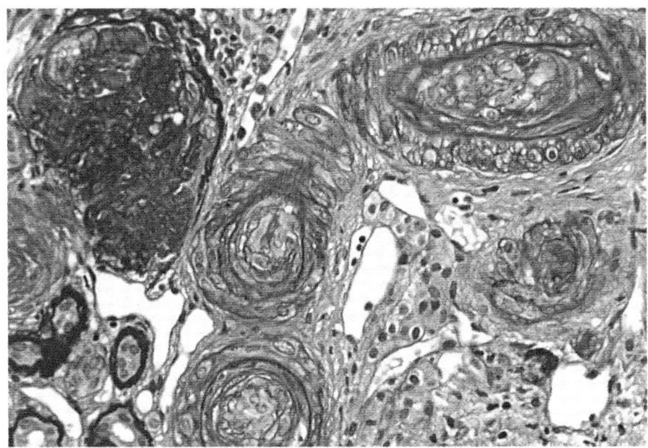

Figure 16-32

MALIGNANT HYPERTENSIVE NEPHROPATHY

Intimal fibrosis of interlobular arteries with multiple layers of PAS-positive material ("onion-skin" changes). Note also the ischemic collapse and sclerosis of the glomerulus on the left, and the tubular atrophy, interstitial fibrosis, and interstitial chronic inflammation.

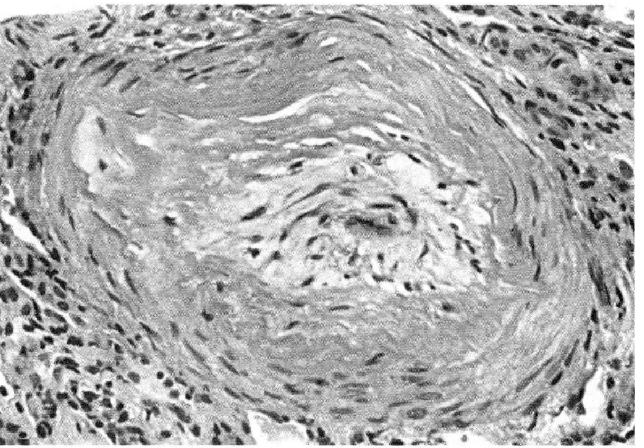

Figure 16-33

EDEMATOUS INTIMAL THICKENING SUPERIMPOSED ON CHRONIC ARTERIOSCLEROSIS

This arcuate artery is from a patient with chronic hypertensive nephrosclerosis who developed malignant hypertension. There is edematous intimal expansion closest to the obliterated lumen. This is internal to the extensive intimal fibrosis that was present before the malignant hypertension developed.

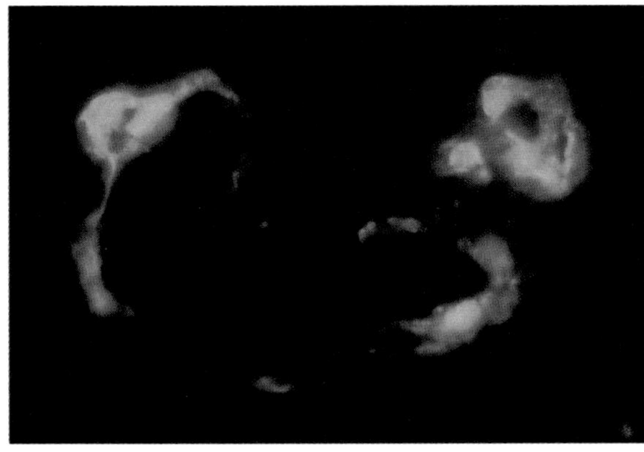

Figure 16-34

MALIGNANT HYPERTENSIVE NEPHROPATHY: VASCULAR FIBRINOID NECROSIS

The walls of the arteriole in the upper right and the interlobular artery in the middle and to the left stain irregularly with an antiserum specific for fibrin. This corresponds to areas of fibrinoid necrosis (direct immunofluorescence, fluoroscein isothiocyanate [FITC] antifibrin).

mesangial cytoplasm into the expanded subendothelial zones and deposition of new basement membrane material. This corresponds to the migration of smooth muscle cells into the edematous intima of arteries, with subsequent production of collagenous matrix.

Areas of fibrinoid necrosis in glomeruli, arterioles, or arteries contain electron-dense material that resembles thrombi, including dense

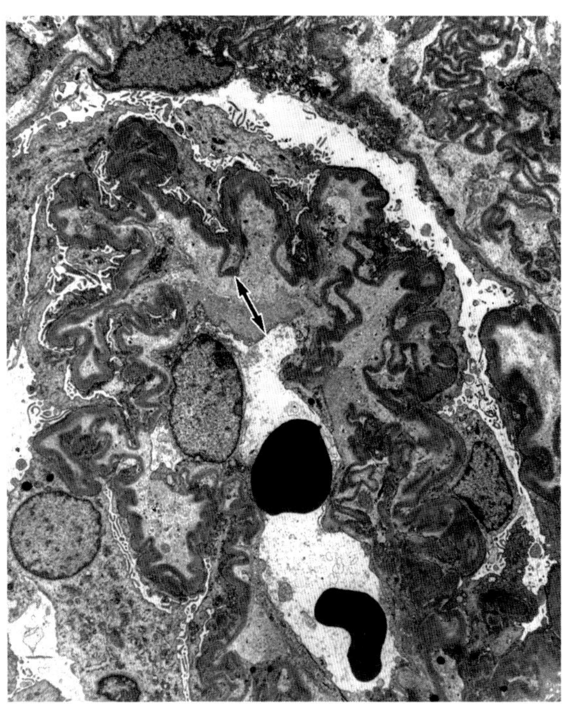

Figure 16-35

MALIGNANT HYPERTENSIVE NEPHROPATHY

Electron micrograph demonstrates glomerular basement membrane wrinkling and lucent expansion of the subendothelial zone (double arrow). There is effacement of visceral epithelial cell foot processes.

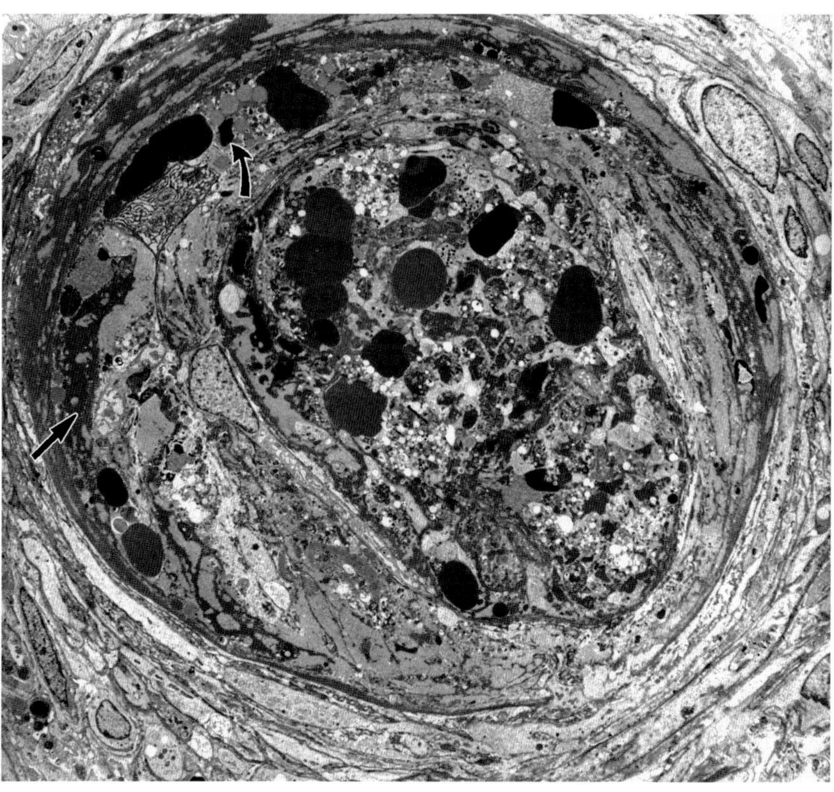

Figure 16-36

MALIGNANT HYPERTENSIVE NEPHROPATHY

This electron micrograph shows an arteriole with fibrinoid necrosis and thrombosis. The lumen contains cellular debris (including schistocytes), platelets, and an electron-dense amorphous coagulum of protein. Most smooth muscle cells are necrotic and the muscularis contains electron-dense fibrinoid material (straight arrow) and schistocytes (curved arrow).

globular and curvilinear bands of polymerized fibrin called fibrin tactoids (figs. 16-36–16-38). As would be expected, the fibrin tactoids often have a fine periodicity that is characteristic of fibrin anywhere (19,28). The fibrinoid material may contain erythrocytes and erythrocyte fragments (schistocytes), and other cellular debris derived from degenerating endothelial cells, smooth muscle cells, and leukocytes (fig. 16-36). Especially in terminal arterioles and glomeruli, fibrinoid necrosis may be accompanied by thrombosis. Thrombotic material and fibrinoid necrosis are distinguishable ultrastructurally primarily by location and presence or absence of tissue debris. For example, material rich in fibrin tactoids (often with admixed platelets) that is in a vascular lumen is a thrombus (fig. 16-38), whereas similar appearing material in an area of injury in the wall of a vessel is fibrinoid necrosis (fig. 16-37).

Differential Diagnosis. The gross and microscopic features of malignant hypertensive nephropathy cannot be distinguished confidently from those caused by any other form of thrombotic microangiopathy, such as hemolytic uremic syndrome, thrombotic thrombocytopenic purpura, systemic sclerosis renal crisis, antiphospholipid antibody syndrome, and acute postpartum renal failure. Thus, unless there is adequate clinical information, a specific diagnosis of malignant hypertensive nephropathy cannot be made. If inadequate clinical data are available, the prudent approach is to make a diagnosis of thrombotic microangiopathy and to note that clinical correlation is required to make a more specific clinicopathologic diagnosis. If clinical data are known to support a diagnosis of malignant hypertension, a pathologic diagnosis of thrombotic microangiopathy consistent with malignant hypertensive nephropathy is warranted. Any form of thrombotic microangiopathy can be accompanied by malignant hypertension, and primary malignant hypertension and malignant hypertension secondary to another thrombotic microangiopathy can be very difficult and sometimes impossible to differentiate.

The renal lesions of overt malignant hypertensive nephropathy are distinct from the lesions of uncomplicated hypertensive nephrosclerosis (Table 16-1), however, there may be minor or poorly defined features suggesting malignant hypertensive injury in specimens that

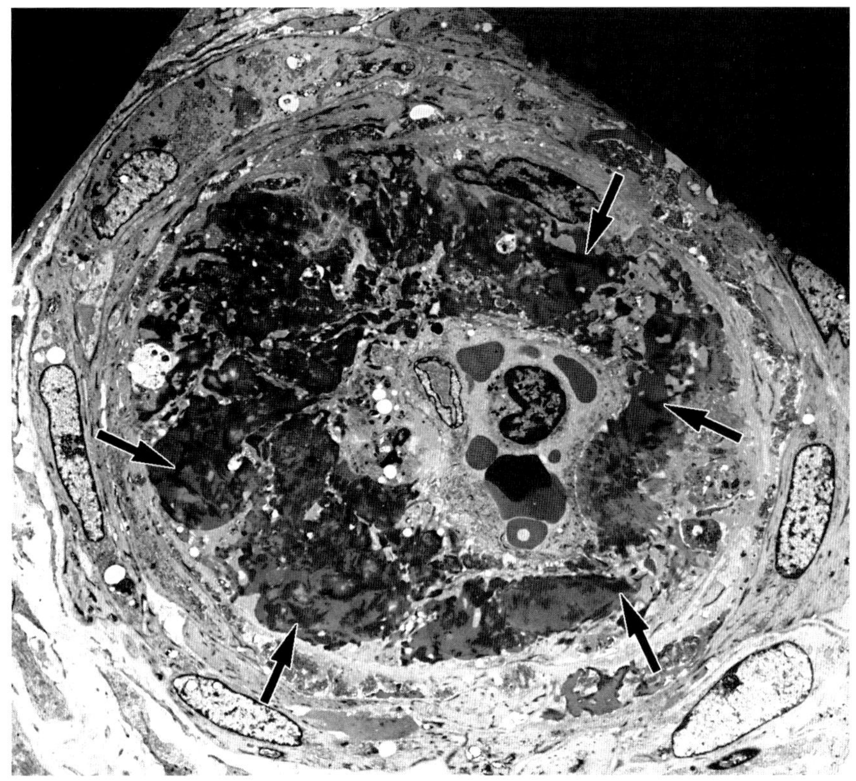

Figure 16-37

MALIGNANT HYPERTENSIVE NEPHROPATHY

This electron micrograph demonstrates a small interlobular artery with circumferential fibrinoid necrosis that is most extensive on the left. The fibrinoid material contains very electron-dense fibrin tactoids (arrows), sometimes surrounded by less dense proteinaceous material.

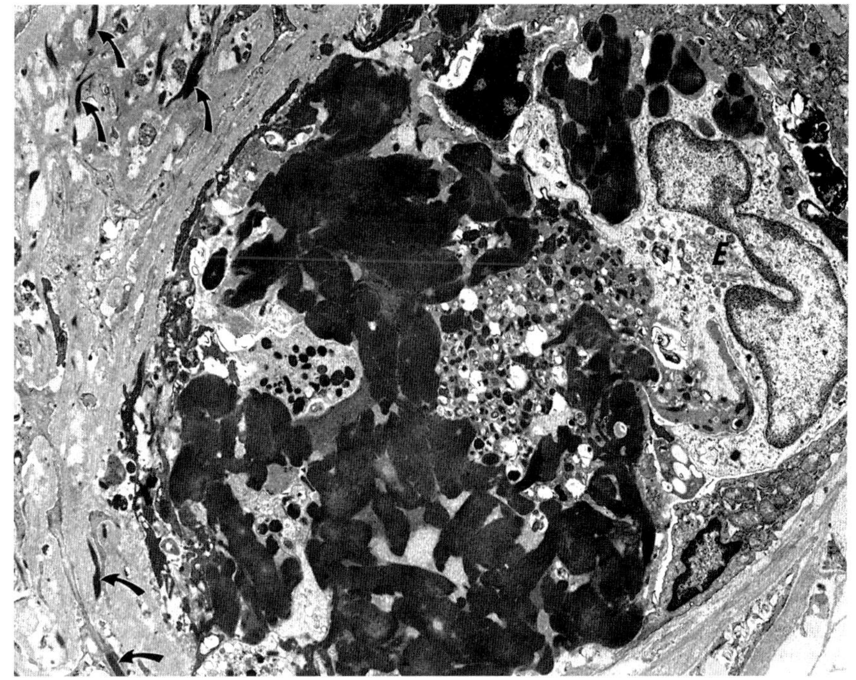

Figure 16-38

MALIGNANT HYPERTENSIVE NEPHROPATHY

This electron micrograph demonstrates thrombosis and mural fibrinoid necrosis in an artery. A somewhat disrupted endothelial cell is to the right (E). The lumen is filled with a thrombus composed predominantly of electron-dense fibrin tactoids admixed with platelets. The wall of the arteriole is to the left and contains scattered fibrin tactoids (curved arrows).

have predominantly features of hypertensive nephrosclerosis. For example, there may be focal edematous intimal thickening in arteries that have predominantly intimal fibrosis, or there may be only rare foci of arteriolar or glomerular fibrinoid necrosis. Patients with incompletely expressed features of malignant hypertensive nephrosclerosis may have clinical evidence of

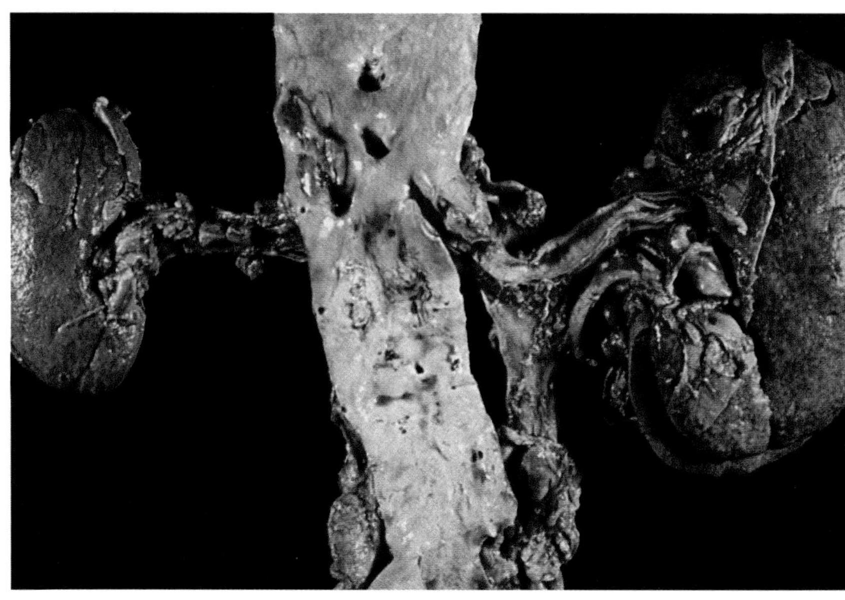

Figure 16-39

RENAL ARTERY STENOSIS

The kidney on the left has marked atrophy secondary to renal artery stenosis. The kidney on the right has a granular surface caused by hypertensive nephropathy, whereas the atrophic kidney has a relatively smooth surface.

Table 16-1

VASCULOPATHIC ISCHEMIC NEPHROPATHY

Diagnostic Terms	Major Pathologic Features
Arterionephrosclerosis, including hypertensive nephrosclerosis and age-related arterionephrosclerosis	Arterial fibrotic intimal thickening, arteriolar hyalinosis, regional (often subcapsular) global glomerular sclerosis with adjacent tubular atrophy, interstitial fibrosis, and chronic inflammation
Malignant hypertensive nephropathy and thrombotic microangiopathy	Arterial edematous and myxoid intimal thickening, arteriolar fibrinoid necrosis, glomerular subendothelial expansion and fibrinoid necrosis, acute ischemic tubular epithelial injury
Renal artery stenosis with chronic ischemic nephropathy	Renal artery stenosis (e.g., caused by atherosclerosis, arteriosclerosis, arteritis, fibromuscular dysplasia, vasculitis, retroperitoneal fibrosis), tubular "endocrine" atrophy, glomerular crowding
Renal atheroembolization (cholesterol crystal embolization)	Cholesterol clefts in vascular lumens with or without adjacent atheromatous debris, thrombosis, leukocytes, or fibrosis.

severe hypertension that does not fulfill all criteria for malignant hypertension. "Accelerated arteriosclerosis" is a term sometimes used for hypertensive renal injury that is more acute than typical hypertensive nephrosclerosis but is less extensive than full-blown malignant hypertensive nephropathy in the same way that "accelerated hypertension" refers to an acute severe elevation in blood pressure that is not as high or sustained as malignant hypertension.

Etiology and Pathogenesis. Severe hypertension alone can cause renal vascular fibrinoid necrosis, as demonstrated by Goldblatt (14). The extremely high blood pressures in patients with malignant hypertension appear to be capable of directly injuring the endothelium of vessels, especially renal vessels, and causing insudation of plasma into the vessel walls. Thus, the fibrin at sites of fibrinoid necrosis comes form transudation of plasma proteins, including coagulation factors, into the extravascular interstitium (19). The coagulation factors contact thrombogenic substances, such as tissue factor, and are activated to form fibrin.

The molecular pathogenesis of malignant hypertension usually involves high-level renin secretion by the kidney that is not down regulated by the rise in blood pressure. This dysregulated renin release causes a vicious cycle of more renin release causing more vascular injury that leads to more renal ischemia and more renin release. The pivotal role of renin in this process is demonstrated by the efficacy of renin system blockers to control malignant hypertension (23).

Treatment and Prognosis. The 1-year survival rate of patients with untreated malignant hypertension is 20 percent compared to 90 percent 5-year survival rate with appropriate treatment (12). Patients must be treated with intravenous hypertensive medications under close supervision. The most commonly used drugs in the initial phase of treatment are intravenous sodium nitroprusside and nitroglycerine. The therapeutic goal is a gradual reduction of mean arterial pressure, for example, by no more than 20 percent over the first hour of therapy, which reduces the risk of organ ischemia caused by reduced perfusion pressure and decreased flow through the vessels that have been narrowed by the vasculopathy of malignant hypertension.

RENAL ARTERY STENOSIS AND CHRONIC ISCHEMIC NEPHROPATHY

Definition. Renal artery stenosis is narrowing of the lumen of the main renal artery. Renal artery stenosis can be asymptomatic or can cause renovascular hypertension, with or without renal insufficiency. This may result in a distinctive pattern of chronic renal parenchymal ischemic injury (chronic ischemic nephropathy) characterized by marked atrophy of cortical tubules. Causes of renal artery stenosis include, but are not limited to, atherosclerosis, fibromuscular dysplasia, dissecting aneurysm, vasculitis (especially Takayasu's arteritis), retroperitoneal fibrosis, neurofibromatosis, and compression by an abdominal neoplasm. Chronic ischemic nephropathy caused by atherosclerotic renal artery stenosis may be accompanied by renal atheroembolization (see later section on atheroembolization).

Clinical Features. Renal artery stenosis is identified in 1 to 5 percent of patients with hypertension (10,16). It is a more frequent cause of hypertension in older adults and children. Between 10 and 40 percent of elderly hypertensive patients have significant renal artery stenosis, usually caused by atherosclerosis (41). Fibromuscular dysplasia is the most common cause of renal artery stenosis in children (8,10, 29). Fibromuscular dysplasia causes approximately 10 percent of renal artery stenosis, is much more frequent in females, and usually is identified between the ages of 15 and 50 years (8,10,33). Fibromuscular dysplasia is most common in the renal arteries, right more than left, but also can affect arteries at other sites (15,22). Neurofibromatosis (von Recklinghausen's disease) and Takayasu's arteritis also are important causes of renovascular hypertension in children (8,32,47). In fact, Takayasu's arteritis is the most common cause of childhood renovascular hypertension in some areas of Asia (32).

Patients with renal artery stenosis may be asymptomatic. The renal perfusion pressure does not decline until more than 50 percent of the renal artery is stenosed (37), and no symptoms are expected until this threshold is exceeded. Renovascular hypertension is the major clinical manifestation of renal artery stenosis. Renal insufficiency may occur, especially if the process is bilateral. Although renal insufficiency that is caused by renal artery stenosis usually is accompanied by hypertension, a minority of patients do not have hypertension (33). Rare patients develop substantial proteinuria, even overt nephrotic syndrome, which is mediated by increased circulating renin and compensatory overwork of nephrons in the contralateral kidney.

The diagnosis is confirmed by aortography and renal artery angiography, Doppler velocimetry, or magnetic resonance angiography. Diagnostic evaluation also includes evaluation of the status of the renin-angiotensin system and of renal perfusion. These data facilitate therapeutic decisions, in particular, the outlook for revascularization (33,41).

Gross Findings. Kidneys of patients with symptomatic chronic renal artery stenosis are small because of chronic ischemic atrophy (fig. 16-39). Most are less than half normal size (24). Unless there is another concurrent process, the external surface is relatively smooth. A granular external surface raises the possibility of another concurrent process, such as arterionephrosclerosis.

Gross examination of the renal artery may suggest the cause of the stenosis. A longitudinal section may be more informative than cross

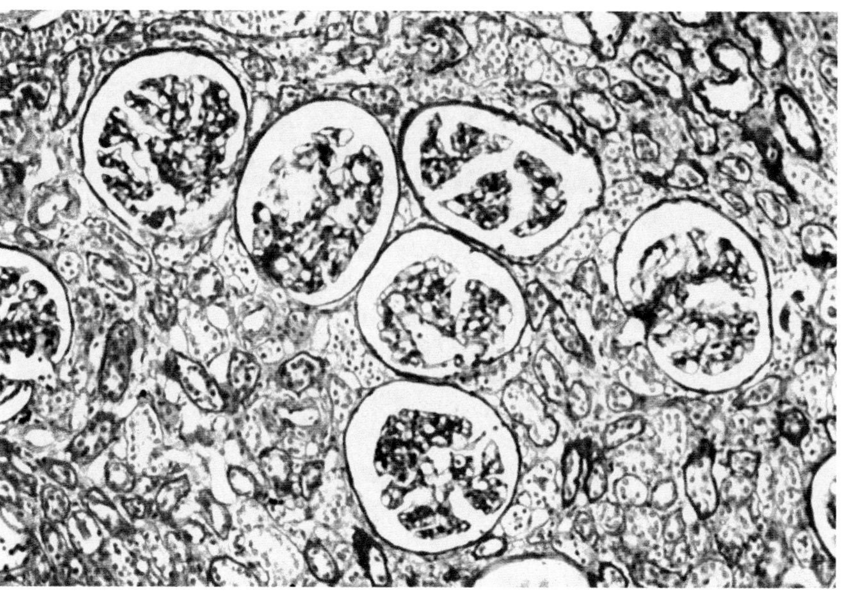

Figure 16-40

CORTICAL TUBULAR ATROPHY CAUSED BY RENAL ARTERY STENOSIS

This specimen is from a patient who developed renal artery stenosis secondary to giant cell arteritis. The glomeruli are crowded together because of a marked reduction in the size of the cortical tubules, especially proximal tubules. There is only slight interstitial fibrosis and chronic inflammation (PAS stain).

sections because it can reveal the site or sites of stenosis. Irregular thickening with varying combinations of friable lipid debris, calcification, and dense fibrosis implicates atherosclerosis. Multiple ridges of hyperplastic tissue alternating with attenuated walls or aneurysms suggests fibromuscular dysplasia, especially the medial variant (15,16). Although most examples of fibromuscular dysplasia have focal or multifocal lesions, some cause more generalized "tubular" thickening of the artery wall (15).

Light Microscopic Findings. The most characteristic histologic finding in a kidney with longstanding renal artery stenosis is a distinctive pattern of tubular atrophy with the resultant crowding of glomeruli (figs. 16-40, 16-41) (24,37). Interstitial fibrosis is much less severe in chronic ischemic nephropathy caused by renal artery stenosis than in hypertensive nephrosclerosis.

A characteristic histologic abnormality in chronic ischemic nephropathy caused by renal artery stenosis is marked atrophy of proximal convoluted tubules, and, to a lesser extent, atrophy of distal tubules (24). There also is injury to selected tubules in the outer medulla, especially the pars recta of the proximal tubule (37). Cortical tubular atrophy caused by renal artery stenosis results in a distinctive pattern of injury distinguished by very small tubules in the cortex (fig. 16-41, left). The usual histologic distinctions between proximal and distal tubules are obscured. This pattern of chronic ischemic atrophy is called "endocrinization" of tubules because the small tubules with inapparent lumens resemble the acinar tissue of endocrine glands. This is different from the nonspecific "thyroidization" pattern of tubular atrophy characterized by dilated atrophic tubule segments filled with cast material (fig. 16-41, right). In chronic ischemic atrophy secondary to renal artery stenosis, there is focal drop out of proximal tubular segments, including segments at the glomerular origin of the proximal tubule. This results in atubular glomeruli (24).

There is variable but usually mild periglomerular and peritubular fibrosis, and interstitial infiltration by mononuclear leukocytes. In general, interstitial fibrosis and chronic inflammation are much more severe in hypertensive nephrosclerosis than in chronic ischemic nephropathy secondary to renal artery stenosis.

Glomeruli are crowded together because of the reduction in size of the tubules, especially proximal tubules that make up the bulk of the cortical tubulointerstitial compartment (fig. 16-40). Glomeruli are slightly smaller than normal, sometimes with an increase in Bowman's space. There often is mild to moderate juxtaglomerular cell hyperplasia. In an analysis by Marcussen (24), approximately half of the glomeruli in kidneys removed for renal artery stenosis did not have a connection between Bowman's space and a proximal tubule. These atubular glomeruli thus do not contribute to excretory

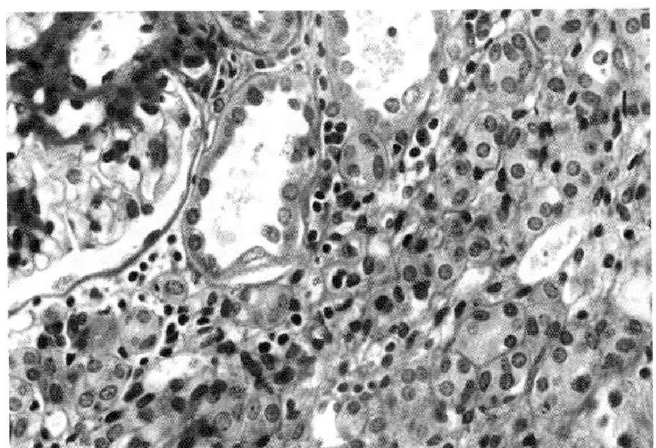
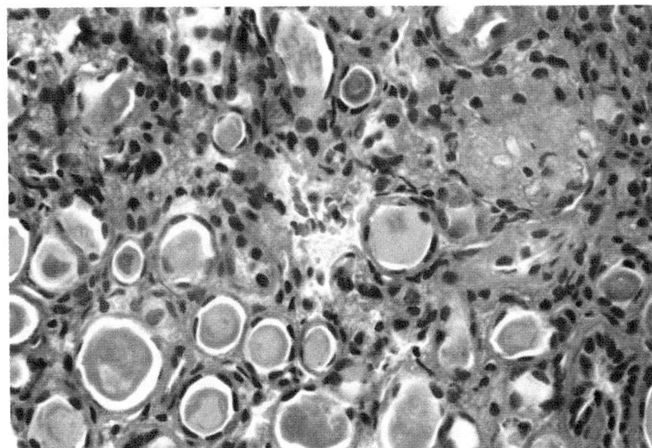

Figure 16-41

ENDOCRINIZATION VERSUS THYROIDIZATION PATTERN OF CORTICAL TUBULAR ATROPHY

Left: This Masson trichrome stain demonstrates how little interstitial fibrosis may be present even in the face of marked tubular atrophy that is caused by renal artery stenosis. Most of the atrophic tubules in this field of view are proximal tubules that have shrunken so small that lumens are difficult to find. This pattern of atrophy is called "endocrinization" because it resembles the acinar parenchyma of endocrine glands. The two larger tubules are probably distal tubules, which are less susceptible to this form of atrophy.

Right: In contrast to the endocrinization pattern of tubular atrophy, this photomicrograph shows the "thyroidization" pattern of atrophy, which is nonspecific and can be seen in any type of chronic renal disease. It is caused by fragmentation of tubules, with the fragments forming isolated spheres. This pattern of atrophy often is a focal component of the chronic changes in advanced hypertensive nephrosclerosis.

function, and probably do not regain function after a surgical revascularization procedure.

When there is unilateral renal artery stenosis, the contralateral kidney is at risk of developing hypertensive nephrosclerosis, focal segmental glomerulosclerosis, or both. This probably results from increased renin secretion from the ischemic kidney, which causes efferent arteriolar constriction in the contralateral kidney, followed by glomerular hyperfiltration and resultant focal segmental glomerulosclerosis (42).

The pathologic changes in the renal artery depend on the underlying cause of the renal artery stenosis. The most common causes are atherosclerosis in adults, and fibromuscular dysplasia and Takayasu's arteritis in children. The pathology of Takayasu's arteritis is discussed in detail in chapter 15.

Atherosclerosis causes more than 90 percent of cases of renal artery stenosis in adults. Chronic ischemic atrophy develops in approximately 20 percent of patients with atherosclerotic renal artery stenosis of greater than 60 percent (33). The pathology of atherosclerosis in the main renal artery is the same as that elsewhere in the arterial tree. Stenosis caused by atherosclerosis usually is at the renal ostium or in the proximal third of the artery (33). Atherosclerosis also can cause renal artery stenosis through the development of a dissection in an atherosclerotic aneurysm of the abdominal aorta that extends into or compresses the main renal artery. Rapid occlusion of the renal artery by a dissecting aneurysm causes renal infarction rather than chronic ischemic nephropathy.

Fibromuscular dysplasia usually affects the distal two thirds of the main renal artery, and preferentially involves one of the three layers of the renal artery, i.e., predominantly the intima, muscularis, or adventitia (15,16,33). The three major types of fibromuscular dysplasia are intimal fibroplasia, medial fibromuscular dysplasia, and periarterial fibroplasia (16). Approximately 95 percent of fibromuscular dysplasia is medial fibromuscular dysplasia, and is further classified into medial fibroplasia, perimedial fibroplasia, medial hyperplasia, and medial dissection.

The most common pattern of medial fibromuscular dysplasia is medial fibroplasia (60 to 70 percent of patients with fibromuscular dysplasia) (15,16). This variant often has a "string of beads" appearance on imaging studies because, histologically, there are areas of medial fibroplasia alternating with areas of medial atrophy

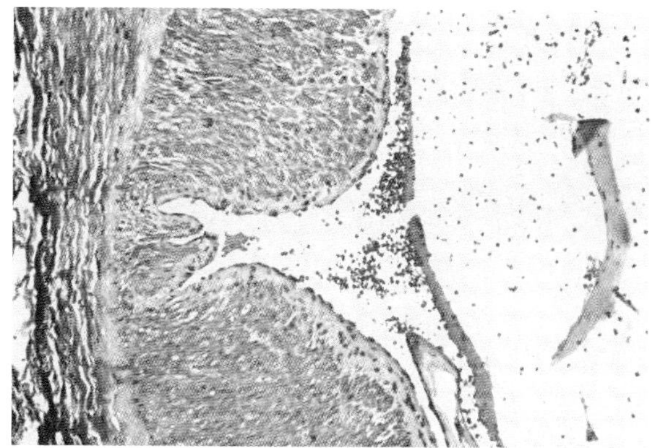

Figure 16-42

FIBROMUSCULAR DYSPLASIA WITH FOCAL MEDIAL ATROPHY

The main renal artery has zones of thickening on either side of a focus of severe medial atrophy and thinning. Alternating thick and thin media causes a "string of beads" appearance radiographically (H&E stain).

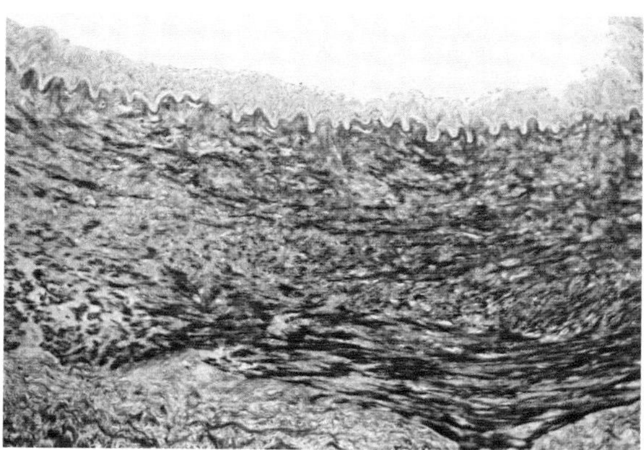

Figure 16-43

FIBROMUSCULAR DYSPLASIA WITH MEDIAL FIBROPLASIA

The muscularis is disorganized and there is extensive replacement of smooth muscle cells by fibroblasts and collagenous matrix. The smooth muscle cells are best preserved in the outer media. There is only slight intimal thickening (Masson trichrome stain).

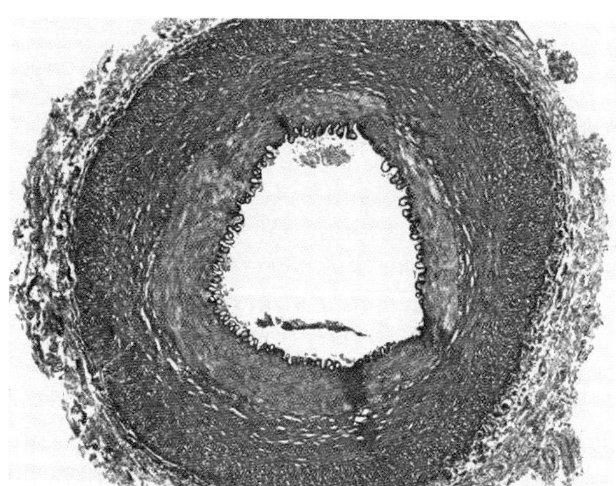

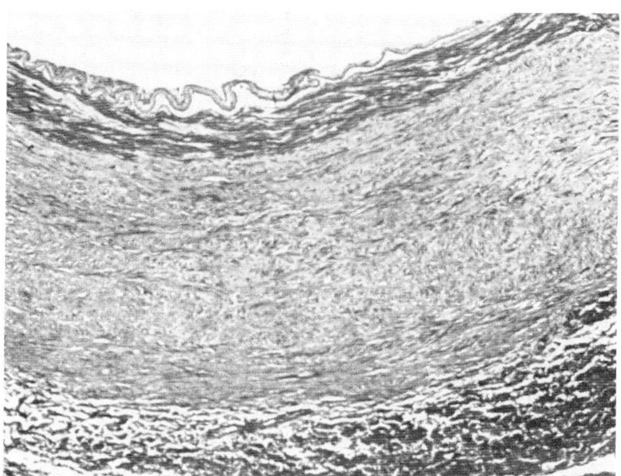

Figure 16-44

FIBROMUSCULAR DYSPLASIA WITH PERIMEDIAL FIBROPLASIA

Left: The Verhoeff van Gieson elastic stain demonstrates that the muscle cells in the outer two thirds of the muscularis are replaced by dense fibrous tissue. The internal elastic lamina is clearly visible but the external elastic lamina is not. (Fig. 2-5 from Churg J, Heptinstall RH, Olsen TS, Sobin LH. Renal disease: classification and atlas. Part I. New York: Igaku-Shoin; 1987:41.)

Right: The Masson trichrome stain clearly demarcates the red (fuchsinophilic), more normal inner muscularis from the blue fibrotic outer muscularis.

and thinning (fig. 16-42). Specimens with medial fibroplasia may have focal transmural replacement of medial smooth muscle cells by fibrous tissue, with varying degrees of interstitial collagen accumulation (fig. 16-43) This is seen best with a trichrome stain. The remaining smooth muscle cells may become disorganized. The internal elastica may be replicated or disrupted.

Perimedial fibroplasia is the second most common form of fibromuscular dysplasia and is characterized by intense fibroplasia in the outer half or more of the muscularis (fig. 16-44) (15,16). The external elastica usually is disrupted.

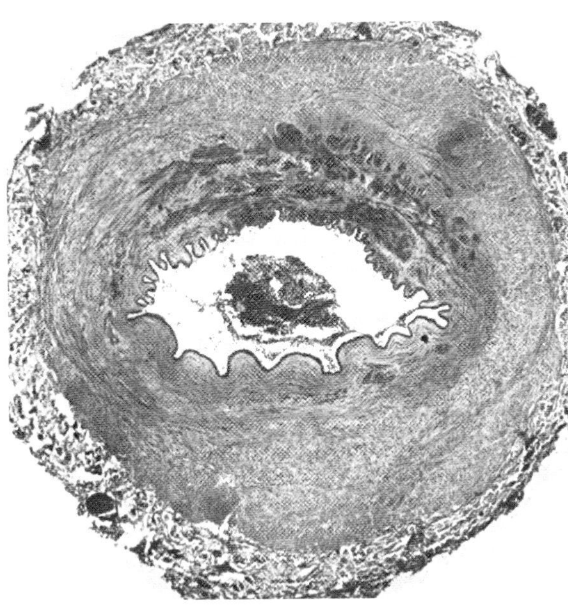

Figure 16-45

FIBROMUSCULAR DYSPLASIA WITH MEDIAL HYPERPLASIA

There is focal disorganization and hyperplasia of smooth muscle cells in the media (H&E stain). (Fig. 2-3 from Churg J, Heptinstall RH, Olsen TS, Sobin LH. Renal disease: classification and atlas. Part I. New York: Igaku-Shoin; 1987:39.)

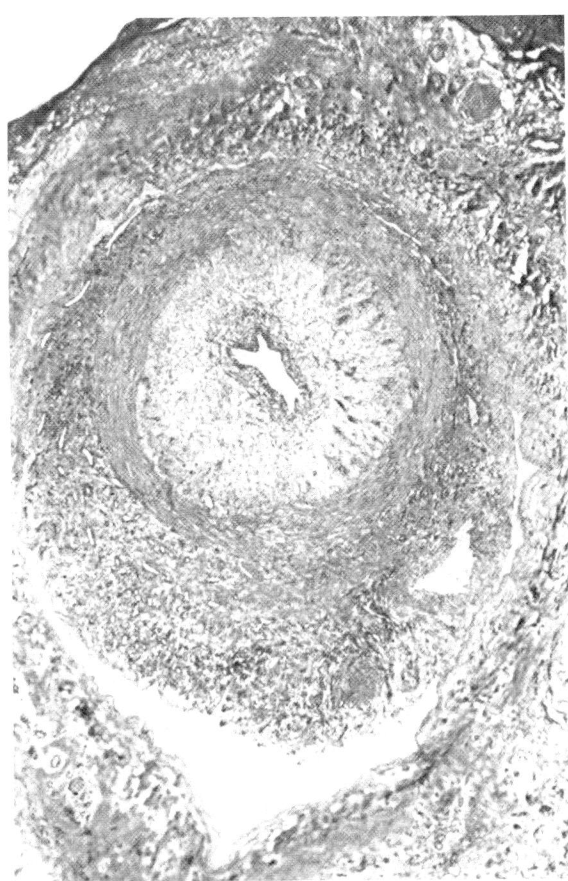

Figure 16-46

FIBROMUSCULAR DYSPLASIA WITH INTIMAL FIBROPLASIA

There is marked circumferential fibrotic thickening of the intima resulting in severe narrowing of the lumen of the renal artery (Masson trichrome stain). (Fig. 2-6 from Churg J, Heptinstall RH, Olsen TS, Sobin LH. Renal disease: classification and atlas. Part I. New York: Igaku-Shoin; 1987:41.)

Medial hyperplasia is less common than medial or perimedial fibroplasia, and is characterized by hyperplasia of medial smooth muscle cells, with little or no fibrosis (fig. 16-45) (15,16). Both the internal and external elastica are intact.

In the medial dissection pattern, blood hemorrhages into the outer media beneath the external elastica. This is accompanied by medial fibroplasia and, usually, intimal fibroplasia (15,16).

Primary intimal fibroplasia accounts for only 1 to 2 percent of patients with fibromuscular dysplasia (16). It must be distinguished from the much more common intimal fibrosis that occurs secondary to many chronic diseases in the kidney, including hypertensive nephrosclerosis. The diagnosis is most appropriate when there are well-circumscribed lesions in the renal artery with no apparent primary cause (fig. 16-46). The fibroplasia sometimes extends into the proximal interlobar arteries, but not into the distal interlobar arteries. Fibrotic intimal thickening in the main renal artery that is similar to generalized fibrotic intimal thickening in interlobar and arcuate arteries is more likely secondary to some other disease, such as hypertensive nephrosclerosis or some other chronic parenchymal disease with secondary hypertension. Fibrous intimal thickening also occurs along with other patterns of fibromuscular dysplasia, possibly as a secondary complication (8).

Periarterial fibroplasia is rare and accounts for less than 1 percent of patients with fibromuscular dysplasia (15,16). It is characterized by marked dense collagenous thickening of the renal artery adventitia, with no substantial infiltration by inflammatory cells. This collagenous adventitial thickening stains intensely

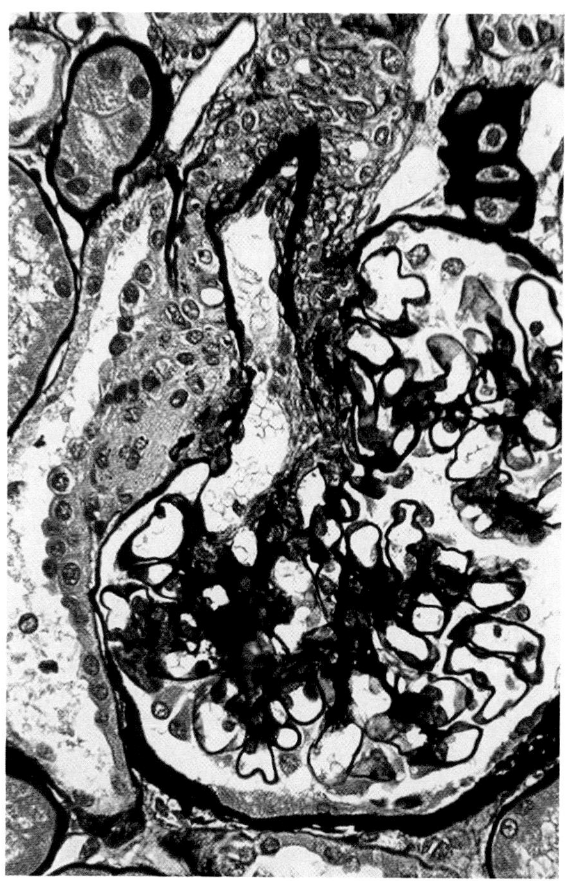

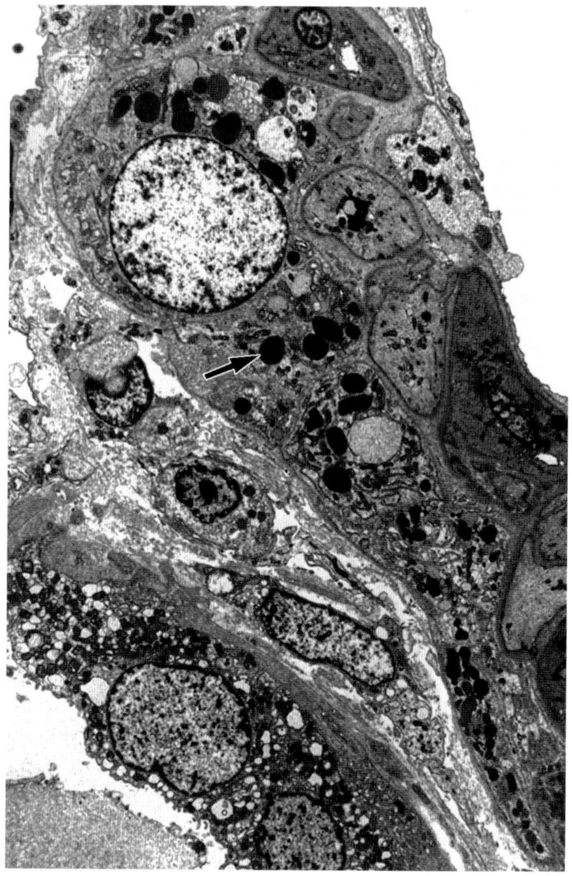

Figure 16-47

JUXTAGLOMERULAR APPARATUS HYPERPLASIA WITH RENAL ARTERY STENOSIS

Left: JMS stain shows hyperplasia of the juxtaglomerular apparatus in a patient with renal artery stenosis.

Right: Electron micrograph shows increased electron-dense renin granules (arrow) in a myoepithelial cell in the muscularis of the afferent arteriole.

with elastic tissue stains, such as the Verhoeff van Gieson stain, even though there is no true increase in elastin. The media is unaffected.

A modified and somewhat simplified pathologic classification of fibromuscular dysplasia includes the following: 1) intimal fibrous dysplasia, 2) medial fibrous dysplasia, 3) medial muscular dysplasia, and 4) perimedial elastic dysplasia (8).

Electron Microscopic Findings. Renal artery stenosis may cause juxtaglomerular cell hyperplasia and increased renin secretion. This is identified by light microscopy as an increase in the extraglomerular mesangial cells and myocytes in the wall of the afferent arteriole adjacent to the lamina densa of the distal tubule (fig. 16-47, left). These changes also are observed by electron microscopy, as well as an increase in electron-dense renin granules in afferent arteriolar granular myoepithelial cells and an increase in the number of these cells (fig, 16-47, right).

A characteristic ultrastructural parenchymal abnormality caused by renal artery stenosis is marked atrophy of proximal tubular epithelial cells. These atrophic tubular epithelial cells are small, with markedly reduced microvilli, reduced basolateral interdigitations, increased numbers of small mitochondria, and a reduction in other cytoplasmic organelles (37). Cortical tubular and glomerular basement membranes are moderately thickened. There is only a slight increase in interstitial tissue.

Differential Diagnosis. The major pathologic differential diagnostic consideration is chronic ischemic injury caused by hypertensive nephrosclerosis. This is more of a problem with small biopsy specimens than when an entire kidney is available for examination. In kidneys with hypertensive nephrosclerosis, there may be focal areas with a pattern of chronic ischemic injury that are indistinguishable from the more generalized parenchymal atrophy caused by renal artery stenosis. This probably results from focal narrowing of relatively large parenchymal arteries, especially interlobar arteries, caused by fibrotic intimal thickening secondary to hypertension. These focal areas of tubular endocrinization and glomerular crowding account for only a minor amount of injury, however. Most of the injury has the typical features of hypertensive nephrosclerosis, including prominent interstitial fibrosis with chronic inflammation, and varying degrees of glomerular sclerosis, including globally sclerotic glomeruli clustered near the capsule.

Etiology and Pathogenesis. The preferential injury to tubules in chronic ischemic nephropathy caused by renal artery stenosis is because of the high energy requirements of the tubules for mitochondrial respiration to support high rates of solute transport (37,40). Sublethal ischemia results in atrophy whereas lethal ischemia causes cell death, probably primarily through apoptosis. Loss of segmental proximal tubule cells through apoptosis or necrosis causes atubular glomeruli. Thus, the often dramatic reduction in renal size caused by renal artery stenosis results from both a reduction in tubular epithelial cell size (atrophy) and loss of tubular epithelial cells.

The etiology and pathogenesis of fibromuscular dysplasia are unknown (8). The term "dysplasia" is not meant to indicate any knowledge about when or how the abnormality developed. This term was selected only for its descriptive Greek roots, that is, "dys" meaning bad and "plasia" meaning molding (15). The vascular lesions may be secondary to congenital abnormalities in composition or structure that manifest only later in life. Alternatively, there could be some unrecognized acquired injury to the vessel wall that stimulates the proliferative and sclerosing injury.

Treatment and Prognosis. Patients with renovascular hypertension caused by atherosclerosis often respond to angiotensin converting enzyme inhibitors or angiotensin receptor blockers (33). The resultant reduced renal perfusion pressure, however, may further worsen renal insufficiency in patients with substantial impairment of renal function (41). When medical treatment fails, balloon angioplasty and revascularization surgery are alternatives. Balloon angioplasty is the first line of interventional therapy for patients with fibromuscular dysplasia, and is successful in approximately 90 percent of patients. Balloon angioplasty is less often a lasting solution for renal artery stenosis caused by atherosclerosis. Surgical revascularization may be required. In the past, aortorenal bypass was the most common surgical approach to revascularization, but there is a current trend toward more bypasses from celiac or mesenteric arteries to the renal artery (33). Surgical intervention for renal artery stenosis in children, most of whom have renal artery fibromuscular dysplasia, usually results in resolution of the renovascular hypertension and, in most of the remaining patients, causes an improvement of the hypertension (7,29).

RENAL ATHEROEMBOLIZATION

Definition. Renal atheroembolization is embolization of atheromatous debris, especially cholesterol crystals, into the renal vasculature, including arteries, arterioles, and glomerular capillaries. A synonym is *cholesterol embolization*.

Clinical Features. Atheroembolization occurs most often in elderly patients with severe atherosclerotic vascular disease (36). Atheroembolization can affect many organs. Symptomatic involvement often affects the skin, kidneys, eyes, gastrointestinal tract, and brain (21,34,36,43). Cutaneous manifestations occur most often in the lower extremities, especially the toes, and include livedo reticularis, cyanosis, and gangrene. Approximately 50 percent of patients with atheroembolization have renal involvement (43). Atheroembolization can cause acute or subacute renal failure that develops immediately after an inciting event (e.g., angiography or aortic surgery) or after a delay of up to several weeks. Laboratory findings include transient hypocomplementemia and eosinophilia, and an elevated erythrocyte sedimentation rate. Renal involvement manifests as renal insufficiency with varying degrees of proteinuria and

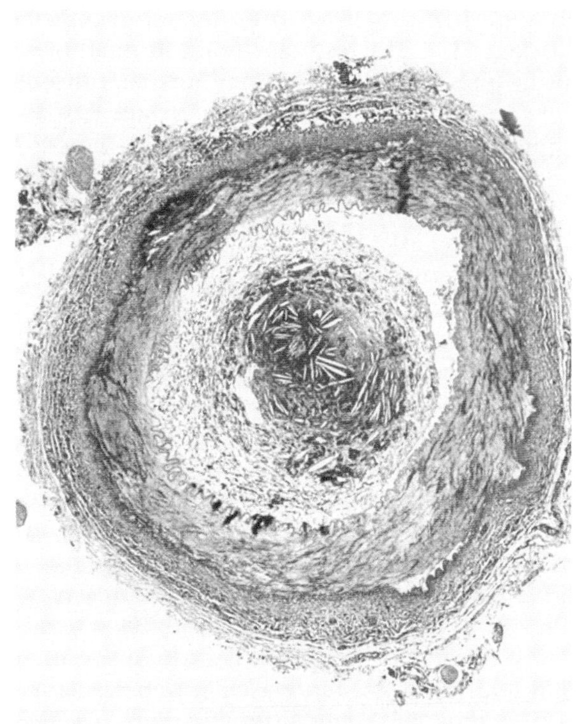

Figure 16-48

ATHEROEMBOLUS IN THE MAIN RENAL ARTERY

Masson trichrome stain demonstrates an acute atheroembolus in the lumen of the main renal artery.

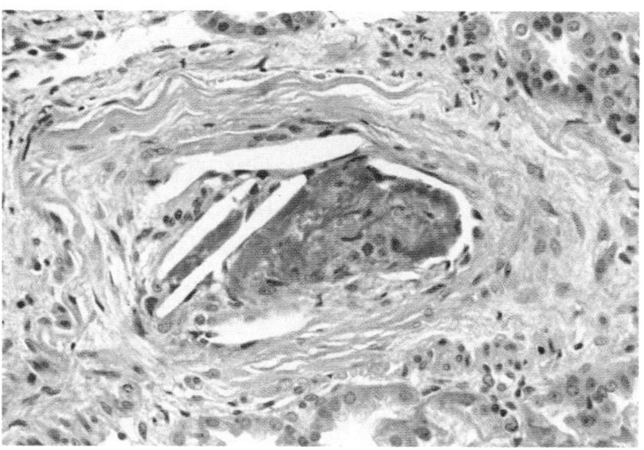

Figure 16-49

ATHEROEMBOLUS IN AN INTERLOBULAR ARTERY

The lumen of this interlobular artery is largely occluded by a recent atheroembolus that adheres to the wall. The cholesterol clefts are embedded in thrombotic material or atheromatous debris. There is a multinucleated giant cell adjacent to one of the clefts (H&E stain).

hematuria. A few patients have nephrotic-range proteinuria, which raises the possibility of glomerular disease. Cutaneous disease usually manifests before evidence of renal disease (36).

Gross Findings. Renal atheroembolization rarely causes grossly discernible renal infarction and thus usually does not produce specific gross lesions. In rare patients, arcuate or larger arteries are occluded, resulting in cortical infarcts with pale centers and red borders.

Light Microscopic Findings. The histologic hallmark of atheroembolization is the presence of elongated clefts in the lumens of vessels, vessel walls, or perivascular tissue that remain after the cholesterol has been dissolved by the standard processing of tissue for light microscopy (figs. 16-48–16-53). In the acute phase, the cholesterol crystals may be naked or surrounded by atheromatous debris or thrombus (figs. 16-48, 16-49). The crystals elicit a leukocyte response and become surrounded by leukocytes, especially macrophages, including multinucleated giant cells (fig. 16-50). Later, there are intimal proliferative reactions that enclose the crystals within a thickened intima (fig. 16-51). Crystals may penetrate or erode into the muscularis of arteries and even into the perivascular tissue. Atheroemboli are seen most often in afferent arterioles (fig. 16-52) and interlobular arteries (fig. 16-49), although larger emboli may lodge in arcuate and interlobar arteries and small emboli find their way into glomerular capillaries (fig. 16-53). There often is associated ischemic glomerular sclerosis, tubular atrophy, interstitial fibrosis, and mild interstitial infiltration of mononuclear leukocytes. In some specimens, eosinophils, macrophages, and multinucleated giant cells accumulate adjacent to cholesterol crystals that have been extruded into the interstitium.

Immunofluorescence Findings. Irregular immunostaining for fibrin, complement components, and immunoglobulins (especially IgM) occurs at sites of acute atheroembolization, especially if the cholesterol crystals are surrounded by thrombotic material. The surface of the crystals are sometimes outlined by a thin layer of staining for complement (fig. 16-54).

Electron Microscopic Findings. Experimental ultrastructural studies of arterial atheroemboli have shown that the noncrystalline atheromatous debris disappears within 2 to 3 days (44, 45). Small crystals are engulfed by macrophages

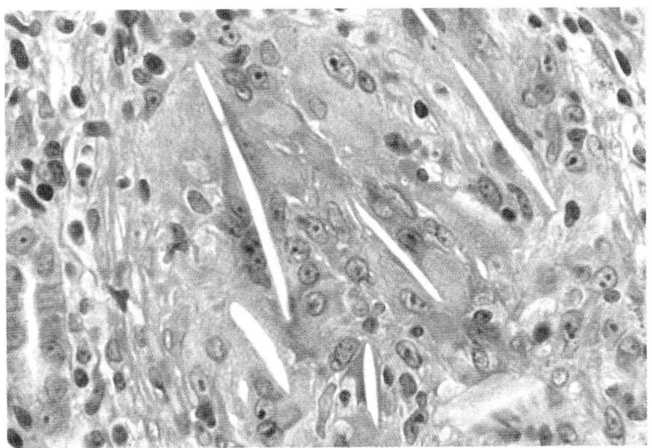

Figure 16-50

CHOLESTEROL CLEFTS IN MULTINUCLEATED GIANT CELLS

There is a marked multinucleated giant cell response to the cholesterol at the old site of atheroembolization. There has been extensive atrophy of the surrounding vessel wall (Masson trichrome stain).

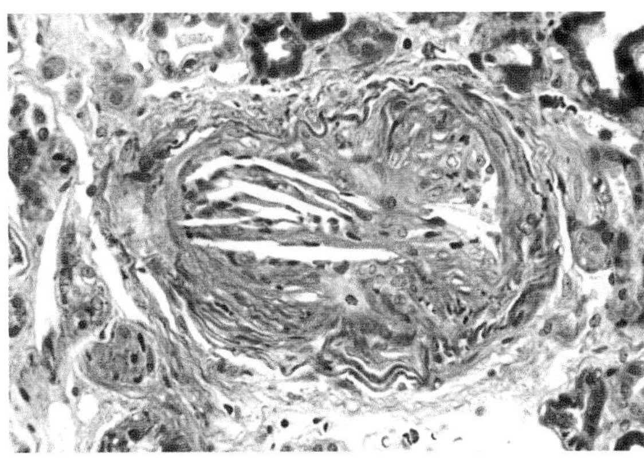

Figure 16-51

ATHEROEMBOLUS IN INTERLOBULAR ARTERY

This interlobular artery is occluded by a proliferative intimal response to an atheroembolus (Masson trichrome stain).

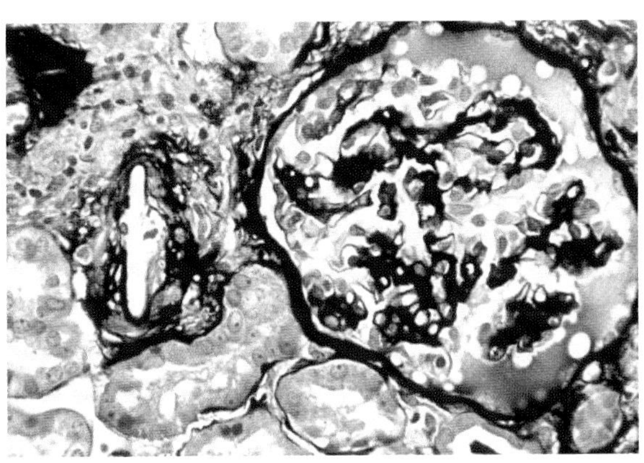

Figure 16-52

ATHEROEMBOLUS IN A HILAR ARTERIOLE

A well-defined cholesterol cleft is distorting the lumen of an afferent arteriole. Note the ischemic collapse of the glomerular tuft (JMS stain with H&E counterstain).

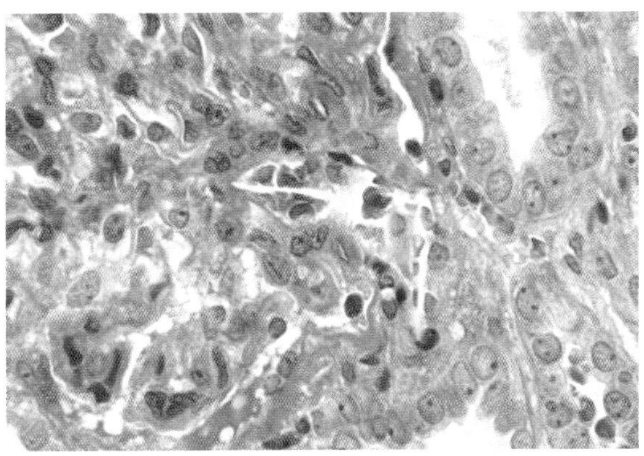

Figure 16-53

ATHEROEMBOLUS IN A GLOMERULAR CAPILLARIES

The cholesterol clefts in the capillary lumens are identifiable primarily by their displacement of erythrocytes and leukocytes (Masson trichrome stain).

and larger crystals engender an adjacent giant cell response. Later, crystals penetrate into vessel walls or are incorporated into vessel walls by endothelialization or intimal fibroblastic proliferation.

Thus, the needle-shaped clefts initially lie within atheromatous or more often thrombotic material (fig. 16-55). Later, they are surrounded by phagocytic leukocytes, such as neutrophils or macrophages (fig. 16-56). The cholesterol crystals may dissect into or through the vessel wall (fig. 16-57). Eventually, the crystals are surrounded by an inflammatory and fibrotic response, either in the vessel lumen, vessel wall, or interstitium.

Differential Diagnosis. Because of evidence of small vessel disease in multiple organs, frequently including kidneys and skin, the clinical differential diagnosis often includes small vessel vasculitis. The older age of the patients raises concern about antineutrophil cytoplasmic antibody (ANCA) small vessel vasculitis, such as microscopic polyangiitis or Wegener's granulomatosis.

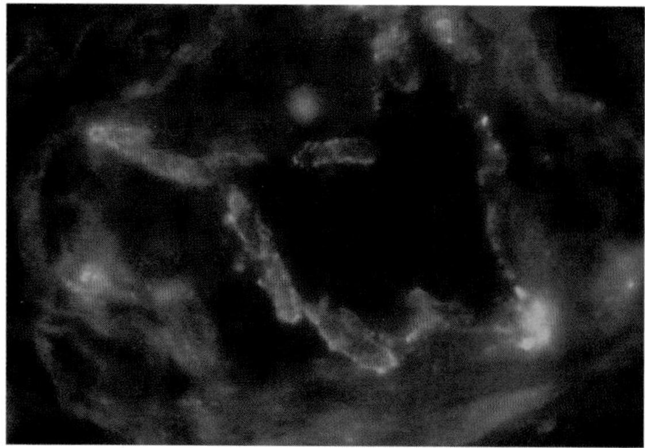

Figure 16-54

COMPLEMENT ON CHOLESTEROL CRYSTALS IN AN ATHEROEMBOLUS

Several cholesterol crystals in the lumen of an interlobular artery are covered by a layer of complement. There also is focal staining of the endothelium (FITC anti-C3).

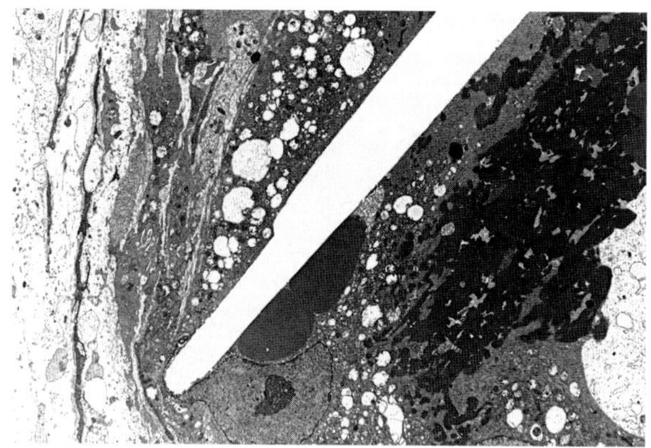

Figure 16-55

ACUTE ATHEROEMBOLUS IN AN ARTERIOLE

By electron microscopy, cholesterol crystal clefts appear as clear angular spaces. To the right of the cleft are electron-dense fibrin tactoids in the lumen of an arteriole.

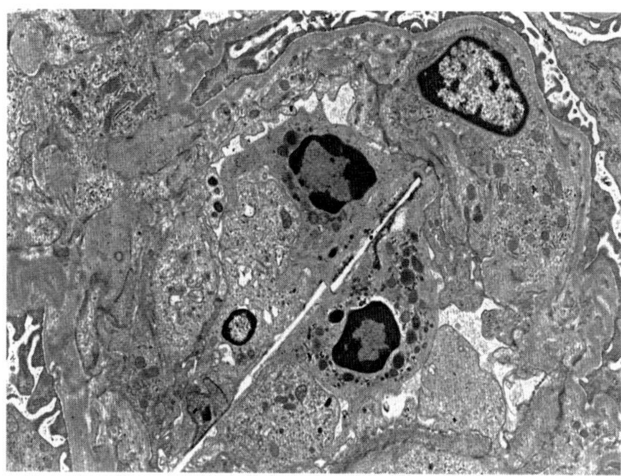

Figure 16-56

ATHEROEMBOLUS IN A GLOMERULAR CAPILLARY

A glomerular capillary lumen contains a neutrophil that has engulfed tiny cholesterol crystals. The lobes of the segmented nucleus are on either side of the crystals. The cytoplasm of the neutrophil contains dense granules.

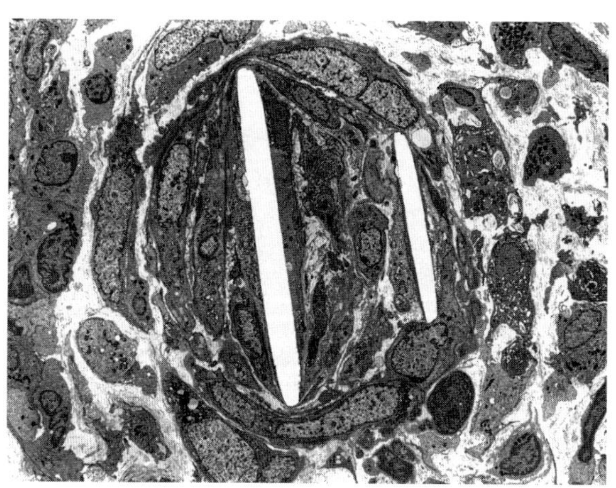

Figure 16-57

ATHEROEMBOLUS IN AN ARTERIOLE

This atheroembolus has cholesterol crystals surrounded by macrophages. The reactive endothelial cells and myocytes, along with the leukocytes, have obliterated the lumen.

Especially if hypocomplementemia is present, cryoglobulinemic vasculitis is a major diagnostic consideration. Serologic testing for ANCA and cryoglobulins is useful but not absolutely definitive for these vasculitides. The concurrence of acute renal failure, rash, and eosinophilia that may occur with atheroembolization raises the possibility of acute hypersensitivity tubulointerstitial nephritis.

Histologically, chance configurations of vascular lumens that resemble cholesterol clefts can be difficult to distinguish from the real thing. Serial sections, and leukocyte or intimal reaction adjacent to crystals, help distinguish between a slit-like lumen and a cholesterol cleft.

Once atheroemboli are identified in renal vessels, the clinical significance must be determined. Are they the principal cause of the renal dysfunction that prompted the renal biopsy? Are they a contributing factor to dysfunction even though there is another more important disease? Or are they merely a clinically insignificant (i.e., incidental) pathologic finding that is accompanying the clinically significant disease? The pathologic and clinical data must be integrated to answer these questions accurately.

Etiology and Pathogenesis. Atheroembolization occurs as a spontaneous process with no apparent initiating event, and secondary to apparent direct causes, such as abdominal trauma, angiography, vascular surgery, or intravenous streptokinase administration (21,34,36). Once the emboli lodge in vessels, they occlude lumens not only by their mere presence, but also by inducing thrombosis, leukocyte aggregation, and eventually an intimal proliferative response (44,45).

Treatment and Prognosis. The prognosis for recovery of renal function is poor. Only rare patients who develop severe renal failure that requires dialysis recover enough native renal function to come off dialysis (21). There is no specific treatment. The risk of atheroembolization should be considered when decisions are made about invasive angiography.

REFERENCES

1. Biava CG, Dyrda I, Genest J, et al. Renal hyaline arteriosclerosis: an electron microscope study. Am J Pathol 1964;44:349–63.
2. Black HR, Zeevi GR, Silten RM, Walker-Smith GJ. Effect of heavy cigarette smoking on renal and myocardial arterioles. Nephron 1983;34:173–9.
3. Bleyer AJ, Shemanski LR, Burke GL, Hansen KJ, Appel RG. Tobacco, hypertension, and vascular disease: risk factors for renal functional decline in an older population. Kidney Int 2000;57:2072–9.
4. Bohle A, Wehrmann M, Greschniok A, Junghans R. Renal morphology in essential hypertension: analysis of 1177 unselected cases. Kidney Int 1998;67(Suppl):S205–6.
5. Bright R. Cases and observations illustrative of renal disease accompanied by albuminous urine. Guy's Hosp Rep 1836;1:338–400.
6. Curtis JJ, Luke RG, Dustan HP, et al. Remission of essential hypertension after renal transplantation. N Engl J Med 1983;309:1009–15.
7. Deschenes G, Zitek M, Gubler MC. [Renal artery pathology and its therapeutic indications in the child.] Ann Pediatr (Paris) 1991;38:387–92.
8. Devaney K, Kapur SP, Patterson K, Chandra RS. Pediatric renal artery dysplasia: a morphologic study. Pediatr Pathol 1991;11:609–21.
9. Diamond JR. Analogous pathobiologic mechanisms in glomerulosclerosis and atherosclerosis. Kidney Int 1991;31(Suppl):S29–34.
10. Fenves AZ, Ram CV. Fibromuscular dysplasia of the renal arteries. Cur Hypertens Rep 1999;1:546–9.
11. Fisher ER, Perez-Stable E, Pardo V. Ultrastructural studies in hypertension. I. Comparison of renal vascular and juxtaglomerular cell alterations in essential and renal hypertension in man. Lab Invest 1966;15:1409–33.
12. Flack JM. Therapy of hypertension. In: Greenberg A, Cheung AK, Coffman TM, Falk RJ, Jennette JC, eds. National Kidney Foundation primer on kidney diseases, 3rd ed. San Diego: Academic Press; 2001:486–97.
13. Fogo A, Breyer JA, Smith MC, et al. Accuracy of the diagnosis of hypertensive nephrosclerosis in African Americans: a report from the African American Study of Kidney Disease (AASK) Trial. Kidney Int 1997;51:244–52.
14. Goldblatt H. The renal origin of hypertension. Physiol Rev 1947;27:120–65.
15. Harrison EG Jr, Hunt JC, Bernatz PE. Morphology of fibromuscular dysplasia of the renal artery in renovascular hypertension. Am J Med 1967;43:97–112.
16. Harrison EG Jr, McCormack LJ. Pathologic classification of renal arterial disease in renovascular hypertension. Mayo Clin Proc 1971;46:161–7.
17. Innes A, Johnston PA, Morgan AG, Davison AM, Burden RP. Clinical features of benign hypertensive nephrosclerosis at time of renal biopsy. Q J Med 1993;86:271–5.
18. Johnson GI. On certain points in the anatomy and pathology of Bright's disease. Trans Med Chir Soc 1868;51:57–78.
19. Kashgarian M. Pathology of small blood vessel disease in hypertension. Am J Kidney Dis 1985;5:A104–10.

20. Kasiske BL. Relationship between vascular disease and age-associated changes in the human kidney. Kidney Int 1987;31:1153–9.
21. Kazancioglu R, Erkoc R, Bozfakioglu S, et al. Clinical outcomes of renal cholesterol crystal embolization. J Nephrol 1999;12:266–9.
22. Kelly TF Jr, Morris GC Jr. Arterial fibromuscular disease. Observations on pathogenesis and surgical management. Am J Surg 1982;143:232–6.
23. Laragh JH. The renin system and new understanding of the complications of hypertension and their treatment. Arzneimittelforschung 1993;43:247–54.
24. Marcussen N. Atubular glomeruli in renal artery stenosis. Lab Invest 1991;65:558–65.
25. McManus JF, Lupton CH Jr. Ischemic obsolescence of renal glomeruli: the natural history of the lesions and their relation to hypertension. Lab Invest 1960;9:413–34.
26. Meyrier A, Hill GS, Simon P. Ischemic renal diseases: new insights into old entities. Kidney Int 1998;54:2–13.
27. Moritz AR, Oldt MR. Arteriolar sclerosis in hypertensive and non-hypertensive individuals. Am J Pathol 1937;13:679–728.
28. Olson JL. Hypertension: essential and secondary forms. In: Jennette JC, Olson JL, Schwartz MM, Silva FG, eds. Heptinstall's pathology of the kidney, 5th ed. Lippincott Raven, Philadelphia; 1998:943–1001.
29. O'Neill JA Jr. Long-term outcome with surgical treatment of renovascular hypertension. J Pediatr Surg 1998;33:106–11.
30. Paronetto F. Immunocytochemical observations on the vascular necrosis and renal glomerular lesions of malignant nephrosclerosis. Am J Pathol 1965;46:901–15.
31. Razzaque MS, Koji T, Kawano H, Harada T, Nakane PK, Taguchi T. Glomerular expression of type III and type IV collagens in benign nephrosclerosis: immunohistochemical and in situ hybridization study. Pathol Res Practice 1994;190:493–9.
32. Rodriguez-Cuartero A, Perez-Blanco FJ, Canora-Lebrato J. Takayasu arteritis and renovascular hypertension. Clin Nephrol 2001;55:176–7.
33. Safian RD, Textor SC. Renal-artery stenosis. N Eng J Med 2001;344:431–42.
34. Saklayen MG, Gupta S, Suryaprasad A, Azmeh W. Incidence of atheroembolic renal failure after coronary angiography. A prospective study. Angiology 1997;48:609–13.
35. Schlessinger SD, Tankersley MR, Curtis JJ. Clinical documentation of end-stage renal disease due to hypertension. Am J Kidney Dis 1994;23:655–60.
36. Scolari F, Bracchi M, Valzorio B, et al. Cholesterol atheromatous embolism: an increasingly recognized cause of acute renal failure. Nephrol Dial Transplant 1996;11:1607–12.
37. Shanley PF. The pathology of chronic renal ischemia. Semin Nephrol 1996;16:21–32.
38. Sommers SC, Melamed J. Renal pathology of essential hypertension. Am J Hypertens 1990;3:583–7.
39. Stoddard LD, Puchtler H. Human renal vascular lesions and hypertension. Pathol Annu 1969;4:253–68.
40. Textor SC. Pathophysiology of renal failure in renovascular disease. Am J Kidney Dis 1994;24:642–51.
41. Textor SC, Wilcox CS. Renal artery stenosis: a common, treatable cause of renal failure? Ann Rev Med 2001;52:421–42.
42. Ubara Y, Hara S, Katori H, Yamada A, Morii H. Renovascular hypertension may cause nephrotic range proteinuria and focal glomerulosclerosis in contralateral kidney. Clin Nephrol 1997;48:220–3.
43. Vacher-Coponat H, Pache X, Dussol B, Berland Y. Pulmonary-renal syndrome responding to corticosteroids: consider cholesterol embolization. Nephrol Dial Transplant 1997;12:1977–9.
44. Warren BA. Vales O. The ultrastructure of the reaction of arterial walls to cholesterol crystals in atheroembolism. Br J Exp Pathol 1976;57:67–77.
45. Warren BA, Vales O. The ultrastructure of the stages of atheroembolic occlusion of renal arteries. Br J Exp Pathol 1973;54:469–78.
46. Weller RO. Vascular pathology in hypertension. Age Ageing 1979;8:99–103.
47. Wiggelinkhuizen J, Cremin BJ. Takayasu arteritis and renovascular hypertension in childhood. Pediatrics 1978;62:209–17.
48. Zucchelli PC, Pavlica P, Zuccala A, Losinno F, Barozzi L. Hypertension-induced renal failure. J Nephrol 2001;14:52–67.

17 DIABETIC NEPHROPATHY

Diabetes mellitus is associated with a number of renal functional and morphologic changes, collectively termed *diabetic nephropathy*. These include *diffuse diabetic glomerulosclerosis, nodular diabetic glomerulosclerosis, exudative or insudative renal changes, advanced nephrosclerosis, papillary necrosis*, and other renal changes (5,8,17,20,28,32,33,39,45,49,52,58,69).

CLINICAL FEATURES

Diabetes mellitus is the most common cause of end-stage renal disease in the United States, accounting for one third to more than half of patients on dialysis (3,10,18,31,35). In terms of cost to the health care system, it constitutes the most important renal disease in the United States. Kidney involvement in patients with diabetes is associated with high morbidity and mortality; death is often due to cardiovascular, cerebrovascular, or renal disease. Approximately 25 to 35 percent of patients with longstanding diabetes mellitus (both types I and II) develop diabetic nephropathy and renal failure (26,34,55,56).

There is an ongoing debate as to the comparability between type I (insulin-dependent, so-called juvenile onset) and type II (noninsulin-dependent, maturity onset) diabetes with respect to the incidence of structural and functional renal abnormalities and progression to end-stage renal disease. Many investigators now believe that there is substantial comparability between these two types of diabetes with respect to their renal complications (29,50,56). Indeed, in many adult patients with diabetes mellitus it is difficult to differentiate type I from type II disease. Contrary to previous beliefs, diabetic nephropathy in older patients is not necessarily milder. It has been suggested that as many as half the patients with type II diabetes in the United States have not been diagnosed, and thus the true disease prevalence is vastly underestimated.

The earliest functional abnormality is microalbuminuria (defined as urinary albumin excretion between 30 and 300 mg/24 hrs) (6,15,16, 41,43,71). It is noted soon after the clinical onset of diabetes, and control of the hyperglycemia may reduce the albumin excretion rates. Microalbuminuria falls below the level of detection by standard urine dipstick and requires more sensitive assays. Microalbuminuria is thought to be an important early marker of developing renal injury, and patients with this finding have an increased likelihood of developing progressive diabetic nephropathy.

Another major early clinical finding in patients with diabetes is an elevation of the glomerular filtration rate (GFR) (associated with enlarged glomeruli) (22); however, because the baseline (normal) GFR is often not known, this abnormality is often considered a "soft" clinical finding. Some investigators believe that increase in GFR is an important harbinger of future progressive diabetic nephropathy.

With the development of clinically overt diabetic nephropathy, proteinuria is detected by standard dipstick analysis (which usually requires about 500 mg/24 hrs of protein). This overt nephropathy occurs an average of more than 20 years after the clinical onset of diabetes mellitus and often heralds the development of progressive end-stage renal disease within a period of 5 years or so (11,24). Type II diabetics often develop nephropathy after a shorter known duration of disease (less than 5 years). Overt nephropathy appears to correlate best with the expansion of the mesangial matrix and possibly the thickening of the glomerular basement membrane (38). Advancing diabetic nephropathy (sometimes termed *Kimmelstiel-Wilson disease*) is manifested later by the onset of hypertension and increasingly severe proteinuria (with 5 to 10 percent of patients having nephrotic syndrome or nephrotic-range proteinuria). It is often quite difficult, if not impossible, to precisely dissect the respective contributions to the renal injury of the diabetes itself versus the accompanying hypertension.

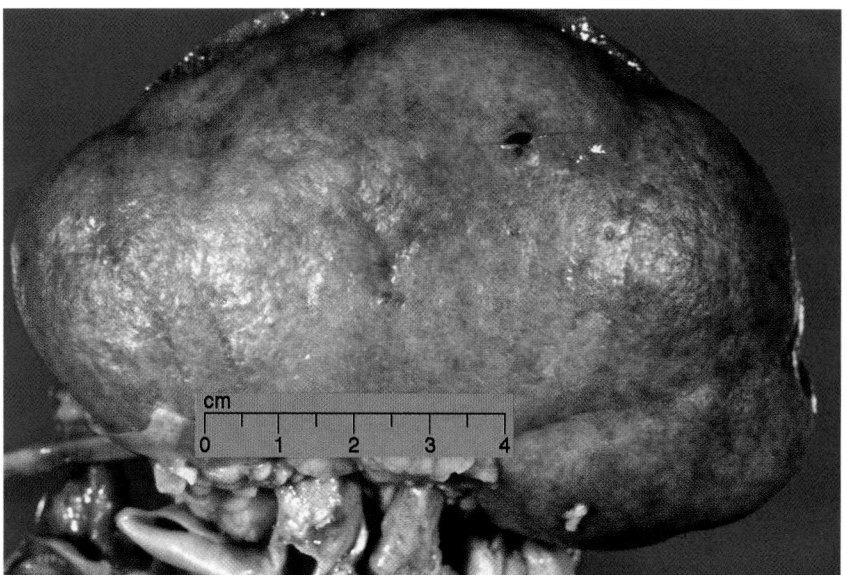

Figure 17-1

DIABETIC NEPHROPATHY

The kidneys are enlarged and have a finely granular surface due to the accompanying arteriolonephrosclerosis. These features give rise to the term "the large contracted kidney" in patients with diabetes.

Microhematuria may be present (50), but is generally considered unusual, unless there is an accompanying renal complication of the nephropathy, such as papillary necrosis or renal stones. Serum urea nitrogen and serum creatinine levels become progressively elevated over time. Other complications of renal insufficiency, such as hyperkalemia or acidosis, can complicate the clinical picture of diabetic nephropathy.

The presence of advanced diabetic conditions has been called the *renal-retinal syndrome* because of the concomitant development of diabetic retinopathy and diabetic nephropathy in most, but not all, patients (14). The occurrence of diabetic retinopathy (especially the exudative forms) correlates well with advanced renal disease (especially in patients with nodular diabetic glomerulosclerosis/Kimmelstiel-Wilson lesions).

Systemic hypertension is often associated with, and may even precede, the development of proteinuria and progressive diabetic nephropathy (4,48). Some investigators have suggested that the risk of renal disease in patients with type I diabetes is linked to a genetic predisposition to high blood pressure (59). This is possibly related to polymorphisms in the genes encoding the proteins of the renin-angiotensin system. The hypertension certainly could add to the susceptibility of developing diabetic renal disease in the presence of poor glycemic control.

PATHOLOGIC FEATURES

Gross Findings. The kidneys may be diffusely and symmetrically enlarged early in the course of the disease (fig. 17-1). Later, kidney size is highly variable, in part because of the concomitant presence of superimposed diseases such as hypertensive vascular disease or pyelonephritis. End-stage kidneys may be small or normal in size, with granular surfaces and irregular, even deep scars. Diabetes is said to be a cause of the "large contracted kidney." Papillary necrosis may be present with loss of the pyramids, but the kidney must be sectioned appropriately to see the papillae and the presence of papillary necrosis.

Light Microscopic Findings. Diabetic nephropathy affects all four components of the kidney: the glomeruli, tubules, interstitium, and the blood vessels.

Glomeruli. Early in the clinical course of diabetes mellitus, there is glomerulomegaly characterized by enlarged glomeruli (probably corresponding to the supernormal GFR). However, unless the glomerular diameter is actually measured, this change may be difficult to appreciate (51). The cause of the hypertrophy/hyperplasia is not certain.

Diffuse diabetic glomerulosclerosis (also called *diffuse intercapillary glomerulosclerosis*) is manifested by diffuse thickening of the glomerular basement membranes and diffuse increase in the amount of mesangial matrix (mesangial

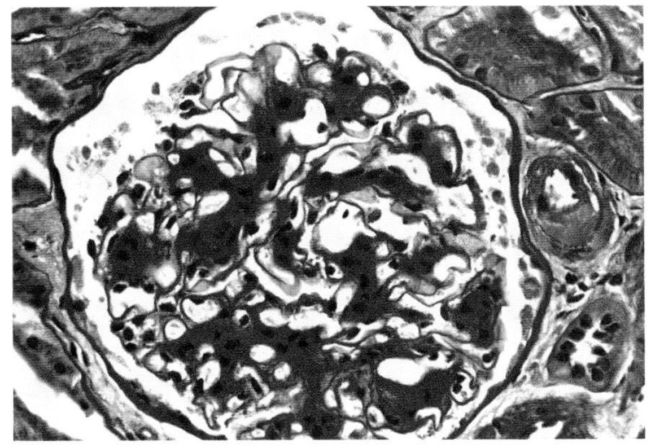

Figure 17-2

DIFFUSE DIABETIC GLOMERULOSCLEROSIS

There is global widening of the glomerular mesangial regions. Moderate to marked enlargement of the glomeruli may be visible. The changes in this glomerulus are representative of the changes in all glomeruli, thus the term "diffuse" glomerulosclerosis. These changes are often associated with an increase in the glomerular filtration rate. There is also accompanying arteriolosclerosis (periodic acid–Schiff [PAS] stain).

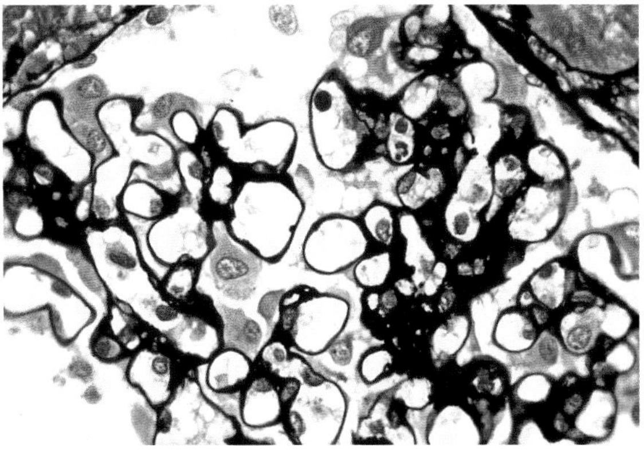

Figure 17-3

DIFFUSE DIABETIC GLOMERULOSCLEROSIS

There is widening of the glomerular mesangial regions, and often, associated diffuse mild thickening of the glomerular basement membranes. The mild to moderately thickened glomerular basement membranes cannot be discerned as thickened in a thin light microscopic section at this stage. In this photomicrograph, there is glomerular capillary ectasia and enlargement of some of the visceral epithelial cells, suggesting proteinuria (Jones methenamine silver [JMS] stain).

sclerosis) (fig. 17-2). Both are difficult to identify in the early or mild stages unless morphometric ultrastructural techniques are utilized. Diffuse diabetic glomerulosclerosis is found in varying degrees of severity in virtually all patients with advancing diabetic nephropathy.

There has been a major debate in the past as to which lesion develops initially and is of greater functional importance: the thickening of the glomerular basement membrane or the increase in mesangial matrix. Recent studies by Mauer et al. (38) suggest that the earliest detectable histologic change is widening of the mesangium due to increased accumulation of the mesangial matrix; this is best demonstrated with the periodic acid–Schiff (PAS) stain (figs. 17-2–17-4). The two lesions are often noted to occur concomitantly (38,61,62). The progressive increase in the volume of the mesangial matrix seems to lag slightly behind the thickening of the glomerular basement membrane, but the matrix becomes more pronounced after one to two decades of diabetes. In some cases there may be a mild proliferation of mesangial cells, although this is usually not marked. Some recent studies in humans and experimental animals have pointed to a process of increased cellular proliferation in the disease process (63).

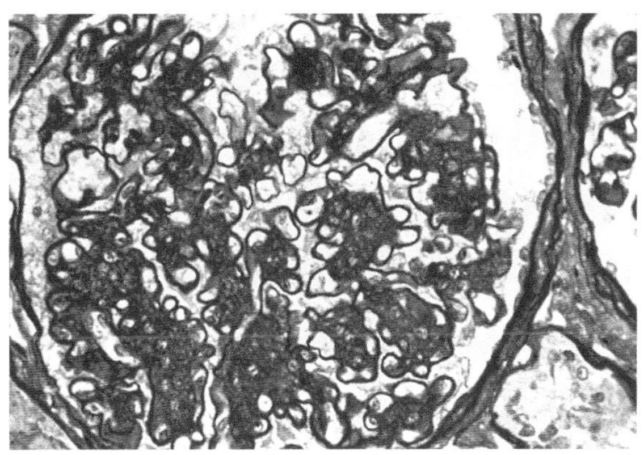

Figure 17-4

DIFFUSE DIABETIC GLOMERULOSCLEROSIS

There is global widening of the glomerular mesangial regions (PAS stain).

Prominent glomerular tuft hypercellularity, however, in a biopsy from a patient with diabetes is usually indicative of a superimposed nondiabetic form of glomerular injury (e.g., acute postinfectious glomerulonephritis, immunoglobulin (Ig)A nephropathy).

In diabetes, thickening of the capillary (and even noncapillary nonvascular) basement membranes is a major underlying structural feature

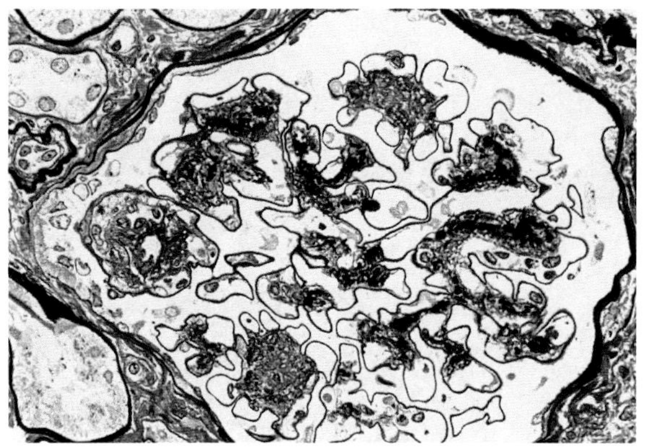

Figure 17-5

NODULAR DIABETIC GLOMERULOSCLEROSIS

There is mild enlargement and rounding of some of the acellular mesangial regions, with the creation of early mesangial Kimmelstiel-Wilson nodules (JMS stain).

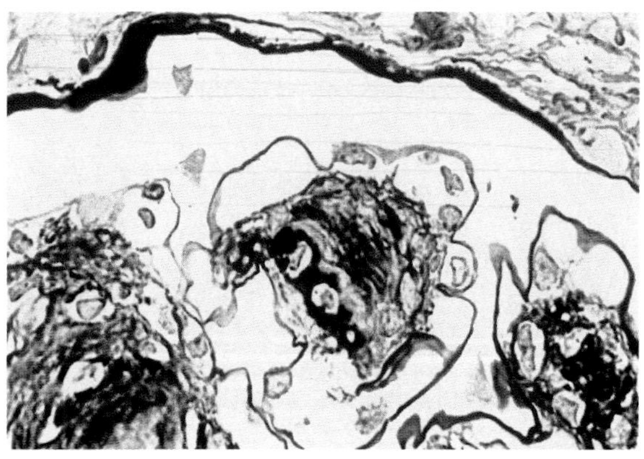

Figure 17-6

NODULAR DIABETIC GLOMERULOSCLEROSIS

A portion of the glomerulus shows increased acellular mesangial matrix and some rounding of the mesangial regions (Kimmelstiel-Wilson lesions) (JMS stain). (Courtesy of Dr. C. Alpers, Seattle, WA.)

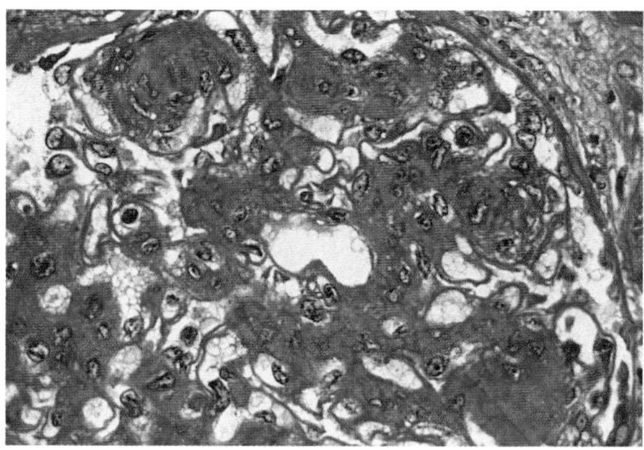

Figure 17-7

NODULAR DIABETIC GLOMERULOSCLEROSIS

A number of rounded, acellular mesangial nodules (Kimmelstiel-Wilson nodules) are noted in the glomerular mesangial regions (Masson trichrome stain).

throughout the body. In the glomerulus, this thickening of the basement membranes is often associated with abnormally permeable (i.e., leaky) capillaries and/or microaneurysm formation. Diffuse thickening of the glomerular capillary basement membranes occurs in virtually all diabetic individuals, even in those without significant proteinuria. Morphometric ultrastructural studies have shown that the glomerular basement membrane thickening begins as early as 2 years after the clinical onset of type I diabetes. At 5 years, the glomerular basement membrane thickening is increased by 30 percent. The glomerular basement membrane is remodeled and changes its composition. Nondiabetic vascular disease can produce similar glomerular lesions. Thus, it is often quite difficult, if not impossible, to determine how much of the mesangial sclerosis and thickening of the glomerular basement membrane is secondary to the hypertension and how much to the diabetes (see Differential Diagnosis).

Nodular diabetic glomerulosclerosis (also called *nodular intercapillary glomerulosclerosis*) is usually superimposed upon the aforementioned diffuse diabetic glomerulosclerosis and is manifest by the occurrence of the characteristic (and formerly pathognomonic) lesion, the Kimmelstiel-Wilson nodule. This rounded, ovoid or spherical, intercapillary lesion is composed of increased mesangial matrix material, often with few mesangial cells (figs. 17-5–17-12). It is eosinophilic and shows the same staining characteristics (by Masson trichrome, Jones methenamine silver [JMS], and PAS) as the mesangial matrix and mesangial sclerotic areas. These mesangial nodules may appear layered or laminated after staining with JMS (figs. 17-13–17-15). At times the silver staining is lost because of the expanded mesangial matrix, consistent with mesangiolysis (65). There is often a cellular rim around the acellular central sclerotic nodular region.

The Kimmelstiel-Wilson nodules are often of varying sizes and they usually number only one

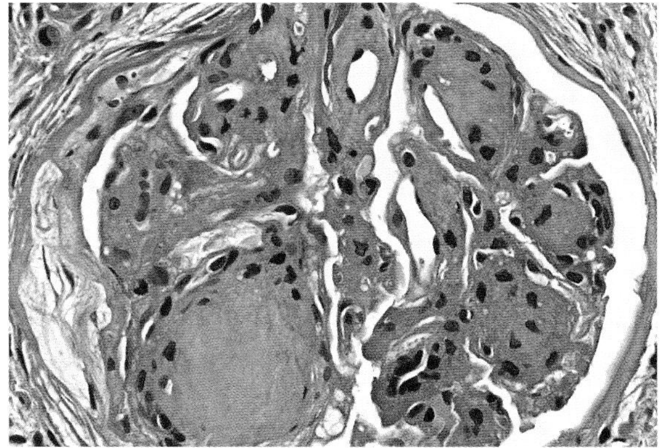

Figure 17-8

NODULAR DIABETIC GLOMERULOSCLEROSIS

A number of rounded, acellular mesangial nodules (Kimmelstiel-Wilson nodules) are present in the glomerular mesangial regions. They vary in size. Most of the cellularity is noted at the edges of the nodules (hematoxylin and eosin [H&E] stain).

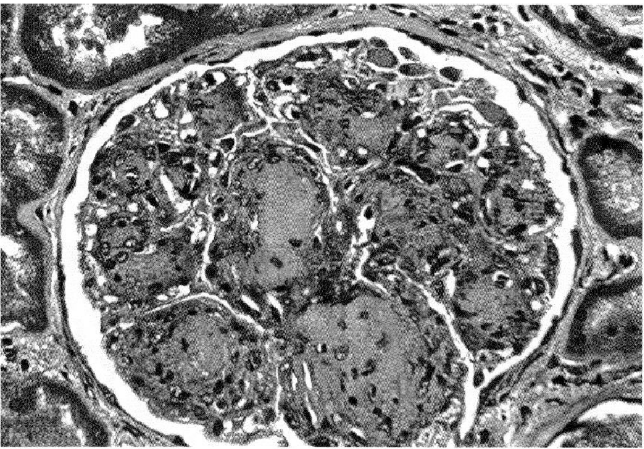

Figure 17-9

NODULAR DIABETIC GLOMERULOSCLEROSIS

A number of rounded, acellular mesangial nodules (Kimmelstiel-Wilson lesions) are present (Masson trichrome stain).

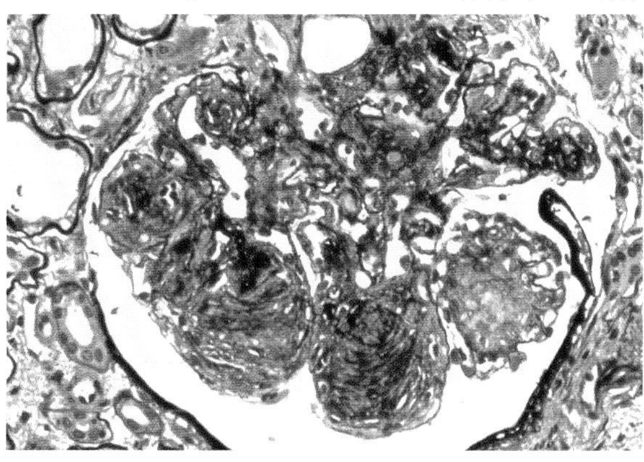

Figure 17-10

NODULAR DIABETIC GLOMERULOSCLEROSIS

Several large Kimmelstiel-Wilson mesangial nodules are present throughout this glomerular tuft (JMS stain).

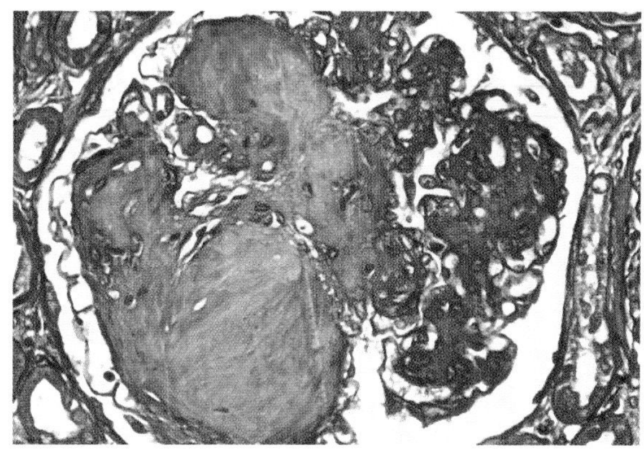

Figure 17-11

NODULAR DIABETIC GLOMERULOSCLEROSIS

Two large, almost confluent, acellular mesangial nodules are present in a specimen from a patient with advanced diabetic nephropathy. The massive nodules have tinctorial properties similar to the other mesangial regions (Masson trichrome stain).

or two per glomerulus, although sometimes they affect more glomerular lobules. They are irregularly distributed among the glomerular tuft regions. If multiple in a glomerulus, they tend to vary in size. Some investigators believe that these sclerotic nodules occur in association with, and in response to, glomerular capillary wall aneurysms, and that repetitive mesangiolysis, microaneurysm formation (figs. 17-16–17-18), and subsequent capillary collapse lead to the formation of the mesangial nodules. Glomerular capillary ectasia is often noted at the periphery of these sclerotic nodules (8,57,65).

Kimmelstiel-Wilson mesangial nodules generally occur 15 to 20 years after the clinical onset of type I diabetes. They may occasionally be encountered in a biopsy from a patient without a documented history of diabetes mellitus, or alternatively, one with a history of diabetes only of short duration. In these cases, it is suggested that the nodular glomerulosclerosis is the result of longer periods of subclinical, undetected

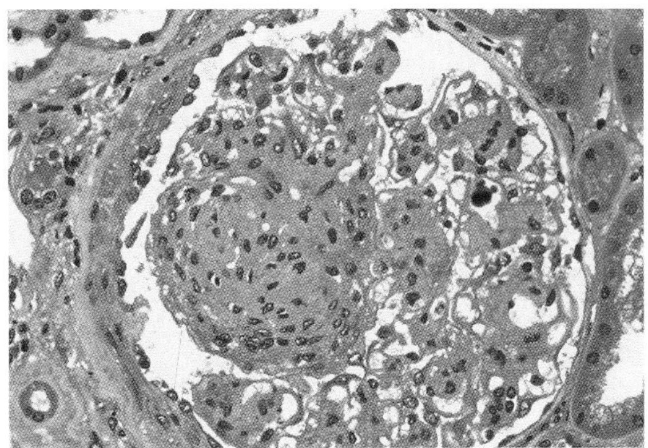

Figure 17-12

NODULAR DIABETIC GLOMERULOSCLEROSIS

This large Kimmelstiel-Wilson mesangial nodule has prominent cellularity. The clinical, laboratory, and other renal morphologic findings, however, were consistent with advancing diabetic nephropathy (H&E stain).

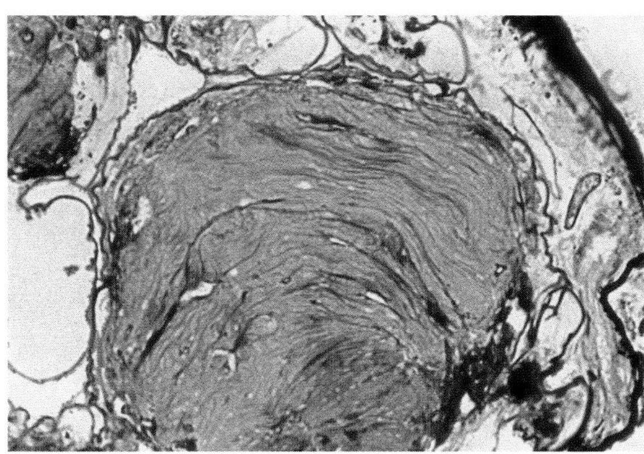

Figure 17-13

NODULAR DIABETIC GLOMERULOSCLEROSIS

The rounded mesangial region is slightly silver positive and shows lamination or layering of the mesangial substances. The adjacent glomerular capillary lumens are compressed (JMS stain). (Courtesy of Dr. C. Alpers, Seattle, WA.)

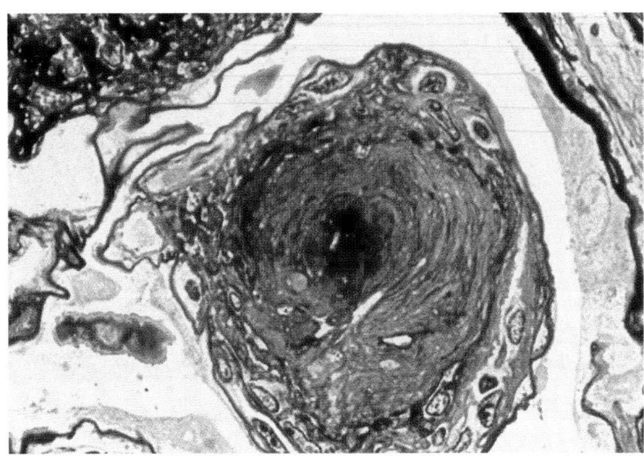

Figure 17-14

NODULAR DIABETIC GLOMERULOSCLEROSIS

The rounded mesangial region is slightly silver positive and shows lamination or layering of the mesangial substances. The adjacent glomerular capillary lumens are compressed (JMS stain). (Courtesy of Dr. C. Alpers, Seattle, WA.)

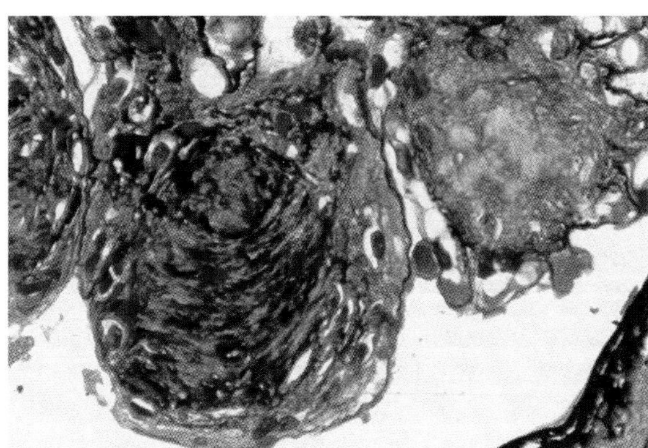

Figure 17-15

NODULAR DIABETIC GLOMERULOSCLEROSIS

The rounded mesangial region is intensely silver positive but shows residual lamination or layering of the mesangial substances. The adjacent capillary lumens are nearly occluded (JMS stain). (Courtesy of Dr. C. Alpers, Seattle, WA.)

diabetes mellitus. Kimmelstiel-Wilson nodule formation has been estimated to occur in approximately 25 percent of renal biopsies in patients with advanced diabetic nephropathy, although the exact prevalence of the lesion is not known (18,38).

The microaneurysms may be the result of mesangiolysis (although mesangiolysis may be difficult to identify). Mesangiolysis is manifested by dissolution, attenuation, fraying, and occasional lamination of the mesangial matrix. It is thought that this causes the glomerular capillary loops to lose their anchor to the mesangial matrix, leading to the microaneurysms. Occasionally, the glomerular capillaries rupture/burst, resulting in synechiae to Bowman's capsule and fibrosis within Bowman's space (57,65).

Microaneurysms are quite characteristic of advancing diabetic nephropathy, although similar lesions are seen in patients with other nondiabetic diseases such as light chain deposition

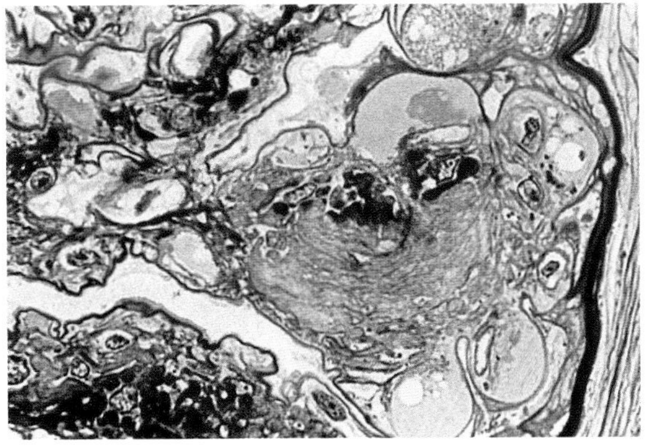

Figure 17-16

NODULAR DIABETIC GLOMERULOSCLEROSIS WITH MICROANEURYSM FORMATION

At the edge of the expanded acellular mesangial nodule are several ectatic glomerular capillaries (microaneurysms) (JMS stain). (Courtesy of Dr. C. Alpers, Seattle, WA.)

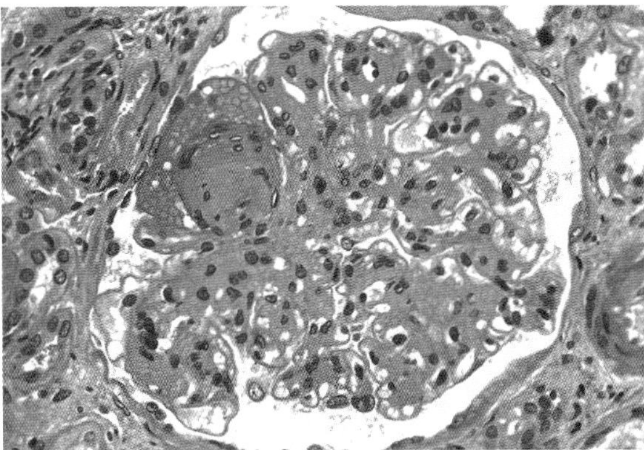

Figure 17-17

GLOMERULAR MICROANEURYSMS

There is a severely ectatic glomerular capillary (microaneurysm) at the edge of the Kimmelstiel-Wilson mesangial nodule (H&E stain).

disease, amyloidosis, and membranoproliferative (mesangiocapillary) glomerulonephritis (see below). As the diabetic nephropathy progresses, the individual nodules enlarge, and eventually compress and efface the nearby glomerular capillaries. Because of the progressive obliteration of the glomerular tuft, there is continuing renal ischemia, tubular atrophy, and interstitial fibrosis.

Another characteristic and advancing lesion seen in diabetic nephropathy is the *exudative* or the more appropriately termed *insudative lesion* (58,66). There are three types. 1) The *fibrin cap* is characterized by accumulations of hyaline-homogeneous eosinophilic acellular material located within the glomerular capillary lumens and often adherent to the glomerular capillary wall (fig. 17-19). This fibrin cap is produced by insudation of plasma proteins into the glomerular capillary wall. By this process, plasma proteins are pushed into the capillary wall and accumulate between the endothelium and the glomerular basement membrane, in a subendothelial location. These lesions vary in size, and may be small or large enough to occlude the glomerular capillary lumen. Although the presence of fibrin caps is not specific for diabetic nephropathy (i.e., they are found in patients with severe glomerulosclerosis of various causes, hypertension, and other diseases) they are most common and severe in patients with advancing diabetic nephropathy.

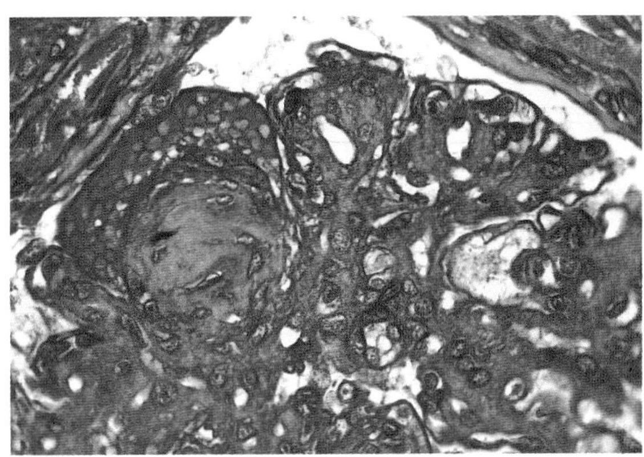

Figure 17-18

GLOMERULAR MICROANEURYSMS

The severely dilated glomerular capillary (microaneurysm) at the edge of the mesangial nodule contains many red blood cells (Masson trichrome stain).

2) The *capsular drop lesion* is noted between the parietal epithelium and Bowman's capsule of the glomerulus (fig. 17-20). Like the fibrin cap, it is a homogenous, eosinophilic, acellular hyaline mass and may represent insudation of plasma proteins. Like the fibrin cap, it is fuchsinophilic with the trichrome stain and is JMS negative (in contradistinction to the staining of mesangial matrix/sclerosis). The capsular drop was thought by many to be not only characteristic but probably pathognomonic of diabetes; however, it has been seen in patients with

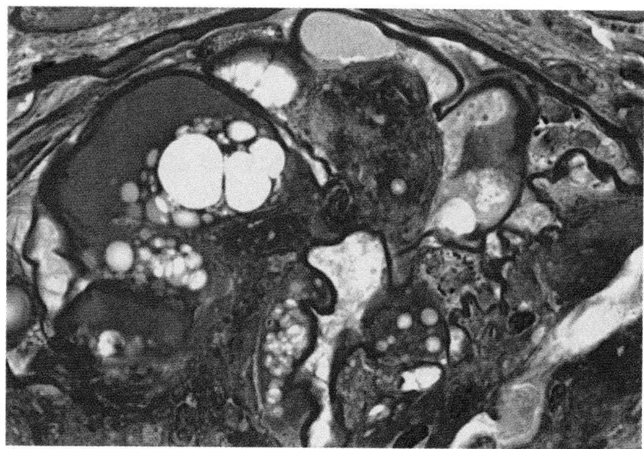

Figure 17-19

ADVANCING DIABETIC NEPHROPATHY: EXUDATIVE/INSUDATIVE LESIONS

There is occlusion of the glomerular capillary by acellular, amorphous hyaline material (with some "bubbles" representing plasma proteins/lipids). The hyaline material is impacted between the glomerular basement membrane and the glomerular endothelium. These are fibrin caps from a patient with severe diabetic nephropathy. They are caused by insudation of plasma proteins between the glomerular endothelium and the basement membrane. Although this lesion is not specific for diabetes, it is seen more commonly and severely in advancing diabetic nephropathy than in other diseases (PAS stain).

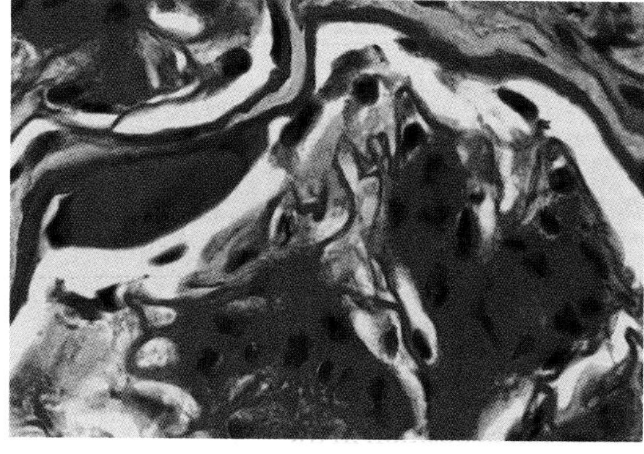

Figure 17-20

ADVANCING DIABETIC NEPHROPATHY: CAPSULAR DROP LESION

The acellular hyaline material is interposed between the glomerular parietal epithelium and Bowman's capsule. Some investigators believe that this lesion is specific for diabetic nephropathy. Although it has occasionally been seen in other severe renal diseases, it is most common in patients with diabetes (H&E stain).

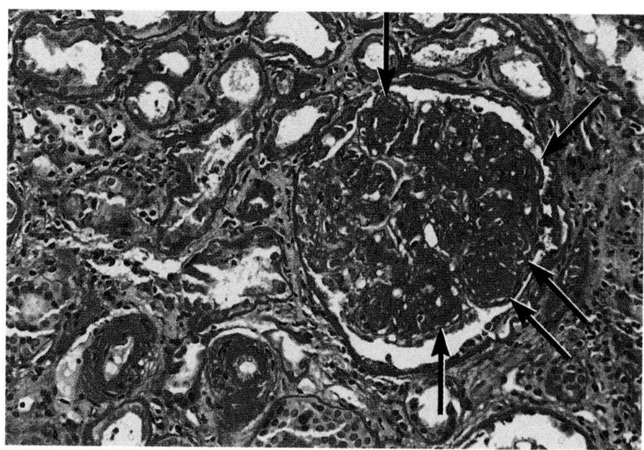

Figure 17-21

PROGRESSIVE DIABETIC NEPHROPATHY

Although there is marked global sclerosis, the originating disease can be discerned because examination of the least involved glomeruli shows residual mesangial nodules (arrows). The severely sclerotic glomerulus is large, signifying that something has been added (i.e., mesangial matrix); this is quite characteristic of advanced diabetic nephropathy (H&E stain).

severe renal disease, without diabetic nephropathy or diabetes itself. The exact pathogenic mechanism(s) leading to this lesion is unclear, but it may be produced either by tracking or movement of the hyaline insudation laterally within Bowman's capsule from a source within the glomerular hilus or the nearby pericapsular arterioles (66).

3) *Hyaline arteriolosclerosis* is described below.

Eventually, the progressive glomerulosclerosis and the accompanying insudative vascular changes lead to *global glomerulosclerosis* (figs. 17-21–17-23). In contradistinction to other causes of global glomerulosclerosis (in which substance is lost and the globally sclerotic glomeruli are small), sclerotic glomeruli in diabetes tend to be large. Even in advanced cases, if the least severely sclerotic glomeruli are studied, remnants of Kimmelstiel-Wilson nodules often are detected.

Tubules. There may be tubular changes secondary to the alterations of the permselectivity of the glomerulus. These include hyaline protein resorption droplets (hyaline change) and lipid droplets within the tubular epithelium. As the renal disease progresses, there may be tubular atrophy with progressively thickened tubular basement membranes (often paralleling the thickening of the glomerular basement membranes) (fig. 17-24). The degree of thickening

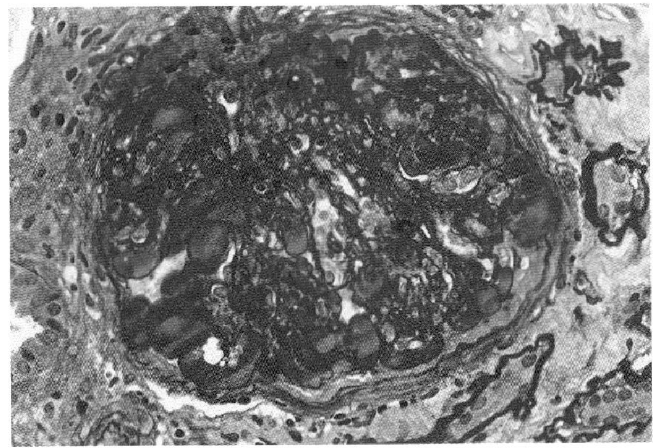

Figure 17-22

PROGRESSIVE DIABETIC NEPHROPATHY

The glomerular capillaries are almost entirely obliterated by increases in mesangial matrix and areas of hyalinosis (plasmatic insudation). Although these changes are not pathognomonic for advancing diabetic nephropathy, they are characteristic (H&E stain).

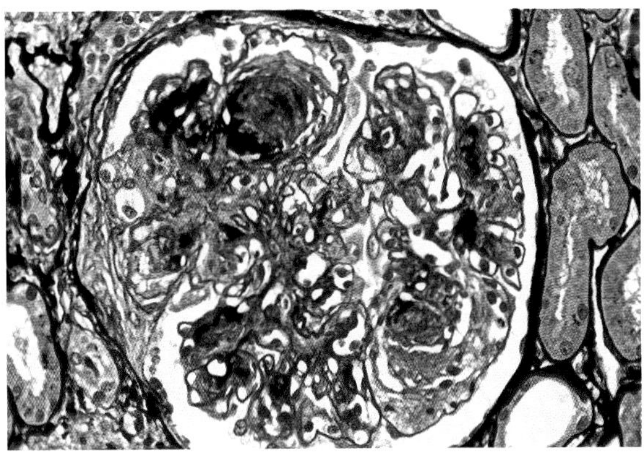

Figure 17-23

ADVANCING DIABETIC NEPHROPATHY

There is severe glomerulosclerosis and segmental adhesions (synechiae) between the glomerular tuft and Bowman's capsule (JMS stain).

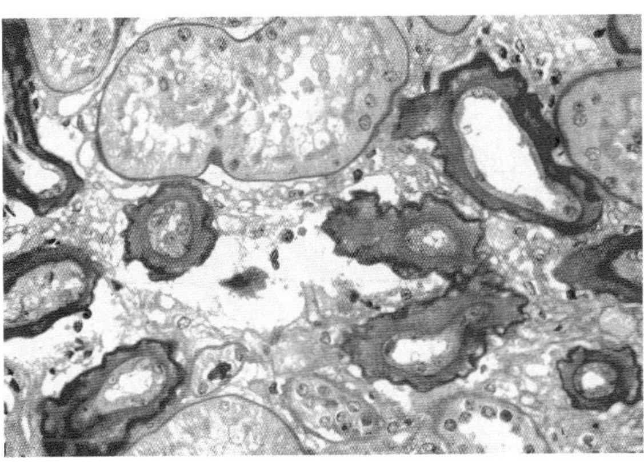

Figure 17-24

ADVANCING DIABETIC NEPHROPATHY

There is severe tubulointerstitial disease secondary to advancing glomerular and vascular disease. The tubular basement membranes are severely thickened (PAS stain).

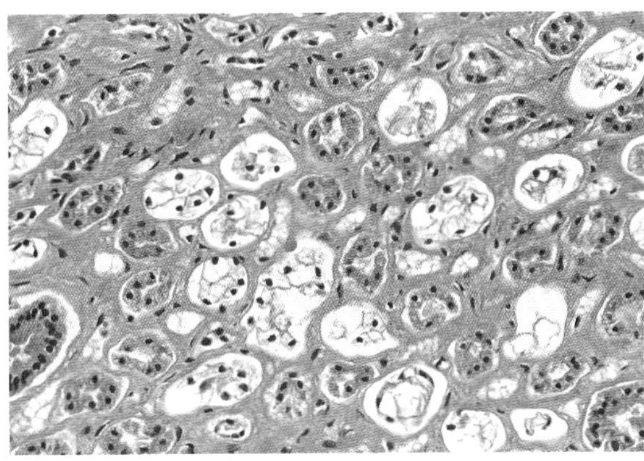

Figure 17-25

DIABETIC NEPHROPATHY: ARMANNI-EBSTEIN LESION

The clearing of the tubular epithelial cell cytoplasm is due to marked glucose deposition in the proximal tubular cells (most often the pars recta of the proximal tubule). This change is rarely seen nowadays because of proper control of blood sugar (H&E stain). (Courtesy of Dr. J. Ormos, Szeged, Hungary, and Dr. J. Pitha, Oklahoma City, OK.)

of the tubular basement membranes in patients with diabetic nephropathy appears greater than is found with similar degrees of tubular atrophy resulting from other causes in nondiabetic patients (12). Occasionally, the tubular basement membranes appear split or laminated at the ultrastructural level. They may be thickened even in the absence of significant tubulointerstitial damage (i.e, tubular atrophy or interstitial fibrosis). The Armanni-Ebstein change (extensive glycogen deposition in the tubular epithelial cells of the pars recta, the last or straight portion of the proximal tubule) is now very rarely seen because of improved glycemic control (fig. 17-25).

Interstitium. The most common change is interstitial fibrosis, often proportional to the severity of the vascular (and sometimes glomerular) changes (27,47,77). Bohle et al. (5) have suggested that interstitial fibrosis is the principal determinant of long-term renal function. The

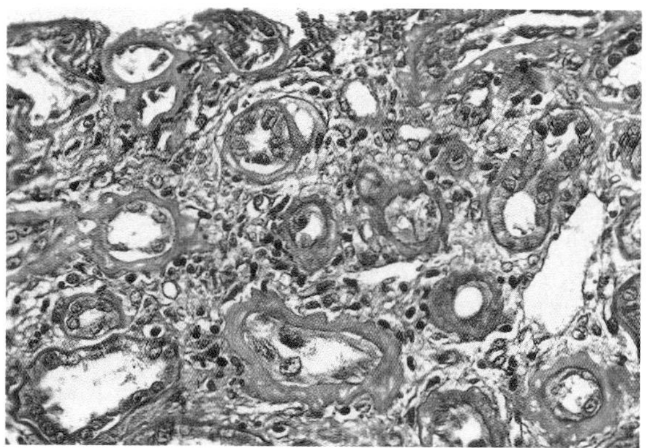

Figure 17-26

ADVANCING DIABETIC NEPHROPATHY

The severe tubulointerstitial disease is secondary to advancing glomerular and vascular disease. There may even be marked interstitial inflammation, but this is usually secondary to the accompanying vascular disease and tubulointerstitial response rather than secondary to an accompanying infection (i.e., pyelonephritis) (Masson trichrome stain).

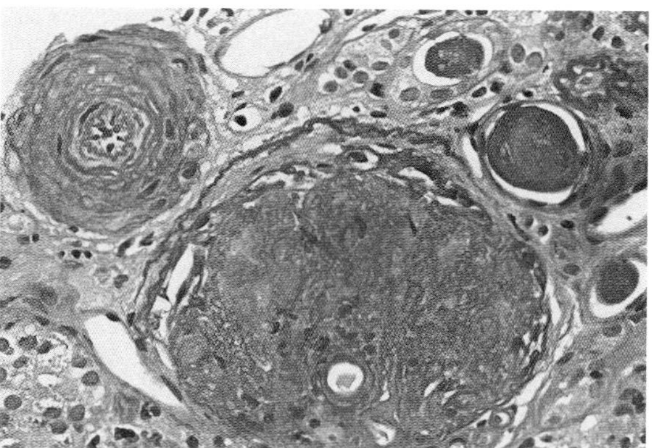

Figure 17-27

ADVANCING DIABETIC NEPHROPATHY

There is severe thickening of the interlobular artery, with marked reduplication of the basement membranes around the medial muscle cells in this form of arteriosclerosis in advancing diabetes. Although this change is most common and severe in patients with diabetes, it is also noted in hypertensive patients as well. Note the large sclerotic glomerulus (PAS stain).

morphometric studies of Lane et al. (36) also suggest a deleterious role for interstitial injury in determining renal function, independent of the glomerular changes. The exact mechanisms that underlie the development of tubulointerstitial injury in diabetic nephropathy are still somewhat unclear. There may be severe interstitial inflammation with interstitial lymphocytes, sometimes suggesting a pyelonephritis or accompanying interstitial nephritis (fig. 17-26). This nonspecific interstitial change (secondary to the severe accompanying vascular disease) led early investigators to suggest that pyelonephritis was a common finding in advancing diabetic nephropathy. However, the lack of confirmatory evidence of infection or a history of abnormalities of the urinary collecting systems failed to confirm this notion.

Blood Vessels. Vascular disease is quite common, and usually quite advanced and widespread, in patients with progressive diabetic nephropathy. Several vascular changes lead to thickening of the vessel walls and narrowing of the vessel lumens. These include intimal fibroplasia in larger arteries (the proximal portions of the interlobular arteries, arcuate arteries, and larger arteries) (fig. 17-27), and hyaline arteriolosclerosis (plasmatic insudation) in small renal arterioles (the terminal portions of the interlobular arteries and arterioles) (figs. 17-28, 17-29). Smaller arteries and arterioles may also show true arterial/arteriolosclerosis, manifested by thickening of the basement membranes of the medial muscle cells.

Hyaline arteriolosclerosis is most commonly noted in the afferent arterioles leading to the glomerular tufts. If the plane of section is such that both afferent and efferent arterioles are seen entering and exiting the glomeruli, then a characteristic change can be recognized, namely, hyalinization of the efferent arteriole (fig. 17-30). This efferent hyalinization is actually quite specific for diabetes mellitus in our experience although others have described it rarely in nondiabetic conditions (60). If only one arteriole is connected to the glomerular structure it is probably impossible to know whether it is an afferent or an efferent arteriole, unless it is in continuity with a larger nearby interlobular artery. Careful study of glomeruli sectioned through the vascular pole increases the chance of detecting this characteristic lesion of combined afferent and efferent arteriolar hyalinosis. Glomeruli downstream from these sites of diminished blood flow may show ischemic changes, collapse, or sclerosis.

Immunofluorescence Findings. The most characteristic immunofluorescence change in advancing diabetic nephropathy is diffuse linear

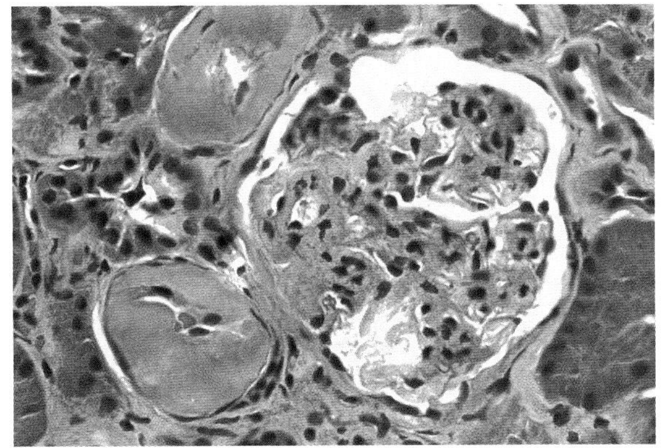

Figure 17-28

ADVANCING DIABETIC NEPHROPATHY: HYALINE ARTERIOLOSCLEROSIS

The vessel walls are thickened by acellular amorphous hyaline material. There is plasmatic insudation of acellular hyaline material into the vessel wall (H&E stain).

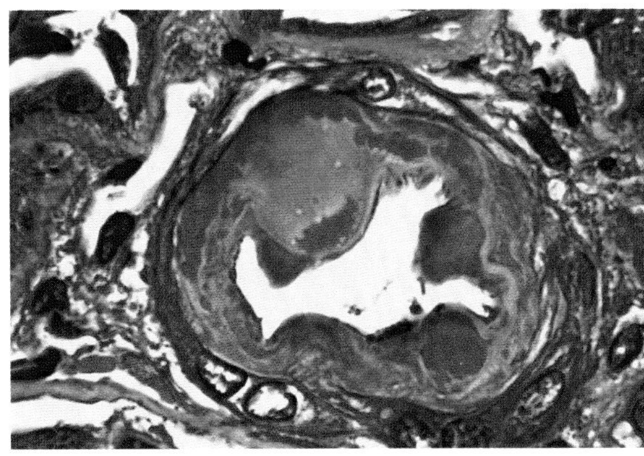

Figure 17-29

ADVANCING DIABETIC NEPHROPATHY: HYALINE ARTERIOLOSCLEROSIS

The arteriolar wall is markedly thickened by amorphous acellular hyaline material (plasmatic insudation). This hyaline material is often red with the Masson trichrome stain.

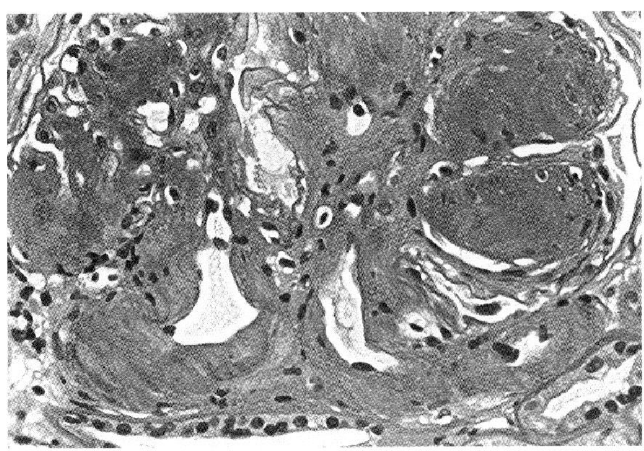

Figure 17-30

ADVANCING DIABETIC NEPHROPATHY: HYALINE ARTERIOLOSCLEROSIS

Both the afferent and the efferent arterioles have vessel walls that are thickened by hyaline insudation. Hyalinization of the efferent arteriole is quite suggestive of diabetic nephropathy (PAS stain).

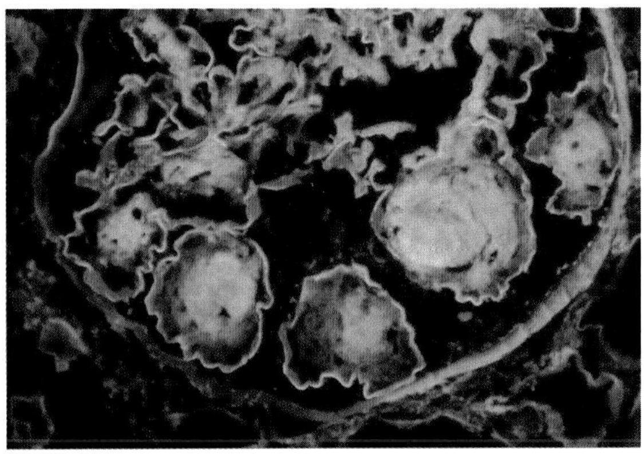

Figure 17-31

DIABETIC NEPHROPATHY

Immunofluorescence microscopy shows global linear staining along the glomerular basement membranes, mesangial nodules, and Bowman's capsule with antibodies to IgG and albumin. This is not antitubular or glomerular basement membrane immunologic disease, but rather nonspecific, nonimmunologic sticking of plasma proteins to the abnormally thickened and diseased basement membranes of diabetic patients (immunofluorescence with fluorescein isothiocyanate [FITC]-labeled anti-IgG antibody).

staining of the tubular basement membranes (and often the glomerular basement membranes) with antisera to albumin and IgG (figs. 17-31, 17-32). Occasionally, other immunoreactants (especially plasma proteins) are positive as well. Complement deposition is typically not present. The deposition of albumin and IgG is thought not to represent a true immunologic deposition, but rather nonimmunologic trapping of these immunoreactants in the thickened and diseased basement membranes, because studies in which the IgG is eluted from the biopsy material fail to demonstrate specific binding of the eluted antibodies to the renal parenchyma (25). This linear staining, which may be fairly intense, is not specific for diabetes, and other important

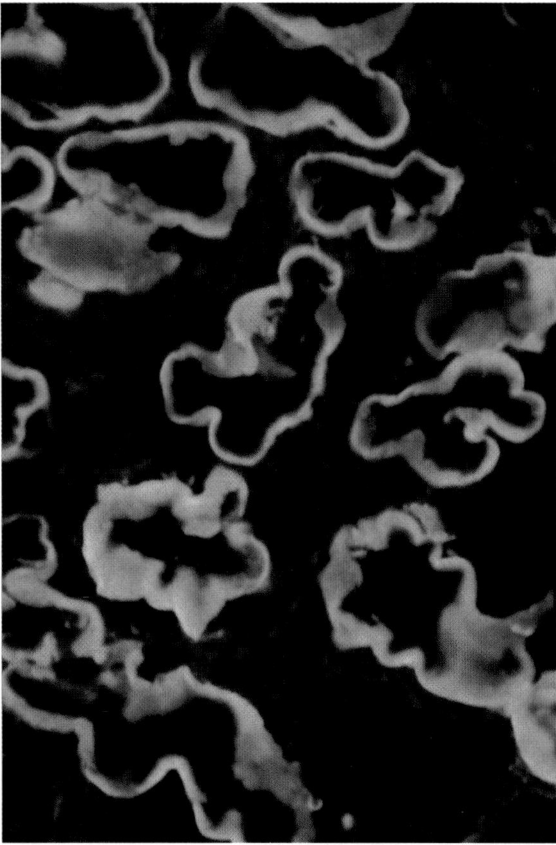

Figure 17-32

DIABETIC NEPHROPATHY

There is diffuse linear staining along the tubular basement membranes (TBM) with antibodies to IgG and albumin. This is not representative of an anti-TBM immunologic disease, but is nonspecific (immunofluorescence with FITC-labeled antialbumin antibody).

conditions, such as Goodpasture's disease (antiglomerular basement membrane [anti-GBM] disease), need to be excluded.

The tubular epithelium often stains for phagocytosed proteins such as albumin (in patients with glomerular disease and proteinuria). The insudative lesions (fibrin caps, hyaline arteriolosclerosis) often show nonspecific, nonimmunologic staining for IgM and complement (C)3.

Electron Microscopic Findings. Ultrastructural studies are most useful to confirm or exclude alternate glomerular diseases, particularly when the clinical history or immunofluorescence findings are ambiguous. The electron microscopic findings of advancing diabetic nephropathy are nonspecific, but as a constellation are fairly typical. The most characteristic ultrastructural changes are diffuse thickening of the glomerular basement membranes, especially the lamina densa, and an increase in the amount of mesangial matrix (mesangial sclerosis) (figs. 17-33–17-35). Kimmelstiel-Wilson nodules are expanded, accentuated, rounded regions of increased mesangial matrix (sclerosis).

The glomerular basement membranes may be mildly to severely thickened. Usually, the thickening cannot be identified by light microscopy until the glomerular basement membranes are three or four times thicker than normal. The contour and texture of the glomerular and tubular basement membranes are usually normal, although lamination may be noted in the latter. Occasionally, there may be mesangial cell interposition and focal widening of the lamina rara interna of the glomerular capillary wall, although these are nonspecific findings. Some investigators have recently noted areas of abnormal thinning of the glomerular basement membranes in patients with advancing diabetic nephropathy (57); the relationship between these changes and the microaneurysms is unclear.

Ultrastructural morphometric studies by Mayer et al. (39) have shown that while most of the expanded mesangial volume is the result of accumulated mesangial matrix, mesangial cell hypertrophy also contributes to this process. As noted before, a greater degree of mesangial expansion is closely associated with a decline in the glomerular filtration rate, increased proteinuria, and more severe hypertension.

The mesangial regions often show accumulations of the matrix and may reveal a finely fibrillar quality. Scattered elements of cell debris with vesicular particles and thread-like structures may be found embedded in the mesangial matrix. There may be some disorganization and fraying of the mesangium at the interface with the glomerular capillary lumen in those glomeruli exhibiting mesangiolysis.

There is often extensive effacement of the foot processes of the glomerular visceral epithelial cells, consistent with the proteinuria. Recent studies focusing on the overall glomerular cell numbers in diabetic nephropathy have shown that although the overall cell density is not significantly altered (63), there may be a

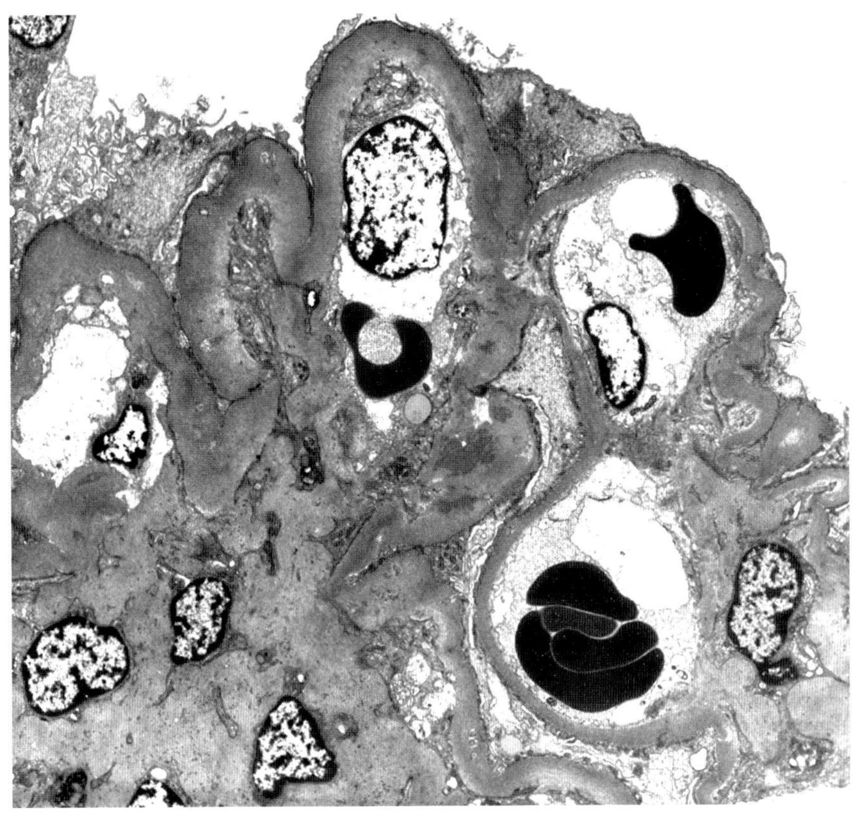

Figure 17-33

ADVANCING DIABETIC NEPHROPATHY

The electron micrograph shows marked thickening of the glomerular basement membranes and widening of the mesangial regions by mesangial sclerosis in a patient with advancing diabetic nephropathy.

selective loss of the visceral epithelial podocytes, which contributes to the proteinuria and progression of the diabetic renal disease (54).

The insudative lesions (fibrin caps, etc.) contain accumulations of amorphous, acellular, electron-dense material, often with lipid droplets (representing evidence of the plasma protein composition of these lesions) (figs. 17-36, 17-37). Smaller accumulations of this type of material also may be found within the mesangial regions and along the glomerular capillary walls. It may be difficult to distinguish such nonimmune hyaline accumulations from granular, electron-dense immune deposits, and the possibility of a superimposed immune complex–mediated glomerular lesion in diabetic patients should be cautiously evaluated. Correlation with the clinical, laboratory, and light and immunofluorescence microscopic findings provides the best opportunity to avoid a misdiagnosis in this setting.

The tubular basement membranes are markedly thickened (fig. 17-38). Lamination or multilayering of these membranes has been noted, and is thought to be secondary to repeated tubular epithelial proliferations (much

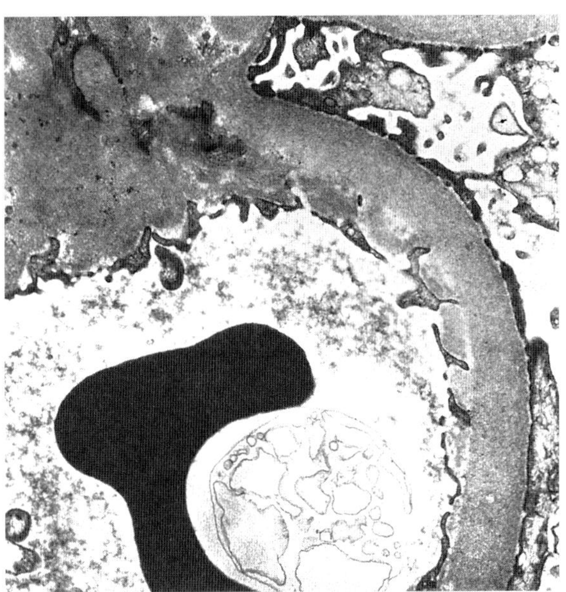

Figure 17-34

DIABETIC GLOMERULOSCLEROSIS

This electron micrograph shows marked thickening of the glomerular basement membrane in a patient with mild diabetic glomerulosclerosis.

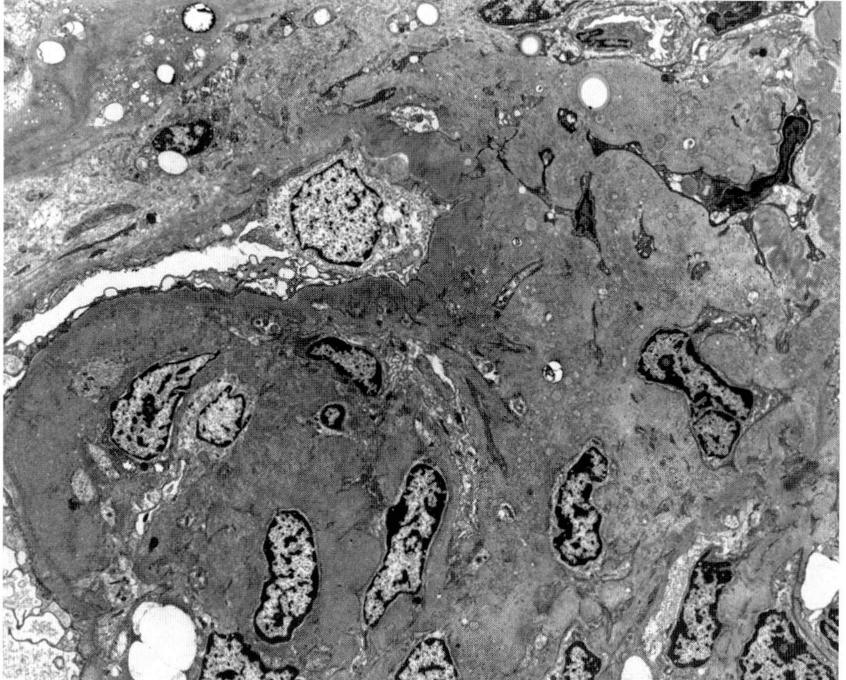

Figure 17-35

DIABETIC NEPHROPATHY

This electron micrograph shows a marked increase of mesangial matrix and the creation of a Kimmelstiel-Wilson nodule in a patient with diabetic nephropathy.

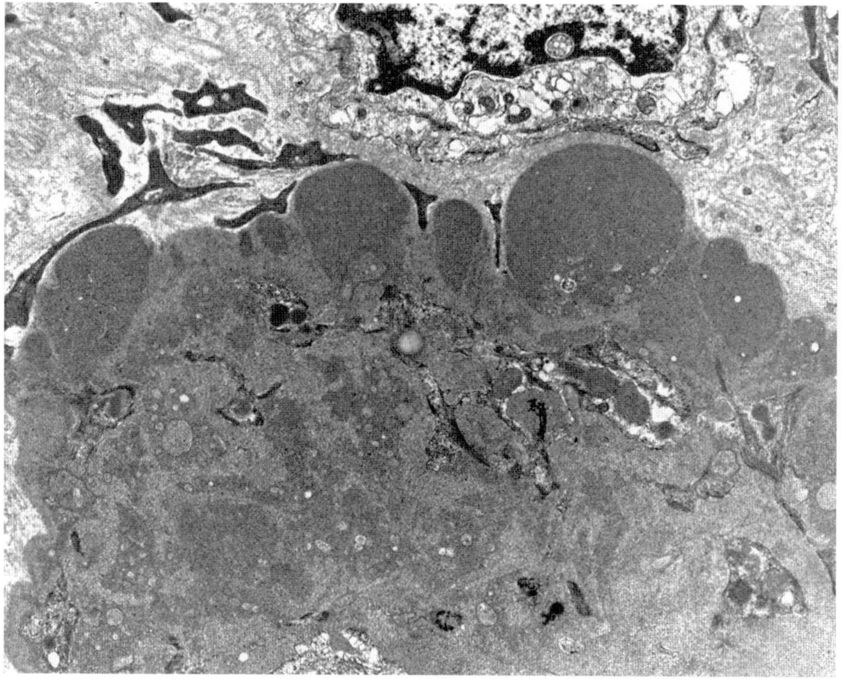

Figure 17-36

ADVANCED DIABETIC NEPHROPATHY

Severe mesangial sclerosis and amorphous electron-dense material representing hyalinosis or regions of nonimmunologic deposition of plasma proteins (plasmatic insudation) are seen in this electron micrograph. These regions of vague electron-dense material need to be distinguished from the more discrete electron-dense immune-type deposits seen in classic immune complex glomerular diseases.

like the growth rings on a tree). Electron microscopic examination of the arterioles shows the deposition of electron-dense material in the vessel walls, thought to represent plasmatic insudation (fig. 17-39).

Immunohistochemical Findings. Although not routinely useful for diagnosis, some experimental studies have added to our knowledge of advancing human diabetic nephropathy. Studies have focused on diminished accumulations

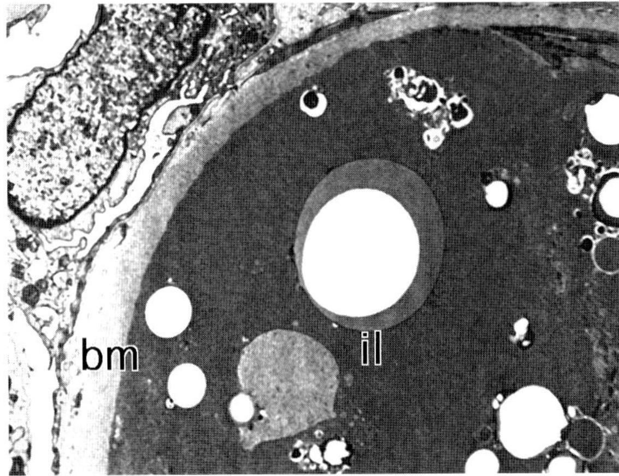

Figure 17-37

FIBRIN CAP

Electron microscopy shows plasmatic insudation (trapping of plasma proteins) between the glomerular endothelium and the basement membrane. Electron-lucent/less osmiophilic regions most likely represent plasma lipids.

of heparan sulfate proteoglycan in the glomerular basement membranes, which may contribute to a charge defect in the glomerular capillary wall permselectivity barrier; this could lead to the proteinuria, alterations of collagen IV alpha-chain subtypes and collagen VI in the mesangial and glomerular capillary walls, and accumulations of the interstitial type collagens (I and III) in areas of mesangial sclerosis and interstitial fibrosis (18,38,70,76). Studies of proteoglycan accumulation, however, have not yet identified a characteristic or specific profile for advancing diabetic nephropathy as compared to other sclerosing glomerular diseases (64). Evidence for the contribution of advanced glycation end products and their receptors in diabetic nephropathy have come from immunohistochemical studies on human tissues (fig. 17-40) (67).

PATHOLOGIC DIFFERENTIAL DIAGNOSIS

There are many distinct glomerular entities that lead to severe proteinuria and the nephrotic syndrome. In a patient with longstanding diabetes mellitus, severe proteinuria is assumed to be secondary to advancing diabetic nephropathy unless the course is atypical. For example, if proteinuria is detected within a few months or years after the apparent clinical onset of diabetes, or if there is a rapid progression to renal failure, renal biopsy is warranted to exclude nondiabetic renal disease. One fourth to half of patients with type II diabetes who undergo renal biopsy have other nondiabetic glomerular diseases, either alone or superimposed on

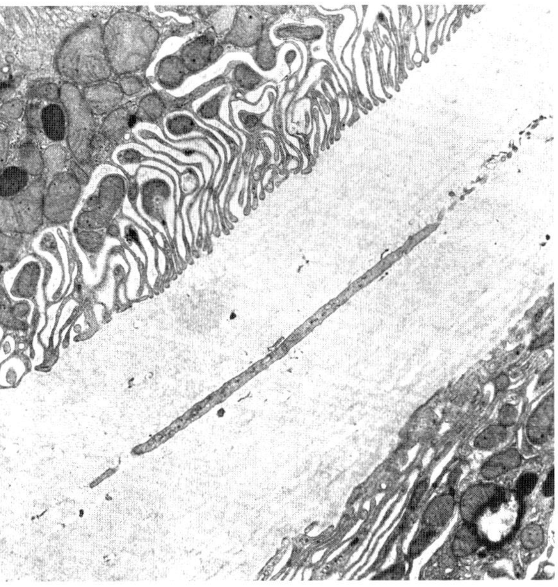

Figure 17-38

ADVANCED DIABETIC NEPHROPATHY: THICKENED TUBULAR BASEMENT MEMBRANES

The tubular basement membranes from this patient with diabetes are thickened.

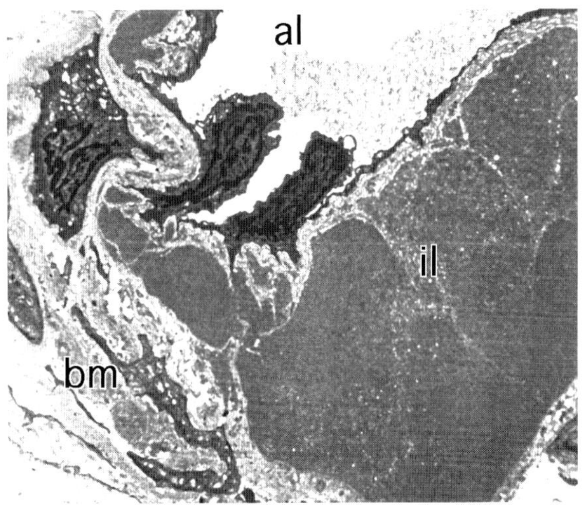

Figure 17-39

DIABETIC NEPHROPATHY

Electron microscopy shows electron-dense material (areas of hyalinosis or plasmatic insudation) in the arteriole wall.

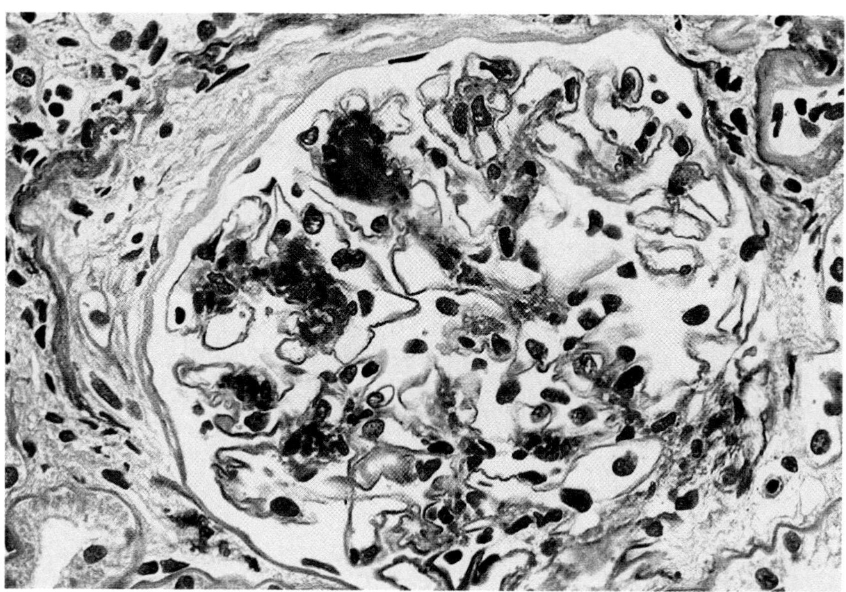

Figure 17-40

DIABETIC NEPHROPATHY

The deposition of advanced glycation end-products is seen via immunohistochemistry in a patient with nodular diabetic glomerulosclerosis (immunohistochemistry with antiadvanced glycation end-products).

the diabetic nephropathy. These include, most commonly, superimposed membranous glomerulopathy or IgA nephropathy, acute postinfectious glomerulonephritis, and less commonly, minimal change nephrotic syndrome, or even membranoproliferative glomerulonephritis, type 1.

A number of glomerular lesions resemble diabetic nephropathy by light microscopy: hypertensive renal disease, light chain deposition disease associated with a plasma cell dyscrasia, membranoproliferative (lobular) glomerulonephritis, and occasionally, amyloidosis. Recently other forms of idiopathic nodular glomerulosclerosis have been described.

Hypertensive renal disease alone, like diffuse diabetic glomerulosclerosis, as noted before, can lead to diffusely thickened glomerular basement membranes and a diffuse increase in the glomerular mesangial matrix. If both hypertension and diabetes mellitus are present, then dissecting out how much of the morphologic change is secondary to hypertension and how much to diabetes is essentially impossible. Of course, other changes, such as the presence of Kimmelstiel-Wilson nodules, hyalinization of the efferent arterioles, and even linear staining of glomerular and tubular basement membranes for IgG and albumin by immunofluorescence, are indicative of the presence of diabetic nephropathy.

The glomerular fibrin cap lesion seen in diabetic nephropathy is not specific for diabetes, and may be noted in a number of other renal diseases, such as focal segmental glomerular sclerosis. Although it is said that the glomerular capsular drop lesion is pathognomonic for diabetic nephropathy, it too, on rare occasion, is noted in other advancing glomerular conditions. Thus, although commonly seen in advancing diabetic renal disease, the hyalinosis lesions of fibrin caps and afferent hyalinosis are nonspecific. The lack of significant mesangial proliferation in diffuse diabetic glomerulosclerosis should aid in its distinction from a mesangioproliferative form of glomerular disease. Alpers et al. (1) have demonstrated an idiopathic lobular glomerulonephropathy with nodular mesangial sclerosis that is a distinct diagnostic entity, and not related to diabetes mellitus. Markowitz et al. (37a) have reported on a series of older, hypertensive patients who smoke who were found to have an idiopathic nodular glomerulosclerosis pattern.

Light chain deposition disease in patients plasma cell dyscrasia may lead to intraglomerular nodular sclerotic lesions resembling Kimmelstiel-Wilson nodules. The nodules in light chain deposition disease are often uniform in size, both within the single glomerulus and between different glomeruli of the same patient. In contrast, true Kimmelstiel-Wilson nodules often vary in size and only usually one or two are present per glomerular tuft. There may be more glomerular cellularity in light chain deposition disease than in diabetes, sometimes approaching a membranoproliferative glomerulonephritis pattern. The JMS stain reveals less argyrophilia in light chain disease glomerular nodules than in the diabetic glomerular mesangial nodules. In light chain disease, either kappa or lambda light chains, but not both, stain immunofluorescently. Discrete immune-type electron-dense deposits are noted in light chain disease (mesangium, glomerular basement membrane, and/or tubular basement membrane); these tend to be generally finer than in most immune-complex glomerular diseases. Usually the severe vascular disease and the diffuse marked thickening of the glomerular basement membranes noted in diabetes are not present in light chain disease.

Patients with membranoproliferative glomerulonephritis (types 1, 2, or 3) sometimes have a lobular accentuation with sclerotic intercapillary nodules that are similar to Kimmelstiel-Wilson nodules. Increased intracapillary hypercellularity, circumferential mesangial cell interposition with diffuse "reduplication" or "tram-tracking" of the glomerular capillary wall, and the presence of discrete glomerular electron-dense immune deposits (detected by immunofluorescence or electron microscopy) favor a true immune-complex membranoproliferative glomerulonephritis, rather than a diabetic nephropathy. There may be tubular basement membrane immune-type discrete deposits in the various types of membranoproliferative glomerulonephritis. Severe vascular disease and thickening of the glomerular basement membranes are more common in patients with advancing diabetic nephropathy.

Amyloidosis involving the glomerulus may have a nodular appearance, resembling the Kimmelstiel-Wilson nodules of diabetes. The amyloid nodules are usually quite acellular and negative with the JMS stain, but stain with Congo red to give the apple-green birefringence of amyloid under polarized light. Thioflavine T is positive in amyloidosis. PAS stains the glomerular amyloid nodules poorly. By electron microscopy, very long, nonbranching, rigid fibrils (8 to 12 nm in diameter) are noted in cases of amyloidosis where only small, nonspecific collagen microfibrils are noted in the sclerotic regions of the diabetic glomerulus.

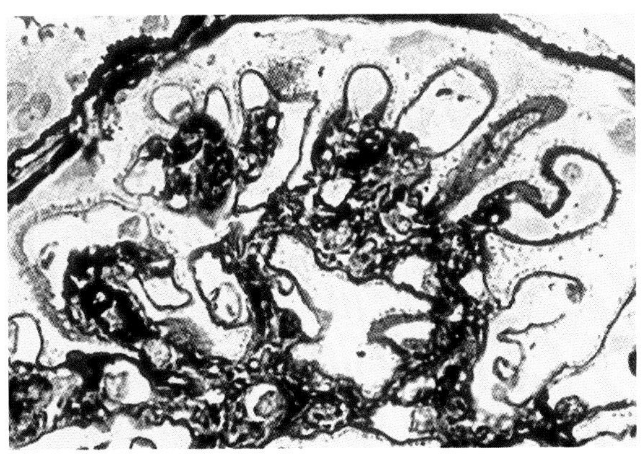

Figure 17-41

MEMBRANOUS GLOMERULONEPHROPATHY SUPERIMPOSED UPON DIABETIC NEPHROPATHY

This is the most common secondary glomerular condition associated with diabetic nephropathy. The JMS stain shows some argyrophilic "spikes" of glomerular basement membrane material protruding from the outer surface of the glomerular basement membrane into Bowman's capsule (JMS stain).

OTHER RENAL DISEASES ASSOCIATED WITH DIABETES

Diabetic patients with atypical clinical features of diabetes and diabetic nephropathy, such as a sudden onset of severe proteinuria and nephrotic syndrome, or alternatively, acute renal failure, may be biopsied in an effort to identify a second, treatable form of renal disease. Virtually all of the common renal diseases have been documented to occur in diabetic patients.

Diabetic nephropathy is probably the most common renal disease to be complicated by another recognizable or distinct form of glomerular disease. Although virtually any other glomerular disease can accompany diabetic nephropathy, the most common is membranous glomerulonephropathy (figs. 17-41–17-43) (2,44,75). Diabetics are predisposed to severe urinary tract infections; papillary necrosis (figs. 17-44, 17-45), acute pyelonephritis, and advanced arterial/arteriolar nephrosclerosis are common and severe complications of advancing diabetic kidney disease. They are considered in other chapters.

ETIOLOGY/PATHOGENESIS

The pathogenesis of diabetic nephropathy is not completely understood (4,18,31,61). It has been known for a long time that poor control of blood sugar, with resultant hyperglycemia,

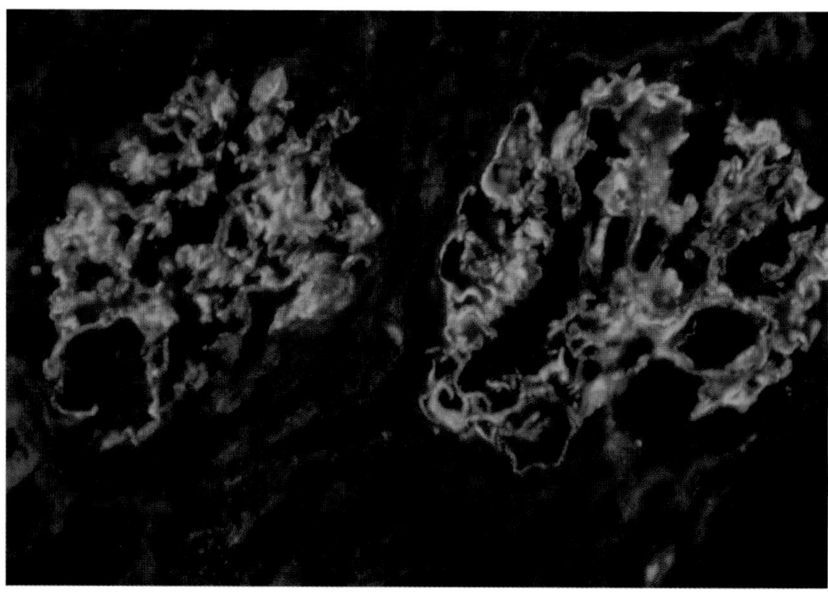

Figure 17-42

MEMBRANOUS GLOMERULONEPHROPATHY SUPERIMPOSED UPON DIABETIC NEPHROPATHY

Immunofluorescence for anti-IgG shows a diffuse granular pattern characteristic of a membranous glomerulonephropathy. There is also a mild "linear" component related to the underlying diabetes mellitus (FITC-labeled anti-IgG antibody).

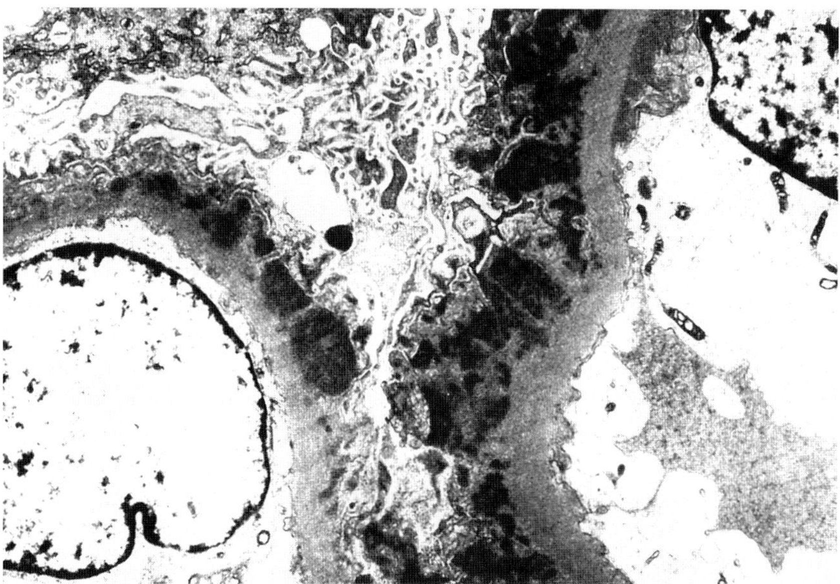

Figure 17-43

MEMBRANOUS GLOMERULONEPHROPATHY SUPERIMPOSED UPON DIABETIC NEPHROPATHY

Electron microscopy shows numerous glomerular, subepithelial, electron-dense immune-type deposits. In addition, there is moderate thickening of the glomerular basement membrane secondary to advancing diabetic nephropathy.

plays an important role. Poor control of blood sugar predisposes to advancing diabetic nephropathy and the other long-term vascular complications of diabetes. Indeed, most evidence now suggests that the diabetic renal changes are caused, in large part, by the underlying diabetic metabolic defects of the hyperglycemia, insulin deficiency, or other related or associated aspects of glucose intolerance. Other factors, such as hemodynamic alterations (hyperfiltration) and systemic hypertension, almost certainly contribute to the onset and progression of diabetic nephropathy. Recently, a number of other possible contributing factors have been suggested.

Many biochemical alterations have been identified in the diabetic basement membranes. There is increased synthesis of collagen type IV and fibronectin, and decreased synthesis of the proteoglycan heparan sulfate. A reduced fixed negative charge has been reported. The anionic charge density of the glomerular basement membranes decreases in proportion to the increase in membrane thickness. The mesangial nodules and glomerular basement membrane changes are

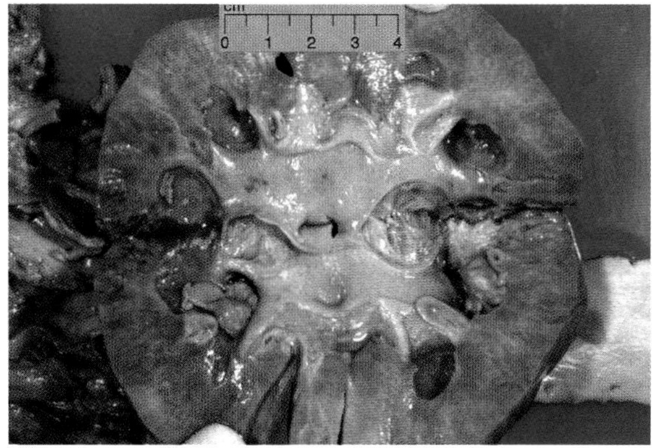

Figure 17-44

DIABETIC NEPHROPATHY: PAPILLARY NECROSIS

There is marked discoloration and whitening of several papillary areas in this kidney from a patient with advancing diabetic nephropathy.

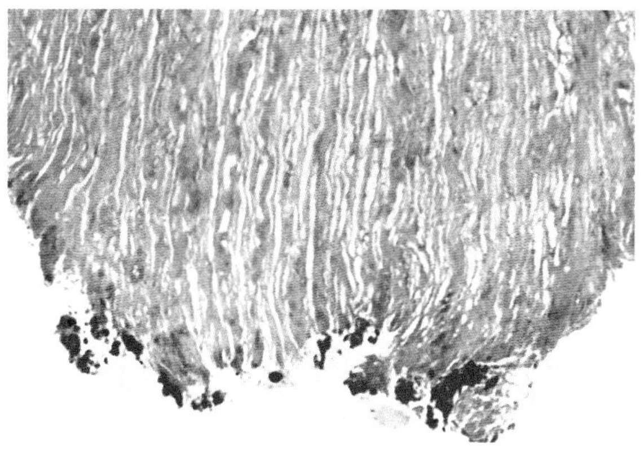

Figure 17-45

DIABETIC NEPHROPATHY: PAPILLARY NECROSIS

The sloughed renal papilla collected from the urine retains some of the medullary tubular outlines, but there is no cellular detail due to the infarction of the papilla.

thought to be due to the increased synthesis and/or decreased removal of these various proteins.

Immunohistochemical studies of the increased glomerular mesangial matrix in patients with diabetes mellitus show increased proteoglycan, collagen, tenascin, and advanced glycation end-products. Mediators of injury include platelet-derived growth factor (PDGF) and transforming growth factor (TGF) beta. Markers of cell proliferation and activation have also been found. In addition to increased glomerular intracapillary pressures, there is evidence of glomerular endothelial dysfunction and altered visceral epithelium.

Hyperglycemia leads to the nonenzymatic glycosylation of various proteins. An example of this is glycosylation of hemoglobin, producing hemoglobin A1C, which serves as a serologic marker. Collagen and other glomerular matrix and basement membrane proteins are also glycosylated, leading to advanced glycation end-products (AGEs) (7,13,72,73). AGEs promote the formation of covalent bonds and the cross-linking of various proteins, including collagen and matrix proteins. These abnormal proteins may also interact with specific cell receptors and lead to basement membrane thickening and other injurious events. Certain drugs, such as aminoguanidine, may lower the AGEs in patients with diabetes mellitus.

Other suggested mechanisms for diabetic nephropathy include: 1) genetic predisposition, 2) the conversion of glucose to sorbitol by the enzyme aldose reductase, and 3) hemodynamic alterations such as increased glomerular filtration rate with glomerulomegaly. Patients with early-onset type I diabetes have glomerulomegaly, increased glomerular filtration rates, increased glomerular filtration areas, and increased glomerular capillary pressures. It has also been shown that inhibition of angiotensin by a converting enzyme inhibitor like captopril has a beneficial effect on renal disease progression, possibly by reversing the increased intraglomerular capillary pressure. Thus, diabetic nephropathy is thought by some to be one of the "hyperfiltration" nephropathies identified by the studies of Dr. Barry Brenner and associates. Mediators such as TGF-beta, nitric oxide (NO), and protein kinase C and other kinins, are undergoing continuing investigation in an attempt to understand and treat this common complication of this important disease.

TREATMENT AND PROGNOSIS

Although the majority of patients with diabetes mellitus do not develop significant clinical renal damage, those with proteinuria usually develop progressive diabetic nephropathy. As noted above, the time interval from the clinical onset of diabetes to clinical proteinuria is usually 10 to 15 years or more. The time from significant proteinuria to end-stage renal disease averages 5 to 10 years, with considerable variability from patient to patient. There is no specific therapy for patients with advancing diabetic nephropathy once it has developed. Hypertension is thought to accentuate the progression of the diabetic renal disease and control of hypertension probably slows the progression. Angiotensin converting enzyme inhibitors such as captopril have been shown both in experimental animals and in man to reduce proteinuria and to slow the progression to renal failure (9,37,42,68).

Experimental studies in diabetic animals suggest that strict control of blood sugar may prevent or even ameliorate the advancing diabetic nephropathy. In animal models, aggressive control of blood glucose may delay or prevent the early onset of microalbuminuria. There is evidence in man that good glycemic control also may delay or prevent the development of nephropathy. Once the diabetic nephropathy is overt, however, there is little evidence that medical control of hyperglycemia affects disease progression (9,30,37,42,68).

Dietary protein restriction decreases the excretion and hyperfiltration of albumin. Progression of the diabetic nephropathy may be slowed.

Dialysis, renal transplantation, and combined pancreas-renal transplantation are the final therapeutic modalities for patients with advancing diabetic nephropathy. Survival rates for diabetic patients undergoing transplantation are better than for those on dialysis. Cardiovascular disease is a common cause of mortality and the most common cause of death in patients with end-stage renal disease.

When nondiabetic kidneys are transplanted into diabetic recipients, features of recurrent diabetic disease are noted within 2 years of transplantation in some patients (23,40). The earliest recurrent morphologic changes are those of hyalinosis and sclerosis of small arteries and arterioles. The incidence/severity of recurrence is not associated with donor source, human leukocyte antigen (HLA) matching, or episodes of rejection. In one large series of 100 diabetic patients receiving a renal allograft, only 2 experienced graft loss as a direct result of the diabetes (46). Most important to patient and renal graft survival was the presence of cardiovascular disease.

There are recent suggestions that diabetic nephropathy may be somewhat reversible. One study showed that after 10 years with a pancreatic transplant, the morphologic signs of diabetic nephropathy may be reversed, including the disappearance of Kimmelstiel-Wilson mesangial nodules (23). Combined pancreas and kidney transplants may retard and even potentially obviate recurrence of the diabetic nephropathy in the allografted kidneys (74). The period of observation needed to substantiate these findings has been too short to be conclusive. Several studies of sequential renal biopsies in patients treated for years with angiotensin converting enzyme inhibitors and good glycemic control have not demonstrated reversibility of the morphologic lesions (19,53).

REFERENCES

1. Alpers CE, Biava CG. Idiopathic lobular glomerulonephritis (nodular mesangial sclerosis): a distinct diagnostic entity. Clin Nephrol 1989;32:68–74.
2. Amoah E, Glickman JL, Malchoff CD, Sturgill BC, Kaiser DL, Bolton WK. Clinical identification of nondiabetic renal disease in diabetic patients with type I and type II disease presenting with renal dysfunction. Am J Nephrol 1988;8:204–11.
3. Andersen AR, Christiansen JS, Andersen JK, Kreiner S, Deckert T. Diabetic nephropathy in type I (insulin-dependent) diabetes: an epidemiological study. Diabetologia 1983;25:496–501.
4. Anderson S, Brenner BM. Pathogenesis of diabetic glomerulopathy: hemodynamic considerations. Diabetes Metab Rev 1988;4:163–77.
5. Bader R, Bader H, Grund KE, Mackensen-Haen S, Christ H, Bohle A. Structure and function of the kidney in diabetic glomerulosclerosis. Correlations between morphological and functional parameters. Pathol Res Pract 1980;167:204–16.
6. Bennett PH, Haffner S, Kasiske BL, et al. Screening and management of microalbuminuria in patients with diabetes mellitus: recommendations to the Scientific Advisory Board of the National Kidney Foundation from an ad hoc committee of the Council on Diabetes Mellitus of the National Kidney Foundation. Am J Kidney Dis 1995;25:107–12.
7. Beyer-Mears A. The polyol pathway, sorbinil, and renal dysfunction. Metabolism 1986;35:46–54.
8. Bloodworth JM Jr. A re-evaluation of diabetic glomerulosclerosis 50 years after the discovery of insulin. Hum Pathol 1978;9:439–53.
9. Bojestig M, Arnqvist HJ, Hermansson G, Karlberg BE, Ludvigsson J. Declining incidence of nephropathy in insulin-dependent diabetes mellitus. N Engl J Med 1994;330:15–8.
10. Borch-Johnsen K. Incidence of nephropathy in insulin-dependent diabetes as related to mortality. In: Mogensen CE, ed. The kidney and hypertension in diabetes mellitus. Boston: Nijhoff; 1988:33–40.
11. Breyer JA. Diabetic nephropathy in insulin-dependent patients. Am J Kidney Dis 1992;20:533–47.
12. Brito PL, Fioretto P, Drummond K, et al. Proximal tubular basement membrane width in insulin-dependent diabetes mellitus. Kidney Int 1998;53:754–61.
13. Brownlee M, Cerami A, Vlassara H. Advanced products of nonenzymatic glycosylation and the pathogenesis of diabetic vascular disease. Diabetes Metab Rev 1988;4:437–51.
14. Chahaz PS, Kohner EM. The relationship between diabetic retinopathy and diabetic nephropathy. Diabetic Nephropathy 1983;2:4.
15. Chavers BM, Bilous RW, Ellis EN, Steffes MW, Mauer SM. Glomerular lesions and urinary albumin excretion in type I diabetes without overt proteinuria. N Engl J Med 1989;320:966–70.
16. Chavers BM, Simonson J, Michael AF. A solid phase fluorescent immunoassay for the measurement of human urinary albumin. Kidney Int 1984;25:576–8.
17. Churg J, Dachs S. Diabetic renal disease: arteriosclerosis and glomerulosclerosis. In: Sommers SC, ed. Pathology annual, Vol. 2. Norwalk, CT: Appleton And Lange; 1966:148.
18. Defronzo RA. Diabetic nephropathy: etiologic and therapeutic considerations. Diabetes Reviews 1995;3:510–64.
19. Effect of 3 years of antihypertensive therapy on renal structure in type 1 diabetic patients with albuminuria: the European Study for the Prevention of Renal Disease in Type I Diabetes (ESPIRIT). Diabetes 2001;50:843–50.
20. Fabre J, Balant LP, Dayer PG, Fox HM, Vernet AT. The kidney in maturity onset diabetes mellitus: a clinical study of 510 patients. Kidney Int 1982;21:730–8.
21. Fioretto P, Mauer SM, Bilous RW, Goetz FC, Sutherland DE, Steffes MW. Effects of pancreas transplantation of glomerular structure in insulin-dependent diabetic patients with their own kidneys. Lancet 1993;342:1193–6.
22. Fioretto P, Steffes MW, Brown DM, Mauer SM. An overview of renal pathology in insulin-dependent diabetes mellitus in relationship to altered glomerular hemodynamics. Am J Kidney Dis 1992;20:549–58.
23. Fioretto P, Steffes MW, Sutherland DE, Goetz FC, Mauer M. Reversal of lesions of diabetic nephropathy after pancreas transplantation. N Engl J Med 1998;339:69–75.
24. Fioretto P, Steffes MW, Sutherland DE, Mauer M. Sequential renal biopsies in insulin-dependent diabetic patients: structural factors associated with clinical progression. Kidney 1995;48:1929–35.
25. Gallo GR. Elution studies in kidneys with linear deposition of immunoglobulin in glomeruli. Am J Pathol 1970;61:377–94.
26. Gambara V, Mecca G, Remuzzi G, Bertani T. Heterogeneous nature of lesions in type II diabetes. J Am Soc Nephrol 1993;3:1458–66.

27. Gilbert RE, Cooper ME. The tubulointerstitium in progressive diabetic kidney disease: more than an aftermath of glomerular injury? Kidney Int 1999;56:1627–37.
28. Glassock RJ, Hirschman GH, Striker GE. Workshop on the use of renal biopsy in research or diabetic nephropathy: a summary report. Am J Kidney Dis 1991;18:589–92.
29. Hasslacher C, Ritz E, Wahl P, Michael C. Similar risks of nephropathy in patients with type I or type II diabetes mellitus. Nephrol Dial Transplant 1989;4:859–63.
30. Hostetter TH. Prevention of end-stage renal disease due to type 2 diabetes. N Engl J Med 2001;345:910–2.
31. Ibrahim HN, Hostetter TH. Diabetic nephropathy. Am Soc Nephrol 1997;8:487–93.
32. Kern WF, Silva FG, Laszik ZG, Bane BL, Nadasdy T, Pitha JV. The kidney in metabolic disorders: diabetes mellitus, hyperuricemia, oxalosis, nephrocalcinosis, and nephrolithiasis. In: Kern WF, ed. Atlas of renal pathology. Philadelphia: Saunders; 1999:97–111.
33. Kimmelstiel PH, Wilson C. Intercapillary lesions in the glomeruli of the kidney. Am J Pathol 1936;12:82–97.
34. Krolewski AS, Warram JH, Christlieb AR, Busick EJ, Kahn CR. The changing natural history of nephropathy in type I diabetes. Am J Med 1985;78:785–94.
35. Krolewski AS, Warram JH, Rand LI, Kahn CR. Epidemiologic approach to the etiology of type I diabetes and its complications. N Engl J Med 1987;317:1390–8.
36. Lane PH, Steffes MW, Fioretto P, Mauer SM. Renal interstitial expansion in insulin-dependent diabetes mellitus. Kidney Int 1993;43:661–7.
37. Manto A, Cotroneo P, Marra G, et al. Effect of intensive treatment on diabetic nephropathy in patients with type I diabetes. Kidney Int 1995;47:231–5.
37a. Markowitz GS, Lin J, Valeri AM, Avila C, Nasr SH, D'Agati VD. Idiopathic nodular glomerulosclerosis is a distinct clinicopathologic entity linked to hypertension and smoking. Hum Pathol 2002;33:826–35.
38. Mauer SM. Structural-functional correlations of diabetic nephropathy. Kidney Int 1994;45:612–22.
39. Mauer SM, Chavers BM, Steffes MW. Should there be an expanded role for kidney biopsy in the management of patients with type I diabetes? Am J Kidney Dis 1990;16:96–100.
40. Michielsen P. Recurrence of the original disease. Does this influence renal graft failure? Kidney Int 1995;52(Suppl):S79–84.
41. Mogensen CE. Microalbuminuria predicts clinical proteinuria and early mortality in maturity-onset diabetes. N Engl J Med 1984;310:356–60.
42. Mogensen CE. The kidney in diabetes: how to control renal and related cardiovascular complications. Am J Kidney Dis 2001;37(Suppl 2):S2–6.
43. Mogensen CE, Christensen CK, Vittinghus E. The stages of diabetic nephropathy. With emphasis on the stage of incipient diabetic nephropathy. Diabetes 1983;32(Suppl 2):64–78.
44. Monga G, Mazzucco G, di Belgiojoso GB, Confalonieri R, Sacchi G, Bertani T. Pattern of double glomerulopathies: a clinicopathologic study of superimposed glomerulonephritis on diabetic glomerulosclerosis. Mod Pathol 1989;2:407–14.
45. Nadasdy T, Silva FG. Nonneoplastic adult renal diseases. In: Sternberg SS, ed. Diagnostic surgical pathology, 3rd ed, vol 1. Philadelphia, Lippincott, Williams & Wilkins; 1999:1701.
46. Najarian JS, Kaufman DB, Fryd DS, et al. Long-term survival following kidney transplantation in 100 type I diabetic patients. Transplantation 1989;47:106–13.
47. Nerlich A, Schleicher E. Immunohistochemical localization of extracellular matrix components in human diabetic glomerular lesions. Am J Pathol 1991;139:889–99.
48. Noth RH, Krolewski AS, Kaysen GA, Meyer TW, Schambelan M. Diabetic nephropathy: hemodynamic basis and implications for disease management. Ann Intern Med 1989;110:795–813.
49. Olson JL. Diabetes mellitus. In: Jennette JC, Olson L, Schwartz MM, Silva FG, eds. Heptinstall's pathology of the kidney, 5th ed. Philadelphia: Lippincott-Raven; 1998:1247–86.
50. O'Neill WM Jr, Wallin JD, Walker PD. Hematuria and red cell casts in typical diabetic nephropathy. Am J Med 1983;74:389–95.
51. Osterby R. Early phases in the development of diabetic glomerulosclerosis. Acta Med Scan 1975;574 (Suppl 1):1–80.
52. Osterby R. Structural changes in the diabetic kidney. Clin Endocrinol Metab 1986;15:733–51.
53. Osterby R, Bangstad HJ, Nyberg G, Rudberg S. On glomerular structural alterations in type-1 diabetes. Companions of early diabetic glomerulopathy. Virchows Arch 2001;438:129–35.
54. Pagtalunan ME, Miller PL, Jumping-Eagle S, et al. Podocyte loss and progressive glomerular injury in type II diabetes. J Clin Invest 1997;99:342–8.
55. Richards NT, Greaves I, Lee SJ, Howie AJ, Adu D, Michael J. Increased prevalence of renal biopsy findings other than diabetic glomerulopathy in type II diabetes mellitus. Nephrol Dial Transplant 1992;7:397–9.

56. Ritz E, Stefanski A. Diabetic nephropathy in type II diabetes. Am J Kidney Dis 1996;27:167–94.
57. Saito Y, Kida H, Takeda S, et al. Mesangiolysis in diabetic glomeruli: its role in the formation of nodular lesions. Kidney Int 1988;34:389–96.
58. Salinas-Madrigal L, Pirani CL, Pollak VE. Glomerular and vascular "insudative" lesions of diabetic nephropathy: electron microscopic observations. Am J Pathol 1970;59:369–97.
59. Seaquist ER, Goetz FC, Rich S, Barbosa J. Familial clustering of diabetic kidney disease. Evidence for genetic susceptibility to diabetic nephropathy. N Engl J Med 1989;320:1161–5.
60. Spear GS, Vitsky BH. Hyalinization of afferent and efferent glomerular arterioles in cyanotic heart disease. Am J Med 1966;41:309–15.
61. Steffes MW. Affecting the decline of renal function in diabetes mellitus. Kidney Int 2001;60: 378–9.
62. Steffes MW, Osterby R, Chavers B, Mauer SM. Mesangial expansion as a central mechanism for loss of kidney function in diabetic patients. Diabetes 1989;38:1077–81.
63. Steffes MW, Schmidt D, Mccrery R, Basgen JM. Glomerular cell number in normal subjects and in type 1 diabetic patients. Kidney Int 2001;59: 2104–13.
64. Stokes MB, Holler S, Cui Y, et al. Expression of decorin, biglycan, and collagen type I in human renal fibrosing disease. Kidney Int 2000; 57:487–98.
65. Stout LC, Kumar S, Whorton EB. Focal mesangiolysis and the pathogenesis of the Kimmelstiel-Wilson nodule. Hum Pathol 1993;24:77–89.
66. Stout LC, Kumar S, Whorton EM. Insudative lesions—their pathogenesis and association with glomerular obsolescence in diabetes: a dynamic hypothesis based on single views of advancing diabetic nephrophathy. Hum Pathol 1994;25:1213–27.
67. Tanji N, Markowitz GS, Fu C, et al. Expression of advanced glycation end products and their cellular receptor RAGE in diabetic nephropathy and nondiabetic renal disease. J Am Soc Nephrol 2000;11:1656–66.
68. Tataranni PA. Changing habits to delay diabetes. N Engl J Med 2001;344:1390–2.
69. Venkataseshan VS, Churg J. Diabetes and other metabolic diseases. In: Silva FG, D'Agati VD, Nadasdy T, eds. Renal biopsy: interpretation. New York: Churchill Livingstone; 1996:221–57.
70. Vernier RL, Steffes MW, Sisson-Ross S, Mauer SM. Heparan sulfate proteoglycan in the glomerular basement membrane in type 1 diabetes mellitus. Kidney Int 1992;41:1070–80.
71. Viberti GC, Hill RD, Jarrett RJ, Argyropoulos A, Mahmud U, Keen H. Microalbuminuria as a predictor of clinical nephropathy in insulin-dependent diabetes mellitus. Lancet 1982;1:1430–2.
72. Vlassara H. Recent progress in advanced glycation end products and diabetic complications. Diabetes 1997;46(Suppl 2):S19–25.
73. Vlassara H, Bucala R, Striker L. Pathogenic effects of advanced glycosylation: biochemical, biologic, and clinical implications for diabetes and aging. Lab Invest 1994;70:138–51.
74. Wilczek HE, Jaremko G, Tyden G, Groth CG. Evolution of diabetic nephropathy in kidney grafts. Evidence that a simultaneously transplanted pancreas exerts a protective effect. Transplantation 1995;59:51–7.
75. Yoshikawa Y, Truong LD, Mattioli CA, Ordonez NG, Balsaver AM. Membranous glomerulonephritis in diabetic patients: a study of 15 cases and review of the literature. Mod Pathol 1990;3:36–42.
76. Zhu D, Kim Y, Steffes MW, Groppoli TJ, Butkowski RJ, Mauer SM. Glomerular distribution of type IV collagen in diabetes by high resolution quantitative immunohistochemistry. Kidney Int 1994;45:425–33.
77. Ziyadeh FN, Goldfarb S. The renal tubulointerstitium in diabetes mellitus. Kidney Int 1991;39: 464–75.

18 THROMBOTIC MICROANGIOPATHIES AND COAGULOPATHIES

The thrombotic microangiopathies and coagulopathies comprise a spectrum of thrombotic and angiopathic lesions that affect small vessels, often including vessels in the kidneys. The three major categories of microangiopathies/coagulopathies are hemolytic uremic syndrome (HUS), thrombotic thrombocytopenic purpura (TTP), and disseminated intravascular coagulation (DIC). Although initially used as a diagnostic term for patients with TTP (3), thrombotic microangiopathy currently is used as a generic category for disease processes that have concurrent microvascular thrombosis, microangiopathic hemolytic anemia, and thrombocytopenia (1,2). Thus, both TTP and HUS are forms of thrombotic microangiopathy.

The archetype patient with HUS has post-diarrheal disease caused by *Escherichia coli,* which produce a Shiga-like toxin that injures the microvascular endothelium and results in an angiopathy with secondary thrombosis. The archetype patient with TTP has the clinical pentad of fever, microangiopathic hemolytic anemia, thrombocytopenia, fluctuating neurological status, and renal disease caused by platelet-rich thrombosis in small vessels of multiple organs including the kidneys. The archetype patient with DIC has sepsis-induced disease in which coagulation factors and platelets are activated to form fibrin-rich thrombi in the microvasculature of many organs, resulting in multiorgan failure. In their purest forms, HUS, TTP, and DIC have distinctive clinical and pathologic features, however, there are so many variations in these features that diagnostic categorization of individual patients may be complicated. In addition, there are multiple genetic and acquired causes for each category that must be identified whenever possible for optimum patient management (Table 18-1).

Table 18-1

THROMBOTIC MICROANGIOPATHIES AND COAGULOPATHIES

Hemolytic Uremic Syndrome (HUS)
- Shiga-like toxin–induced HUS (e.g., *Escherichia coli, Shigella dysenteriae*)
- Neuraminidase-induced HUS (e.g., *Streptococcus pneumoniae*)
- Iatrogenic HUS
  - Drug-induced HUS (e.g., cyclosporine, tacrolimus, mitomycin-C, cisplatin, oral contraceptives, quinine)
  - Bone marrow transplantation–induced HUS
  - Radiation-induced HUS
- Systemic sclerosis renal crisis HUS
- Pregnancy-associated HUS
- Familial HUS (e.g., autosomal recessive, autosomal dominant, factor H mutations)
- Malignant hypertensive nephropathy
- Radiation nephritis
- Idiopathic HUS

Antiphospholipid Antibody Syndrome (APS)
- Primary APS
- Secondary APS (e.g., secondary to systemic lupus erythematosus, rheumatoid arthritis)

Toxemia of Pregnancy
- Preeclampsia
- Eclampsia
- HELLP (hemolysis, elevated liver enzymes, low platelets) syndrome

Thrombotic Thrombocytopenic Purpura (TTP)
- Familial TTP (e.g., defects in or absence of vWF multimerase)[a]
- Autoimmune TTP (e.g., autoantibodies to vWF multimerase)
- Drug-induced TTP (e.g., ticlopidine, clopidogrel)
- Idiopathic TTP

Disseminated Intravascular Coagulation (DIC)
- Bacterial sepsis with DIC (e.g., Gram-negative sepsis)
- Viral hemorrhagic fever with DIC (e.g., Dengue, Marburg, Ebola)
- Neoplasia-induced DIC (e.g., pancreatic carcinoma–induced DIC)
- Pregnancy-related DIC (e.g., with retained dead fetus, placental separation)
- Trauma-induced DIC (e.g., penetrating head injury)
- Venom-induced DIC (e.g., snakebite)

[a]vWF = von Willebrand factor.

HEMOLYTIC UREMIC SYNDROME

Definition. HUS is characterized clinically by the concurrence of microangiopathic hemolytic

Table 18-2

PREDOMINANT PATHOLOGIC FEATURES AND MAJOR PATHOGENIC EVENTS IN THE THROMBOTIC MICROANGIOPATHIES AND COAGULOPATHIES

	Predominant Pathology	Major Pathogenic Event
Hemolytic uremic syndrome	Glomerular capillary subendothelial expansion, arteriolar fibrinoid necrosis, arterial edematous intimal expansion, vascular thrombosis	Endothelial injury caused by many different etiologies, predominantly in renal vessels, causing focal occlusion, thrombosis, and renal ischemia
Thrombotic thrombocytopenic purpura	Platelet-rich thrombi in many organs	Enhanced platelet aggregation, e.g., caused by abnormal vWF-cleaving metalloproteinase activity[a]
Disseminated intravascular coagulation	Fibrin-rich thrombi in many organs	Enhanced coagulation and fibrinolysis, e.g., caused by increased circulating tissue factor
Antiphospholipid antibody syndrome	Thrombosis in veins, arteries, arterioles, and capillaries; glomerular subendothelial expansion and GBM remodeling[a]	Antibodies to phospholipids or phospholipid-binding proteins that bind to endothelial cells or platelets to foster thrombosis
Preeclampsia/eclampsia	Glomerular capillary endothelial swelling (endotheliosis)	Abnormal placentation with generation of humoral factors that injure maternal endothelial cells

[a]vWF = von Willebrand factor; GMB = glomerular basement membrane.

anemia and acute renal failure, and pathologically by a distinctive, although not completely specific, renal angiopathy (Table 18-2). HUS is distinguished from TTP by more severe renal involvement and by less multiorgan involvement, however, there are overlapping clinical and pathologic features.

Clinical Features. Patients with all forms of HUS typically have features of microangiopathic hemolytic anemia, including anemia, schistocytosis, and thrombocytopenia (5,22,26). In addition to the anemia and schistocytosis, evidence of hemolysis includes reticulocytosis, elevated serum lactic dehydrogenase levels and reduced haptoglobin. Giant platelets may be seen on blood smears. Almost all patients have some degree of hematuria and proteinuria, and about a third have oliguria. The microangiopathy is the primary abnormality and the hemolytic anemia and thrombocytopenia are secondary. Thus, it is not surprising that some patients with unequivocal pathologic evidence of HUS lack significant anemia or thrombocytopenia (8). This could be due to mild disease without extensive erythrocyte fragmentation and platelet consumption, or very severe disease that prevents enough blood from flowing through injured vessels to cause erythrocyte fragmentation and platelet consumption.

Patients with HUS who do not have diarrhea have a higher incidence of hypertension (approximately 50 percent) than do patients with HUS associated with diarrhea (approximately 25 percent). Patients with thrombotic microangiopathy due to malignant hypertensive nephropathy and systemic sclerosis renal crisis tend to have a less severe form of anemia and thrombocytopenia than those with other forms of HUS. Leukocytosis may be present, especially in patients with postdiarrheal HUS (19). Occasional patients have hypocomplementemia (31a). Manifestations of central nervous system involvement may develop, such as seizures and coma, but are less frequent than with TTP. Unlike DIC, patients with HUS usually have normal prothrombin times and partial thromboplastin times. Although the pathology is indistinguishable, there are a number of etiologically distinct categories of HUS that cause characteristic clinical features, such as an association with infection, pregnancy, autoimmune disease, or drug therapy (Table 18-1).

Postdiarrheal HUS is the most common cause of acute renal failure in young children in North America. In the United States, up to 90 percent of HUS in children is caused by Shiga-like toxin–producing *E. coli* (19,31a); this type of HUS is sometimes designated D+ HUS to distinguish it from HUS that is not associated with diarrhea (D- HUS) (26). D+ HUS most often is caused by O157:H7 *E. coli* (7). Approximately 5 to 10 percent of patients with Shiga-like toxin–producing *E. coli* infections develop HUS (19). The microangiopathic hemolytic anemia and acute renal failure develop abruptly about 1 week after the onset of the acute gastroenteritis and diarrhea.

The most common form of pregnancy-associated HUS is acute postpartum HUS, which typically develops 1 to 2 weeks after an apparently normal pregnancy (32). HUS also may develop during pregnancy, however, this is rare compared to postpartum HUS and must be distinguished from severe preeclampsia/eclampsia and HELLP (hemolysis, elevated liver enzymes, and low platelets) syndrome (6,12).

Treatment with cytotoxic drugs, calcineurin inhibitors, radiation, and bone marrow transplantation can induce HUS (4,10,35). *Bone marrow transplant nephropathy* may in fact be caused by the combined or independent effects of chemotherapy and radiation (10). There may be a long latency period between exposure to radiation and the development of *radiation nephritis*. Thus, this possibility must be considered even with a relatively remote history of radiation exposure.

Systemic sclerosis renal crisis is caused by an acute episode of thrombotic microangiopathy that usually is superimposed on chronic systemic sclerosis vascular injury. Patients present with sudden onset of malignant hypertension, rapid loss of renal function, and high levels of circulating renin (9,14). An episode of renal crisis in a patient with systemic sclerosis can be precipitated by conditions that reduce renal blood flow, such as cold, dehydration, sepsis, or cardiac disease (14). Compared to most other forms of thrombotic microangiopathy, systemic sclerosis renal crisis is associated with a lower frequency of, and less severe, microangiopathic hemolytic anemia. Most patients have characteristic features of systemic sclerosis, including scleroderma, however, some do not, and the findings on renal biopsy are the first suggestion of the disease (9). Serology for antitopoisomerase antibodies (anti-Scl-70) is very useful for supporting a diagnosis of systemic sclerosis in a patient with atypical clinical features. Distinguishing this variant of thrombotic microangiopathy from other forms is important because patient prognosis and therapy differ. For example, angiotensin converting enzyme inhibitors dramatically improve the renal outcome if patients are treated promptly (9,14). Although severe hypertension often contributes to the renal vascular injury in systemic sclerosis, there are mechanisms other than hypertension that cause vascular injury, and a few patients with acute vasculopathy do not have severe hypertension (21).

Patients with malignant hypertensive nephropathy have a thrombotic microangiopathy that can be pathologically indistinguishable from other causes of HUS, especially systemic sclerosis. Clinically, however, the hemolytic anemia and thrombocytopenia often are less severe, and, pathologically, chronic hypertensive vasculopathy usually is in the background (36). Malignant hypertensive nephropathy is covered in detail in chapter 16.

Gross Findings. In the acute phase of HUS, the kidneys typically are enlarged (9a). There may be petechial and purpuric hemorrhages on the external and cut surfaces (fig. 18-1), however, this is less frequent than with TTP and DIC. In severe cases, widespread or focal cortical necrosis appears as slightly bulging pale zones (22). The zones of necrosis usually are not wedge shaped (i.e., are not broader at the capsule), which differs from the typical wedge-shaped infarcts caused by more localized occlusion of larger arteries (e.g., polyarteritis nodosa and other vasculitides, and thromboembolic disease). In the chronic phase in patients who have sustained substantial irreversible injury, the kidneys are small and may have scattered, depressed scars and calcifications at sites of earlier cortical necrosis. The external surface may be coarsely granular as a result of alternating zones of greater and lesser degrees of ischemic atrophy or scarring (fig. 18-2).

Light Microscopic Findings. Histologic abnormalities may be isolated to glomeruli, arterioles, or small arteries, or, most often, involve varying combinations of these structures (Table 18-2) (5,9a,16,20,22,25,31). HUS of different causes (Table 18-1) has pathologic changes that are indistinguishable from each other, although there are characteristic trends in some categories.

The most ubiquitous glomerular lesion is capillary wall thickening, caused in the acute phase

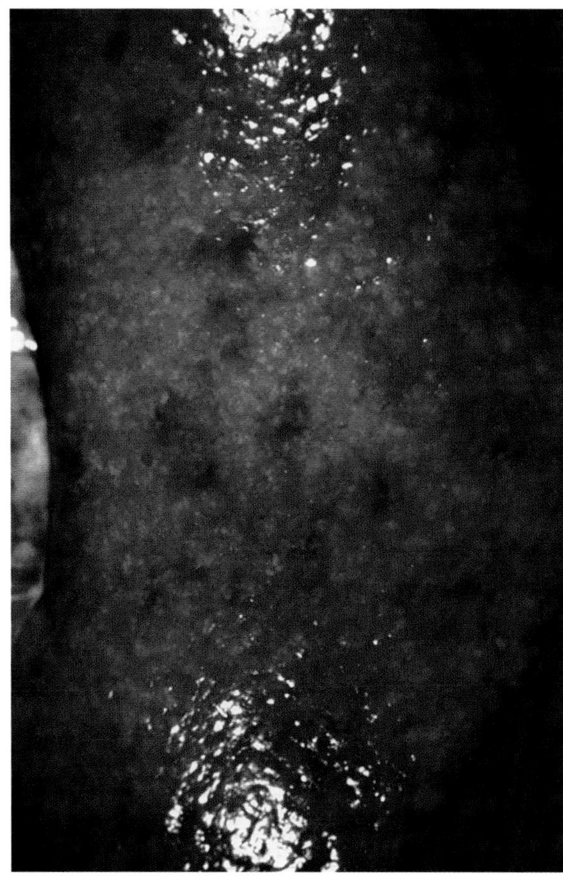

Figure 18-1

ACUTE THROMBOTIC MICROANGIOPATHY INDUCED BY SYSTEMIC SCLEROSIS RENAL CRISIS

There are scattered hemorrhages as well as many small pale areas corresponding to foci of infarction (focal cortical necrosis).

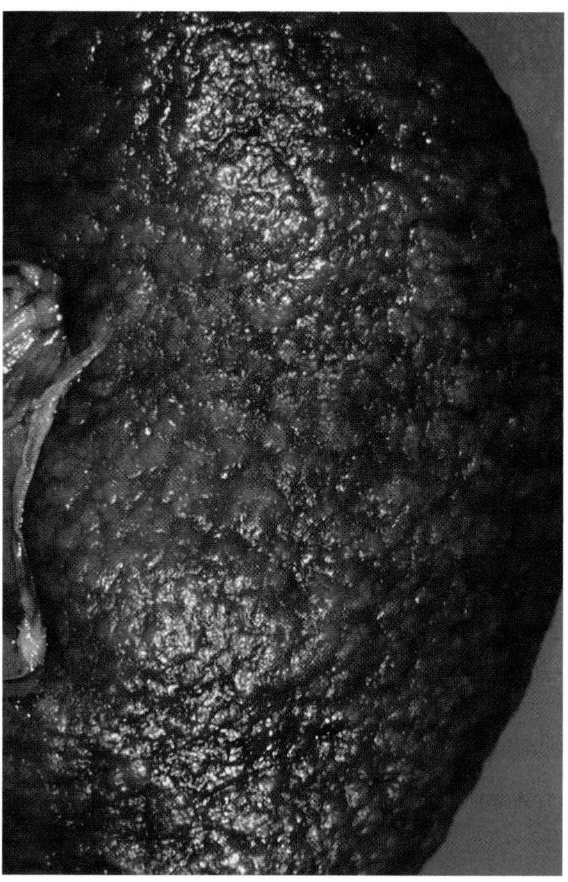

Figure 18-2

CHRONIC ISCHEMIC INJURY CAUSED BY SYSTEMIC SCLEROSIS

The external surface is coarsely granular as a result of focal disproportionate retraction in the areas of most severe ischemic atrophy and scarring.

by expansion of the subendothelial zone (figs. 18-3, 18-4). Subendothelial expansion often is readily apparent by light microscopy (fig. 18-4), but when mild may only be identified by electron microscopy. Some glomeruli or glomerular segments appear bloodless because of the obliteration of lumens by the thickened capillary walls, whereas others are markedly congested, possibly because of downstream occlusion of blood flow. Within days of the initial acute injury, extensions of mesangial cytoplasm grow into the expanded subendothelial zones and lay down new basement membrane material. This results in a complex replication of basement membrane material seen well with the periodic acid–Schiff (PAS) and Jones methenamine silver (JMS) stains (fig. 18-5). Wrinkling of the glomerular basement membranes may occur, especially when there is extensive arterial disease causing glomerular ischemia (fig. 18-6).

Mesangiolysis usually is present, at least focally, and is very conspicuous in some specimens (figs. 18-6, left; 18-7; 18-8, left) (20). Mesangiolysis may be the mesangial counterpart of subendothelial expansion. Acute mesangiolysis is characterized by expansion of the matrix by poorly staining material and coalescence of capillary loops (capillary aneurysm formation) as a result of separation of segments of paramesangial basement membrane from the mesangial matrix. This is analogous to the separation of the capillary wall basement membrane from the endothelial cells. In both instances, edematous zones that have reduced collagenous matrix material separate the cells from the basement membrane. The expanded mesangial areas may have almost no staining with JMS or PAS. Capillary walls and mesangial areas at sites of subendothelial expansion and mesangiolysis may contain fragmented erythrocytes (schistocytes). Mesangiolysis is particularly prominent in some examples of HUS caused by radiation or chemotherapeutic drugs (fig. 18-8, left). Additional features of radiation, and to a lesser extent chemotherapy, injury include tubular and glomerular epithelial cell atypia and nucleomegaly caused by perturbations in cell division and polyploidy (fig. 18-8, right).

Eventually, the mesangial areas that are expanded by mesangiolysis fill with increasing amounts of collagen, giving the glomerular tuft a somewhat lobular appearance. This lobular pattern along with the replication of glomerular basement membranes that develops as a consequence of the subendothelial expansion gives a light microscopic pattern that mimics membranoproliferative glomerulonephritis, albeit with less glomerular hypercellularity (fig. 18-5, right); however, the findings by immunofluorescence and electron microscopy allow differentiation between the two.

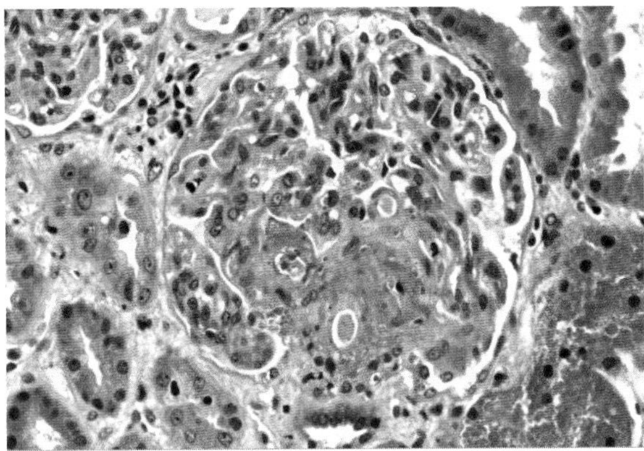

Figure 18-3

HEMOLYTIC UREMIC SYNDROME

The glomerular capillary walls are variably thickened, resulting in focal narrowing or obliteration of lumens. The hilum shows fibrinoid necrosis containing schistocytes (hematoxylin and eosin [H&E] stain).

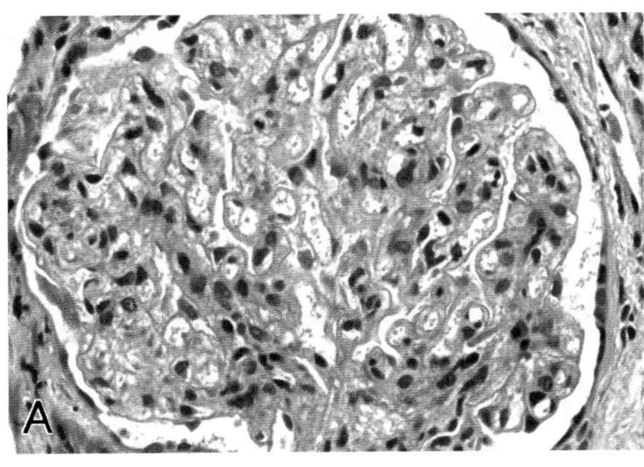

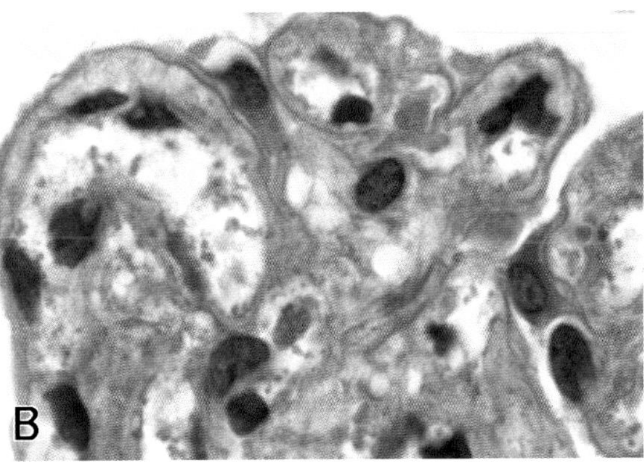

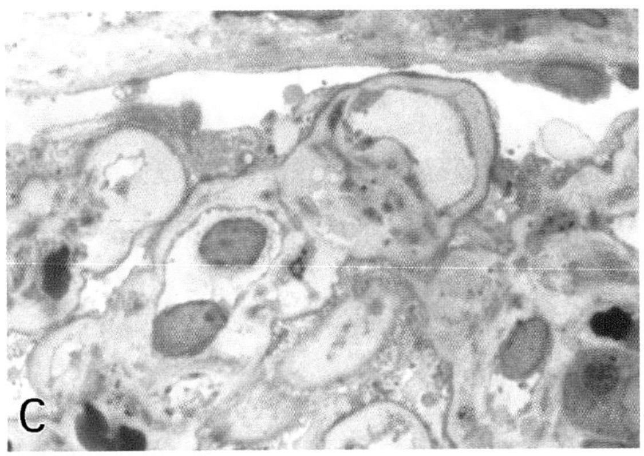

Figure 18-4

HEMOLYTIC UREMIC SYNDROME

A: There is global thickening of glomerular capillary walls caused by expansion of the subendothelial zone.

B: The global thickening can be seen in the paraffin section with an H&E stain at high magnification.

C: The thickening is seen best in the 1-µm plastic section stained with toluidine blue.

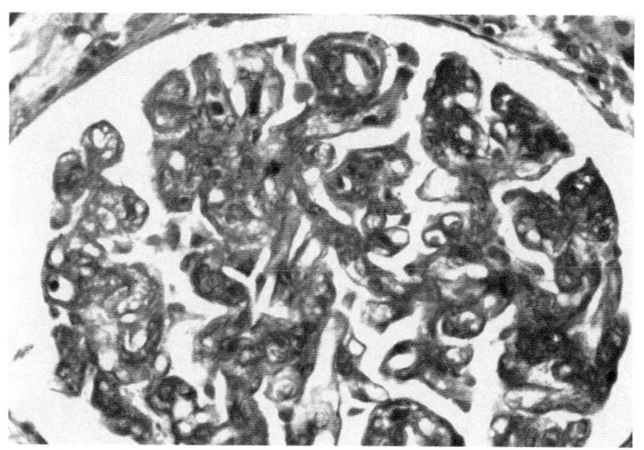

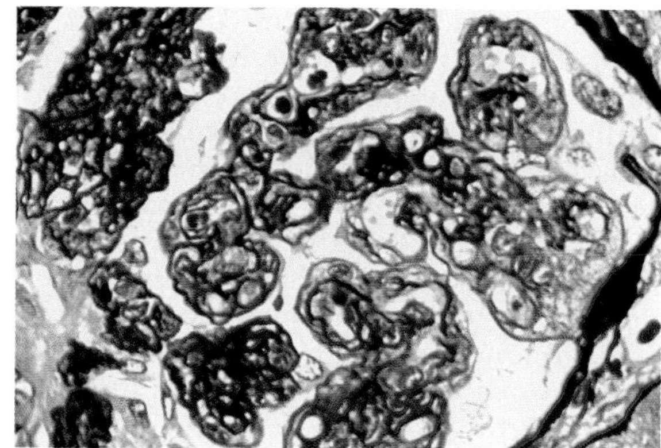

Figure 18-5

HEMOLYTIC UREMIC SYNDROME

Extensive glomerular basement membrane remodeling has produced complex replication that can be seen with a PAS stain (left) or Jones methenamine silver (JMS) stain (right). The mesangial matrix also is expanded.

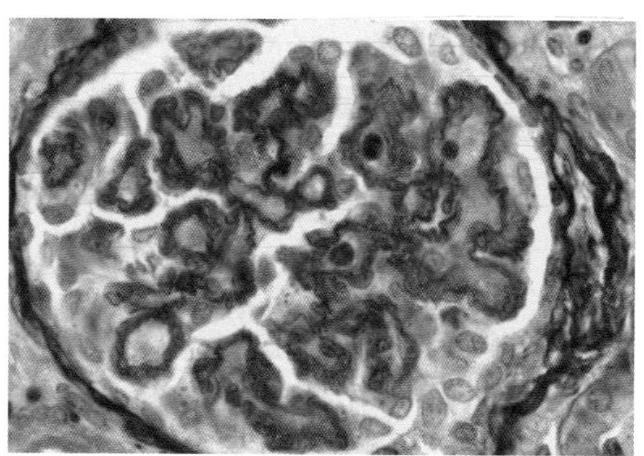

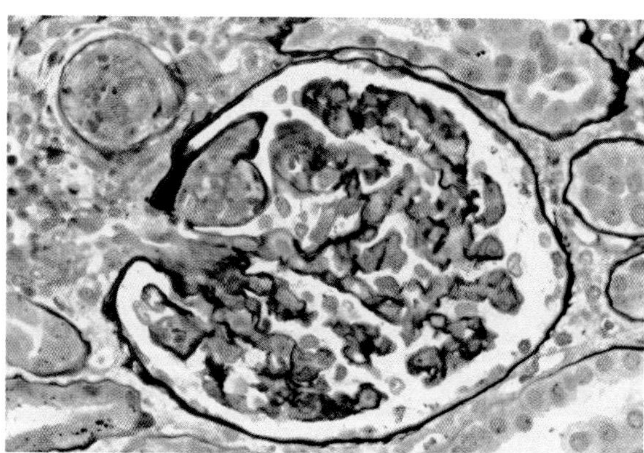

Figure 18-6

HEMOLYTIC UREMIC SYNDROME

Glomeruli from two different specimens both show glomerular basement membrane wrinkling and mesangiolysis. Compared to figure 18-3, much of the mesangial areas do not stain with the PAS (left) or JMS (right) stain. Some capillaries have coalesced to produce abnormally large lumens, especially in the left figure. Thrombosis in a hilar arteriole is seen in the right figure.

Specimens may have numerous glomerular capillary thrombi, or few or no capillary thrombi identifiable by light microscopy. Identification of thrombi is not necessary to make a pathologic diagnosis of HUS. Thrombi in HUS usually are red (fuchsinophilic) with the Masson trichrome stain (fig. 18-9A). Focal segmental glomerular fibrinoid necrosis may be identified (figs. 18-3, 18-7, 18-9, 18-10). Global fibrinoid necrosis is rare. Global coagulative necrosis also may occur, usually in or near zones of cortical necrosis (fig. 18-11). Foci of fibrinoid necrosis often are in the hilum and contiguous with fibrinoid necrosis in hilar arterioles. Whole and fragmented erythrocytes (schistocytes), and apoptotic or necrotic cells, often are in the foci of fibrinoid necrosis (figs. 18-3, 18-10); there may be a few marginated neutrophils as well. Crescent formation occurs in approximately 5 percent of HUS specimens (fig. 18-9C), but usually affects less than a quarter of glomeruli. When present, crescent formation often is adjacent to segments with thrombosis, extensive mesangiolysis, fibrinoid necrosis, or combinations of these lesions.

Acute arteriolar lesions include subendothelial expansion, fibrinoid necrosis, and thrombosis. Larger arterioles with a well-defined elastica are more likely to have subendothelial edematous intimal expansion, and smaller arterioles adjacent to the glomerular hilum are more likely to have fibrinoid necrosis. The fibrinoid necrosis is deeply acidophilic and usually has ragged outer borders that may extend for a short distance beyond the vessel wall (fig. 18-12). The fibrinoid material may contain erythrocytes and schistocytes. The fibrinoid necrosis of HUS differs from that of a necrotizing vasculitis because it lacks an associated conspicuous infiltrate of inflammatory cells. However, apoptotic nuclear debris and a few neutrophils often are within the fibrinoid material. Fibrinoid material is red (fuchsinophilic) with the Masson trichrome staining. Fibrinoid necrosis may be continuous with segmental fibrinoid necrosis in the hilum of the glomerulus. There may be dilation of the vessel at a site of fibrinoid necrosis. Fibrinoid necrosis often is accompanied by thrombosis in the lumen (fig. 18-13). As the fibrinoid necrosis ages, it is progressively replaced by collagenous matrix, resulting in arteriolar sclerosis. The sclerotic material is less deeply acidophilic and is blue or green with a Masson trichrome stain rather than red. An intermediate stage of cellular organization of vessel wall fibrinoid necrosis and thrombosis may produce a spherical mass of cells called a "glomeruloid" lesion or body (fig. 18-14).

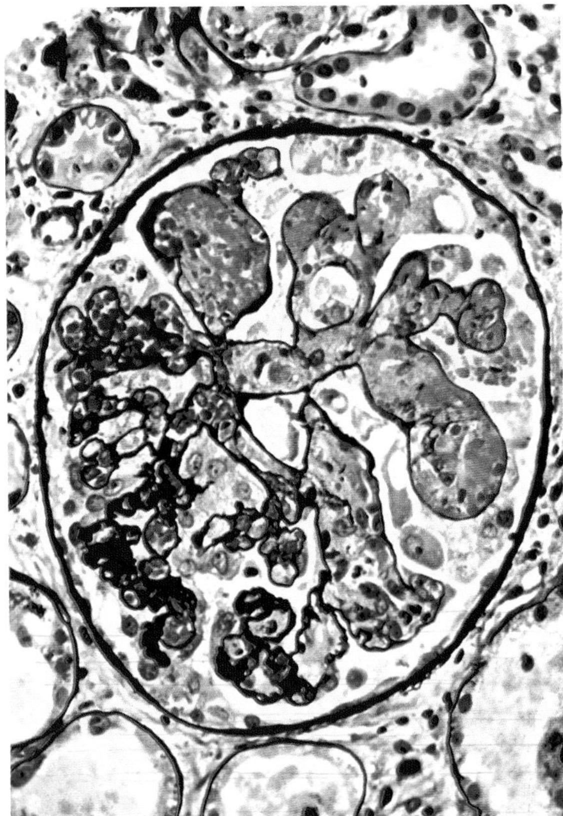

Figure 18-7

HEMOLYTIC UREMIC SYNDROME INDUCED BY ABRUPTIO PLACENTA

There is segmental necrosis with thrombosis and mesangiolysis. Complete loss of silver-positive mesangial matrix is seen in the segments at the upper right and top that have extensive mesangiolysis (JMS stain).

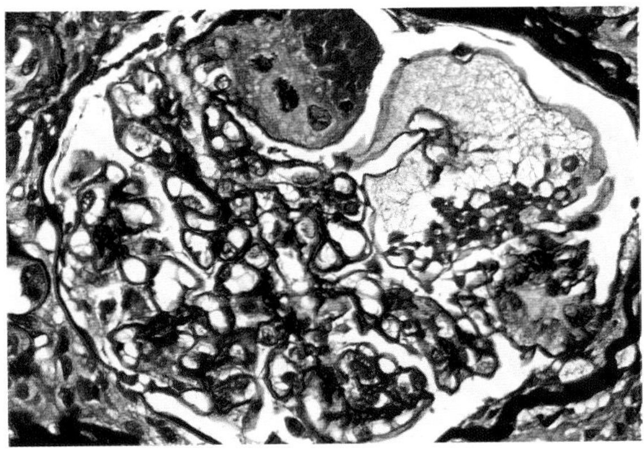

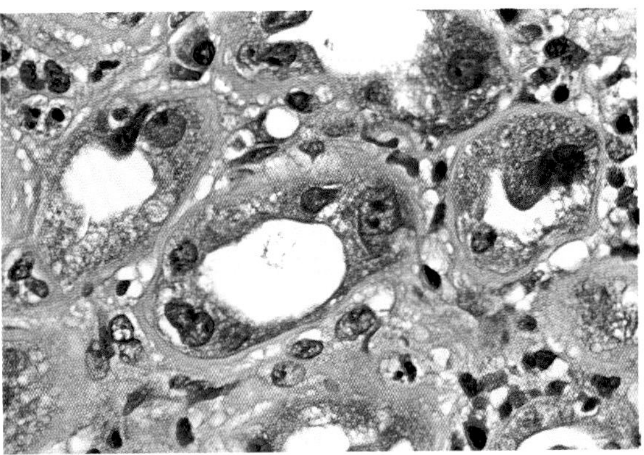

Figure 18-8

RADIATION NEPHRITIS

The glomerulus has prominent segmental mesangiolysis with formation of capillary microaneurysms (left, JMS stain); the tubular epithelial cells have atypia and nucleomegaly (right, H&E stain).

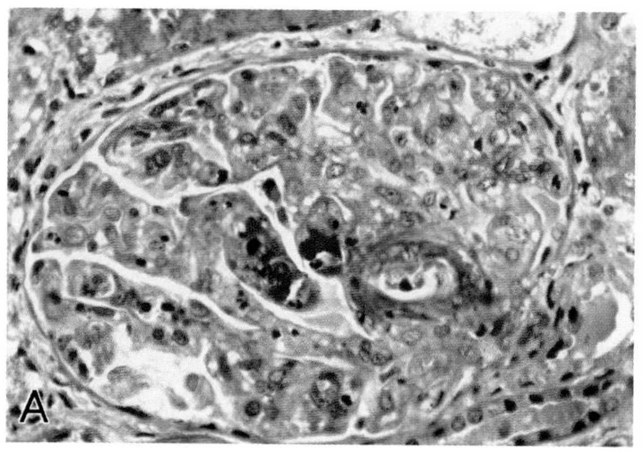

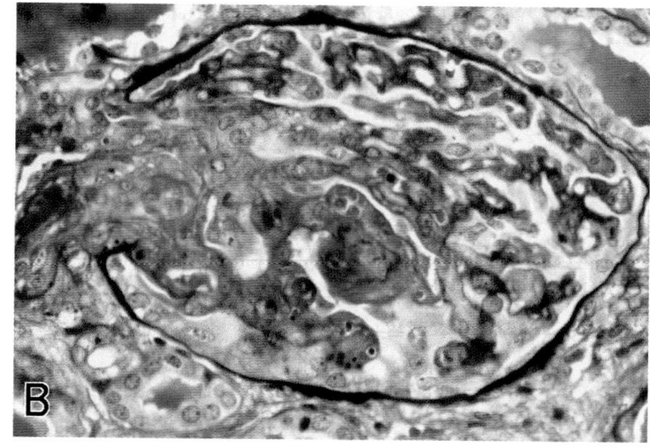

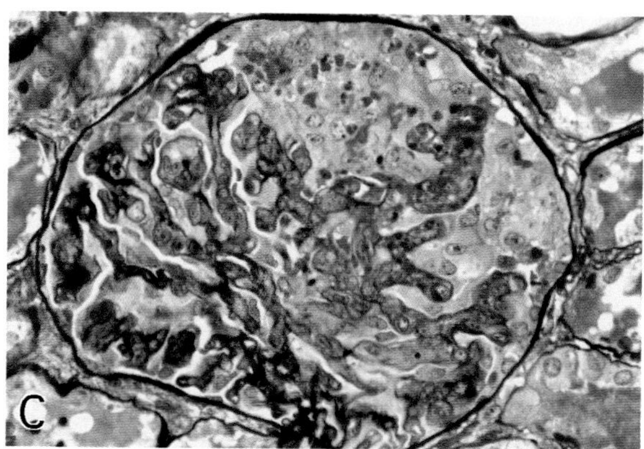

Figure 18-9

ACUTE POSTPARTUM HEMOLYTIC UREMIC SYNDROME

In addition to capillary wall thickening and focal obliteration of lumens, there are capillary thrombi (dark red material in capillary lumens in panel A with Masson trichrome stain), segmental fibroid necrosis (A, B, and C), and crescent formation adjacent to segmental fibrinoid necrosis (C). Note also the scattered apoptotic nuclei probably derived from endothelial cells (B and C, stained with the JMS stain and H&E counterstain).

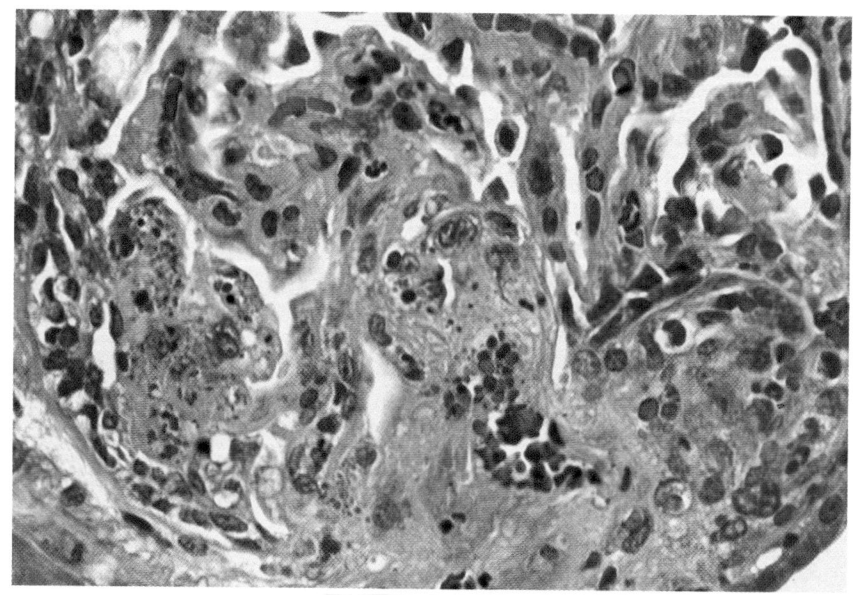

Figure 18-10

HEMOLYTIC UREMIC SYNDROME

This glomerular hilum has areas of fibrinoid necrosis, which contain numerous schistocytes, within areas of mesangiolysis.

The most common acute lesion in arcuate and interlobular arteries is edematous or mucoid intimal thickening (figs. 18-15, 18-16). In acute lesions, the expanded intima is clear or stains poorly with the hematoxylin and eosin (H&E) stain. Often, however, the expanded intima has a slightly basophilic appearance because of the accumulation of acid mucopolysaccharides (glycosaminoglycans), which can be detected with an alcian blue stain (fig. 18-17).

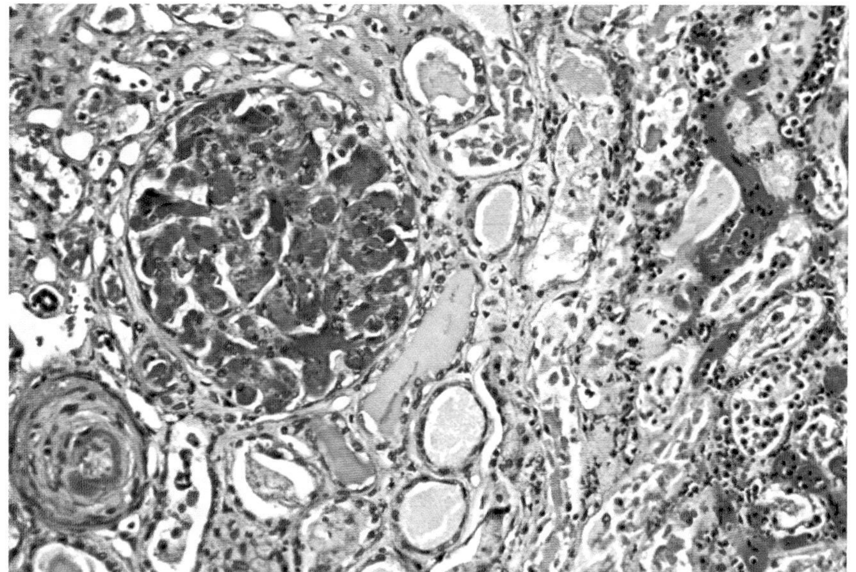

Figure 18-11

HEMOLYTIC UREMIC SYNDROME WITH FOCAL CORTICAL NECROSIS

In this patient with systemic sclerosis renal crisis, there is cortical necrosis on the right with secondary infiltration of neutrophils. There is extensive thrombosis and necrosis of the glomerulus. The artery at the lower left has intimal thickening and luminal thrombosis.

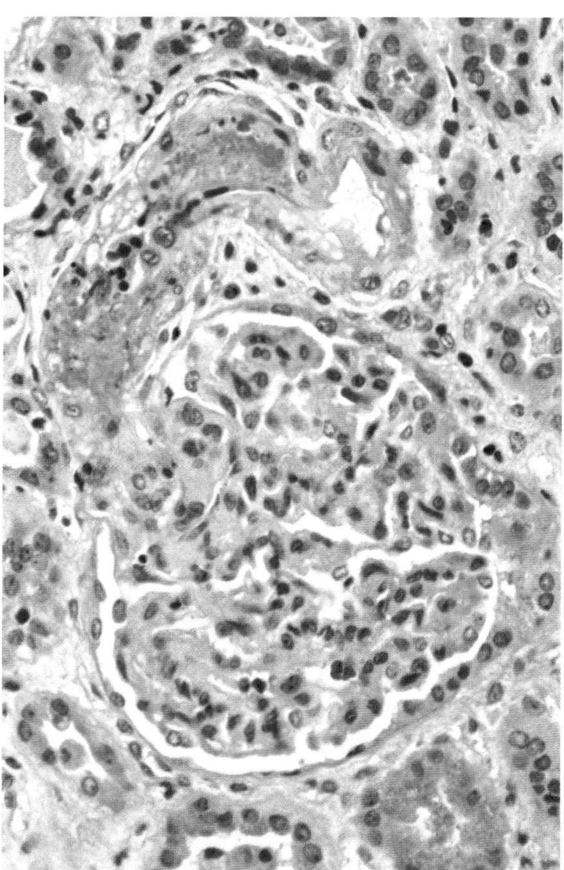

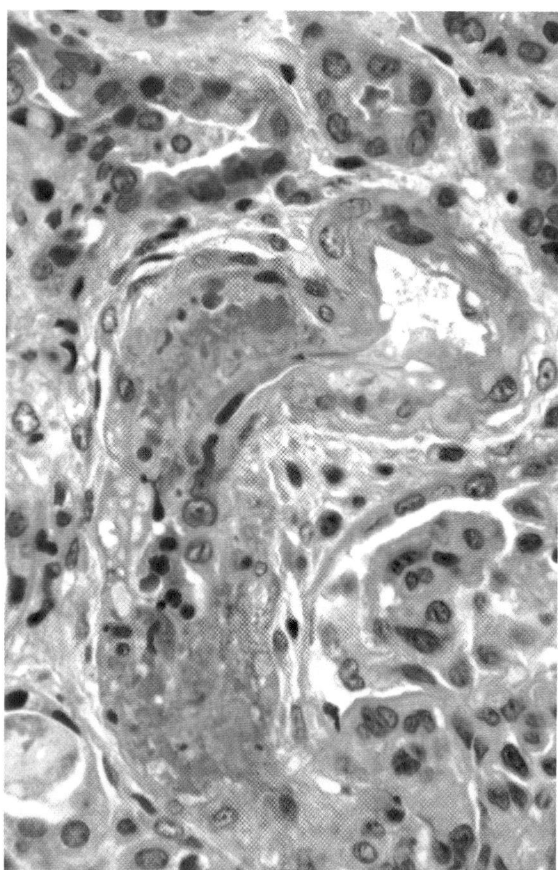

Figure 18-12

HEMOLYTIC UREMIC SYNDROME

The areas of fibrinoid necrosis in the hilar arteriole contain erythrocytes, schistocytes, and apoptotic debris probably derived primarily from endothelial cells and myocytes (H&E stain).

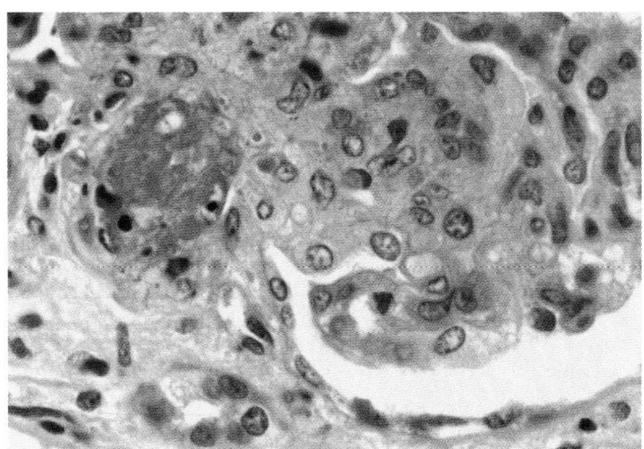
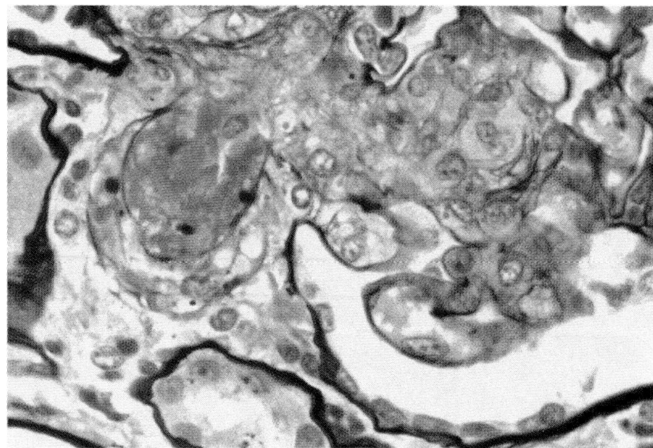

Figure 18-13

HEMOLYTIC UREMIC SYNDROME

The hilar arteriole contains a thrombus. Endothelial cells are gone and some myocytes are apoptotic/necrotic. The low intensity staining of the mesangium with the JMS stain in the right figure is indicative of mesangiolysis. The H&E stain (left) accentuates a few schistocytes in the zone of mesangiolysis.

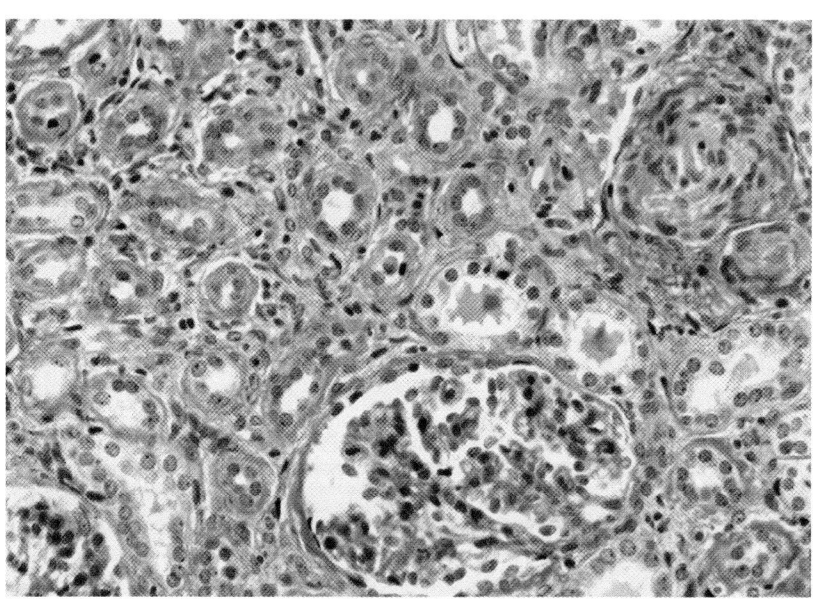

Figure 18-14

HEMOLYTIC UREMIC SYNDROME

This is a late lesion with ischemic glomerular and tubulointerstitial changes; a glomeruloid structure is at the upper right. The glomeruloid structure is produced by proliferating endothelial cells, smooth muscle cells, and myofibroblasts in response to arteriolar injury. The basement membranes of the glomerulus are wrinkled. There is diffuse tubular atrophy and interstitial fibrosis.

Thus, the intimal alteration sometimes is called "mucoid" intimal expansion. The expanded intima may contain schistocytes (fig. 18-16) and the narrowed lumen may become thrombosed (fig. 18-18).

As the lesion ages, the basophilic, amphophilic, or acidophilic staining varies in intensity. There is progressive ingrowth of spindle cells (smooth muscle cells, myofibroblasts, fibroblasts) into the thickened intima, and progressive accumulation of matrix. The early phase of intimal organization resembles undifferentiated mesenchymal tissue, with few cells and a somewhat basophilic or amphophilic matrix that is sometimes called "mucoid" or "myxoid" intimal thickening. As more collagen is deposited, the thickened intima becomes more acidophilic and eventually is overtly fibrotic. Acute arterial lesions are superimposed on chronic fibrotic intimal thickening, especially in malignant nephrosclerosis and progressive systemic sclerosis renal crisis (fig. 18-19). In both of these diseases, there have been reports of antecedent chronic phases of the vasculopathies going on for years that become

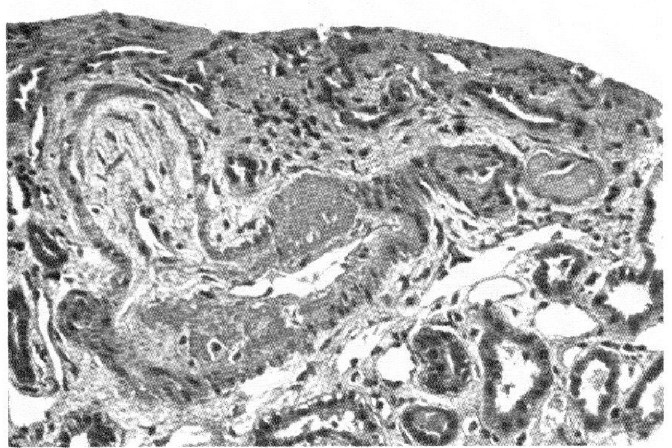

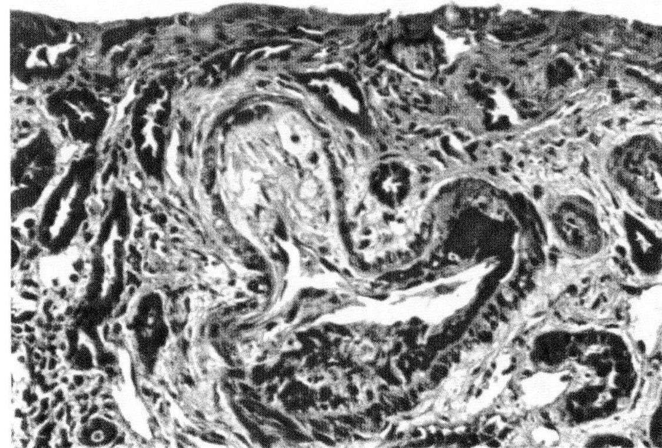

Figure 18-15

HEMOLYTIC UREMIC SYNDROME

Left: This oblique section through an interlobular artery and arteriole shows marked edematous intimal expansion in the portion of the artery farthest from the arteriole, and fibrinoid change in the artery wall closest to the arteriole and in the arteriole.

Right: The fibrinoid material is red (fuchsinophilic) with the Masson trichrome stain.

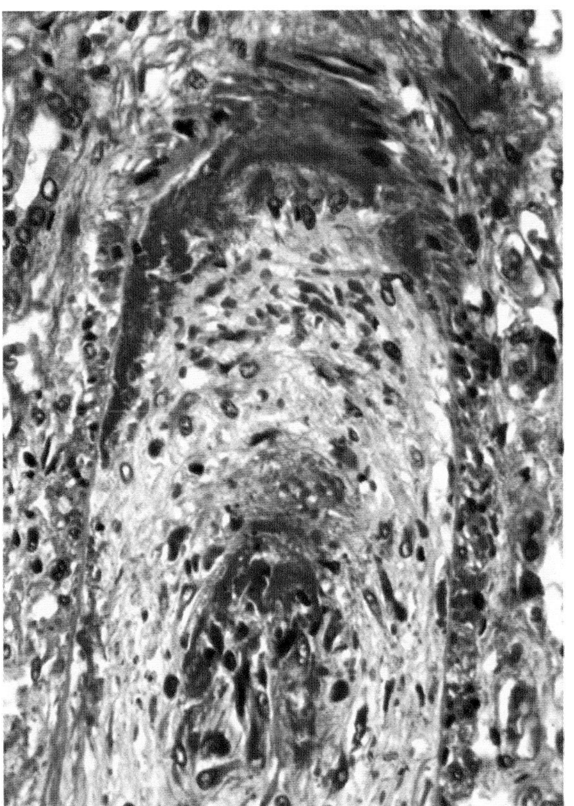

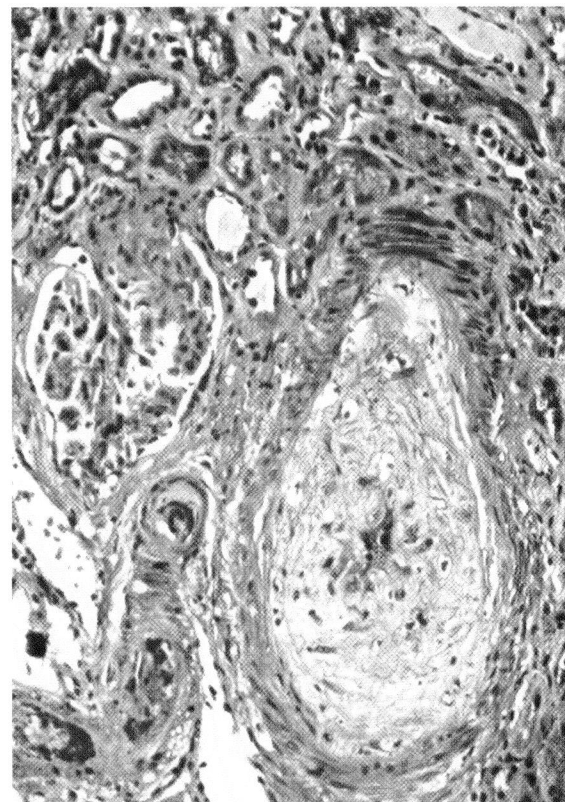

Figure 18-16

SYSTEMIC SCLEROSIS RENAL CRISIS HEMOLYTIC UREMIC SYNDROME

Both figures show severe edematous intimal expansion in an interlobular artery with almost total occlusion of the lumen.

Left: Focal fibrinoid material and scattered schistocytes are seen in the intima (H&E stain).

Right: There is fibrinoid necrosis and thrombosis in the arteriole in the lower left, segmental consolidation of the glomerulus, and ischemic simplification of some tubular epithelial cells (Masson trichrome stain).

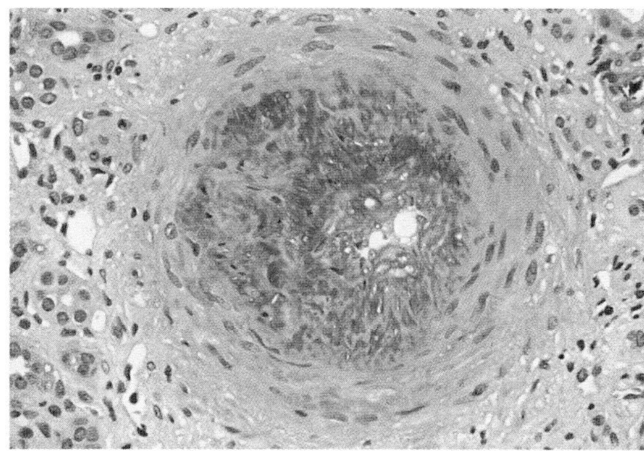

Figure 18-17

SYSTEMIC SCLEROSIS RENAL CRISIS
HEMOLYTIC UREMIC SYNDROME

There is severe intimal expansion of an interlobular artery, with almost total occlusion of the lumen. This alcian blue stain documents the presence of acid mucopolysaccharides in the extracellular matrix of the intima.

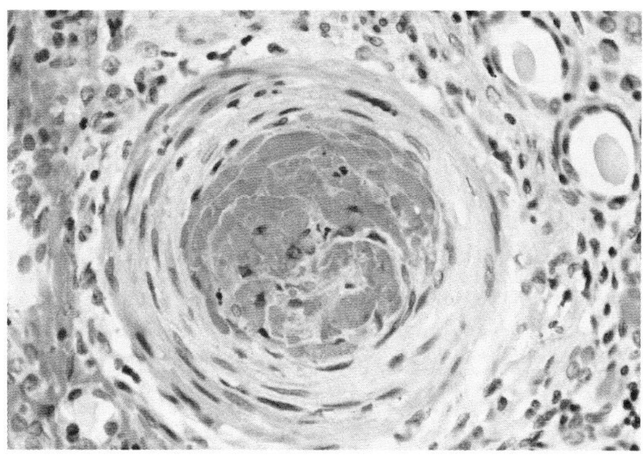

Figure 18-18

HEMOLYTIC UREMIC SYNDROME

There are severe arterial changes with marked intimal expansion and luminal thrombosis (H&E stain).

complicated by accelerated acute phases. The acute vascular lesions of HUS eventually evolve into chronic arteriolosclerosis and arteriosclerosis. The intimal fibrosis may form concentric laminations producing an "onion skin" pattern (fig. 18-20).

In the acute phase, the cortical tubulointerstitial tissue may be relatively normal, or, more often, has varying degrees of interstitial edema, tubular epithelial simplification (ischemic flattening with loss of brush border), and focal coagulative necrosis (focal cortical necrosis). Interstitial neutrophilic infiltration accompanies the ischemic necrosis. There may be scattered interstitial hemorrhages. As the disease progresses, more chronic ischemic changes develop, such as tubular atrophy, interstitial fibrosis, and usually mild focal interstitial infiltration of mononuclear leukocytes (figs. 18-14–18-16, 18-20, 18-21). In patients who develop substantial chronic sequelae of HUS, in addition to chronic tubulointerstitial and chronic arterial and arteriolar disease, the glomeruli have varying degrees of focal segmental to global sclerosis (figs. 18-20, 18-21).

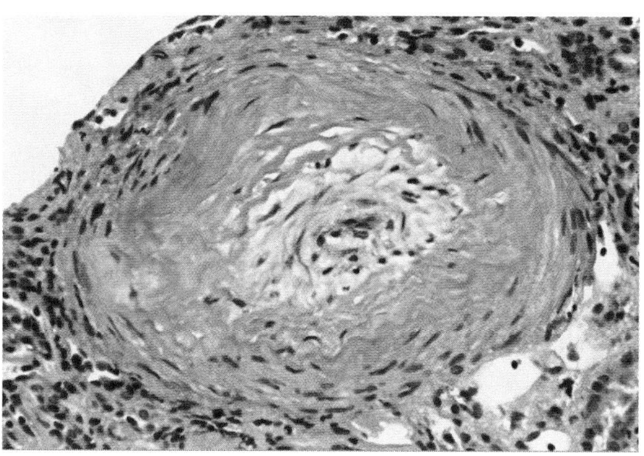

Figure 18-19

SYSTEMIC SCLEROSIS VASCULOPATHY

The acute edematous intimal expansion is superimposed on preexisting chronic fibrotic intimal thickening.

Immunofluorescence Findings. Immunohistology demonstrates fibrin and fibrinogen in thrombi within glomerular capillaries (fig. 18-22), arterioles, and arteries (9a,13,20,25). Foci of fibrinoid necrosis and edematous intimal expansion stain irregularly for fibrin and fibrinogen, as well as immunoglobulin (Ig)M, complement (C)3, and C1q (figs. 18-22–18-24). Staining for IgG and IgA typically is negative.

Electron Microscopic Findings. The findings by electron microscopy confirm the features seen by light microscopy (9a,22,24). In glomerular capillaries, the most ubiquitous finding is irregular, electron-lucent expansion of the subendothelial zone (figs. 18-25–18-27). This may be so extensive that the capillary lumen is completely obliterated. Endothelial cells may be swollen, but this is less pronounced than in the endotheliosis of preeclampsia/eclampsia. Thrombi, which contain varying mixtures of platelets and fibrin, may be seen in the lumens

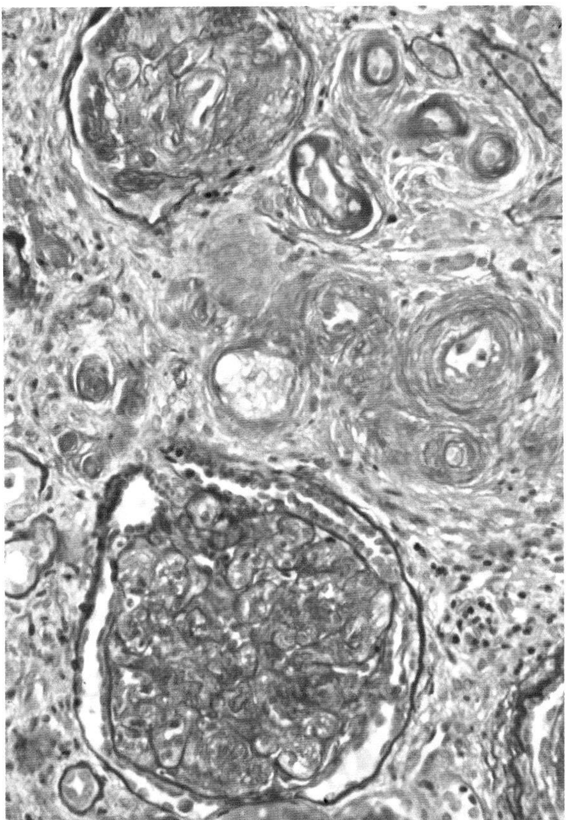

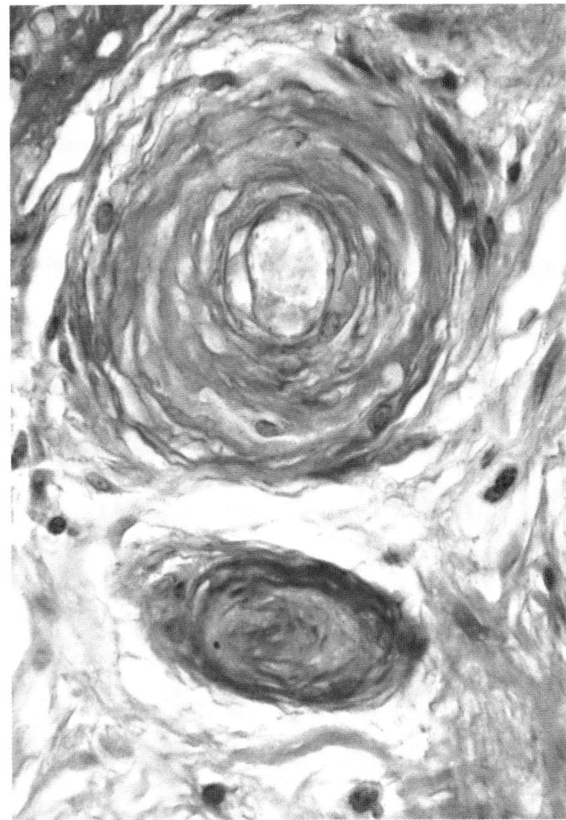

Figure 18-20

CHRONIC VASCULOPATHY CAUSED BY HEMOLYTIC UREMIC SYNDROME

There are extensive sclerotic changes in glomeruli, arterioles, and arteries, as well as interstitial fibrosis, tubular atrophy, and slight interstitial infiltration by mononuclear leukocytes. Laminations in the fibrotic intima give the arteries an "onion skin" pattern (PAS stain).

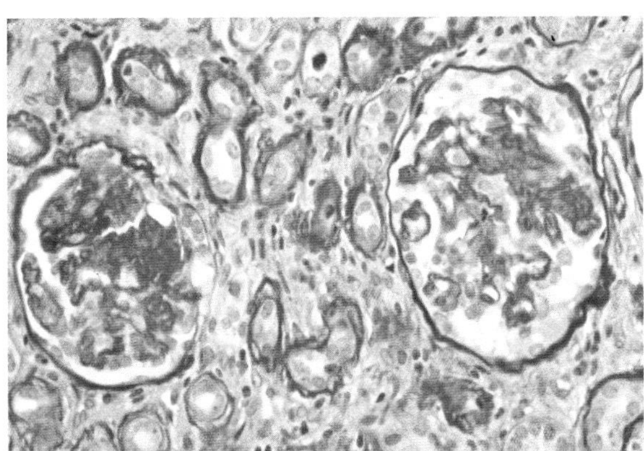

Figure 18-21

CHRONIC SEQUELAE OF HEMOLYTIC UREMIC SYNDROME

There is wrinkling of glomerular basement membranes, segmental glomerular sclerosis, tubular atrophy, interstitial fibrosis, and slight interstitial infiltration by mononuclear leukocytes.

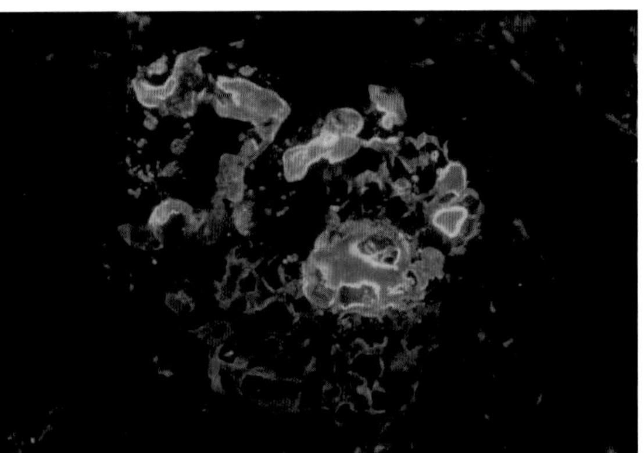

Figure 18-22

HEMOLYTIC UREMIC SYNDROME

A glomerulus has capillary thrombi and a zone of fibrinoid necrosis that stain with a fluoresceinated antiserum specific for fibrinogen.

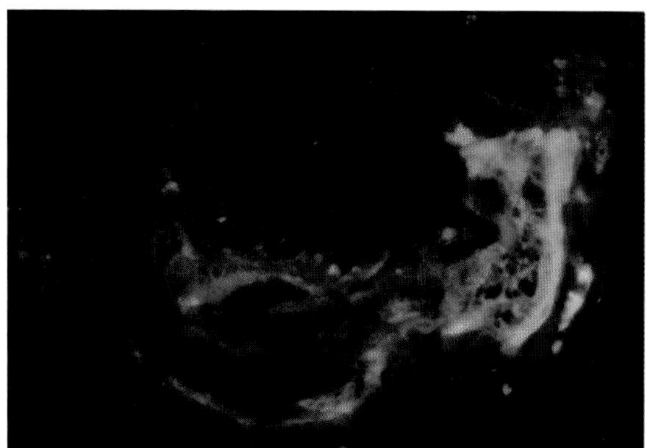

Figure 18-23

HEMOLYTIC UREMIC SYNDROME

Fluoresceinated antiserum specific for fibrin and fibrinogen irregularly stains the fibrinoid necrosis of a hilar arteriole.

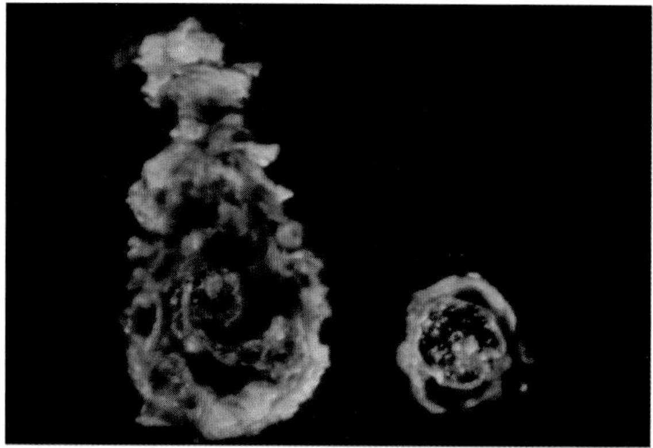

Figure 18-24

HEMOLYTIC UREMIC SYNDROME

The vessel walls of an interlobular artery and arteriole are stained irregularly with a fluoresceinated antiserum specific for IgM.

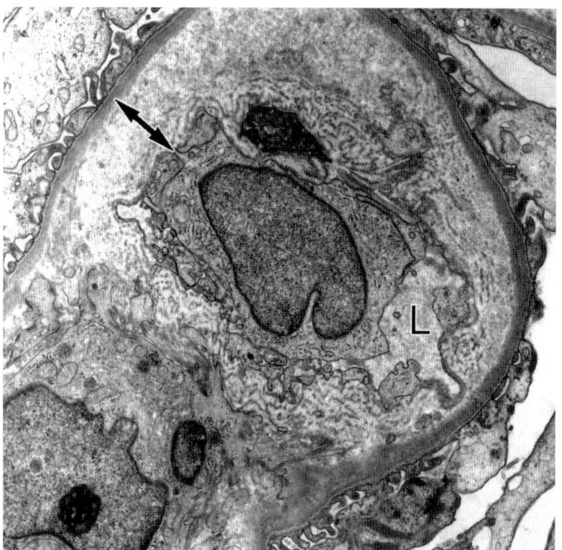

Figure 18-25

HEMOLYTIC UREMIC SYNDROME

The glomerular capillary lumen (L) is markedly narrowed by electron-lucent expansion of the subendothelial zone (double arrow).

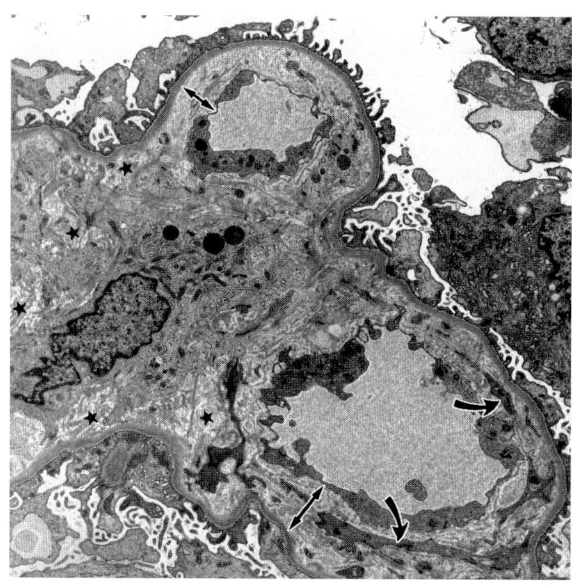

Figure 18-26

HEMOLYTIC UREMIC SYNDROME

Two capillary loops and adjacent mesangium show lucent expansion of the subendothelial zone (double arrows), subendothelial interposition of mesangial cytoplasm (curved arrows), and increased lucency of the mesangial matrix indicative of mesangiolysis (stars). There is slight swelling of the endothelial cytoplasm.

(fig. 18-28). The expanded subendothelial zone may contain flocculent, moderately electron-dense material, fibrin tactoids, or schistocytes. Extension of the electron-lucent zone into the mesangium, thus expanding the distance between the mesangial cells and the paramesangial basement membrane, is the ultrastructural counterpart of the mesangiolysis seen by light microscopy (figs. 18-26, 18-27). The mesangial matrix that is immediately beneath the paramesangial basement membrane is most prone to becoming electron lucent (mesangiolysis)

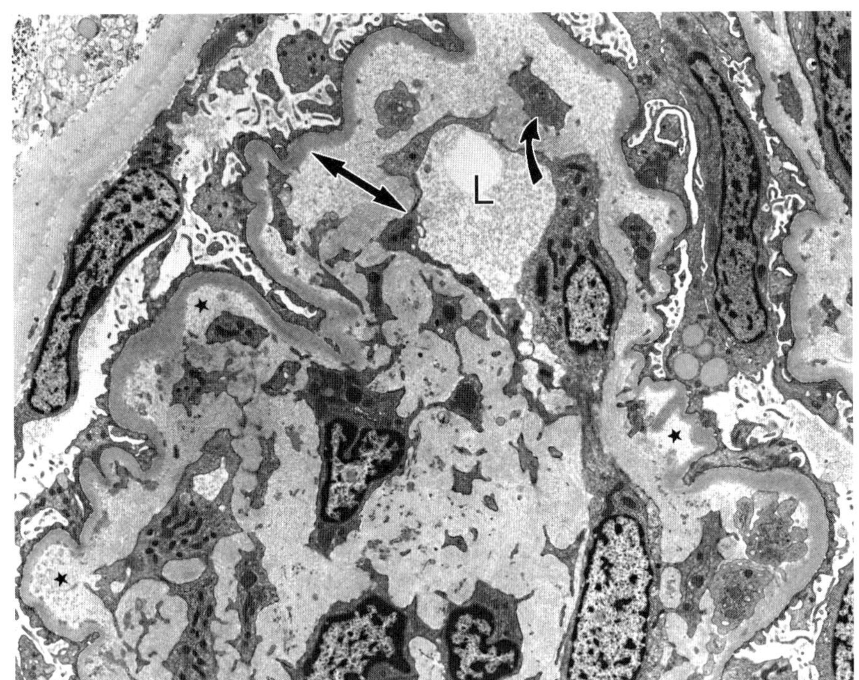

Figure 18-27

HEMOLYTIC UREMIC SYNDROME

There is marked electron-lucent expansion of the subendothelial zone (double arrow) and increased electron lucency of the mesangial matrix beneath the paramesangial basement membrane (mesangiolysis; stars). The central mesangial matrix also is increased. Note the effacement of podocyte foot processes and subendothelial extensions of mesangial cytoplasm (curved arrow).

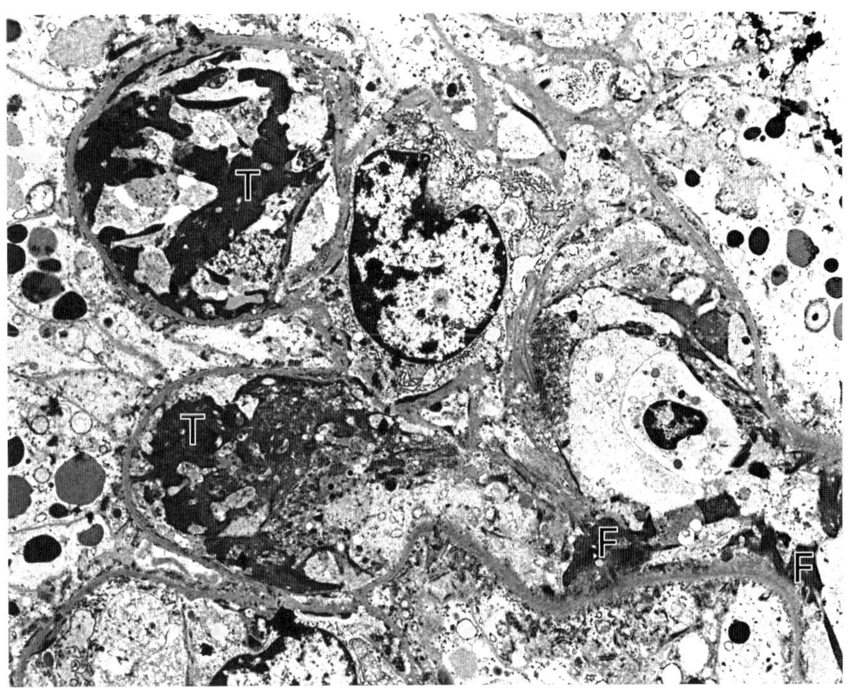

Figure 18-28

***STREPTOCOCCUS PNEUMONIAE*-INDUCED HEMOLYTIC UREMIC SYNDROME**

Two capillary lumens to the left are occluded by thrombi (T) composed of electron-dense fibrin admixed with degranulated platelets. Electron-dense fibrinous material also extends into the mesangium (F), indicative of fibrinoid necrosis. Endothelial cells are absent or necrotic.

(fig. 18-27). When this mesangiolysis is severe, the paramesangial basement membrane loses contact with the mesangium and balloons out to form part of the wall of a capillary aneurysm. Fragments of erythrocytes, platelets, and fibrin tactoids occasionally are identified in the zone of mesangiolysis. Focal effacement of podocyte foot processes is common. As the glomerular lesions age, there is mesangial interposition (fig. 18-26) and deposition of new matrix material in the capillary walls as well as increased matrix accumulation in the mesangium.

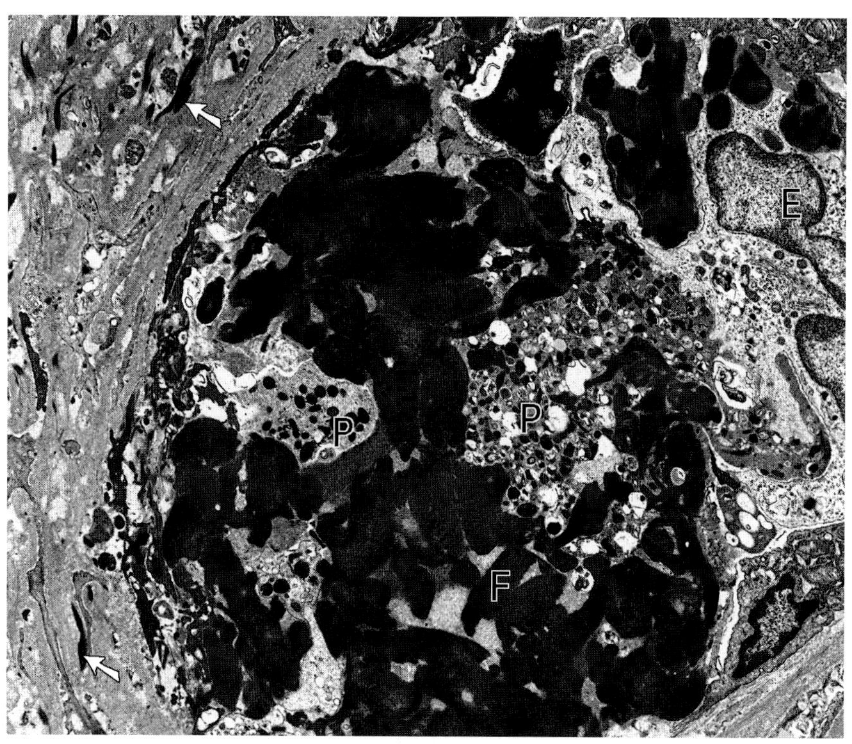

Figure 18-29

HEMOLYTIC UREMIC SYNDROME

This hilar arteriole contains a thrombus and has mural fibrinoid necrosis. There are electron-dense fibrin tactoids (F) admixed with platelets (P) in the lumen. A swollen endothelial cell (E) is to the right but the luminal surface on the left is denuded. On the left, the muscularis contains fibrin tactoids (arrows), indicative of fibrinoid necrosis.

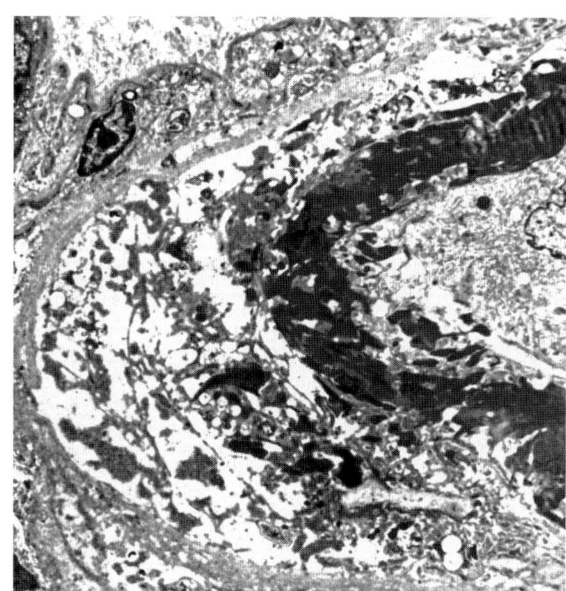

Figure 18-30

HEMOLYTIC UREMIC SYNDROME

The wall of this arteriole contains a band of irregular dense material that includes angular fibrin tactoids, indicative of fibrinoid necrosis.

The most widespread arteriolar and arterial lesion is expansion of the subendothelial zone (intima) by electron-lucent or electron-dense material. Thrombi may be identified that contain varying proportions of platelets and fibrin (fig. 18-29). The fibrin appears as amorphous dense material or curvilinear fibrin tactoids. Focal endothelial cell swelling or denudation often is seen at the sites of thrombosis, and occasionally elsewhere. At sites of fibrinoid necrosis, there is degeneration of myocytes and accumulation of electron-dense material in the muscularis that may form angular fibrin tactoids (fig. 18-30). At sites of edematous intimal thickening, there is an electron-lucent zone between the endothelium and the internal elastic lamina; this zone contains varying amounts of flocculent or fibrillar dense material, erythrocyte fragments, and elongated cells consistent with fibroblasts and myofibroblasts. As the intimal lesion evolves, the numbers of cells and interstitial collagen fibrils increase.

Differential Diagnosis. The various categories of HUS listed in Table 18-1 cannot be confidently distinguished from each other based on pathologic findings alone. As discussed in more detail later in this chapter, TTP and DIC have some pathologic features that overlap with HUS. TTP, and especially DIC, however, are characterized primarily by vascular thrombosis whereas HUS is characterized not only by thrombosis in the lumen but also by prominent vessel wall damage, even at sites where there is no thrombosis. Unfortunately, in many specimens there are substantial overlapping features because primary vessel wall injury may induce secondary thrombosis and primary thrombosis may induce secondary responses in vessel walls. For example, either pathway can eventually result in an artery with a thrombus in the lumen and an adjacent thickened intima. Thus, the pathologic findings in a tissue specimen should be correlated with clinical features before making a final interpretation.

The glomerular lesion of HUS (capillary wall thickening, glomerular basement membrane replication, and mesangial expansion) can resemble membranoproliferative glomerulonephritis although with less hypercellularity. The findings by immunofluorescence and electron microscopy readily rule out the latter. The chronic sclerotic phase of HUS may be difficult or impossible to distinguish from severe chronic hypertensive nephropathy. Knowledge of earlier pathologic or clinical features is required to conclude that the chronic vasculopathy evolved from acute HUS. HUS specimens with arteriolar fibrinoid necrosis, segmental glomerular fibrinoid necrosis, and crescent formation (which occurs rarely with HUS) can raise the possibility of pauci-immune necrotizing and crescentic glomerulonephritis and vasculitis. The absence of numerous leukocytes at sites of vascular necrosis and the presence of the typical glomerular capillary and arterial lesions of HUS rule out a diagnosis of glomerulonephritis or vasculitis.

Etiology and Pathogenesis. All forms of HUS appear to result from endothelial injury, however, there are multiple etiologic agents that can produce endothelial injury, leading to a final common pathway of pathologic changes and clinical manifestations that typify the HUS patient (19,22,26,31a). Injury to endothelial cells causes the cell surface to shift from an antithrombotic to a prothrombotic state, and if severe enough, causes endothelial apoptosis or necrosis that exposes or releases thrombogenic tissue components (e.g., tissue factor). Injury may result from the synergistic interactions of many factors, including various combinations of toxins (e.g., bacterial toxins), antibodies (e.g., antiendothelial antibodies, antiphospholipid antibodies), vasculotoxic therapeutic agents (e.g., calcineurin inhibitors, chemotherapeutic drugs), radiation, lipopolysaccharides, proinflammatory cytokines, complement components, and coagulation factors.

Injury to endothelial cells allows plasma and even blood cells to breach the endothelial layer. In glomeruli, this causes an edematous expansion of the subendothelial zone and mesangium (mesangiolysis) but is largely contained by the glomerular basement membrane. In arterioles that have thin basement membranes and no internal elastica, the increased permeability allows plasma and its constituents to enter the muscularis where the coagulation factors come in contact with enough tissue factor and other thrombogenic substances to form fibrin, resulting in the histologic finding of arteriolar fibrinoid necrosis. In larger arterioles and arteries that have an internal elastica, the increased endothelial permeability allows fluid to build up in the intima between the endothelial cell and elastica, but usually there is little overt fibrin formation. This intimal fluid initially seems to derive from the plasma but quickly accrues products from cells within the intima, including mucopolysaccharides and collagen. Within days of the acute injury, the expanded subendothelial zones are infiltrated by smooth muscle cells (mesangial cells in glomerular capillaries and smooth muscle cells from the muscularis in arteries) and myofibroblasts, which lay down new collagenous matrix, resulting in basement membrane replication in the glomerular capillaries, sclerosis of arterioles, and intimal fibrosis in arteries.

The etiology and pathogenesis of the endothelial injury in postdiarrheal HUS are understood best. D+ HUS is caused by Shiga-like toxin (SLT) that is produced by *E. coli* and *Shigella dysenteriae* (17,19). Endothelial cells, especially endothelial cells in the glomeruli, have receptors for SLT. Once SLT binds to these receptors, protein synthesis is halted, resulting in cell injury or death. This pathogenic step can be facilitated by various co-factors, such as proinflammatory cytokines. For example, tumor necrosis factor-alpha increases the number of receptors on endothelial cells and thus enhances SLT toxicity (31a).

HUS secondary to *Streptococcus pneumoniae* infection is caused by a neuraminidase that is produced by the bacteria (26,27). By removing N-acetylneuraminic acid residues, the neuraminidase exposes the Thomsen-Freidenreich (TF) cryptic antigen on the surface of erythrocytes, platelets, and glomerular endothelial cells. Once exposed, this antigen reacts with "naturally occurring" IgM anti-TF antibodies, resulting in HUS. Patients have a positive Coombs test because the anti-TF antibodies bind to erythrocytes. The reaction of the antibodies with platelets, erythrocytes, and endothelial cells results in a particularly aggressive expression of HUS, with a mortality rate of approximately 50 percent.

HUS is a cause of acute renal failure in patients with human immunodeficiency virus (HIV) infection (11,28). The basis for this relationship is unknown. Possibilities include a direct effect of the infection, an indirect effect of immune dysregulation, or the result of an intercurrent infection.

The etiology of HUS that is not associated with infections is not well understood. Vasculotoxic drugs and radiation appear to cause direct injury to endothelial cells and medial smooth muscle cells. Toxic antiendothelial antibodies may initiate endothelial injury in some patients (23). Antiendothelial antibodies are detected most often in patients with systemic sclerosis. Drug-induced HUS, such as that caused by calcineurin inhibitors, probably results from direct toxicity to endothelial cells and smooth muscle cells in small vessels and capillaries (15).

Hereditary HUS occurs as an autosomal recessive or autosomal dominant disease, and secondary to complement factor H mutations (18, 22). Hereditary HUS recurs in renal transplants, which confirms an extrarenal cause. HUS may recur from 2 weeks to many years after transplantation. Some patients with hereditary HUS have mutations in genes that code for factor H (29,30). Factor H is a plasma protein that controls the activation of the alternative complement activation pathway in the fluid phase and on cell surfaces. Factor H provides protection to cells from the damage of alternative pathway complement (29). C3b is constantly deposited on the surface of endothelial cells in contact with blood (30). Factor H competes with factor B for binding to C3b and also is a co-factor with factor I for breakdown of C3bBb, which is the C3 convertase of the alternative pathway. Thus, a deficiency of functional factor H predisposes endothelial cells to injury mediated by the alternative complement activation pathway. The association of factor H defects and HUS suggests that the mediation of at least some forms of HUS involves injury to endothelial cells by the alternative complement activation pathway.

Genetic defects in factor H also have been identified in 10 to 30 percent of patients with nonfamilial (idiopathic) HUS that is not associated with diarrhea (29,30). This supports a possible role for alternative pathway complement activation in sporadic (idiopathic) HUS as well.

Overall, the evidence indicates that multiple etiologies can initiate a final common pathogenic pathway that probably always involves endothelial injury and results in the pathologic and clinical manifestations of HUS.

Treatment and Prognosis. The prognosis for patients with D+ HUS is good compared to those with other forms of HUS (26,31a,33). Treatment focuses primarily on supportive care, with management of fluids and balance of electrolytes, administration of blood product when necessary, control of hypertension, and initiation of dialysis if renal failure is severe (26). Antibiotic treatment is not recommended because this may result in the increased production and release of SLT (31a). The value of enteral or parenteral adsorbents that bind SLT are under investigation. Most patients with D+ HUS, especially children, completely recover within several weeks, although 3 to 5 percent of patients die during the acute phase (31a). Approximately a third have persistent mild proteinuria and about a quarter have some degree of renal insufficiency that usually is not clinically significant (33). Oliguria that lasts for longer than 2 weeks is a predictor of poor renal outcome.

Patients with HUS who have exclusively glomerular involvement have a better prognosis than those with HUS with arterial involvement (9a,31a). Exclusive glomerular involvement is most common in mild D+ HUS and is least common in idiopathic D- HUS.

Patients with HUS that is not associated with diarrhea (D- HUS) have a 10 to 30 percent mortality rate and often have significant permanent renal dysfunction (26,29). Plasma exchange has been used to treat patients who do not have HUS antecedent diarrhea, but the effectiveness in this setting is uncertain and controversial (26). Plasma exchange is of very questionable value for patients with HUS caused by drugs, bone marrow transplantation, or cancer (6). Drug-induced HUS often resolves, or improves and stabilizes, after discontinuation of the etiologic drug (35,37). HUS arising during pregnancy improves with delivery, thus delivery should be induced as early as possible. HUS caused by *S. pneumoniae* should not be treated with fresh frozen plasma because plasma often contains anti-TF antibodies, or with erythrocytes or platelets because these have the TF antigen and may cause additional hemolysis and thrombosis (26,27). The 1-year survival rate in patients with systemic sclerosis renal crisis HUS has dramatically improved from 15 percent to 76 percent with treatment with angiotensin converting enzyme inhibitors (34). The pathologist should always consider the possibility of systemic sclerosis in appropriate patients with HUS, such as an older patient with a positive antinuclear antibodies (ANA) and acute HUS changes superimposed on chronic vasculopathy. All types of HUS other than D+ HUS (which rarely results in renal transplantation anyway) may recur in renal transplants and can cause graft failure.

ANTIPHOSPHOLIPID ANTIBODY SYNDROME

Definition. Antiphospholipid antibody syndrome (APS) is the association of circulating antiphospholipid antibodies with venous, arterial, arteriolar, or capillary thrombosis; pregnancy loss; or both (38,46). APS may occur as a primary (idiopathic) process or secondary to a systemic disease, usually systemic lupus erythematosus or rheumatoid arthritis (40,43). Approximately 40 percent of lupus patients have antiphospholipid antibodies and up to 15 percent have evidence of secondary APS (42). Antiphospholipid antibodies include lupus anticoagulant and anticardiolipin antibodies (39), and may react with proteins that are associated with lipids, such as beta-2 glycoprotein and prothrombin (40). Lupus anticoagulant is detected by observing an increased clotting time in a phospholipid-dependent coagulation test that is partially corrected by mixing with normal plasma. Anticardiolipin antibodies are detected by an immunoassay using the phospholipid cardiolipin as the target antigen.

Clinical Features. An international consensus statement proposes that a diagnosis of APS requires the identification of one clinical and one laboratory criterion (46). The clinical criterion can be either vascular thrombosis or pregnancy morbidity, and the laboratory criterion can be either identification of anticardiolipin antibodies or lupus anticoagulant. Both tests should be performed because only about half of patients with APS have both antibodies and thus half will not be identified if only one test is performed (40). Pregnancy morbidity includes unexplained death of a morphologically normal fetus and premature births of morphologically normal neonates before the 35th week of gestation.

The most frequent clinical manifestations are thrombosis of medium-sized and large arteries and veins, and recurrent spontaneous abortions (40). The most frequent site of arterial thrombosis is the cerebral vessels. The most common clinically apparent venous thrombosis is deep venous thrombosis of the legs. Ischemia results from both primary thrombosis and thromboembolization. The latter may derive from sterile thrombotic endocarditis. Other clinical manifestations include stroke, multi-infarct dementia, epilepsy, retinal artery occlusion, gangrene of the extremities, gut pain or infarction, Budd-Chiari syndrome, pulmonary thromboembolism, and livedo reticularis. Thrombocytopenia occurs in up to half of patients. Overt microangiopathic hemolytic anemia is uncommon. A rare expression of APS is the HELLP (hemolysis, elevated liver enzymes, and low platelets) syndrome that occurs during pregnancy (45), however, HELLP usually occurs in patients with severe preeclampsia/eclampsia who do not have antiphospholipid antibodies. Although clinically apparent thrombotic and thromboembolic events are sporadic, laboratory findings, such as elevated circulating prothrombin fragments and fibrinopeptides, suggest more persistent coagulation activation.

Renal injury ranges from thrombotic microangiopathy affecting small renal vessels, including glomerular capillaries, to focal or total infarction caused by thrombosis of the main renal

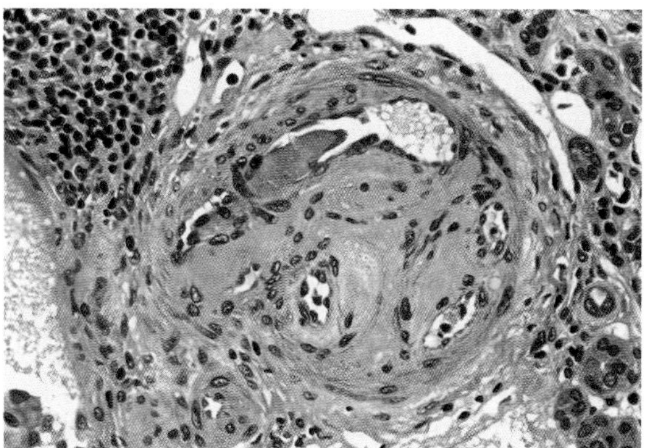

Figure 18-31

ANTIPHOSPHOLIPID ANTIBODY SYNDROME

An interlobular artery from a patient with anticardiolipin antibodies shows an old recanalized organized thrombus with superimposed acute thrombosis in one of the new channels (H&E stain).

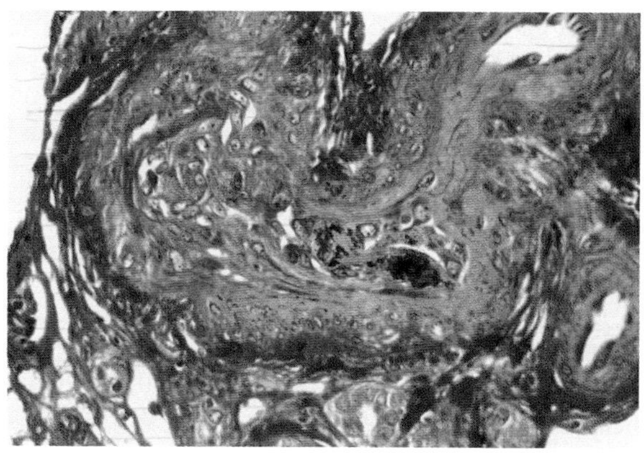

Figure 18-32

ANTIPHOSPHOLIPID ANTIBODY SYNDROME

An artery from a patient with anticardiolipin antibodies was stained with phosphotungstic acid-hematoxylin (PTAH) and shows acute thrombosis, with dark blue fibrin strands in a thrombus near the center of the image. There is a background of chronic intimal thickening.

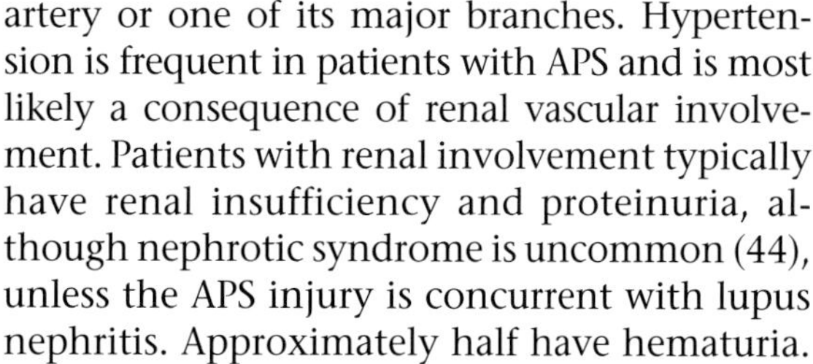

artery or one of its major branches. Hypertension is frequent in patients with APS and is most likely a consequence of renal vascular involvement. Patients with renal involvement typically have renal insufficiency and proteinuria, although nephrotic syndrome is uncommon (44), unless the APS injury is concurrent with lupus nephritis. Approximately half have hematuria.

Gross Findings. In the acute phase, severely affected kidneys are swollen and mottled red or pale (42a). Cut sections may reveal varying degrees of cortical necrosis or infarction that manifest as zones of pale cortex, often with a thin subcapsular rim of residual, viable, red parenchyma. In the chronic phase, kidneys are reduced in size and may have scattered, irregular, depressed scars at sites of earlier cortical necrosis.

Light Microscopic Findings. Light microscopic abnormalities include one or more of the following: acute and organized thrombotic lesions (figs. 18-31–18-33), prominent arteriosclerosis with fibrotic intimal thickening, and acute and chronic thrombotic microangiopathy lesions that resemble those of HUS (38,41,42,44), which have already been illustrated.

The most common pathologic finding in the kidneys of patients with APS is marked arteriosclerosis, with intimal thickening and narrowing of the lumen, primarily affecting the arcuate and interlobular arteries (44). This usually is accompanied by hyaline sclerosis of arterioles. The intimal thickening in arteries tends to be more cellular than the more densely fibrotic intimal thickening most often seen with chronic hypertensive nephropathy. Edematous (mucoid) intimal thickening occurs less often and is usually accompanied by thrombotic microangiopathy changes in arterioles and glomerular capillaries. The HUS-like thrombotic microangiopathy lesions of APS (38,41,42,44) are indistinguishable from those produced by HUS. In one study of 16 patients with primary APS who had renal dysfunction, 5 had features of HUS-like thrombotic microangiopathy, including arteriolar fibrinoid necrosis, intramural entrapment of schistocytes, and subendothelial expansion in glomerular capillaries with obliteration of lumens, mesangiolysis, and arteriolar and capillary thrombosis (44). The acute glomerular injury progresses to prominent remodeling and replication of glomerular basement membranes (38, 41). The multiple complex basement membrane layers are seen best with the PAS or JMS stain.

In the later phases of renal involvement, there is progressive glomerular and vascular scarring. Arteries and arterioles may contain thrombi in varying stages of organization or may have well-developed recanalization. Asymmetric intimal thickening may be the result of remodeled organized thrombi. Most patients

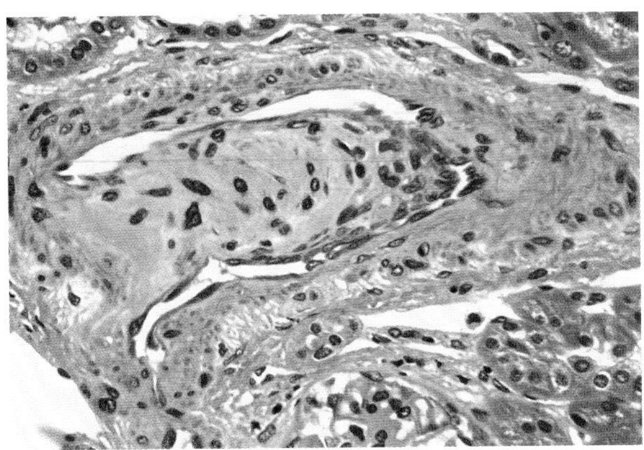

Figure 18-33

ANTIPHOSPHOLIPID ANTIBODY SYNDROME

An interlobular artery from a patient with anticardiolipin antibodies shows a newly organized thrombus partly obstructing the lumen.

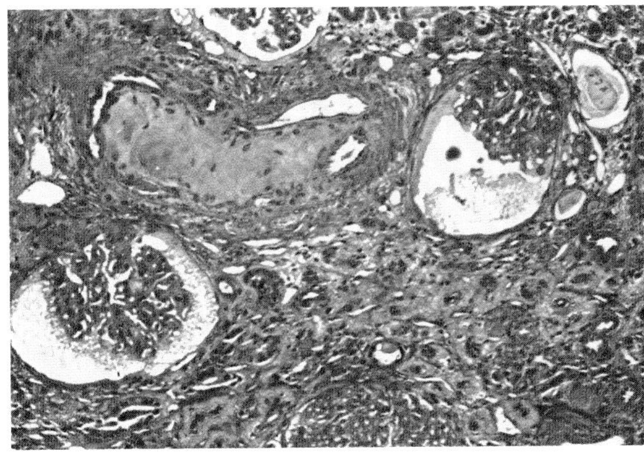

Figure 18-34

ANTIPHOSPHOLIPID ANTIBODY SYNDROME

There is an organized thrombus in the interlobular artery, as well as chronic ischemic changes, including tubular atrophy, interstitial fibrosis, and wrinkling of glomerular basement membranes (Masson trichrome stain).

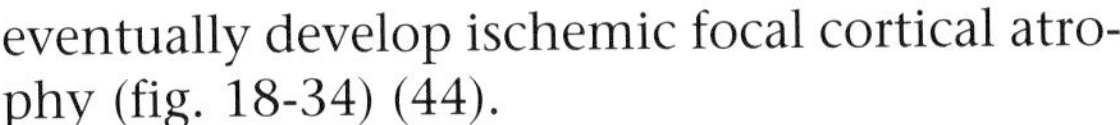

eventually develop ischemic focal cortical atrophy (fig. 18-34) (44).

Patients with secondary APS have the lesions of primary APS superimposed on the features of the underlying primary disease, which most often is lupus or a lupus-like process (38,39).

Immunofluorescence Findings. In primary APS, immunofluorescence microscopy demonstrates fibrin in thrombi (44). Foci of edematous intimal thickening and arteriolar fibrinoid necrosis stain variably for fibrin, C3, and IgM. There is no significant staining for IgG or IgA. Specimens with secondary APS superimposed on lupus nephritis have the expected frequency of staining with antisera specific for IgG, IgA and IgM for glomerular and extraglomerular immune complex deposits.

Electron Microscopic Findings. The ultrastructural features of APS with an acute microangiopathy are indistinguishable from those of HUS (38,41). The most distinctive changes are in the glomeruli. There is irregular lucent expansion of the subendothelial zone, which may extend into the mesangium as mesangiolysis. Glomerular basement membranes often are focally wrinkled. Strands of new basement membrane material are laid down in the expanded subendothelial zones, sometimes accompanied by extensions of mesangial cytoplasm or projections of endothelial cytoplasm. In patients with APS secondary to systemic lupus erythematosus, there usually are background features of immune complex glomerulonephritis, such as electron-dense deposits and endocapillary hypercellularity.

Differential Diagnosis. A diagnosis of APS should be considered in a patient whose biopsy demonstrates thrombosis in arteries or veins, or a thrombotic microangiopathy, especially if both are present. Based on pathology alone, however, the renal injury of APS cannot be unequivocally distinguished from other thrombotic microangiopathies. Nevertheless, the recognition of APS versus some other form of thrombotic microangiopathy is important because of the high risk for recurrent extrarenal and renal thrombotic disease, and the importance of prophylactic anticoagulant therapy. The suspicion should be especially high if there are thrombi in renal veins or arteries that have no underlying angiopathic changes, such as fibrinoid necrosis or edematous intimal thickening. APS also should be suspected if thrombi are of markedly varying ages, that is, some are relatively young with no organization and others are well organized with prominent growth of cells or recanalization (fig. 18-31). Secondary APS should be suspected in a patient with pathologic changes of lupus nephritis with superimposed thrombotic or microangiopathic changes. Even if the pathologic findings in a renal biopsy specimen look like typical HUS, APS should be an important differential diagnostic consideration if the patient has a history of arterial or venous thrombotic events, stroke, or pregnancy morbidity.

Etiology and Pathogenesis. Lupus anticoagulant is a misnomer because this autoantibody actually promotes thrombosis in vivo even though it prolongs coagulation in standard in vitro, phospholipid-dependent assays of coagulation (e.g., activated partial thromboplastin time). At least some antiphospholipid antibodies are specific for beta-2 glycoprotein I (apolipoprotein H), which binds to anionic phospholipids and has anticoagulant properties (40). However, there are other targets for antiphospholipid antibodies, such as prothrombin that is bound to lipid membranes and even phospholipids themselves.

The basis for the hypercoagulability in patients with APS is not well understood. There may be multiple mechanisms, such as interference with the anticoagulant properties of beta-2 glycoprotein I or antithrombin, direct activation of platelets, and injury to endothelial cells caused by binding of antibodies to cell membrane surfaces, either directly or via linking proteins (40,41).

Treatment and Prognosis. Patients with ischemic stroke caused by APS have a high morbidity and potential mortality rate, as well as a high recurrence rate (40). Other arterial and venous thromboses, and the various renal manifestations, also cause morbidity and mortality. Renal involvement can lead to end-stage renal disease in patients with primary APS because of the renal thrombosis and microangiopathy alone, and can worsen the prognosis in patients with APS superimposed on lupus nephritis (39). Therapy involves various strategies for anticoagulation, however, this must be regulated based on the risk of thrombosis versus the risk of hemorrhage. The latter is particularly problematic in patients who have thrombocytopenia caused by the APS.

PREECLAMPSIA AND ECLAMPSIA

Definition. Toxemia of pregnancy includes preeclampsia and eclampsia (48,49,52). Preeclampsia is characterized by the presence of hypertension, edema, proteinuria, and renal insufficiency after 20 weeks of pregnancy in a previously normotensive woman. Eclampsia is defined by the occurrence of convulsions in a woman with preeclampsia. Preeclampsia/eclampsia can be superimposed on chronic hypertensive disease; it also can manifest before 20 weeks' gestation in a woman with a molar pregnancy.

Clinical Features. Preeclampsia/eclampsia affects 5 to 10 percent of pregnancies in the United States (48,51). Approximately 30 percent of pregnant women who have hypertension before they become pregnant develop superimposed preeclampsia/eclampsia during pregnancy (52). Many different specific clinical diagnostic criteria for preeclampsia/eclampsia have been published (52). One simple definition is gestational hypertension with proteinuria (51,52). Hypertension in pregnancy is defined as diastolic pressure of 90 or more mm Hg and systolic pressure of 140 or more mm Hg (52,53). Proteinuria in pregnancy is defined as 300 mg or more/24 hours. The proteinuria may reach nephrotic range and may be accompanied by mild hematuria. The edema is most pronounced in the hands and face. Often the glomerular filtration rate is reduced, however, this may be masked because of the elevated creatinine clearance that normally occurs during pregnancy. Thrombocytopenia and schistocytosis may occur but are less pronounced than in full-blown thrombotic microangiopathy. Overt microangiopathic hemolytic anemia raises the possibility of a pregnancy-associated HUS or TTP rather than preeclampsia/eclampsia.

The HELLP syndrome occurs during pregnancy, may accompany preeclampsia/eclampsia, and may be an expression of more severe vasculopathy than usually seen with preeclampsia/eclampsia (47). Some pregnant patients have complex features that illustrate the complicated interrelationships between preeclampsia/eclampsia, HELLP syndrome, and HUS. For example, a patient with preeclampsia may develop features of HELLP syndrome and progress to overt HUS following delivery (50).

Light Microscopic Findings. The most characteristic histologic lesion is glomerular endothelial swelling that results in narrowing or occlusion of lumens and a "bloodless" appearance to the glomeruli (fig. 18-35) (48,49,54,55). This distinctive appearance is called *endotheliosis* (55). Glomerular lesions usually are diffuse and global but may be focal and segmental in less severely affected kidneys. An occasional finding is marked vacuolation of endothelial cells,

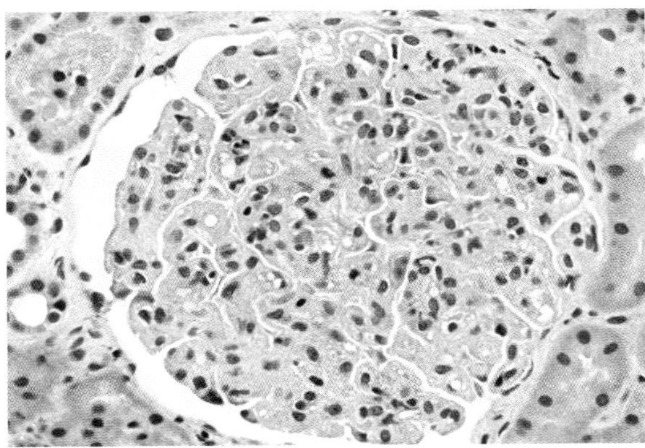

Figure 18-35

PREECLAMPSIA

The glomerulus has a "bloodless" consolidated appearance caused by swelling of endothelial cells (endotheliosis). The endothelial cytoplasm is slightly vacuolated. Most lumens cannot be identified, and those that can are markedly narrowed (H&E stain).

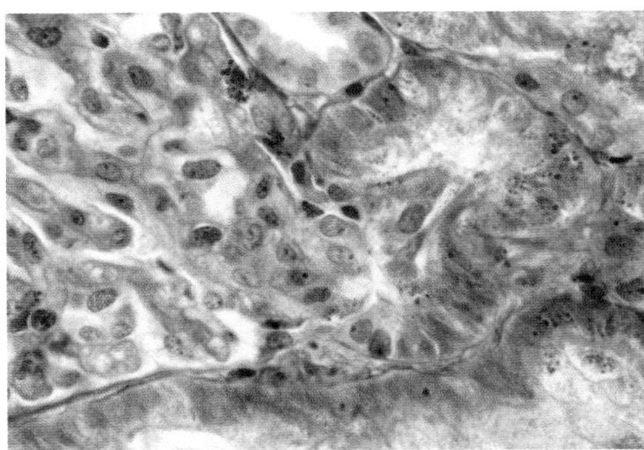

Figure 18-36

PREECLAMPSIA

Masson trichrome stain shows herniation of the glomerular tip into the origin of the proximal tubule.

which produces foam cells in capillaries. Glomeruli are enlarged beyond what is expected for gestation. Capillaries, especially in the glomerular tip adjacent to the origin of the proximal tubule, may be particularly dilated or elongated (49,54). Occasionally, the swollen tip of the glomerulus herniates into the lumen of the proximal tubule (fig. 18-36). The protruding tips often contain foam cells (54). Glomerular mesangial regions may be slightly expanded by matrix deposition and slight hypercellularity. Overt glomerular capillary thrombi are rare. If thrombi are conspicuous, concurrent endotoxic shock or antiphospholipid antibody syndrome should be suspected (49). Visceral epithelial cells are occasionally swollen, and may contain prominent lipid or protein droplets (fig. 18-37).

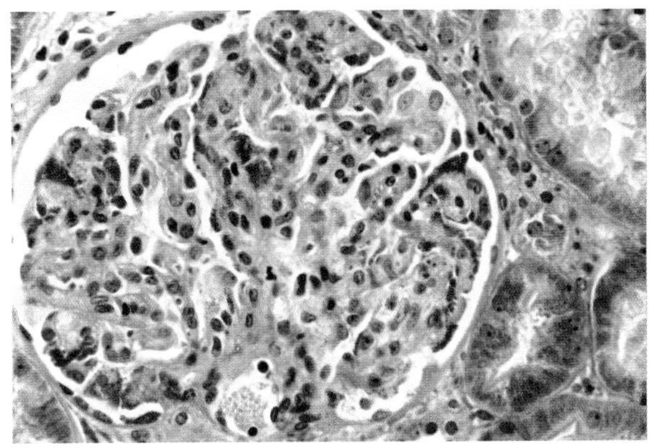

Figure 18-37

PREECLAMPSIA

The protein resorption droplets in podocytes stain red with the Masson trichrome stain. Capillary lumens are obliterated by endothelial swelling.

Although the glomerular basement membranes initially appear normal, within a week special stains often demonstrate layering of basement membrane material beneath and between the swollen endothelial cells, producing a pattern of basement membrane replication or fine trabeculation (fig. 18-38), often called a "laddering" or "string of beads" effect (fig. 18-38, left) (49). Mesangial matrix expansion is rarely conspicuous.

The glomerulus is the primary site of the pathologic changes of preeclampsia/eclampsia. Any arteriolar or arterial lesions should suggest either antecedent disease (e.g., hypertensive vasculopathy) or an alternative diagnosis (e.g., pregnancy-associated HUS). For example, the finding of arteriolar fibrinoid necrosis and thrombosis in a patient with pregnancy, proteinuria, and renal insufficiency shifts the diagnosis away from preeclampsia/eclampsia towards the thrombotic microangiopathy of HUS.

The endothelial swelling typically resolves within 2 weeks of delivery (54). The subendothelial irregularities in the glomerular basement membrane may persist for months. The most

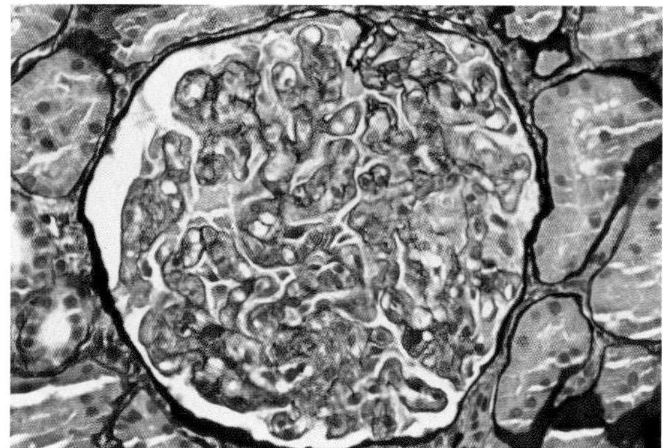

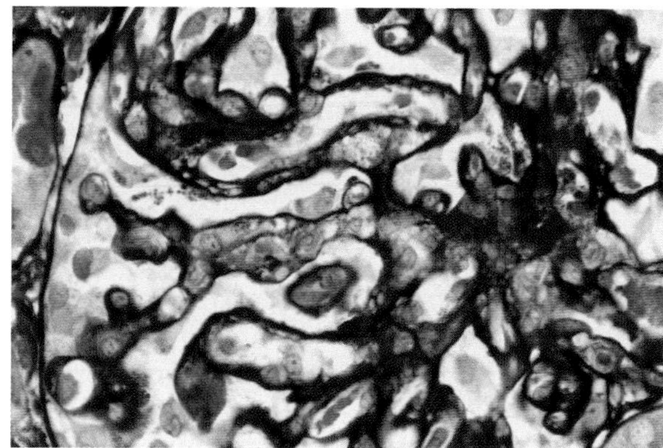

Figure 18-38

PREECLAMPSIA

The different specimens from a patient with preeclampsia are stained with JMS and H&E counterstain.

Left: Lower magnification shows global basement membrane remodeling with extensive trabeculation, replication of capillary wall basement membranes, and slight mesangial matrix expansion.

Right: Higher magnification also shows basement membrane remodeling, including a "string of beads" appearance along the wall of the elongated capillary lumen near the top of the image.

persistent lesions are small adhesions, most often to portions of Bowman's capsule that are near the origin of the proximal tubule (54). Small segmental increases in matrix within the glomerular tuft lie adjacent to the adhesions. Larger segmental scars are rare. Typical progressive focal segmental glomerulosclerosis can arise from preeclampsia/eclampsia, however, in most patients with combined features of focal segmental glomerulosclerosis and preeclampsia/eclampsia, the former appears to have been present prior to the onset of the latter (49). If enough nephrons are lost or injured due to preeclampsia/eclampsia, secondary focal segmental glomerulosclerosis may be induced by nephron overwork.

Immunofluorescence Findings. There are no specific immunohistologic features. Immunostaining for fibrin, IgM, and complement components is identified in approximately half of specimens, although this is usually of low intensity (49). The staining is seen in glomerular capillary walls and mesangium, and less frequently in afferent arterioles. Staining for IgG and IgA is negative.

Electron Microscopic Findings. The most conspicuous and most specific ultrastructural finding is glomerular capillary endothelial swelling (endotheliosis) (fig. 18-39) (48,49,55). Lumens often appear completely occluded, although this probably is not a functional reality because many patients with pronounced endotheliosis have little or no renal insufficiency. Swollen endothelial cells often contain increased numbers of clear or dense vacuoles. The latter have the appearance of phagolysosomes containing lipid, and may have a whorled myeloid-figure pattern. Extensive lipid accumulation occasionally occurs and causes endothelial cells to have a "foam cell" appearance (fig. 18-40). The fenestrations of swollen endothelial cells usually are lost. Occasional cells have focal ruffled or waffled projections of cytoplasm from their luminal surfaces (fig. 18-41). There may be irregular expansion of the subendothelial zone, but this is much less conspicuous than in HUS. The expanded subendothelial zone may contain flocculent, granular or amorphous, moderately electron-dense material (figs. 18-42, 18-43). In general, the expanded subendothelial zone in preeclampsia/eclampsia has more electron-dense material in it than the more lucent expanded subendothelial zone in HUS. This dense material, however, has the appearance of protein insudation rather than immune complex localization. In older lesions, bands of basement membrane material that surround projections of endothelial cytoplasm into the subendothelial zone produce the layering of basement membranes seen by light microscopy. There may be a slight increase in mesangial matrix and cells. Podocyte

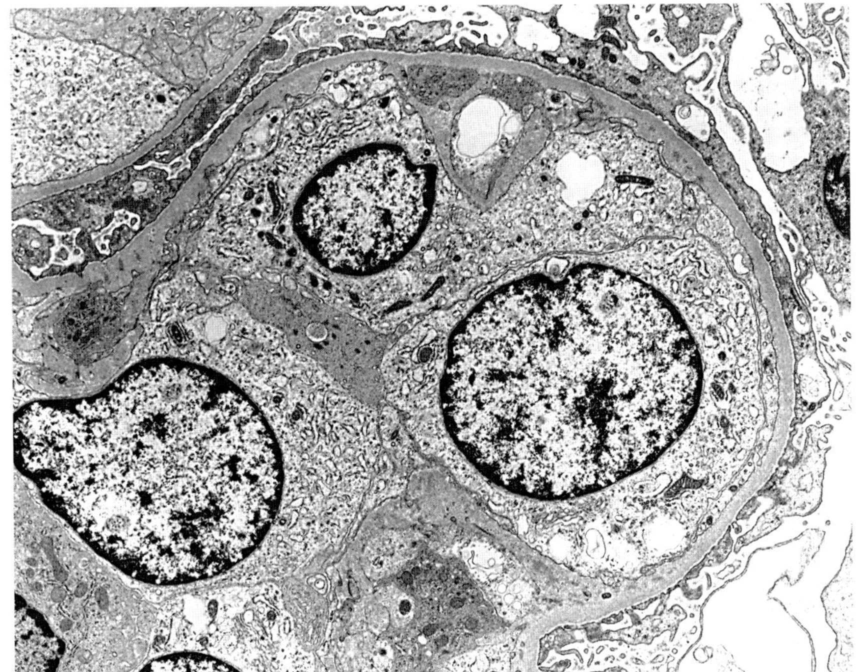

Figure 18-39

PREECLAMPSIA

A capillary lumen is obliterated by swollen endothelial cells (endotheliosis). Note the absence of significant subendothelial expansion in this specimen. There is effacement of podocyte foot processes.

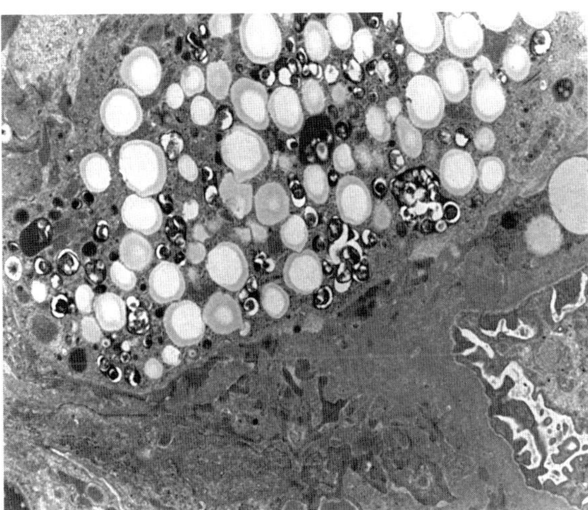

Figure 18-40

PREECLAMPSIA

The endothelial cytoplasm at the top of the image contains numerous lipid vacuoles, including some with myelin figures. There is slight expansion of the mesangial matrix at the bottom of the image.

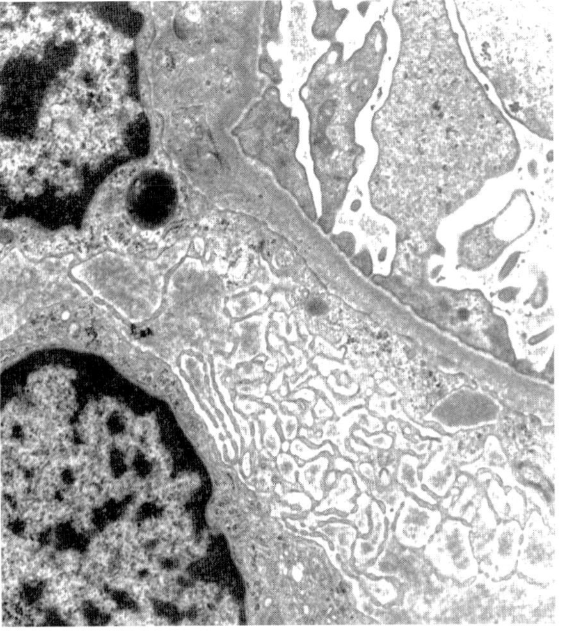

Figure 18-41

PREECLAMPSIA

Numerous endothelial cytoplasmic extensions project into the capillary lumen.

foot processes often are focally effaced. Podocyte cytoplasm may contain increased numbers of lucent or electron-dense vacuoles.

Differential Diagnosis. The major clinical differential diagnostic consideration is between preeclampsia/eclampsia and a thrombotic microangiopathy (especially HUS) (53). This is an important distinction to make because of the very different prognoses and therapies. A diagnosis

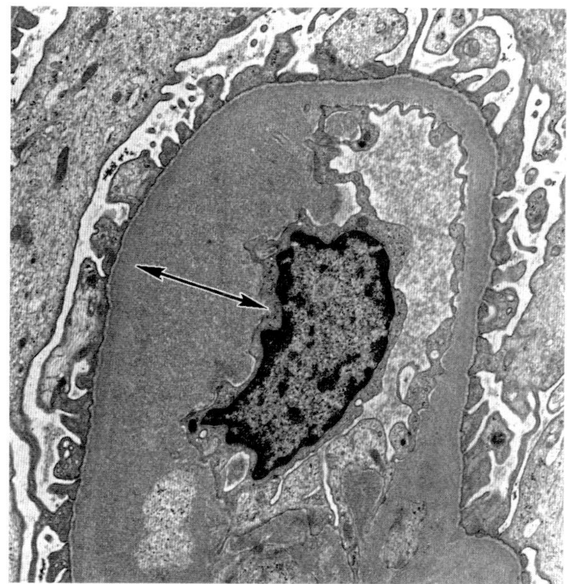

Figure 18-42

PREECLAMPSIA

Granular, moderately electron-dense material accumulates in the subendothelial zone (double arrow).

of preeclampsia/eclampsia prompts consideration of early delivery and the patient has a relatively good prognosis. A diagnosis of thrombotic microangiopathy has a much worse prognosis and prompts consideration of plasma exchange (53). A further diagnostic complication is the HELLP syndrome, which may occur with severe preeclampsia/eclampsia or thrombotic microangiopathy. When microangiopathic hemolytic anemia and thrombocytopenia occur during the first trimester, preeclampsia/eclampsia is ruled out by definition. However, over three quarters of women who develop thrombotic microangiopathy during pregnancy do so after 20 weeks (53). In some patients, the overlap in clinical and laboratory features among preeclampsia/eclampsia, HELLP syndrome, HUS, and TTP prevents a definitive clinical diagnosis and leads to renal biopsy.

Renal biopsy evaluation in hypertensive pregnant patients changes the clinical diagnosis in 25 percent of nulliparous and over 50 percent of multiparous women (49). Pathologically, preeclampsia/eclampsia can be distinguished from

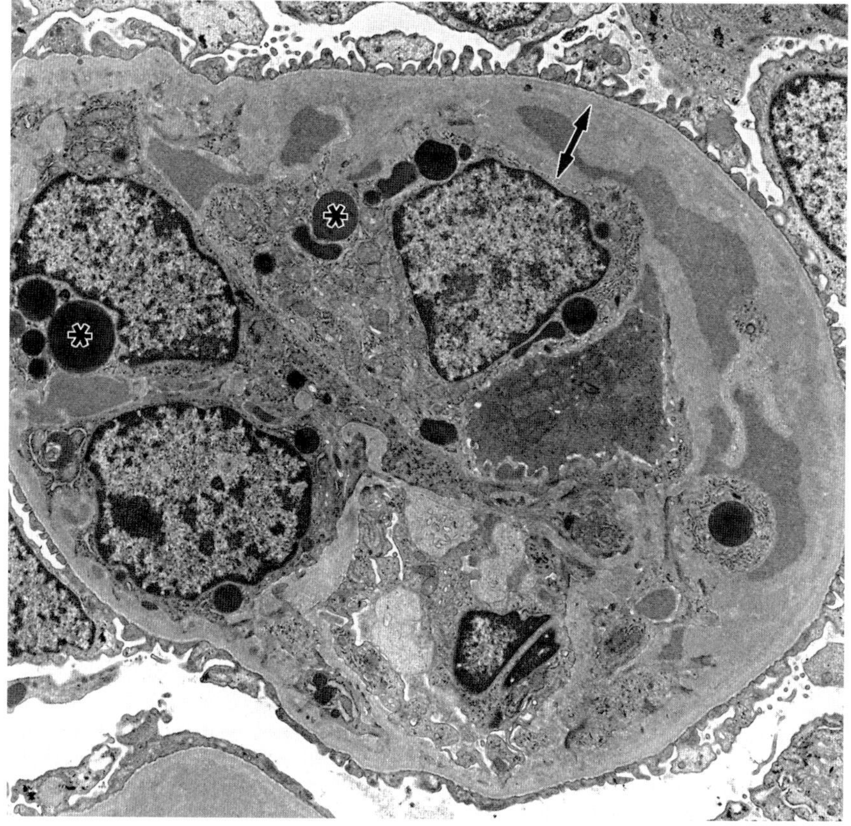

Figure 18-43

PREECLAMPSIA

A capillary is obliterated by a combination of endothelial swelling and accumulation of subendothelial material of variable density (double arrow). The endothelial cells contain dense vacuoles (asterisks).

HUS by the presence of predominant endotheliosis in the former and the distinctly different pattern of vessel wall injury in the latter, discussed in detail earlier in this chapter (48,49). For example, arteriolar fibrinoid necrosis and obliteration of glomerular capillary lumens by marked expansion of the subendothelial zone supports a diagnosis of HUS, whereas obliteration of glomerular capillary lumens by endothelial cytoplasmic swelling and no acute pathologic changes in arteries or arterioles supports a diagnosis of preeclampsia/eclampsia. Conspicuous microvascular platelet-rich thrombi, with minor vessel wall changes, raise the possibility of TTP. Conspicuous microvascular fibrin-rich thrombi with no underlying vessel wall changes raise the possibility of DIC.

The clinical differential diagnosis is very large in pregnant women who have hypertension and proteinuria without microangiopathic hemolytic anemia. The renal biopsy often reveals preeclampsia/eclampsia, but any glomerular disease may be found (49). Focal segmental glomerulosclerosis is found most frequently. It usually can be readily distinguished from preeclampsia/eclampsia. The greatest problem arises with the glomerular tip lesion variant of focal segmental glomerulosclerosis, which may have consolidated segments that herniate into the origin of the proximal tubule. This mimics the herniation of the glomerular tip into the proximal tubule that may occur in preeclampsia/eclampsia. The distinction between the tip lesion variant of focal segmental glomerulosclerosis and preeclampsia/eclampsia requires identification of widespread endotheliosis in the latter.

Etiology and Pathogenesis. The etiology and pathogenesis of preeclampsia/eclampsia are incompletely understood. The leading theory is that abnormal placentation results in release or generation of toxic factors in the maternal circulation, which cause maternal renal endothelial dysfunction in many organs, including the kidney, liver, brain, and lungs (51,52). Abnormal placentation is accompanied by defective uterine artery remodeling, causing reduced perfusion and impaired barrier function, allowing the escape of fetal and trophoblastic materials into the maternal circulation. The occurrence of preeclampsia/eclampsia in molar pregnancies demonstrates that products from the fetus are not required. Toxic factors may include cytokines or oxidants. Synergistic environmental or genetic factors that affect homeostatic systems, such as vasoactive hormones, coagulation factors, inflammatory mediators, or immune responses, may play a role. Different patients may have different causes that all lead to a final common pathway of pathologic injury and clinical manifestations.

Treatment and Prognosis. Maternal mortality from eclampsia is low in countries with good prenatal care, but in countries with poor prenatal care eclampsia accounts for 40 to 80 percent of maternal mortality (51). The definitive treatment for preeclampsia is delivery. Approximately 10 percent of preeclampsia/eclampsia occurs before the 34th week of gestation and the consequent early delivery of the fetus accounts for 15 percent of preterm births in the United States (51). Magnesium sulfate is effective for controlling the hypertension of patients with preeclampsia, for reducing the risk of progressing from preeclampsia to eclampsia (i.e., developing convulsions), and for reducing the number of recurrent convulsions in women with eclampsia (52).

THROMBOTIC THROMBOCYTOPENIC PURPURA

Definition. The classic clinical pentad of manifestations in patients with TTP is fever, microangiopathic hemolytic anemia, thrombocytopenic, fluctuating neurological abnormalities, and renal disease (56,58,59,63). This multiorgan dysfunction is caused by platelet-rich thrombosis in small vessels in many organs.

Clinical Features. The clinical features of patients with TTP overlap with those of HUS and DIC (63). Compared to HUS, patients with TTP usually have more pronounced neurologic manifestations, and less pronounced hemolysis, and less severe renal insufficiency. Patients with TTP rarely undergo renal biopsy, thus most renal pathologic material is from autopsies. The most common clinical presentation is with fever, fluctuating neurologic dysfunction, and bleeding. Neurologic abnormalities include confusion, headache, somnolence, aphasia, and focal motor or sensory defects. Thrombocytopenia is a constant finding. The blood smear typically shows schistocytes and reduced platelets. When

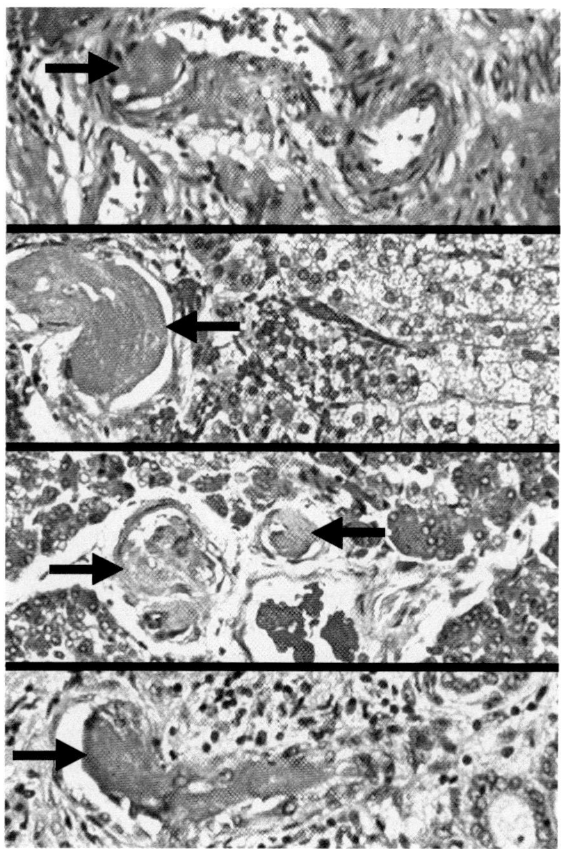

Figure 18-44

THROMBOTIC THROMBOCYTOPENIC PURPURA

From top to bottom, thrombi are seen in small vessels in the renal sinus, adrenal cortex, pancreas, and thyroid. The thrombi do not completely fill the lumens and are partly covered by endothelial cells.

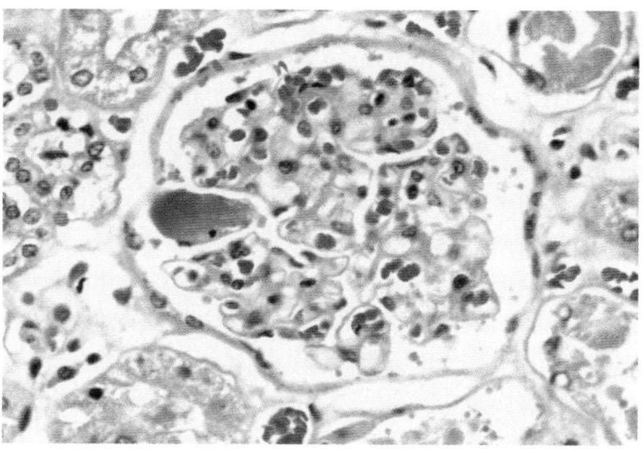

Figure 18-45

THROMBOTIC THROMBOCYTOPENIC PURPURA

Glomerulus with one capillary lumen occluded by a thrombus. The overall architecture of the glomerulus is otherwise unremarkable.

renal failure occurs, it often is late in the course of the disease and usually mild, unless complicated by the acute renal failure that is a component of severe generalized multiorgan failure. Approximately three quarters of patients with TTP have mild hematuria and proteinuria (62), approximately two thirds have mild azotemia, and less than one fifth have severe renal failure.

Gross Findings. The kidneys may appear normal or pale. Small petechial hemorrhages often are present over the external and cut surfaces of the kidney, and on the urothelial surface of the pelvis and calyces (63). Unlike HUS, infarcts or zones of cortical necrosis are rarely seen even when there is severe renal failure.

Light Microscopic Findings. The pathologic hallmark of TTP is thrombosis (fig. 18-44), as opposed to the pathologic hallmark of HUS which is vessel wall damage (58,63). The classic finding in the kidney is scattered thrombi within arterioles and glomerular capillaries (figs. 18-45, 18-46) (56,63). The thrombi are acidophilic and usually amorphous or finely granular, and less often hyaline (glassy) or fibrillar. Especially in arterioles and small arteries, the thrombi may not appear to completely fill the lumen (fig. 18-44). Endothelial cells may cover such eccentric thrombi, and eventually infiltrate thrombi and undergo hyperplasia adjacent to thrombi. When this endothelial proliferation is prominent, especially at a site of arteriolar dilation, the lesion takes on a "glomeruloid" appearance (fig. 18-47). Glomeruloid lesions or bodies, which also occur in HUS, are more common in TTP (58). The larger thrombotic lesions undergo progressive organization and fibrosis, eventually resulting in eccentric intimal thickening. Such secondary changes in vessel walls produce features that overlap with HUS. Foci of acidophilic, PAS-positive hyaline material may occur beneath the endothelial cells in arterioles and arteries, especially in patients who have had prolonged or recurrent clinical manifestations (fig. 18-48). This probably represents insudative lesions at former sites of thrombosis or late phase organization of thrombi.

Because of the consumptive coagulopathy, there may be foci of hemorrhage scattered throughout the tubulointerstitial tissue (fig. 18-

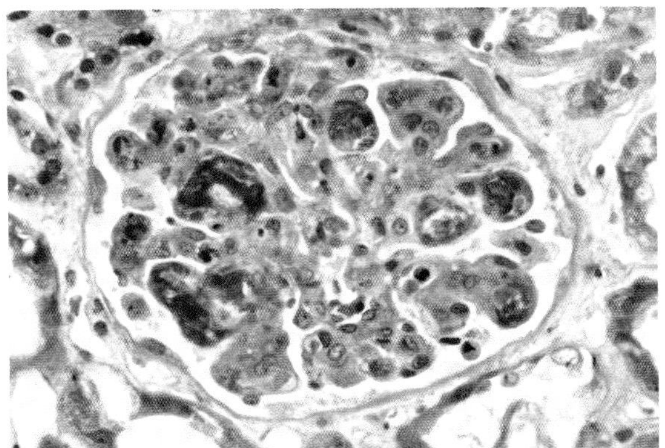

Figure 18-46

THROMBOTIC THROMBOCYTOPENIC PURPURA

Glomerulus with numerous capillary thrombi that stain red (fuchsinophilic) with the Masson trichrome stain.

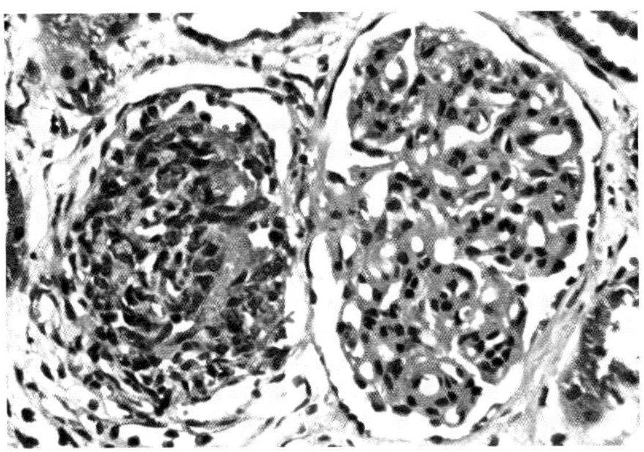

Figure 18-47

THROMBOTIC THROMBOCYTOPENIC PURPURA

The glomeruloid lesion (glomeruloid body) on the left presumably was once a thrombosed arteriole in which smooth muscle and endothelial cells proliferated in an attempt to organize the thrombus.

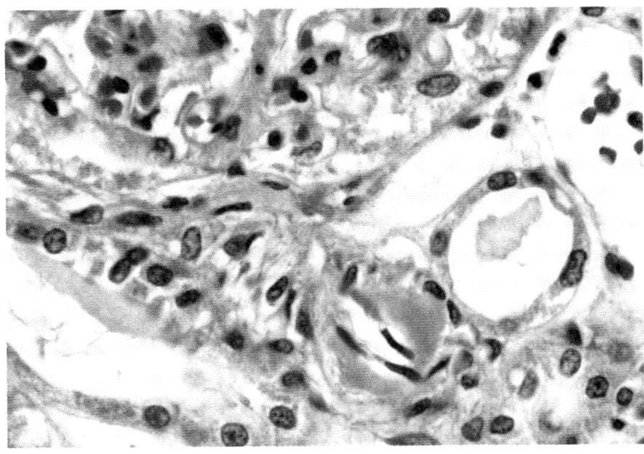

Figure 18-48

THROMBOTIC THROMBOCYTOPENIC PURPURA

A hilar arteriole from a patient who died of thrombotic thrombocytopenic purpura (TTP) has amorphous acidophilic material beneath the endothelial cells.

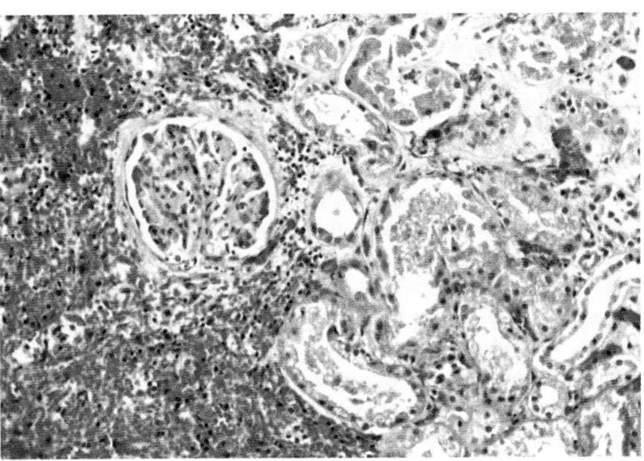

Figure 18-49

THROMBOTIC THROMBOCYTOPENIC PURPURA

This autopsy specimen from a patient who died of TTP shows focal interstitial hemorrhage caused by the coagulopathy.

49). Features of ischemic acute renal failure, such as simplification or necrosis of proximal tubular epithelial cells, may occur (fig. 18-50), but cortical necrosis is uncommon.

Immunofluorescence Findings. The major finding is staining of thrombi for fibrin and fibrinogen (fig. 18-51) (63,65). Unlike HUS, there is little or no staining for complement components. There is no significant staining for immunoglobulins.

Electron Microscopic Findings. The most characteristic finding is microvascular thrombosis, although this may be difficult to find if it is focal. Most thrombi have an admixture of platelets and fibrin, with platelets predominating, but some aggregates of platelets have no ultrastructurally identifiable fibrin (fig. 18-52) (65). In addition to the presence of thrombi, the other major ultrastructural finding is slight focal accumulation of electron-dense material beneath endothelial cells in glomerular capillaries, arterioles, and arteries (63,65). This injury is observed beneath the thrombi and also at sites where there are no thrombi (although

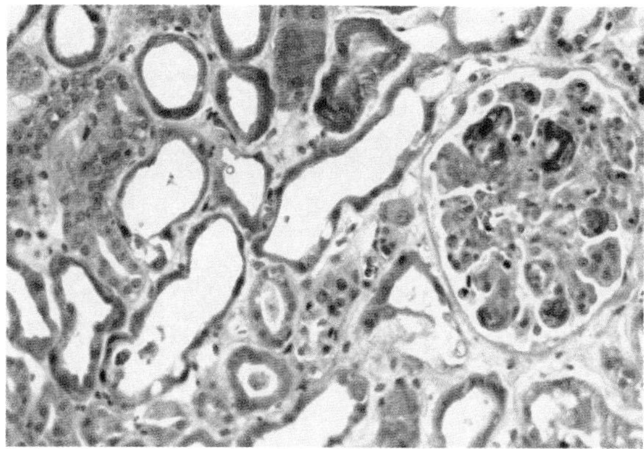

Figure 18-50

THROMBOTIC THROMBOCYTOPENIC PURPURA

The same specimen as seen in figure 18-46 shows numerous glomerular capillary thrombi. Acute ischemic changes are seen in tubular epithelial cells, specifically the flattening (simplification) of proximal tubular epithelial cells.

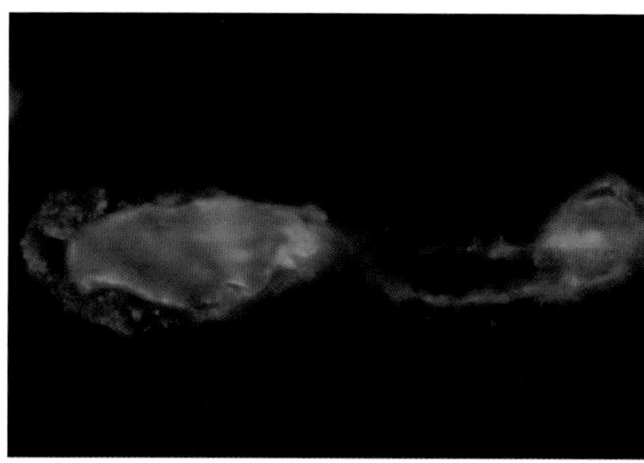

Figure 18-51

THROMBOTIC THROMBOCYTOPENIC PURPURA

Immunofluorescence microscopy using an antiserum specific for fibrin shows thrombi in an arteriole in the renal cortex.

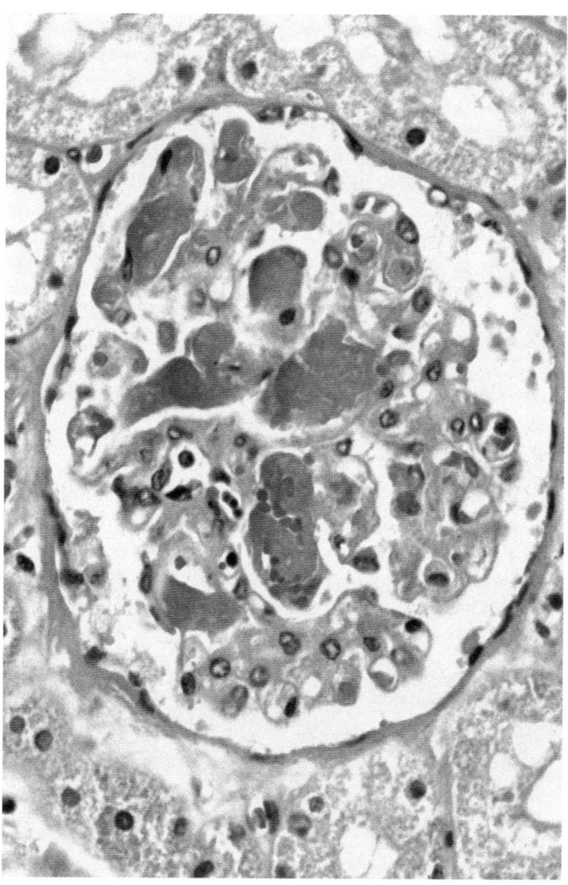

Figure 18-52

THROMBOTIC THROMBOCYTOPENIC PURPURA

A platelet-rich thrombus is in a glomerular capillary. There is slight swelling of the underlying endothelial cell cytoplasm, but no significant expansion of the subendothelial zone.

thrombi may have been at these sites earlier). The subendothelial lesions are more dense but much smaller and fewer than the more lucent subendothelial lesions of HUS. In glomerular capillaries, endothelial cells adjacent to thrombi are swollen and without fenestrations.

Differential Diagnosis. None of the histologic features of TTP are specific. They all can be seen in kidneys affected by DIC and HUS. DIC is distinguished from TTP by clinical and laboratory data discussed elsewhere in this chapter. Pathologically, TTP has thrombi with more platelets than fibrin, whereas DIC has thrombi that consist of more fibrin than platelets. HUS is distinguished from TTP by a combination of clinical, laboratory, and pathologic data. TTP has thrombosis as the major pathologic lesion whereas HUS has vessel wall changes as the dominant feature. However, especially as the lesions evolve, the pathologic features of TTP and HUS may overlap because primary thrombosis causes secondary vessel wall changes and primary vessel wall injury causes secondary thrombosis. Thus, both processes eventually result in concurrent vessel wall changes (e.g., intimal thickening/subendothelial expansion) and thrombosis.

Etiology and Pathogenesis. The etiology and pathogenesis of TTP is very different from that of HUS. Defects in the function of von Willebrand factor (vWF) are implicated in the pathogenesis of TTP (60,64,66). vWF is synthesized in megakaryocytes and endothelial cells as very large multimers, ranging from 500 to 10,000 kDa. These large multimers are normally reduced in size by partial proteolysis by vWF-cleaving metalloproteinase. This metalloproteinase is a member of the ADAMTS (a distintegrin-like and metalloprotease with thrombospondin type 1 motif) protein family (64). Patients with TTP have high levels of large vWF multimers in their circulation, which predispose to platelet aggregation and resultant thrombosis. Patients with TTP also have a defect in the vWF-cleaving metalloproteinase (61,64). Those with nonfamilial TTP have a circulating inhibitor of vWF-cleaving metalloproteinase (e.g., an autoantibody) and those with familial TTP have an inherited abnormality in vWF-cleaving metalloproteinase ADAMTS-13 activity. Patients with HUS do not have comparable abnormalities in vWF or the vWF-cleaving metalloproteinase (61,64,66).

Treatment and Prognosis. In the past, patients with TTP had a mortality rate of 80 to 90 percent. This has been reduced dramatically to less than 25 percent with plasma exchange therapy using fresh frozen plasma or cryosupernatant (57). Severe renal failure is a poor prognostic sign (59). The effectiveness of plasma exchange probably results from the removal of vWF-cleaving protease inhibitors (e.g., antiprotease antibodies), replacement of vWF-cleaving proteases, or both. The value of plasma infusion without plasma exchange is controversial.

A variety of adjunctive therapies have been used, especially in patients who do not respond well to plasma exchange. These include the use of corticosteroids, vincristine, intravenous gamma globulin, and antiplatelet drugs, as well as splenectomy. TTP recurs in approximately a quarter of patients.

DISSEMINATED INTRAVASCULAR COAGULATION

Definition. DIC is a consumptive coagulopathy in which the homeostatic system is activated within the microvasculature of many organs, resulting in numerous microthrombi, depletion of coagulation factors, and activation of the fibrinolytic system (68). Both humoral coagulation factors and platelets are consumed, although there is a predominance of coagulation factor consumption. This contrasts with HUS and TTP in which a predominance of platelets is consumed.

Clinical Features. The primary manifestations are hemorrhage and multiorgan failure. Hemostatic defects may manifest as oozing from venous and arterial puncture sites, and spontaneous hemorrhage such as petechiae, purpura, ecchymoses, bleeding into the gut, epistaxis, hematuria, adrenal hemorrhage, and hemoptysis. Organ dysfunction caused by microvascular thrombosis includes cutaneous acrocyanosis, renal failure, respiratory distress, and neurologic abnormalities. Laboratory abnormalities include prolonged thrombin and prothrombin times, decreased fibrinogen, increased fibrin split products, and thrombocytopenia. Schistocytes are observed in about half of patients but are usually less numerous than in TTP or HUS. Occasional patients with histologic features of DIC do not have the clinical features of the disease (67).

Gross Findings. The external and cut surfaces of the kidneys often have numerous petechiae and, occasionally, larger purpuric lesions. Grossly discernable cortical necrosis or infarction is rare.

Light Microscopic Findings. The most specific pathologic feature of DIC is numerous fibrin-rich thrombi in capillaries, venules, and arterioles. In the kidney, these are most prevalent in hilar arterioles and glomerular capillaries. In H&E-stained sections, the thrombi are acidophilic and most often have a fine fibrillary texture, although they may be granular, amorphous, or hyaline (fig. 18-53). Because of the activation of fibrinolytic mechanisms, the number of thrombi identified in biopsy tissue or at postmortem examination may not accurately reflect the extent of thrombosis that has occurred. Organized thrombi are much less frequent than in TTP or HUS. The vessels that contain thrombi usually have unremarkable walls or only slight endothelial swelling. Prominent staining of the thrombi of DIC is demonstrated with fibrin stains such as phosphotungstic acid-hematoxylin (PTAH) (fig. 18-54) (67). Acute ischemic changes, such as proximal tubular epithelial simplification or necrosis, may be present. Scattered interstitial hemorrhages are common.

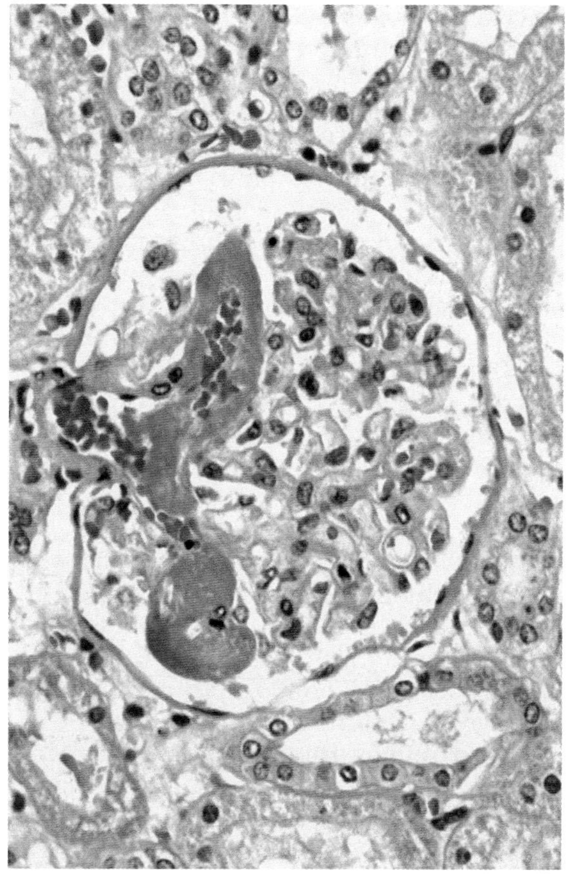

Figure 18-53

DISSEMINATED INTRAVASCULAR COAGULATION

There are multiple thrombi in glomerular capillaries from a patient with sepsis-induced disseminated intravascular coagulation (DIC). The underlying glomerular architecture is unremarkable.

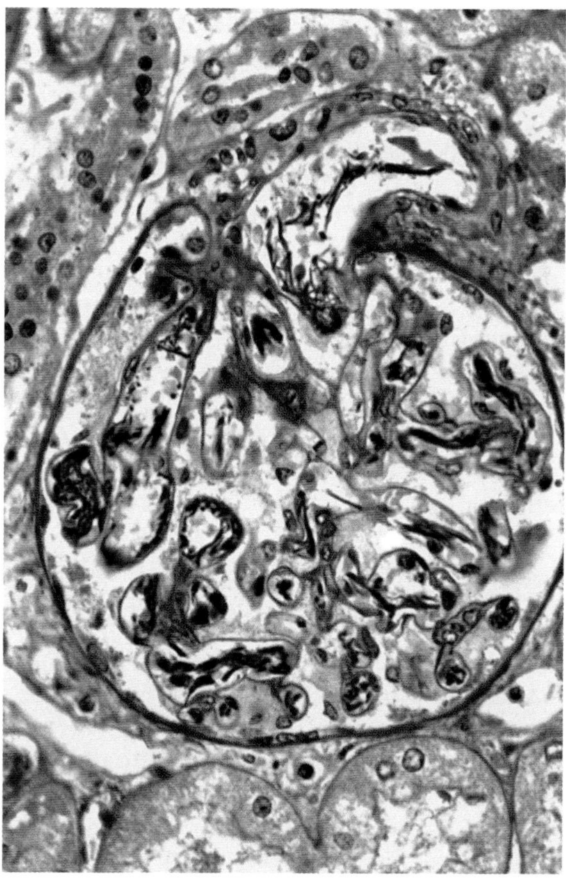

Figure 18-54

DISSEMINATED INTRAVASCULAR COAGULATION

PTAH stain demonstrates numerous dark blue fibrin strands in glomerular capillaries from a patient with sepsis-induced DIC. The afferent arteriole and glomerular capillaries are histologically unremarkable.

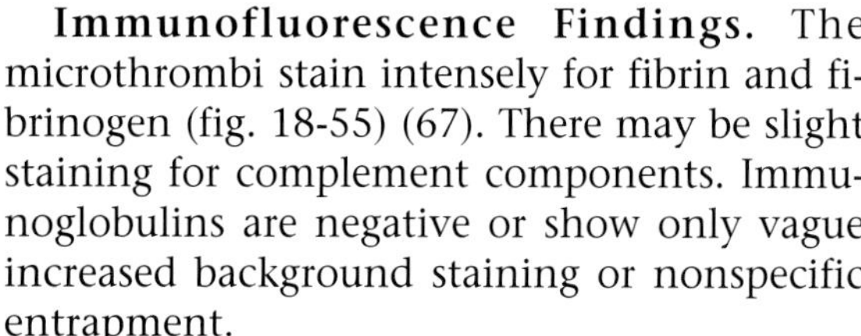

Immunofluorescence Findings. The microthrombi stain intensely for fibrin and fibrinogen (fig. 18-55) (67). There may be slight staining for complement components. Immunoglobulins are negative or show only vague increased background staining or nonspecific entrapment.

Electron Microscopic Findings. The major ultrastructural finding is thrombi in capillaries, venules, and arterioles. These thrombi contain predominantly fibrin (fig. 18-56), which differs from the platelet-rich thrombi of HUS and TTP. A high proportion of platelets should raise the possibility of TTP. The underlying vessel walls typically are unremarkable in DIC. Extensive subendothelial expansion should raise the possibility of HUS.

Differential Diagnosis. The major differential considerations when thrombi are identified within otherwise unremarkable renal arterioles and glomerular capillaries are DIC and TTP. HUS and related diseases are unlikely if there are no vascular lesions, such as marked subendothelial expansion in glomerular capillaries, fibrinoid necrosis in arterioles, or edematous intimal thickening in arteries. If the microthrombi are numerous in the kidney, DIC is more likely than TTP. Although not absolutely specific, the composition of the thrombi points toward DIC if a PTAH stain revels numerous fibrin strands

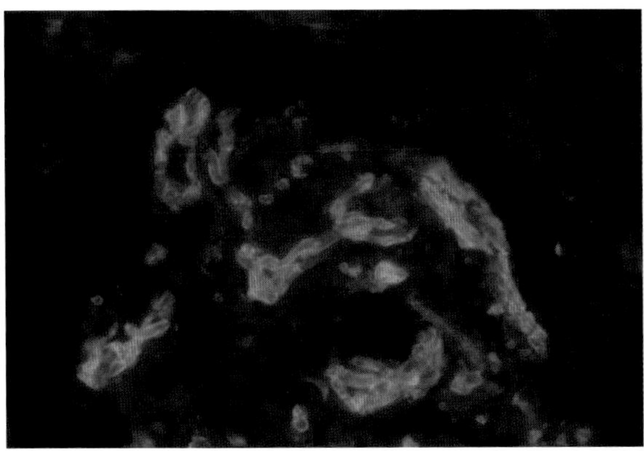

Figure 18-55

DISSEMINATED INTRAVASCULAR COAGULATION

Immunofluorescence microscopy using an antiserum specific for fibrin demonstrates numerous thrombi in glomerular capillaries of a patient with sepsis-induced DIC.

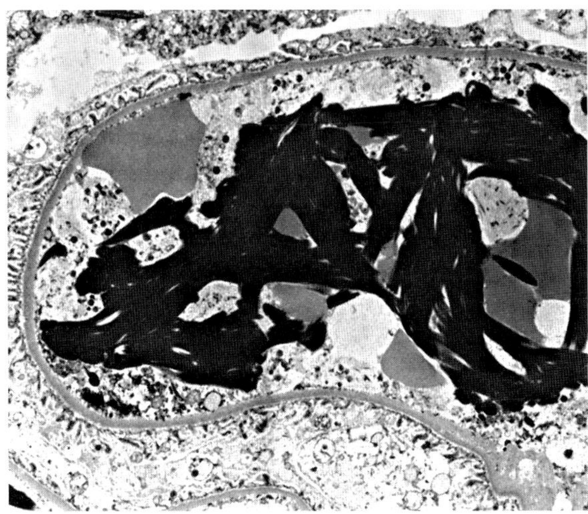

Figure 18-56

DISSEMINATED INTRAVASCULAR COAGULATION

Fibrin tactoids in a thrombus in the lumen of a glomerular capillary in a postmortem specimen from a patient with sepsis-induced DIC. The cellular elements have autolysis artifact.

throughout the thrombi and toward TTP or HUS if the central core of the thrombi shows little or no PTAH staining because it is composed predominantly of platelets rather than fibrin.

Etiology and Pathogenesis. The major events in normal hemostasis are platelet adhesion and aggregation, coagulation factor cascade activation with fibrin formation, and coagulation cascade regulation by antagonists and fibrinolysis. In DIC, both coagulation and fibrinolysis are increased, but there is an imbalance that favors thrombosis.

There are multiple disease processes that induce DIC (see Table 18-1). The processes may share an ability to increase circulating levels of tissue factor. Coagulation in DIC is mediated primarily through the tissue factor-factor VIIa complex of the extrinsic pathway (68). A variety of pathogenic processes induce endothelial cells to express tissue factor, such as endotoxins, cytokines, and viral infections. This results in a shift from an anticoagulant to a procoagulant state in the microvasculature. The widespread microvascular thrombosis causes multiorgan failure. The thrombosis also causes consumption of coagulation factors and platelets, and generation of fibrin split products that are inhibitors of hemostasis. This results in widespread bleeding, especially from the microvasculature, as well as ischemia in multiple organs.

Treatment and Prognosis. More than half of patients with DIC die, either as a direct result of the multiorgan failure caused by the DIC or because of the combined morbidity of the DIC and the cause of the DIC, such as sepsis, trauma, or neoplasia. Any identifiable underlying cause (see Table 18-1) should be treated. Supportive care is very important: appropriate blood product replacement therapy (e.g., platelets, cryoprecipitate, fresh frozen plasma), fluid balance maintenance, and care of respiratory and cardiac dysfunction. Dialysis may be required for renal failure. Heparin therapy may be beneficial but should not be used in patients with platelet counts below 50,000/uL. Experimental protocols are investigating the efficacy of specific inhibitors of tissue factor and other coagulation factors that are involved in the microvascular thrombosis (68).

REFERENCES

Introduction

1. Churg J, Strauss L. Renal involvement in thrombotic microangiopathies. Semin Nephrol 1985;5:46-56.
2. Ruggenenti P, Noris M, Remuzzi G. Thrombotic microangiopathy, hemolytic uremic syndrome, and thrombotic thrombocytopenic purpura. Kidney Int 2001;60:831–46.
3. Symmers W St C. Thrombotic microangiopathic haemolytic anaemia (thrombotic microangiopathy). Br Med J 1952;2:897–903.

Hemolytic Uremic Syndrome

4. Abraham KA, Little MA, Dorman AM, Walshe JJ. Hemolytic-uremic syndrome in association with both cyclosporine and tacrolimus. Transpl Int 2000;13:443–7.
5. Argyle JC, Hogg RJ, Pysher TJ, Silva FG, Siegler RL. A clinicopathological study of 24 children with hemolytic uremic syndrome. A report of the Southwest Pediatric Nephrology Study Group. Pediatr Nephrol 1990;4:52–8.
6. Bosch T, Wendler T. Extracorporeal plasma treatment in thrombotic thrombocytopenic purpura and hemolytic uremic syndrome: a review. Ther Apher 2001;5:182–5.
7. Boyce TG, Swerdlow DL, Griffin PM. Escherichia coli O157:H7 and the hemolytic-uremic syndrome. N Engl J Med 1995;333:364–8.
8. Brilliant SE, Lester PA, Ohno AK, Carlon MJ, Davis BJ, Cushner HM. Hemolytic-uremic syndrome without evidence of microangiopathic hemolytic anemia on peripheral blood smear. South Med J 1996;89:342–5.
9. Canet JJ, Castañé J, Alvarez M, Nava JM, Llibre J. Scleroderma renal crisis sine scleroderma. Nephron 2002;90:119–20.

9a. Churg J, Strauss L. Renal involvement in thrombotic microangiopathies. Semin Nephrol 1985;5:46–56.

10. Cruz DN, Perazella MA, Mahnensmith RL. Bone marrow transplant nephropathy: a case report and review of the literature. J Am Soc Nephrol 1997;8:166–73.
11. D'Agati V, Appel GB. Renal pathology of human immunodeficiency virus infection. Semin Nephrol 1998;18:406–21.
12. Dashe JS, Ramin SM, Cunningham FG. The long-term consequences of thrombotic microangiopathy (thrombotic thrombocytopenic purpura and hemolytic uremic syndrome) in pregnancy. Obstet Gynecol 1998;91:662–8.
13. Fennell RH Jr, Reddy CR, Vazquez JJ. Progressive systemic sclerosis and malignant hypertension: immunohistochemical study of renal lesions. Arch Pathol 1961;72:209.
14. Generini S, Fiori G, Moggi Pignone A, Matucci Cerinic M, Cagnoni M. Systemic sclerosis. A clinical overview. Adv Exp Med Biol 1999;455:73–83.
15. Griffiths MH, Crowe AV, Papadaki L, et al. Cyclosporin nephrotoxicity in heart and lung transplant patients. QJM 1996;89:751–63.
16. Habib R, Mathieu H, Royer P. Maladie thrombotique artériolocapillaire du rein chez l'enfant. Rev Fr Etud Clin Biol 1958;3:891.
17. Kaplan BS, Cleary TG, Obrig TG. Recent advances in understanding the pathogenesis of the hemolytic uremic syndromes. Pediatr Nephrol 1990;4:276–83.
18. Kaplan BS, Papadimitriou M, Brezin JH, Tomlanovich SJ, Zulkharnain. Renal transplantation in adults with autosomal recessive inheritance of hemolytic uremic syndrome. Am J Kidney Dis 1997;30:760–65.
19. King AJ. Acute inflammation in the pathogenesis of hemolytic-uremic syndrome. Kidney Int 2002;61:1553–64.
20. Koitabashi Y, Rosenberg BF, Shapiro H, Bernstein J. Mesangiolysis: an important glomerular lesion in thrombotic microangiopathy. Mod Pathol 1991;4:161–6.
21. Kovalchik MT, Guggenheim SJ, Silverman MH, Robertson JS, Steigerwald JC. The kidney in progressive systemic sclerosis: a prospective study. Ann Intern Med 1978;89:881–7.
22. Laszik Z, Silva FG. Hemolytic-uremic syndrome, thrombotic thrombocytopenic purpura, and systemic sclerosis (systemic scleroderma). In: Jennette JC, Olson JL, Schwartz MM, Silva FG, eds. Heptinstall's pathology of the kidney. Philadelphia: Lippincott-Raven; 1998:1003–57.
23. Leung DY, Moake JL, Havens PL, Kim M, Pober JS. Lytic anti-endothelial cell antibodies in haemolytic-uraemic syndrome. Lancet 1988;2:183–6.
24. Martinoli C, Bertolotto M, Pretolesi F, Crespi G, Derchi LE. Kidney: normal anatomy. Eur Radiol 1999;9(Suppl 3):S389–93.
25. McCoy RC, Tisher CC, Pepe PF, Cleveland LA. The kidney in progressive systemic sclerosis: immunohistochemical and antibody elution studies. Lab Invest 1976;35:124–31.
26. Meyers KE, Kaplan BS. Hemolytic-uremic syndromes. In: Barratt TM, Avner ED, Harmon WE, eds. Pediatric nephrology, 4th ed. Baltimore: Lippincott, Williams & Wilkins; 1999:811–22.

27. Myers KA, Marrie TJ. Thrombotic microangiopathy associated with Streptococcus pneumoniae bacteremia: case report and review. Clin Infect Dis 1993;17:1037–40.
28. Peraldi MN, Maslo C, Akposso K, Mougenot B, Rondeau E, Sraer JD. Acute renal failure in the course of HIV infection: a single-institution retrospective study of ninety-two patients and sixty renal biopsies. Nephrol Dial Transplant 1999;14:1578–85.
29. Perez-Caballero D, Gonzalez-Rubio C, Gallardo ME, et al. Clustering of missense mutations in the C-terminal region of factor H in atypical hemolytic uremic syndrome. Am J Hum Genet 2001;68:478–84.
30. Richards A, Buddles MR, Donne RL, et al. Factor H mutations in hemolytic uremic syndrome cluster in exons 18-20, a domain important for host cell recognition. Am J Hum Genet 2001;68:485–90.
31. Richardson SE, Karmali MA, Becker LE, Smith CR. The histopathology of the hemolytic uremic syndrome associated with verocytotoxin-producing Escherichia coli infections. Hum Pathol 1988;19:1102–8.
31a. Ruggenenti P, Noris M, Remuzzi G. Thrombotic microangiopathy, hemolytic uremic syndrome, and thrombotic thrombocytopenic purpura. Kidney Int 2001;60:831–46.
32. Segonds A, Louradour N, Suc JM, Orfila C. Postpartum hemolytic uremic syndrome: a study of three cases with a review of the literature. Clin Nephrol 1979;12:229–42.
33. Siegler RL, Milligan MK, Burningham TH, Christofferson RD, Chang SY, Jorde LB. Long-term outcome and prognostic indicators in the hemolytic-uremic syndrome. J Pediatr 1991;118:195–200.
34. Steen VD, Costantino JP, Shapiro AP, Medsger TA Jr. Outcome of renal crisis in systemic sclerosis: relation to availability of angiotensin converting enzyme (ACE) inhibitors. Ann Intern Med 1990;113:352–7.
35. Trimarchi HM, Truong LD, Brennan S, Gonzalez JM, Suki WN. FK506-associated thrombotic microangiopathy: report of two cases and review of the literature. Transplantation 1999;67:539–44.
36. Weller RO. Vascular pathology in hypertension. Age Ageing 1979;8:99–103.
37. Zent R, Katz A, Quaggin S, et al. Thrombotic microangiopathy in renal transplant recipients treated with cyclosporin A. Clin Nephrol 1997;47:181–6.

Antiphospholipid Antibody Syndrome

38. D'Agati V, Kunis C, Williams G, Appel GB. Anticardiolipin antibody and renal disease: a report of three cases. J Am Soc Nephrol 1990;1:777–84.
39. Daugas E, Nochy D, Huong du LT, et al. Antiphospholipid syndrome nephropathy in systemic lupus erythematosus. J Am Soc Nephrol 2002;13:42–52.
40. Greaves M. Antiphospholipid antibodies and thrombosis. Lancet 1999;353:1348–53.
41. Griffiths MH, Papadaki L, Neild GH. The renal pathology of primary antiphospholipid syndrome: a distinctive form of endothelial injury. QJM 2000;93:457–67.
42. Hughson MD, McCarty GA, Brumback RA. Spectrum of vascular pathology affecting patients with the antiphospholipid syndrome. Hum Pathol 1995;26:716–24.
42a. Laszik Z, Silva FG. Hemolytic-uremic syndrome, thrombotic thrombocytopenic purpura, and systemic sclerosis (systemic scleroderma). In: Jennette JC, Olson JL, Schwartz MM, Silva FG, eds. Heptinstall's pathology of the kidney. Philadelphia: Lippincott-Raven; 1998:1003–57.
43. Merkel PA, Chang Y, Pierangeli SS, Convery K, Harris EN, Polisson RP. The prevalence and clinical associations of anticardiolipin antibodies in a large inception cohort of patients with connective tissue diseases. Am J Med 1996;101:576–83.
44. Nochy D, Daugas E, Droz D, et al. The intrarenal vascular lesions associated with primary antiphospholipid syndrome. J Am Soc Nephrol 1999;10:507–18.
45. Ornstein MH, Rand JH. An association between refractory HELLP syndrome and antiphospholipid antibodies during pregnancy; a report of 2 cases. J Rheum 1994;21:1360–4.
46. Wilson WA, Gharavi AE, Koike T, et al. International consensus statement on preliminary classification criteria for definite antiphospholipid syndrome: report of an international workshop. Arthritis Rheum 1999;42:1309–11.

Preeclampsia and Eclampsia

47. Beller FK, Dame WR, Ebert C. Pregnancy induced hypertension complicated by thrombocytopenia, haemolysis and elevated liver enzymes (HELLP) syndrome. Renal biopsies and outcome. Austral N Z J Obstet Gynaecol 1985;25:83–6.
48. Fogo AB. Renal disease in pregnancy. In: Jennette JC, Olson JL, Schwartz MM, Silva FG, eds. Heptinstall's pathology of the kidney, 5th ed. Philadelphia: Lippincott-Raven; 1998:1097–130.

49. Gaber LW, Spargo BH, Lindheimer MD. Renal pathology in pre-eclampsia. Baillieres Clin Obstet Gynecol 1994;8:443–68.
50. Kahra K, Draganov B, Sund S, Hovig T. Postpartum renal failure: a complex case with probable coexistence of hemolysis, elevated liver enzymes, low platelet count, and hemolytic uremic syndrome. Obstet Gynecol 1998;92:698–700.
51. Lain KY, Roberts JM. Contemporary concepts of the pathogenesis and management of preeclampsia. JAMA 2002;287:3183–6.
52. Lindheimer MD, Davison JM, Katz AI. The kidney and hypertension in pregnancy: twenty exciting years. Semin Nephrol 2001;21:173–89.
53. McMinn JR, George JN. Evaluation of women with clinically suspected thrombotic thrombocytopenic purpura-hemolytic uremic syndrome during pregnancy. J Clin Apheresis 2001;16:202–9.
54. Sheehan HL. Renal morphology in preeclampsia. Kidney Int 1980;18:241–52.
55. Spargo BH, McCartney CP, Winemiller R. Glomerular capillary endotheliosis in toxemia of pregnancy. AMA Arch Pathol 1959;68:593–9.

Thrombotic Thrombocytopenic Purpura

56. Berkowitz LR, Dalldorf FG, Blatt PM. Thrombotic thrombocytopenic purpura: a pathology review. JAMA 1979;241:1709–10.
57. Bosch T, Wendler T. Extracorporeal plasma treatment in thrombotic thrombocytopenic purpura and hemolytic uremic syndrome: a review. Ther Apher 2001;5:182–5.
58. Churg J, Strauss L. Renal involvement in thrombotic microangiopathies. Semin Nephrol 1985;5:46-56.
59. Eknoyan G, Riggs SA. Renal involvement in patients with thrombotic thrombocytopenic purpura. Am J Nephrol 1986;6:117–31.
60. Fujikawa K, Suzuki H, McMullen B, Chung D. Purification of human von Willebrand factor-cleaving protease and its identification as a new member of the metalloproteinase family. Blood 2001;98:1662–6.
61. Furlan M, Robles R, Galbusera M, et al. von Willebrand factor-cleaving protease in thrombotic thrombocytopenic purpura and the hemolytic-uremic syndrome. N Engl J Med 1998;339:1578–84.
62. Holdsworth S, Boyce N, Thomson NM, Atkins RC. The clinical spectrum of acute glomerulonephritis and lung haemorrhage (Goodpasture's syndrome). Q J Med 1985;55:75–86.
63. Laszik Z, Silva FG. Hemolytic-uremic syndrome, thrombotic thrombocytopenic purpura, and systemic sclerosis (systemic scleroderma). In: Jennette JC, Olson JL, Schwartz MM, Silva FG, eds. Heptinstall's pathology of the kidney. Philadelphia: Lippincott-Raven; 1998:1003–57.
64. Moake JL. von Willebrand factor, ADAMTS-13, and thrombotic thrombocytopenic purpura. Semin Hematol 2004;41:4–14.
65. Symmers W St C. Thrombotic microangiopathic haemolytic anaemia (thrombotic microangiopathy). Br Med J 1952;2:897–903.
66. Veyradier A, Obert B, Houllier A, Meyer D, Girma JP. Specific von Willebrand factor-cleaving protease in thrombotic microangiopathies: a study of 111 cases. Blood 2001;98:1765–72.

Disseminated Intravascular Coagulation

67. Kawasaki H, Hayashi K, Awai M. Disseminated intravascular coagulation (DIC). Immunohistochemical study of fibrin-related materials (FRMs) in renal tissues. Acta Pathol Jpn 1987; 37:77–84.
68. van Gorp EC, Suharti C, ten Cate H, et al. Review: infectious diseases and coagulation disorders. J Infect Dis 1999;180:176–86.

19 DISEASES OF THE RENAL TUBULES

Most diseases that affect the tubules also affect the interstitial regions (hence the term "tubulointerstitial disease/nephritis") (see chapter 21). In this section, we consider diseases primarily affecting the tubules.

ACUTE TUBULAR NECROSIS

Definition. Acute tubular necrosis (ATN) is a clinical-pathologic entity that is manifested morphologically by the primary destruction or alteration of the renal tubular epithelium (6,9, 13,24,39–41,48,49,54). Clinically, it is the most common cause of acute renal failure, resulting in elevations of blood urea nitrogen (BUN) and serum creatinine, and often causing oliguria or anuria (Table 19-1). The deterioration of renal function occurs over a period of hours to days.

The two major forms of ATN are ischemic and toxic. Unlike toxic ATN, the form of ATN associated with ischemia may be quite difficult to detect on histologic grounds; there may not be frank or widespread tubular epithelial necrosis, but only subtle cellular changes of sublethal tubular injury. This results in a discordance between the severity of the clinical findings and the morphologic changes that accompany it. Therefore, the terms *acute vasomotor nephropathy, shock kidney, ischemic acute tubular nephropathy,* and *ischemic acute tubular nephrosis or necrosis* are used alternatively for ischemic ATN. There is considerable difference in opinion over the definition of terms and how the term "ATN" should be applied.

Clinical Features. As noted above, ATN is the most common cause of acute renal failure, especially before the age of 60 years. The frequency of acute renal failure depends on the clinical setting (2,3,25,28,31,33). In many instances, there is one or more detectable precipitating events which may operate at multiple times and which precede the clinical onset of renal failure by several days to 1 week. ATN is commonly encountered in hospitalized patients. Although the ischemic episodes and/or the presence of a nephrotoxin, either endogenous or exogenous, can be identified, often the exact cause of the tubular injury is not known (Table 19-2). In half the patients with ATN, the clinical onset is signaled by an abrupt onset of oliguria (less than 400 mL/day of urine); in the other half or more of patients, there is nonoliguric renal failure. There is usually a rapid deterioration of renal function over a short period of time (hours to days). BUN and serum creatinine levels are elevated and the urinalysis usually shows only hyaline, granular, or pigmented casts. The urine

Table 19-1

CAUSES OF ACUTE RENAL FAILURE

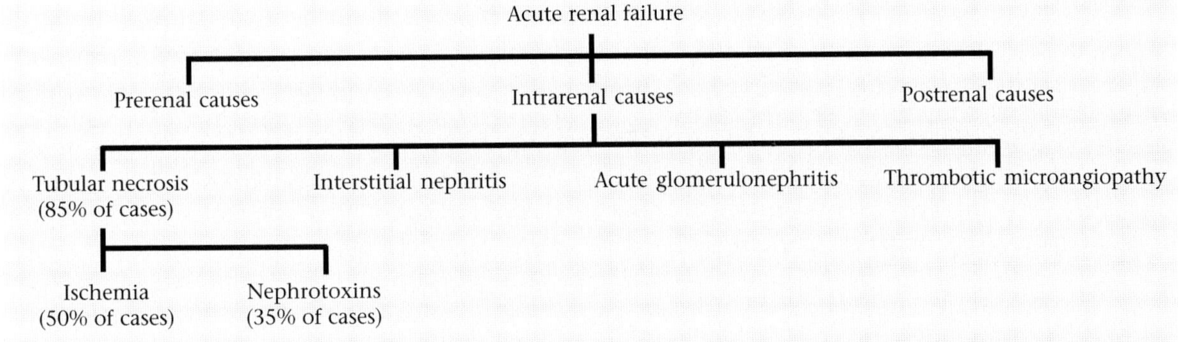

Acute renal failure
- Prerenal causes
- Intrarenal causes
  - Tubular necrosis (85% of cases)
    - Ischemia (50% of cases)
    - Nephrotoxins (35% of cases)
  - Interstitial nephritis
  - Acute glomerulonephritis
  - Thrombotic microangiopathy
- Postrenal causes

[a]Modified from reference 51.

Table 19-2

NEPHROTOXINS LEADING TO ACUTE TUBULAR NECROSIS

Endogenous/Tissue Toxins	Exogenous/Drugs
Excessive light chains of immunoglobulins (as in multiple myeloma)	Aminoglycosides
Myoglobin (skeletal muscle injuries with rhabdomyolysis)	Radiocontrast agents
Hemoglobin (mismatched blood transfusion reaction)	Chemotherapeutic agents (e.g., cisplatin)
Heme pigments (hemolysis, blood transfusions)	Heavy metals (e.g., mercury)
	Organic solvents (e.g., carbon tetrachloride)

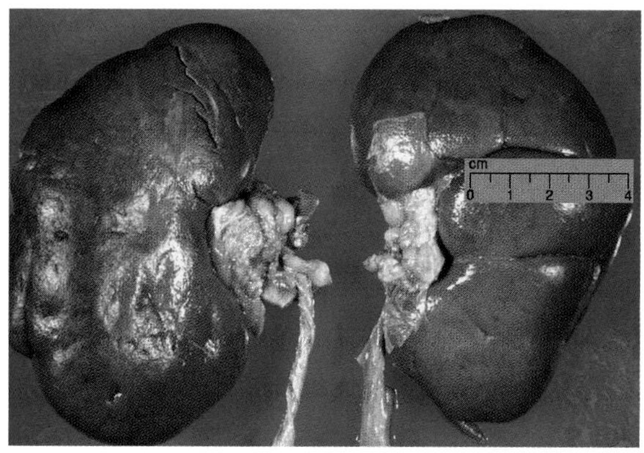

Figure 19-1

ACUTE TUBULAR NECROSIS

The kidneys are swollen and somewhat pale.

is dilute (isosthenuric or hyposthenuric compared to the serum) and the urine sodium and fractional excretion of sodium are high (compared to patients with prerenal azotemia). This is consistent with the decreased reabsorptive capacity of the damaged tubular epithelium. There is a sudden inability to maintain normal fluid and electrolyte homeostasis.

The clinical course of patients with ATN can be divided into three stages: initiation, maintenance, and recovery (53). In the ischemic form (2,20), the initiating stage is manifested by the inciting medical, surgical, or obstetric event. Often, the only clinical indication is a decline of urine output with an elevation of BUN/serum creatinine. During this stage, the decline of urine output is secondary to decreased blood flow to the kidneys. In the maintenance stage, there is a sustained decline in urine volume (between 40 and 400 mL/day), with rising BUN, salt and water overload, metabolic acidosis, and hyperkalemia. The recovery stage shows a steady increase in urine volume (which may reach several liters/day). Because the tubular epithelium is still damaged, there is a loss of large amounts of water, sodium, potassium, and other solutes in the urine. Hypokalemia can become a major clinical problem. Eventually, with recovery, there is restoration of renal tubular function and improvement in urinary concentrating ability. BUN and serum creatinine return to baseline levels; however, it may take several months for the tubular functions to normalize. The morbidity and mortality of patients with ATN are largely the result of the many possible accompanying complications and clinical settings (see Treatment and Prognosis).

A renal biopsy is generally not performed for the evaluation and management of patients with clinically obvious ATN; however, when the signs, symptoms, or laboratory values are ambiguous or fail to support a clinical diagnosis of ATN, renal biopsy may be of help. In a recent prospective renal biopsy study of patients with acute renal failure, knowledge of the morphologic findings altered management in almost three fourths of patients (43,45,54). Also, other conditions may be clinically indistinguishable from ATN (30,38). ATN is a common finding in the kidney at autopsy, although its diagnosis is more difficult in autopsy than in biopsy specimens because of autolytic changes that can mimic tubular changes of ischemic ATN (see below).

Gross Findings. The kidneys are enlarged, tense, and pale (fig. 19-1). On cross section, the renal parenchyma is swollen and may bulge from the capsule. The cortex is widened and there may be accentuation of the corticomedullary junction, with the medulla appearing dark or deep red in contrast to the paler cortex

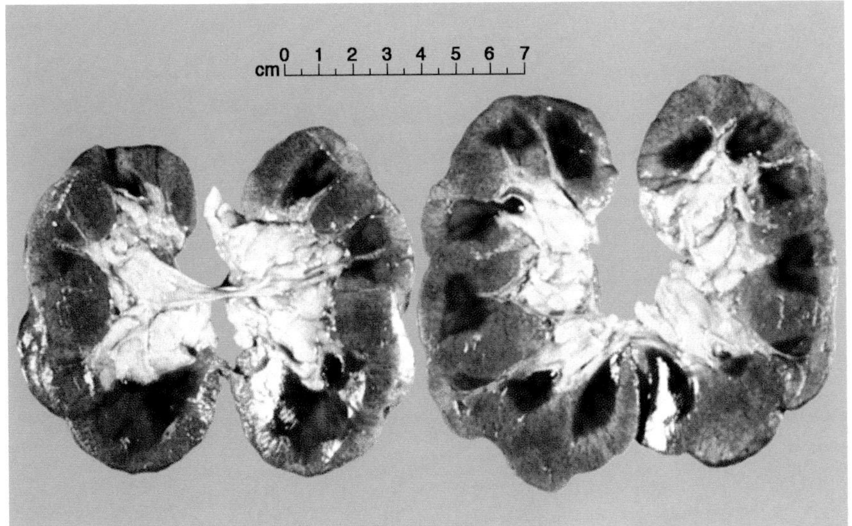

Figure 19-2

ACUTE TUBULAR NECROSIS

Cross section of the kidneys with "lower nephron nephrosis" secondary to myoglobinuric acute tubular necrosis.

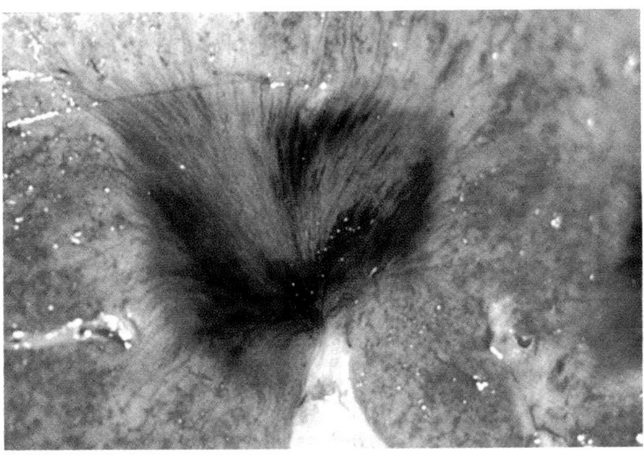

Figure 19-3

ACUTE TUBULAR NECROSIS

Cross section of the medulla of a kidney from a patient with "lower nephron nephrosis," or myoglobinuric acute tubular necrosis.

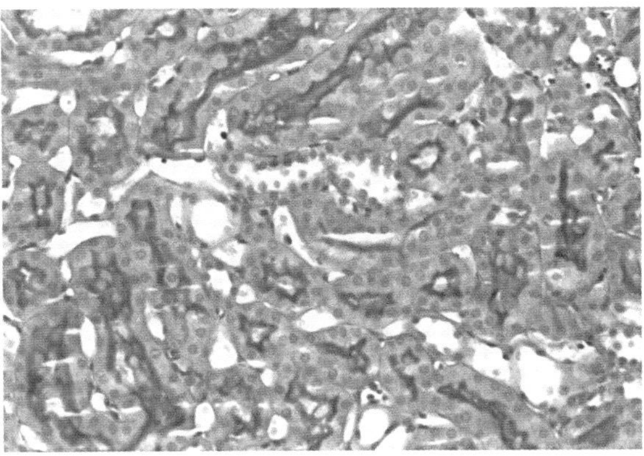

Figure 19-4

NORMAL RENAL CORTEX

The brush borders of the proximal tubular epithelium are seen (periodic acid–Schiff [PAS] stain).

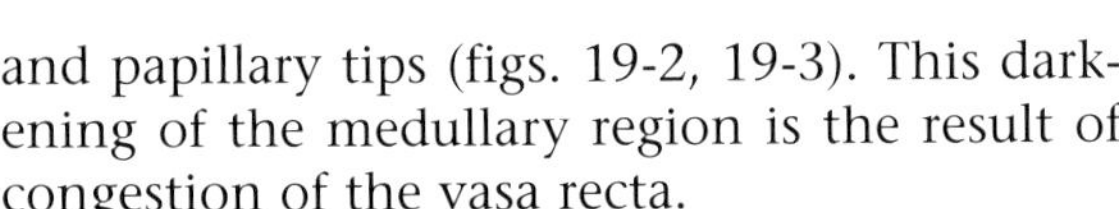

and papillary tips (figs. 19-2, 19-3). This darkening of the medullary region is the result of congestion of the vasa recta.

Light Microscopic Findings. Knowledge of the histology of the renal tubules in the normal renal cortex and medulla is essential (fig. 19-4). The major changes of ATN are noted initially in the renal tubules (fig. 19-5); these range from subtle to severe, but are usually patchy (figs. 19-6–19-15). Frank tubular epithelial necrosis is not always evident by light microscopy, especially in ischemic injuries. Ischemic changes are characteristically focal and mild.

The many changes that may be evident by light microscopy are: 1) injury, with degeneration and necrosis of the individual tubular epithelial cells (coagulation necrosis [loss of cell nuclei but partial preservation of cell outlines], karyorrhexis, pyknosis) (figs. 19-6, 19-7); 2) formation of blebs in the apical membranes of proximal tubular cells with shedding into the tubular lumens (early ischemic change) (fig. 19-8); 3) swelling of the tubular epithelium (fig. 19-10). This severe ballooning of the cytoplasm is especially seen with toxins; 4) separation (detachment) of the tubular epithelial cells from

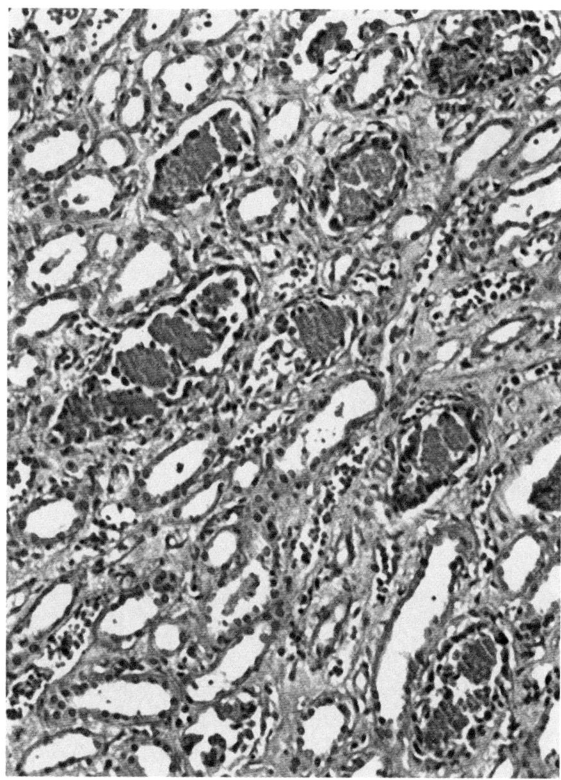

Figure 19-5

ACUTE TUBULAR NECROSIS: SHOCK KIDNEY

There are a large number of casts in the tubules. Note the extreme thinning of the tubular epithelium (hematoxylin and eosin [H&E] stain).

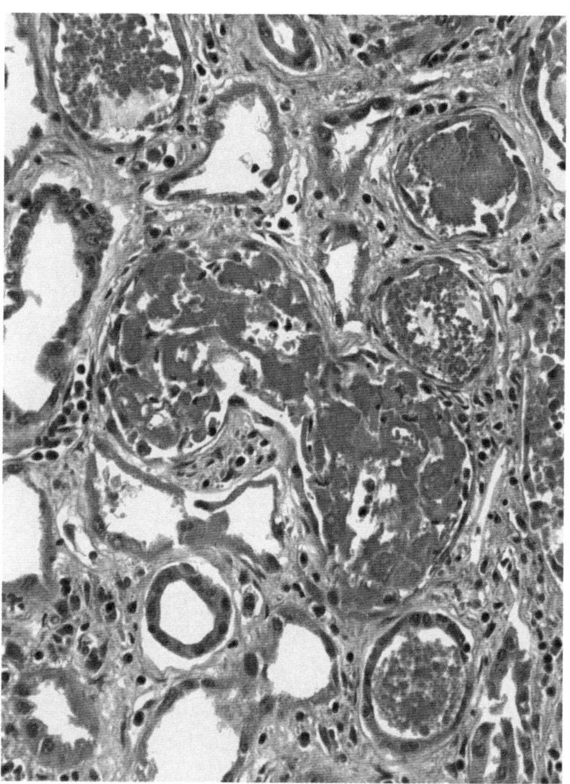

Figure 19-6

ACUTE TUBULAR NECROSIS

There is destruction of the tubular epithelium, with coagulation necrosis (loss of cell nuclei with some preservation of cell outlines). There is loss or thinning of the tubular epithelium and cast formation (H&E stain).

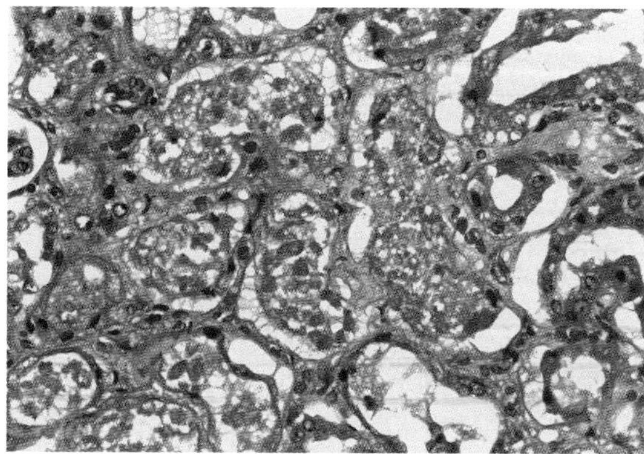

Figure 19-7

ACUTE TUBULAR NECROSIS

Widespread tubular epithelial necrosis in a patient with toxic nephropathy secondary to aminoglycoside antibiotic therapy (H&E stain).

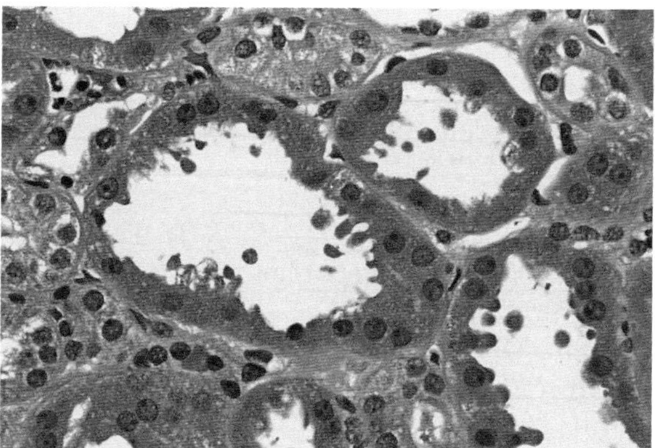

Figure 19-8

ACUTE TUBULAR NECROSIS (ISCHEMIC TUBULAR NEPHROPATHY)

One of the earliest changes in ischemic nephropathy is tubular epithelial surface "blebbing" of the apical cell membrane, seen here in some of the proximal tubules (H&E stain).

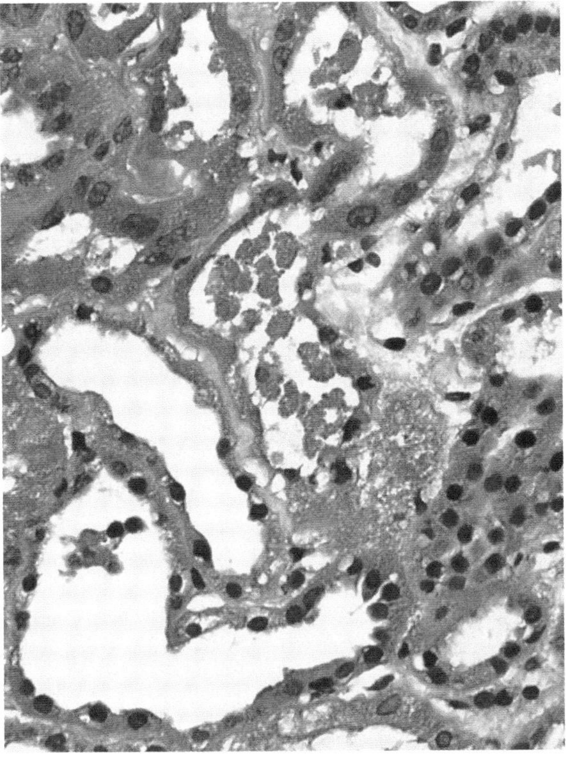

Figure 19-9

ACUTE TUBULAR NECROSIS

There is necrosis of the tubular epithelium, with separation of tubular cells from the tubular basement membrane. In addition to denudation of the tubular epithelium, several necrotic epithelial cells are noted in the tubular lumens (H&E stain).

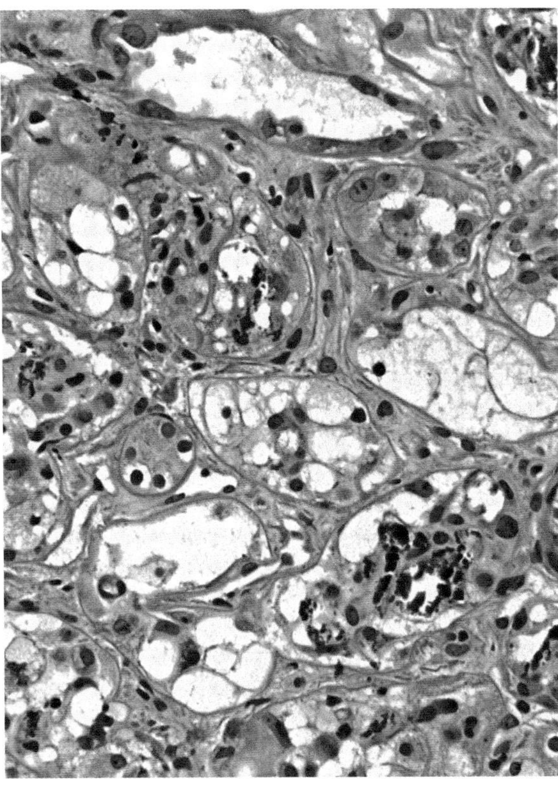

Figure 19-10

ACUTE TUBULAR NECROSIS

Acute tubular necrosis in a patient poisoned with ethylene glycol. There is marked vacuolization of the tubular epithelial cells. In one area there is complete necrosis and loss of the tubular epithelial cells (H&E stain).

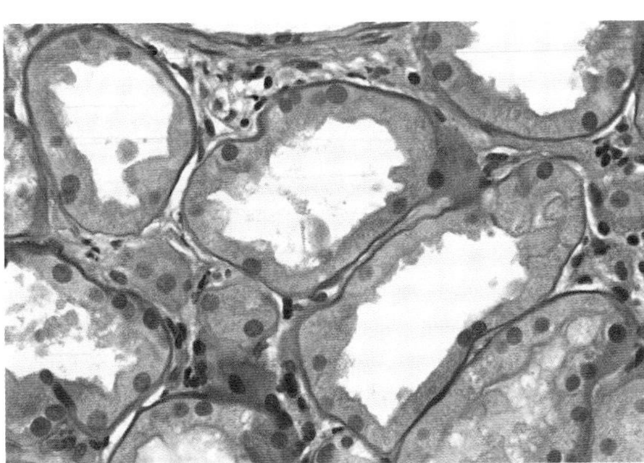

Figure 19-11

ACUTE TUBULAR NECROSIS
(ACUTE TUBULAR ISCHEMIC NEPHROPATHY)

There is moderate thinning of the proximal tubular epithelial cells and widening of the tubular lumens. There is loss of the normally present PAS-positive brush borders in this transplant patient with ischemia (PAS stain).

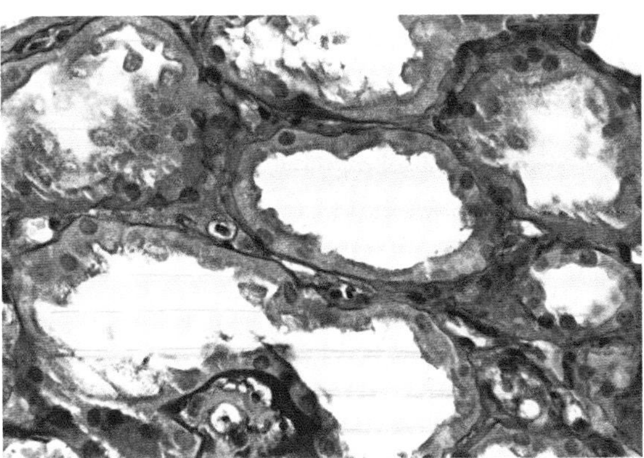

Figure 19-12

ACUTE TUBULAR NECROSIS

There is marked thinning of the tubular epithelium (and in areas, loss of the epithelium) and dilatation of the tubular lumens. A few casts were noted elsewhere (PAS stain).

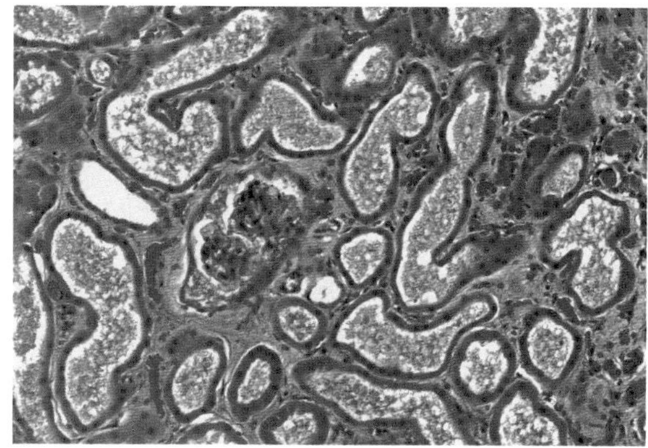

Figure 19-13

ACUTE TUBULAR NECROSIS

There is marked thinning of the tubular epithelium with dilatation of the tubular lumens (H&E stain).

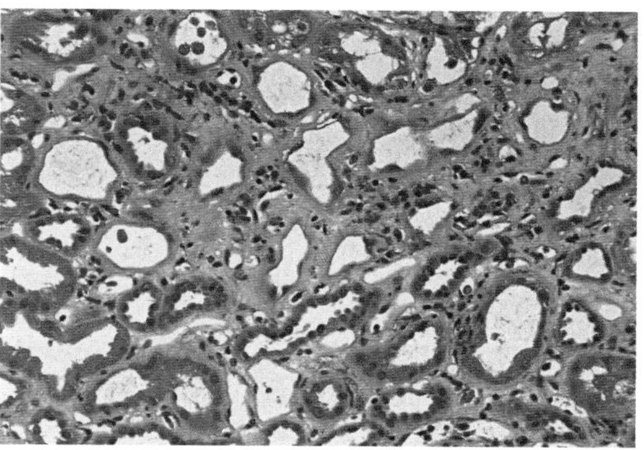

Figure 19-14

ACUTE TUBULAR NECROSIS

There is marked thinning of the tubular epithelium with dilatation of the tubular lumens (H&E stain).

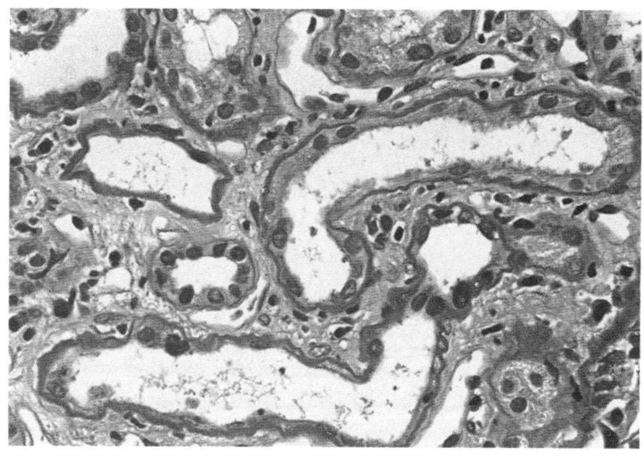

Figure 19-15

ACUTE TUBULAR NECROSIS

There is thinning of the tubular epithelium with dilatation of the tubular lumens (H&E stain).

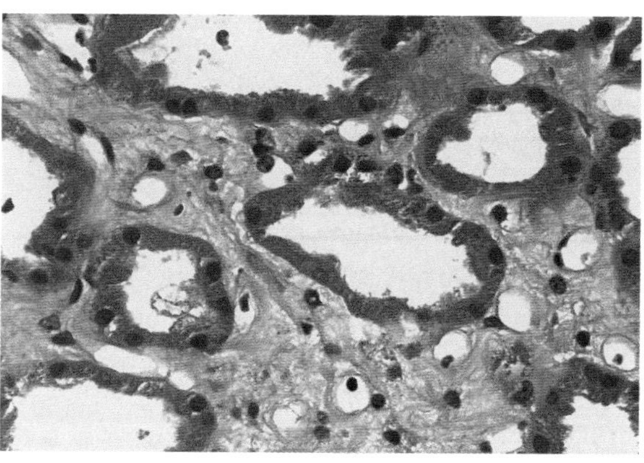

Figure 19-16

ACUTE TUBULAR NECROSIS

There is separation of the tubules by interstitial edema (H&E stain).

the underlying tubular basement membranes (fig. 19-9); 5) loss or attenuation of the periodic acid–Schiff (PAS)–positive brush border of the proximal tubular epithelial cells (fig. 19-11; compare with fig. 19-4); 6) thinning ("simplification") of the tubular epithelium (figs. 19-12–19-15); 7) dilatation (enlargement) of the tubular lumens (figs. 19-12–19-15); 8) interstitial edema with widening of the normally sparse interstitium and separation of the tubules from each other (fig. 19-16); 9) presence of casts (hyaline, pigmented, eosinophilic, cellular, or granular debris), especially in the distal tubules (figs. 19-17–19-20). Deeply pigmented casts suggest hemolysis or rhabdomyolysis (i.e., hemoglobin or myoglobin); 10) tubular lumens containing sloughed epithelial cells (which are both viable and dead), leukocytes, and cellular debris (figs. 19-6, 19-7, 19-9); 11) numerous nucleated (mononuclear) cells in the vasa recta of the outer medulla (probably mostly myeloid precursors) (fig. 19-21). Early in the course these mononuclear cells may be lymphocytes, and eventually the myeloid cells are replaced by nucleated red blood cells and red blood cell precursors; 12) scant peritubular inflammation (lymphocytes, monocytes,

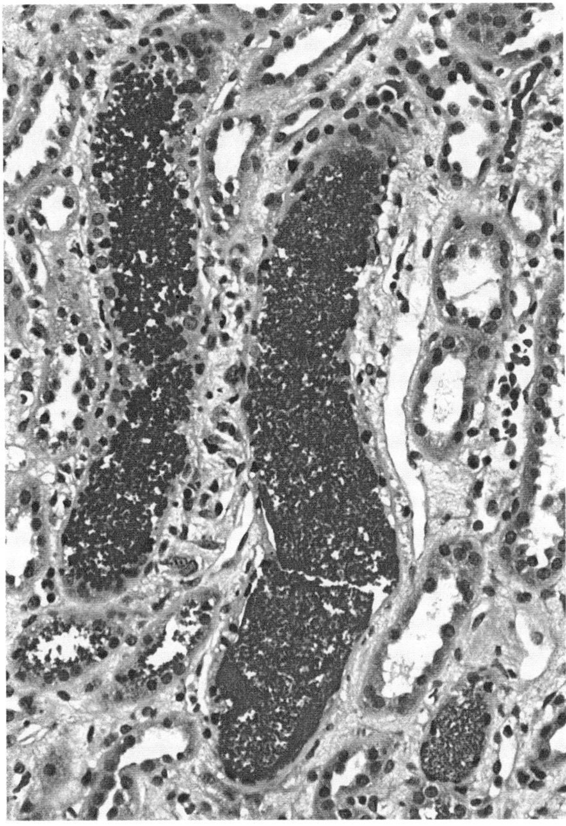

Figure 19-17

ACUTE TUBULAR NECROSIS

Casts of various types (hyaline, granular, pigmented) may be seen in patients with acute tubular necrosis. This patient had hemoglobinuric acute tubular necrosis following a mismatched blood transfusion (H&E stain).

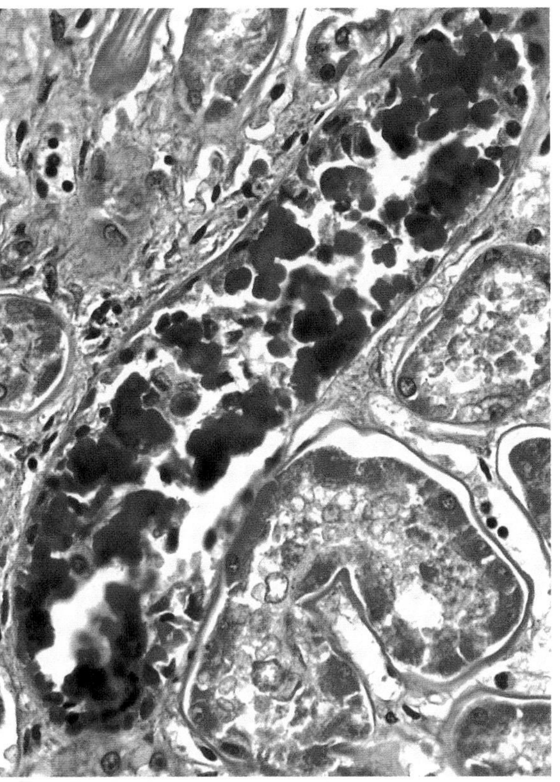

Figure 19-18

ACUTE TUBULAR NECROSIS

Large pigmented cast from a patient with myoglobin nephropathy (crush injury) (H&E stain).

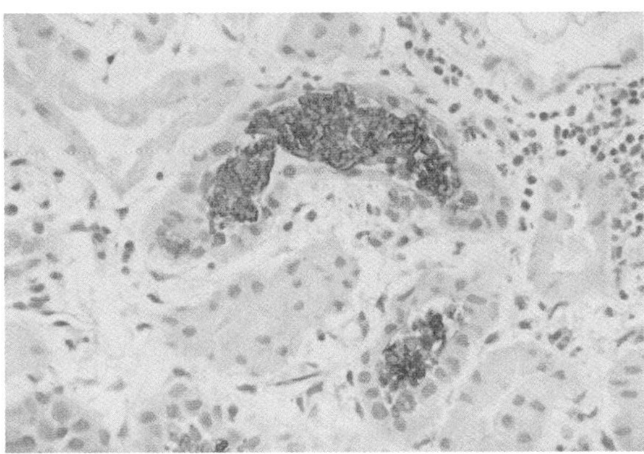

Figure 19-19

ACUTE TUBULAR NECROSIS

Immunoperoxidase staining with an antibody to myoglobin. (Courtesy of Dr. R. Verani, Houston, TX.)

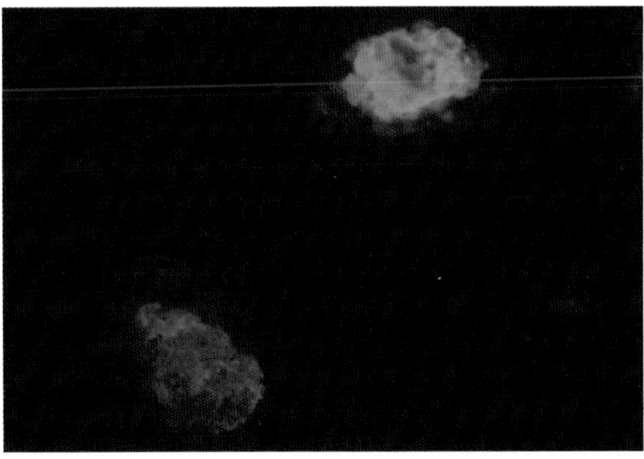

Figure 19-20

CHRONIC RENAL FAILURE

Renal casts often stain nonspecifically with a number of immunoreactants that are normal or abnormally filtered proteins. Casts are akin to "ink blotters" that soak up many of the fluids noted in the ultrafiltrate. Immunofluorescence microscopy delineates nonspecific staining for the various immunoglobulins, complement components, and other nonspecific immunoreactants (anti-C3 stain).

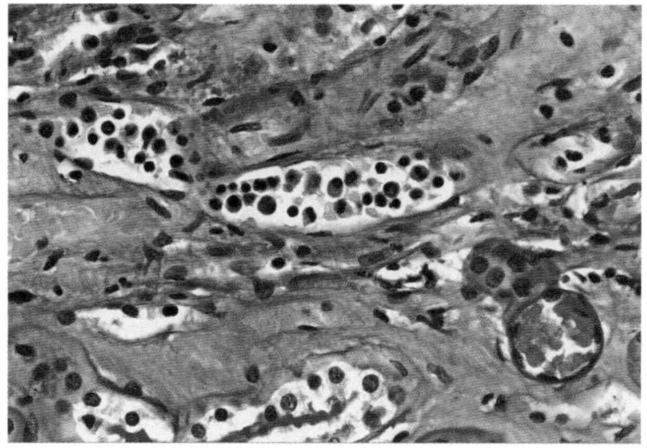

Figure 19-21

ACUTE TUBULAR NECROSIS

This section of renal medulla shows a large number of mononuclear hematopoietic cells in the vasa recta, which is good morphologic evidence of acute tubular necrosis. The nature of the mononuclear cells has been debated but these probably mostly represent hematopoietic cells of the myeloid series (with margination) (H&E stain).

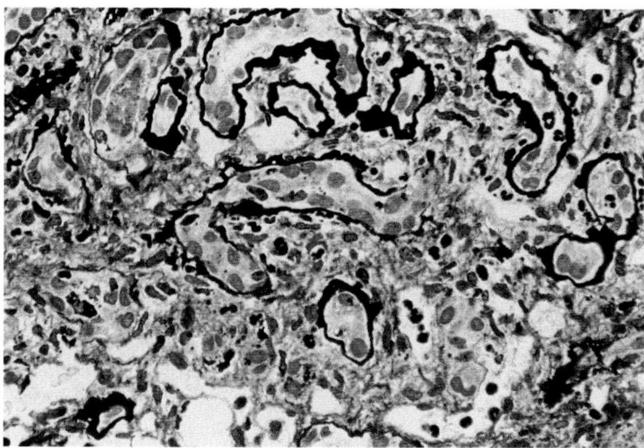

Figure 19-22

ACUTE TUBULAR NECROSIS

This patient had nephrotoxicity secondary to treatment with cisplatin. There may be secondary changes in and around the degenerating and necrotic tubules, such as mild interstitial inflammation and disruption or breaks of the tubular basement membrane (Jones methenamine silver [JMS] stain).

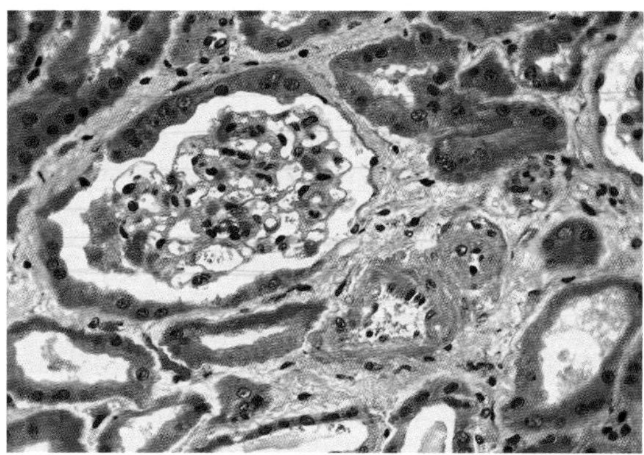

Figure 19-23

ACUTE TUBULAR NECROSIS

Sometimes there is "proximalization," or proximal tubular epithelial cell change, in the lining cells of Bowman's capsule (parietal epithelial cells) (H&E stain).

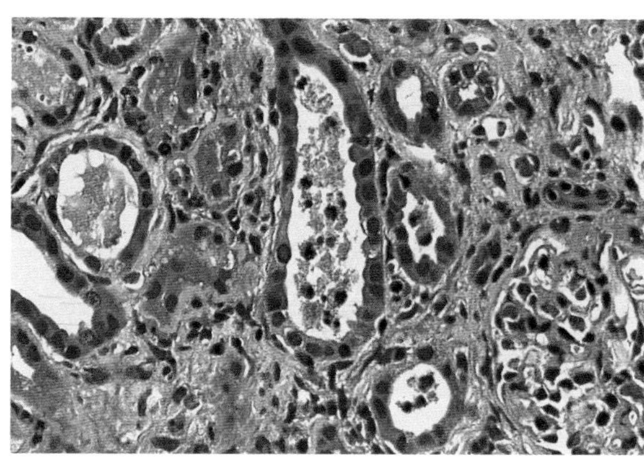

Figure 19-24

ACUTE TUBULAR NECROSIS: REGENERATIVE PHASE

After the acute episode of acute tubular necrosis, the tubular epithelial cells regenerate. At this stage, proximal tubular epithelium cannot be distinguished from distal tubular epithelium by conventional light microscopy (H&E stain).

and occasional polymorphonuclear leukocytes). These inflammatory cells are usually clustered around necrotic and/or ruptured tubular segments. There may be nearby Tamm-Horsfall extrusion (see chapters 20 and 24). Even occasional scattered eosinophils (usually low in number) can be found, usually in the recovery stage; 13) rupture of the tubular basement membranes (tubulorrhexis) (fig. 19-22). There may be small adjacent granulomatous interstitial lesions; 14) apoptosis (cell shrinkage with nuclear fragmentation); 15) prominent parietal epithelium of Bowman's capsule with herniation of proximal tubular epithelium into Bowman's space (fig. 19-23); 16) focal calcification of necrotic tubular material (especially noted with certain toxins); and 17) occasional foamy tubular epithelial cell changes ("hydropic degeneration,"

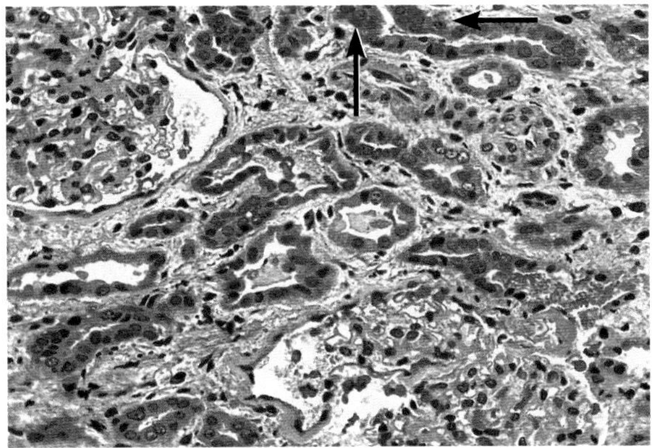

Figure 19-25

ACUTE TUBULAR NECROSIS: REGENERATIVE PHASE

In the regenerative phase, it appears that there has been epithelial cellular overgrowth. Eventually, the tubules are completely reconstituted (H&E stain).

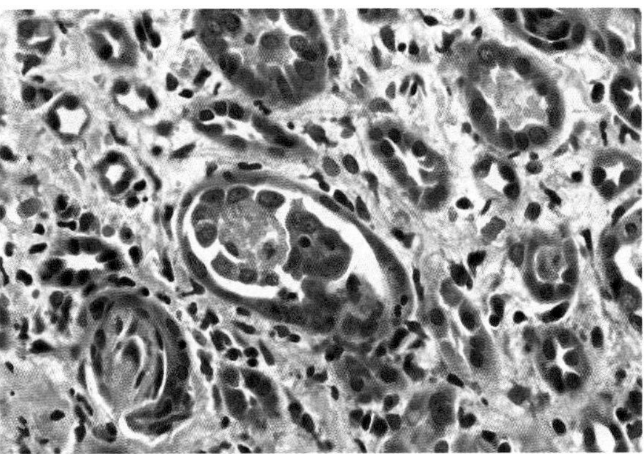

Figure 19-26

ACUTE TUBULAR NECROSIS: REGENERATIVE STAGE

Nucleomegaly is often seen in the regenerative stage of acute tubular necrosis. This patient did not have evidence of any of the viral infections that can lead to large nuclei (H&E stain).

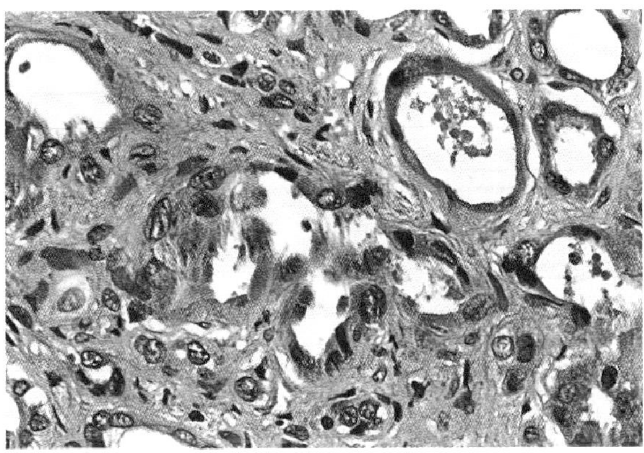

Figure 19-27

ACUTE TUBULAR NECROSIS: REGENERATIVE PHASE

Nucleomegaly can be seen in the regenerating epithelium and needs to be distinguished from viral nucleopathic effects (H&E stain).

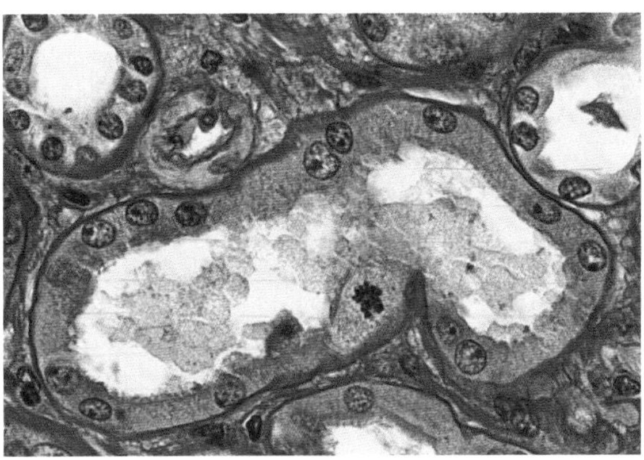

Figure 19-28

ACUTE TUBULAR NECROSIS

A mitotic figure is noted in one of the tubular epithelial cells. Normally, mitotic figures are not seen in the tubular epithelium because the turnover of tubular epithelium is quite low (about one mitotic figure/tubule/day). The mitotic count is increased in acute tubular injury with regeneration (H&E stain).

fatty change, etc.). This is especially noted in various toxic forms (7,12,13,24,27,36, 39,41,48).

Later, in the reactive/reparative/regenerative stage, the following histologic changes may be seen: 1) basophilic staining of tubular epithelial cytoplasm (figs. 19-24–19-26); 2) large hyperchromatic nuclei (often with prominent nucleoli) (figs. 19-26, 19-27); 3) mitotic figures in the tubular epithelial cells (fig. 19-28); 4) peritubular inflammation/granulomata, secondary to extruded casts (Tamm-Horsfall protein in the interstitial areas); 5) tubularization of the parietal epithelium of Bowman's capsule; and 6) flattening of the tubular epithelial cells.

Some of the morphologic changes in these two groups (the initial and the reactive/reparative/regenerative) are superimposed upon each other. The regenerative changes in the tubular epithelium recapitulate certain aspects of renal epithelial cell development in embryogenesis,

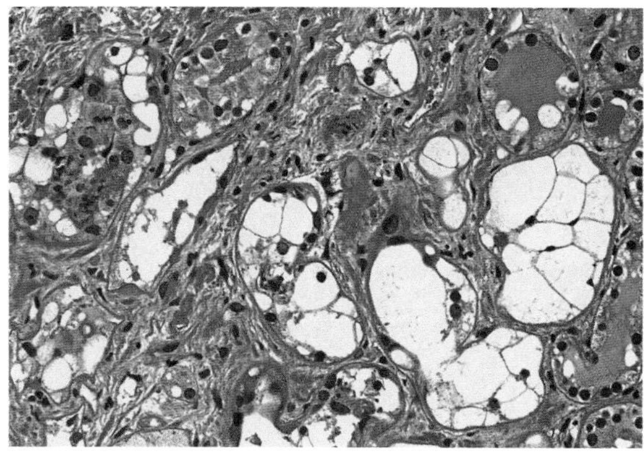

Figure 19-29

ACUTE TUBULAR NECROSIS: ETHYLENE GLYCOL TOXICITY

The tubular epithelial cells are markedly ballooned (H&E stain).

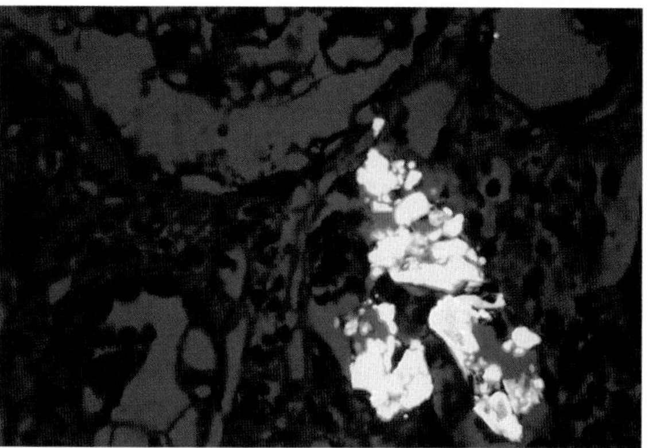

Figure 19-30

ACUTE TUBULAR NECROSIS: ETHYLENE GLYCOL POISONING

The oxalate crystals are polarized.

such as the expression of certain proteins normally present only early in development. The sequelae of acute tubule injury or necrosis may be progressive interstitial fibrosis (37).

The distribution of the lesions (i.e., proximal or distal segment[s]) of the nephron involved depends on the etiology of the ATN. Ischemic ATN is manifested by tubular epithelial damage along multiple patchy segments of the nephron, often with what seems like large skip areas in between (11). There may be breaks in the tubular basement membranes (tubulorrhexis) (fig. 19-22) and the presence of tubular luminal casts (figs. 19-17, 19-18). As noted before, the necrosis may be quite subtle and easily missed by histologic examination. The thick ascending limb of Henle and the last or straight portion of the proximal tubules seem to be especially vulnerable sites for ischemia. Cortical nephrons appear to be more extensively damaged than juxtamedullary nephrons. Obviously, it is difficult to differentiate superficial cortical from juxtamedullary nephrons in a biopsy specimen, unless there is an attached medulla or renal capsule. The distal tubules can be filled with casts as well. Large, very eosinophilic casts (possibly even pigmented casts, often representing myoglobin or hemoglobin) are seen in the distal tubules and collecting ducts. These casts are comprised mainly of Tamm-Horsfall protein, sometimes in association with hemoglobin, myoglobin, or other proteins from the plasma. The exact nature of the casts depends on the initiating cause of the injury (e.g., crush injury with resultant myoglobinuria).

The toxic form of ATN often shows more obvious and extensive tubular epithelial cell necrosis by light microscopy (see Table 19-2) (3,5). Because the proximal tubular segment of the nephron is the site most commonly responsible for the excretion of organic acids and ions (such as drugs and other toxins), this is the segment most commonly injured (18,19,36). Heavy metals and organic toxins often lead to extensive involvement of all nephron segments, with a greater predilection for cortical nephrons.

With certain poisons there are characteristic morphologic findings (24). *Mercuric chloride* causes large acidophilic inclusions in severely injured cells. The third portion (S3) or pars recta of the proximal tubule is the most commonly involved segment of the nephron. Later there may be severe calcification of the tubules/cells in the lumens. *Carbon tetrachloride* results in an accumulation of neutral lipids in the injured tubular cells, followed by necrosis. *Ethylene glycol* causes marked ballooning and hydropic/vacuolar changes in the proximal tubular cells, with calcium oxalate crystals in the tubular lumens (figs. 19-29, 19-30). *Diethylene glycol* leads to tubular injury and cellular atypia without the oxalate crystals.

Other renal injuries are caused by other exposures, including a variety of industrial exposures, accidental/intentional ingestions (such as

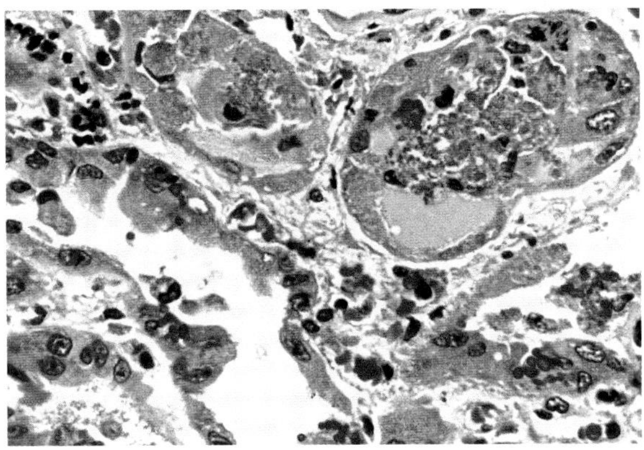

Figure 19-31

ACUTE TUBULAR NECROSIS: ARSENIC POISONING

There is marked necrosis of the tubular epithelium (H&E stain).

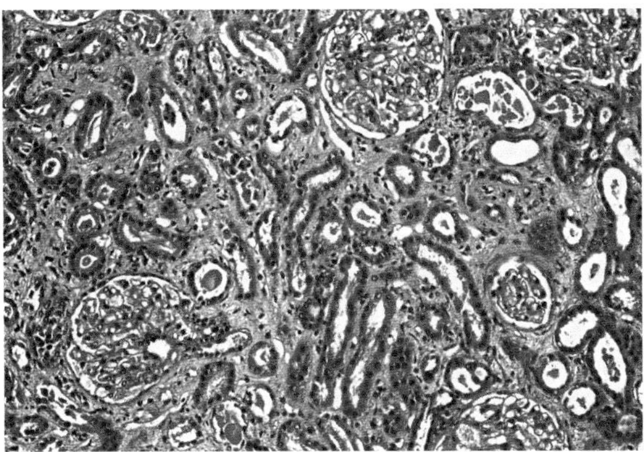

Figure 19-32

ACUTE TUBULAR NECROSIS: PENTAMIDINE AND BACTRIM TOXICITY

The tubular lumens are dilated and the epithelium is thinned (H&E stain).

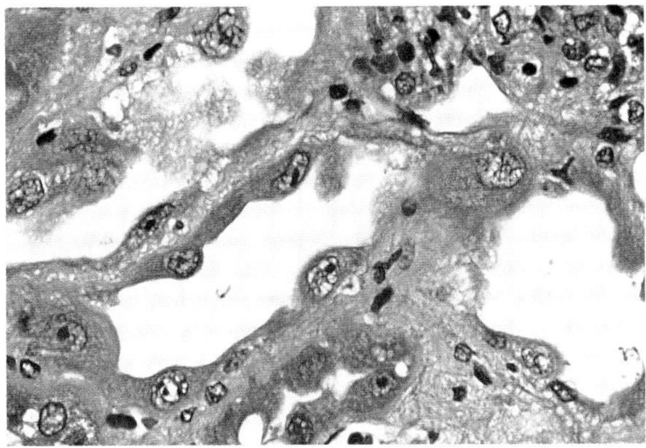

Figure 19-33

ACUTE TUBULAR INJURY: FOSCARNET TOXICITY

Foscarnet is an antiviral drug. At times it is difficult to distinguish between acute tubular cell injury and interstitial injury. Other regions of this kidney showed interstitial fibrosis (H&E stain).

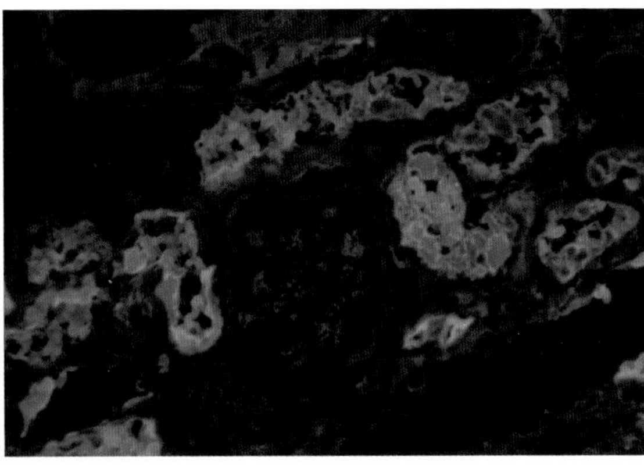

Figure 19-34

ACUTE TUBULAR NECROSIS

Some investigators have noted that necrotic tubular epithelium may show nonspecific, nonimmunologic immunofluorescence staining, as is seen here (anti-IgG).

arsenic [fig. 19-31]), therapeutic agents (such as the aminoglycoside antibiotics [fig. 19-32], antineoplastic and antiviral agents [fig. 19-33], and herbal remedies [especially aristocholic acid/Chinese herbal teas]), and ischemic/microcirculatory disturbances leading to rhabdomyolysis (the latter also seen in cocaine abuse). All of these exhibit the spectrum of morphologic changes described for toxic ATN. Myoglobin-induced tubulopathy is usually associated with not only large amounts of myoglobinuria but also an accompanying ischemia.

Immunofluorescence Findings. These studies are usually negative or nonspecific. Some have suggested that endogenous fluorescence can be noted in the necrotic tubules (i.e., positive fluorescent staining without the application of fluoresceinated antisera to cyrostat sections) (see fig. 19-21). Tubular casts may show nonspecific nonimmunologic binding of immunoglobulins and other serum proteins (fig. 19-34).

Electron Microscopic Findings. Glomeruli show minimal changes. The luminal surfaces of the tubular epithelium are simplified (after

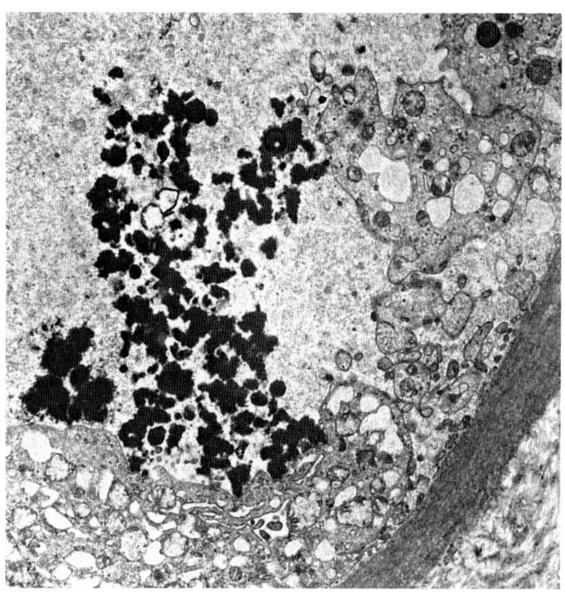

Figure 19-35

ACUTE TUBULAR NECROSIS

There is degeneration and mummification of some tubular epithelial cells, some of which are detached from the underlying tubular basement membrane. There is loss of the brush border and dilatation of the endoplasmic reticulum. A large amorphous cast is seen in the tubule (electron micrograph).

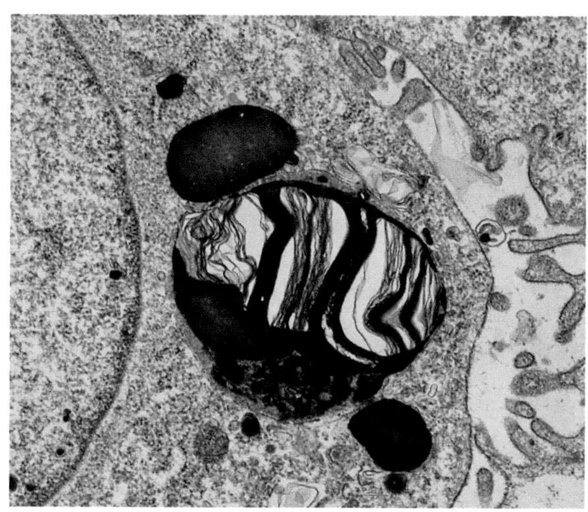

Figure 19-36

AMINOGLYCOSIDE-INDUCED ACUTE TUBULAR NECROSIS

There are large myeloid bodies in the proximal tubular epithelium. Any patient (irrespective of whether they have tubular injury or not) may have myeloid bodies if they have received aminoglycosides, however. Thus the presence of myeloid bodies is only indicative that the patient has been receiving this antibiotic, not whether it has induced cellular injury.

early apical ballooning of the cell membrane in ischemia). There is often loss or blunting of the brush border of the proximal tubular epithelial cells. The basolateral interdigitations become simplified. There are various cytoplasmic vacuolization changes, including dilatation of the endoplasmic reticulum, mitochondrial swelling, and increased numbers of lipofuscin granules. Small gaps may be seen in the lining of the tubular epithelium (a nonreplacement phenomenon) (fig. 19-35). The tubular epithelium may loosen from the tubular basement membrane. Gentamicin inclusions are often noted in patients receiving this antibiotic, although the presence of inclusions does not directly correlate with drug toxicity (i.e., every patient receiving gentamicin has these inclusions in their renal epithelial cells) (fig. 19-36).

Special Studies. Various nephron site-specific lectins and antibodies may be employed to demonstrate the site of the nephron affected; however, these are not in general diagnostic use (34,47).

Differential Diagnosis. The clinical differential diagnosis of ATN includes all causes of acute renal failure including interstitial nephritis, acute severe glomerulonephritis (e.g., acute poststreptococcal or crescentic pauci-immune or immunoglobulin [Ig]A glomerulonephritis), bilateral renal cortical necrosis, thrombotic microangiopathy, and urinary tract obstruction (bilateral) (see Table 19-1). The most important histologic differential diagnosis is between primary acute interstitial nephritis with secondary involvement of the nearby tubules, and primary severe acute tubular necrosis with secondary surrounding and reactive inflammation. Because the histologic features of these two conditions may overlap, differentiation is based upon the clinical and morphologic features. The presence of major, extensive or severe interstitial inflammation and associated tubulitis (the latter defined as infiltration of inflammatory cells in the tubular epithelial regions) favors primary acute interstitial nephritis rather than primary acute tubular necrosis. The presence of many neutrophils (especially associated with the tubules or in aggregates [abscesses]) indicates an acute pyelonephritis rather than ATN; the presence of a number of eosinophils and tubulitis suggests a primary allergic interstitial nephritis.

Etiology and Pathogenesis. The two major causes of ATN are ischemia and toxicity. Both lead to ATN via tubular epithelial cell damage (10,26). Prolonged renal ischemia is the most common cause of ATN. The tubular epithelium is susceptible to hypoxia/anoxia, usually secondary to a variety of conditions (hypotension, shock, blood loss, burns, extensive trauma, sepsis), leading to a period of inadequate blood flow to visceral or peripheral organs (55). Certain toxins normally excreted by the kidneys may cause renal injury. It is thought that there are several factors that predispose the tubules to toxic injury, such as active renal transport systems for organic ions/organic acids and various other renal toxins, the capacity for renal concentration of toxic agents, and a large surface for renal tubular reabsorption of potential toxins (23). Impaired glomerular permselectivity allows the escape of tubulotoxic substances into the urinary space and uptake by the tubular epithelium.

ATN in hospitalized patients is often due to more than one insult. For example, the exposure of septic patients to aminoglycosides and the administration of radiocontrast agents in those patients treated with angiotensin converting enzyme inhibitors are frequent combinations that lead to acute renal insult. As noted elsewhere, nephrotoxins (endogenous or exogenous) and accompanying ischemia often combine to lead to ATN in severely ill patients (such as those with sepsis, hematologic cancers, or acquired immunodeficiency syndrome [AIDS]). Ischemia leads to many functional and structural alterations in the tubular epithelium, such as loss of cell polarity, which are considered later (22). Because the kidney (especially the renal medulla and corticomedullary junction) normally has a tenuously supplied blood flow, it is especially susceptible to further ischemia; these renal regions are thought to be preferentially affected by diminished blood flow (11). In the outer medullary regions where the renal tubules have high oxygen requirements because of solute reabsorption, ischemia causes swelling of tubular epithelial and endothelial cells as well as complement-dependent and -independent (e.g., intercellular adhesion molecule [ICAM]-1–mediated) adherence of neutrophils to capillaries and venules (with release of their injurious products including reactive oxygen species, proteases, elastases, myeloperoxidases, and other tissue damaging enzymes). This leads to congestion and diminution of flood flow, further disturbing the tenuous balance between oxygen needs and oxygenation.

Once the initial severe tubular injury has occurred, there may be progression to acute renal failure and ATN via a number of pathways: 1) obstruction of the tubular lumens by casts, cells, and other debris; 2) transtubular backleak of the glomerular filtrate through the tubular epithelium and tubular basement membranes, with coursing of the ultrafiltrate into the renal interstitium; and 3) vasoconstriction with a decreased glomerular filtration rate due to tubuloglomerular feedback events at the level of the juxtaglomerular apparatus (JGA) (15). This last mechanism is due to activation of the renin-angiotensin system, although other vasoconstrictive agents are thought to also play a role. Intrarenal vasoconstriction caused by an imbalance between systemic or local vasoconstrictive (e.g., endothelin) and vasodilative (e.g., nitric oxide [NO], prostaglandins) factors is important (24). Alternatively, some investigators have suggested a direct effect of certain toxins on the ultrafiltration coefficient of the glomerular capillary wall. It is likely that all these play a part, at different times or with various tubulotoxic agents, in the pathogenesis of ATN. The injury in ATN appears to be multistep and sequential. Patients with preexisting renal insufficiency (including prerenal azotemia) are predisposed to acute renal failure (and ATN) by drugs that alter intrarenal hemodynamics (e.g., nonsteroidal anti-inflammatory agents) or reach high concentrations in renal tissues (e.g., aminoglycoside antibiotics or radiocontrast agents). Patients with diabetes mellitus or hyperbilirubinemia also appear predisposed to acute renal failure of this type. Because the aging kidney loses functional reserve, its ability to withstand a variety of acute insults may be compromised.

Regardless of the cause of the ATN, there are changes in the structure and function of the renal tubular epithelial cells. Injured proximal tubular epithelium shows alterations of cellular polarity (of Na^+/K^+-adenosine triphosphatase [ATPase]), with a redistribution from the basolateral to the apical membrane contributing to altered sodium-coupled vectorial active transport across the cells (24). This may lead to the enhanced delivery of Na^+ to the distal tubules, with tubuloglomerular feedback and subsequent renal vasoconstriction. Other cellular components involved in the establishment and maintenance of cellular polarity are disturbed; disruption of the cytoskeletal complex (1) leads to relocation of the apical and basolateral membrane-specific proteins into abnormal positional domains (24). There may also be internalization and blebbing of the apical brush border membranes. Disruption of the basal membrane proteins leads to impaired adhesion of the tubular cells to the underlying matrix. Programmed cell death (apoptosis) is induced. Integrins are redistributed to the apical surface. The integrity of the tubular epithelial tight junctions is disrupted, perhaps secondary to the accompanying alterations in the microtubule and cytoskeletal networks (e.g., actin, ankyrin, and fodrin) (24). This contributes to backleak of the glomerular filtrate.

Biochemical changes after ischemic injury include depletion of cellular ATP, which leads to an increase in cytosolic calcium, and a subsequent activation of proteases (e.g., calpain) and phospholipidases; these break down or rearrange the cytoskeleton (1) and interfere with mitochondrial energy metabolism. With the restoration of blood flow and oxygenation after a period of ischemia, there is often a rapid burst of oxidant formation and generation of reactive oxygen species (either from the hypoxic renal epithelium or the infiltrating leukocytes). The breakdown of ATP and the formation of adenosine, inosine, and hypoxanthine can leak from cells and lead to vasoconstriction and further formation of reactive oxygen species. Apoptosis has been noted in experimental and human ATN (secondary to activation of a variety of caspases). In addition, the ischemic tubular epithelium expresses a number of cytokines and adhesion molecules which recruit leukocytes that may participate in subsequent injury (24).

Less is known about tubular epithelial repair than injury. During recovery, the cytoskeleton assemblies (e.g., ankyrin) codistribute and interact with Na^+/K^+-ATPase, to return it to the basolateral membrane. Recycling of misplaced Na^+/K^+-ATPases, rather than increased synthesis, accounts for repolarization. The brush border is restored. Repair or re-epithelialization of the tubules appears to be mediated by a complex symphony of growth factors and cytokines, produced by the tubular cells themselves and/or by the accompanying inflammatory infiltrate. Epidermal growth factor (EGF), transforming growth factor (TGF)-alpha, hepatocyte growth factor, and insulin-like growth factor have all been identified as important repair proteins for the regeneration of renal tubular epithelium. It appears that heat shock proteins (HSP), such as HSP 70 and HSP 72 (acting as chaperones to protect misfolded/misplaced proteins from degradation until ATP levels are restored) play a major role in protection and recovery. Repair is associated not only with mitogenesis but also with down-regulation of genes governing cellular differentiation (as occurs during embryonic development). Thus, the pathogenesis of ATN and its resolution are complex and involve cellular events that regulate cell polarity, cell-matrix interactions, cell proliferation, and cell differentiation, and the accompanying inflammatory responses (24).

Treatment and Prognosis. Once ATN is established, there is no preventive treatment for it (14,21,29). Patients with oliguria have a worse prognosis than those with normal urine flow. Persistent prerenal azotemia is the most common predisposing factor in ischemia-induced ATN (33). Restoration of renal blood flow during the prerenal azotemia phase of renal ischemia may prevent the ischemic form of ATN. However, once ischemic ATN occurs, treatment is only supportive. Patients can be supported for prolonged periods of time with various types of dialysis, followed by eventual recovery of renal tubular function. Depending on the published series and the type of renal injury, from 20 to 60 percent of patients with ATN require dialysis. The tubules have a great capacity to regenerate if the patient is maintained on dialysis. Patient survival is more often a function of other organ system involvement and complications, such as accompanying sepsis or respiratory failure. Mortality rates vary widely dependent upon the patient populations studied. The increasing frequency of coexisting

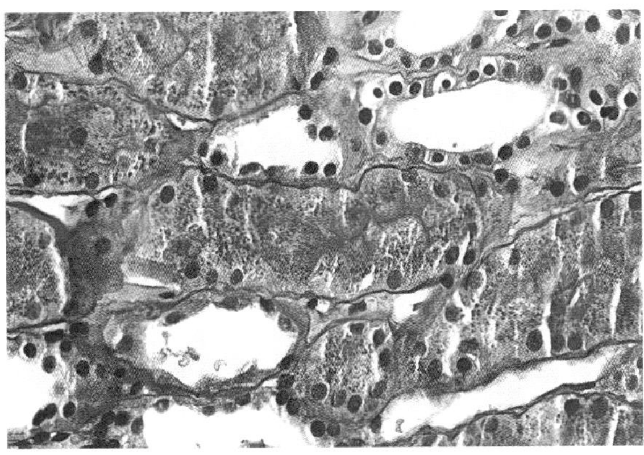

Figure 19-37

HYALINE DROPLET CHANGE (PROTEIN DROPLET REABSORPTION)

There are a large number of droplets within the tubular epithelium. This occurs as a result of increased protein loss by the glomerulus and secondary reabsorption by the proximal tubular epithelium. This microscopic change indicates an altered and diseased glomerulus (H&E stain).

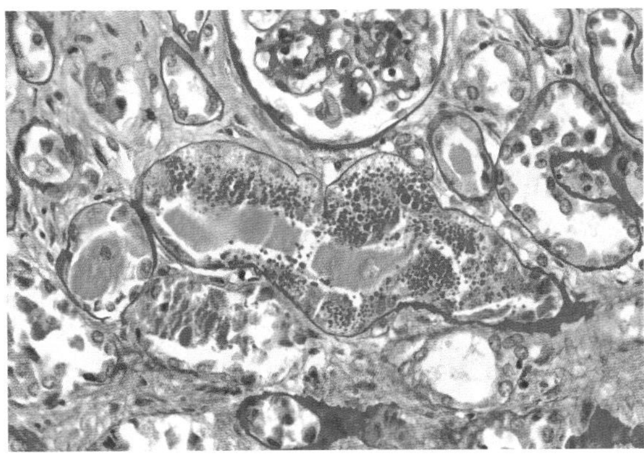

Figure 19-38

HYALINE DROPLET CHANGE (PROTEIN DROPLET REABSORPTION)

There are large numbers of PAS-positive droplets in the tubular epithelial cells, evidence generally of breakdown of the permselective barrier of the glomerulus (i.e., glomerular leakage of proteins) (PAS stain).

serious illnesses and aging (42) probably accounts for the increasing, or at best stable, mortality rate.

Renal failure often lasts only 1 or 2 weeks. The chance of recovery decreases after 1 month, although recovery has been noted after 1 year. Harbingers of a poor prognosis include severe oliguria, prolonged renal insufficiency/failure, multiple organ failure, and advanced age. Trauma and major surgery are associated with high mortality rates whereas pregnant patients with ATN have a much lower mortality rate.

OTHER RENAL TUBULAR CHANGES

Hyaline Droplet Change

This lesion of the proximal tubular epithelium consists of protein reabsorption droplets that result from increased protein filtration by the glomeruli. The droplets vary in size from small to large (fig. 19-37) (46) and are eosinophilic when stained with hematoxylin and eosin (H&E), pink with PAS, and black with Jones methenamine silver (JMS) stains (figs. 19-37–19-39). The droplets may be seen only in the apical regions of the cells, or may completely fill the expanded proximal tubular epithelium. The distribution is often focal or patchy. By immunofluorescence, the droplets may stain for albumin, immunoglobulins, and occasionally other immunoreactants that

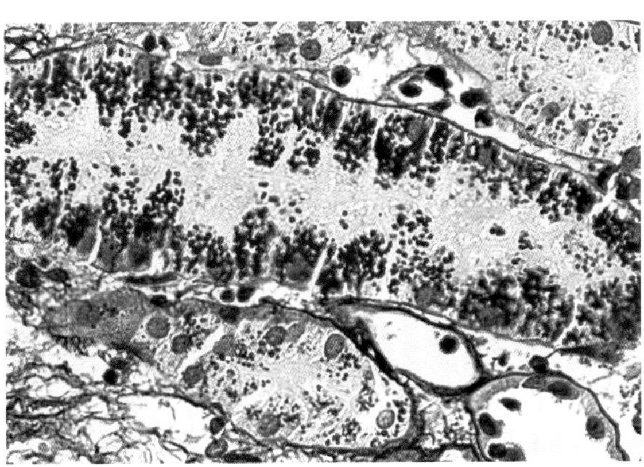

Figure 19-39

HYALINE DROPLET CHANGE (PROTEIN DROPLET REABSORPTION)

JMS-positive protein resorption droplets are seen in the proximal tubular epithelial cells (JMS stain).

have been allowed to pass through the diseased glomerulus (fig. 19-40).

Hyaline droplet changes are similar, functionally, to those seen in the visceral epithelium of glomeruli which are diseased, and lead to severe proteinuria and even nephrotic syndrome. The droplets represent reabsorbed protein (fig. 19-41). The abnormally filtered protein (by the damaged glomerulus) is absorbed by pinocytosis and then taken up by the lysosomes, which attempt to dispose of the protein. The droplets disappear as the proteins are hydrolyzed and returned to the circulation. Although almost always indicative of a severely damaged (and leaky) glomerulus, there is an imperfect correlation between the extent of the hyaline droplet formation and the severity of the proteinuria. Recent studies on the effect of the resorbed proteins on tubular function and their role in the production of tubulointerstitial disease have suggested that they may play a role in progressive renal disease.

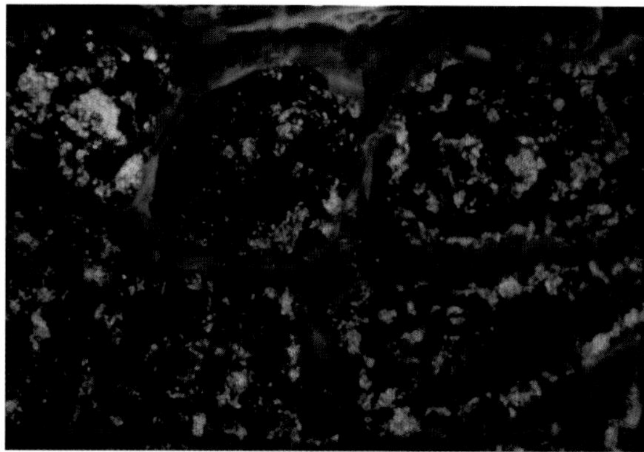

Figure 19-40

HYALINE DROPLET CHANGE

Numerous protein droplets are seen in the proximal tubular epithelial cells (immunofluorescence with anti-albumin antibodies).

Hydropic Change (Osmotic Nephrosis)

Hydropic change is a fine and usually diffuse vacuolar clearing of the cytoplasm of the proximal tubular epithelium (figs. 19-42–19-46) (46). These finely granular changes contrast with the much coarser and irregular vacuolation seen with hypokalemia (see below). Hydropic change may be histologically similar to the finely dispersed, clear vacuolar fatty change seen in paraffin sections from patients with the nephrotic syndrome (because lipid cannot be well detected unless one uses frozen sections which retain fat) (fig. 19-47). The brush border is generally well preserved.

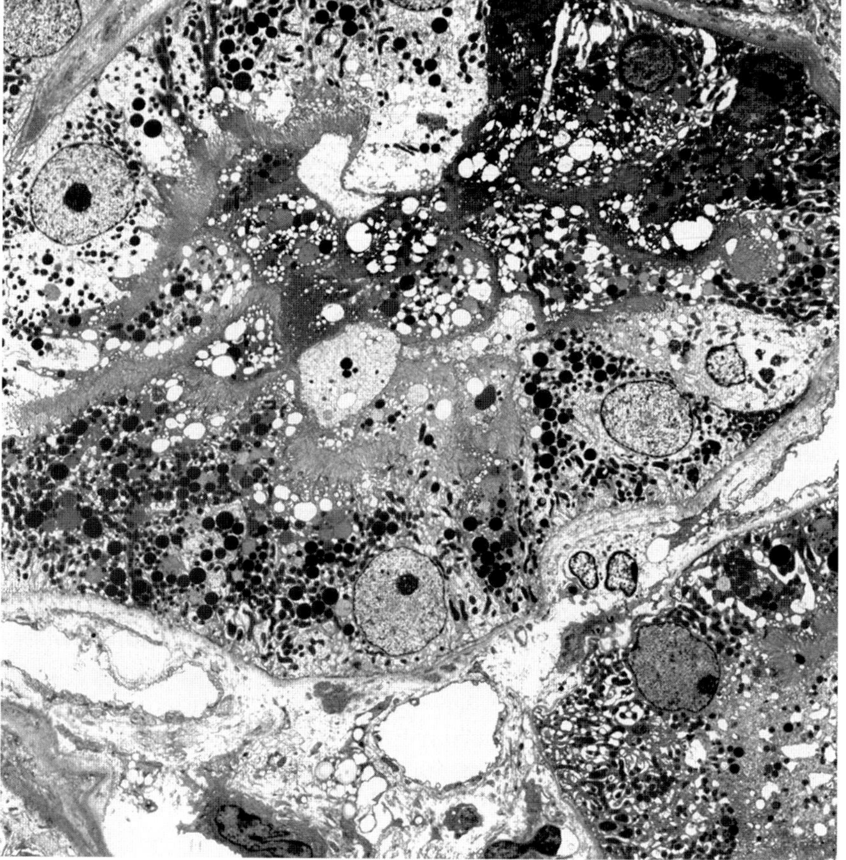

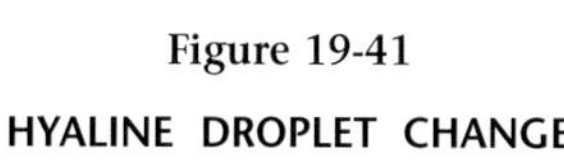

Figure 19-41

HYALINE DROPLET CHANGE

Large numbers of phagolysosomes are seen within the tubular epithelium (electron micrograph).

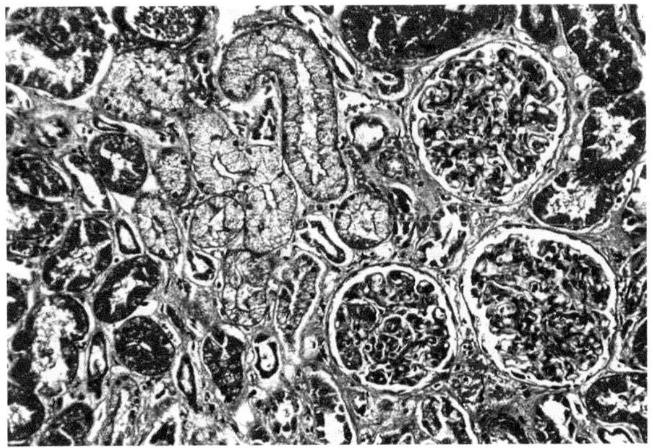

Figure 19-42

HYDROPIC CHANGE (OSMOTIC NEPHROSIS)

There is fine diffuse vacuolization within the tubular epithelial cells. This change is seen in patients receiving hypertonic solutions such as sucrose, mannitol (as with this patient), high molecular weight dextrans, or radiopaque contrast materials (Masson trichrome stain).

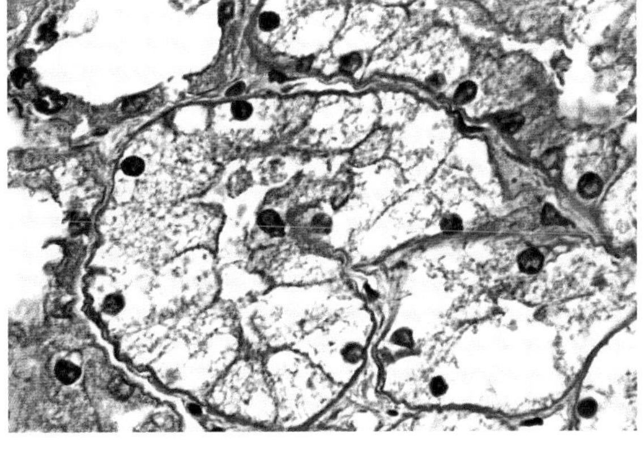

Figure 19-43

HYDROPIC CHANGE (OSMOTIC NEPHROSIS)

The cause of the hydropic change in this patient was the administration of low molecular weight dextran (H&E stain).

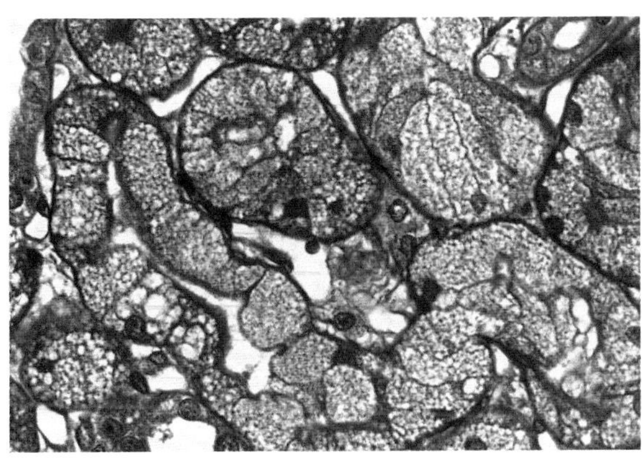

Figure 19-44

HYDROPIC CHANGE (OSMOTIC NEPHROSIS)

There is fine, diffuse vacuolization within the tubular epithelium. These changes are entirely reversible (Masson trichrome stain).

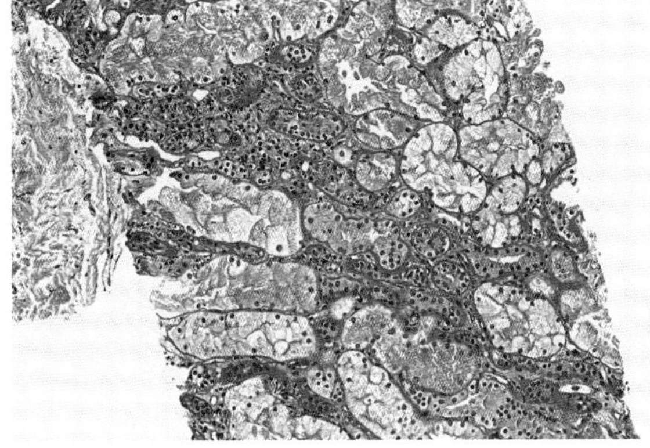

Figure 19-45

HYDROPIC CHANGE (OSMOTIC NEPHROSIS)

The cause of this patient's hydropic change was the intravenous administration of immunoglobulin (H&E stain).

Hydropic change may be seen in patients who have received hypertonic sucrose solutions, mannitol, high molecular weight dextrans, radiopaque contrast material, or intravenous immunoglobulin (IVIG)(12). The alternative term, osmotic nephrosis, is not favored by some, because hydropic change can be seen in patients who have not received any hypertonic substances. Renal function can be normal. Hydropic change may occur in the renal allograft of patients treated with cyclosporin A or tacrolimus ("isometric or isotonic vacuolization").

The vacuolation is secondary to the distension of cytosomes, probably membrane-bound lysosomes (fig. 19-46). There may be dilatation of the endoplasmic reticulum. Extension of the extracellular compartments by fluid seems to account for the separation of the cell membranes at the base of the tubular cells in experimental animals.

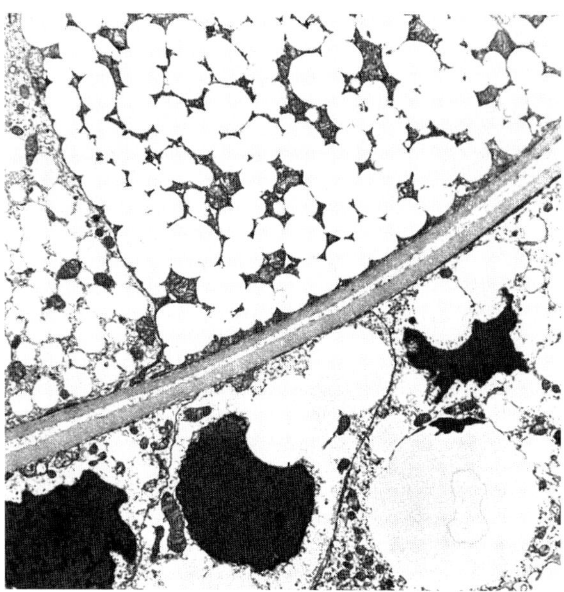

Figure 19-46

HYDROPIC CHANGE (OSMOTIC NEPHROSIS)

Electron micrograph shows multiple clear vacuoles throughout the tubules.

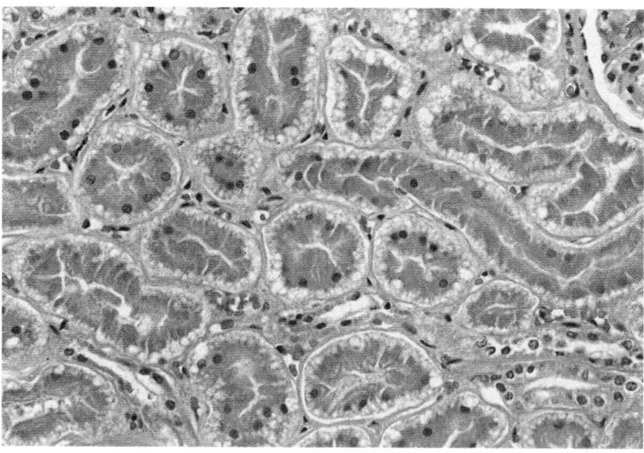

Figure 19-47

FATTY CHANGE

Basally placed fine vacuolization of the proximal tubular epithelium is seen in this patient with the nephrotic syndrome. The basal vacuolization represents fat deposition, not osmotic change, which may be histologically similar. In hydropic change the small vacuoles are usually evenly dispersed throughout the cell cytoplasm whereas in the early or mild stages of fatty change the homogeneous vacuoles are usually basally distributed. Fat stains (such as Sudan black or oil red-O) can be performed on fresh frozen sections in order to demonstrate the lipid droplets (H&E stain).

Recent studies have shown that intravenous immunoglobulin (IVIG), as noted before, can produce a morphologic appearance which resembles forms of osmotic nephrosis (12). Some authors have suggested that this change is due to the sucrose present in most IVIG preparations, and some recent IVIG preparations are not thought to be as nephrotoxic as others.

Fatty Change

Fatty change is most commonly seen in patients with severe proteinuria or nephrotic syndrome (with its accompanying hyperlipidemia/hyperlipiduria). The cytoplasm is finely vacuolated, with clear vacuoles often best seen at the base of the proximal tubular epithelium (fig. 19-47). These lipid droplets are small but they displace the eosinophilic cytoplasm. Small fat droplets are similar to the changes seen with hydropic change. Unless fat stains are performed on frozen sections (lipid is lost during the preparation of paraffin sections), they may be missed. In general, the more fat that is present, the more the fat is basally placed. This change is also noted in patients receiving phosphorus or carbon tetrachloride, and in patients with Reye's syndrome.

Foam Cells

In addition to the fine clearing or vacuolization of fatty change noted in routinely processed formalin-fixed paraffin-embedded sections (in which the fat is dissolved by the alcohol in the tissue sections), there may be large foamy cells in both the tubular epithelium and the renal interstitium (figs. 19-48, 19-49). These foamy cells are usually in patients with longstanding nephrotic syndrome and resultant hyperlipidemia/hyperlipiduria. If they occur in patients without significant proteinuria, then the diagnosis of Alport's hereditary nephropathy should be considered. The foam cells have large intracellular collections of cholesterol esters and other lipids.

Hypokalemic Nephropathy

In hypokalemic nephropathy, large, various sized, coarse, empty vacuoles are in the cytoplasm of renal tubular epithelial cells, especially the distal tubular cells (fig. 19-50) (4,17,32,44,46,52). The vacuolation appears to be secondary to dilatation of the extracellular spaces, with ballooning of the basolateral cell membranes. Cytoplasmic vacuoles are also noted by electron microscopy. Hypokalemic nephropathy is caused

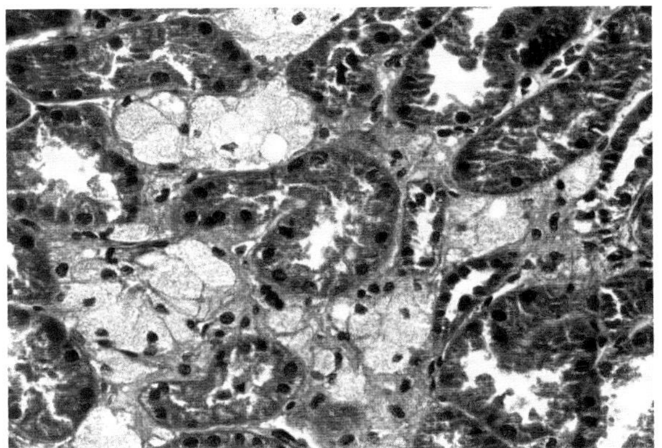

Figure 19-48

FOAM CELLS

Generally seen in patients with severe proteinuria (and secondary hyperlipidemia/hyperlipiduria), these cholesterol esters and other fats are noted within both the tubular epithelium and interstitial cells. If these foam cells are present in a patient without proteinuria/nephrotic syndrome, then hereditary Alport's syndrome should be considered (Masson trichrome stain).

by chronic longstanding loss of potassium due to several conditions, including chronic laxative abuse, potassium-losing rectosigmoid polyps, or various intrinsic renal conditions (such as chronic glomerulonephritis). It can be seen in the recovery phase of ATN. Indeed, there are a large number of gastrointestinal, adrenal, renal, and metabolic conditions that can lead to this pattern of disease. There is an imperfect correlation between the morphologic changes and the defects in renal concentrating ability.

Patients with longstanding potassium loss have muscular weakness, thirst, polyuria, and polydipsia. Characteristic electrocardiographic and neurologic changes occur. Serum potassium levels are generally low; however, normal serum levels can be found in the presence of decreased intracellular potassium. The clinical findings are reversible by cautious potassium administration. The long-term effects of longstanding potassium loss are unclear, but there is some indication that this condition might lead to interstitial fibrosis and inflammation; this has not been extensively confirmed.

Hemosiderin and Other Pigments in Renal Tubular Epithelium

Hemosiderin deposition in the tubular epithelium is seen in a variety of conditions that

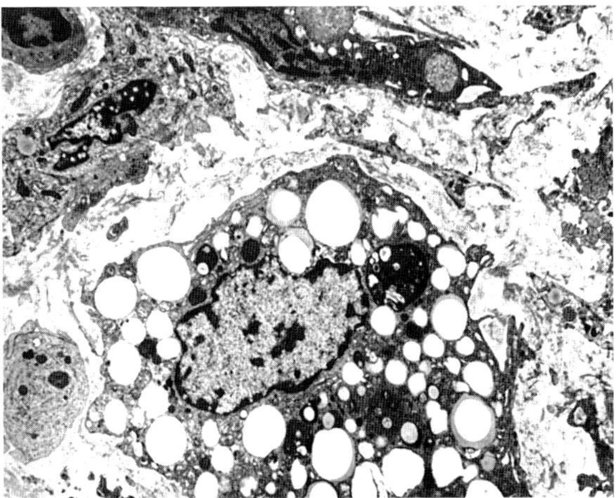

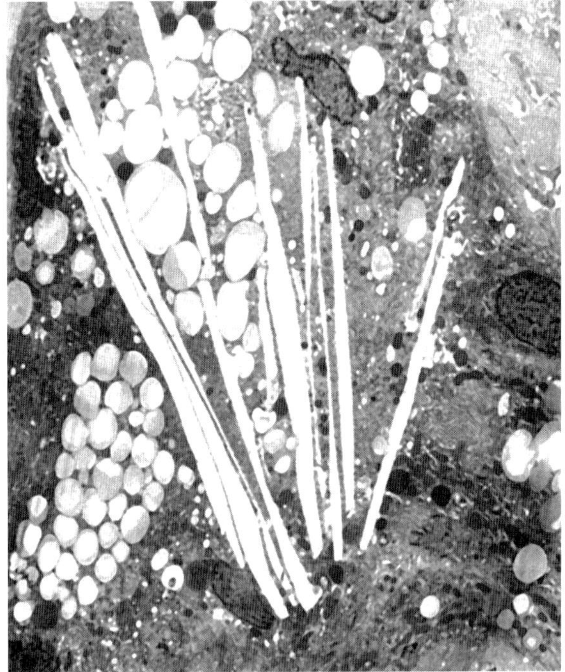

Figure 19-49

FOAM CELLS

Electron micrographs demonstrate fat in the interstitium and tubular epithelium from a patient with nephrotic syndrome.

lead to intravascular hemolysis, such as erythrocyte destruction by mechanical heart valves. Prussian blue staining of iron is noted in the renal tubular epithelium on histologic sections (figs. 19-51, 19-52). Staining of iron in the urine sediment is a diagnostic test for iron in tubular epithelial cells since these cells shed into the urine. The morphologic appearance may seem

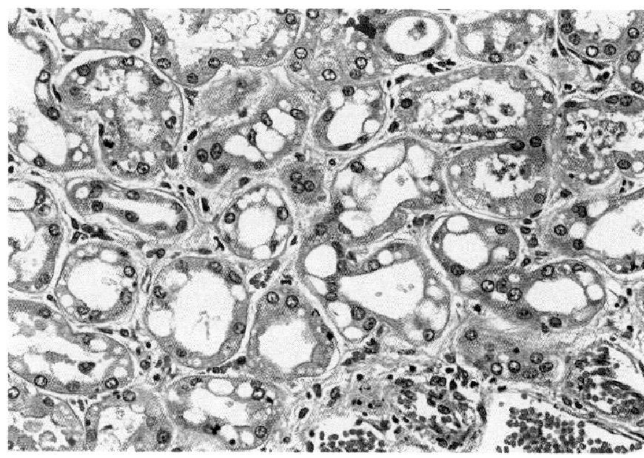

Figure 19-50

HYPOKALEMIC NEPHROPATHY

There are large, coarse vacuoles of various sizes in the tubular epithelium. These clear vacuoles are larger and more irregular than those noted in hydropic change. These changes, indicative of hypokalemia, are generally found in patients with severe, longstanding loss of potassium (H&E stain). (Courtesy of Dr. J. Pitha, Oklahoma City, OK.)

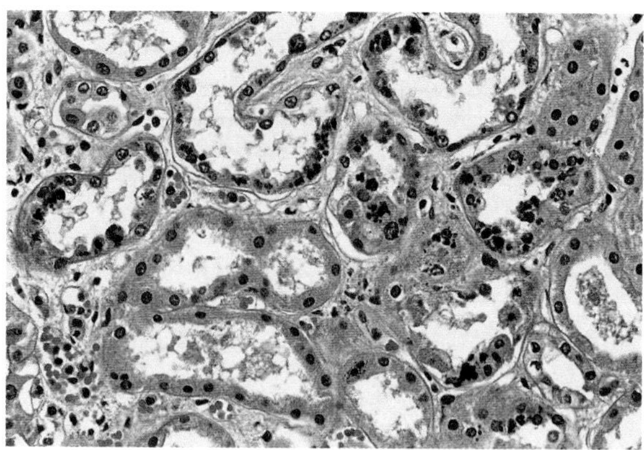

Figure 19-51

IRON PIGMENTATION

This patient had hemosiderosis and iron deposition in the tubular epithelium. There was no evidence of major renal dysfunction. An artificial metallic heart valve led to microangiopathic hemolytic anemia (H&E stain).

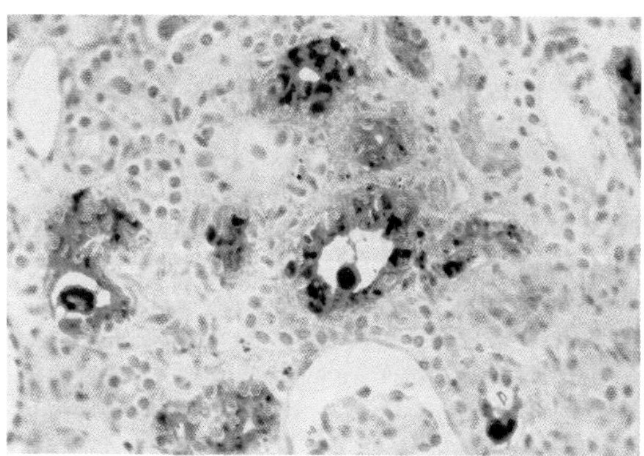

Figure 19-52

IRON PIGMENTATION

Prussian blue iron stain shows iron deposition in this patient with the hemolytic uremic syndrome.

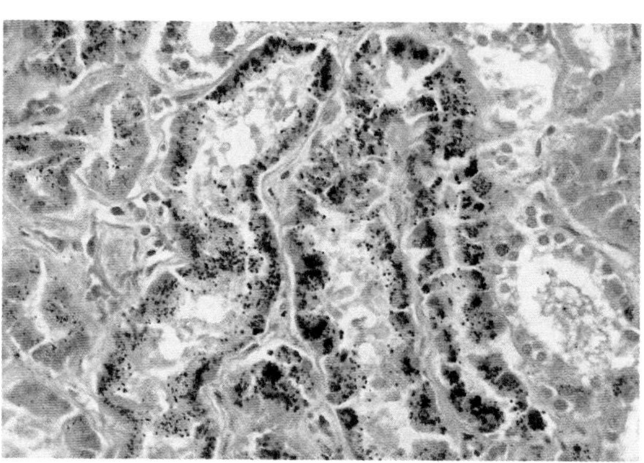

Figure 19-53

OTHER PIGMENTS IN THE TUBULAR EPITHELIUM

Melanin pigmentation is seen in this patient with disseminated melanoma. There was no evidence of renal dysfunction (slightly stained with eosin).

severe, but it is usually associated with little functional renal tubular injury.

Hemosiderin must be distinguished from other pigments. Melanin from patients with disseminated melanoma (fig. 19-53) can be seen in the tubular epithelium, often without major clinical tubular dysfunction; lead nephropathy may be detected by large intranuclear inclusions (figs. 19-54–19-56) (8,16); and gold nephropathy is detected by the presence of filamentous inclusions noted by electron microscopy in the cytoplasm of tubular cells (fig. 19-57).

Tubular Atrophy

Tubular atrophy is an end-stage morphologic pattern seen with a variety of severe renal injuries (including those of glomerular, tubular, interstitial, or vascular diseases). The tubular basement membranes are usually quite thickened and wrinkled, and the tubular epithelial cells

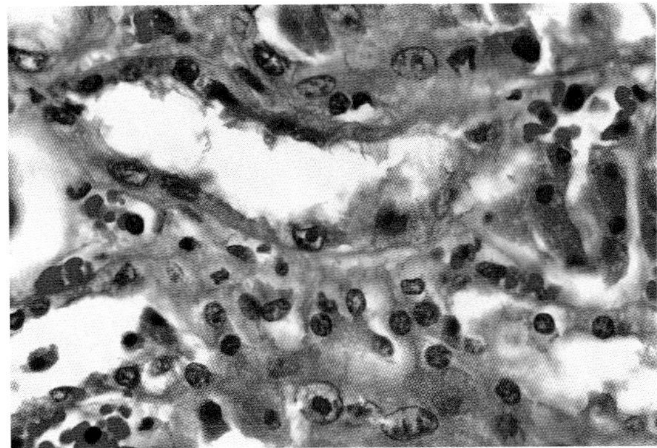

Figure 19-54

LEAD NEPHROPATHY

The large intranuclear inclusions (which can be accentuated by the acid-fast stain used for mycobacteria) can be a sign of lead nephropathy (H&E stain).

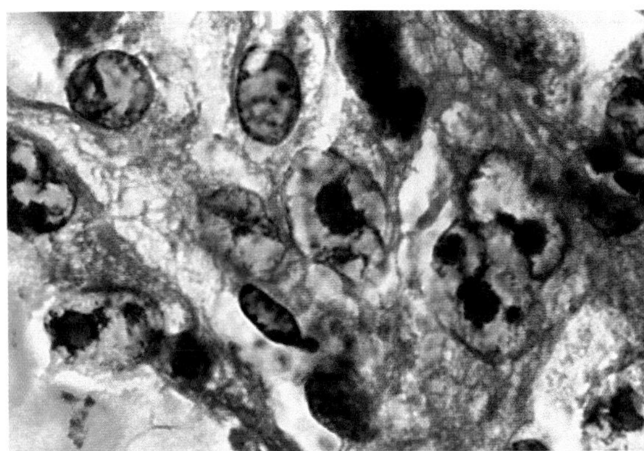

Figure 19-55

LEAD NEPHROPATHY

The large intranuclear inclusions are often seen in patients with lead toxicity.

have lost most of the defining histologic characteristics that distinguish proximal tubules from distal tubules by H&E staining.

Renal function appears to more closely correlate with the preservation of the tubulointerstitial compartment than with the structural alterations of the glomeruli or blood vessels, irrespective of the underlying renal disease. There are at least three subtypes of atrophic tubules according to their light microscopic appearance: 1) "classic" atrophic tubules with thick, wrinkled, occasionally lamellated tubular basement membranes and simplified tubular epithelium (figs. 19-58, 19-59); 2) "endocrine" tubules with narrow or no tubular lumens, clear epithelial cells, and relatively thin basement membranes (figs. 19-60–19-62); and 3) tubules showing "thyroidization" (round tubules with simplified epithelium and uniform casts) (figs. 19-63, 19-64) (35). Endocrine tubules are frequently organized in clusters. Light microscopically, these tubules are somewhat reminiscent of endocrine glands (hence, Hans Selye's term "endocrine kidney"). Conversely, other renal tubules may be enlarged and dilated with large hypertrophic epithelial cells. It is unclear whether these enlarged tubules are primarily hypertrophic or hyperplastic, and have been designated as "super" tubules. These dilated super tubules are thought to develop as a consequence of compensatory growth mechanisms or obstruction.

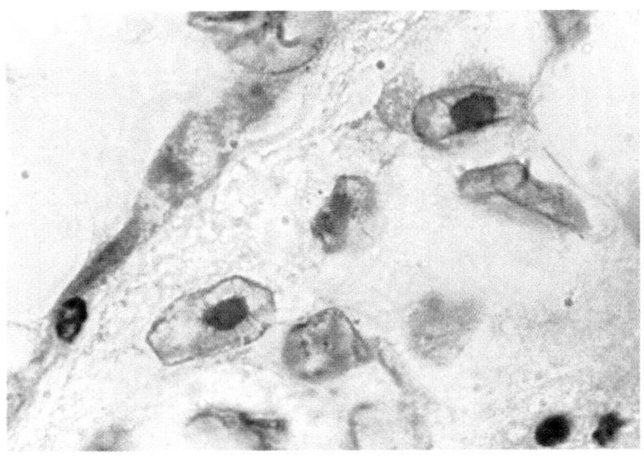

Figure 19-56

LEAD NEPHROPATHY

The large intranuclear inclusions are seen in patients with lead toxicity (acid-fast stain).

The mechanisms leading to tubular atrophy are unclear. Certainly long-term ischemia, secondary to vascular disease or altered glomerular hemodynamics, can injure nephrons. This can occur via intraglomerular hypertension/mesangial sclerosis and subsequent diminution of flow out the efferent arteriole, with decreased blood flow to the vasa recta and the cortical interstitial capillaries. It has recently been suggested that impaired glomerular permselectivity allows escape into the urinary space of substances toxic to the tubular epithelium. The mechanisms of tubulointerstitial disease are considered in

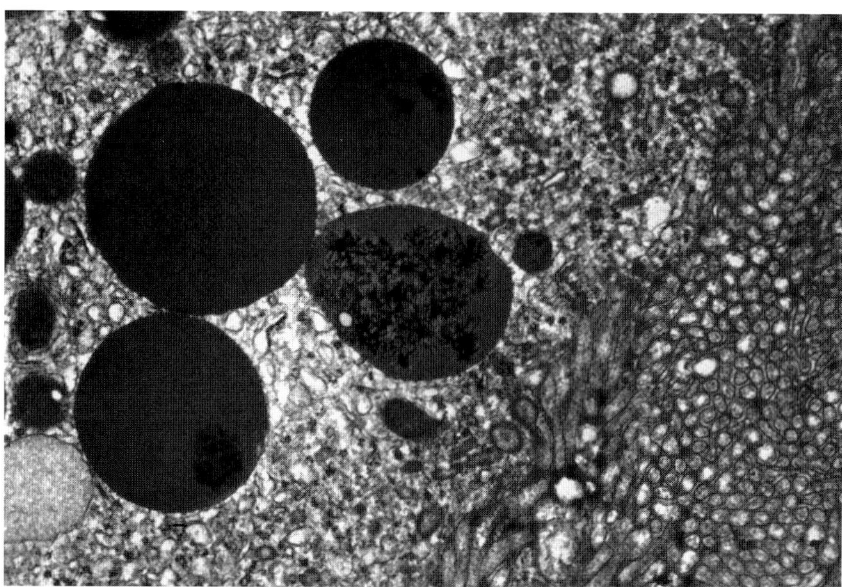

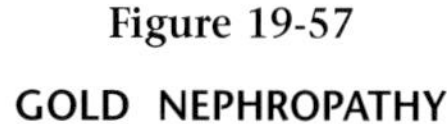

Figure 19-57

GOLD NEPHROPATHY

Electron micrograph shows particulate gold in the tubular epithelium. This patient, with rheumatoid arthritis, received a large amount of gold therapy.

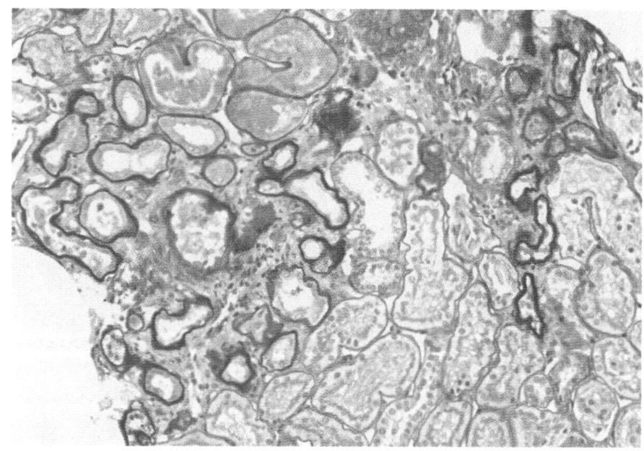

Figure 19-58

TUBULAR ATROPHY (CLASSIC TYPE)

There is patchy thickening of the tubular basement membranes and simplification of the tubular epithelial cells (PAS stain).

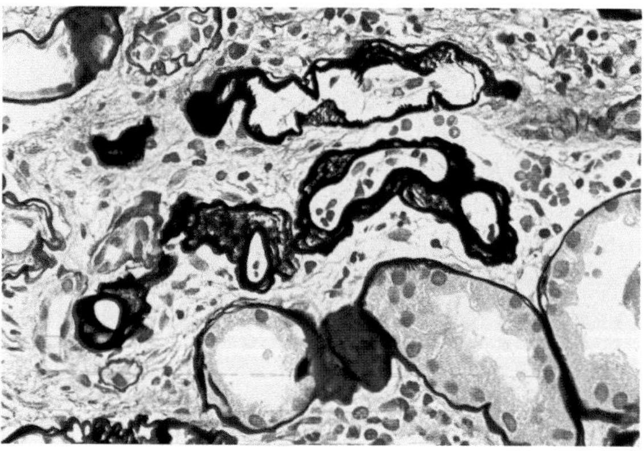

Figure 19-59

TUBULAR ATROPHY (CLASSIC TYPE)

JMS stain.

chapters 20 and 21. Because of the close association between the renal tubules and the supporting interstitium, there is an intimate relationship between what happens in the interstitium and the tubules (see fig. 19-38) (31).

Other Causes of Tubular Atrophy. A number of other agents can cause severe tubular changes and atrophy (fig. 19-65). In patients with HIV-associated nephropathy, the tubules show marked microcystic dilatation (fig. 19-66). A large number of etiologic agents and processes also lead to tubular atrophy and accompanying interstitial fibrosis (see chapters 20 and 21). Some progressive renal disorders thought to be of a hereditary nature lead to significant cortical tubular atrophy and interstitial fibrosis. These include the nephronophthisis-uremic medullary cystic disease complex and the mitochondriopathies.

The *nephronophthisis-uremic medullary cystic disease complex (NUMCD)* is a group of progressive renal disorders that usually have their onset in childhood. Although there are cysts in the medulla, ranging in size from 1 to 10 mm in diameter, the progressive cortical tubulointerstitial damage is the cause of the eventual renal insufficiency (figs. 19-67, 19-68). Several variants of NUMCD are known. As with other

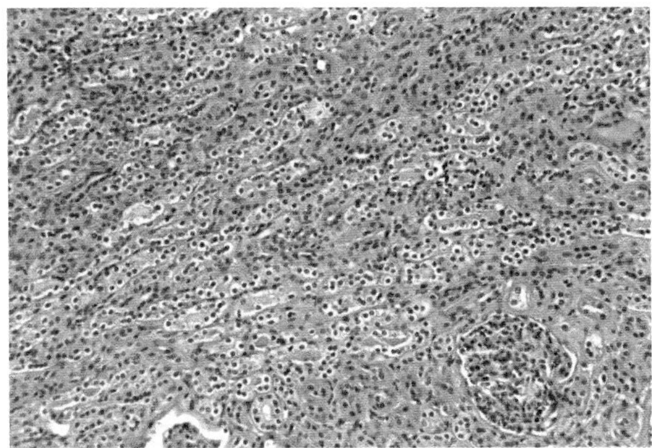

Figure 19-60

TUBULAR ATROPHY ("ENDOCRINE" TUBULES)

There is close approximation of a large number of glomeruli. Normally, about 90 percent of the renal cortex is composed of renal tubules, however, the loss of intervening tubules allows the glomeruli to closely approximate each other (H&E stain).

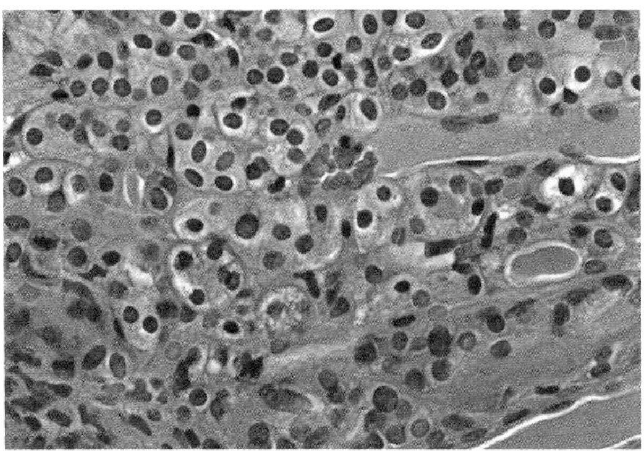

Figure 19-61

TUBULAR ATROPHY ("ENDOCRINE" TUBULES)

The diffusely uniform tubules appear similar to endocrine cells, such as parathyroid cells. There are few tubular lumens (H&E stain).

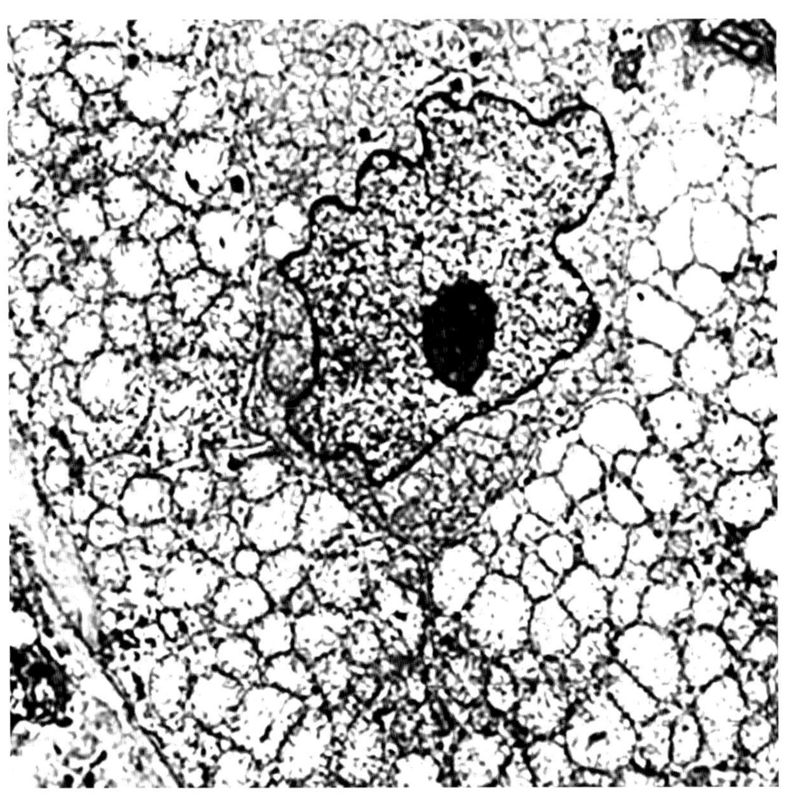

Figure 19-62

TUBULAR ATROPHY ("ENDOCRINE" TUBULES)

The simplified tubular epithelial cells contain many mitochondria.

tubulointerstitial diseases, the clinical features of polyuria and polydipsia reflect a marked tubular defect in concentrating ability. Transmission often involves an autosomal recessive or dominant mode of inheritance.

Grossly, the kidneys are small, with contracted granular surfaces and cysts in the medulla (especially at the corticomedullary junction). The widespread cortical atrophy and interstitial fibrosis are usually associated with well-

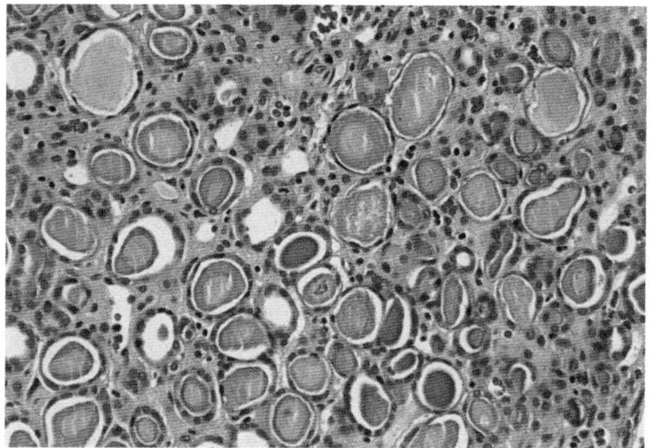

Figure 19-63

TUBULAR ATROPHY ("THYROIDIZATION")

Most of the tubules have a very thin epithelium and contain large uniform hyaline casts within their lumens. Although this pattern is most classically noted in patients with chronic pyelonephritis, thyroidization can be seen in any renal condition leading to tubulointerstitial injury (H&E stain).

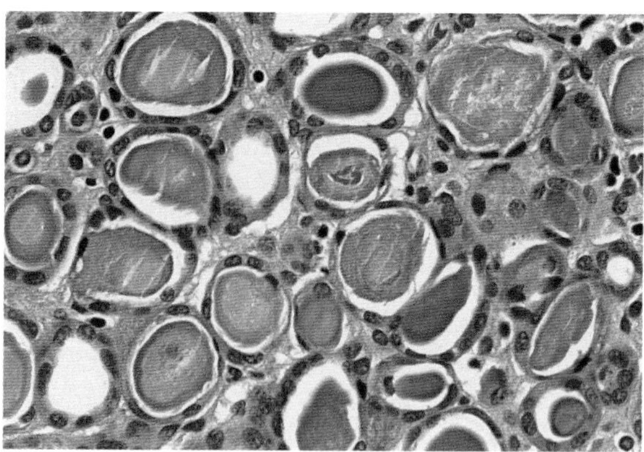

Figure 19-64

TUBULAR ATROPHY ("THYROIDIZATION")

Although commonly seen in patients with chronic pyelonephritis, this morphologic change can be seen with other renal diseases (PAS stain).

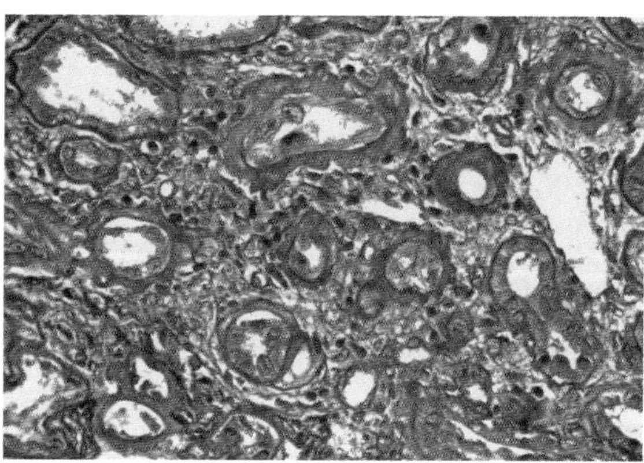

Figure 19-65

TUBULAR ATROPHY IN A PATIENT WITH ADVANCED DIABETIC NEPHROPATHY AND VASCULAR INJURY

In addition to the tubular atrophy, there is a pronounced interstitial inflammatory infiltrate. This patient did not have evidence of chronic pyelonephritis. The inflammation is secondary to the severe vascular injury (Masson trichrome stain).

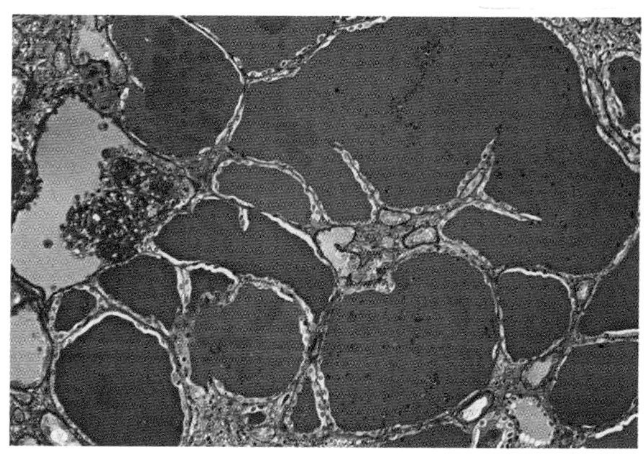

Figure 19-66

MICROCYST FORMATION (TUBULAR DILATATION) IN A PATIENT WITH HUMAN IMMUNODEFICIENCY VIRUS (HIV)-ASSOCIATED NEPHROPATHY

There is marked dilatation of the tubules with extreme thinning of the tubular epithelium. Although this morphologic change is not pathognomonic of HIV, the severe tubular change is often noted in patients with HIV-associated nephropathy (PAS stain).

preserved glomeruli. The tubular basement membranes show characteristic changes of thinning, splitting into lamellae, net-like transformation, disintegration, or collapse (fig. 19-69). Immunofluorescence studies are negative.

The *mitochondriopathies,* which lead to progressive tubular atrophy and interstitial fibrosis, have been recently described (50). These renal lesions are often associated with other lesions of the central nervous system such as growth retardation and ophthalmoplegia, and the skeletal, cardiac muscular, pancreatic, and hematopoietic systems (50). Later in the course of the disease the liver, endocrine system, and kidney are affected. This widespread distribution of lesions is probably secondary to the large number of mitochondria in these tissues. Clinically, the patient

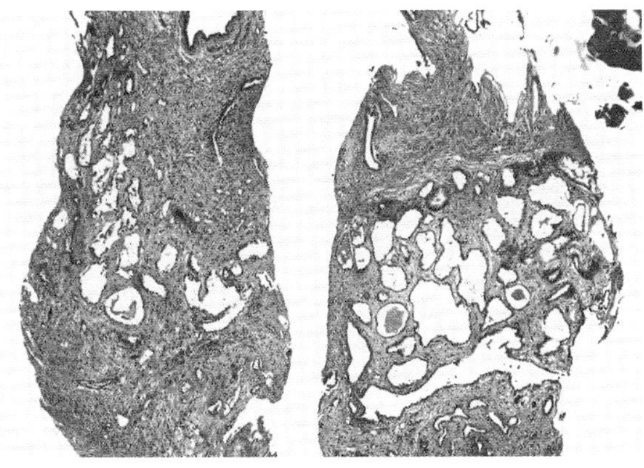

Figure 19-67

NEPHRONOPHTHISIS

There is marked dilatation of the tubules near the corticomedullary junction (H&E stain).

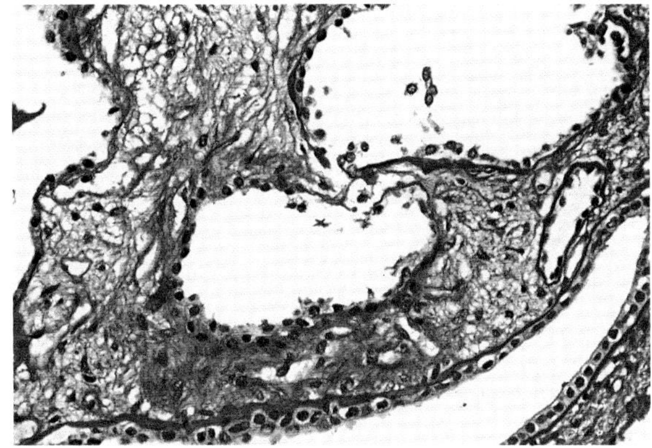

Figure 19-68

NEPHRONOPHTHISIS

There is marked dilatation of the tubules at the corticomedullary junction (PAS stain).

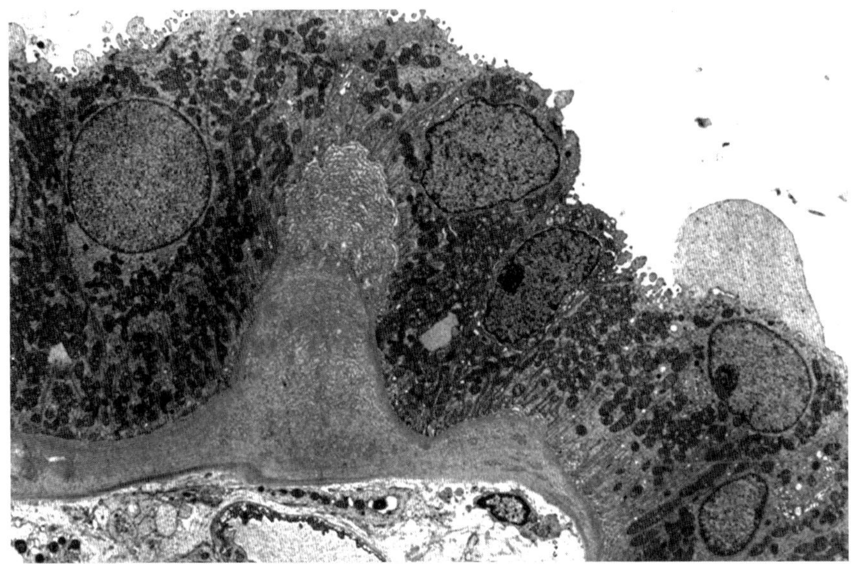

Figure 19-69

NEPHRONOPHTHISIS

Ultrastructural study of the tubular basement membranes shows marked thickening as well as abnormal contours of the tubules.

may show evidence of partial Fanconi's syndrome. Although the tubulointerstitial changes are characteristic of a mitochondriopathy, they are not specific for this disorder (fig. 19-70). Electron microscopy may show tubular cell mitochondria with an extremely dysmorphic appearance: prominent size variation, abnormal arborization, disorientation of the cristae, and osmiophilic inclusions (figs. 19-71, 19-72). Studies of mitochondrial enzymes can be performed on cryostat renal sections, and with molecular analysis of the mtDNA of the kidney and peripheral blood using Southern blot and polymerase chain reaction (PCR) analyses (50).

VIRUSES IN TUBULAR EPITHELIUM

Many viruses can infect the renal tubular epithelium without leading to severe or specific histologic changes. The morphologic evidence of virally-induced renal tubular injury depends on the virus and the patient's response to the viral infection. Often the patients are immunosuppressed. Large intranuclear (Cowdry type A) and intracytoplasmic inclusions are characteristic (actually pathognomonic) of infection with cytomegalovirus (CMV) (see chapter 26).

Necrosis of the tubular epithelium, with large, sometimes "smudgy," nuclei is characteristic for adenovirus (figs. 19-73–19-75)

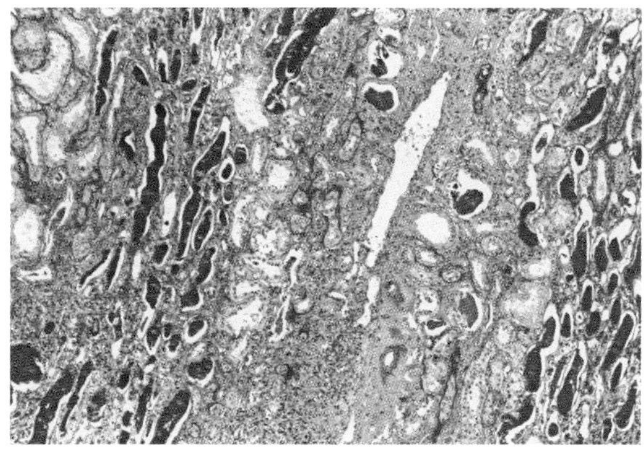

Figure 19-70

TUBULAR ATROPHY SECONDARY TO A MITOCHONDRIAL DNA DELETION

PAS stain.

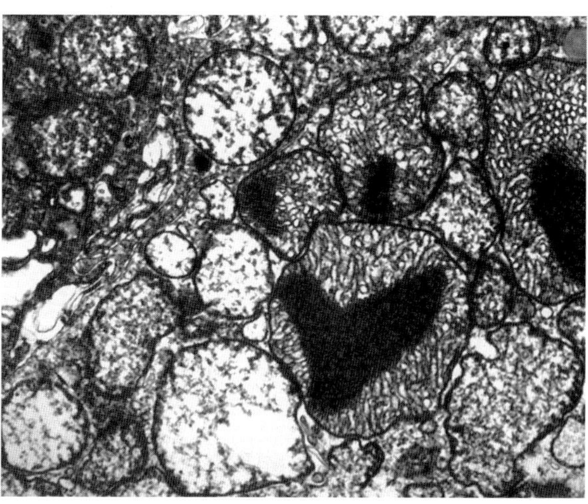

Figure 19-72

TUBULOINTERSTITIAL DISEASE SECONDARY TO A MITOCHONDRIAL DNA DELETION

The mitochondria are abnormally shaped.

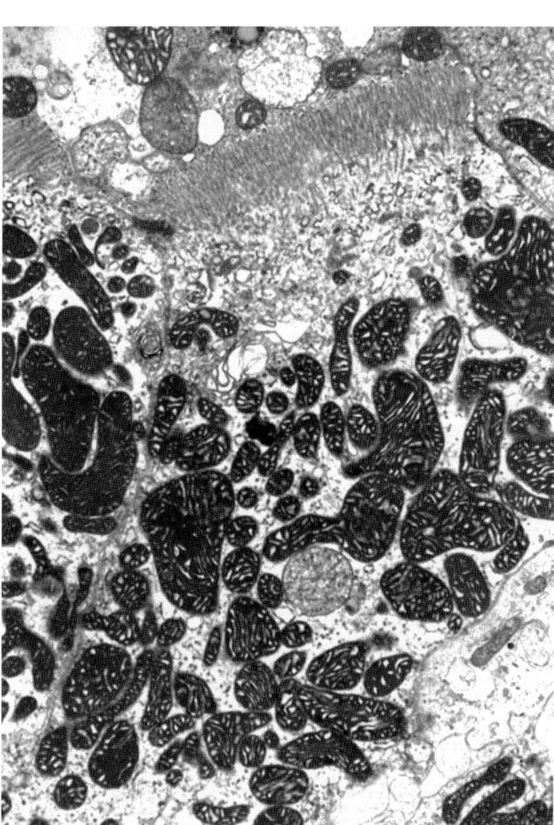

Figure 19-71

TUBULOINTERSTITIAL DISEASE SECONDARY TO A MITOCHONDRIAL DNA DELETION

There are a large number of abnormal (in size and shape) mitochondria.

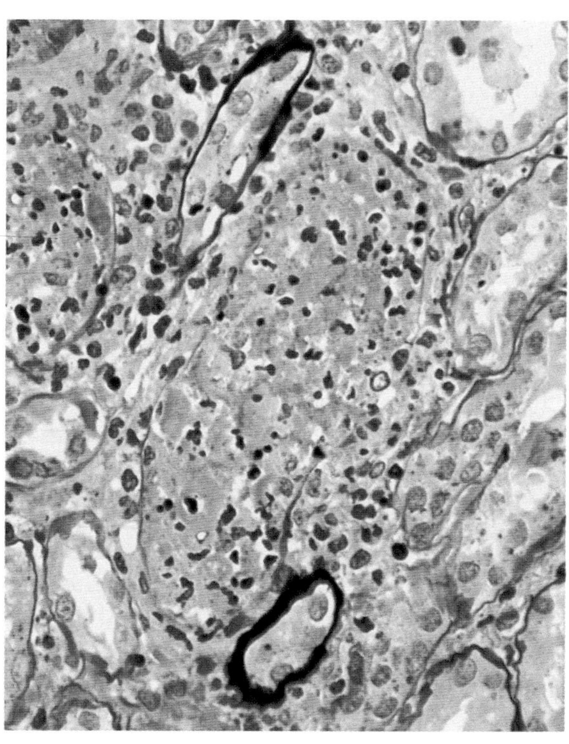

Figure 19-73

ADENOVIRUS INFECTION OF THE TUBULAR EPITHELIUM

The large areas of tubular necrosis suggest an acute process, possibly infectious. This immunosuppressed patient had received a renal allograft (JMS stain). (Figs. 19-73 and 19-74 are from the same patient.)

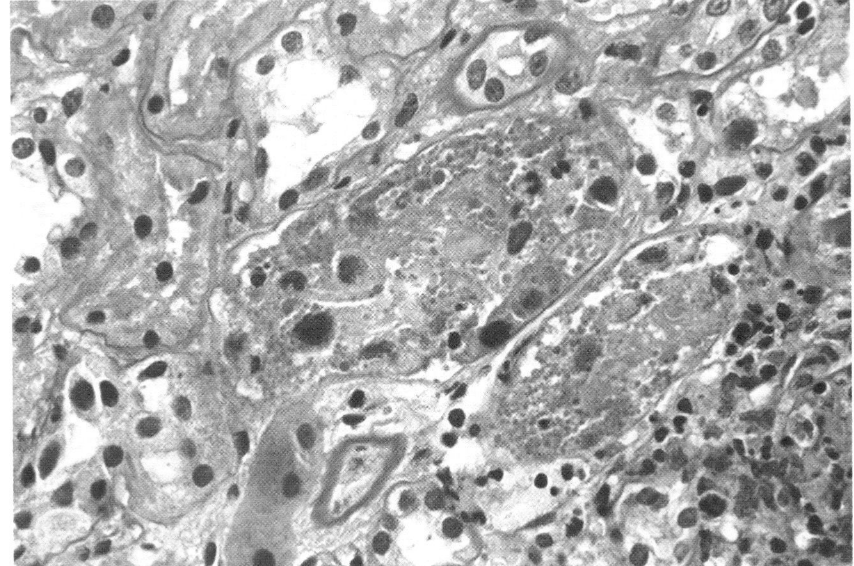

Figure 19-74

ADENOVIRUS INFECTION OF THE TUBULAR EPITHELIUM

The large smudged nuclei are microscopic evidence of a viral infection (PAS stain).

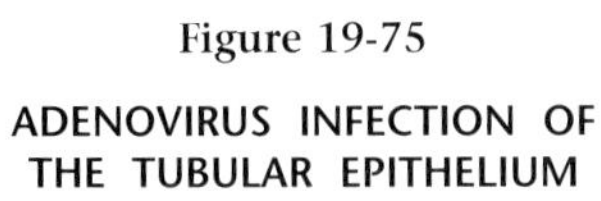

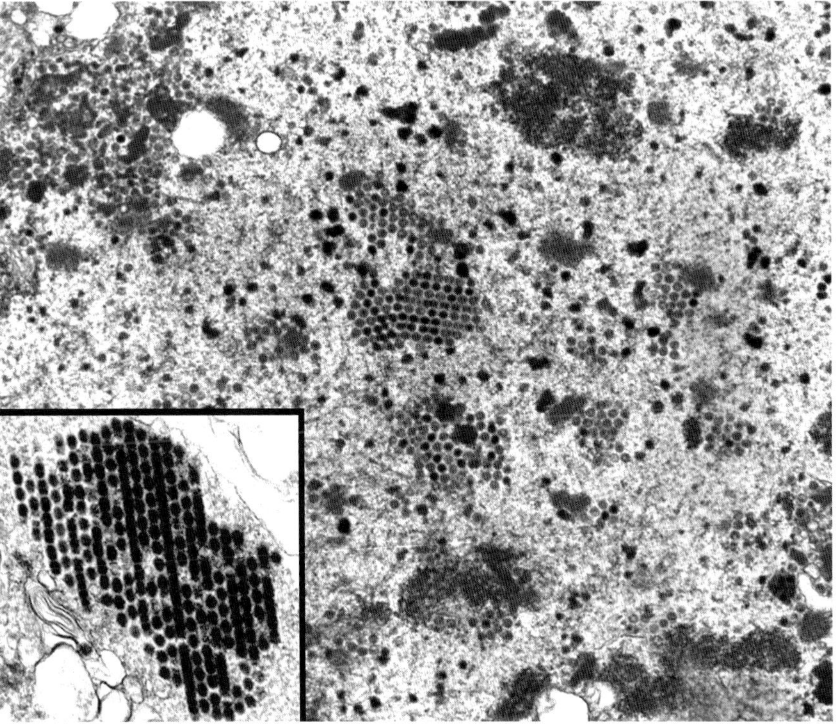

Figure 19-75

ADENOVIRUS INFECTION OF THE TUBULAR EPITHELIUM

Electron microscopy shows a large number of viral particles within the tubular epithelium in this patient with adenovirus infection.

whereas polyoma (BK) virus is often associated with an intense interstitial lymphoplasmacytic infiltrate (figs. 19-76–19-78), which can be mistaken for cellular/interstitial allograft rejection. Thus the nuclei of the tubular epithelial cells should be carefully examined using the H&E stain for the presence of intranuclear inclusions. It should be noted, however, that large nuclei (i.e., nucleomegaly) can most often be seen in regenerative renal tubular epithelial cells (after bouts of acute tubular injury, such as with ATN). Studies by electron microscopy, immunohistochemistry, and in situ hybridization using specific viral probes play a major role in the identification of these viruses (figs. 19-77, 19-78) (see chapter 26).

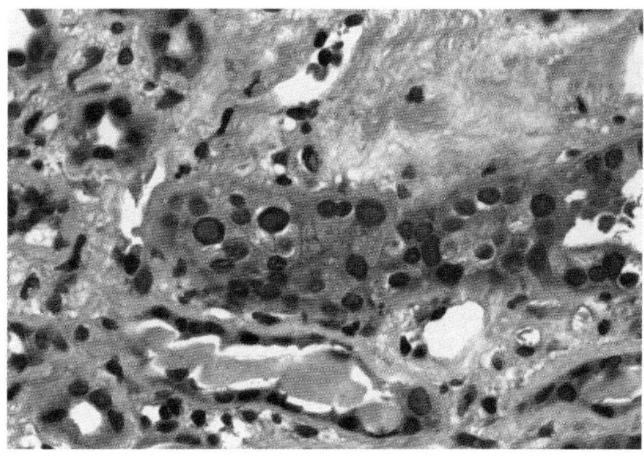

Figure 19-76

POLYOMA VIRUS INFECTION

This patient was immunosuppressed following a renal allograft transplantation. Note the large atypical nuclei with some central clearing.

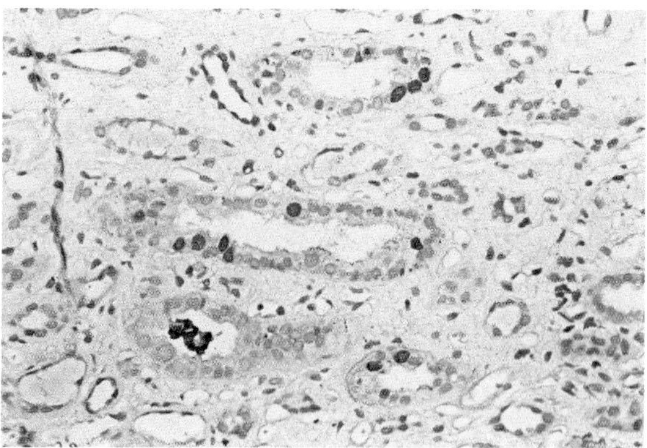

Figure 19-77

POLYOMA VIRUS INFECTION

Immunocytochemistry with antibody to polyoma virus.

Figure 19-78

POLYOMA VIRUS INFECTION

Electron micrograph of the intranuclear viral particles. Insert: High magnification of virus in the nucleus.

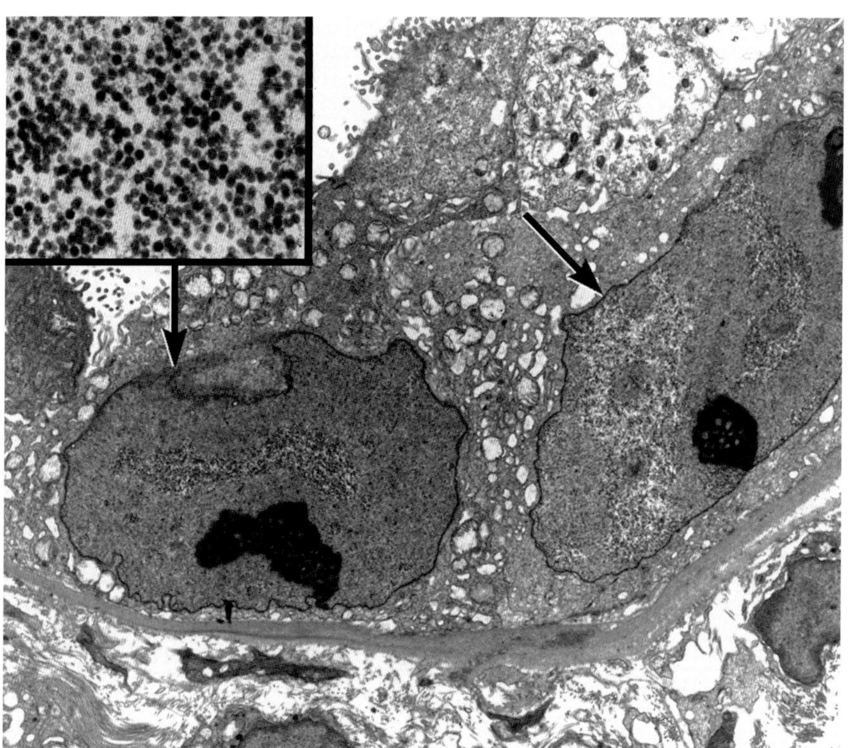

REFERENCES

1. Abbate M, Bonventre JV, Brown D. The microtubule network of renal epithelial cells is disrupted by ischemia and reperfusion. Am J Physiol 1994;267:F971–8.
2. Abuelo JG. Diagnosing vascular causes of renal failure. Ann Intern Med 1995;123:601–14.
3. Abuelo JG. Renal failure caused by chemicals, foods, plants, animal venoms, and misuse of drugs. An overview. Arch Intern Med 1990;150:505–10.
4. Agnoli GC, Borgatti R, Cacciari M, et al. Studies on renal function in healthy women with different degrees of induced potassium depletion. 2). Patterns of hypokalemic renal dysfunction. Boll Soc Ital Biol Sper 1993;69:557–62.
5. Ahijado F, Garcia de Vinuesa S, Luno J. Acute renal failure and rhabdomyolysis following cocaine abuse. Nephron 1990;54:268.
6. Anderson RJ, Schrier RW. Acute tubular necrosis. In: Schrier RW, Gottschalk CW, eds. Diseases of the kidney, 5th ed. Boston: Little, Brown; 1988:1413.
7. Antonovych TT. Drug-induced nephropathies. Pathol Annu 1984;19(Pt 2):165–96.
8. Bennett WM. Lead nephropathy. Kidney Int 1985;28:212–20.
9. Bohle A, Jahnecke J, Meyer D, Schubert GE. Morphology of acute renal failure: comparative data from biopsy and autopsy. Kidney Int 1976;10(Suppl):S9–16.
10. Bonventre JV. Mechanisms of ischemic acute renal failure. Kidney Int 1993;43:1160–78.
11. Brezis M, Rosen S. Hypoxia of the renal medulla—its implications for disease. N Engl J Med 1995;332:647–55.
12. Cantu TG, Hoehn-Saric EW, Burgess KM, Racusen L, Scheel PJ. Acute renal failure associated with immunoglobulin therapy. Am J Kidney Dis 1995:25:228–34.
13. Churg J, Cotran RS, Sinniah R, et al. Renal disease. Classification and atlas of tubulointerstitial disease. New York: Igaku-Shoin; 1984.
14. Conger JD. Interventions in clinical acute renal failure: what are the data? Am J Kidney Dis 1995;26:565–76.
15. Conger JD, Robinette JB, Hammond WS. Differences in vascular reactivity in models of ischemic acute renal failure. Kidney Int 1991;39:1087–97.
16. Cory-Slechta DA. Lead exposure during advanced age: alterations in kinetics and biochemical effects. Toxicol Appl Pharmacol 1990;104:67–78.
17. Cremer W, Bock KD. Symptoms and course of chronic hypokalemic nephropathy in man. Clin Nephrol 1977;7:112–9.
18. Cronin RE, Henrich WL. Toxic nephropathy. In: Brenner BM, ed. Brenner & Rector's the kidney, 5th ed. Philadelphia: Saunders; 1996:1680.
19. Depierreux M, Van Damme B, Vanden Houte K, Vanherwegham JL. Pathologic aspects of a newly described nephropathy related to the prolonged use of Chinese herbs. Am J Kidney Dis 1994;24:172–80.
20. Flameenbaum W. Pathophysiology of acute renal failure. In: Solez K, Whelton A, eds. Acute renal failure: correlations between morphology and function. New York: Dekker; 1984:149.
21. Finn WF. Diagnosis and management of acute tubular necrosis. Med Clin North Am 1990;74:873–91.
22. Fish EM, Molitoris BA. Alterations in epithelial polarity and the pathogenesis of disease states. N Engl J Med 1994;330:1580–8.
23. Humes H. Aminoglycoside nephrotoxicity. Kidney Int 1988;33:900–11.
24. Kashgarian M. Acute tubular necrosis and ischemic renal injury. In: Jeanette JC, Olson JL, Schwartz MM, Silva FG, eds. Hepinstall's pathology of the kidney, 5th ed. Philadelphia, Lippincott-Raven; 1998:863–89.
25. Kaufman J, Dhakal M, Patel B, Hamburger R. Community-acquired acute renal failure. Am J Kidney Dis 1991;17:191–8.
26. Kelly CJ, Neilson EG. Tubulointerstitial diseases. In: Brenner BM, ed. Brenner & Rector's the kidney, 5th ed. Philadelphia: Saunders; 1996:1655–79.
27. Kern WF, Laszik ZG, Nadasdy T, Silva FG, Bane BL, Pitha JV. Disorders of the tubules. In: Kern WF, ed. Atlas of renal pathology. Philadelphia: Saunders; 1999:126–35.
28. Liano F, Garcia-Martin F, Gallego A, et al. Easy and early prognosis in acute tubular necrosis: a forward analysis of 228 cases. Nephron 1989;51:307–13.
29. Lieberthal W. Levinsky NG. Treatment of acute tubular necrosis. Semin Nephrol 1990;10:571–83.
30. Markowitz GS, Radhakrishnan J, Kambham N, Valeri AM, Hines WH, D'Agati VD. Lithium nephrotoxicity: a progressive combined glomerular and tubulointerstitial nephropathy. J Am Soc Nephrol 2000;11:1439–48.
31. Mathew TH. Drug-induced renal disease. Med J Aust 1992;156:724–8.
32. Mujais SK, Katz AI. Potassium deficiency. In: Seldin DW, Giebisch GH, eds. The kidney: physiology and pathophysiology, 2nd ed. New York: Raven Press; 1992:2249.
33. Myers BD, Moran SM. Hemodynamically mediated acute renal failure. N Engl J Med 1986; 314:97–105.
34. Nadasdy T, Laszik Z, Blick KE, et al. Human acute tubular necrosis: a lectin and immunohistochemical study. Hum Pathol 1995;26:230–9.
35. Nadasdy T, Laszik Z, Blick KE, Johnson DL, Silva FG. Tubular atrophy in the end-stage kidney: a lectin and immunohistochemical study. Hum Pathol 1994;25:22–8.

36. Nadasdy T, Racusen LC. Renal injury caused by therapeutic and diagnostic agents and abuse of analgesics and narcotics. In: Jeanette JC, Olson JL, Schwartz MM, Silva FG, eds. Hepinstall's pathology of the kidney, 5th ed. Philadelphia: Lippincott-Raven; 1998:811–61.
37. Nath KA. The tubulointerstitium in progressive renal disease. Kidney Int 1998;54:992–4.
38. Norman RW, Mack FG, Awad SA, Belitsky P, Schwartz RD, Lannon SG. Acute renal failure secondary to bilateral ureteric obstruction: review of 50 cases. Can Med Assoc J 1982;127:601–4.
39. Olsen S, Burdick JF, Keown PA, Wallace AC, Racusen LC, Solez K. Primary acute renal failure ("acute tubular necrosis") in the transplanted kidney: morphology and pathogenesis. Medicine (Baltimore) 1989;68:173–87.
40. Olsen S, Solez K. Acute renal failure in man: pathogenesis in light of new morphological data. Clin Nephrol 1987;27:271–7.
41. Olsen S, Solez K. Acute tubular necrosis and toxic renal injury. In: Tisher CC, Brenner BM, eds. Renal pathology with clinical and functional correlations, 2nd ed. Philadelphia: Lippincott-Raven; 1994:769–809.
42. Pascual J, Liano F, Ortuno J. The elderly patient with acute renal failure. J Am Soc Nephrol 1995; 6:144–53.
43. Richards NT, Darby S, Howie AJ, Adu D, Michael J. Knowledge of renal histology alters patient management in over 40% of cases. Nephrol Dial Transplant 1994;9:1255–9.
44. Riemenschneider T, Bohle A. Morphologic aspects of low-potassium and low-sodium nephropathy. Clin Nephrol 1983;19:271–9.
45. Schena FP, Gesualdo L. Renal biopsy—beyond histology and immunofluorescence. Nephrol Dial Transplant 1994;9:1541–4.
46. Schwartz MM. Prologue to section III. In: Jennette JC, Olson JL, Schwarz MM, Silva FG, eds. Heptinstall's pathology of the kidney, 5th edition. Philadelphia: Lippincott-Raven; 1998:657–65.
47. Silva FG, Nadasdy T, Laszik Z. Immunohistochemical and lectin dissection of the human nephron in health and disease. Arch Pathol Lab Med 1993;117:1233–9.
48. Solez K, Morel-Maroger L, Sraer JD. The morphology of "acute tubular necrosis" in man: analysis of 57 renal biopsies and a comparison with the glycerol model. Medicine (Baltimore) 1997;58:362–76.
49. Solez K, Racusen LC. Acute renal failure: the heart of the matter. In: Solez K, Racusen LC, eds. Acute renal failure: diagnosis, treatment, and prevention. New York: Dekker; 1991:501.
50. Szabolcs M, Seigle R, Shanske S, Bonilla E, DiMauro S, D'Agati V. Mitochondrial DNA deletion: a cause of chronic tubulointerstitial nephropathy. Kidney Int 1994;45:1388–96.
51. Thadhani R, Pascual M, Bonventre JV. Acute renal failure. N Engl J Med 1996;334:1448–60.
52. Toyoshima H, Watanabe T. Rapid regression of renal medullary granular change during reversal of potassium depletion nephropathy. Nephron 1988;48:47–53.
53. Turney JH, Marshall DH, Brownjohn AM, Ellis CM, Parsons FM. The evolution of acute renal failure, 1956-1988. Q J Med 1990;74:83–104.
54. Wilson DM, Turner DR, Cameron JS, Ogg CS, Brown CB, Chantler C. Value of renal biopsy in acute intrinsic renal failure. Br Med J 1976;2:459–61.
55. Zager RA. Endotoxemia, renal hypoperfusion, and fever: interactive risk factors for aminoglycoside and sepsis-associated acute renal failure. Am J Kidney Dis 1992;20:223–30.

20 INFECTIOUS TUBULOINTERSTITIAL NEPHRITIS

ACUTE (BACTERIAL) PYELONEPHRITIS

Definition. The term pyelonephritis has different meanings to different pathologists. Pyelonephritis can be used to mean an infection of the renal parenchyma secondary to an ascending infection that has gained access to the kidney via ureters, and the renal pelvis and calyces. Other nephrologists and pathologists include in the term infections reaching the kidney by the bloodstream (hematogenous infection), irrespective of whether the pyelocalyceal system is involved. Regardless of the route, infection of the renal parenchyma is the essential feature of both definitions (16,17,20).

The authors use the term acute pyelonephritis to indicate all bacterial infections of the renal parenchyma, irrespective of the route of the infectious agent. Ninety-five percent of the cases of acute pyelonephritis are secondary to ascending infections, with the bacteria gaining access to the kidneys via retrograde flow up the ureters. In the remaining 5 percent of cases, the bacteria reach the kidney through the blood, from a source outside of the kidney (i.e., hematogenous infection) (16,17).

Clinical Features. Acute pyelonephritis primarily affects three age groups: 1) infants, usually with structural defects of the urinary tract, 2) young women, and 3) older men. In the neonatal period, congenital anomalies of the urinary tract account for most cases; in women, it is thought that trauma through sexual intercourse predisposes to infection; whereas in older men, enlarged prostates seem to obstruct the urine outflow and lead to infection (10,16,17,20,21,31,32).

The classic clinical symptoms are fever, malaise, back pain (costovertebral angle tenderness), and evidence of urinary bladder/urethral irritation, such as frequency, urgency, and dysuria. The urine contains many leukocytes (pyuria). The presence of granular leukocyte (pus) casts proves renal parenchymal involvement since casts can only be formed in the renal tubules. There also may be hematuria. Quantitative urine culture demonstrates more than 10^5 colony-forming units (CFU)/mL in most patients. Blood urea nitrogen (BUN) and serum creatinine levels are usually normal unless the patient is volume depleted or has a preexisting renal disease. The peripheral white blood cell count is elevated, often with a left shift toward band forms (16,17,21,31).

Gross Findings. Because the majority of patients recover without complications, the kidneys are rarely examined by pathologists. The kidneys are enlarged and edematous, with yellow or white microabscesses on the surface (figs. 20-1, 20-2). On bisection, these microabscesses are usually confined to the cortex; pale streaks may extend from the medulla into the cortex, representing collecting ducts that are filled and lined by purulent material (polymorphonuclear leukocytes) (fig. 20-3). The distribution of these lesions is somewhat random and patchy, but may involve primarily the upper and lower poles of the kidney (for reasons noted below) (fig. 20-4). There may be large wedge-shaped areas of suppurative coalescence. The mucosa of the pyelocalyceal system is erythematous, edematous, and often involved with and covered by a purulent exudate. The pelvis may be dilated, and the papillae may be blunted, flattened, or even overtly necrotic (16,17,20).

Light Microscopic Findings. The major morphologic findings are patchy interstitial inflammation by polymorphonuclear leukocytes and acute tubular injury (figs. 20-5–20-8). Often there is initial acute inflammation involving the renal medulla. The interstitium, initially the medulla and then the cortex, shows a dense inflammatory infiltrate composed of neutrophils, lymphocytes, and even plasma cells and occasional eosinophils (figs. 20-6–20-10). The neutrophilic infiltrate can be quite evanescent, giving way within days to lymphocytes and plasma cells (fig. 20-11). Neutrophils may occur in microabscesses, a characteristic feature of acute

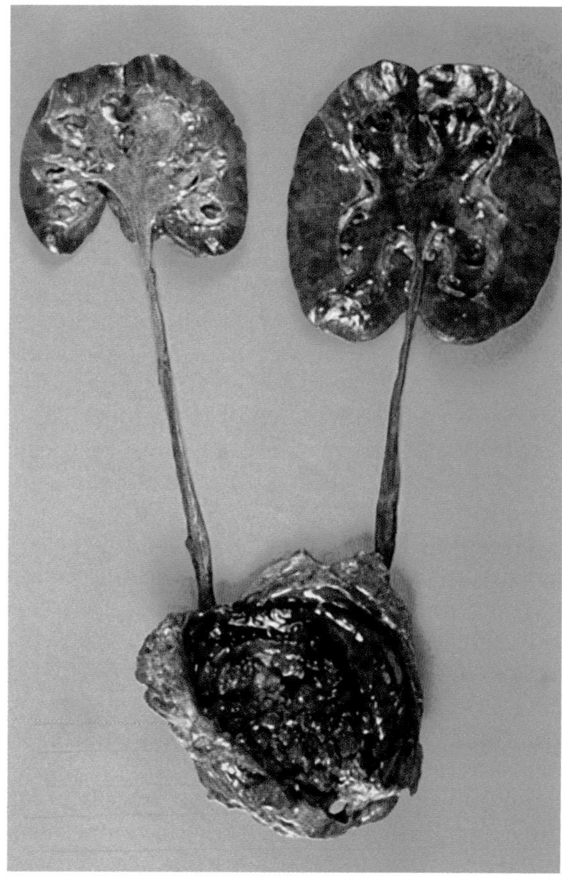

Figure 20-1

ACUTE HEMORRHAGIC CYSTITIS

Acute infection of the urinary bladder is often the precursor of ascending bacterial infection of the kidney. The urinary bladder also contains a transitional cell carcinoma. There is inflammation of the renal pelvis (pyelitis) and the left kidney is scarred. (Courtesy of Dr. J. Ormos, Szeged, Hungary.)

pyelonephritis. The neutrophils often track up the collecting tubules from the medullary tips; they are found within the tubular lumens, filling and distending them, as well as ringing the outer aspect of the tubules, just between the tubular basement membranes and the interstitium. In areas of severe inflammation, tubules may be destroyed. This patchy parenchymal involvement is usually somewhat circumscribed, separated by zones of relatively normal-appearing renal parenchyma. If sections of the pyelocalyceal system are included (and they need to be), severe inflammation of the pelvic mucosa is found in cases of ascending infection. Characteristically, in ascending pyelonephritis, the glomeruli and larger blood vessels are spared this inflammatory insult. However, if the source of infection is hematogenous, septic arteritis and glomerular neutrophilic infiltrates (and even glomerular abscesses) may be seen (16,17).

Immunofluorescence/Electron Microscopic Findings. These are not helpful in the diagnosis other than to exclude a separate coexisting renal disease.

Special Studies. A variety of pathogens can be identified using stains for bacteria (Gram and the Brown-Brenn) (fig. 20-12) and fungi (periodic acid–Schiff [PAS], Grocott methenamine silver).

Differential Diagnosis. Because the kidney reacts in a limited way to a thousand different injuries, the tubulointerstitial damage is quite nonspecific. Other noninfectious conditions can lead to similar morphologic findings. These include allergic or drug-induced (hypersensitivity) interstitial nephritis, and the "secondary" interstitial inflammation associated with marked glomerular inflammation, such as in association with crescentic or acute glomerulonephritis. The presence of marked neutrophilic invasion of the tubular lumens or microabscesses, however, is quite characteristic of acute bacterial pyelonephritis. The clinical history is often of assistance.

Etiology and Pathogenesis. As noted above, 95 percent of cases of acute pyelonephritis are secondary to ascending bacterial infection emanating from a primary infection in the urinary bladder (16,17,21). Most infections are due to Gram-negative bacteria which are normal flora of the gastrointestinal tract. By far, the most common infectious agent is *Escherichia coli*, although other organisms such as *Proteus, Klebsiella, Enterobacter* sp, *Streptococcus faecalis*, and staphylococci can all contribute. Virtually any bacterial and fungal agent can cause renal infection. Most patients with urinary tract infection are infected by an organism from their own fecal flora (a form of endogenous infection) (16,17,21,30,31).

In hematogenous forms, bacteria reach the kidney through the blood stream from distant foci of infection in the course of septicemia or visceral infections (such as endocarditis). This occurs primarily in patients with ureteral obstruction, debilitated patients, immunosuppressed patients, or patients with other conditions predisposing the kidney to direct blood-borne

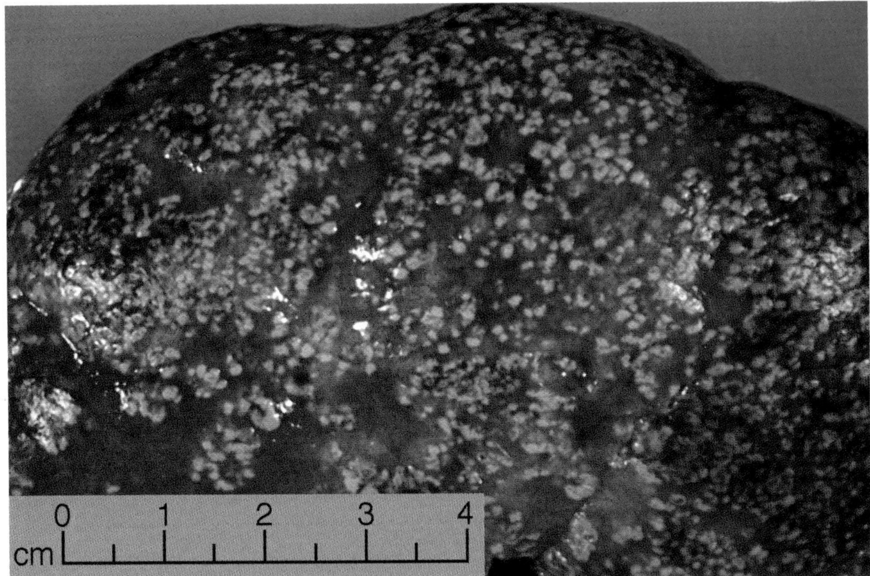

Figure 20-2

ACUTE PYELONEPHRITIS

The surface of the kidney from a patient with severe acute pyelonephritis shows a large number of yellow microabscesses. The patient had an ascending bacterial infection.

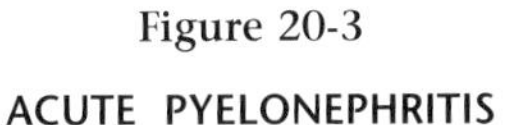

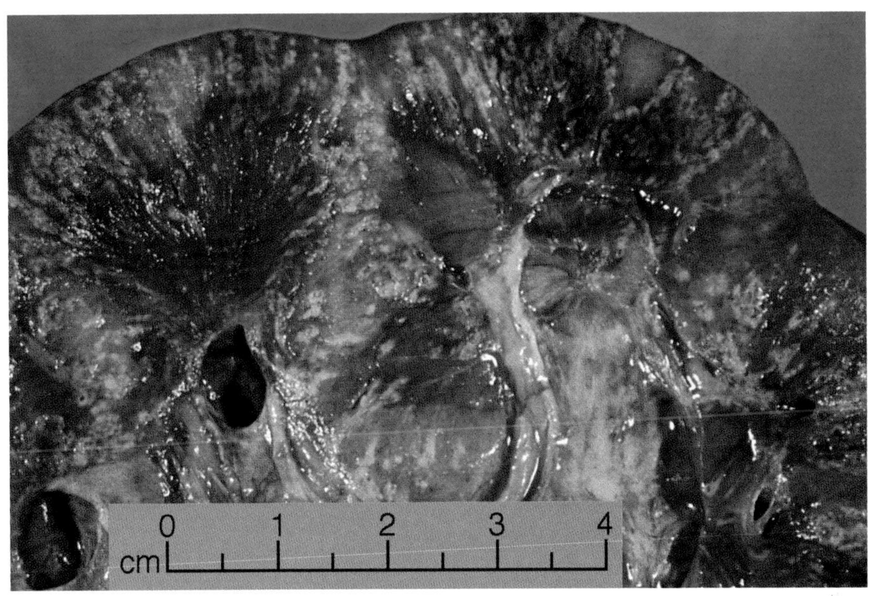

Figure 20-3

ACUTE PYELONEPHRITIS

The cut surface of the kidney seen in figure 20-2 shows many small abscesses in the renal cortex and medulla.

infection. Hematogenous infections are often caused by virulent nonenteric bacteria (such as staphylococci).

In the ascending form, the most common route is retrograde flow up the ureters (16,17,21, 30,31). This process appears to require a sequence of events: in the female, colonization of the introitus and distal urethra by endogenous coliform bacteria is a common prerequisite. The ability of the bacteria to adhere to vaginal/urethral mucosa is via the P-fimbriae (pili) of bacteria and other adhesion molecules which bind with urothelial cell receptors. Certain types of fimbriae have been shown to promote renal tropism, an enhanced inflammatory bacterial response, and/or persistence of the infection. Recently, special adhesins have been associated with acute infection. The ureteral organisms may gain entrance into the urinary bladder by catheterization or other instrumentation. Trauma (by sexual intercourse) and the short urethra in the female are thought to predispose this group of patients to infection. Hormonal changes may affect the adherence of bacteria to the urothelium.

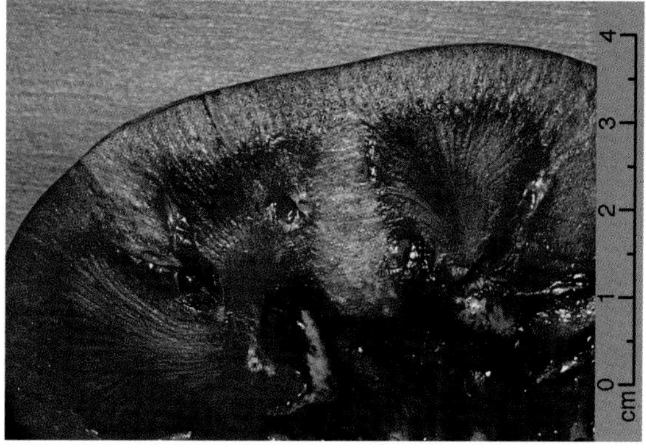

Figure 20-4

ACUTE PYELONEPHRITIS

The cut surface of this kidney shows a wedge-shaped lighter region of the cortex that represents acute pyelonephritis.

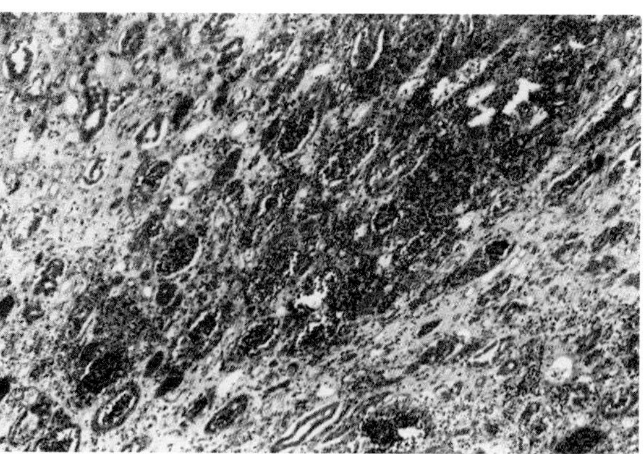

Figure 20-5

ACUTE INFECTIOUS (BACTERIAL) PYELONEPHRITIS

Ascending bacterial infection (due to *Escherichia coli*) involves many of the collecting ducts in the medulla. Note the patchy nature of the infiltrate (hematoxylin and eosin [H&E] stain).

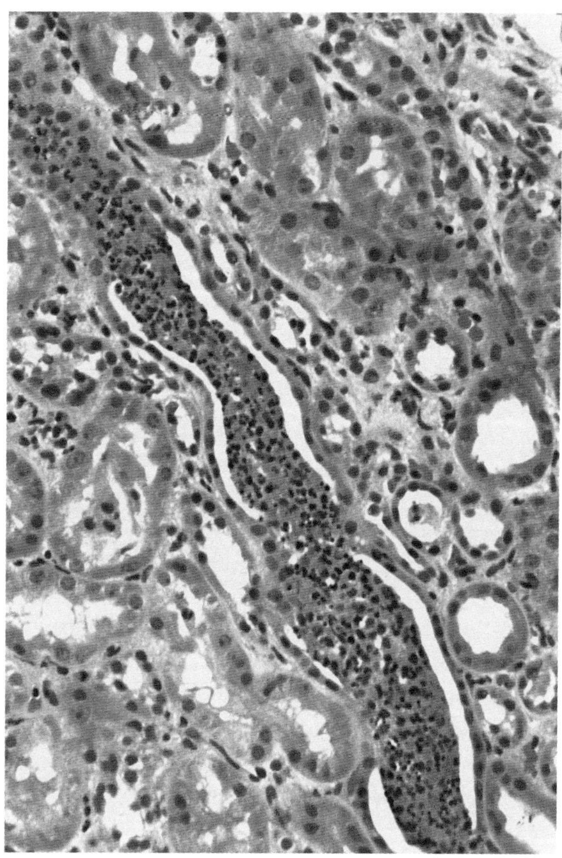

Figure 20-6

ACUTE PYELONEPHRITIS

One duct contains a cast of polymorphonuclear leukocytes; the pus cast may be seen in the urine of a patient with acute pyelonephritis (H&E stain).

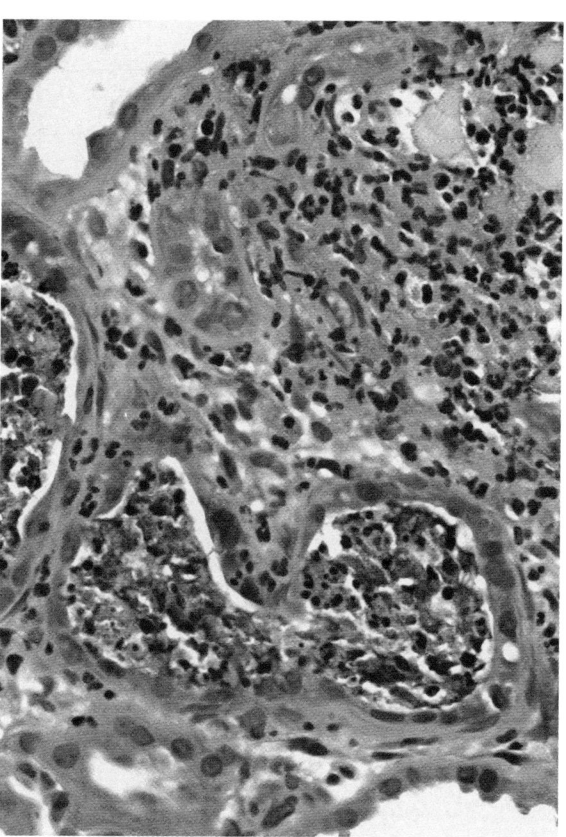

Figure 20-7

ACUTE PYELONEPHRITIS

There is intense infiltration of acute inflammatory cells. The polymorphonuclear leukocytes are noted both within the tubule and in the adjacent interstitium.

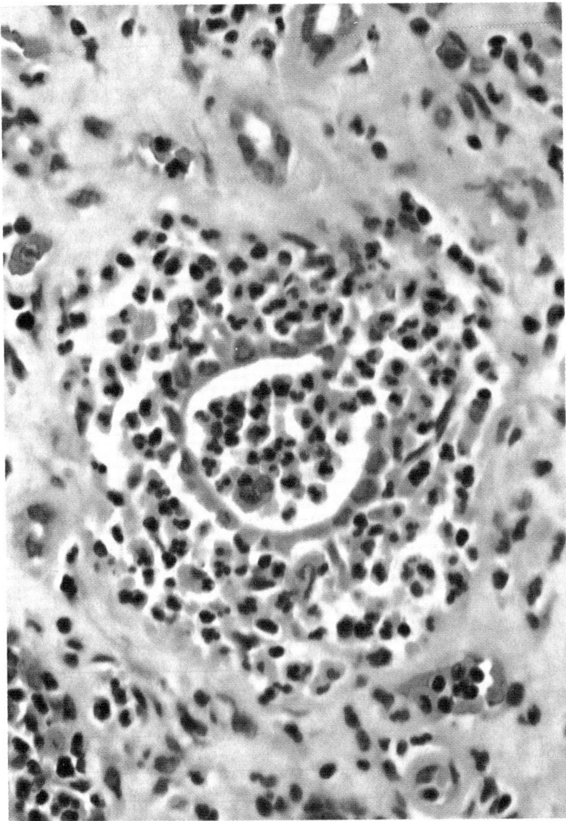

Figure 20-8

ACUTE PYELONEPHRITIS

Polymorphonuclear leukocytes infiltrate through the renal collecting tubule with disruption of the tubular epithelium. Bacterial organisms and the accompanying polymorphonuclear leukocytes often track up the renal collecting tubules in this way.

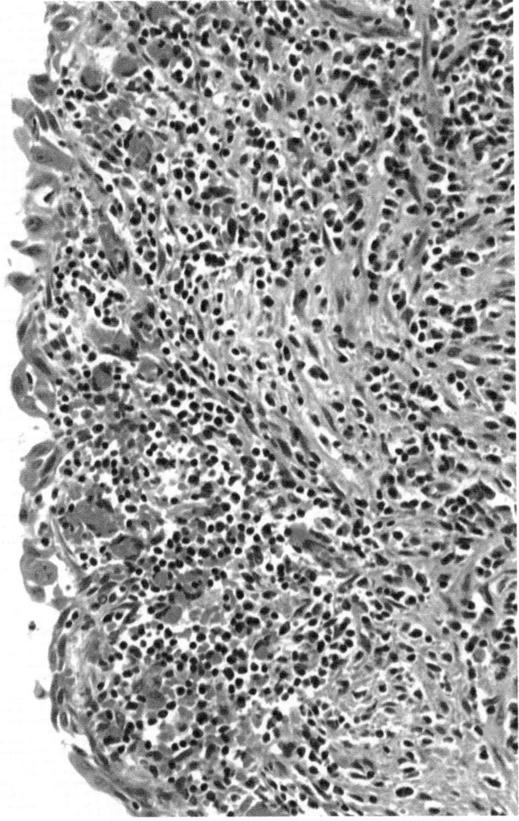

Figure 20-9

ACUTE PYELITIS

There is acute inflammation/infection of the renal pyelocalyceal system. Note the intense acute inflammation by polymorphonuclear leukocytes in the renal papillary tips with erosion or loss of the overlying transitional epithelium (urothelium). The renal pelvis is the first area of involvement in a typical ascending bacterial infection.

Normally, any bacterial organisms introduced into the urinary bladder are rapidly cleared by micturition and by the presence of other antibacterial mechanisms. However, urinary outflow obstruction and urinary bladder dysfunction may result in incomplete emptying of the bladder and retention of urine. Urinary stasis favors bacterial growth. Ordinarily, urine is not allowed to ascend the ureters during micturition because of one-way valves in the ureterovesicle orifices. Incompetence of the ureterovesicle orifice (by a congenitally short intravesical portion of the ureter or dysfunction secondary to inflammation), however, allows reflux of infected urine up the ureter. Infected urine can be propelled up to the renal pyelocalyceal regions and into the renal medulla through patent collecting ducts at the tips of the papillae (i.e., intrarenal reflux). Intrarenal reflux is more common in the upper and lower poles of the kidney where the papillae are compound and do not close under the pressure of refluxing urine (21,27,28). These compound papillae have flattened or concave tips rather than the convex pointed papillae present in the midzones of the kidney; these convex papillae do close under pressure and largely prevent intrarenal reflux. Reflux can be demonstrated by a voiding cystourethrogram and is seen in up to half of children with bacterial cystitis.

The major mechanisms predisposing to acute pyelonephritis are, therefore, urinary obstruction, instrumentation, vesicoureteric reflux,

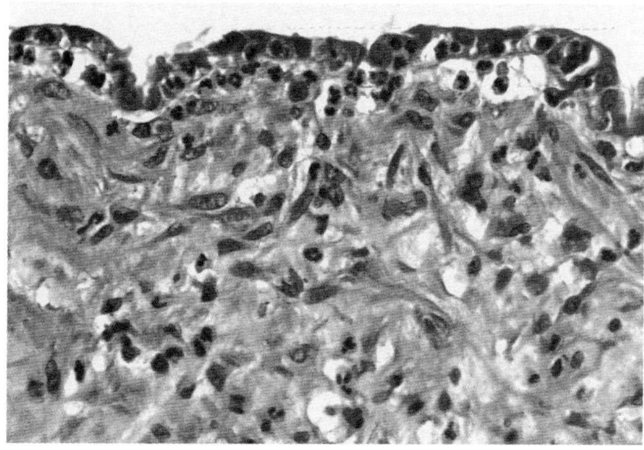

Figure 20-10

ACUTE PYELITIS

There is loss of the transitional epithelium, with an acute and chronic inflammatory cell infiltrate, in this region of the kidney (H&E stain).

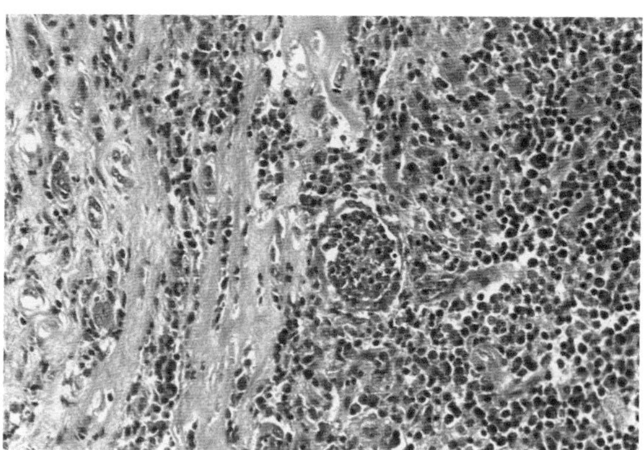

Figure 20-11

ACUTE ASCENDING BACTERIAL PYELONEPHRITIS

Large numbers of chronic inflammatory cells (plasma cells and lymphocytes) are in the renal interstitium in this patient with acute bacterial pyelonephritis. Chronic inflammatory cells, such as plasma cells, can be found early in the disease process (H&E stain).

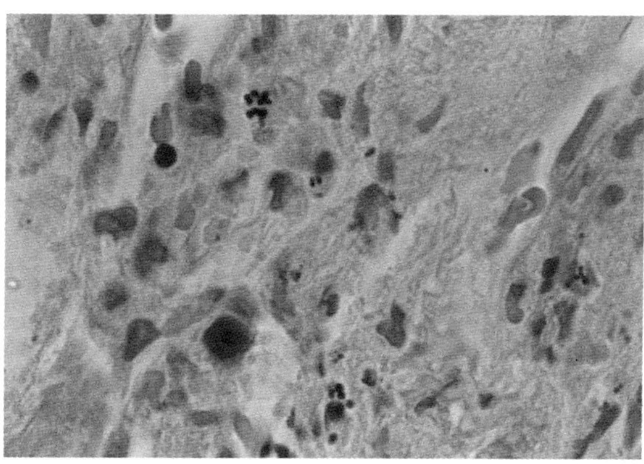

Figure 20-12

ACUTE PYELONEPHRITIS

This bacterial (Gram) stain shows several, small, rounded bacterial organisms in the renal parenchyma. Usually it is difficult to demonstrate bacterial organisms in acute pyelonephritis, even in a virulent case.

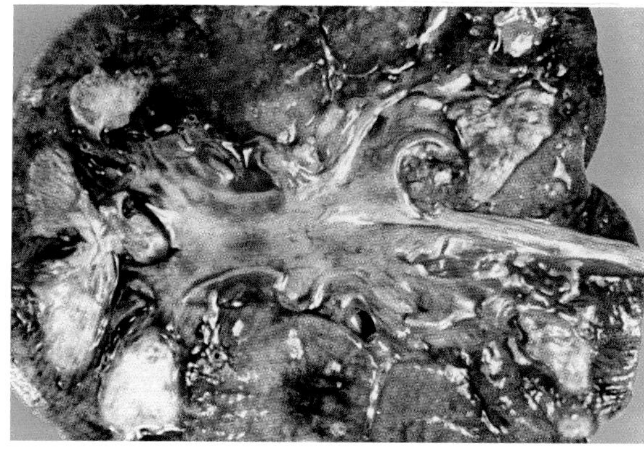

Figure 20-13

PAPILLARY NECROSIS (NECROTIZING PAPILLITIS)

The renal pelvis shows multiple infarcted renal papillae in association with dilated renal calyces. The necrotic renal papillae are yellow. (Courtesy of Dr. J. Ormos, Szeged, Hungary.)

pregnancy, preexisting renal diseases (such as scarring and obstruction), diabetes mellitus (leading to neurogenic bladder), immunosuppression, and immunodeficiency (10,16,17,20,21,31).

Treatment and Prognosis. Proper antibiotic therapy usually is effective in eradicating the acute bacterial infection. If there are multiple recurrent bacterial infections, then abnormalities of the urinary tract are searched for and corrected. Most patients do well (21,31,32).

Specific Complications of Acute Pyelonephritis. *Papillary Necrosis.* This is a severe complication of acute pyelonephritis and may even lead to acute renal failure (figs. 20-13, 20-14). It is often associated with urinary tract obstruction and infection or diabetes. It may be bilateral or unilateral (depending on the site of the obstruction and infection). One, few, or all the papillae may be involved. On cross-section, the papillary tips of the distal two thirds of the papillae have a gray-white to yellow discoloration which represents necrosis/infarction.

Microscopically, there is coagulation necrosis early on, with loss of tubular epithelial cell nuclei but preservation of cell outlines (fig. 20-14). Later, the medulla has a ghost-like appearance, with the tubular epithelium lost and only the conduits (remnants of the ducts of Bellini) left in place. These sloughed papillae may be shed into the urine. Thus, any tissue found in the urine needs to be submitted for histologic evaluation (after straining of the urine in suspected cases). The acute inflammatory infiltrate is limited to the junctions between the histologically preserved and the necrotic regions.

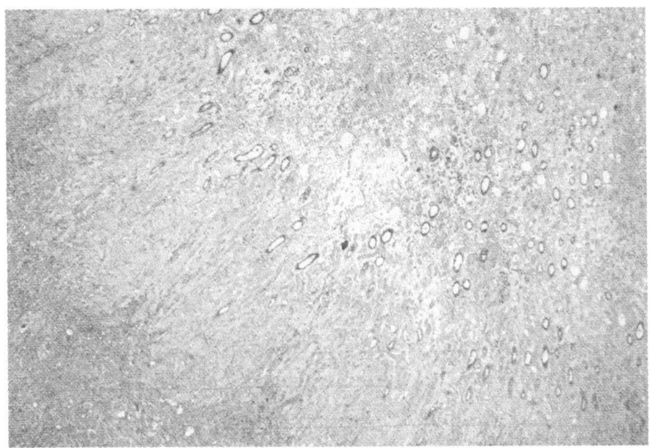

Figure 20-14

PAPILLARY NECROSIS

The necrotic renal papillae show histologic evidence of infarction, with coagulation necrosis and retention of the medullary tubular outlines, but little cellular epithelial detail (H&E stain).

Pyonephrosis. Pyonephrosis occurs when there is total or almost total obstruction, especially if high, in the urinary tract. The pockets of pus (polymorphonuclear leukocytes) are unable to drain out and fill the renal pyelocalyceal system and ureter (fig. 20-15).

Perinephric Abscess. Perinephric abscess occurs when the suppurative inflammation extends through the renal cortex and renal capsule into the adjacent perinephric fat (fig. 20-16). This may be clinically difficult to diagnose.

CHRONIC PYELONEPHRITIS

Definition. The use of the term chronic pyelonephritis is somewhat controversial. In the past it was defined as a chronic tubulointerstitial disorder that was diagnosed liberally whenever any significant degree of lymphocytic infiltration was noted in the renal interstitium; it was presumed to indicate the sequelae of chronic inflection. After it was discovered that chronic interstitial inflammation may be found in conditions lacking evidence of past or present infection (by history or culture of the renal parenchyma), the diagnostic criteria for this diagnosis were made more stringent (6,16,20,27,28, 30). Today, chronic pyelonephritis is defined as a chronic tubulointerstitial disease in which there is chronic interstitial inflammation and

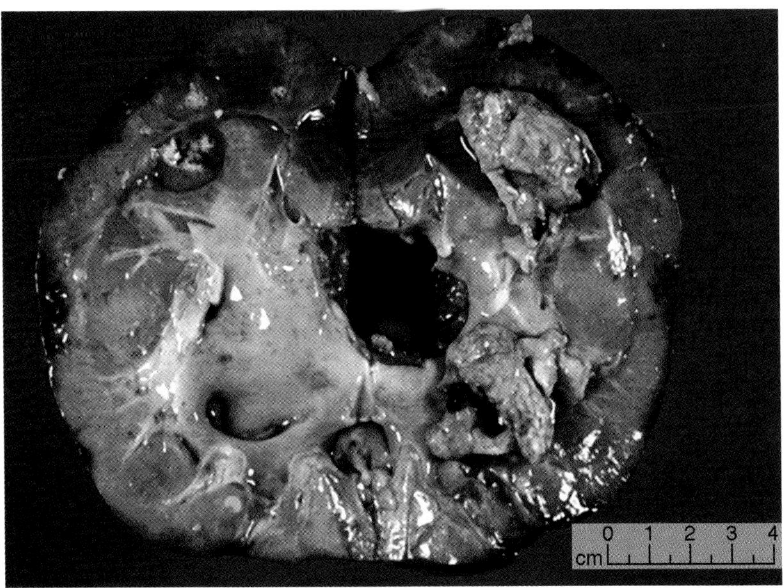

Figure 20-15

PYONEPHROSIS

There is marked destruction of the renal parenchyma, with dilatation of the renal pyelocalyceal systems. These cystic dilatations were filled with purulent material and a large renal stone.

renal scarring associated with severe morphologic involvement of the renal calyces and pelvis. Pyelocalyceal damage is required.

Clinical Features. Chronic pyelonephritis occurs in all age groups; women are more often affected than men. Some patients have a prior history of repeated urinary tract infections, whereas others do not. A history of urinary tract anomalies or obstruction, or a history of urologic surgical repair when the patient was young is not unusual (16,30,32).

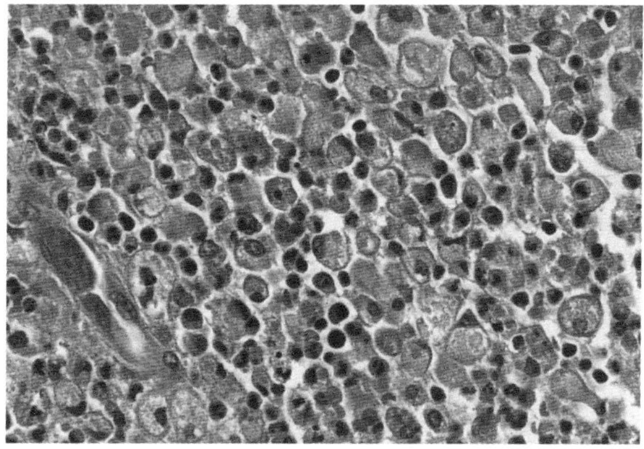

Figure 20-16

PERINEPHRIC ABSCESS WITH XANTHOGRANULOMATOUS PYELONEPHRITIS

Micrograph of a region outside the kidney shows a large collection of foamy macrophages and lymphocytes (H&E stain).

The clinical course of chronic pyelonephritis is often insidious, with a silent, distant onset. In other cases, the presentation is acute, secondary to recurrent bouts of acute pyelonephritis, and manifesting with back pain, fever, toxemia, pyuria, and bacteruria. Many patients present later in the course of their disease with the gradual onset of renal insufficiency. Hypertension is often present at diagnosis. BUN and serum creatinine levels may be normal or increased. Proteinuria may be present; the urinary findings are not specific. Loss of tubular function, especially of urinary concentrating ability, gives rise to polyuria and nocturia. Radiologic studies show asymmetrically contracted and deformed kidneys, with characteristic coarse, patchy, cortical scars and blunting/deformity of the calyceal system. Bacteriuria may be absent in the late stages of the disease.

Gross Findings. The characteristic gross pathologic finding is irregularly scarred renal cortices (figs. 20-17–20-19). The cortical scars are typically single or multiple, large, broad-based, and U-shaped, overlying the dilated, blunted, or deformed calyces (fig. 20-17). The scars vary in size and number, and may involve any region of the kidney, but especially the upper and lower poles (fig. 20-18). They are often sharply demarcated from the normal renal parenchyma. The remainder of the cortical surface may be smooth or granular (if there is accompanying

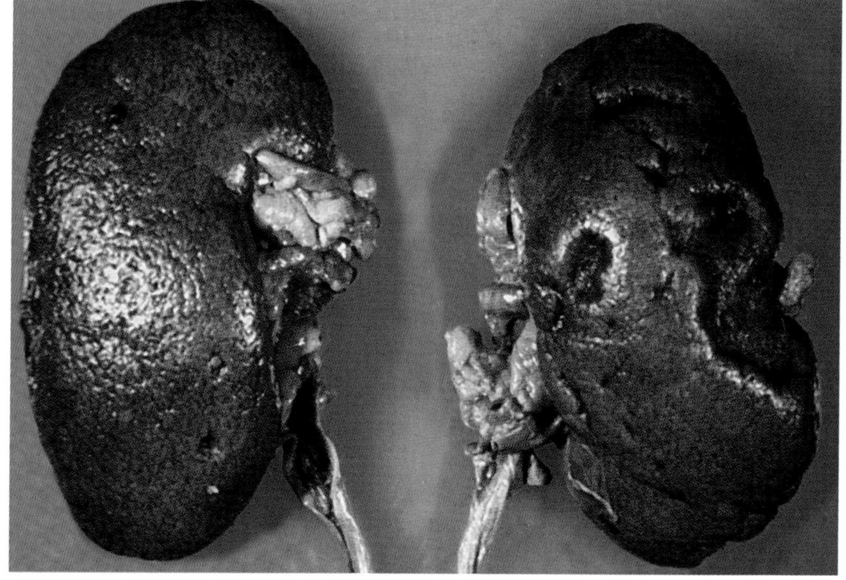

Figure 20-17

CHRONIC PYELONEPHRITIS

Unilateral, deep, U-shaped, broad-based cortical scars are seen in the right kidney of this patient with documented chronic pyelonephritis. These types of large cortical scars need to be distinguished from cortical scars due to vascular disease of larger arteries of the kidney. The renal pelvises need to be examined for evidence of past or present chronic inflammation with destruction or deformation of the convex renal papillary tips.

arterial and arteriolar nephrosclerosis secondary to hypertension) (16,17,20,27,28,30).

Light Microscopic Findings. The light microscopic changes are quite nonspecific and patchy. The tubules and interstitium are predominantly involved, both in the medulla and the cortex (figs. 20-20–20-27). There is focal, often extreme, thinning of the renal cortex and medulla, which may reach a parenchymal thickness as small as 1 to 2 mm (fig. 20-23). Tubular atrophy is often manifested by uniformly dilated renal tubules with marked thinning of the tubular epithelium and uniform colloid hyaline casts ("thyroidization") (fig. 20-25). Although thyroidization is most often associated with chronic pyelonephritis, it is certainly not pathognomonic for it. There are varying degrees of patchy chronic interstitial inflammation with lymphocytes and plasma cells involving the cortex and/or medulla. Interstitial fibrosis is present. Periglomerular fibrosis is noted, but the glomeruli are usually spared major morphologic injury. The arteries may be thickened, secondary to associated hypertension. Glomeruli may be quite close together due to loss of the intervening tubular parenchyma. Importantly, a diagnosis of true chronic pyelonephritis requires that the pyelocalyceal regions be sampled and that they show evidence of severe chronic inflammation (figs. 20-20, 20-21). There is lymphocytic infiltration of the submucosa, sometimes with germinal centers, and deformation of the pyelocalyceal regions with fibrosis. Destruction of these final drainage routes (ducts of Bellini) accounts for the patchy cortical scars described above (fig. 20-21). The presence of polymorphonuclear leukocytes in the tubular lumens (pus casts) and the surrounding interstitium may denote the presence of an accompanying superimposed acute renal infection.

In chronic pyelonephritis with reflux or obstruction, there may be eosinophilic, PAS-positive

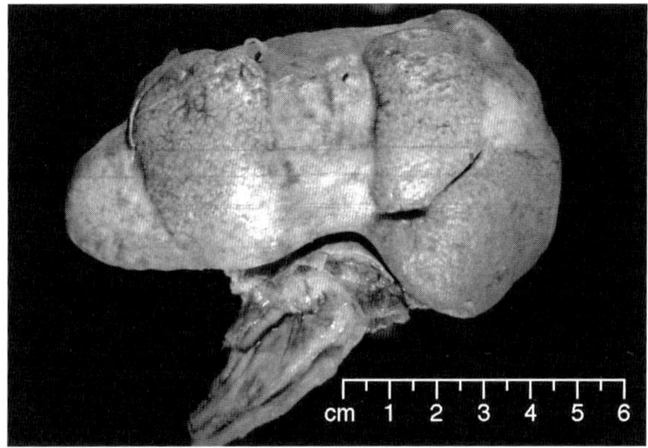

Figure 20-18

CHRONIC PYELONEPHRITIS

Many patchy regions of renal scarring are seen in a case of advanced renal parenchymal scarring caused by severe chronic pyelonephritis. (Courtesy of Dr. Stejskal, Prague, Czech Republic.)

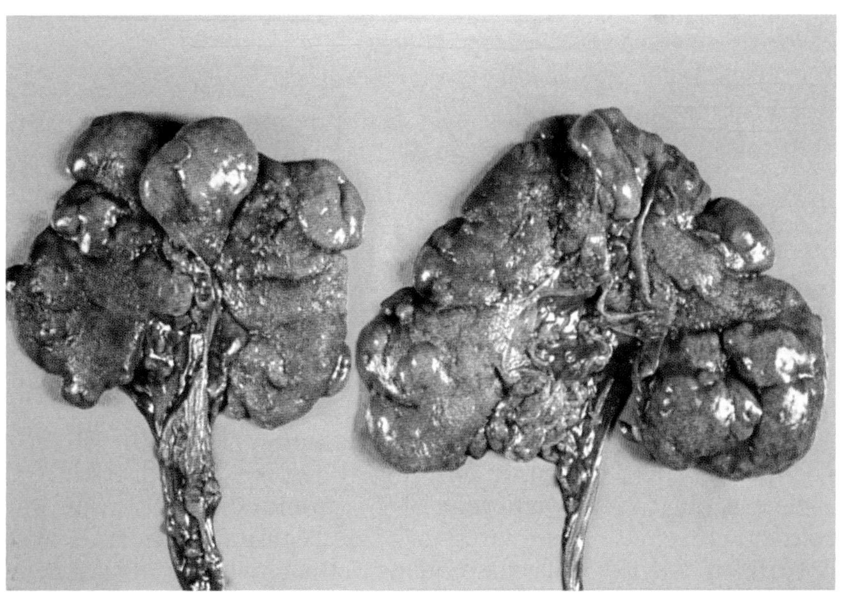

Figure 20-19

END-STAGE KIDNEY DISEASE DUE TO CHRONIC PYELONEPHRITIS

There is widespread atrophy of the renal cortex in this patient with longstanding renal infections. (Courtesy of Dr. J. Ormos, Szeged, Hungary.)

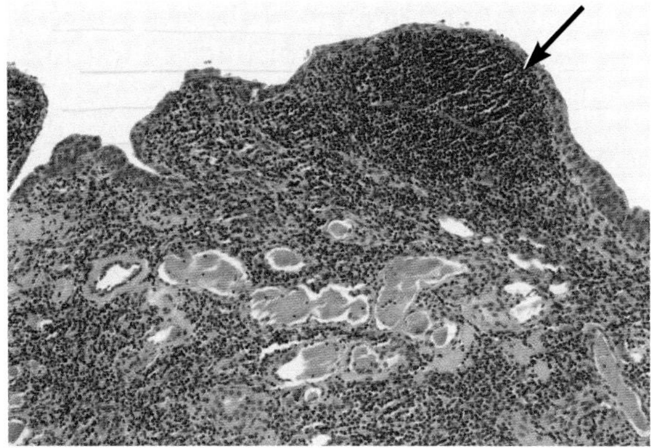

Figure 20-20

CHRONIC PYELONEPHRITIS

The renal pelvis shows marked chronic inflammation with plasma cells and lymphocytes. There is a suggestion of rudimentary germinal center formation (arrow) (H&E stain).

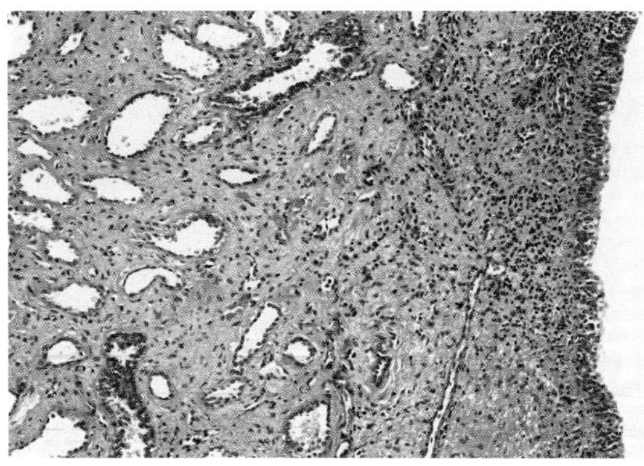

Figure 20-21

CHRONIC PYELONEPHRITIS

A section of the renal medulla shows loss of the normal convexity of the renal pelvis, which is replaced by a slight concavity. There is deformation of the collecting tubules and fibrosis of the medullary regions (H&E stain).

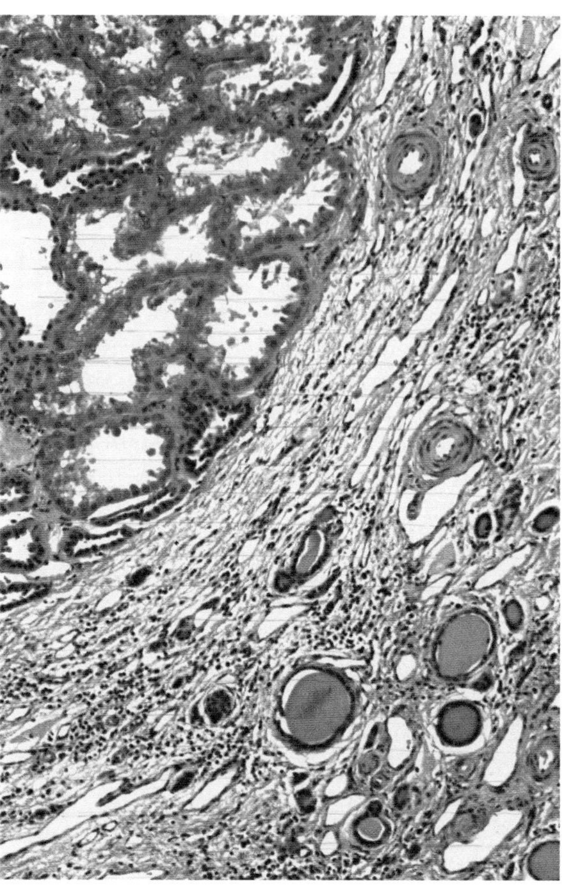

Figure 20-22

CHRONIC PYELONEPHRITIS

A focal or segmental scar (interstitial fibrosis and tubular atrophy) is seen in the kidney of a patient with chronic pyelonephritis. Both vascular and pyelonephritis scars can be quite focal and well delineated. The tubular structures on the top left show marked hyperplasia (H&E stain).

tubular cast material, representing extravasated Tamm-Horsfall protein, in the interstitium (see chapter 24). There is often an inflammatory infiltrate around these extravasated proteins (4,16,17,20).

Patients with chronic pyelonephritis may, over the course of years, develop severe proteinuria and in some cases even the nephrotic syndrome; these patients often develop secondary focal segmental glomerulosclerosis due to the loss of renal mass and hyperfiltration in remnant nephrons (fig. 20-28). Patients with chronic pyelonephritis and focal sclerosis often progress more rapidly to end-stage renal disease than patients without this glomerular lesion (3,9,23). Severe vascular lesions may be present, secondary to hypertension.

In chronic obstructive pyelonephritis (see below), there is generalized atrophy of the renal parenchyma and generalized dilatation of the pelvis. Calculi may form within the dilated pelvic structures (16).

Immunofluorescence/Electron Microscopic Findings. These are noncontributory. There may be nonimmunologic, nonspecific "sticking" of various immunoreactants and plasma proteins to the renal casts (fig. 20-29).

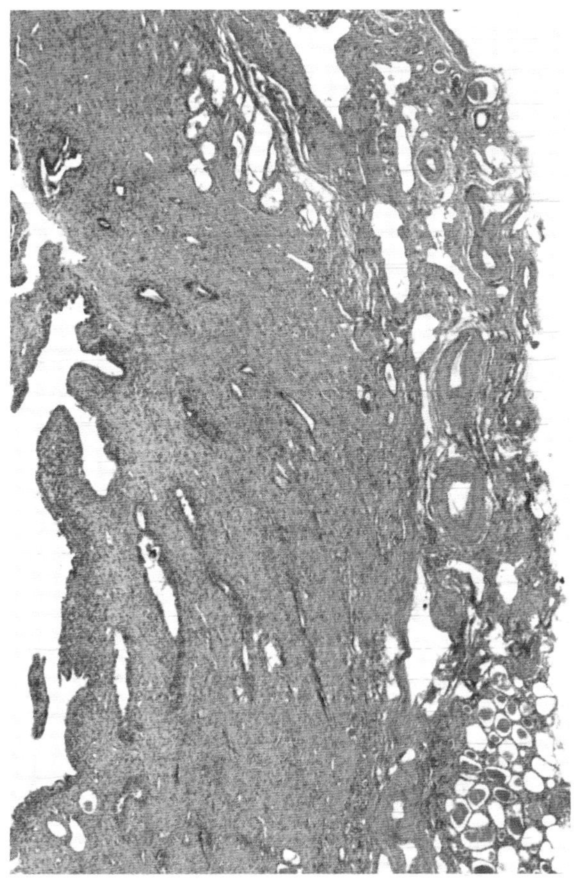

Figure 20-23

CHRONIC PYELONEPHRITIS

There is marked thinning of the renal cortex overlying the inflamed and scarred renal pelvis in this patient with longstanding chronic pyelonephritis.

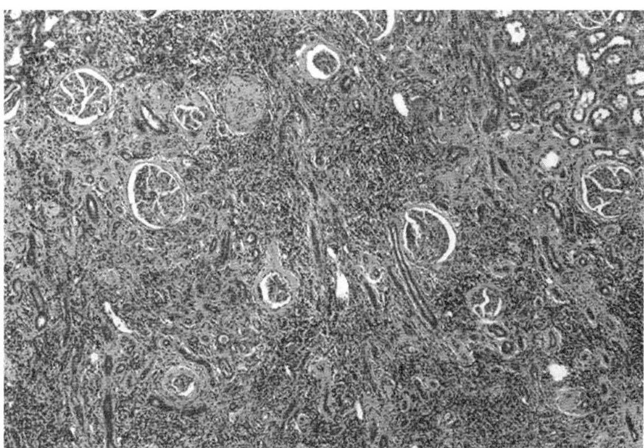

Figure 20-24

CHRONIC PYELONEPHRITIS

There is intense interstitial inflammation by lymphocytes but fairly good preservation of the glomeruli in this patient with chronic pyelonephritis. The glomeruli are frequently quite well preserved in patients with chronic pyelonephritis, even in those with severe advanced renal disease (H&E stain).

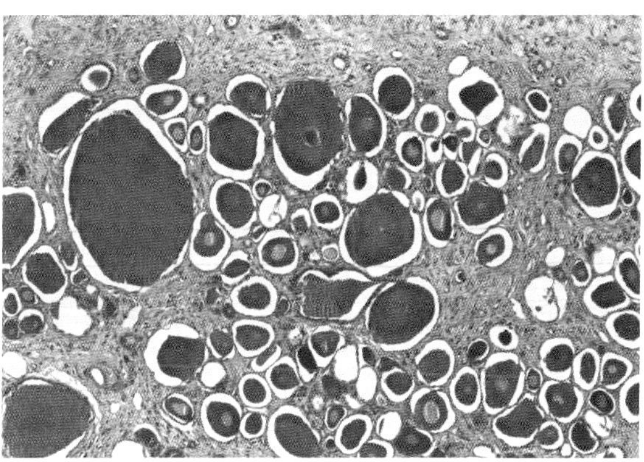

Figure 20-25

CHRONIC PYELONEPHRITIS: "THYROIDIZATION" OF THE RENAL TUBULES

This atrophic tubular change, with homogeneous eosinophilic casts and diffusely thinned renal tubular epithelium, is typical of chronic pyelonephritis, although it can be seen in virtually any advanced (or advancing) renal parenchymal disorder (periodic acid-Schiff [PAS] stain).

Differential Diagnosis. Because the histologic findings are so nonspecific, the clinical and surgical history as well as evidence of pyelocalyceal destruction and deformation (by either radiologic studies or gross examination) are essential for the definitive diagnosis of chronic pyelonephritis. Vascular diseases (arterial nephrosclerosis) can lead to large, wedge-shaped (even U-shaped) cortical scars resembling those of chronic pyelonephritis; however, in vascular diseases the underlying medullary and calyceal areas are usually normal, in contrast to the striking alterations in chronic pyelonephritis. If the whole kidney is available, it is important to section it in such a way as to be able to study completely all the pyelocalyceal regions and papillae. Kidneys are diffusely, symmetrically scarred in patients with chronic glomerulonephritis (see chapter 25) (16). With a biopsy specimen, the clinical history and radiologic studies are required to solidify the diagnosis of chronic pyelonephritis.

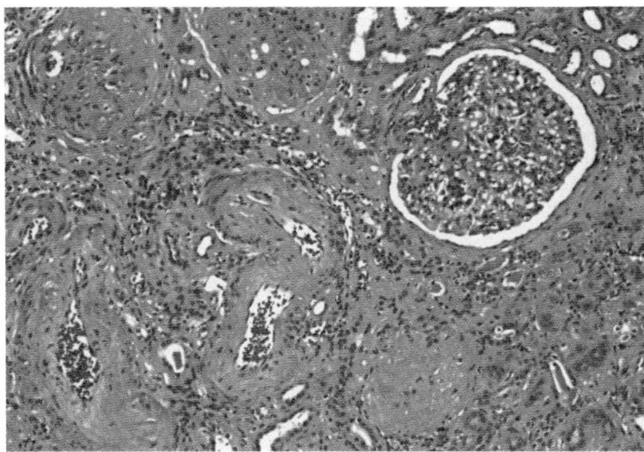

Figure 20-26

CHRONIC PYELONEPHRITIS

This low-power magnification micrograph shows the typical, although not pathognomonic, histologic pattern of chronic pyelonephritis: interstitial fibrosis and inflammation, severe secondary vascular disease (with intimal thickening), tubular atrophy, and relative preservation of the glomeruli, although a few globally sclerotic glomeruli are noted (H&E stain).

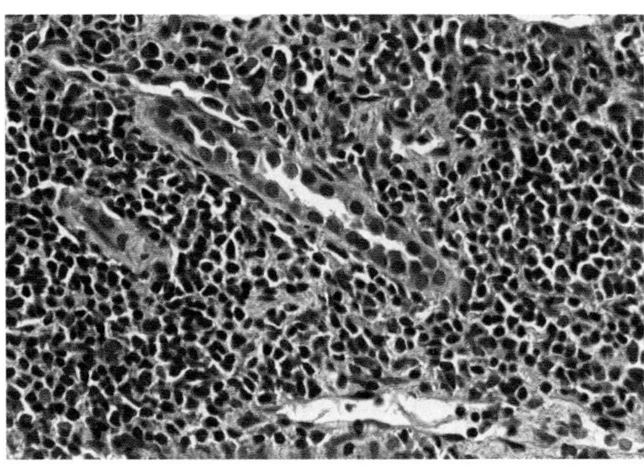

Figure 20-27

CHRONIC PYELONEPHRITIS

There is marked interstitial inflammation by mostly lymphocytes. This morphologic picture is nonspecific and can be associated with many conditions other than chronic pyelonephritis (see text) (H&E stain).

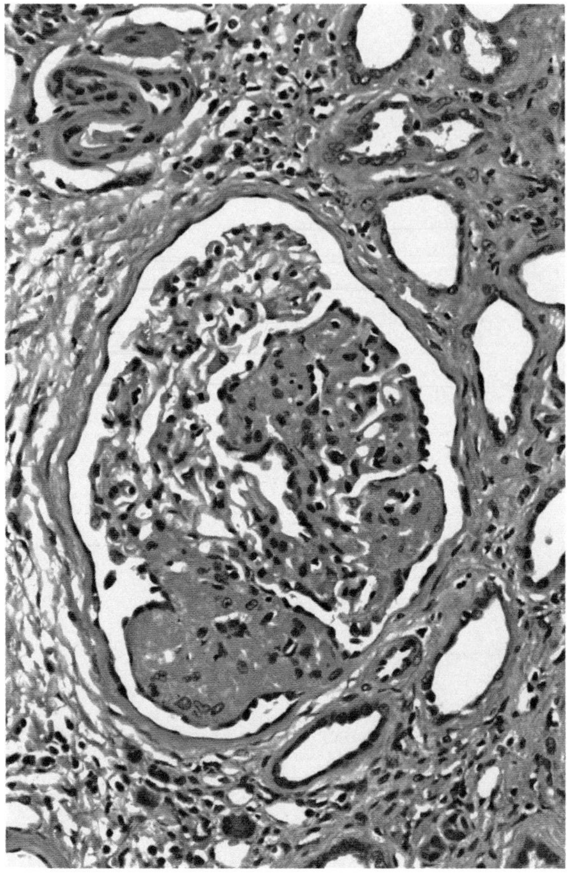

Figure 20-28

CHRONIC PYELONEPHRITIS

This patient with bonafide chronic pyelonephritis developed severe proteinuria and advancing renal insufficiency. Histologic examination of the kidney revealed a secondary focal segmental and global glomerulosclerosis (focal sclerosis). This glomerular pattern can occur secondary to chronic pyelonephritis and is often a harbinger of a poor prognosis.

Etiology and Pathogenesis. Two variants of chronic pyelonephritis have been described: 1) *chronic obstructive pyelonephritis*, secondary to obstruction of the urinary tract, and 2) *chronic nonobstructive pyelonephritis* (16,29). In the chronic obstructive form, obstructive anomalies of the urinary tract contribute to the renal parenchymal atrophy. It is often impossible to differentiate the effects of obstruction alone from the effects of complicating bacterial infection. In the nonobstructive form, vesicoureteral and intrarenal reflux are essential pathogenetic mechanisms; hence the term *reflux nephropathy* has been applied commonly to this entity. The role of infection in the pathogenesis of nonobstructive pyelonephritis remains controversial.

Reflux Nephropathy (Chronic Nonobstructive Pyelonephritis)

Severe ureterovesicle (UV) reflux, caused by structural and/or functional disorders of the UV valve, may result in permanent renal scarring (3,4,

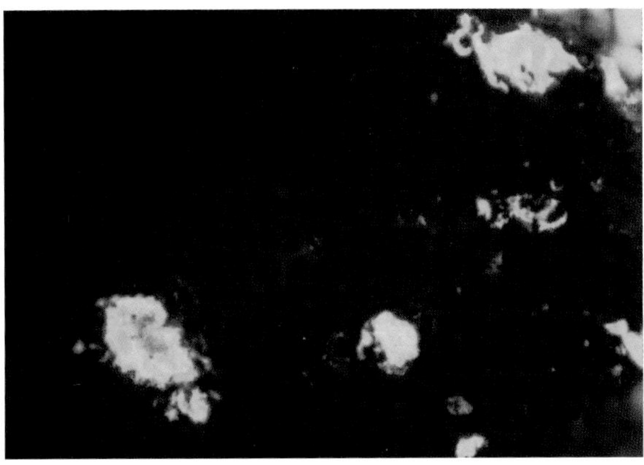

Figure 20-29

CHRONIC PYELONEPHRITIS

By direct immunofluorescence, the renal casts stain nonspecifically for a variety of immunoreactants applied to the snap-frozen renal tissues. Renal casts often stain in this nonspecific, nonimmunologic pattern (anti-IgG).

8,9,13,16,23,27–30). The renal scarring often occurs during infancy, when the kidney is rapidly growing, and probably represents failure of that segment of the kidney to develop normally, rather than scarring of a portion of the kidney that has already formed fully, although progressive renal parenchymal scarring (starting at the pyelocalyceal system) can occur later in life over time if the reflux is severe.

Intrarenal reflux seems to be required for renal scarring to occur. Intrarenal reflux usually occurs in compound papillae, where two or three pyramids are normally fused together. These compound papillae have rounded/oval openings into the ducts of Bellini, which allows reflux of urine into the renal parenchyma. They are generally found at the poles of the kidney (which are the most common sites of the scars in chronic pyelonephritis). Whether the reflux by itself can lead to the scarring seen in chronic pyelonephritis, or concomitant bacterial infection is required for such changes, is unclear. Some investigators believe that if the reflux is severe enough, the changes of reflux nephropathy can still be produced even in the presence of sterile urine. Focal segmental sclerosis may develop as a secondary complication of reflux nephropathy. Antibiotic prophylaxis in children with UV reflux may decrease the incidence of subsequent scarring and pyelonephritis.

The so-called Ask-Upmark kidney has generated much controversy over the years. The Ask-Upmark kidney has one or more narrow, diverticulum-like outpouchings of the renal pelvis which extend far into the renal parenchyma; the renal tissues are atrophic at the tip of these outpouchings, leading to deep grooving of the subcapsular surface. A somewhat similar lesion has been described as "segmental hypoplasia." The patients are usually under 15 years of age, with a predominance of females. Dysplastic elements are absent. Most now consider this an acquired lesion that falls best into the category of reflux nephropathy for a number of reasons: 1) many patients have vesicoureteral reflux; 2) cases are described in which the normal kidneys have transformed during the period of observation; 3) studies using microangiographic methods have demonstrated the spiraling of the interlobular arteries, suggesting secondary atrophy of the renal parenchymal tissues; and 4) all of the changes are characteristic of those seen in human reflux nephropathy and the experimental models of reflux in the pig (which is multipapillate).

Xanthogranulomatous Pyelonephritis

Definition. This uncommon variant of pyelonephritis is characterized by a severe pyelocalyceal inflammation, with prominent, foamy, lipid-laden macrophages (2,12,15).

Clinical Features. Adults in their 50s and 60s are most commonly affected. The disease is more common in women than men and the renal involvement is virtually always unilateral. Obstruction of the urinary tract is almost always present, and renal calculi are frequent. Bacterial infection and obstruction are thought to play definitive roles.

Flank pain, fever, weight loss, and malaise are present, sometimes years before the clinical diagnosis. Most patients have a history of previous renal calculi, urinary tract obstruction, or diabetes mellitus. The involved kidney may be palpable. Urinalysis demonstrates mild proteinuria and pyuria. Renal failure is uncommon.

Gross Findings. The kidney is large and often adherent to the perirenal fat. There is a thickened capsule. On cross-sectioning of the kidney, the pelvicalyceal system is dilated, with lost or very deformed papillae. Staghorn calculi

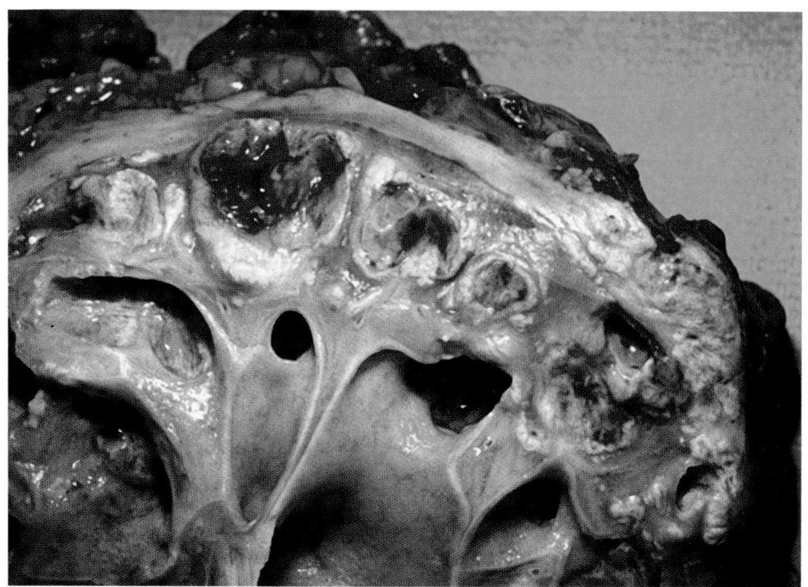

Figure 20-30

XANTHOGRANULOMATOUS PYELONEPHRITIS

Large portions of the renal medulla (and cortex) are replaced by pale tan-yellow areas of severe acute and chronic inflammation. The renal calyces are dilated and partially destroyed.

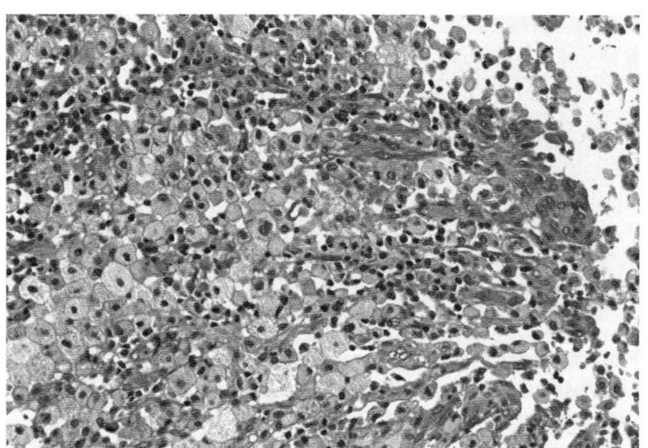

Figure 20-31

XANTHOGRANULOMATOUS PYELONEPHRITIS

There is widespread inflammatory destruction of the renal pelvic areas by large numbers of lymphocytes and foamy histiocytes (H&E stain).

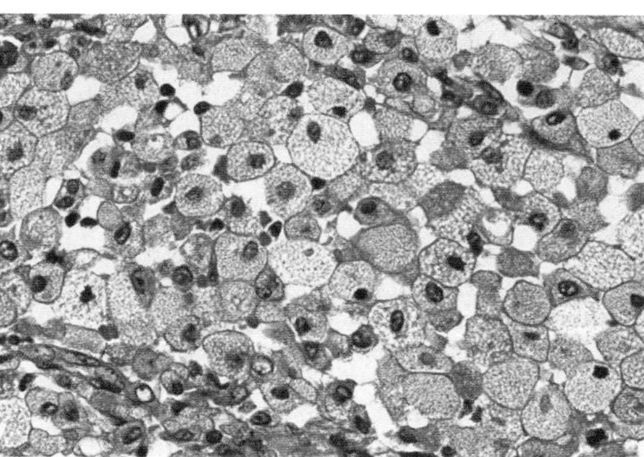

Figure 20-32

XANTHOGRANULOMATOUS PYELONEPHRITIS

A high magnification view shows the large collections of foamy histiocytes. These need to be distinguished from collections of neoplastic clear cells, as in a clear cell carcinoma of the kidney (H&E stain).

may be present. The most characteristic changes are alterations of the calyces by yellow, friable material; this material may also be present in the cortex, along with discrete abscesses (fig. 20-30). Grossly, the lesions may be confused with renal cell carcinoma (see below) (2,12,15,16) as well as renal medullary tuberculosis.

Light Microscopic Findings. The yellow areas of the calyces described above are composed of sheets of large, lipid-laden, foamy macrophages, often mixed with smaller mononuclear cells (macrophages), lymphocytes, plasma cells, and occasional neutrophils (figs. 20-31, 20-32). Multinucleated giant cells may be present but are not required for the diagnosis of xanthogranulomatous pyelonephritis. The adjacent renal parenchyma shows diffuse tubular atrophy/interstitial inflammation and fibrosis.

Immunofluorescence Findings. These are noncontributory.

Electron Microscopic Findings. The foamy macrophages contain bacteria and numerous phagolysosomes. Electron microscopy is not required for a definitive diagnosis.

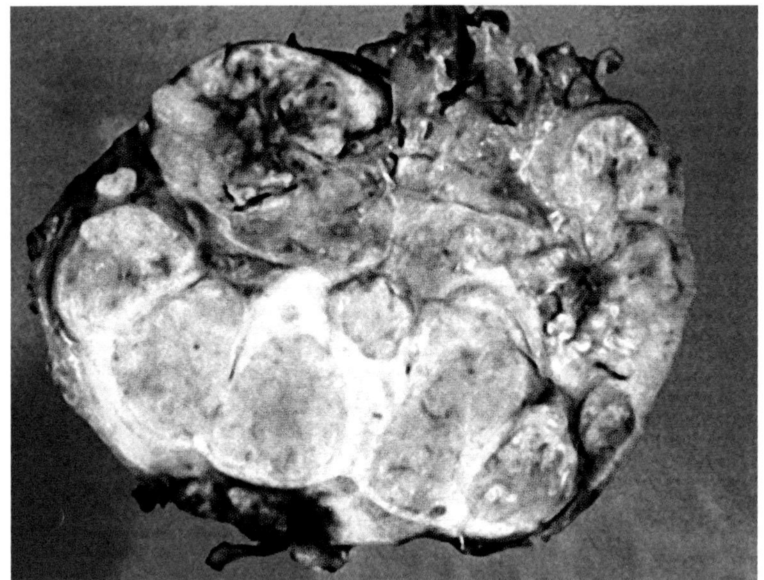

Figure 20-33

RENAL MALAKOPLAKIA

There is replacement of the renal parenchyma by the amorphous mass representing malakoplakia. (Courtesy of Dr. J. Ormos, Szeged, Hungary.)

Special Studies. Presumably, immunohistochemical markers that distinguish macrophages from renal tubular epithelial neoplasms could be helpful in the rare instances that distinction between this infectious pattern and a renal cell adenoma/carcinoma is necessary (see below).

Differential Diagnosis. The most important entity in the differential diagnosis is clear cell renal cell carcinoma (2,12,15). The xanthogranulomatous inflammatory lesions sometimes produce large yellowish nodules which may be confused microscopically with clear cell carcinoma. Arteriography can demonstrate a constant difference between the two. Microscopically, the key is to identify the foamy cells as macrophages and not malignant epithelial cells.

Etiology and Pathogenesis. The exact cause of xanthogranulomatous pyelonephritis is unknown. Bacterial infection and obstruction appear to play important roles. The most common bacterial organisms associated with this lesion are *E. coli, Proteus* sp, *Klebsiella* sp, and *Pseudomonas* sp; other organisms are associated on occasion.

Treatment and Prognosis. Unilateral nephrectomy is indicated. Because the disease is unilateral, renal function is maintained.

Malakoplakia

Definition. Malakoplakia is a non-neoplastic (reactive) space-occupying lesion (or lesions) found in many different organs and probably represents altered/imperfect intracellular processing of engulfed bacteria by histiocytes (1,11,12,14,22).

Clinical Features. Malakoplakia, which is most commonly found in the urinary bladder, may also involve the renal pelvis and the renal parenchyma. It is most often diagnosed in the fifth decade of life. It is more common in women than men and is frequently associated with bacterial infection. Calculi are seldom found. *E. coli* is the most common bacterial organism cultured from the urine.

Malakoplakia may lead to obstruction when it involves the renal pelvis. Bilateral disease is not uncommon. Approximately half of patients have an immunodeficiency or autoimmune disorder (such as malignancies, acquired immunodeficiency syndrome [AIDS], rheumatoid arthritis, or immunosuppressive therapy).

Symptoms include fever, chills, and flank pain. Urinalysis shows proteinuria, pyuria, and hematuria. Renal failure may be seen. Like xanthogranulomatous pyelonephritis, malakoplakia may be mistaken for a neoplasm.

Gross Findings. The kidney may be involved focally or diffusely (fig. 20-33). The lesions are raised, yellow plaques. They may be multiple and occur on the pelvic lining, on the capsular surface, or extend into the renal parenchyma (1,11,12,14,22).

Light Microscopic Findings. There are clusters of mononuclear cells (macrophages) with

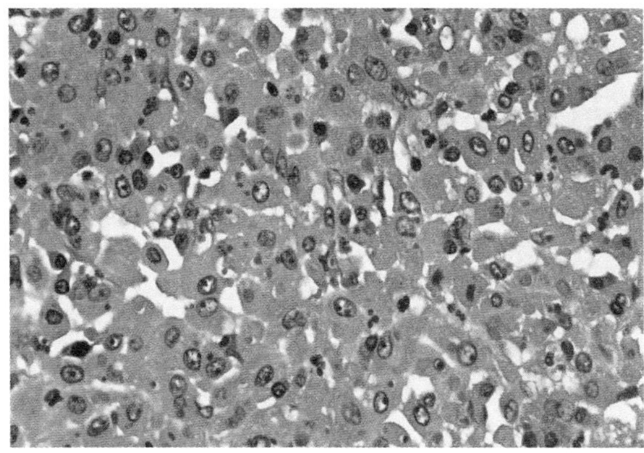

Figure 20-34

RENAL MALAKOPLAKIA

Histologic examination shows many rounded histiocytes (von Hanseman cells) (H&E stain).

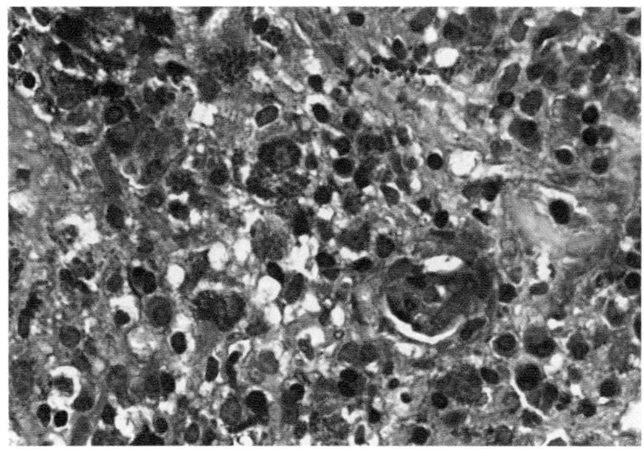

Figure 20-35

RENAL MALAKOPLAKIA

There are a large number of polygonal cells with PAS-positive cytoplasmic granules in the interstitium in this patient with malakoplakia.

foamy, eosinophilic cytoplasm (von Hanseman cells) (fig. 20-34). Cytoplasmic granules and inclusions (4 to 10 µm) are present. These Michaelis-Gutmann bodies stain for calcium (von Kossa stain) and iron (Prussian blue), and are hematoxylin and eosin (H&E) and PAS (with/without diastase) positive (figs. 20-35, 20-36). Michaelis-Gutmann bodies may be homogenous or laminated. The adjacent renal parenchyma may be infiltrated by the macrophages or compressed by the expanding nodules.

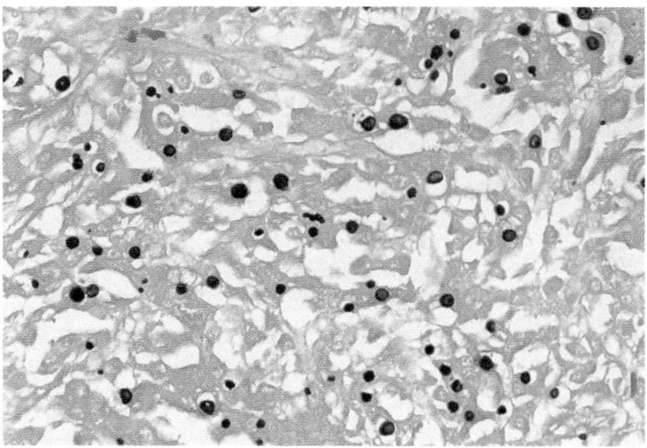

Figure 20-36

RENAL MALAKOPLAKIA

Calcium deposition in a number of cells (Michaelis-Gutmann bodies) in a patient with renal malakoplakia (von Kossa calcium stain).

Immunofluorescence Findings. These are noncontributory.

Electron Microscopic Findings. The intracytoplasmic inclusions show a crystalline structure with a central dense core, an intermediate halo, and a peripheral lamellated ring (lysosomal membrane) (fig. 20-37). Rod-shaped structures resembling bacteria are often present within phagolysosomes.

Differential Diagnosis. This lesion is easily misdiagnosed as a neoplasm if malakoplakia is not considered in the differential diagnosis of a space-occupying mass or severe interstitial inflammation.

Etiology and Pathogenesis. Malakoplakia probably occurs because of a defect in macrophage bactericidal function. The exact pathogenetic mechanism remains unclear.

Megalocytic Interstitial Nephritis

Megalocytic interstitial nephritis is a rare condition that resembles malakoplakia. Indeed, some investigators believe that it represents an early stage of malakoplakia. The clinical findings overlap with those of malakoplakia, and like malakoplakia, chronic bacterial infection and urinary tract obstruction play important roles in its pathogenesis (1,14).

There may be diffuse involvement of the kidney, with multiple foci of yellow-gray lesions of various sizes; there may be discrete nodules within the cortex. Histologically, there are large

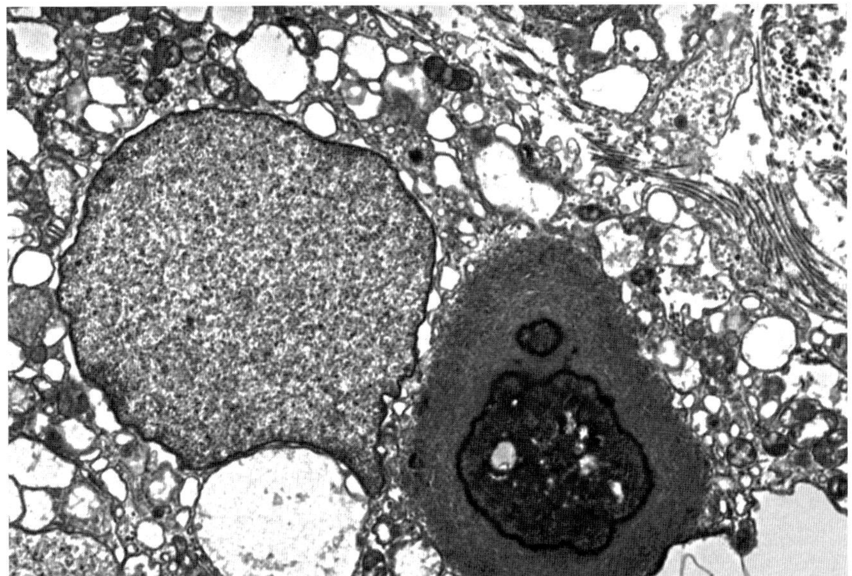

Figure 20-37

RENAL MALAKOPLAKIA

Electron micrograph shows one of the renal malakoplakia cells containing a Michaelis-Gutmann body. Note its crystalline structure, with a central dense core and outer ring (usually comprised of calcium and iron).

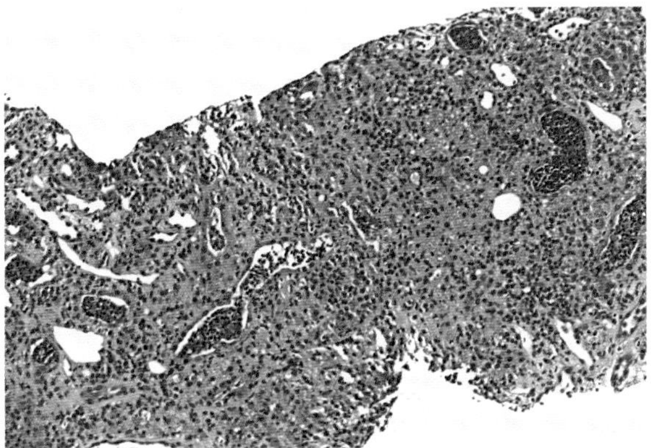

Figure 20-38

MEGALOCYTIC INTERSTITIAL NEPHRITIS

The renal interstitium is expanded by a moderately cellular infiltration of histiocytic cells. Such cells are also noted in the tubular lumens (H&E stain).

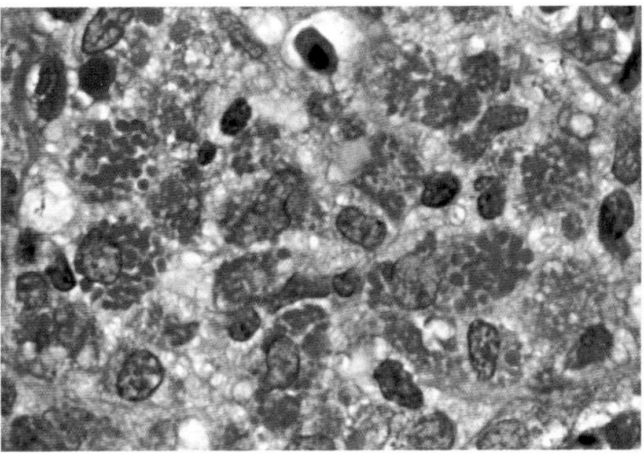

Figure 20-39

MEGALOCYTIC INTERSTITIAL NEPHRITIS

Large, numerous PAS-positive macrophages are present. Some investigators believe that megalocytic interstitial nephritis is a form of renal malakoplakia.

numbers of plump polygonal cells with an eosinophilic granular cytoplasm (fig. 20-38). These granules stain intensely for PAS (figs. 20-38, 20-39) (1,14,16). Occasionally, Gram-positive bacterial organisms are demonstrated (fig. 20-40).

The major distinction between this entity and malakoplakia is the presence of Michaelis-Gutmann bodies in malakoplakia. There may be some overlap between these two lesions in the literature (i.e, some investigators have labeled cases with characteristic Michaelis-Gutmann bodies as megalocytic interstitial nephritis).

TUBERCULOSIS OF THE KIDNEY

Definition. The genitourinary tract is the most common site of extrapulmonary tuberculosis (TB), representing about one fifth of extrapulmonary cases. The kidney is affected by about 10 percent of the extrapulmonary cases (12,16,17,25).

Clinical Features. There is often a long latent period between the development of pulmonary TB and the diagnosis of genitourinary TB. Symptoms may be mild or absent. Fever and night sweats are rare. Most symptoms relate to

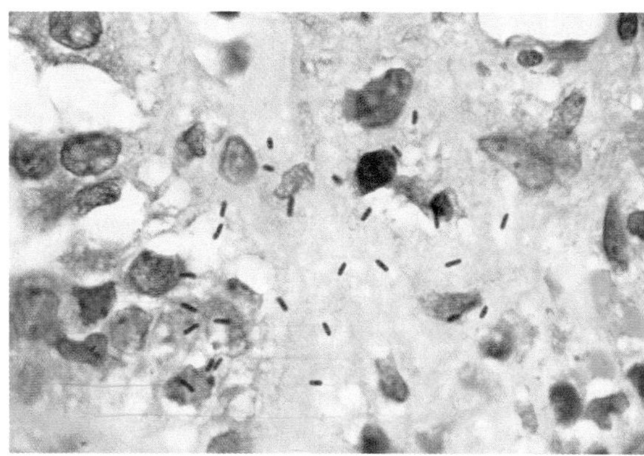

Figure 20-40

MEGALOCYTIC INTERSTITIAL NEPHRITIS

Rarely, the bacterial organism (in this case *E. coli*) is identified in the lesion (Gram stain).

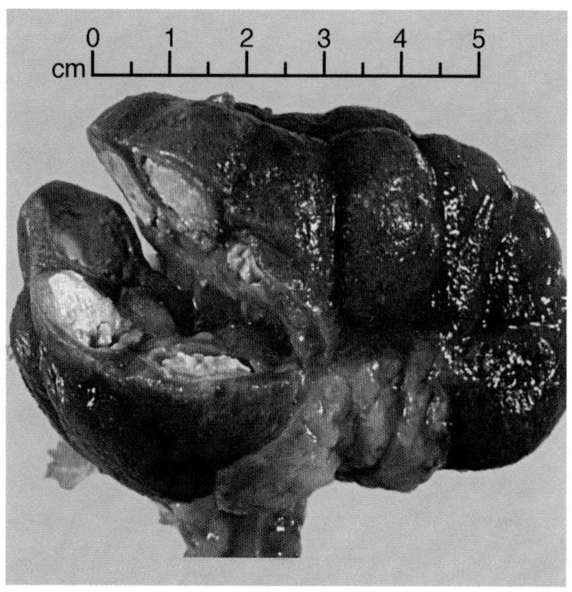

Figure 20-41

RENAL TUBERCULOSIS

The large caseating nodules markedly distort the renal architecture. (Courtesy of Dr. Stejskal, Prague, Czech Republic.)

urinary bladder infection, such as frequency, dysuria, loin pain, and hematuria. The purified protein derivative (PPD) tuberculin test is positive and there is usually evidence of previous pulmonary TB on the chest X ray.

Although renal insufficiency and hypertension are rare, most patients have an abnormal urinalysis. The most common and characteristic findings are sterile pyuria and microscopic hematuria. The first morning urine should be cultured for TB organisms. Acid-fast stains of the urine are fraught with hazard because of the common false-positive results due to nonpathogenic forms of mycobacteria that can be present in the urine.

Gross Findings. The initial lesions occur in the renal medulla, with ulceration of the transitional epithelium lining the papillae. The papillae become deformed and clubbed, and are replaced progressively by caseous necrosis. Caseous material spreads throughout the mucosal lining, eventually filling and obliterating the calyces (figs. 20-41, 20-42). The ureteropelvic junction also can become obstructed by caseous material, producing hydronephrosis (fig. 20-43). The overlying renal cortex can become atrophic, with extensive parenchymal destruction (12,17,25). Renal medullary TB and xanthogranulomatous pyelonephritis are easily confused on gross examination.

Light Microscopic Findings. The early findings demonstrate neutrophils and macrophages in the renal medulla. This is followed by production of granulomata, often with central caseous necrosis. The renal cortex may be focally to diffusely involved by severe tubulointerstitial disease (tubular atrophy, interstitial fibrosis, and inflammation). The infiltrating cells are mostly composed of lymphocytes, plasma cells, and monocytes. Rarely, there is extensive interstitial fibrosis or destruction of the renal parenchyma.

Persistent infection in the medulla results in a severe caseating granulomatous reaction. Large tumor-like masses ("tuberculomas") may form or calyceal amputation may occur.

Immunofluorescence/Electron Microscopic Findings. These are noncontributory.

Special Studies. The mycobacterial organisms are usually identified with acid-fast stains such as the Ziehl-Neelsen or Fite. Fluorochromes such as auramine rhodamine are also used to demonstrate the organisms.

Etiology and Pathogenesis. Spread to the kidney probably occurs hematogenously during the primary infection with TB (before the development of cell-mediated immunity against the organism). In most cases, the organism is controlled and the lesions heal. In a small number

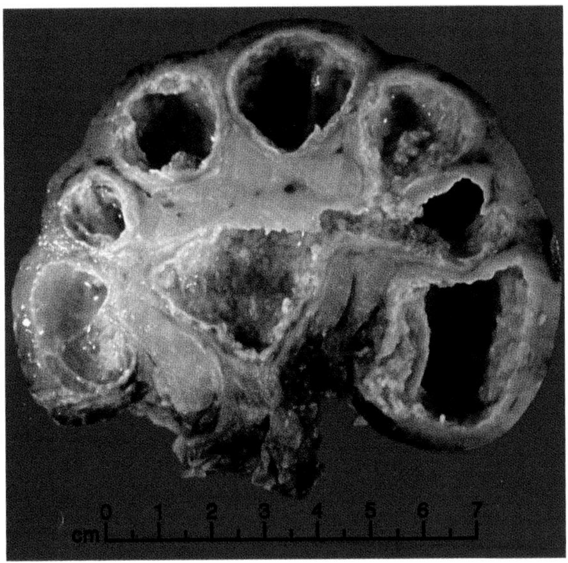

Figure 20-42

RENAL TUBERCULOSIS

Cross section of the kidney shows destruction and dilatation of the renal pelvic system, with white regions of caseous necrosis. (Courtesy of Dr. Stejskal, Prague, Czech Republic.)

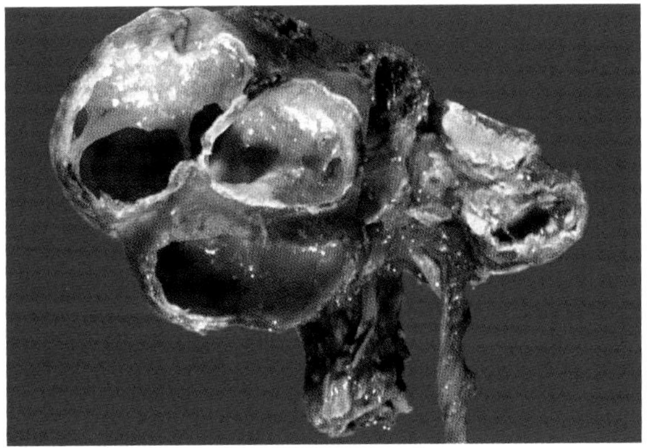

Figure 20-43

RENAL TUBERCULOSIS

A kidney is almost totally destroyed by renal tuberculosis. (Courtesy of Dr. T. Nadasdy, Rochester, New York.)

of patients, infection persists in the medulla, resulting in a caseating granulomatous reaction.

It is likely that the incidence of renal TB will increase. This is due to the increased risk of TB in immunocompromised patients (as in AIDS) and the immigration of individuals from areas of high prevalence, such as the Far East. The recent development of drug resistance in patients with TB infections is worrisome.

OTHER SPECIFIC RENAL INFECTIONS (NONBACTERIAL)

Fungal Infections Directly Involving the Kidney

Primary fungal infections of the renal parenchyma are rare. One of the most common fungal agents that can involve the kidney is *Candida* (Table 20-1). Fungi most often infect the kidney by hematogenous routes from a systemic infection. The source may be nosocomial (5,6,8,16,21).

Candidiasis. Most infections from this fungal agent are opportunistic, usually originating in the mucosal surfaces of the upper aerodigestive tract or the vagina. Hematogenous dissemination then occurs. Immunosuppressed patients are most at risk; neonates and granulocytopenic patients also are at risk.

Table 20-1

FUNGAL/ACTINOMYCETAL INFECTIONS INVOLVING THE KIDNEY

Candidiasis
Torulopsosis
Aspergillosis
Cryptococcosis
Histoplasmosis
Coccidioidomycosis
Blastomycosis
Paracoccidioidomycosis
Mucormycosis
Actinomycosis
Nocardiosis

The clinical presenting signs and symptoms are those of a severe renal infection. There may be ureteral colic or even anuria if the fungus ball obstructs the ureter(s). Detection of *Candida* organisms in the urine is diagnostic.

The kidneys may show little involvement, or conversely, show miliary abscesses, extensive necrosis, and even papillary necrosis. Mycotic aneurysms may be present in glomerular capillaries and arterioles (figs. 20-44–20-46).

Histologically, the fungal organism has nonbranching chains of tubular cells, pseudohyphae and rounded yeast forms, 2 to 4 µm in

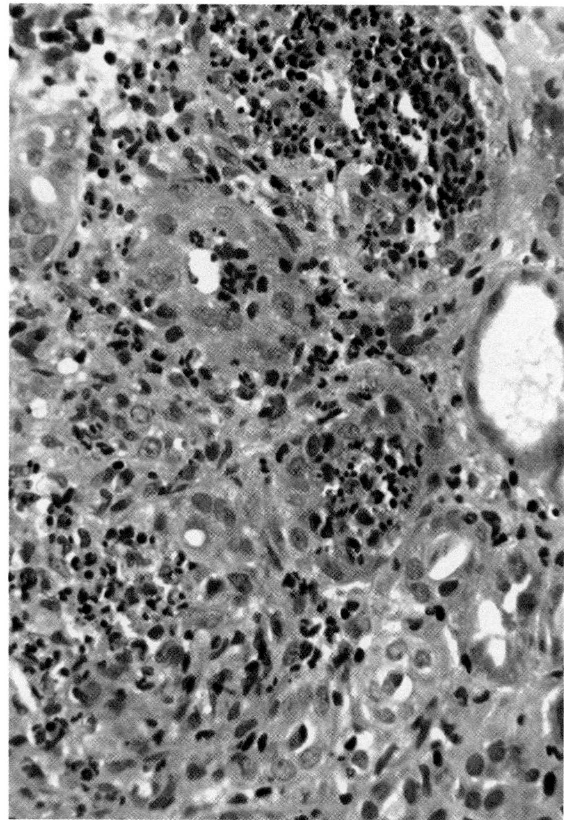

Figure 20-44

RENAL CANDIDIASIS

Disseminated candidiasis in a kidney from a patient who was immunosuppressed. With the H&E stain the section looks like acute (bacterial) pyelonephritis with many intratubular and interstitial neutrophils. (Figs. 20-44 to 20-46 are from the same patient.)

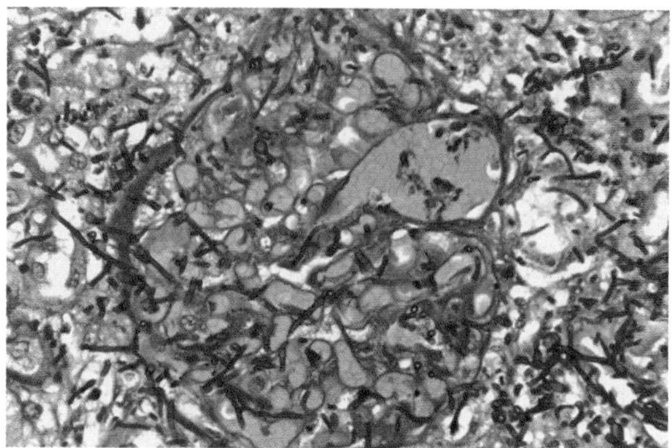

Figure 20-45

DISSEMINATED CANDIDIASIS

The PAS stain shows many hyphal forms and occasional yeast forms.

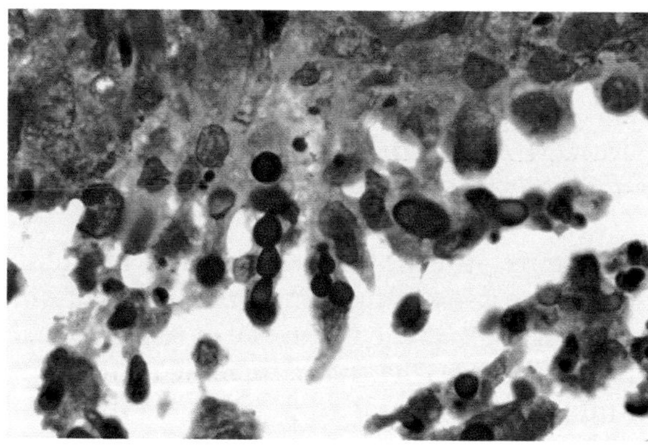

Figure 20-46

DISSEMINATED CANDIDIASIS (YEAST FORMS)

PAS stain.

diameter. They usually invoke (except for severely immunocompromised patients) an accompanying inflammatory response. They may be visualized by the H&E stain, but are more readily identified with the PAS or Grocott silver stain. Their ability to colonize surface epithelia, and invade tissues and blood vessels, involves the elaboration of a panoply of cytokines, adhesion molecules, and surface receptors (5,8,16).

Torulopsosis. *Torulopsis glabrata* is an opportunistic yeast-like fungus present in the normal oral pharynx, gastrointestinal tract, skin, and genitourinary tract. This is the second most common fungal pathogen of the urinary tract. Usually, the kidneys are involved as part of the disseminated infection, but they can be the site of a primary infection through the ascending route.

There may be microscopic renal involvement or miliary or extensive abscess formation. Papillary necrosis and perinephric abscess formation have been noted. The *T. glabrata* organisms are 2- to 4-μm, budding, round to oval, nonencapsulated, yeast-like organisms, best demonstrated with the Grocott methenamine silver stain (5,8,16).

Other Fungal Organisms. Other fungi show changes in the kidney that are similar to those in other organs (figs. 20-47–20-49). The reader is referred to Heptinstall (16), the Armed Forces Institute of Pathology (AFIP) infectious disease Fascicle (5), and other sources (8) for further reading. If there is a focal or localized region of renal inflammation characterized by tubulointerstitial

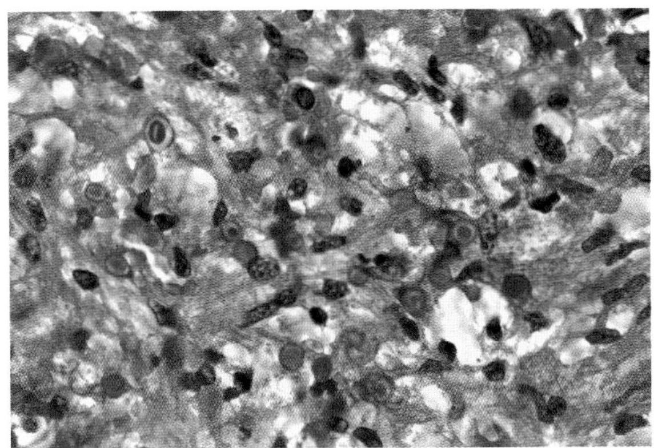

Figure 20-47

CRYPTOCOCCAL INFECTION OF THE KIDNEY

Amid the inflammation are a number of clear spaces which represent the cryptococcal organisms (H&E stain).

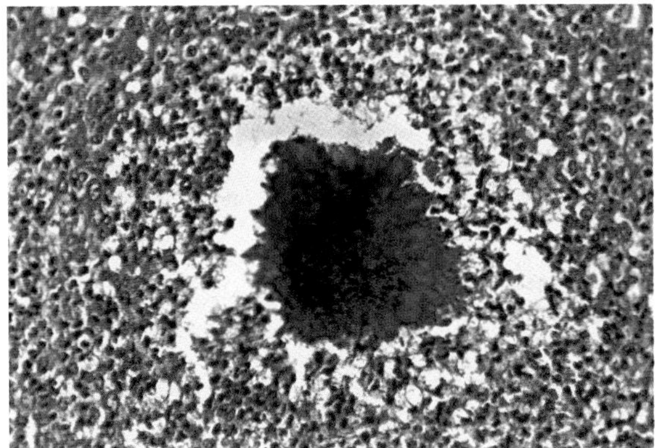

Figure 20-48

RENAL INFECTION BY *ACTINOMYCES*

Renal infection by *Actinomyces* in this immunocompromised patient. The large sulfur granule is surrounded by acute and chronic inflammation (H&E stain).

inflammation, one should question, especially in an immunocompromised host, whether special stains (PAS, Grocott silver) should be performed in order to accentuate the visualization of fungal organisms (figs. 20-46, 20-49).

Viral Infections

Cytomegalovirus (CMV) Infection. This opportunistic pathogen causes severe infection in immunocompromised hosts (26). It is the most common viral infection in pediatric transplant recipients 1 month beyond transplantation and is also a cause of congenital and neonatal tubulointerstitial nephritis. It is also seen in AIDS patients.

There is characteristically a tubulointerstitial nephritis with interstitial mononuclear cells, tubulitis, and viral inclusions in the nuclei and/or cytoplasm of various renal epithelial (tubular and glomerular) cells. The intranuclear inclusions are large, amorphous, and separated from the nuclear membrane. Typical Cowdry type A inclusions are present (fig. 20-50). If the typical intranuclear and cytoplasmic inclusions are seen, then the diagnosis of CMV is unequivocally made (8). If the intranuclear inclusions are atypical, immunocytochemistry or in situ hybridization can be performed to detect CMV (fig. 20-51). Alternatively, polymerase chain reaction (PCR) can be used to detect CMV organisms, although the exact site (infiltrating inflammatory cells versus native renal cells) cannot be determined by this sensitive assay. Recovery of renal function occurs with the use of antiviral agents.

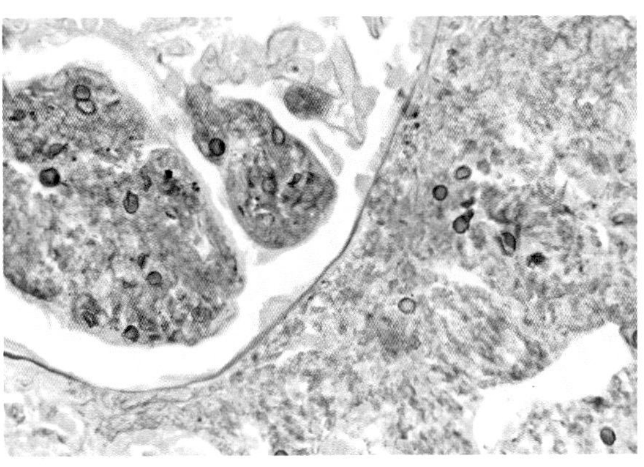

Figure 20-49

PNEUMOCYSTIS IN THE KIDNEY OF A PATIENT WITH ACQUIRED IMMUNODEFICIENCY SYNDROME

"Ping-pong ball"-like structures are seen within the glomeruli and the interstitium (Grocott silver stain).

Polyomavirus (BK) Infection. This was first described in a patient with a renal allograft and ureteric obstruction. It is an opportunistic pathogen and a cause of tubulointerstitial nephritis, especially seen in the renal transplant population. Polyomavirus has a tropism for urothelium and may persist there for a long time. The diagnosis can be made by isolating the BK virus from the urine (18,24).

The kidneys usually show severe mononuclear-lymphoplasmacytic interstitial infiltration with tubular cell injury. There may be acute tubular necrosis, hematoxyphilic inclusions in

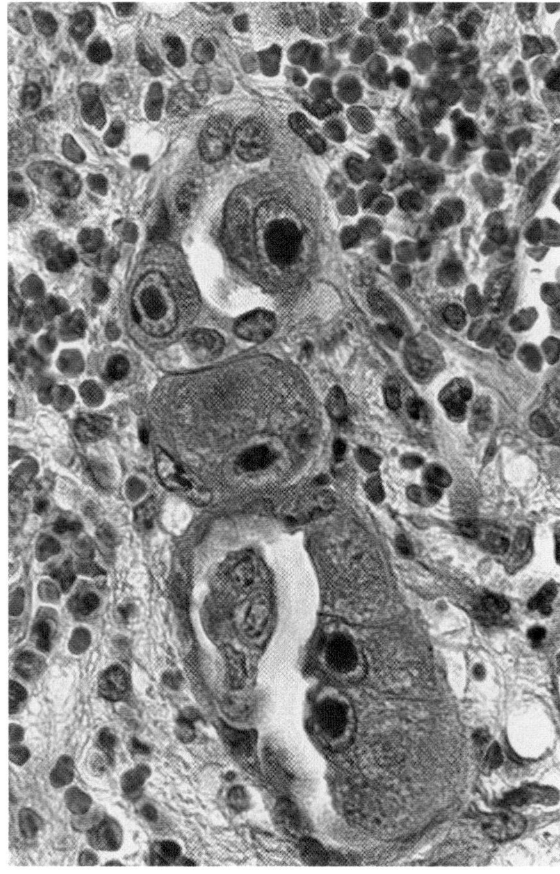

Figure 20-50

CYTOMEGALOVIRUS INFECTION IN THE KIDNEY

Large, Cowdry type A intranuclear eosinophilic inclusions are present in this immunosuppressed patient.

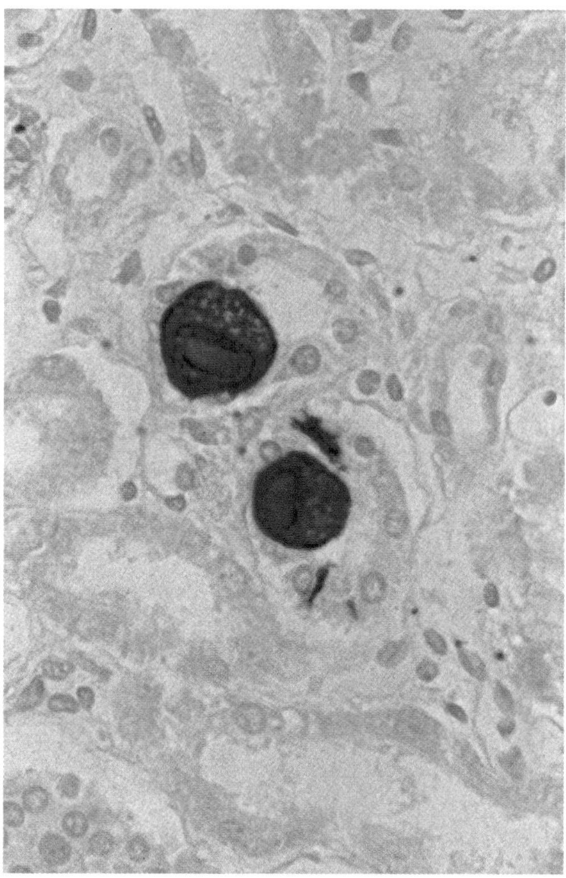

Figure 20-51

CYTOMEGALOVIRUS INFECTION IN THE KIDNEY

Immunocytochemical demonstration of organisms with Texas Red–labeled antibody to cytomegalovirus.

the nuclei of the tubular epithelial cells, and foci of interstitial fibrosis. The enlarged tubular epithelial cells have irregular and variably enlarged and dark-staining nuclei (8). The BK virus is detected by immunocytochemistry or in situ hybridization. By electron microscopy, typical arrays of viral particles are identified both within and on the surface of tubular epithelial cells (see chapters 19 and 26).

Adenovirus Infection. This opportunistic virus is a rare cause of tubulointerstitial nephritis; more commonly, there is widespread tubular necrosis (19). Most infected patients are immunocompromised/immunosuppressed. Adenovirus tends to target the transplanted kidney. It may been seen in AIDS patients. Hemorrhagic cystitis, renal insufficiency, or acute renal failure occur.

Histologically, the major findings are tubulointerstitial mononuclear infiltrates (cortex and/or medulla) and nuclear inclusions ("smudge cells") in the tubular epithelium (8,18,19). There may be quite severe necrotizing tubular necrosis. Immunocytochemistry demonstrates the adenovirus antigens and electron microscopy shows the crystalline arrays of viral particles (see chapter 19).

The diagnosis depends on the detection of the typical intranuclear inclusions, which impart a glassy appearance to the nucleus. Immunocytochemistry, in situ hybridization, and electron microscopy or PCR aid in the diagnosis. Fatality is high and graft loss is common.

Hantavirus Infection. Tubulointerstitial nephritis is common in eastern Asia and some countries in Europe. Hantaan viruses (named after the river in the demilitarized zone between North and South Korea) cause epidemic hemorrhagic fever, renal disease, and often acute renal failure (33). Reservoirs for the virus are the field mouse and the bat. Infection is by inhalation of aerosols of rodent secretions (8,33). There is an acute viral illness with fever, headache, hemorrhagic shock with thrombocytopenia, and proteinuria/hematuria, followed by acute renal failure.

The most common morphologic changes occur in the medulla and the corticomedullary junction and consist of isolated to diffuse necrosis of the tubules with various degrees of interstitial hemorrhage. Interstitial inflammation occurs as well. It is thought that the virus causes renal disease by direct invasion of renal tissues, although immunologic mechanisms (such as immune complex formation) can occur and endothelial injury/platelet consumption leads to a bleeding diathesis with disseminated intravascular coagulation (DIC).

A number of other viruses (e.g., Puumala) cause somewhat similar patterns of response. In the United States and Mexico, a serologically related virus, the Prospect Hill virus (the cause of Hantavirus pulmonary syndrome), does not have renal disease as part of the clinical syndrome; however, viral RNA has been detected in the tubular epithelium and endothelium of the kidney in some of these patients (8,16).

Human immunodeficiency virus (HIV) (7) and Epstein-Barr virus (EBV) (8) infections are considered in chapters 6 and 26, respectively.

Rickettsial Infections

Rickettsia are transmitted through a variety of vectors; there is obligatory intracellular microorganism infection. All rickettsia are zoonoses that are found in arthropods, and humans are incidental hosts that do not normally maintain these organisms in nature. Rocky Mountain spotted fever, Mediterranean spotted fever, scrub typhus, and epidemic typhus all cause major clinical disease. Most lead to renal involvement, with mild to severe renal insufficiency. There may be acute renal failure and death. The reader is referred to Heptinstall (16) and others (5,8).

Table 20-2

INFECTIOUS TUBULOINTERSTITIAL NEPHRITIS

Acute (Bacterial) Pyelonephritis and Urinary Tract Infections
General (ascending types)
Associated with systemic infection
Specific complications: papillary necrosis, pyelonephrosis, perinephric abscess
Chronic Pyelonephritis
Chronic pyelonephritis (chronic obstructive pyelonephritis)
Reflux nephropathy (chronic nonobstructive pyelonephritis)
Other types: xanthogranulomatous, malakoplakia, megalocytic interstitial nephritis
Tuberculosis
Other Specific Renal Infections (Nonbacterial)
Fungal organisms (eg., *Candida*)
Viral infections
Cytomegalovirus (CMV)
Polyoma (BK) virus
Adenovirus
Hanta virus
Epstein-Barr virus (EBV), human immunodeficiency virus (HIV)

Parasitic Infections

At least three major parasitic organisms can lead to a granulomatous tubulointerstitial nephritis: *Plasmodium* sp (malaria), *Schistosoma* sp (schistosomiasis), and *Filaria* (filariasis). The renal inflammatory response is caused by localization of the parasites (e.g., *Filaria*) or their eggs (e.g., *Schistosoma*). The tubulointerstitial lesions may be due to the interactions of various factors, including ischemia and inflammatory mediators. Evidence of the organism or eggs should be searched for in the histologic sections. Glomerular immune complex disease can occasionally be seen, presumably the result of a combination of the parasitic antigen and the antibody response to that antigen. The reader is referred to Heptinstall (16), the AFIP infectious disease Fascicle (5), and other sources (8) for further demonstration of these organisms and lesions.

Table 20-2 summarizes the major types of infectious tubulointerstitial nephritis.

REFERENCES

1. al-Sulaiman MH, al-Khader AA, Mousa DH, al-Swailem RY, Dhar J, Haleem A. Renal parenchymal malacoplakia and megalocytic interstitial nephritis: clinical and histological features. Report of two cases and review of the literature. Am J Nephrol 1993;13:483–8.
2. Antonakopoulos GN, Chapple CR, Newman J, et al. Xanthogranulomatous pyelonephritis. A reappraisal and immunohistochemical study. Arch Pathol Lab Med 1988;112:275–81.
3. Becker GJ, Kincaid-Smith P. Reflux nephropathy: the glomerular lesion and progression of renal failure. Pediatr Nephrol 1993;7:365–9.
4. Bhagavan BS, Wenk RE, Dutta D. Pathways of urinary backflow in obstructive uropathy. Demonstration by pigmented gelatin injection and Tamm-Horsfall uromucoprotein markers. Hum Pathol 1979;10:669–83.
5. Binford CH, Connor DH, eds. Pathology of tropical and extraordinary diseases, vols 1, 2. Washington, DC: Armed Forces Institute of Pathology; 1976.
6. Cavallo T. Tubulointerstitial nephritis. In: Jennette JC, Olson JL, Schwartz MM, Silva FG, eds. Heptinstall's pathology of the kidney, 5th ed. Philadelphia: Lippincott-Raven; 1998:667–723.
7. Cohen AH, Nast CC. Renal injury caused by human immunodeficiency virus infection. In: Jennette JC, Olson JL, Schwartz MM, Silva FG, eds. Heptinstall's pathology of the kidney, 5th ed. Philadelphia: Lippincott-Raven; 1998:785–810.
8. Connor, DH, Chandler, FW, Schwartz DA, et al, eds. Pathology of infectious diseases. Stanford, Conn: Appleton & Lange; 1997.
9. Cotran RS. Nephrology Forum. Glomerulosclerosis in reflux nephropathy. Kidney Int 1982;21: 528–34.
10. Curhan GC, Zeidel ML. Urinary tract obstruction. In: Brenner BM, ed. Brenner & Rector's the kidney, 5th ed. Philadelphia: WB Saunders; 1996:1820–43.
11. Dobyan DC, Truong LD, Eknoyan G. Renal malacoplakia reappraised. Am J Kidney Dis 1993;22:243–52.
12. Eble JN. Unusual renal tumors and tumor-like conditions. In: Eble JN, ed. Tumors and tumor-like conditions of the kidneys and ureters. New York: Churchill Livingstone; 1990:145–76.
13. El-Khatib MT, Becker GJ, Kincaid-Smith PS. Morphometric aspects of reflux nephropathy. Kidney Int 1987;32:261–6.
14. Esparza AR, McKay DB, Cronan JJ, Chazan JA. Renal parenchymal malakoplakia. Histologic spectrum and its relationship to megalocytic interstitial nephritis and xanthogranulomatous pyelonephritis. Am J Surg Pathol 1989;13:225–36.
15. Goodman M, Curry T, Russell T. Xanthogranulomatous pyelonephritis (XGP): a local disease with systemic manifestations. Report of 23 patients and review of the literature. Medicine (Baltimore) 1979;58:171–81.
16. Heptinstall RH. Urinary tract infection, pyelonephritis, reflux nephropathy. In: Jennette JC, Olson JL, Schwartz MM, Silva FG, eds. Heptinstall's pathology of the kidney, 5th ed. Philadelphia: Lippincott-Raven; 1998:725–83.
17. Hill GS. Renal infection. In: Hill GS, ed. Uropathology. New York: Churchill Livingstone; 1989:333–429.
18. Howell DN, Smith SR, Butterly DW, et al. Diagnosis and management of BK polyomavirus interstitial nephritis in renal transplant recipients. Transplantation 1999;68:1279–88.
19. Ito M, Hirabayashi N, Uno Y, Nakayama A, Asai J. Necrotizing tubulointerstitial nephritis associated with adenovirus infection. Hum Pathol 1991;22:1225–31.
20. Kern WF, Silva FG, Laszik ZG, Bane BL, Nadasdy T, Pitha JV, eds. Disorders of the interstitium: interstitial nephritis, pyelonephritis, papillary necrosis, analgesic nephropathy, and obstructive nephropathy (hydronephrosis). In: Atlas of renal pathology. Philadelphia: W.B. Saunders; 1999:136–57.
21. Kunin CM. Urinary tract infections: detection, prevention, and management, 5th ed. Baltimore: Williams & Wilkins; 1997.
22. McClure J. Malakoplakia. J Pathol 1983;140:275–330.
23. Morita M, Yoshiara S, White RH, Raafat F. The glomerular changes in children with reflux nephropathy. J Pathol 1990;162:245–53.
24. Nickeleit V, Hirsch HH, Binet IF, et al. Polyomavirus infection of renal allograft recipients: from latent infection to manifest disease. J Am Soc Nephrol 1999;10:1080–9.
25. Peterson JC, Tisher CC. Tuberculosis of the kidney. In: Tisher CC, Brenner BM, eds. Renal pathology: with clinical and functional correlations, 2nd ed. Philadelphia: JB Lippincott; 1994:895–904.
26. Platt JL, Sibley RK, Michael AF. Interstitial nephritis associated with cytomegalovirus infection. Kidney Int 1985;28:550–2.

27. Ransley PG, Risdon RA. The renal papilla, intrarenal reflux and chronic pyelonephritis. In: Hodson J, Kincaid-Smith P, eds. Reflux nephropathy. New York: Masson; 1979:126–33.
28. Risdon RA. Pyelonephritis and reflux nephropathy. In Tisher CC, Brenner BM, eds. Renal pathology: with clinical and functional correlations, 2nd ed. Philadelphia: Lippincott-Raven; 1994:832–62.
29. Roberts JA. Mechanisms of renal damage in chronic pyelonephritis (reflux nephropathy). Curr Top Pathol 1995;88:265–87.
30. Rubin RH, Cotran RS, Tolkoff-Rubin NE. Urinary tract infection, pyelonephritis and reflux nephropathy. In: Brenner BM, ed. Brenner & Rector's the kidney, 5th ed. Philadelphia: WB Saunders; 1996:1597–650.
31. Stamey TA. Pathogenesis and treatment of urinary tract infection. Baltimore: Williams & Wilkins; 1980.
32. Tolkoff-Rubin NE, Rubin RH. Urinary tract infection. In: Cotran RS [guest ed], Brenner BM, Stern JH, eds. Tubulointerstitial nephropathies. Contemporary issues in nephrology. New York: Churchill Livingstone; 1983:49–82.
33. van Ypersele de Strihou C, Mery JP. Hantavirus-related acute interstitial nephritis in western Europe. Expansion of a world-wide zoonosis. Q J Med 1989;73:941–50.

21 NONINFECTIOUS TUBULOINTERSTITIAL NEPHROPATHIES

TUBULOINTERSTITIAL NEPHRITIS INDUCED BY DRUGS AND TOXINS

"Man is the only animal that has an incessant desire to take drugs." William Osler

Various toxins and drugs cause tubulointerstitial injury. The diverse morphologic patterns of injury they produce reflect equally diverse pathogenetic mechanisms of disease. Interstitial immunologic reactions include: 1) an acute hypersensitivity nephritis caused by drugs such as antibiotics (e.g., methicillin); 2) acute renal failure appearing as acute tubular necrosis; and 3) chronic sublethal injury that affects the tubules in a cumulative manner over the years.

Acute Allergic Drug-Induced Interstitial Nephritis

Acute allergic drug-induced interstitial nephritis is caused by a large variety of drugs, including a number of antibiotics (e.g., beta-lactam antibiotics), nonsteroidal anti-inflammatory drugs (NSAID), diuretics, anticonvulsants, and an ever expanding list of new drugs (Table 21-1). First reported after the administration of sulfonamides, interstitial nephritis is the most common type of drug-induced renal injury (2,4–6,9,15,17,18,20,23,32,34,36,37,45–48,50,53,55,58,59,63,67,72,73).

Clinical Features. The clinical evidence of renal disease begins about 2 weeks (range, 2 to 40 days) after exposure to the drug. It is characterized classically by the triad of fever, rash, and eosinophilia (6,17,23,32,50,58,63,73). Urinary abnormalities such as hematuria, mild proteinuria, and sterile leukocyturia (with eosinophils) (24) are identified. Azotemia, with rising blood urea nitrogen (BUN) and serum creatinine levels, leads to signs and symptoms of acute renal failure such as nausea and vomiting. Oliguria is present in about half of patients.

The renal sonogram usually reveals normal-sized or enlarged swollen kidneys, reflecting the acute nature of the injury. Renal biopsy is the only means of definitive diagnosis (37,67). In some cases, accidental reexposure to the causative agent precipitates prompt recrudescence of the disease and provides circumstantial evidence of causality. Some investigators co-culture the patient's lymphocytes with the purported drug of injury to search for evidence of lymphocyte stimulation.

Table 21-1

MEDICATIONS ASSOCIATED WITH INTERSTITIAL NEPHRITIS[a]

Antibiotics	**Diuretics**
Penicillins	Thiazides
Cephalosporins	Furosemide
Rifampin	Triamterene
Ciprofloxacin	Chlorthalidone
Vancomycin	
Erythromycin	**Miscellaneous**
Sulfonamides	Acetaminophen
Trimethoprim-Sulfamethoxazole	Captopril
Aminoglycosides	Cimetidine
Ethambutol	Ranitidine
Tetracyclines	Phenobarbital
	Dilantin
Nonsteroidal Anti-Inflammatory Drugs	Phenytoin
	Phenacetin
Acetylsalicylic acid	Phenindione
Naproxen	Allopurinol
Ibuprofen	Interferon
Indomethacin	Lithium
Phenylbutazone	Cyclosporine
Sulindac	
Tolmetin	
Mefenamic acid	
Fenoprofen	

[a]Modified from table 13-2 from reference 51.

Gross Findings. The kidneys may be slightly enlarged due to interstitial inflammation and edema.

Light Microscopic Findings. The major histologic abnormalities are in the interstitium, which demonstrates intense edema and infiltration by inflammatory cells of various types, including lymphocytes, plasma cells, macrophages, eosinophils, and polymorphonuclear leukocytes (figs. 21-1–21-5) (15,18,20,23,26,41,42,51,55,67). Although eosinophils are a distinctive finding in drug-induced allergic interstitial nephritis,

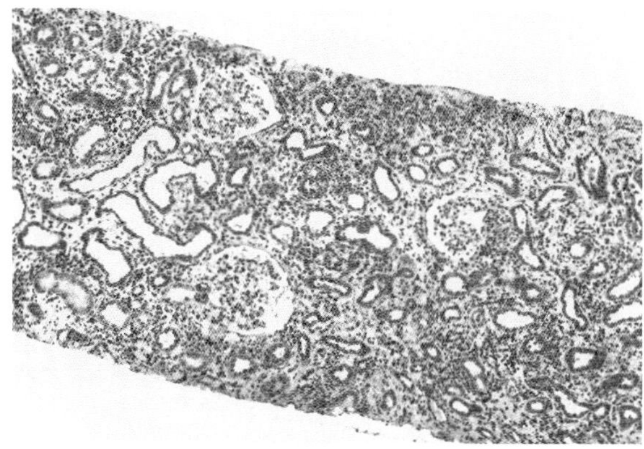

Figure 21-1

ACUTE (ALLERGIC) INTERSTITIAL NEPHRITIS

Expansion of the interstitium because of inflammatory infiltrates separates the tubules. The glomeruli appear unremarkable (hematoxylin and eosin [H&E] stain).

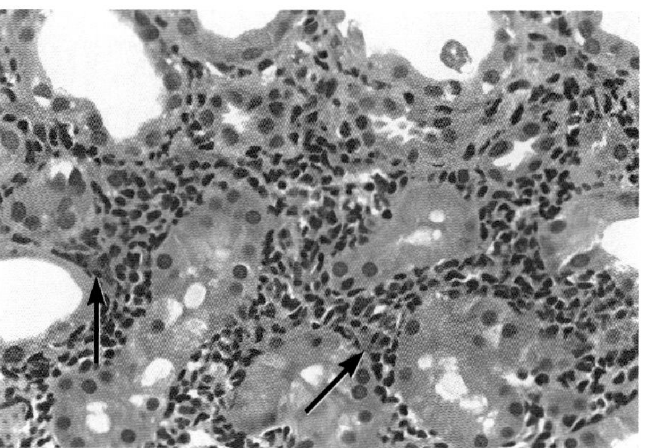

Figure 21-2

ACUTE (ALLERGIC) INTERSTITIAL NEPHRITIS

Expansion of the interstitium secondary to inflammation separates the cortical tubules. In addition to the interstitial lymphocytes, there are plasma cells and eosinophils; the eosinophils are difficult to identify in this figure (arrows). The presence of interstitial eosinophils in primary interstitial nephritis suggests an allergic (hypersensitivity) response, most commonly to a drug (H&E stain).

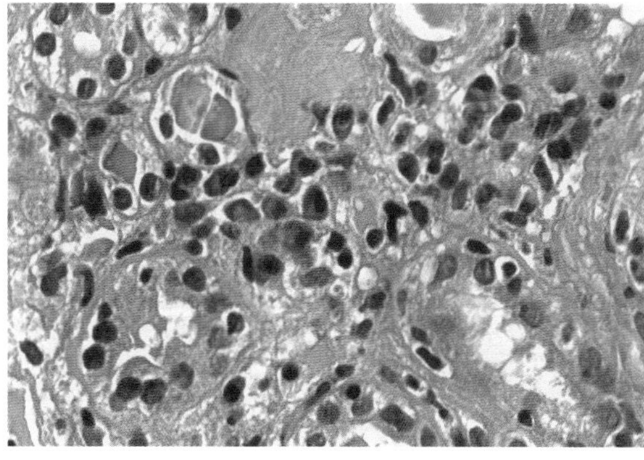

Figure 21-3

ACUTE (ALLERGIC) INTERSTITIAL NEPHRITIS

The infiltrate is composed of a predominance of plasma cells and plasmacytoid inflammatory cells (H&E stain).

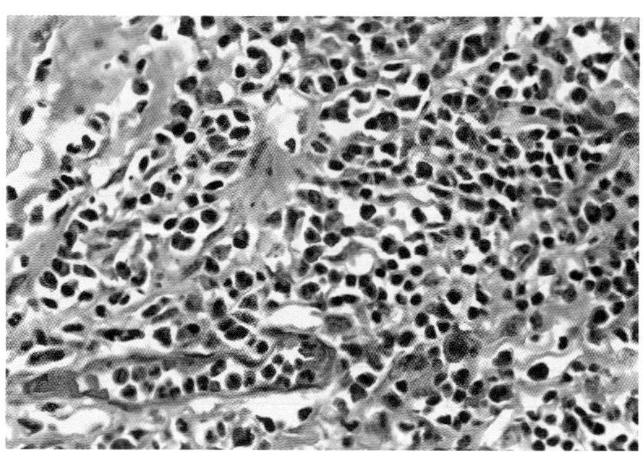

Figure 21-4

ACUTE INTERSTITIAL NEPHRITIS

The renal interstitium is expanded by a number of inflammatory cells, lymphocytes, plasma cells, and importantly, eosinophils. The presence of interstitial inflammation with many eosinophils suggests a hypersensitivity (allergic) response, most commonly secondary to a drug (H&E stain).

they usually only comprise a minority (less than 10 percent) of the total interstitial leukocytes. Leukocyte infiltration of the tubular epithelium (i.e., tubulitis) is a characteristic morphologic finding in the active phase (figs. 21-6, 21-7). Variable amounts of tubular injury (tubular necrosis, desquamation, flattening, degeneration, regeneration,) often accompany the interstitial inflammation and tubulitis (figs. 21-8, 21-9). Interstitial granulomata with epithelioid histiocytes and a few giant cells are seen in some cases (figs. 21-10, 21-11). The glomeruli are normal except in those patients taking NSAIDs, which may produce a minimal change nephrotic syndrome (1,52,84). Examples of various drug-induced acute interstitial nephritides are demonstrated in figures 21-12 to 21-21. As noted, one of the most common injurious agents leading to a hypersensitivity (allergic) drug allergy is some type of antibiotic.

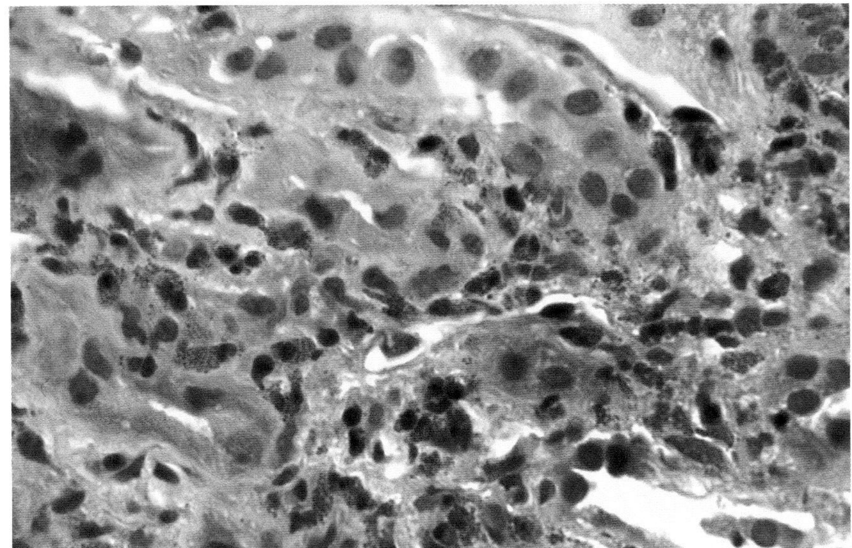

Figure 21-5

ACUTE INTERSTITIAL NEPHRITIS

The large number of interstitial eosinophils suggests a drug allergy. This patient had ampicillin-induced acute interstitial nephritis.

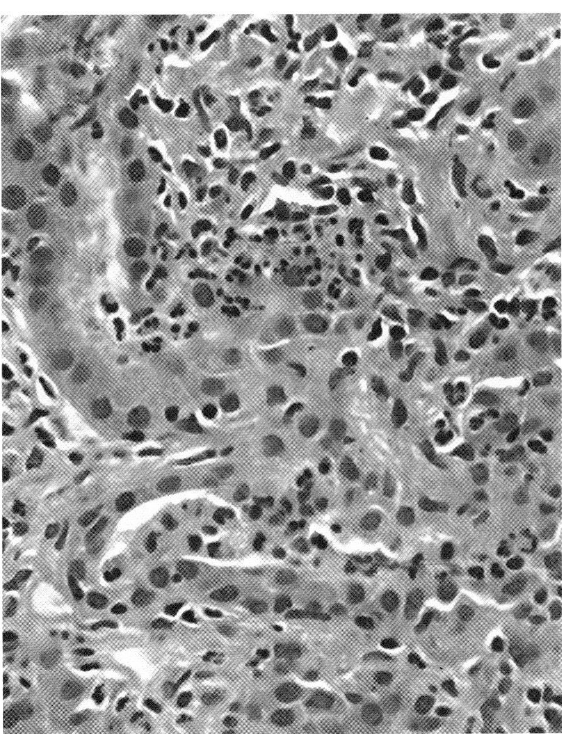

Figure 21-6

ACUTE INTERSTITIAL NEPHRITIS

In addition to the interstitial expansion by a number of lymphocytes and other inflammatory cells (including polymorphonuclear leukocytes), there is invasion of the tubular epithelium ("tubulitis"). The differential diagnosis includes primary interstitial nephritis with secondary tubulitis and acute tubular necrosis with secondary nearby inflammation. With a neutrophilic tubulitis and some intratubular neutrophils, it is sometimes difficult to exclude an infectious etiology (H&E stain).

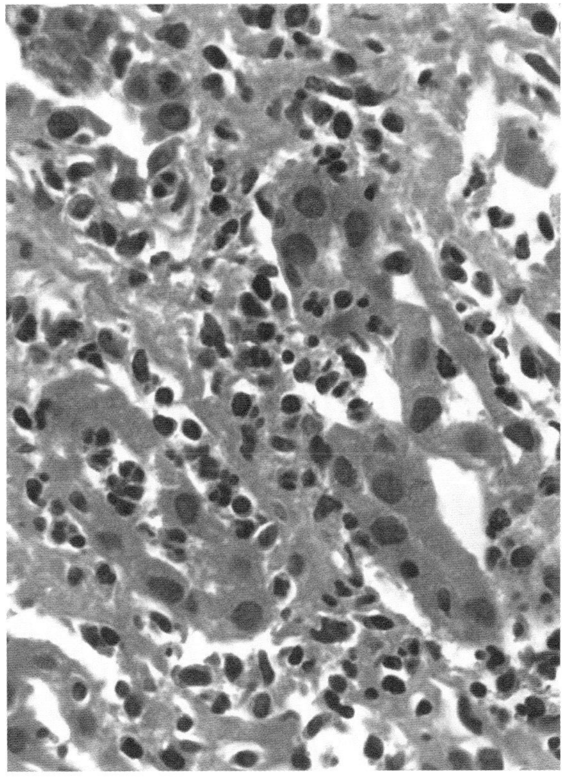

Figure 21-7

ACUTE INTERSTITIAL NEPHRITIS SECONDARY TO DRUG ALLERGY

There is severe acute tubulointerstitial disease. Involvement of one of the compartments (tubules or interstitium) often leads to secondary involvement of the other because of the close association between the interstitial compartment and the adjacent tubules. At times, the best diagnosis is that of "tubulointerstitial disease or nephropathy" (H&E stain).

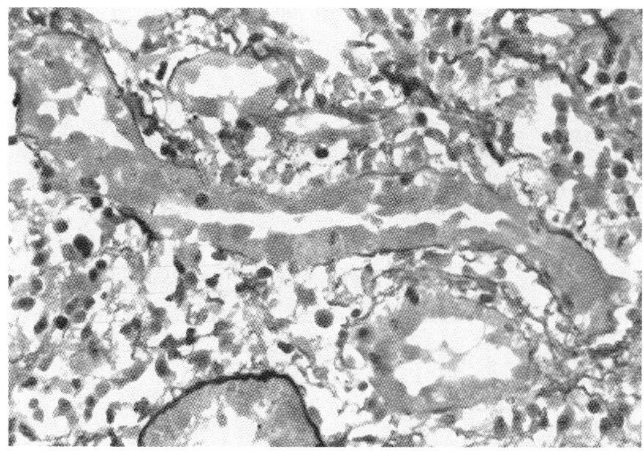

Figure 21-8

ACUTE INTERSTITIAL NEPHRITIS

There is severe tubulointerstitial disease with rupture or loss of the tubular basement membranes, breakdown of the tubular basement membranes, and nearby secondary interstitial inflammation. These changes can be seen with any severe tubulointerstitial disease process. The intratubular luminal contents (casts, etc) can leak outside the tubules into the interstitium (Jones methenamine silver [JMS] stain).

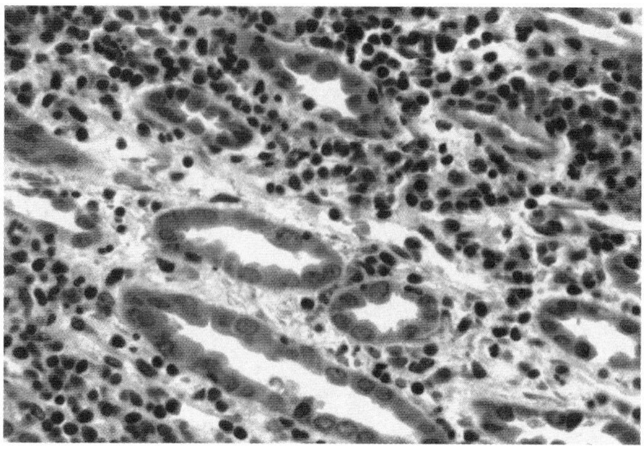

Figure 21-9

ACUTE INTERSTITIAL NEPHRITIS

Lymphocytes and other inflammatory cells, with accompanying edema, expand the renal interstitium. The tubules appear undifferentiated and are regenerating (H&E stain).

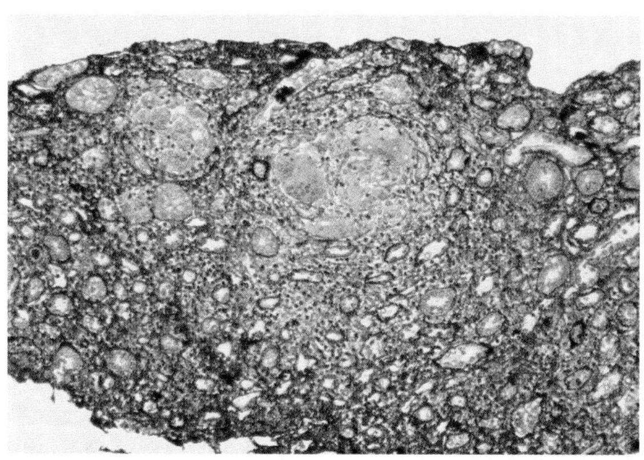

Figure 21-10

GRANULOMATOUS INTERSTITIAL NEPHRITIS

The renal interstitium is expanded by inflammation. In one large area, a large granulomatous collection of histiocytes and giant cells is seen. This patient had Dilantin-induced granulomatous interstitial nephritis (JMS stain).

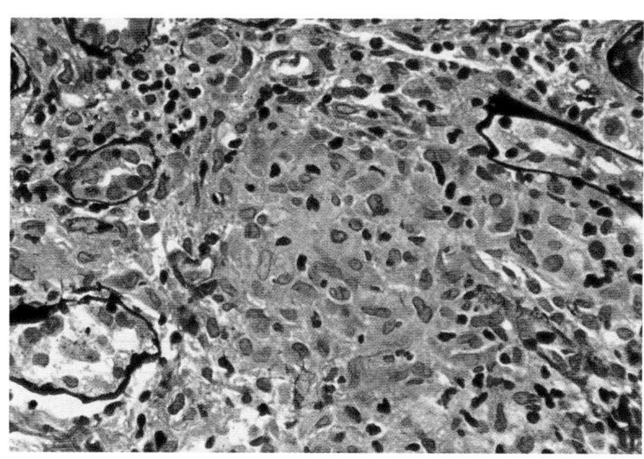

Figure 21-11

GRANULOMATOUS INTERSTITIAL NEPHRITIS

Sometimes the granulomas are not well formed and are discernable only by their somewhat localized regions of interstitial expansion. There are a number of histiocytoid mononuclear cells (JMS stain).

Immunofluorescence Findings. Immunofluorescence is generally negative. Nonspecific granular positivity for C3 may be present in some tubular basement membranes; rarely are immune deposits identified. Intense linear staining for immunoglobulin (Ig)G along tubular basement membranes has been reported in cases of methicillin-induced interstitial nephritis (34).

Electron Microscopic Findings. Electron microscopy does not contribute to the diagnosis except to exclude other conditions. However, there is widespread effacement of glomerular visceral epithelial cell foot processes in NSAID-related minimal change nephrotic syndrome. Discrete electron-dense immune-type deposits are found on rare occasion along the tubular basement membranes.

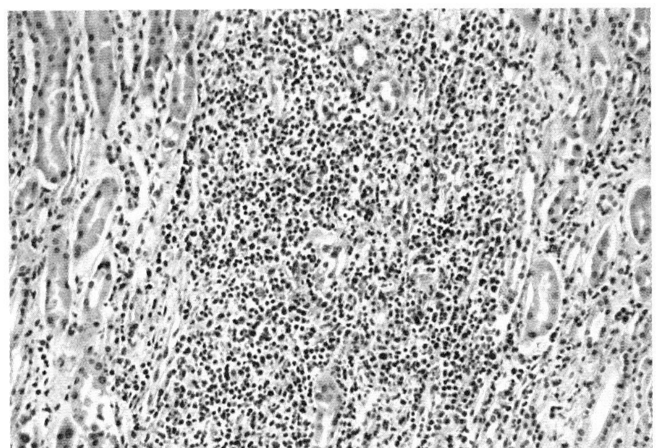

Figure 21-12

ACUTE INTERSTITIAL NEPHRITIS
SECONDARY TO PENICILLIN HYPERSENSITIVITY

There is widespread expansion of the renal interstitium by large sheets of inflammatory cells (H&E stain). (Figs. 21-12 to 21-14 are from the same patient.)

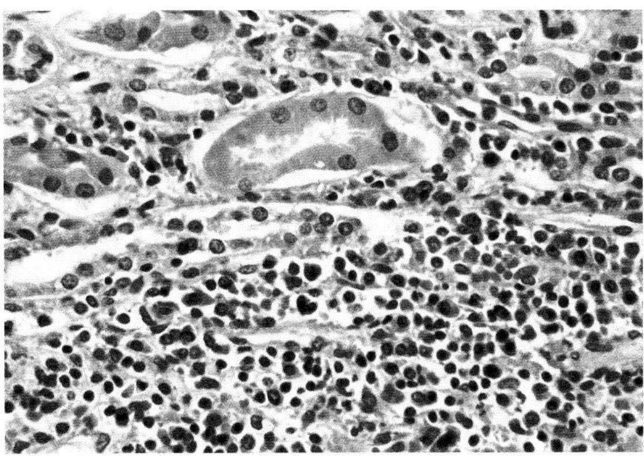

Figure 21-13

ACUTE INTERSTITIAL NEPHRITIS
SECONDARY TO PENICILLIN HYPERSENSITIVITY

Large numbers of small lymphocytes expand the renal interstitium (H&E stain).

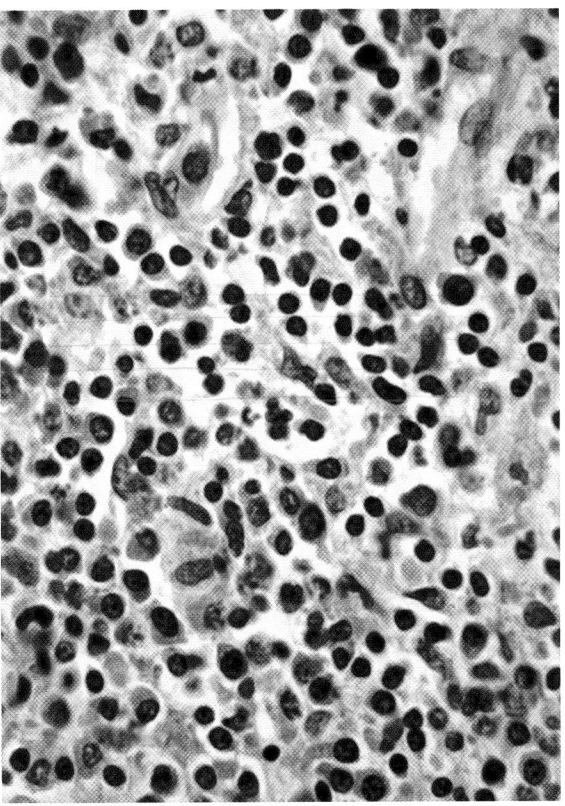

Figure 21-14

ACUTE INTERSTITIAL NEPHRITIS
SECONDARY TO PENICILLIN HYPERSENSITIVITY

In addition to the interstitial lymphocytes, there are numbers of eosinophils, making this infiltrate highly suggestive of a drug allergy (H&E stain).

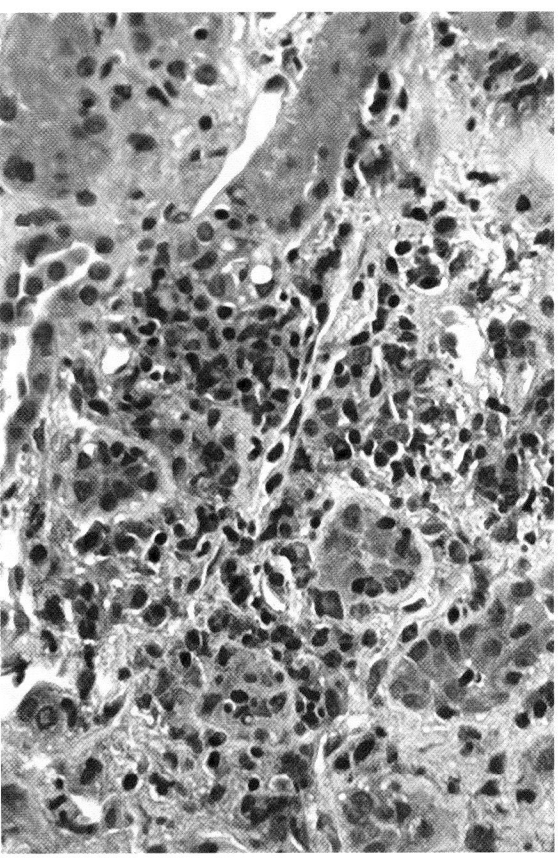

Figure 21-15

ACUTE INTERSTITIAL NEPHRITIS
SECONDARY TO AMPICILLIN ALLERGY

In addition to the interstitial inflammatory infiltrate, there is severe tubulitis (H&E stain).

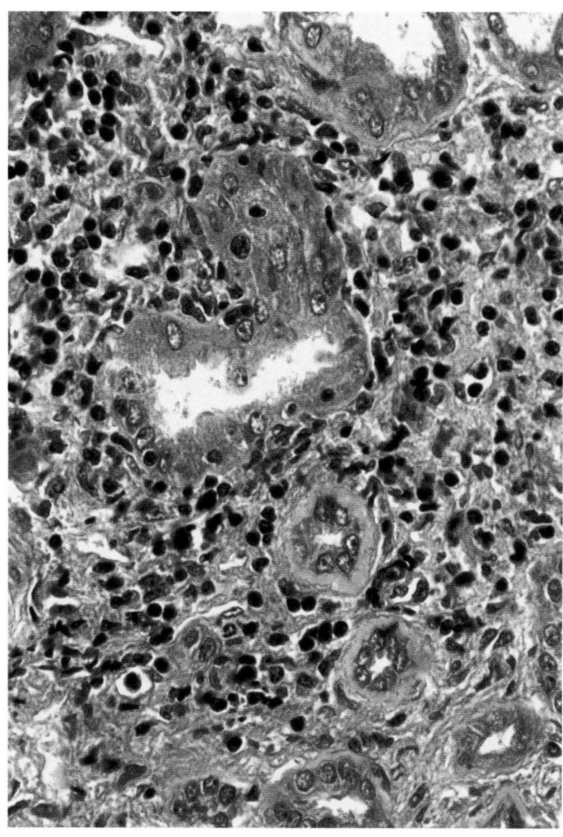

Figure 21-16

ACUTE INTERSTITIAL NEPHRITIS SECONDARY TO BACTRIM HYPERSENSITIVITY

The interstitial infiltrate involves the adjacent tubules (H&E stain).

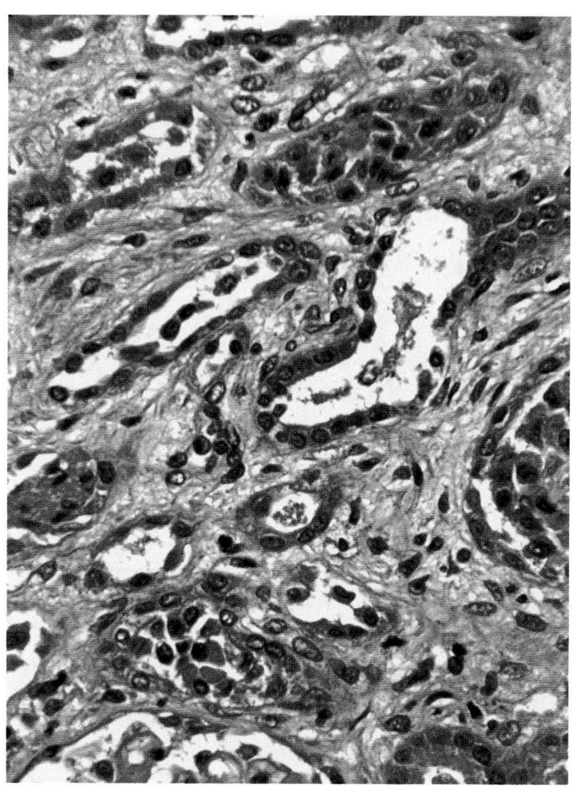

Figure 21-17

CHRONIC INTERSTITIAL NEPHRITIS SECONDARY TO BACTRIM AND PENTAMIDINE ADMINISTRATION

Chronic interstitial nephritis in a patient with acquired immunodeficiency syndrome treated with bactrim and pentamidine. The term chronic interstitial nephritis is used here because of the interstitial fibrosis, not the character of the interstitial inflammatory infiltrate (H&E stain).

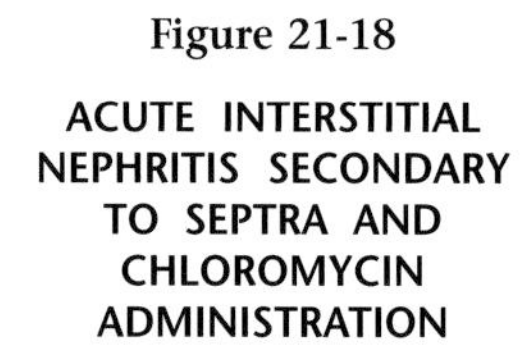

Figure 21-18

ACUTE INTERSTITIAL NEPHRITIS SECONDARY TO SEPTRA AND CHLOROMYCIN ADMINISTRATION

Inflammatory cells expand the interstitium (H&E stain).

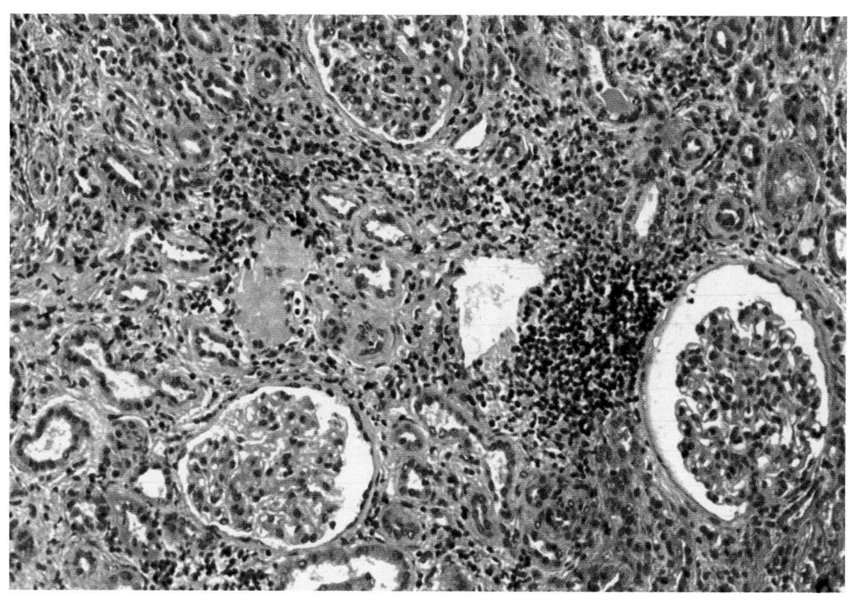

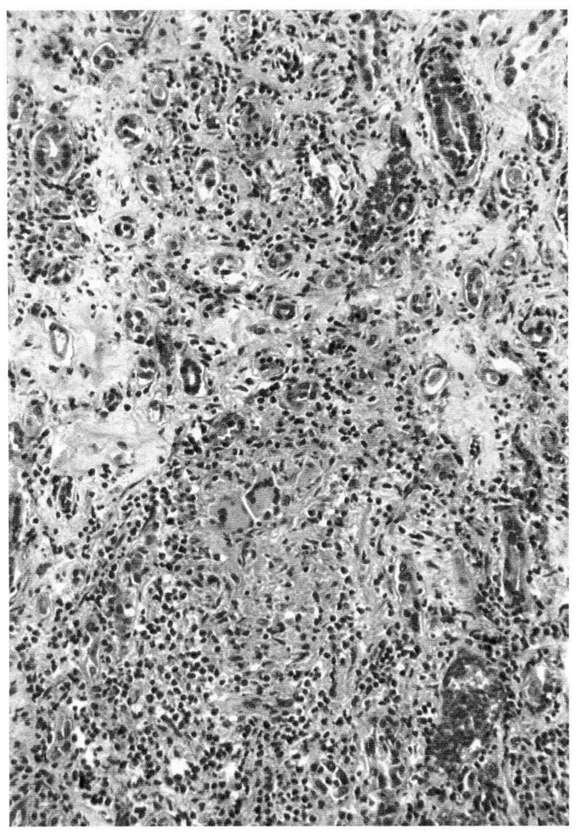

Figure 21-19

ACUTE INTERSTITIAL NEPHRITIS SECONDARY TO CARBENICILLIN ADMINISTRATION

In some regions of the figure the interstitial inflammation is organized as granulomata (H&E stain). (Figs. 21-19 and 21-20 are from the same patient.)

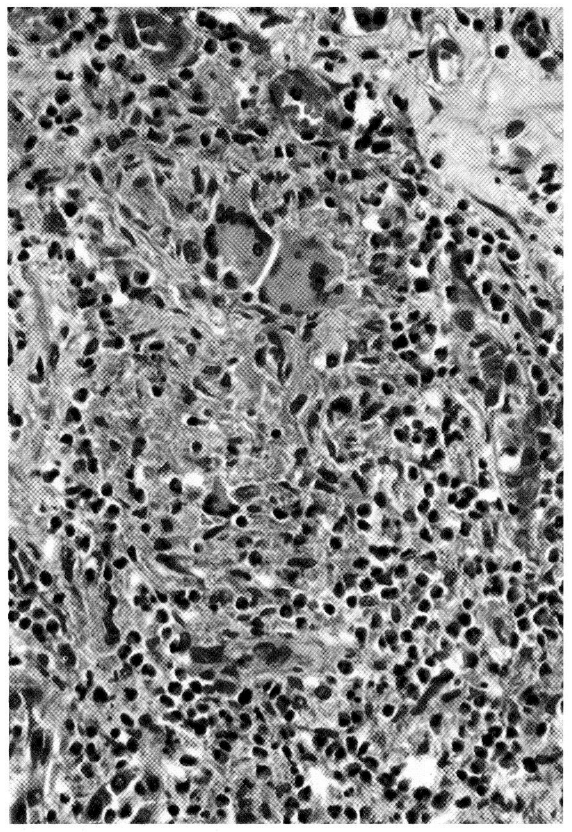

Figure 21-20

ACUTE INTERSTITIAL NEPHRITIS SECONDARY TO CARBENICILLIN ADMINISTRATION

Higher magnification of figure 21-19 shows the granulomatous interstitial inflammation (H&E stain).

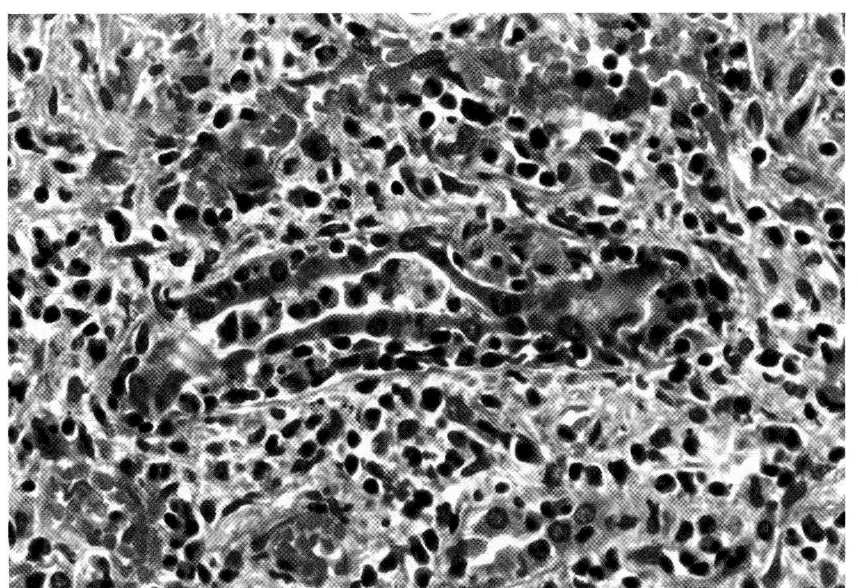

Figure 21-21

ACUTE INTERSTITIAL NEPHRITIS SECONDARY TO CARBENICILLIN ADMINISTRATION

There is severe tubulointerstitial disease with interstitial inflammation and alteration of the adjacent tubules with tubulitis (H&E stain).

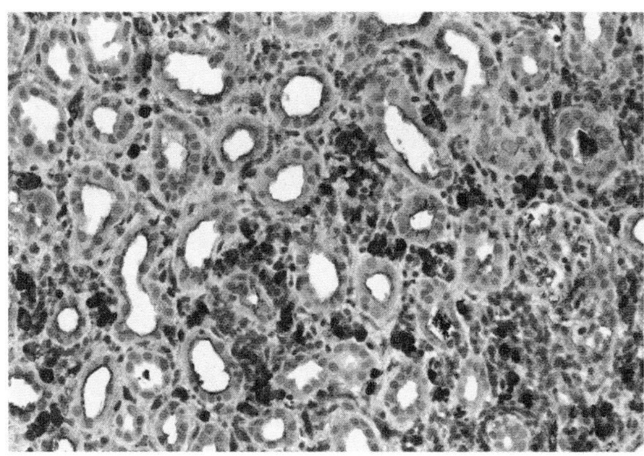
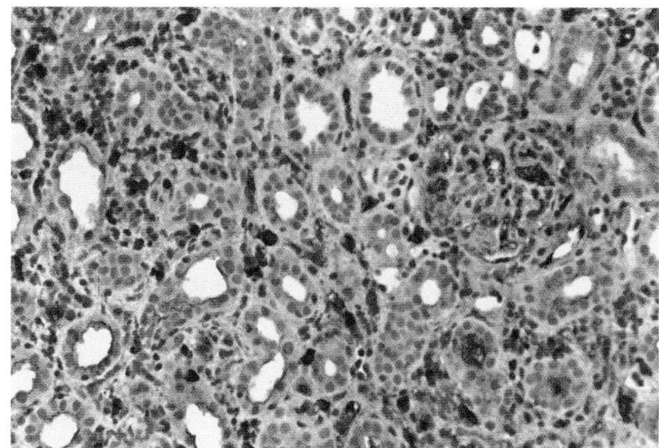

Figure 21-22

ACUTE INTERSTITIAL NEPHRITIS

Left: Immunocytochemistry using an antibody to kappa light chains (H&E stain).
Right: Immunocytochemistry using an antibody to lambda light chains. The similar distribution of cytoplasmic positivity for kappa and lambda light chains supports a polyclonal (reactive) plasma cell infiltrate (H&E stain).

Table 21-2

DIFFERENTIAL DIAGNOSIS OF ACUTE INTERSTITIAL NEPHRITIS AND ACUTE TUBULAR NECROSIS

Acute Interstitial Nephritis	Acute Tubular Necrosis
Interstitial inflammation (with eosinophils)	Thinning of periodic acid–Schiff (PAS)-positive brush border
Tubulitis (lymphocytes in the tubules)	Tubular epithelial necrosis
Granulomatous infiltration	Leukocyte accumulation in vasa recta
Tubular casts (may be granular)	Tubular casts (hyaline, granular, other types)

Special Studies. Immunophenotyping of the interstitial infiltrate has been performed by many investigators, but this is rarely of diagnostic utility (fig. 21-22) (7,14,18,27,50). The infiltrate usually has a predominance of CD4-positive T lymphocytes, and there is often enhanced expression of human leukocyte antigen (HLA) class II antigens by the tubular epithelial cells (19). The segment of the nephron involved in cases of interstitial nephritis has been studied with nephron-specific lectins and immunohistochemical agents. A few studies have shown predominant inflammatory involvement of the distal portions of the nephron but this needs to be confirmed (40,44).

Differential Diagnosis. One of the major problems is the differentiation between a primary interstitial nephritis with secondary accompanying tubulitis and tubular injury (45) versus primary acute tubular necrosis with secondary accompanying interstitial inflammation (Table 21-2 and chapter 19). This distinction is especially difficult if a biopsy is performed after the initiation of steroid therapy or relatively late in the course of the interstitial nephritis, at which time most of the infiltrate and tubulitis may have resolved but the damaged tubules have not yet recovered.

The presence of any eosinophils in the renal interstitium is suggestive of drug-induced/allergic interstitial nephritis (although interstitial eosinophils can be seen in severe cases of Wegener's granulomatosis and other severe necrotizing glomerular lesions) (fig. 21-23). Eosinophils may also be seen adjacent to disrupted tubules (e.g., Tamm-Horsfall protein casts in the interstitium). Various forms of severe acute glomerulonephritis, such as glomerulonephritis due to Wegener's granulomatosis, may produce a surprisingly severe interstitial inflammation, even with large numbers of eosinophils (fig. 21-23). The so-called granulomata in the renal interstitium of patients with Wegener's granulomatosis

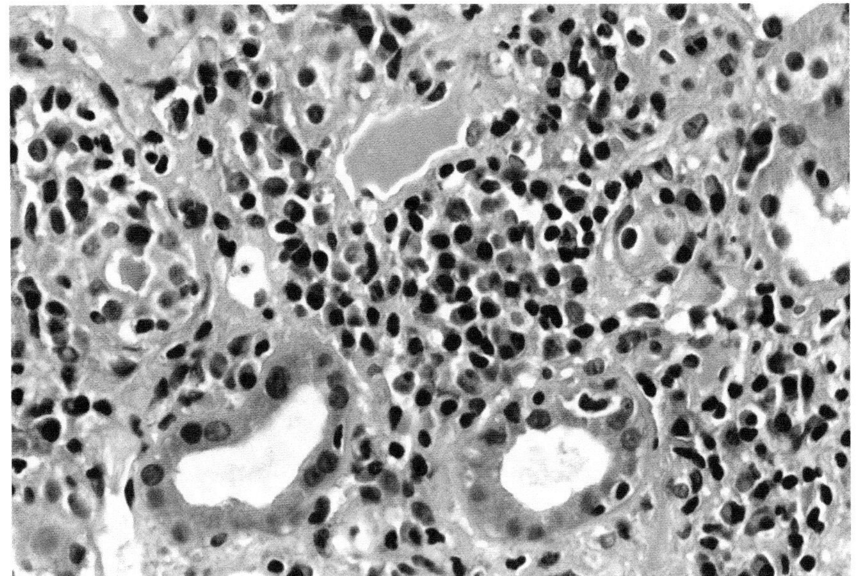

Figure 21-23

"SECONDARY" INTERSTITIAL NEPHRITIS

The renal interstitium is expanded by plasma cells and eosinophils (the latter are not seen in this picture). This patient had severe crescentic glomerulonephritis associated with ANCAs (antineutrophil cytoplasmic antibodies) and polyangiitis. The severe interstitial inflammation is considered secondary to the underlying glomerular process.

are virtually always tangential sections of the granulomatous crescents that have destroyed Bowman's capsule and other glomerular landmarks. Of course, infectious etiologic agents need to be excluded in any case of interstitial nephritis (see chapter 20) (35,38,54).

Histologic changes resembling those of drug-induced interstitial nephritis can be found in patients with lupus nephritis in the absence of known drug exposure. Granular immune deposits are often identified in the tubular basement membranes and interstitium by immunofluorescence and electron microscopy in such cases. Similar lesions are seen in patients with antitubular basement membrane antibodies as well; however, antitubular basement membrane (anti-TBM) nephritis is distinguished by linear staining for IgG. A special type of acute interstitial nephritis is seen in patients with uveitis and bone marrow and lymph node granulomata; this syndrome (Dobrin's syndrome) occurs primarily in adolescent girls and young women (16,79). Like drug-induced allergic interstitial nephritis, immunofluorescence and electron microscopy do not show immune deposits in patients with Dobrin's syndrome.

Etiology and Pathogenesis. Many lines of evidence support an immune mechanism (2,5, 6,13,14,17–19,23,25,34,47,50,53,59). Clinical evidence of a hypersensitivity type of response includes the latent period between administration of the drug and the onset of clinical signs/symptoms, the presence of peripheral eosinophilia, eosinophilic infiltration of the kidney, and rash. This adverse reaction is not dose related and recurrence of the disease may follow inadvertent reexposure to the same or a related drug. Serum IgE levels are elevated in some patients, and in some cases, IgE-containing plasma cells and basophils are found in the renal interstitium; this is suggestive of an IgE-mediated, late phase hypersensitivity response. Positive skin tests to certain drug haptens and the presence of mononuclear cells and granulomata also suggest various types of delayed-hypersensitivity phenomena (e.g., type IV hypersensitivity reaction).

The most likely sequence of immunologic events is that the drug acts as a hapten. During secretion of the drug by the appropriate segment of the nephron (which usually occurs in the distal portion of the proximal tubules, which secrete organic ions/acids), the offending drug is covalently bound to cytoplasmic or extracellular components of the tubular epithelial cells, rendering them immunogenic (34). This process incites IgE- and cell-mediated immune reactions to the tubular epithelium or the tubular basement membranes.

The NSAIDs (COX-1 and COX-2 inhibitors) may lead to renal disease (papillary necrosis with secondary interstitial inflammation/fibrosis) through alterations in the production of prostaglandins and secondary changes in the renal medullary blood flow (see below).

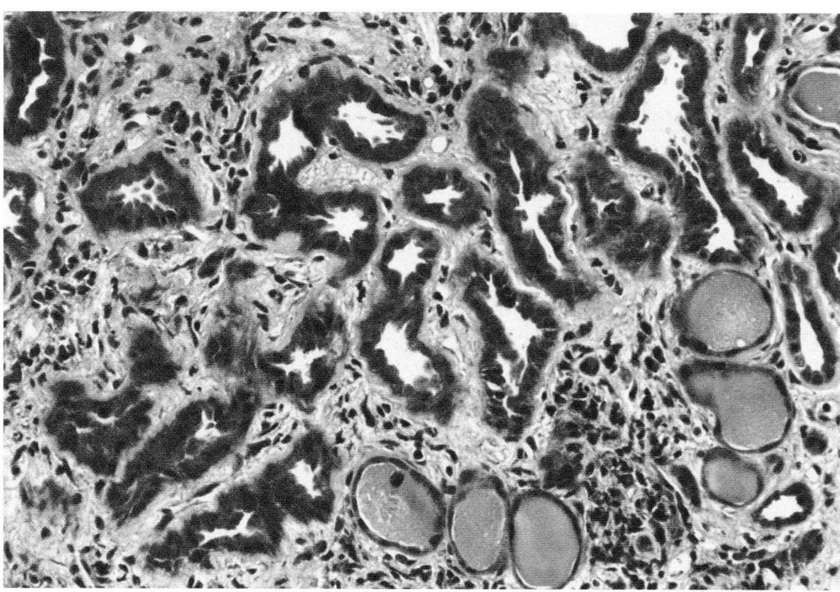

Figure 21-24

CHRONIC INTERSTITIAL NEPHRITIS

The interstitial fibrosis separates the tubules. The character of the interstitial expansion (in this case fibrosis more than inflammation) leads to the designation of "chronic" interstitial nephritis in this patient. The cause of the primary interstitial injury (or tubulointerstitial nephropathy) was unclear (Masson trichrome stain).

Treatment and Prognosis. It is important to recognize this disorder promptly because cessation of the offending drug is usually followed by recovery, although it may take several months for renal function to return toward normal. Failure to recognize the cause of injury may allow irreversible progressive renal damage. Steroid therapy may hasten the recovery according to anecdotal reports, however its role has not been defined in large controlled studies (71).

If the inciting drug is identified and withdrawn, the prognosis should be excellent (6,9, 17,23,40,63,64,71). If the cause of the interstitial nephritis is not identified, then progression to chronic renal insufficiency may occur.

Chronic Toxin/Drug-Induced Tubulointerstitial Nephritis

Definition. This insidious, slowly progressive disease of the tubular and interstitial regions is caused by a number of toxins or drugs. The term chronic (as opposed to acute) is predicated on the finding of a fibrotic renal interstitium (as opposed to one that is edematous and inflamed). Interstitial fibrosis is sometimes best noted with the trichrome stain (fig. 21-24). The terminology "acute" or "chronic" is applied depending on whether interstitial edema or fibrosis is present, respectively, rather than on the temporal clinical course or the type of interstitial infiltrate (23,41,42,48).

Clinical Features. This lesion can mimic other primary renal diseases and may manifest clinically by minor functional renal abnormalities or by severe renal insufficiency. The course is usually one of gradually progressive renal failure and hypertension. Specific tubular defects that are associated with this condition include renal concentrating defects (nephrogenic diabetes insipidus), renal tubular acidosis, and Fanconi's syndrome (5,10,15,31,50,65). The urinary excretion of beta-2-microglobulin has been used as a marker of progressive renal tubular damage. It has been used to screen individuals at risk for the nephrotoxic effects of various occupational exposures.

Etiology and Pathogenesis. A wide variety of toxins and drugs may lead to this condition (see Table 21-1) (20,23,26,42,43,48,57,58,64,65, 68,76,78). It is difficult to definitively identify an exact causative agent in some cases. Identification of increased renal tissue levels of the suspect toxin by sophisticated methods, including mass spectrophotometry, may not be sufficient evidence of cause because increased levels of the toxin could be due to lack of excretion in a patient with renal failure, rather than indicative of an increased exposure. The cause is often idiopathic; therefore, the exact pathogenic mechanisms of disease are also uncertain. Chronic exposures to lead, cadmium, gold, platinum, mercury, lithium, silver, copper, and iron

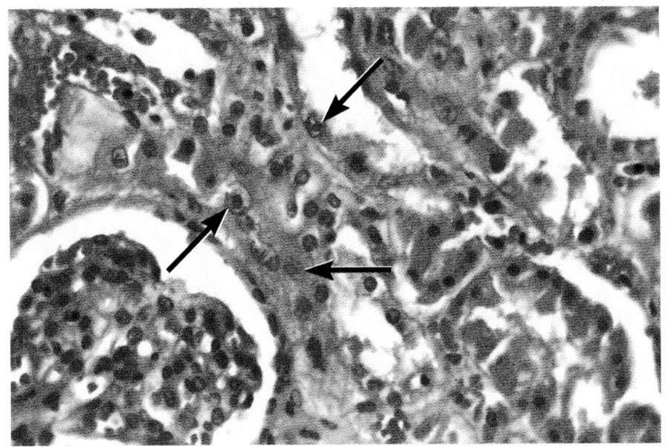

Figure 21-25

LEAD NEPHROTOXICITY

There is tubulointerstitial disease with interstitial fibrosis and tubular injury. Many tubular nuclei have large intranuclear inclusions (arrows), characteristic of lead toxicity (see chapter 19) (H&E stain).

have all been associated with the development of chronic tubulointerstitial disease (see below). Endemic Balkan nephropathy is thought by some to be related to chronic exposure to a fungal toxin. A number of other drugs also have been implicated in the genesis of the nonspecific lesion in Balkan nephropathy.

NSAIDs typically are thought to lead to renal disease by reducing renal medullary blood flow due to cyclooxygenase inhibition, reducing synthesis of prostaglandins, and altering renal blood flow (to the already tenuously supplied renal corticomedullary and medullary regions). It now appears that even the COX-2 inhibitors may lead to renal injury.

Specific Toxins Leading to Tubulointerstitial Disease

Lead Nephropathy. In adults, lead nephropathy is usually an occupational illness, whereas in children, soil and paint ingestion are major sources of lead exposure. The clinical diagnosis is based on a history of exposure, evidence of renal dysfunction, and usually a positive calcium disodium edetate (EDTA) mobilization test. Various other tests are also available (18).

Acute lead exposure leads to dysfunction of the proximal tubules. The complex of proximal tubular dysfunction, including glycosuria, phosphaturia, aminoaciduria, and renal tubular acidosis, is known as *Fanconi's syndrome*. The predominant renal histologic change is the presence of lead inclusions in the nuclei of renal tubular cells (sometimes with cytoplasmic inclusions) (fig. 21-25). The inclusions are red with the Giemsa stain and quite acidophilic (or red) with acid-fast stains. Other stains may accentuate these lead inclusions as well. Electron microscopy shows a characteristic intranuclear deposition of fibrils and enlarged mitochondria with osmiophilic densities between the cristae (18).

Chronic lead exposure and intoxication are widespread. The decreased renal function is proportional to the increased lead concentration in the blood. Chronic lead intoxication is manifested clinically by renal proximal tubular defects; decreased glucose reabsorptive capacity is an early indicator of tubular cell injury. Most patients have recurrent gout, hyperuricemia, and hypertension. Histologically, there is multifocal tubular atrophy and interstitial fibrosis. Nuclear inclusions are not a common feature at this late stage.

The mechanism of lead toxicity is via interactions of this heavy metal with renal membranes and enzymes, leading to disruption of energy production and interference with calcium metabolism and ion transport. Lead can also be complexed to other proteins, causing intranuclear transport, chromatin binding, and alterations of gene expression (see chapter 19) (18).

Cadmium Nephropathy. Cadmium exposure is primarily an occupational illness of workers employed in the manufacture of pigment, plastic, electric storage batteries, and metal alloys. Exposure also occurs through contaminated water and food, or even cigarette smoking. Cadmium toxicity is manifested clinically by gradually progressive renal insufficiency and the urinary excretion of low and high molecular weight proteins, enzymes, prostanoids, glycosaminoglycans, sialic acid, glucose, and amino acids. Fanconi's syndrome may be present. Cadmium exposure also leads to hypercalciuria, nephrolithiasis, and osteomalacia (18).

Grossly, the kidneys are red-brown, hard, and small and shrunken. Morphologically, there is extensive tubular atrophy and interstitial fibrosis, preferentially involving the outer cortex. Inflammatory cells are present in only small numbers. In some cases there are no significant tissue abnormalities despite functional tubular toxicity. Morphologic tissue injury is proportionate to the quantity of the cadmium deposition.

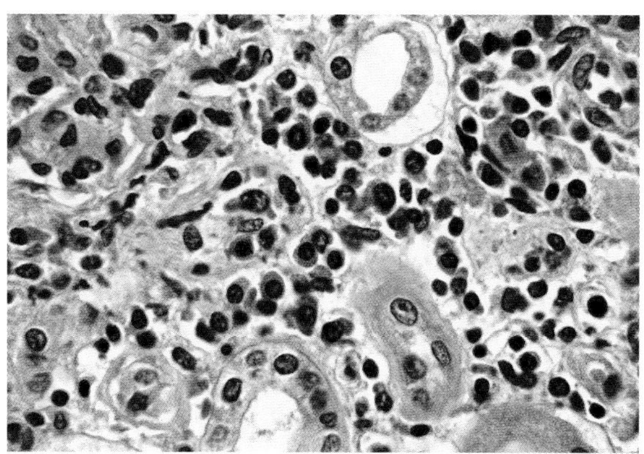

Figure 21-26

GOLD TOXICITY

There is marked interstitial inflammation and expansion secondary to gold injury. No other cause of the interstitial nephritis was apparent in this patient (H&E stain).

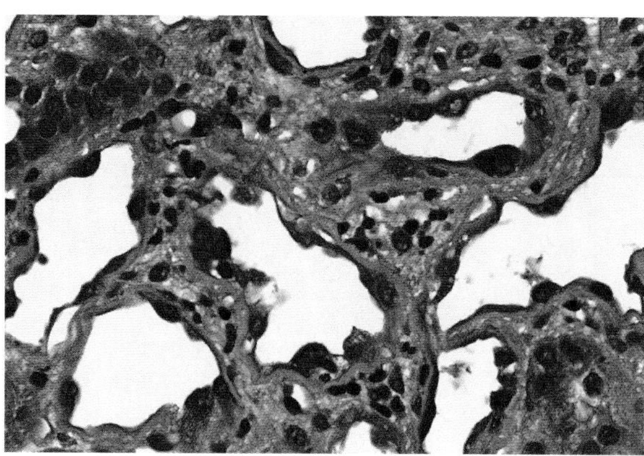

Figure 21-27

CISPLATIN-INDUCED TUBULOINTERSTITIAL INJURY

The tubules show marked alteration, with extreme thinning of the tubular epithelium. The tubules are beginning to be separated by the expanded interstitium (H&E stain).

Cadmium is initially bound to metallothionein-forming complexes in the liver after absorption by the gastrointestinal tract. Filtered by the glomeruli, these cadmium-metallothionein complexes are absorbed by the proximal tubular epithelium and degraded in lysosomes, leading to altered lysosomal biogenesis, decreased lysosomal protease activity, and increased urinary excretion of low molecular weight proteins (tubular proteinuria), calcium, and enzymes.

Mercury Nephropathy. Mercury toxicity can result from a variety of sources, including occupational and therapeutic exposures. Ingestion of inorganic mercurial compounds can lead to chronic mercury toxicity manifesting as the nephrotic syndrome (due to a membranous glomerulonephropathy), or proximal tubular cell dysfunction. Mercury can be quantitated in the kidneys by means of X-ray fluorescence analysis (18).

Mercuric chloride ingestion results in an enlarged and pale kidney. Microscopically, there is severe and extensive necrosis of tubular cells (primarily in the middle and straight portions of the proximal tubules), leading to tubular simplification and desquamation. Interstitial edema and inflammatory infiltration by mononuclear cells accompany the tubular damage. Later there is progressive loss of tubules and interstitial fibrosis.

Inorganic mercury affects the proximal tubular epithelium, and leads to vesiculation and exfoliation of the brush border. Intracellular calcium influx and cell death ensue. Mercury inhibits water permeability (induced by vasopressin) and also depolarizes the inner mitochondrial membrane, leading to increased reactive oxygen metabolites and loss of respiratory function.

Miscellaneous Heavy Metal Nephropathy. *Gold.* Gold inclusions are found in the cytoplasm of tubular epithelial cells and free in the interstitium. Patients may develop proteinuria (due to membranous glomerulonephropathy), hematuria, acute tubular necrosis, or chronic tubulointerstitial nephritis (fig. 21-26; see chapter 19) (18).

Copper/Iron. These may deposit in the tubular cells, inducing tubular cell necrosis and acute renal failure when ingested in large doses (see chapter 19). Copper has been reported to cause tubulointerstitial nephritis (18).

Cisplatin. This may result in renal dysfunction and tubular cell injury, with flattening of the epithelium, dilatation of tubules, and necrosis; focal interstitial edema and fibrosis can be found (figs. 21-27, 21-28) (18).

Arsenic. Reports of coagulative necrosis of the proximal tubular epithelium and chronic renal injury have been reported. There may be interstitial fibrosis manifesting with Fanconi's syndrome and renal insufficiency (fig. 21-29; see chapter 19) (18).

Miscellaneous. Other agents leading to chronic tubulointerstitial nephropathy include NSAIDs (fig. 21-30), lithium (figs. 21-31–21-33), and antiviral agents such as foscarnet (figs. 21-34, 21-35).

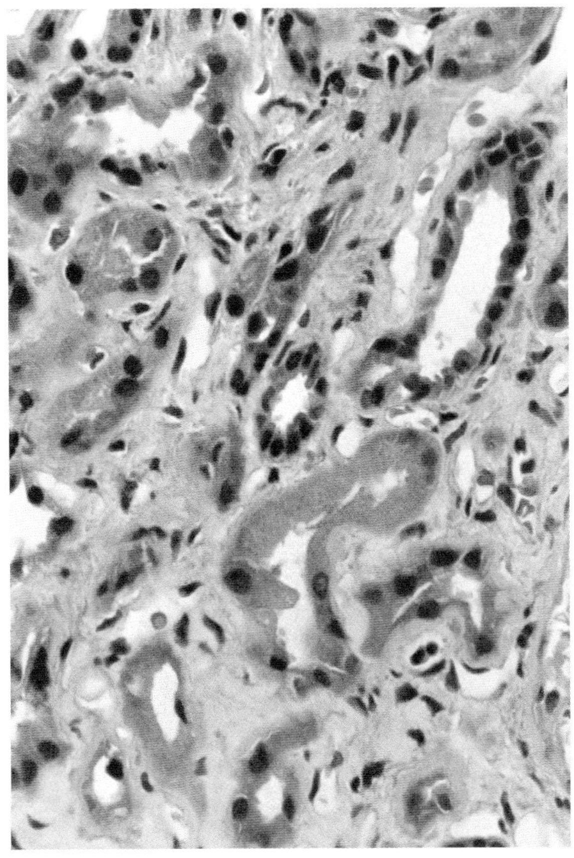

Figure 21-28

CISPLATIN-INDUCED TUBULOINTERSTITIAL INJURY

The interstitial fibrosis is more apparent in this patient than in the patient seen in figure 21-27 (H&E stain).

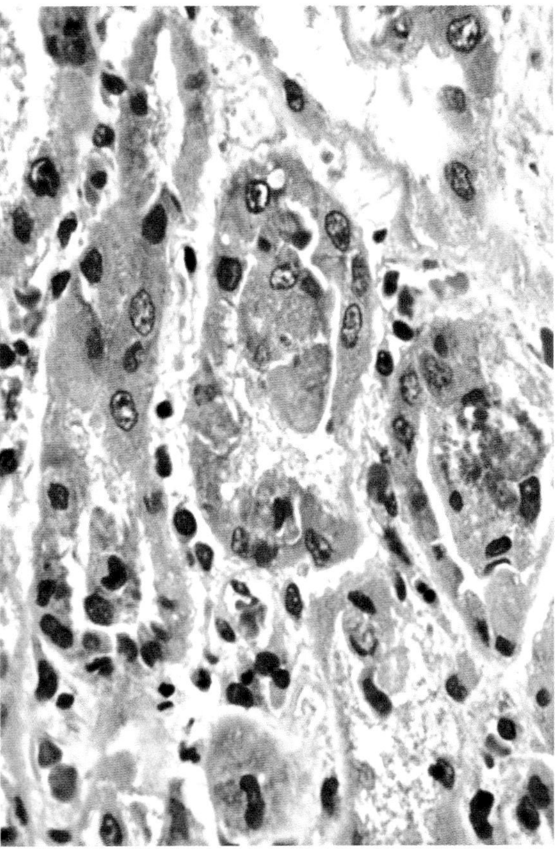

Figure 21-29

ARSENIC-INDUCED TUBULOINTERSTITIAL INJURY

There is severe degeneration of the tubular epithelium and some interstitial edema and inflammation (H&E stain).

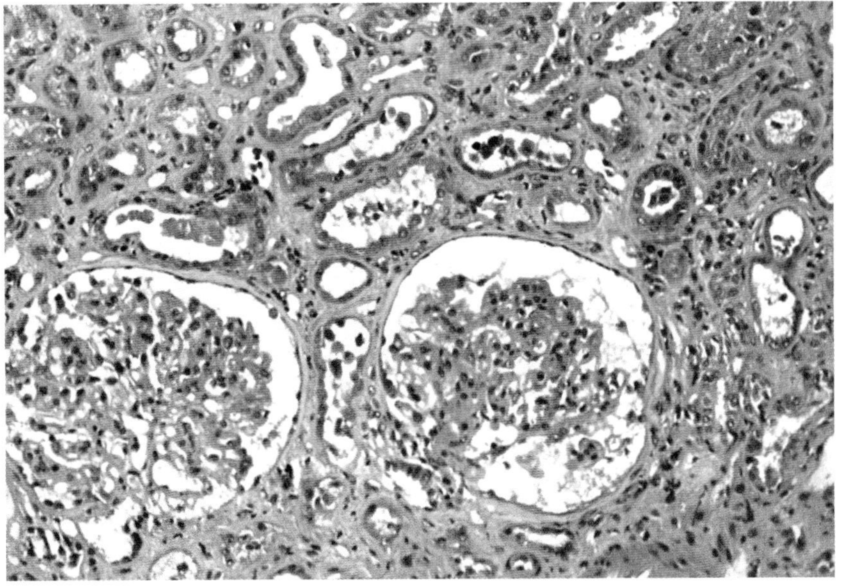

Figure 21-30

NONSTEROIDAL ANTI-INFLAMMATORY DRUG–INDUCED TUBULOINTERSTITIAL DISEASE

The tubules are separated by interstitial fibrosis and, more focally, inflammation. This patient also had minimal change nephrotic syndrome (H&E stain).

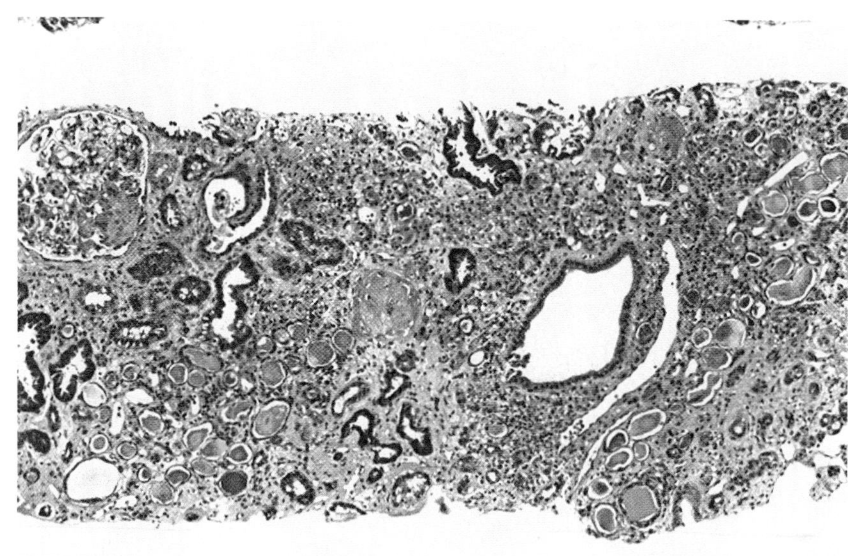

Figure 21-31

LITHIUM TOXICITY: CHRONIC INTERSTITIAL NEPHRITIS

The tubules are separated by the interstitial fibrosis. Several tubules are dilated. The glomerulus at the upper left appears to show segmental sclerosis, which has also been reported with lithium toxicity (H&E stain).

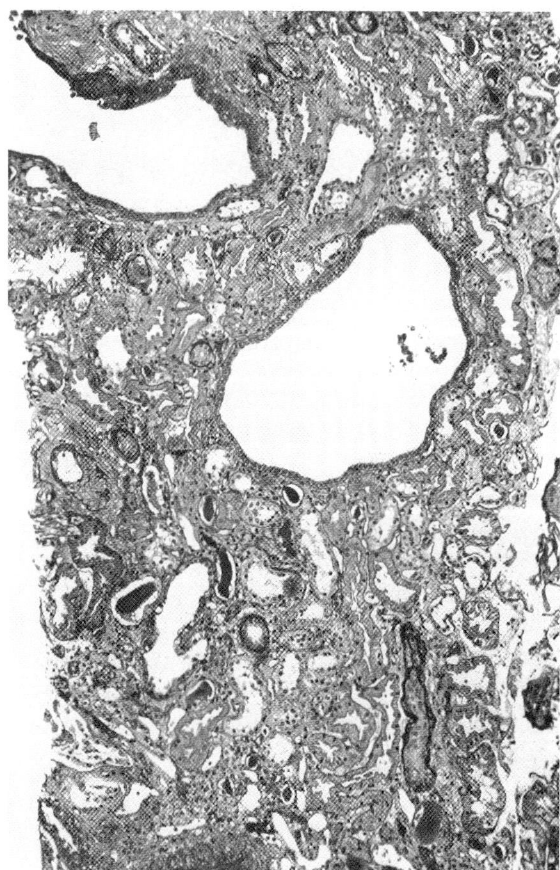

Figure 21-32

LITHIUM TOXICITY: CHRONIC INTERSTITIAL NEPHRITIS

The tubules are separated by the interstitial fibrosis. There are several dilated tubules (H&E stain).

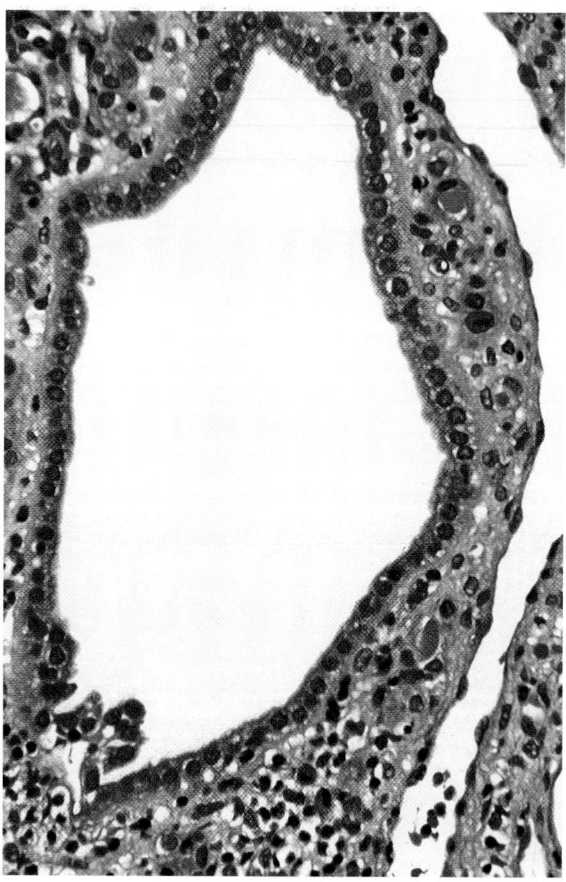

Figure 21-33

LITHIUM TOXICITY: CHRONIC INTERSTITIAL NEPHRITIS

A large dilated tubule with thinned epithelium is adjacent to inflamed and fibrotic interstitium (H&E stain).

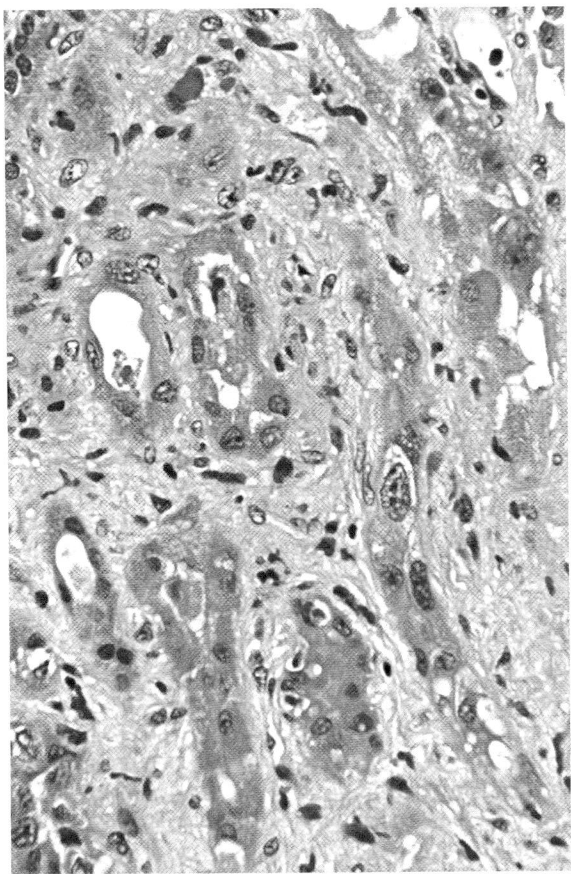

Figure 21-34

FOSCARNET TOXICITY:
CHRONIC INTERSTITIAL NEPHRITIS

The interstitium is expanded by fibrosis and the tubules show marked degenerative changes (H&E stain). (Figs. 21-34 and 21-35 are from the same patient.)

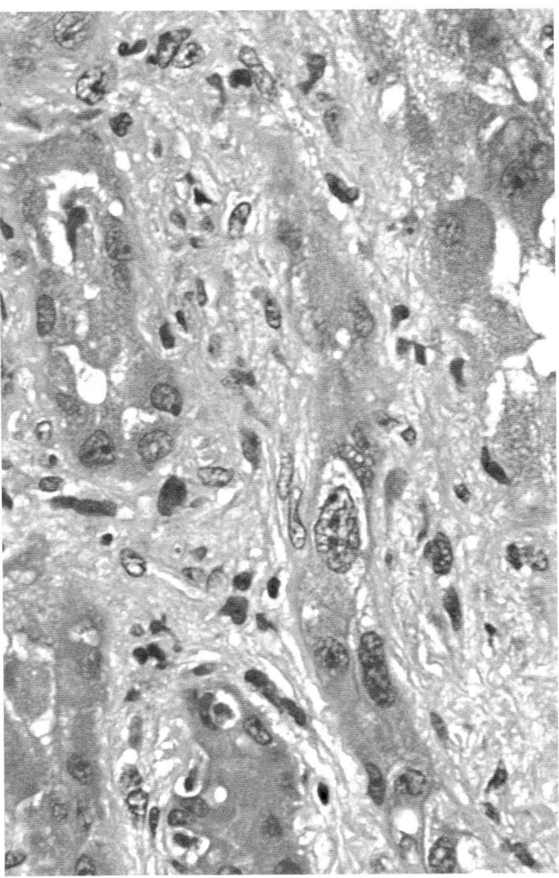

Figure 21-35

FOSCARNET TOXICITY:
CHRONIC INTERSTITIAL NEPHRITIS

There is severe interstitial fibrosis (H&E stain).

Analgesic Abuse Nephropathy

Definition. This form of chronic renal disease is caused by excessive ingestion of certain analgesic mixtures (first described in patients taking phenacetin-aspirin-caffeine). It is characterized morphologically by chronic tubulointerstitial nephritis and papillary necrosis (28,30,33, 61,62,64,69,70).

Clinical Features. Although initially phenacetin-aspirin-caffeine was the compound most frequently implicated as the cause of chronic renal failure due to chronic tubulointerstitial nephritis (28,30,33,61,62,64,65,70), later reports implicated a number of common analgesics, including acetaminophen (a metabolite of phenacetin) and even NSAIDs (1,7,27,52,74,83,84). Patients who develop analgesic nephropathy have usually ingested large amounts of combination analgesic compounds over the years (more than 2 kg of aspirin or phenacetin over a 3-year period).

Analgesic abuse nephropathy is more common in women than men. It is especially prevalent in patients complaining of recurrent headaches and muscular pain. There is gradual cumulative renal injury that only becomes clinically manifest when significant chronic renal insufficiency has occurred.

As the chronic renal insufficiency progresses, the clinical presentation varies. Nocturia and polyuria are common manifestations of the loss of concentrating ability of the injured nephron. This is due to severe medullary damage and frequent renal papillary necrosis. There may be an

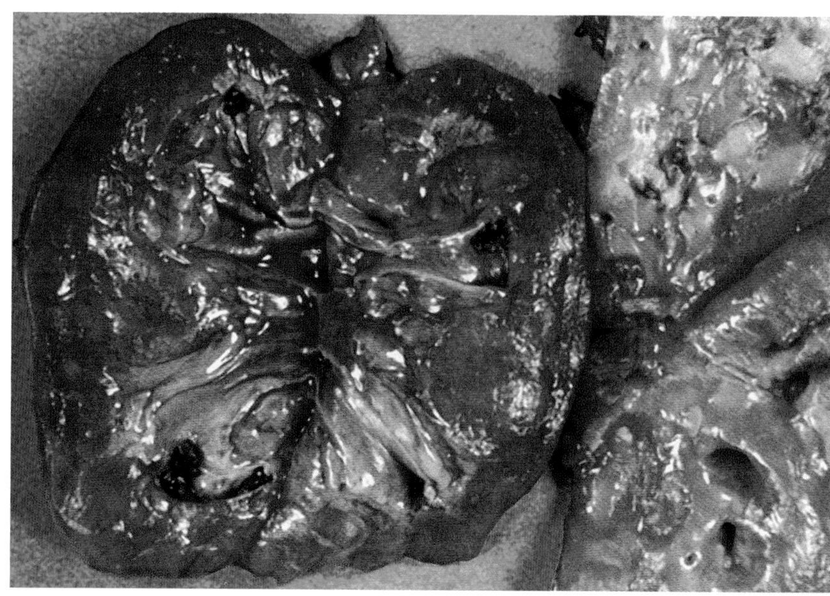

Figure 21-36

ANALGESIC NEPHROPATHY: PAPILLARY NECROSIS

The opened kidney shows several deformed or absent papillary regions. This was secondary to chronic analgesic abuse (aspirin and other drugs). (Courtesy of Dr. P. Kincaid-Smith, Melbourne, Australia.)

acquired distal tubular acidosis (which can contribute to renal stones). Anemia (out of proportion to the degree and duration of the renal insufficiency), gastrointestinal symptoms, and hypertension are common. About half of patients have a urinary tract infection. Sloughing of the renal papillae can lead to gross hematuria or painful renal colic secondary to ureteral obstruction. Papillary necrosis can be detected utilizing computerized tomographic imaging. Papillary transitional cell carcinoma of the renal pelvis has been noted in several patients with longstanding analgesic abuse nephropathy (8). The mechanism leading to this neoplasm is unknown.

Analgesic nephropathy occurs worldwide. Its frequency depends on the degree of analgesic consumption in various parts of the world (being high in the past in parts of Australia and Western Europe) and the ability of the pathologist (or surgical pathologist) to adequately section the kidney and inspect the collecting systems/papillae. In the United States, the incidence is highest in the southeast regions. Where over-the-counter sale of analgesic mixtures have been restricted, there has been a reduction in the incidence of this disease.

Etiology and Pathogenesis. Animal models of papillary necrosis have been studied by administering a mixture of aspirin and phenacetin, often with water depletion. In humans, cases ascribed to ingestion of a single agent are uncommon and most patients with this disease have consumed combination analgesic compounds. Although there was initial confusion over which renal insult, the interstitial disease or the papillary necrosis, was primary, it is now clear that papillary necrosis is the primary event; the cortical interstitial nephritis occurs secondary to the destruction of portions of the papillae (and their collecting ducts). It appears that the phenacetin metabolite, acetaminophen, injures medullary cells by both its covalent binding and oxidative damage. Aspirin potentiates the effects of phenacetin by inhibiting the vasodilatory effects of prostaglandin, thus predisposing the already tenuously blood-supplied renal medulla (and especially papillae) to further ischemia and damage. Thus, the combination of direct renal toxic damage and ischemic injury harms both tubular cells and the vascularity (28,52,61,64,69,83).

Gross Findings. The renal surfaces often show depressed cortical regions, representing the cortical atrophy overlying the necrotic papillae. The necrotic papillae may demonstrate necrosis, fragmentation, sloughing, or calcification. It is typical to see papillae in varying stages of injury. Often, the necrotic papillae remain attached to the renal cortex/medulla (fig. 21-36).

Light Microscopic Findings. Because a renal biopsy rarely samples the inner medulla, it is often difficult (and probably impossible) to determine whether the nonspecific cortical

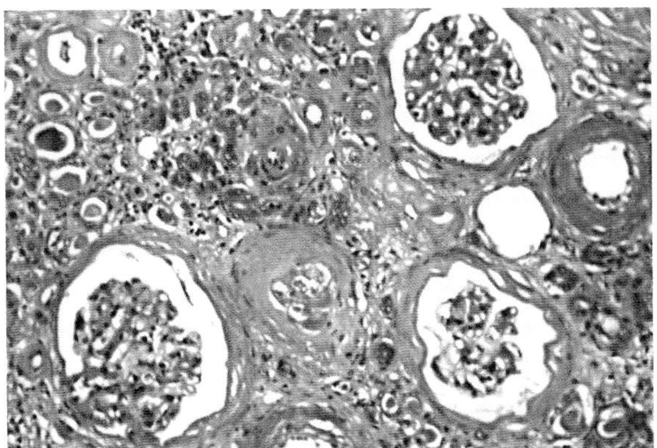

Figure 21-37

ANALGESIC NEPHROPATHY

The renal cortex shows widespread interstitial fibrosis and tubular atrophy, usually secondary to the underlying papillary necrosis (H&E stain).

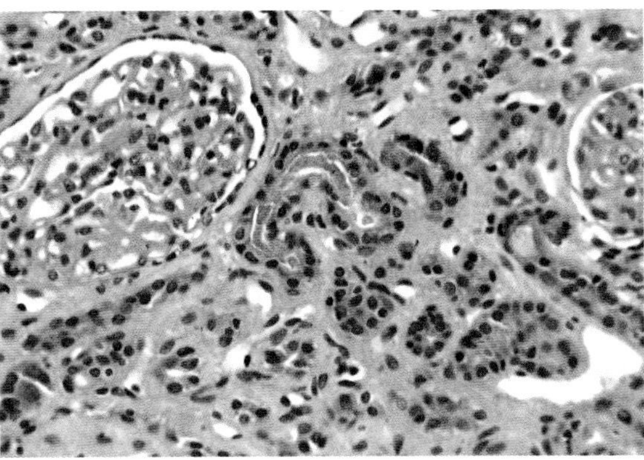

Figure 21-38

ANALGESIC NEPHROPATHY: CHRONIC INTERSTITIAL NEPHRITIS

Severe tubular atrophy and interstitial fibrosis are seen in this patient who chronically ingested analgesics (aspirin, phenacetin, etc) (H&E stain).

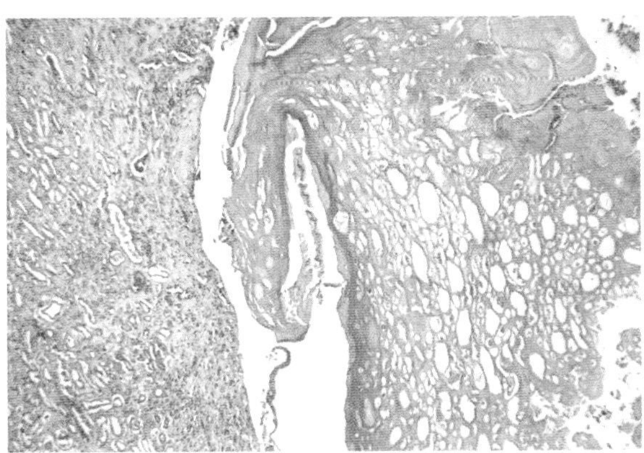

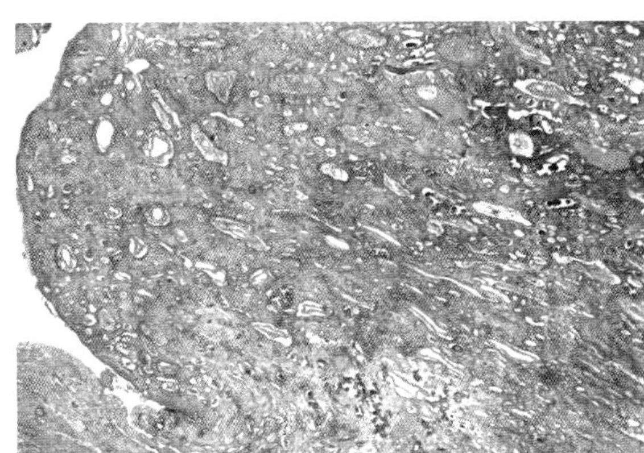

Figure 21-39

ANALGESIC NEPHROPATHY

The two figures show papillary necrosis with loss of tubular epithelial nuclei, but some preservation of the tubular outlines. (left, H&E stain; right, Masson trichrome stain).

tubulointerstitial nephritis is secondary to papillary necrosis. There is usually extensive interstitial fibrosis with few inflammatory cells. Tubular atrophy is usually present (figs. 21-37–21-39). The renal cortical columns of Bertin are spared from cortical atrophy (7,20,27,42,52,61,62,64,74).

The papillary necrosis may be patchy, but in the advancing form of analgesic nephropathy, the entire papillary structure may be necrotic. There are often ghosts of tubules and areas of dystrophic calcification. In certain cases the entire papilla may be sloughed into the urine.

Periodic acid–Schiff (PAS)-positive material is often noted around the small arterioles in the renal pelvic and peripelvic (ureteric) submucosal structures (analgesic microangiopathy). This represents thickening of the basement membranes in these areas.

Immunofluorescence/Electron Microscopy/Special Studies. These are noncontributory.

Differential Diagnosis. The cortical changes are entirely nonspecific. Therefore, radiologic evidence of papillary necrosis and calcification are valuable diagnostic aids. The differential

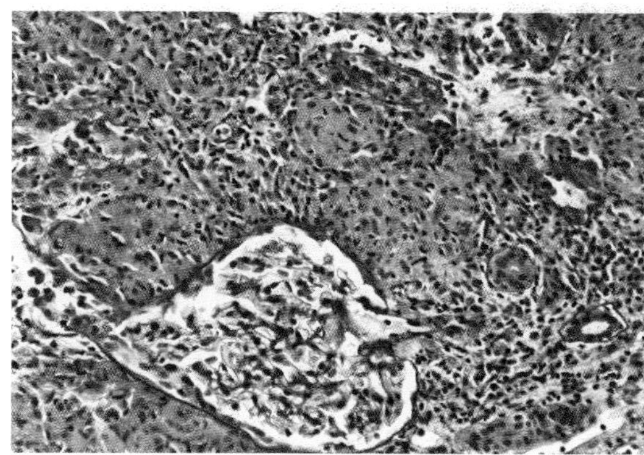

Figure 21-40

GRANULOMATOUS INTERSTITIAL NEPHRITIS

There is marked separation of the tubules by interstitial expansion. The cause of the granulomatous interstitial nephritis was uncertain (H&E stain).

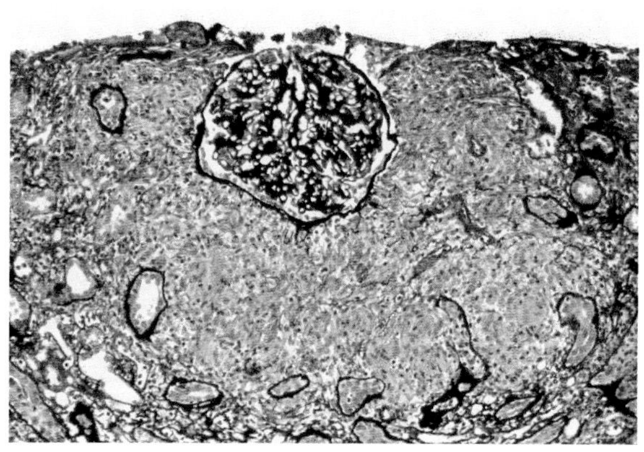

Figure 21-41

GRANULOMATOUS INTERSTITIAL NEPHRITIS

There is separation of the tubules by a localized collection of inflammatory cells. Note the "bending" of the tubules around these inflammatory cells. This patient was treated with tofranil, the apparent cause of the granulomatous interstitial nephritis (JMS stain). (Figs. 21-41 and 21-42 are from the same patient.)

diagnosis of papillary necrosis includes diabetes mellitus, sickle cell disease, and obstruction/infection.

Treatment and Prognosis. If most of the papillae have not sloughed off and the offending agents are no longer administered, then renal function may remain stable (or even improve in some patients). In some cases, the treatment of the accompanying infection (secondary to ureteral obstruction by the necrotic sloughed papillae) leads to improved renal function.

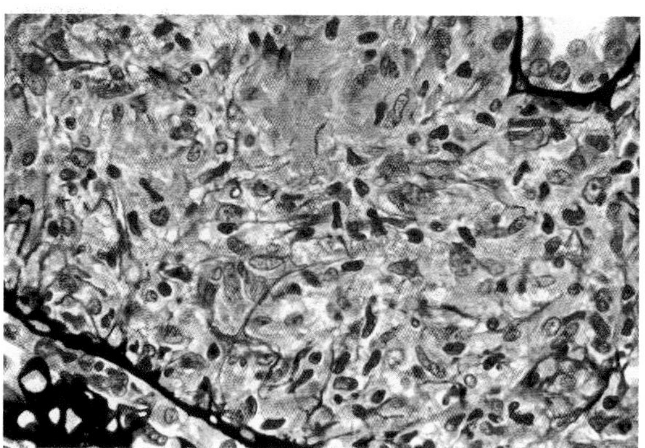

Figure 21-42

GRANULOMATOUS INTERSTITIAL NEPHRITIS

A higher magnification of the biopsy seen in figure 21-41 shows the histiocytoid monocytes forming the noncaseating granulomata (JMS stain).

Granulomatous Interstitial Nephritis

Definition. Granulomatous interstitial nephritis is defined histologically as a primary interstitial nephritis manifesting interstitial granulomata.

Clinical Features. These are the same as those of any other primary tubulointerstitial nephritis of the kidney (22,39,56,60,75,80,81).

Gross Findings. These are nonspecific.

Light Microscopic Findings. Intersitial clusters or collections of epithelioid histiocytes and giant cells forming granulomata, with varying numbers of small lymphocytes and other interstitial leukocytes, are seen microscopically (figs. 21-40–21-47). Caseous necrosis generally only occurs in patients with mycobacterial or fungal infections (22,39,56,60,75,80,81).

Immunofluorescence/Electron Microscopic Findings. These are not helpful.

Special Studies. Special stains for organisms including (Ziehl-Neelsen, PAS, and Grocott or Gomori silver stains) should be performed in all cases.

Differential Diagnosis. Granulomata associated with mycobacterial or fungal infections usually, but not always, show central caseous necrosis. Thus, special stains for mycobacterial or fungal organisms should be performed (with appropriate positive controls). Sarcoidosis can be suspected when the granulomata are small, well defined, and noncaseating, and when they contain Schaumann bodies (laminated intracytoplasmic concretions) or asteroid bodies.

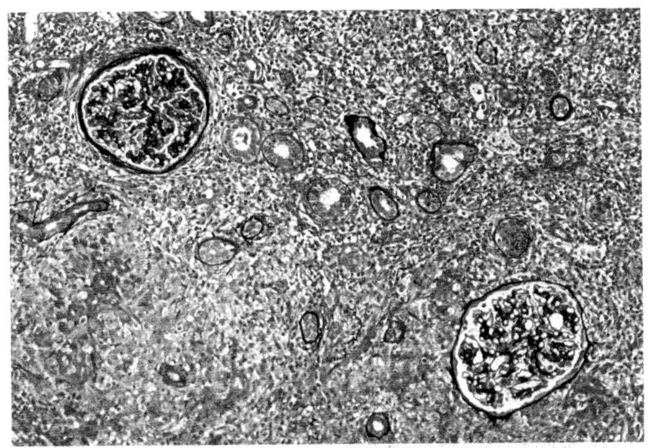

Figure 21-43

GRANULOMATOUS INTERSTITIAL NEPHRITIS SECONDARY TO AZULFIDINE THERAPY

JMS stain.

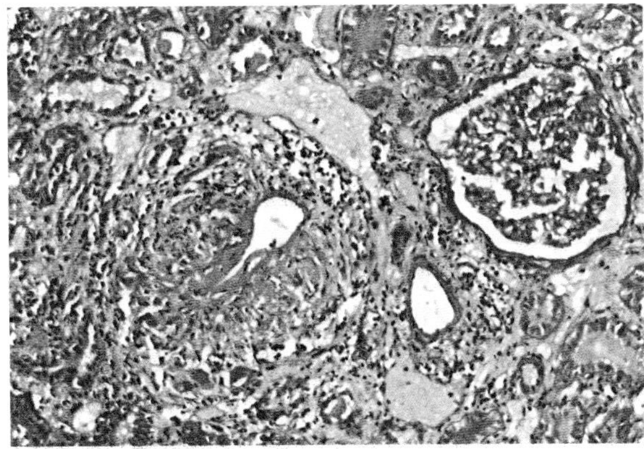

Figure 21-44

GRANULOMATOUS INTERSTITIAL NEPHRITIS SECONDARY TO DILANTIN THERAPY

The granulomatous reaction appears to be centered around a blood vessel (H&E stain).

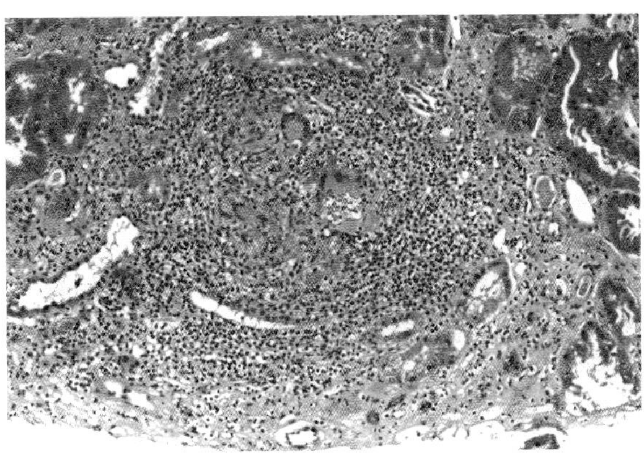

Figure 21-45

GRANULOMATOUS INTERSTITIAL NEPHRITIS SECONDARY TO SARCOIDOSIS

The noncaseating granulomata are not pathognomonic for sarcoidosis; however, the central calcified body (Schaumann body) is (H&E stain).

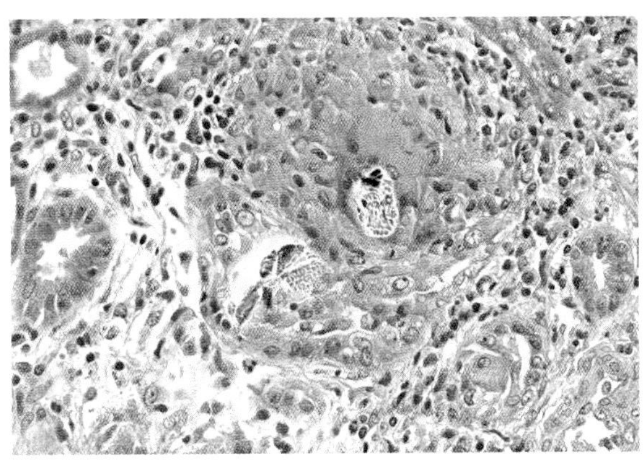

Figure 21-46

GRANULOMATOUS INTERSTITIAL NEPHRITIS

The oxalate crystals are surrounded by a granulomatous reaction. This pattern is sometimes seen in oxalate deposition in the kidney, in patients with gastric bypass surgery (for obesity), and other causes of faulty oxalate metabolism (H&E stain). (Courtesy Dr. W. Kern, Oklahoma City, OK.)

Calcifications may be seen in the tubules in sarcoidosis. The morphologic changes are not pathognomonic, however, and clinicopathologic correlations may aid in the diagnosis (i.e., disease in other sites such as the lung, lymph nodes, etc). Wegener's granulomatosis can lead to a granulomatous infiltration in the interstitium; however, most of these apparently interstitial granulomata actually represent granulomatous crescents that have destroyed Bowman's capsule. Nonetheless, true interstitial granulomata may be identified in a minority of cases of Wegener's granulomatosis.

Etiology and Pathogenesis. Granulomatous interstitial nephritis can be caused by a wide variety of conditions. The most common cause is probably hypersensitivity/allergic reactions to a variety of medications (such as anticonvulsant drugs, antibiotics, antihypertensive agents). Other causes include infectious organisms (mycobacterial or fungal), sarcoidosis, and Wegener's granulomatosis.

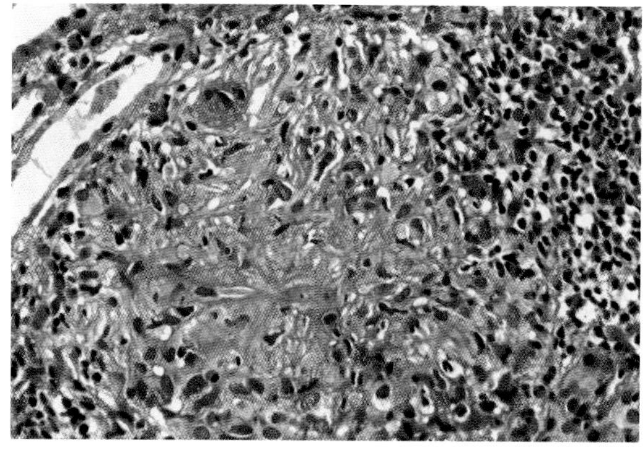

Figure 21-47

GRANULOMATOUS INTERSTITIAL REACTION IN A PATIENT WITH ANCA-RELATED CRESCENTIC GLOMERULONEPHRITIS

This is not a true interstitial granuloma, but instead the very edge of a glomerulus with crescent formation and severe disruption of Bowman's capsule (granulomatous crescent formation) (H&E stain).

TUBULOINTERSTITIAL NEPHRITIS CAUSED BY PRIMARY DIRECT IMMUNOLOGIC MECHANISMS

Primary tubulointerstitial nephritis can be mediated by antibodies, immune complexes, or T cells. Although a number of immune glomerular diseases involve the tubulointerstitial regions, only those diseases that primarily affect the tubulointerstitial regions (with minimal or no glomerular involvement) are considered here (13, 18). It should not be forgotten that progressive tubulointerstitial injury occurs in most forms of chronic renal disease, regardless of the nature of the primary or initial inciting agent (10,11,31,66).

Antitubular Basement Membrane Antibody Injury Due to Drugs

The presence of intense linear deposits of immunoreactants (especially immunoglobulins and complement) along the tubular basement membranes that is associated with tubulointerstitial inflammation is suggestive of anti-TBM nephritis (12,13,18,25,49). Methicillin-induced anti-TBM nephritis is the classic drug-induced form (34). Methicillin was removed from the market years ago because of this toxicity. The differential diagnosis includes the nonimmunologic linear deposition of IgG and albumin of diabetic nephropathy. Weak linear IgG staining of tubular basement membranes also occurs as "background staining" in the normal human kidney.

Primary Antitubular Basement Membrane Antibody Nephritis

Primary anti-TBM nephritis is a rare condition characterized by intense linear deposits of IgG and complement along the tubular basement membranes due to circulating anti-TBM antibodies in the serum (12,18). There is mononuclear and neutrophilic infiltration of the tubules and interstitium, associated with tubular cell injury and interstitial edema. Glomeruli and vessels are unremarkable. Only a few cases have been reported. Some occur in young children with membranous glomerulopathy (see chapter 7) (49). More commonly, anti-TBM antibody deposits occur secondary to primary glomerular antiglomerular basement membrane (anti-GBM) antibody disease (Goodpasture's disease).

Immunofluorescence studies show intense linear staining of the tubular basement membranes for IgG, often associated with complement. At least three major antigens have been found to play an immunogenic role in the induction of this disorder. They are described elsewhere (18). Interaction of the antigen and antibody results in complement activation and deposition of complement (C)3 in the tubular basement membrane. Leukocytic infiltration is enhanced by the expression of intracellular adhesion molecule (ICAM)-1 beta-2-integrin; there is upregulation of various interleukins and tumor necrotic factor. The tubulointerstitial injury results from the release of proteases and various reactive oxygen species.

Immune Complex Injury

This form of interstitial nephritis is defined by granular deposits of immunoglobulins and complement in the tubular basement membranes, interstitial regions, or both (figs. 21-48–21-55). The immune complex deposits are most often associated with an underlying primary glomerular disease, such as a lupus nephropathy, membranous glomerulonephropathy, membranoproliferative glomerulonephritis, crescentic glomerulonephritis, acute postinfectious glomerulonephritis, or shunt nephritis (18). Primary tubulointerstitial injuries with little or no glomerular deposition or damage have been

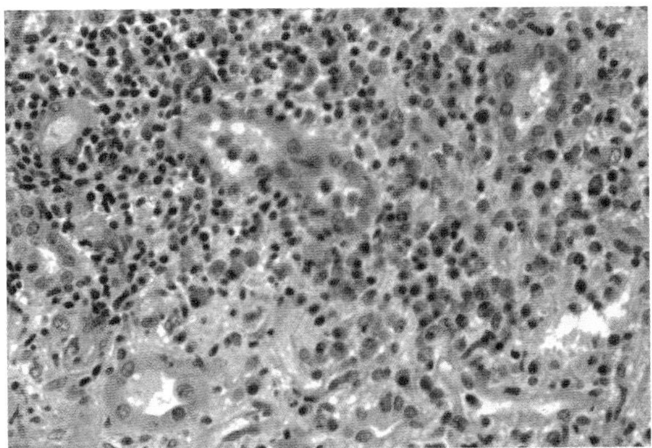

Figure 21-48

TUBULOINTERSTITIAL NEPHRITIS SECONDARY TO PRIMARY DIRECT IMMUNOLOGIC MECHANISMS

This patient with systemic lupus erythematosus had immunofluorescent granular deposits of IgG along the tubular basement membranes (H&E stain).

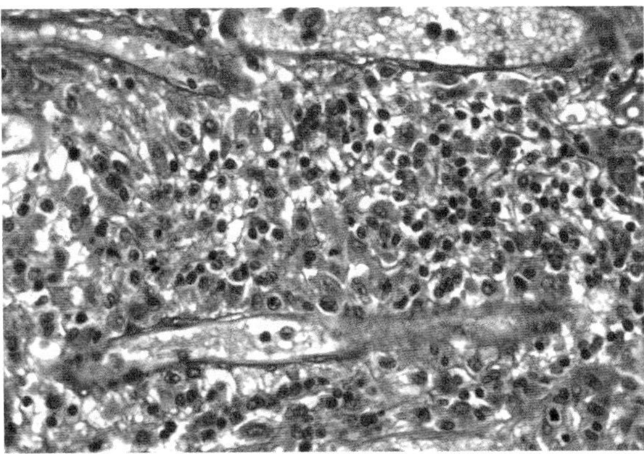

Figure 21-49

TUBULOINTERSTITIAL NEPHRITIS

This patient with systemic lupus erythematosus had immune deposits along the tubular basement membranes. Note the marked expansion of the interstitium by a severe interstitial inflammation comprised primarily of plasma cells (periodic acid–Schiff [PAS] stain).

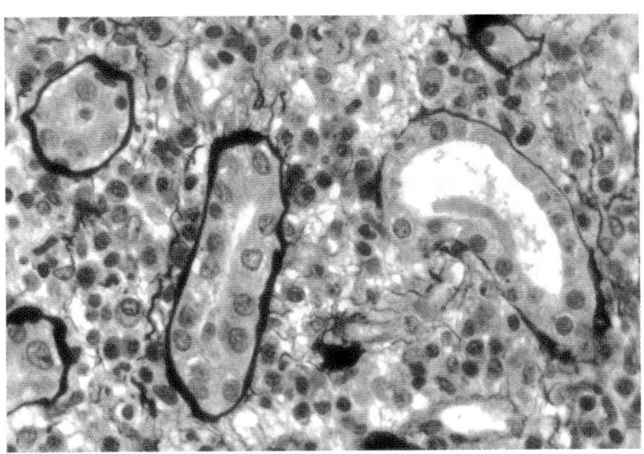

Figure 21-50

TUBULOINTERSTITIAL NEPHRITIS

The interstitium is severely expanded by a large collection of inflammatory cells and tubular basement membrane deposits in a patient with severe systemic lupus erythematosus. There was also a class IV lupus nephritis (diffuse proliferative glomerulonephritis) (JMS stain).

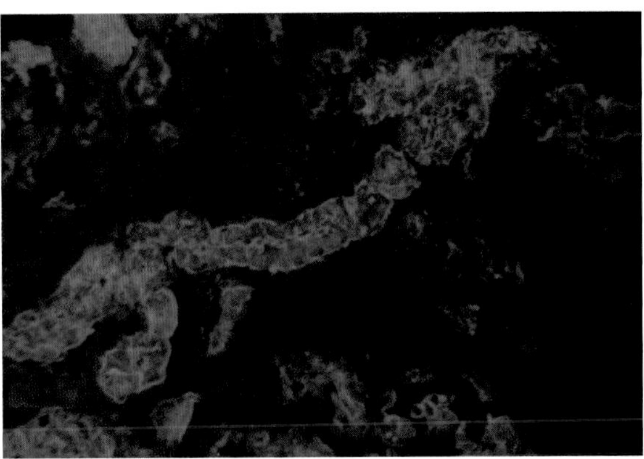

Figure 21-51

TUBULOINTERSTITIAL NEPHRITIS SECONDARY TO SYSTEMIC LUPUS ERYTHEMATOSUS

Immune complexes are deposited in the tubular basement membranes (anti-IgG; immunofluorescence micrograph).

reported, however. In these cases, focal interstitial infiltrates with lymphocytes, and tubular atrophy associated with granular C3, Clq, and electron-dense deposits along the tubular basement membranes, are seen by electron microscopy. There may be clinical evidence of proximal tubule dysfunction. There are at least two cases in which the granular deposits were of IgE; the pathogenesis in these cases is unclear (18).

The nature of the antigens involved, with a few possible exceptions, is unknown (18,23,50). It is likely that the antigen targets differ. Some of the antigens proposed include gp330 (megalin) present in the brush border of proximal tubules and the foot processes of rat podocytes (thought to be involved in the production of experimental membranous glomerulonephropathy), and Tamm-Horsfall protein normally synthesized in the thick ascending limb of

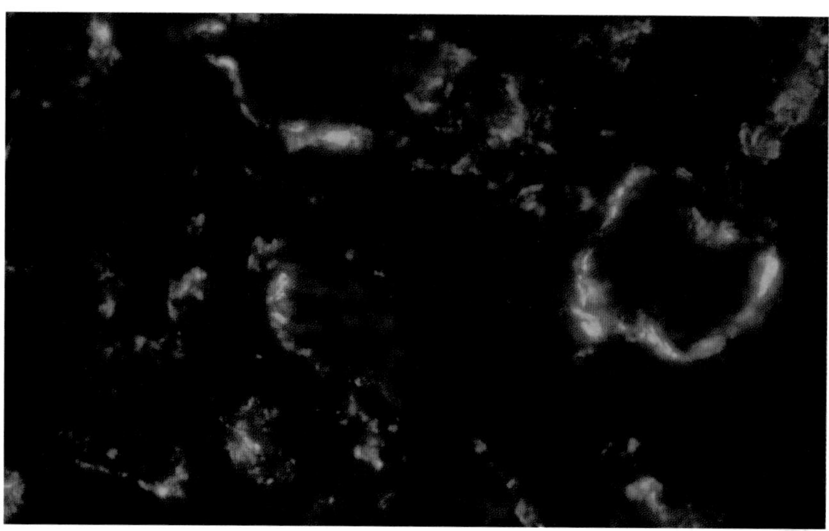

Figure 21-52

TUBULOINTERSTITIAL NEPHRITIS SECONDARY TO SYSTEMIC LUPUS ERYTHEMATOSUS

Immune complexes are deposited in the tubular basement membranes (anti-IgG; immunofluorescence micrograph).

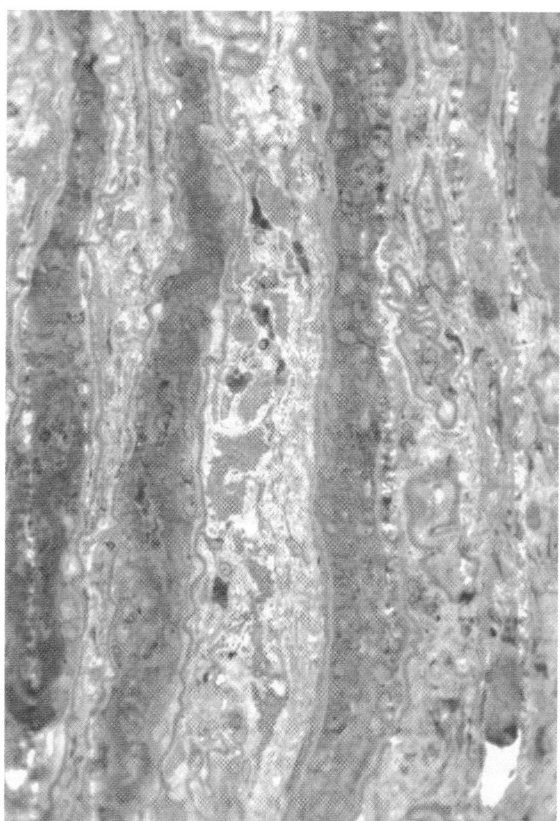

Figure 21-53

INTERSTITIAL DEPOSITS

This patient with plasma cell dyscrasia had nodular glomerulosclerosis secondary to light chain deposition. The plastic section shown here (in preparation for electron microscopic studies) shows large interstitial immune (kappa light chain) deposits. There was a sprinkling of interstitial inflammatory cells, mostly lymphocytes and plasma cells (Epon embedded).

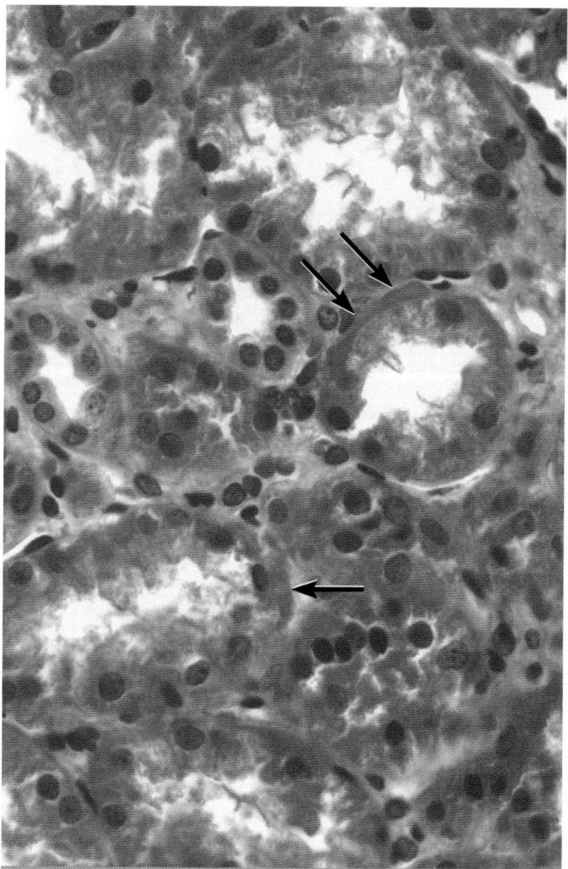

Figure 21-54

TUBULAR BASEMENT MEMBRANE DEPOSITS

This patient with dense deposit disease has large fuchsinophilic deposits along some of the tubular basement membranes (arrows) (Masson trichrome stain).

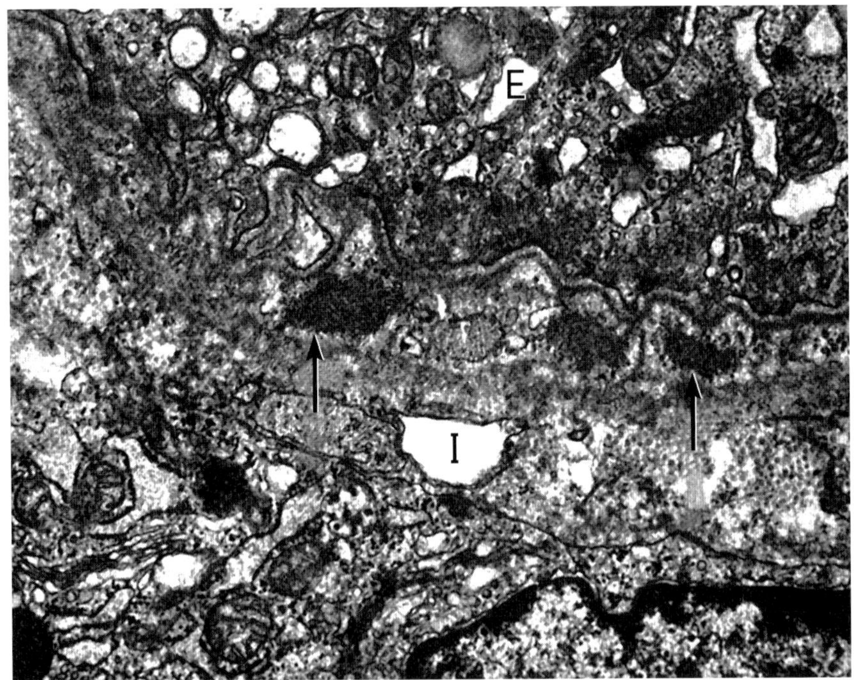

Figure 21-55

TUBULAR BASEMENT MEMBRANE DEPOSITS

This patient had infectious endocarditis. Electron microscopy shows immune deposits in the kidney because of drug allergy secondary to the antibiotic amoxicillin. (I = interstitium; E = tubular epithelial cell.)

Henle. The immune deposits may result from immune complexes formed in the peripheral circulation or from local interactions between the blood-borne free antibody with deposited/planted/normal antigens in the renal tissues. Cell-mediated injury may be complement dependent, leading to activation of leukocytes, and release of various proteases and toxic oxygen radicals (18).

T-Cell Injuries

The primary example of T-cell–mediated tubulointerstitial injury is allograft rejection, which results from a disparity in the major histocompatability (MHC) antigens between the donor and the recipient (18). Allograft rejection is detailed in chapter 26.

Some forms of tubulointerstitial nephritis in the native kidney are also mediated by T cells. This was first described in 1975 by Dobrin in patients with acute renal failure due to tubulointerstitial nephritis, associated with anterior uveitis and granulomas in the bone marrow and lymph nodes. The patients were young adolescent females. Subsequent studies of this disorder have shown that the kidney contains interstitial infiltrates of mononuclear cells, including large numbers of lymphocytes, and smaller numbers of plasma cells, macrophages, and eosinophils. Immunofluorescent studies are usually negative. Immunophenotyping of the cells show mostly T cells with variable numbers of CD4 and CD8 subsets. Some patients also have chronic sialoadenitis. The cause of the disease is unknown, but an autoimmune pathogenesis is likely (18).

Other forms of T-cell–mediated tubulointerstitial injury include sarcoidosis and some cases of granulomatous tubulointerstitial nephritis (see above). Chronic interstitial disease with interstitial fibrosis and tubular atrophy is present in virtually all forms of progressive glomerular and vascular diseases. Cell-mediated immunity appears to play a major role in the pathogenesis of progressive tubulointerstitial disease. In these instances, inflammatory cells accumulate in the interstitium in response to deposition or local formation of immune complexes, or in response to cytokines and other mediators released from injured glomeruli. In response to these various cytokines and other mediators, adhesion molecules and growth factors are overexpressed, and inflammatory cells accumulate in the interstitium. The mechanisms by which inflammatory cells induce fibrosis have been reviewed, but the effects of tumor growth factor (TGF)-beta and interleukin (IL)-4 or indirect stimulation of fibroblasts through monocyte/macrophage activation seem to be primary and important (18,23,50).

The morphologic findings consist of inflammatory infiltrates of lymphocytes, plasma cells, and a few eosinophils; lymphocytes account for most of the infiltrating cells. Tubular epithelial changes include tubulitis, degeneration, and regeneration, and casts are often present. Tubular atrophy and interstitial fibrosis are seen later in the disease course. Immunofluorescence is generally negative, unless the tubulointerstitial changes are secondary to an underlying (primary) immune glomerular disease (18).

Because the pathogenesis of tubulointerstitial nephritis due to T-cell mechanisms can only be demonstrated with the transfer of T cells from one donor to a recipient (i.e., adoptive transfer), the definitive diagnosis in humans must be inferential and based upon the animal models studied in which T cells have been demonstrated to play a major pathogenic role. It seems that mononuclear cells can mediate tubulointerstitial disease in at least two major ways: 1) delayed-type hypersensitivity involving prior exposure and sensitization of the host caused by CD4-positive T cells and macrophages. This leads to the production of lymphokines and a granulomatous reaction, and is seen in some drug reactions and sarcoidosis; 2) cytotoxic T-cell injury not requiring prior sensitization of CD4 and CD8 cells. Allograft rejections appear to result from this mechanism (18).

TUBULOINTERSTITIAL NEPHROPATHIES ASSOCIATED WITH METABOLIC DISORDERS

Urate Nephropathy

There are three types of urate nephropathy that occur in patients with hyperuricemic disorders: acute uric acid nephropathy, chronic urate nephropathy, and nephrolithiasis.

Acute Uric Acid Nephropathy. This is caused by the precipitation of uric acid crystals in the kidney tubules, especially the collecting ducts. It leads to obstruction and the development of acute renal failure. It is particularly common in patients undergoing chemotherapy for leukemia or lymphoma; the cytoreductive therapy lyses the tumor cells, followed by the release of nucleotides, which are catabolized to uric acid. An acid pH favors the precipitation of uric acid in the collecting ducts (18).

Chronic Urate Nephropathy (Gouty Nephropathy). This occurs in patients with protracted forms of hyperuricemia. There is predominantly medullary deposition of monosodium urate crystals in the acidic milieu of the distal tubules and collecting ducts, and the interstitial regions of the medulla (fig. 21-56; see chapters 19 and 23).

The urate crystals have a distinctive morphologic appearance. They are birefringent, needle-like crystals in the tubular lumens and/or interstitium. They induce a "tophus" surrounded by foreign body giant cells (fig. 21-56). There may be tubular obstruction by the urates, which leads to tubular atrophy and interstitial fibrosis. Hypertension and vascular disease are often present.

Nephrolithiasis (Secondary to Uric Acid Stones). This is discussed in chapter 23 .

Balkan (Endemic) Nephropathy

Balkan nephropathy is an unusual disease found in Croatia, Bosnia, Serbia, Bulgaria, and Romania. It occurs in families and may be endemic, involving up to 10 percent of the population of a region. It occurs along the tributaries of the Danube River basin and usually involves patients more than 20 years of age. It appears to take years to develop (20,77).

Clinical onset is manifested by insidious weakness, anorexia, anemia, weight loss, lumbar pain, albuminuria, hypertension, edema, and copper yellow skin of the palms and soles. There is tubular proteinuria (up to 2 g/24 hours) and increased excretion of beta-2-microglobulin, both signs of tubular damage and early nephropathy.

In advanced conditions, the kidneys are reduced in size and can weigh 20 g each. The major morphologic changes are interstitial fibrosis, variable amounts of interstitial inflammation, and tubular atrophy. There seems to be more involvement of the superficial cortex than the deeper cortex, at least early on. Papillary necrosis is not common; however, transitional cell carcinomas have been discovered in the renal pelvis and the ureters. The tumors may be multiple and bilateral. Squamous cell carcinomas have also been described.

The pathogenetic mechanisms involved in the tubulointerstitial disease are unknown. A number of purported etiologic agents have been

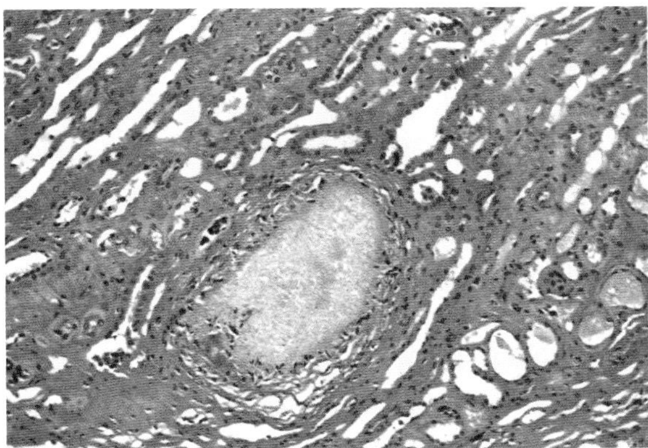

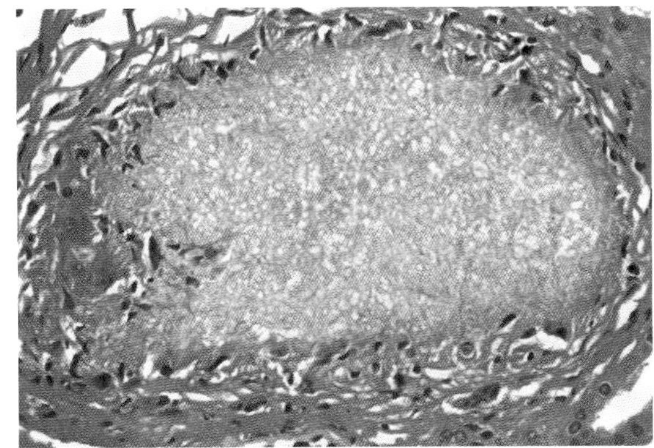

Figure 21-56

TUBULOINTERSTITIAL NEPHRITIS SECONDARY TO URATE NEPHROPATHY

There is a large, pale stained, amorphous and acellular cast in the distal collecting system. Note the nearby giant cell formation (H&E stain).

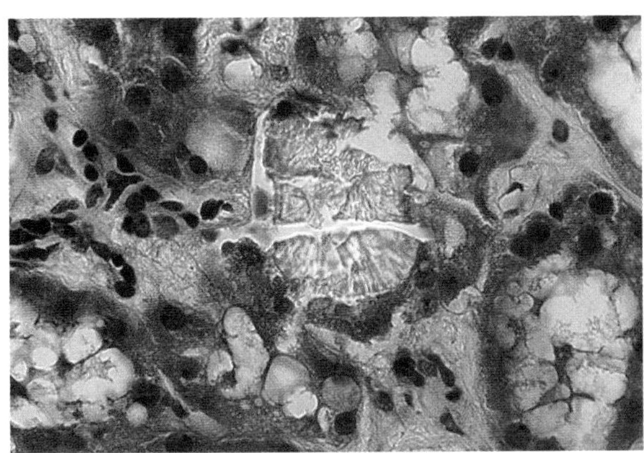

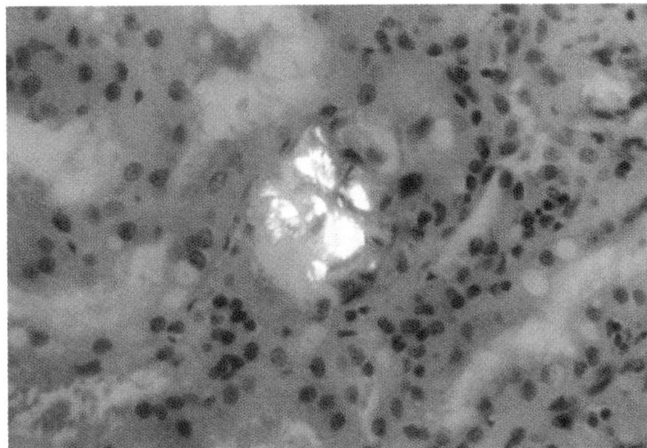

Figure 21-57

TUBULOINTERSTITIAL NEPHRITIS SECONDARY TO OXALATE DEPOSITION

There are large refractile acellular deposits in several of the tubular lumens. They are doubly refractile under the polarized lens (H&E stain).

suggested including fungi (ochratoxin A), heavy metals, silica, and low molecular weight proteins (20,77). None have been substantiated. There is a similarity between Balkan nephropathy and Chinese herbs nephropathy (29), the latter implicating aristolochic acid.

Oxalate Nephropathy (Crystal Nephropathy)

Oxalate crystals are frequently seen in the tubular lumens of patients with hyperoxaluric states (including glycol poisoning, excessive ingestion of oxalate-containing foods, chronic intestinal disease, primary genetic hyperoxaluria) and end-stage kidney disease. The morphologic findings are the nonspecific findings of tubular atrophy and interstitial fibrosis. The distinctive feature is the presence of crystal deposition (82,85). The identification of these crystals can sometimes be accentuated by the use of a polarizing microscope (fig. 21-57; see chapter 23).

Radiation Nephropathy

Definition. Inadvertent or unavoidable exposure of the kidney to ionizing radiation in the course of radiologic treatment of malignant tumors may lead to renal damage (3,21). The delivery of total body irradiation in preparation for bone marrow transplantation in patients with leukemia/lymphoma is another potential cause of radiation injury to the kidney. Although the recent introduction of techniques to minimize acute organ radiation toxicity has made this disorder rare, the increasing use of whole body radiation with bone marrow transplantation for the treatment of malignant neoplasms and autoimmune diseases has rekindled interest in this condition (3,21).

Clinical Features. *Acute Radiation Nephritis/Acute Radiation Nephropathy.* This develops over several months (6 to 12 months) after irradiation. There is a gradual onset of renal insufficiency, edema, hypertension (which may be malignant), anemia, headaches, proteinuria, and urinary casts. There is sometimes a microangiopathic hemolytic type of anemia (and other changes consistent with a thrombotic microangiopathy, which is considered in chapter 18). Chemotherapeutic agents (such as actinomycin D, doxorubicin, bleomycin, vinblastine, vincristine, and cyclophosphamide) often shorten the latency period between the exposure to irradiation and the onset of nephropathy. These agents may also increase the overall risk of developing radiation nephropathy. Harbingers of a poor renal prognosis include generalized edema, severe hypertension (with hypertensive retinopathy), and a BUN above 100 mg/100 mL in the first 3 months of the disease (3,21).

Chronic Radiation Nephritis/Chronic Radiation Nephropathy. There are two types of patients with chronic radiation nephritis: 1) those who present initially with acute radiation nephritis which then evolves into chronic nephropathy, and 2) those who give no history of acute symptomatology but present for the first time with proteinuria and chronic renal failure years after the original exposure to radiation. The BUN and serum creatinine levels are elevated and patients are hypertensive. Chronic uremia of long duration is common. Both patient groups appear at great risk for the development of renal failure and end-stage kidney disease (3,21).

Gross Findings. The kidneys are normal or contracted in size. There may be a thickened renal capsule, but this is nonspecific. The subcapsular surface is smooth in young patients, but is granular if blood vessels are involved.

Light Microscopic Findings. There are several different types of lesions. One involves primarily the glomeruli and smaller arteries/arterioles; it is mainly a thrombotic microangiopathy and is considered in chapter 18. Lesions affecting primarily the tubulointerstitial regions are considered here (3,21).

Although there is no specific or distinctive type of tubular or interstitial pattern of injury in radiation nephritis, there is often severe involvement of the interstitial and tubular regions. The considerable loss of tubules is usually paralleled by the concomitant degree of interstitial fibrosis. There is often accompanying global glomerular sclerosis. Other, nonspecific changes include tubular epithelial cell vacuolization and desquamation of the tubular epithelium.

Immunofluorescence/Electron Microscopy/Special Studies. These are usually noncontributory. Certain glomerular and vascular changes are noted, and these are detailed in chapter 18.

Differential Diagnosis. Because the exposure to radiation is often distant, a careful clinical history is required. The potential contribution of other nephrotoxins, such as chemotherapeutic, antineoplastic, and other agents, must be considered. A diagnosis of radiation nephropathy is supported by any evidence of acute or chronic thrombotic microangiopathy.

Etiology and Pathogenesis. The exact pathogenic mechanisms in radiation nephropathy remain unclear, despite extensive animal experimentation. Studies in certain species of mammals (especially rodents [rats and mice] and canines) suggest a major toxicity to the tubular epithelium, followed by tubular necrosis and regeneration. More recent studies in other species (especially pigs and monkeys) suggest primary injury to the vascular endothelium (especially glomeruli and the peritubular capillaries), with secondary tubular injury. The exact primary site of injury in man is not certain at the present time (3,21).

Treatment and Prognosis. The dosage of radiation required to elicit renal cellular damage approaches 2,300 R, delivered to both kidneys. A number of considerations are important when considering specific organ (renal) tolerance to radiation, including the use of potentiating renal nephrotoxins and the portal and methods of irradiation.

IDIOPATHIC TUBULOINTERSTITIAL NEPHRITIS

Idiopathic tubulointerstitial nephritis represents a number of diverse conditions. Obviously, this diagnosis can only be made by the exclusion of the various etiologic agents previously considered. It may be acute, granulomatous, or chronic, as described in the preceding sections. Because the morphologic changes are nonspecific, close clinicopathologic correlation is mandatory before the diagnosis of idiopathic tubulointerstitial nephritis is entertained; it is a diagnosis of exclusion and defeat (18).

REFERENCES

1. Abraham PA, Keane WF. Glomerular and interstitial disease induced by nonsteroidal anti-inflammatory drugs. Am J Nephrol 1984;4:1–6.
2. Adler SG, Cohen AH, Border WA. Hypersensitivity phenomenon and the kidney: role of drugs and environmental agents. Am J Kidney Dis 1985;5:75–96.
3. Alpers CE. Irradiation injury. In: Jennette JC, Olson JL, Schwartz MM, Silva FG, eds. Heptinstall's pathology of the kidney, 5th ed. Philadelphia: Lippincott-Raven; 1998:1131–48.
4. Antonovych TT. Drug-induced nephropathies. Pathol Annu 1984;19:165–96.
5. Appel GB. Acute interstitial nephritis. In: Nielsen EE, Couser WG, eds. Immunologic renal disease. Philadelphia: Lippincott-Raven; 1997:1221–34.
6. Appel GB, Kunis CL. Acute tubulo-interstitial nephritis. In: Cotran RS [guest ed.], Brenner BM, Stein JH, eds. Tubulointerstitial nephritis. Contemporary issues in nephrology, vol. 10. New York: Churchill Livingstone; 1983:151–85.
7. Bender WL, Whelton A, Beschorner WE, Darwish MO, Hall-Craggs M, Solez K. Interstitial nephritis, proteinuria, and renal failure caused by nonsteroidal anti-inflammatory drugs. Immunologic characterization of the inflammatory infiltrate. Am J Med 1984;76:1006–12.
8. Bengtsson U, Johansson S, Angervall L. Malignancies in the urinary tract and their relation to analgesic abuse. Kidney Int 1978;13:107–13.
9. Bertani T, Remuzzi G, Garattini S, eds. Drugs and kidney, vol 33. Serono Symposia Publications. New York: Raven Press; 1986.
10. Bohle A, Mackensen-Haen S, von Gise H. Significance of tubulointerstitial changes in the renal cortex for the excretory function and concentration ability of the kidney: a morphometric contribution. Am J Nephrol 1987;7:421–33.
11. Bohle A, Mackenseon-Haen S, von Gise H, et al. The consequences of tubulo-interstitial changes for renal function in glomerulopathies. A morphometric and cytological analysis. Pathol Res Pract 1990;186:135–44.
12. Brentjens JR, Matsuo S, Fukatsu A, et al. Immunologic studies in two patients with antitubular basement membrane nephritis. Am J Med 1989;86:603–8.
13. Brentjens JR, Noble B, Andres GA. Immunologically mediated lesions of kidney tubules and interstitium in laboratory animals and in man. Springer Semin Immunopathol 1982;5:357–78.
14. Brunati C, Brando B, Confalonieri R, Belli LS, Lavagni MG, Minetti L. Immunophenotyping of mononuclear cell infiltrates associated with renal disease. Clin Nephrol 1986;26:15–20.
15. Buysen JG, Houthoff HJ, Krediet RT, Arisz L. Acute interstitial nephritis: a clinical and morphological study in 27 patients. Nephrol Dial Transplant 1990;5:94–9.
16. Cacoub P, Deray G, Le Hoang P, et al. Idiopathic acute interstitial nephritis associated with anterior uveitis in adults. Clin Nephrol 1989;31:307–10.
17. Cameron JS. Allergic interstitial nephritis: clinical features and pathogenesis. Q J Med 1988;66:97–115.
18. Cavallo T. Tubulointerstitial nephritis. In: Jennette JC, Olson JL, Schwartz MM, Silva FG, eds. Heptinstall's pathology of the kidney, 5th ed. Philadelphia: Lippincott-Raven; 1998:667–723.
19. Cheng HF, Nolasco F, Cameron JS, et al. HLA-DR display by renal tubular epithelium and phenotype of infiltrate in interstitial nephritis. Nehrol Dial Transplant 1989;4:205–15.
20. Churg J, Cotran RS, Sinniah R, et al. Renal disease. Classification and atlas of tubulointerstitial disease. New York: Igaku-Shoin; 1985.
21. Cohen EP. Radiation nephropathy after bone marrow transplantation. Kidney Int 2000;58: 903–18.
22. Cohen MS. Granulomatous nephritis. Urol Clin North Am 1986;13:647–59.
23. Colvin RB, Fang LS. Interstitial nephritis. In: Tisher CC, Brenner BM, eds. Renal pathology: with clinical and functional correlations, 2nd ed. Philadelphia: Lippincott; 1994:723–68.
24. Corwin HL, Korbet SM, Schwartz MM. Clinical correlates of eosinophiluria. Arch Intern Med 1985;145:1097–9.
25. Cotran RS, Galvenek E. Immunopathology of the human tubulo-interstitial diseases: localization of immunoglobulins, complement, and Tamm-Horsfall protein. Contrib Nephrol 1979;16:126–31.

26. Cotran RS, Thiru S, Verani R, et al. Tubulointerstitial nephropathies. In: Brenner BM, Rector FC, eds. The kidney. Philadelphia: WB Saunders; 1988.
27. D'Agati VD, Theise ND, Pirani CL, Knowles DM, Appel GB. Interstitial nephritis related to nonsteroidal anti-inflammatory agents and beta-lactam antibiotics: a comparative study of the interstitial infiltrates using monoclonal antibodies. Mod Pathol 1989;2:390–6.
28. De Broe ME, Elseviers MM. Analgesic nephropathy. N Engl J Med 1998;338:446–52.
29. Diamond JR, Pallone TL. Acute interstitial nephritis following use of tung shueh pills. Am J Kidney Dis 1994;24:219–21.
30. Dubach UC, Rosner B, Pfister E. Epidemiologic study of abuse of analgesics containing phenacetin. Renal morbidity and mortality (1968-1979). N Engl J Med 1983;308:357–62.
31. Eknoyan G, McDonald MA, Appel D, Truong LD. Chronic tubulo-interstitial nephritis: correlation between structural and functional findings. Kidney Int 1990;38:736–43.
32. Ellis D, Fried WA, Yunis J, Blau EB. Acute interstitial nephritis in children: a report of 13 cases and review of the literature. Pediatrics 1981;67: 862–70.
33. Feinstein AR, Heinemann LA, Curhan GC, et al. Relationship between nonphenacetin combined analgesics and nephropathy: a review. Ad Hoc Committee of the International Study Group on Analgesics and Nephropathy. Kidney Int 2000;58:2259–64.
34. Galpin JE, Shinaberger JH, Stanley TM, et al. Acute interstitial nephritis due to methicillin. Am J Med 1978;65:756–65.
35. Grcevska L, Polenakovic M, Oncevski A, Zografski D, Gligic A. Different pathohistological presentations of acute renal involvement in Hantaan virus infection: report of two cases. Clin Nephrol 1990;34:197–201.
36. Greising J, Trachtman H, Gauthier B, Valderrama E. Acute interstitial nephritis in adolescents and young adults. Child Nephrol Urol 1990;10:189–95.
37. Haas M, Spargo BH, Wit EJ, Meehan SM. Etiologies and outcome of acute renal insufficiency in older adults: a renal biopsy study of 259 cases. Am J Kidney Dis 2000;35:433–47.
38. Haines JD Jr, Calhoon H. Interstitial nephritis in a patient with Legionnaires' disease. Postgrad Med 1987;81:77–9.
39. Hannedouche T, Grateau G, Noel LH, et al. Renal granulomatous sarcoidosis: report of six cases. Nephrol Dial Transplant 1990;5:18–24.
40. Hawkins EP, Berry PL, Silva FG. Acute tubulointerstitial nephritis in children: clinical, morphologic, and lectin studies. A report of the Southwest Pediatric Nephrology Study Group. Am J Kidney Dis 1989;14:466–71.
41. Heptinstall RH. Interstitial nephritis. A brief review. Am J Pathol 1976;83:214–36.
42. Heptinstall RH. Interstitial nephritis. In: Heptinstall RH, ed. Pathology of the kidney, 4th ed. Boston: Little, Brown and Co; 1992:1315–68.
43. Houghton DC, English J, Bennett WM. Chronic tubulointerstitial nephritis and renal insufficiency associated with long-term "subtherapeutic" gentamicin. J Lab Clin Med 1988;112:694–703.
44. Ivanyi B, Marcussen N, Kemp E, Olsen TS. The distal nephron is preferentially infiltrated by inflammatory cells in acute interstitial nephritis. Virchows Arch A Pathol Anat Histopathol 1992;420:37–42.
45. Ivanyi B, Olsen S. Tubulitis in renal disease. Curr Top Pathol 1995;88:117–43.
46. Jaradat M, Phillips C, Yum MN, Cushing H, Moe S. Acute tubulointerstitial nephritis attributable to indinavir therapy. Am J Kidney Dis 2000;35: E16.
47. Kambham N, Markowitz GS, Tanji N, Mansukhani MM, Orzi A, D'Agati, VD. Idiopathic hypocomplementemic interstitial nephritis with extensive tubulointerstitial deposits. Am J Kidney Dis 2001;37:388–99.
48. Kashgarian M. Tubulointerstitial diseases. In: Silva FG, D'Agati VD, Nadasdy T, eds. Renal biopsy interpretation. New York: Churchill Livingstone; 1996:309–31.
49. Katz A, Fish AJ, Santamaria P, Nevins TE, Kim Y, Butkowski RJ. Role of antibodies to tubulointerstitial nephritis antigen in human anti-tubular basement membrane nephritis associated with membranous nephropathy. Am J Med 1992;93:691–8.
50. Kelly CJ, Neilson EG. Tubulointerstitial diseases. In: Brenner BM, ed. Brenner & Rector's the kidney, 5th ed. Philadelphia: WB Saunders; 1986:1655–79.
51. Kern WF, Silva FG, Laszik ZG, Bane BL, Nadasdy T, Pitha JV, eds. Disorders of the interstitium: interstitial nephritis, pyelonephritis, papillary necrosis, analgesic nephropathy, and obstructive nephropathy (hydronephrosis). In: Kern WF, ed. Atlas of renal pathology. Philadelphia: W.B. Saunders; 1999:136–57.
52. Kleinknecht D. Interstitial nephritis, the nephrotic syndrome, and chronic renal failure secondary to nonsteroidal anti-inflammatory drugs. Semin Nephrol 1995;15:228–35.
53. Kleinknecht D, Kanfer A, Morel-Maroger L, Mery JP. Immunologically mediated drug-induced acute renal failure. Contrib Nephrol 1978;10:42–52.
54. Kunin CM. Urinary tract infections: detection, prevention, and management, 5th ed. Baltimore: Williams & Wilkins; 1997.
55. Laberke HG, Bohle A. Acute interstitial nephritis: correlations between clinical and morphological findings. Clin Nephrol 1980;14:263–73.

56. Lien YH, Hansen R, Kern WF, et al. Ciprofloxacin-induced granulomatous interstitial nephritis and localized elastolysis. Am J Kidney Dis 1993;22:598–602.
57. Markowitz GS, Radhakrishnan J, Kambham N, Valeri AM, Hines WH, D'Agati VD. Lithium nephrotoxicity: a progressive combined glomerular and tubulointerstitial nephropathy. J Am Soc Nephrol 2000;11:1439–48.
58. Mathew TH. Drug-induced renal disease. Med J Aust 1992;156:724–8.
59. Michel DM, Kelly CJ. Acute interstitial nephritis. J Am Soc Nephrol 1998;9:506–15.
60. Mignon F, Mery JP, Mougenot B, Ronco P, Roland J, Morel-Maroger L. Granulomatous interstitial nephritis. Adv Nephrol Necker Hosp 1984;13:219–45.
61. Mihatsch MJ, Brunner FP, Gloor FJ. Analgesic nephropathy and papillary necrosis. In: Tisher CC, Brenner BM, eds. Renal pathology: with clinical and functional correlations, 2nd ed. Philadelphia: Lippincott; 1994:905–36.
62. Mihatsch MJ, Torhorst J, Steinmann E, et al. The morphologic diagnosis of analgesic (phenacetin) abuse. Pathol Res Pract 1979;164:68–79.
63. Murray KM, Keane WR. Review of drug-induced acute interstitial nephritis. Pharmacotherapy 1992;12:462–7.
64. Nadasdy T, Racusen LC. Renal injury caused by therapeutic and diagnostic agents and abuse of analgesics and narcotics. In: Jennette JC, Olson JL, Schwartz MM, Silva FG, eds. Heptinstall's pathology of the kidney, 5th ed. Philadelphia: Lippincott-Raven; 1998:811–61.
65. Neelakantappa K, Gallo GR, Lowenstein J. Ranitidine-associated interstitial nephritis and Fanconi syndrome. Am J Kidney Dis 1993;22:333–6.
66. Ong AC, Fine LG. Loss of glomerular function and tubulointerstitial fibrosis: cause or effect? Kidney Int 1994;45:345–51.
67. Ooi BS, Jao W, First MR, Mancilla R, Pollak VE. Acute interstitial nephritis. A clinical and pathologic study based on renal biopsies. Am J Med 1975;59:614–28.
68. Ottosen PD, Sigh B, Kristensen J, Olsen S, Christensen S. Lithium induced interstitial nephropathy associated with chronic renal failure. Reversibility and correlation between functional and structural changes. Acta Pathol Microbiol Immunol Scand (A) 1984;92:447–54.
69. Perneger TV, Whelton PK, Klag MJ. Risk of kidney failure associated with the use of acetaminophen, aspirin, and nonsteroidal antiinflammatory drugs. N Engl J Med 1994;331:1675–9.
70. Pommer W, Bronder E, Greiser E, et al. Regular analgesic intake and the risk of end-stage renal failure. Am J Nephrol 1989;9:403–12.
71. Pusey CD, Saltissi D, Bloodworth L, Rainford DJ, Christie JL. Drug associated acute interstitial nephritis: clinical and pathological features and the response to high dose steroid therapy. Q J Med 1983;52:194–211.
72. Rashed A, Azadeh B, Abu Romeh SH. Acyclovir-induced acute tubulointerstitial nephritis. Nephron 1990;56:436–8.
73. Rossert J. Drug-induced acute interstitial nephritis. Kidney Int 2001;60:804–17.
74. Schlondorff D. Renal complications of nonsteroidal anti-inflammatory drugs. Kidney Int 1993;44:643–53.
75. Schwarz A, Krause PH, Keller F, Offermann G, Mihatsch MJ. Granulomatous interstitial nephritis after nonsteroidal anti-inflammatory drugs. Am J Nephrol 1988;8:410–6.
76. Spoendlin M, Moch H, Brunner F, et al. Karyomegalic interstitial nephritis: further support for a distinct entity and evidence for a genetic defect. Am J Kidney Dis 1995;25:242–52.
77. Stefanovic V, Polenakovic MH. Balkan nephropathy. Kidney disease beyond the Balkans? Am J Nephrol 1991;11:1–11.
78. Szabolcs MJ, Seigle R, Shanske S, Bonilla E, DiMauro S, D'Agati V. Mitochondrial DNA deletion: a cause of chronic tubulointerstitial nephropathy. Kidney Int 1994;45:1388–96.
79. Vanhaesebrouck P, Carton D, De Bel C, Praet M, Proesmans W. Acute tubulointerstitial nephritis and uveitis syndrome (TINU syndrome). Nephron 1985;40:418–22.
80. Verani R, Nasir M, Foley R. Granulomatous interstitial nephritis after a jejunoileal bypass: an ultrastructural and histochemical study. Am J Nephrol 1989;9:51–5.
81. Viero RM, Cavallo T. Granulomatous interstitial nephritis. Hum Pathol 1995;26:1347–53.
82. Wandzilak TR, Williams HE. The hyperoxaluric syndromes. Endocrinol Metab Clin North Am 1990;19:851–67.
83. Whelton A. Nephrotoxicity of nonsteroidal anti-inflammatory drugs: physiologic foundation and clinical implications. Am J Med 1999;106:13S–24S.
84. Whelton A, Hamilton CW. Nonsteroidal anti-inflammatory drugs: effects on kidney function. J Clin Pharmacol 1991;31:588–98.
85. Williams AW, Wilson DM. Dietary intake, absorption, metabolism, and excretion of oxalate. Semin Nephrol 1990;10:2–8.

22 PLASMA CELL DYSCRASIA: TUBULOINTERSTITIAL INVOLVEMENT

MYELOMA CAST NEPHROPATHY

Definition. A number of different morphologic patterns of injury can be seen in the kidney of patients with one of the various plasma cell dyscrasias. These include myeloma cast nephropathy, monoclonal immunoglobulin deposition disease (including light chain deposition disease [LCDD], light/heavy chain deposition disease [LHCDD], heavy chain deposition disease [HCDD]), amyloidosis of the light (AL) or heavy chain (AH) type, and neoplastic infiltration of the renal parenchyma (27,32,38, 48). This section deals with the pattern known as myeloma cast nephropathy (*Bence Jones cast nephropathy* or *myeloma kidney)*, which is defined as extensive involvement of the kidney by renal tubular casts composed of monoclonal light chains, often associated with interstitial inflammation, fibrosis, infiltration of casts by polymorphonuclear leukocytes, giant cell reaction, and eventually tubular atrophy (8,9,12, 14,15,17,18,49,50,53,58,63).

Clinical Features. The plasma cell dyscrasias, or the dysproteinemias, represent an excessive neoplastic proliferation of a clone of plasma cells or B lymphocytes (2,23–25,29,44,61). This clone of cells often produces a monoclonal immunoglobulin (paraprotein) protein (M protein), which is detected as an M spike on electrophoresis of the serum or urine. Immunoelectrophoresis, followed by immunofixation, is usually required to determine the composition of the monoclonal protein. The paraprotein produced in large excess may be: 1) an intact immunoglobulin, including heavy/light chains, 2) a free light chain, 3) an intact immunoglobulin with excess free light chains, or 4) a free heavy chain. There are rare cases in which no M protein is detected (so called nonsecretory myeloma). The monoclonal immunoglobulins from a single patient share an identical heavy or light chain (either kappa or lambda light chain, but not both).

The most common plasma cell dyscrasia is a *monoclonal gammopathy of undetermined significance (MGUS)*, formerly termed *benign monoclonal gammopathy* (21,22). This is defined as an M spike on electrophoresis in patients who do not fulfill the clinical criteria for multiple myeloma. Only about one fourth of these patients develop overt multiple myeloma, often unpredictably. *Multiple myeloma* is the second most common monoclonal gammopathy. Although definitions of multiple myeloma vary in individual centers, most include a combination of features including: an M spike detected in serum and/or urine, plasmacytosis of at least 10 percent on bone marrow biopsy, hypercalcemia, and bony lesions (either sharply punched-out osteolytic lesions or diffuse osteopenia without discrete lesions). Other monoclonal gammopathies are caused by Waldenström's macroglobulinemia (immunoglobulin [Ig]M) and various forms of B-cell lymphoma (5).

Patients with multiple myeloma are usually older and present with back pain (due to the local effects of the tumor in the bone and often bone fractures), anemia, and hypercalcemia and hyperuricemia. The serum creatinine is elevated in most patients at the time of diagnosis (10,11,60). Acute renal failure is common and may be precipitated by episodes of dehydration or by intravenous radiographic contrast studies (11). Proteinuria is present in most patients, but the nephrotic syndrome is rare, unless there is an accompanying glomerular lesion (such as amyloidosis or monoclonal immunoglobulin deposition disease). The proteinuria is usually tubular (rather than glomerular) due to leakage of the monoclonal light chains into the urine (see Pathogenesis for further explanation). Because the proteinuria is nonalbuminuric, urine tested by dipstick for protein is usually only weakly positive, whereas urine tested for quantitated protein is substantially positive. This discrepancy, which can be an initial clue to the diagnosis of myeloma kidney, is explained by the fact that the dipstick method detects albumin only, and not light chain protein. Renal tubular dysfunction can result in

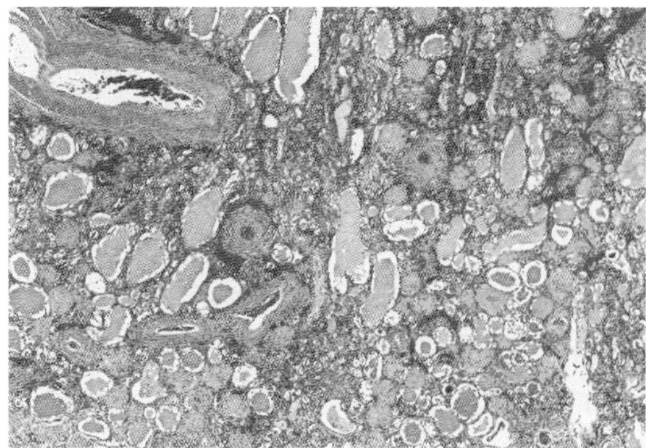

Figure 22-1

MYELOMA CAST NEPHROPATHY

There are a massive number of large, refractile, hyaline casts in the dilated renal cortical tubules (hematoxylin and eosin [H&E] stain).

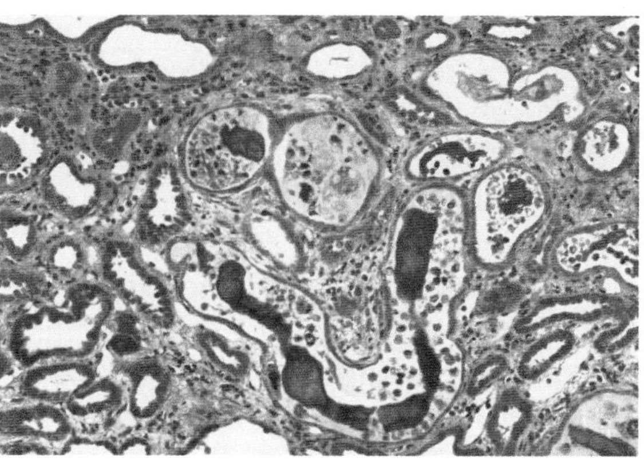

Figure 22-2

MYELOMA CAST NEPHROPATHY

There is a large noncellular hyaline cast present in the dilated and tortuous tubule. The cast has different tinctorial properties, implying multiple layers or deposition of material (Masson trichrome stain).

abnormal acidification, with renal tubular acidosis, defects in the ability to concentrate the urine, nephrogenic diabetes insipidus, and especially, Fanconi's syndrome. Hematuria is rare.

A monoclonal immunoglobulin protein (M spike or M component) is found in the serum or urine by protein electrophoresis in most patients with myeloma cast nephropathy. (Not all patients with myeloma cast nephropathy, however, have multiple myeloma; some may have MGUS). Although the nature of the serum protein varies, it is common to detect free light chains (Bence Jones protein) in the urine. Quantitated total serum immunoglobulin is often depressed. Immunocytochemical studies to examine bone marrow using antisera to kappa and lambda light chains often show an imbalance of the normal 2–3 to 1 ratio of kappa to lambda light chains in the plasma cell cytoplasm, consistent with a clonal proliferation, even in cases that lack plasmacytosis. Serum immunoglobulins of the nonplasma cell dyscrasia type are typically depressed. The only way to determine the exact type of renal disease in a patient with a plasma cell dyscrasia is to perform a renal biopsy.

Gross Findings. The kidneys are usually normal in size and show no distinctive gross features. They may be enlarged in some cases, but the cortical surface is generally smooth (unless there is some accompanying arterio/arteriolonephrosclerosis). On cross section, the cortex is pale but the corticomedullary distinctions are preserved.

Light Microscopic Findings. The most characteristic and virtually pathognomic lesion in myeloma cast nephropathy is in the tubules. There are extensive, large, long and straight, hyaline refractile casts in the tubular system, most commonly the distal tubules and collecting ducts (figs. 22-1, 22-2). In some cases, casts also involve proximal tubules and Bowman's space. These are the largest known casts. These distinctive casts often give the appearance of being brittle or hard and "crackable," and fragment on sectioning (figs. 22-3, 22-4).

The casts are dense, strongly eosinophilic, acellular, and may appear multilamellar. They are usually only weakly positive with the periodic acid–Schiff (PAS) stain, if at all, and often negative with the Jones methenamine silver (JMS) stain. With the trichrome stain, the casts appear polychromatic, with a mixed red-blue coloration in distinct lamellations. The tubular casts may have a fibrillar or crystalloid-like structure (figs. 22-5, 22-6). Some casts exhibit apple-green birefringence following Congo red staining, as seen with the polarizing light microscope, but this finding does not merit the diagnosis of renal amyloidosis since the amyloid is exclusively intratubular and not deposited in the renal parenchyma (figs. 22-7, 22-8) (6,59). The accompanying tubules are dilated and the epithelium often is degenerated, with thinning, atrophy, and the presence of cytoplasmic protein droplets

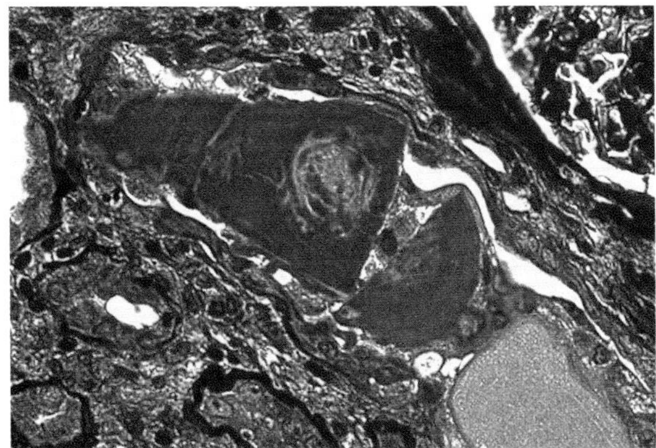

Figure 22-3

MYELOMA CAST NEPHROPATHY

The large, acellular, hyaline cast shows a cleavage plane or "fracture" which is quite characteristic, although perhaps not pathognomonic, for myeloma cast nephropathy (Masson trichrome stain).

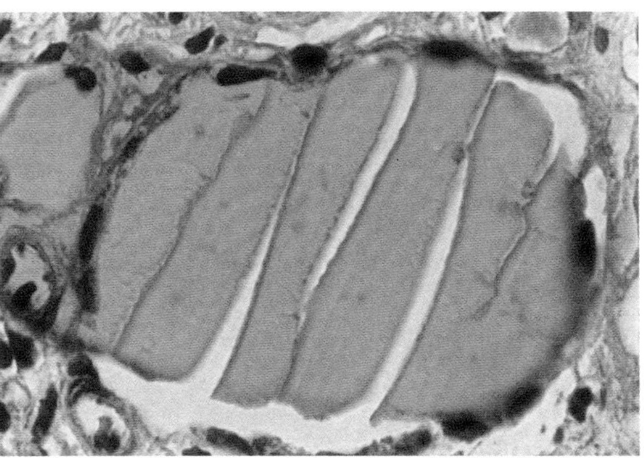

Figure 22-4

MYELOMA CAST NEPHROPATHY

The large, acellular, glassy, hyaline refractile cast gives a "crackable" look when sectioned with the microtome. It is apparently so hard that the microtome blade has displaced the cast from the tubular lumen (H&E stain).

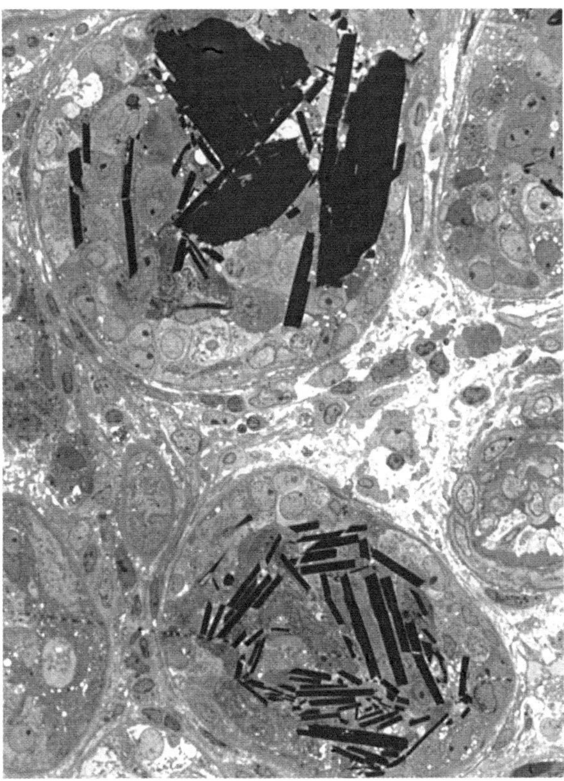

Figure 22-5

MYELOMA CAST NEPHROPATHY

This plastic-embedded section (Epon for electron microscopic studies) shows that the large casts appear "crackable," with jagged edges. This is characteristic, although probably not pathognomonic, of a plasma cell dyscrasia–induced myeloma cast nephropathy.

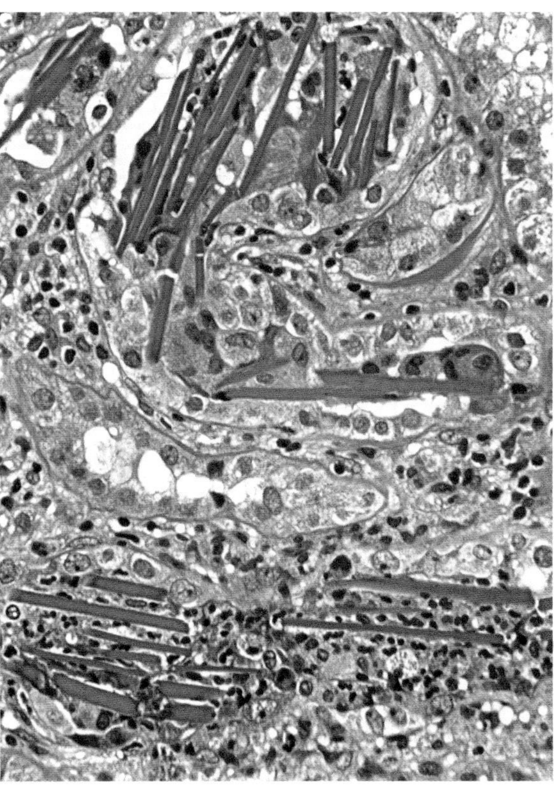

Figure 22-6

MYELOMA CAST NEPHROPATHY

The casts are composed of multiple elongated spicular crystals which appear to erode the thinned tubular epithelium. There are a number of polymorphonuclear leukocytes on the edges of these elongated casts (periodic acid–Schiff [PAS] stain).

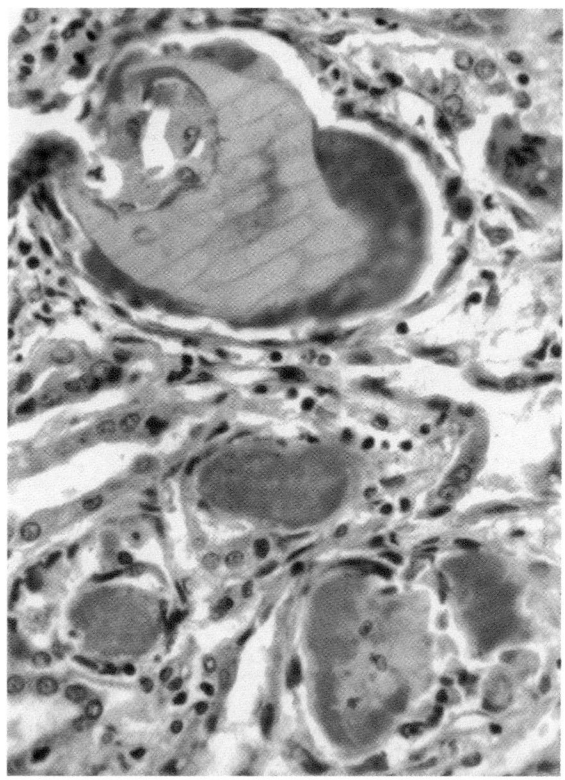

Figure 22-7

MYELOMA CAST NEPHROPATHY

There are a number of large casts in the extremely dilated tubular system. The multiple layers or lamination of the stained area suggests successive deposition of acellular material (Congo red stain).

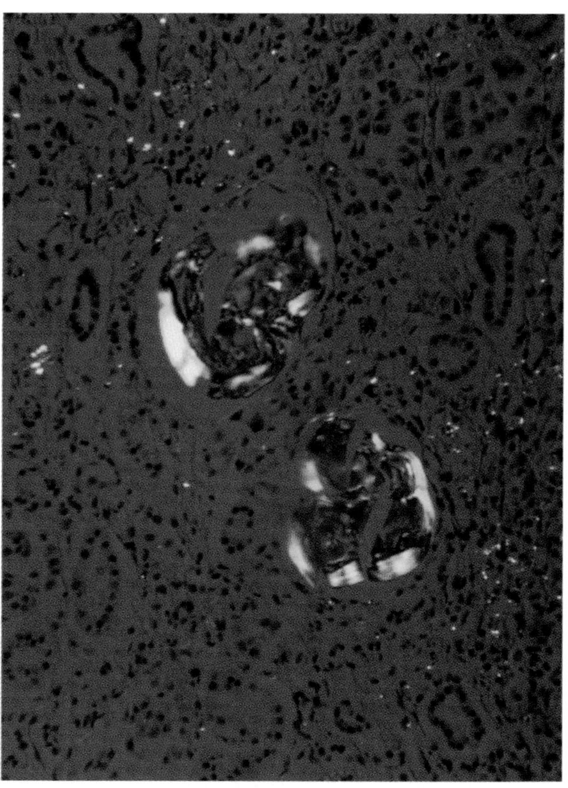

Figure 22-8

MYELOMA CAST NEPHROPATHY

Apple green birefringence of the amyloid-positive cast is seen in this patient with classic myeloma cast nephropathy. This is not considered tissue deposition of amyloid and the diagnosis of renal amyloidosis is not warranted (Congo red stain with polarization).

or even large hyperchromatic nuclei (fig. 22-9). There may be sloughing of the tubular epithelium and focal denudation of the tubular basement membranes.

The widespread tubular degeneration and atrophy is not only confined to the tubules containing the casts. Occasionally, a thinned layer of dehisced cells (probably tubular epithelium) overlies and covers some of the acellular cast material; however, this is not specific for a plasma cell dyscrasia. The casts are thought to increase in size with time, leading to intratubular obstruction and renal failure. Most investigators, however, have not found good evidence of a direct relationship between the extent of cast formation and the degree of tubular atrophy and interstitial fibrosis.

The casts are often surrounded by mononuclear cells and, especially, characteristic multinucleated giant cells and polymorphonuclear leukocytes, which often give the appearance of trying to engulf or phagocytize the cast material (figs. 22-10, 22-11). In the past, there was some debate whether the origin of the multinucleated giant cells was tubular or hematopoietic. Immunocytochemical and lectin studies have shown that these multinucleated cells are indeed hematopoietic (monocyte/macrophage lineage), entering the renal tubular lumen probably through gaps in the tubular basement membranes and then fusing to form the characteristic giant cells (1,51,52,56). Polymorphonuclear leukocytes are often found in relatively large numbers at the edge of these casts; indeed, this is one of the few conditions other than acute bacterial pyelonephritis or fulminant viral infection of the tubules in which moderate to large numbers of

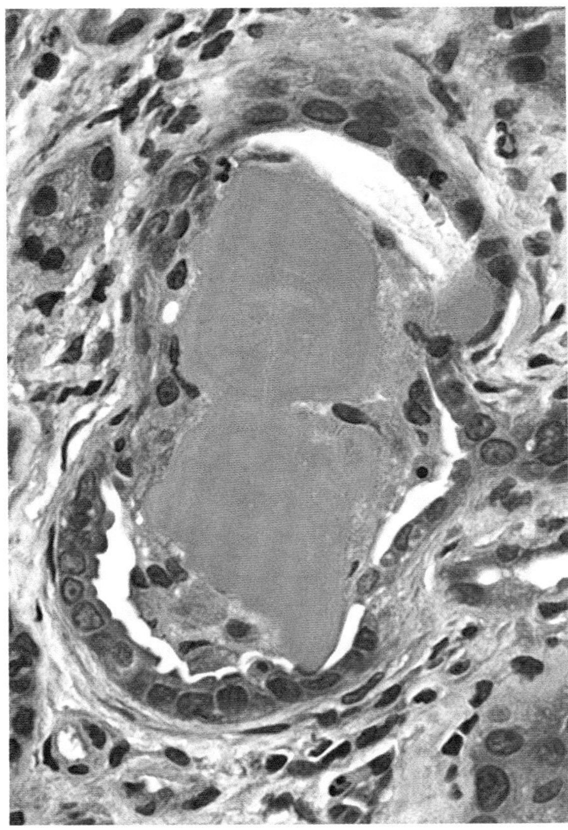

Figure 22-9

MYELOMA CAST NEPHROPATHY

The large cast is associated with alteration of the tubular epithelium and focal thinning. In other areas, the altered tubular epithelium is cuboidal (H&E stain).

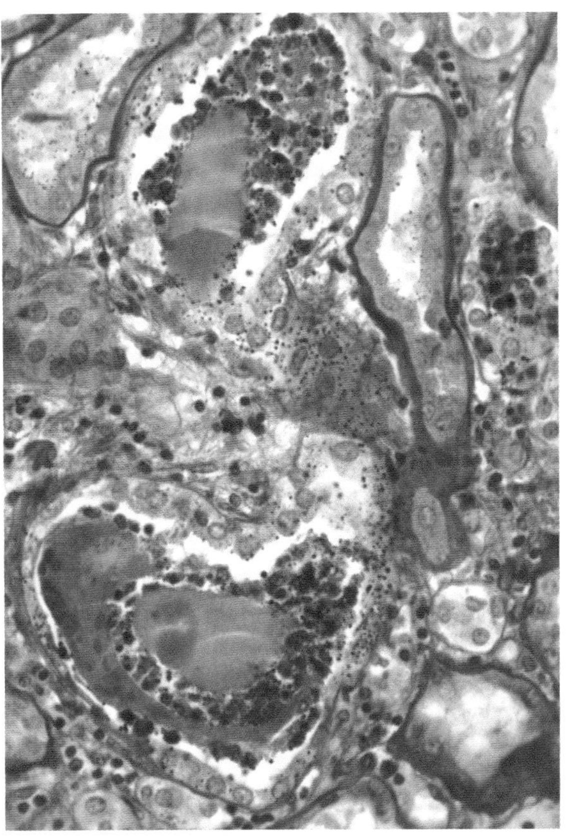

Figure 22-10

MYELOMA CAST NEPHROPATHY

The casts and the giant cell are surrounded by polymorphonuclear leukocytes. This is characteristic of myeloma cast nephropathy (PAS stain).

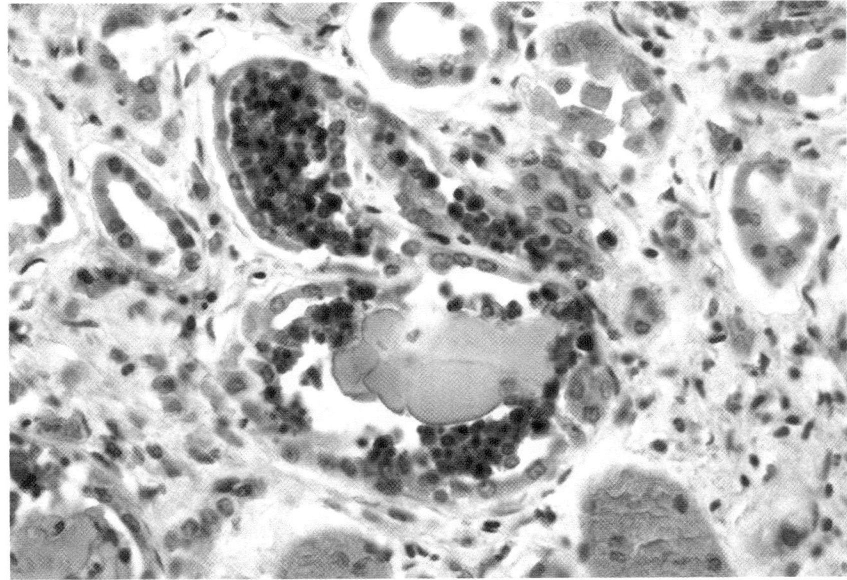

Figure 22-11

MYELOMA CAST NEPHROPATHY

The large casts are surrounded by many polymorphonuclear leukocytes. Polymorphonuclear leukocytes are not only found in patients with acute infection (acute bacterial pyelonephritis) but can also be seen, characteristically, in myeloma cast nephropathy (Leder stain).

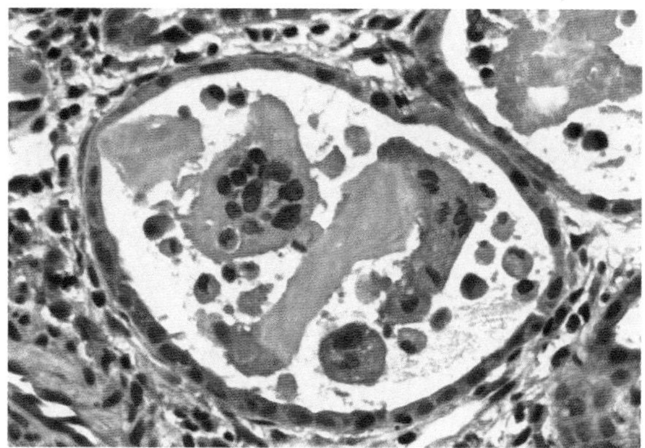

Figure 22-12

MYELOMA CAST NEPHROPATHY

The casts are surrounded by large multinucleated giant cells. This is quite characteristic of myeloma cast nephropathy, although it has on rare occasion (as a result of a certain drug or a pancreatic neoplasm) been described in patients apparently without a plasma cell dyscrasia (H&E stain).

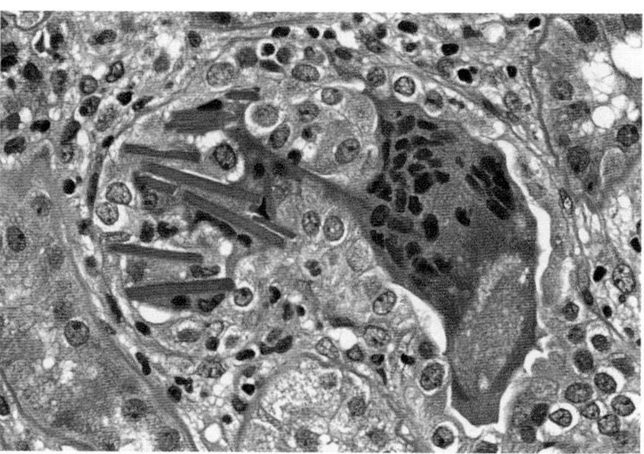

Figure 22-13

MYELOMA CAST NEPHROPATHY

The cast is surrounded by a large multinucleated giant cell. The origin/nature of these giant cells has been controversial in the past (H&E stain).

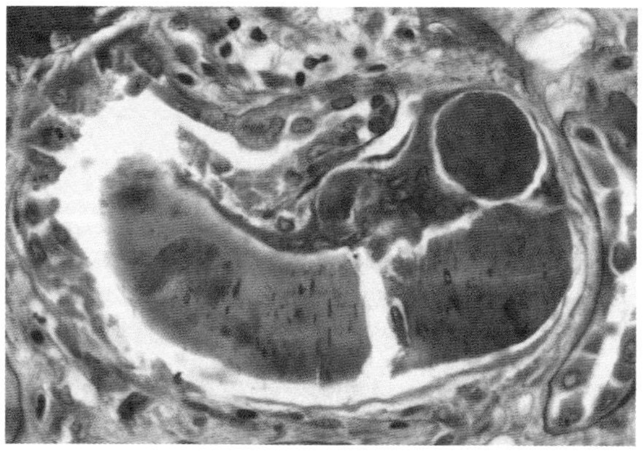

Figure 22-14

MYELOMA CAST NEPHROPATHY

Giant cells surround and appear to adhere to the large acellular cast material (H&E stain).

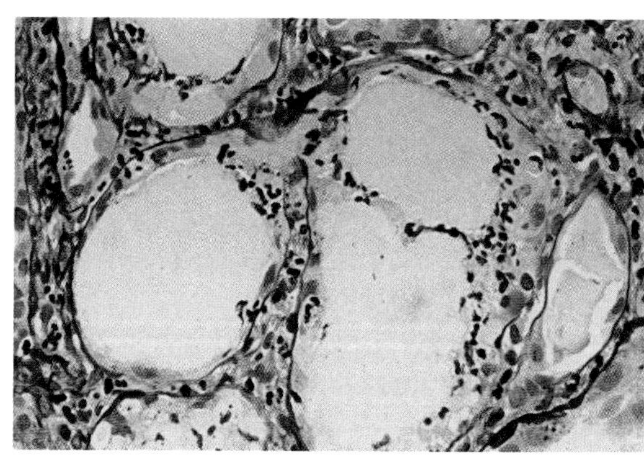

Figure 22-15

MYELOMA CAST NEPHROPATHY

The large casts are surrounded by giant cells and neutrophils and appear to be breaking through the nearby tubular basement membrane. Note the surrounding interstitial inflammation. The loss of the tubular basement membrane staining is consistent with tubulorrhexis (Jones methenamine silver [JMS] stain).

polymorphonuclear leukocytes can be seen in the renal tubules (figs. 22-10, 22-11). The combination of fractured hard casts, giant cells, and polymorphonuclear infiltrates is quite distinctive of myeloma cast nephropathy (figs. 22-12–22-14).

Renal interstitial changes may be present and include interstitial fibrosis, edema, and inflammation. If the large hyaline casts exude or extravasate into the adjacent interstitium, there may be severe inflammation, even with the formation of giant cells in the interstitium (figs. 22-15–22-17). Rarely, the crystal-like cast formations extravasate into the renal interstitium.

Glomerular changes are often minor, with only a slight increase in mesangial matrix or thickening of the glomerular basement membranes. Light chain deposition disease and other glomerular plasma cell dyscrasias are covered elsewhere (35). A small percentage of patients with plasma cell dyscrasia may have both

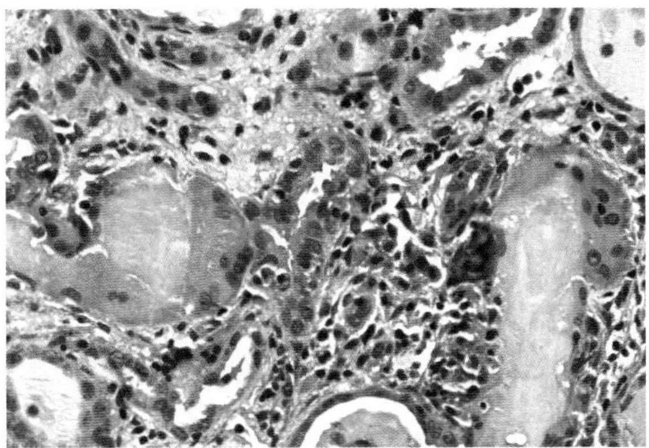

Figure 22-16

MYELOMA CAST NEPHROPATHY

The large casts extravasate outside the tubular lumens. Giant cells are attached to the large acellular cast (H&E stain).

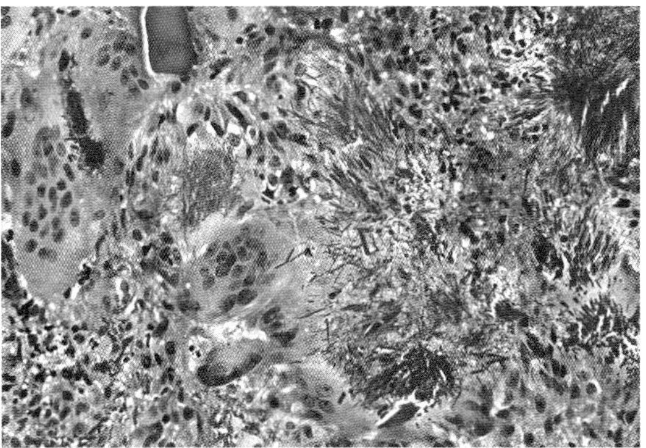

Figure 22-17

PLASMA CELL DYSCRASIA

Extratubular deposition of light chain material is seen. The trichrome-red spicular material breaks through the tubular basement membrane and is deposited in the renal interstitium (Masson trichrome stain). (Courtesy of Dr. A. Cohen, Los Angeles, CA.)

myeloma cast nephropathy and a monoclonal immunoglobulin deposition disease, usually light chain deposition disease (usually kappa). In these patients, light chains are deposited in the glomerular mesangium, and the glomerular and tubular basement membranes (fig. 22-18). An even smaller percentage of patients have myeloma cast nephropathy and amyloidosis, which can affect any renal compartment. Cases with overlapping pathologic patterns are usually distinguished by the presence of severe albuminuria due to the glomerular lesion.

Because most cases of myeloma cast nephropathy occur in older patients, there may be associated advancing lesions of arterionephrosclerosis and arteriolonephrosclerosis. There may be morphologic evidence of hypercalcemia with nephrocalcinosis (fig. 22-19) or myelomatous infiltration of the renal parenchyma (figs. 22-20, 22-21).

Immunofluorescence Findings. In contradistinction to earlier studies (26,53), there is general consensus now that the characteristic finding on immunofluorescence is strong, dominant staining of the casts for a single light chain (either kappa or lambda) (12,27), especially in early disease or in cases where "acute" casts have not been covered by Tamm-Horsfall protein or a variety of tubular fluids (figs. 22-22, 22-23). Some cases may stain weakly for the other light chain, but the discrepancy in intensity is usually obvious. Staining for other immune reactants (such as albumin or immunoglobulins) may be found in some casts, especially ordinary (nonmyeloma) casts, or in the setting of concomitant glomerular disease with enhanced ultrafiltration of various serum proteins, thus leading to "contamination" of the tubular casts by the abnormally filtered serum proteins. In cases with myeloma cast nephropathy and overlapping with monoclonal

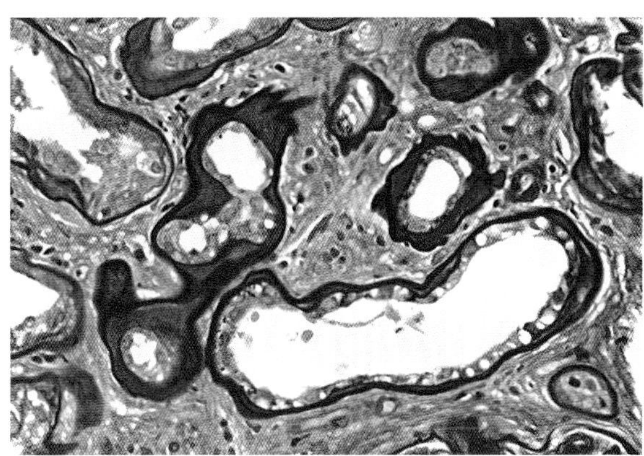

Figure 22-18

PLASMA CELL DYSCRASIA

There is marked thickening of the tubular basement membranes. This represents kappa light chain deposition. Both electron and immunofluorescence microscopy showed tubular basement membrane deposits. This patient had light chain deposition disease (PAS stain).

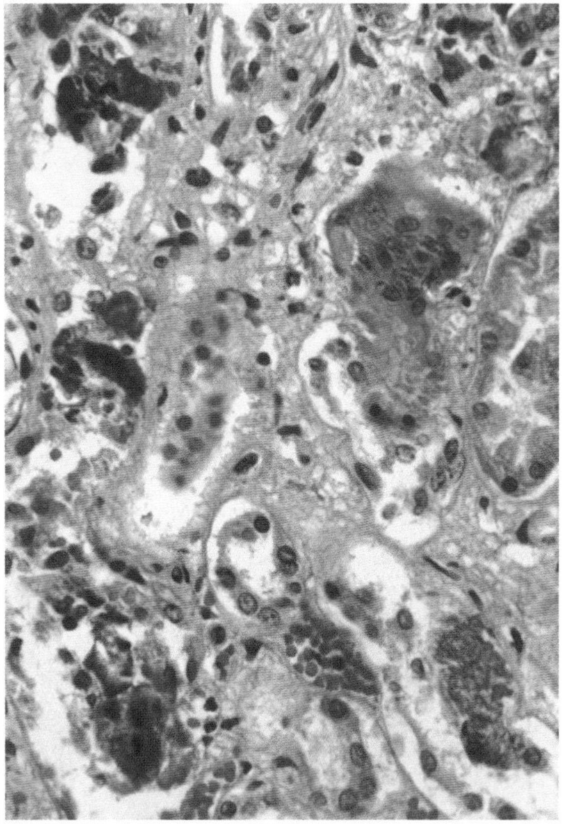

Figure 22-19

MYELOMA CAST NEPHROPATHY

There is marked deposition of calcium in this hypercalcemic patient with plasma cell dyscrasia and myeloma cast nephropathy.

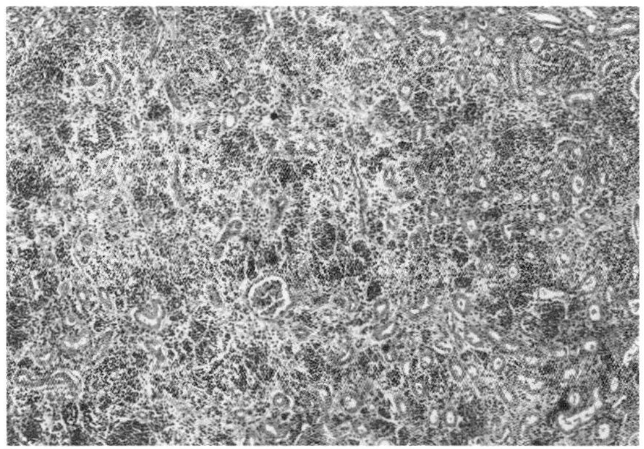

Figure 22-20

MYELOMATOUS INFILTRATION OF THE RENAL PARENCHYMA IN PATIENT WITH PLASMA CELL DYSCRASIA

There are several fairly well-localized nodules composed almost entirely of neoplastic plasma cells (H&E stain).

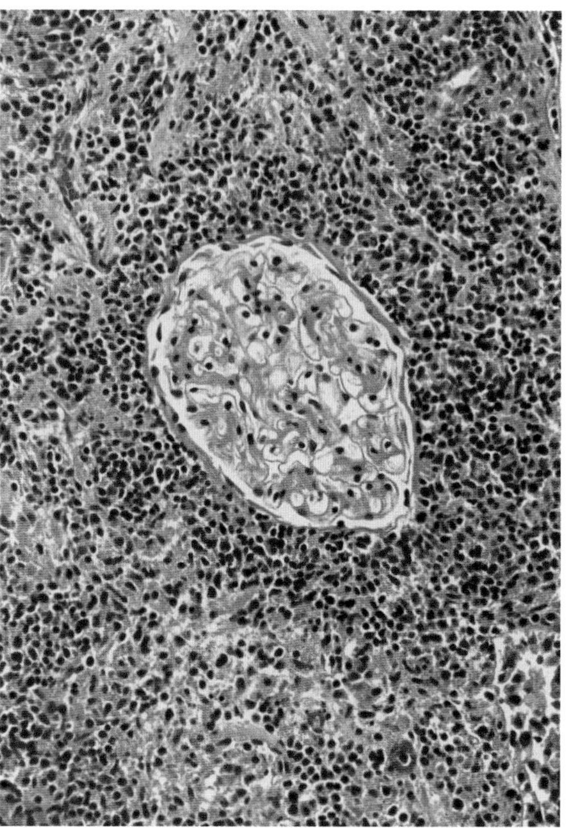

Figure 22-21

LYMPHOMA INVOLVING THE RENAL PARENCHYMA DIRECTLY

A large number of neoplastic lymphoid cells infiltrate into the renal interstitium.

immunoglobulin deposition disease, there is also linear staining of tubular (and sometimes glomerular) basement membranes for monoclonal light chains (figs. 22-24, 22-25) (12,27).

Electron Microscopic Studies. The ultrastructural appearance of the casts is variable. Most are highly electron dense and crackable (showing fractures upon sectioning) (figs. 22-26–22-29). They may be homogeneous, coarsely clumped, or fibrillar, and some contain large parallel linear arrays of fibrils or needle-like, round or rhomboid crystalloid structures. The latter are often described as a "linear lattice." Highly organized crystalline casts are quite distinctive of myeloma cast nephropathy. Fibrillar casts, however, are less specific and must be differentiated from Tamm-Horsfall casts. Electron-dense immune-type deposits may be noted in the tubular basement membranes and renal interstitium in some cases

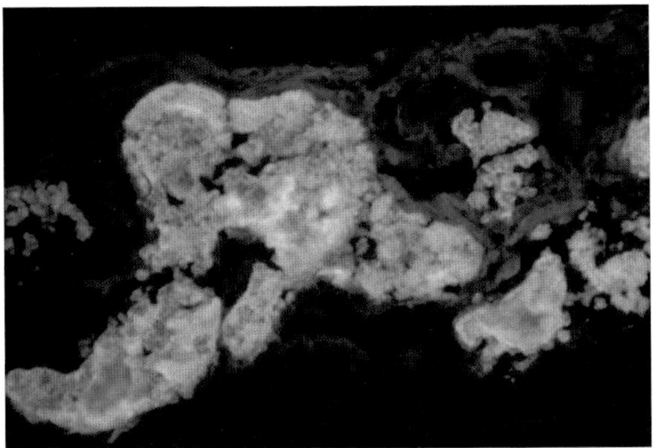

Figure 22-22

MYELOMA CAST NEPHROPATHY

The large confluent casts in the tubular lumens stain brightly for lambda light chain by immunofluorescence (antilambda light chain).

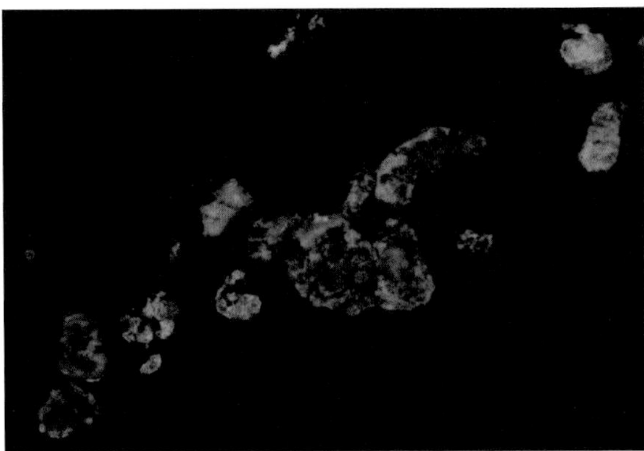

Figure 22-23

MYELOMA CAST NEPHROPATHY

Immunofluorescence with the antikappa light chain stain shows little or no staining of the same region and same casts as noted in figure 22-22. This is highly suggestive of lambda light chain deposition in the casts. This patient had myeloma cast nephropathy of the lambda light chain type.

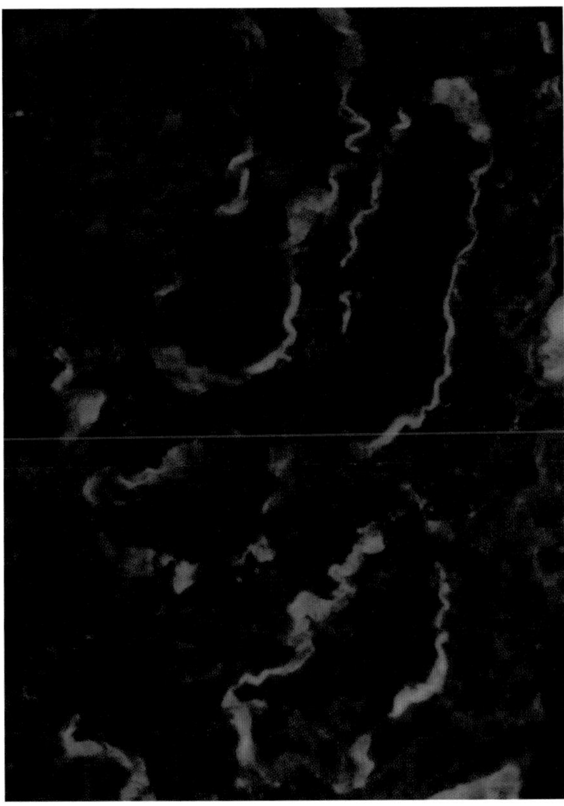

Figure 22-24

PLASMA CELL DYSCRASIA

Immunofluorescence using an antibody to kappa light chains shows strong linear staining along the tubular basement membranes in this patient with plasma cell dyscrasia. This patient had light chain deposition disease (antikappa light chain).

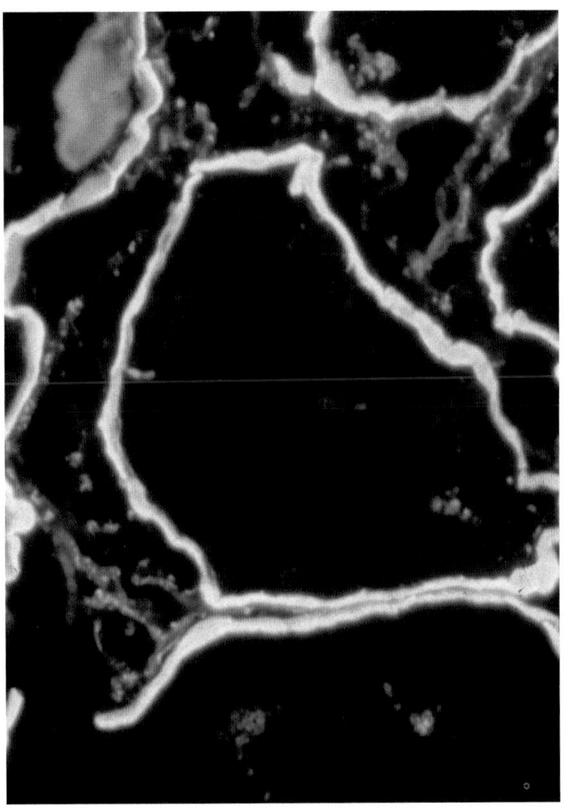

Figure 22-25

PLASMA CELL DYSCRASIA

Intense tubular basement membrane staining for antikappa light chain in this patient with plasma cell dyscrasia and a classic myeloma cast nephropathy (antikappa light chain).

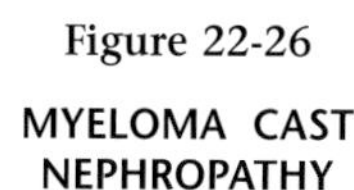

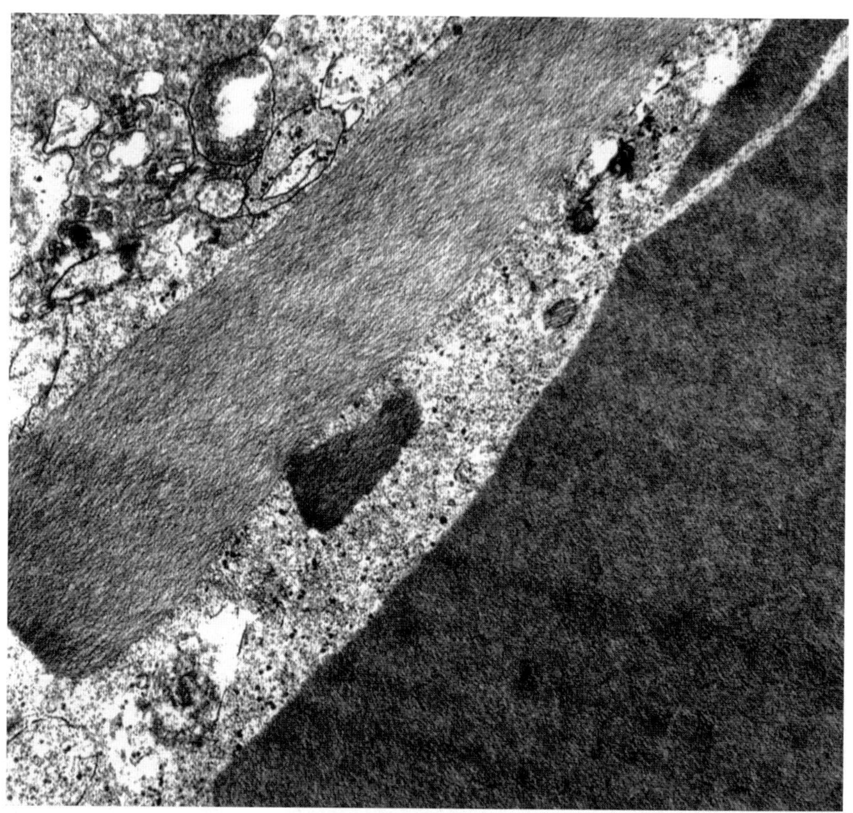

Figure 22-26

MYELOMA CAST NEPHROPATHY

Ultrastructural studies of the large hyaline casts show a fine fibrillar structure. Although this change is often seen in the casts of patients with myeloma cast nephropathy, it is probably not pathognomonic.

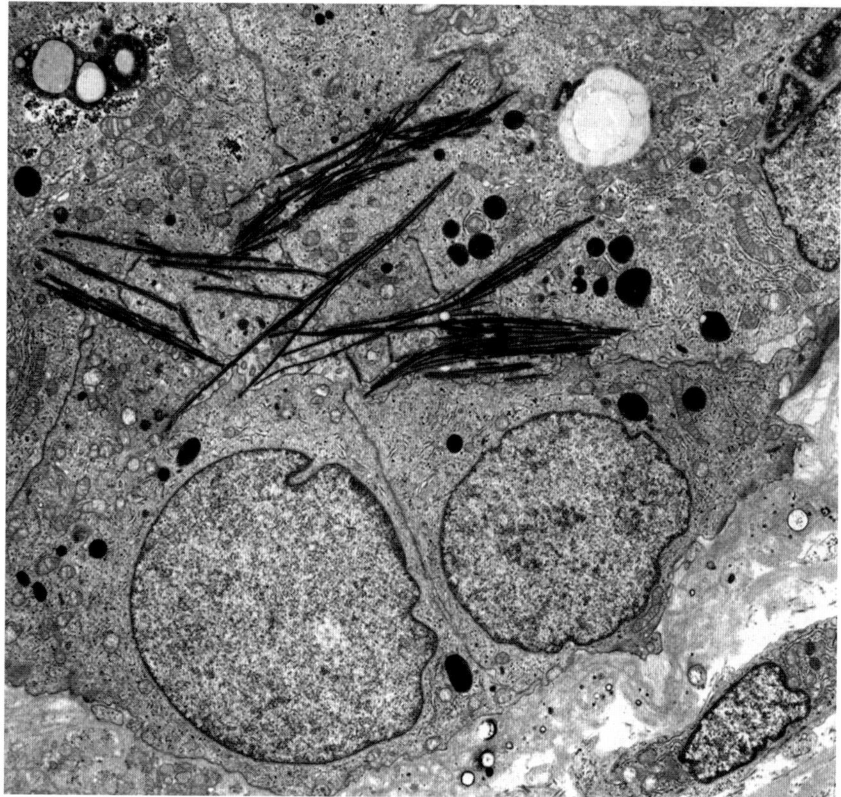

Figure 22-27

MYELOMA CAST NEPHROPATHY

Electron micrograph shows elongated, sharp-ended, spicular structures in myeloma cast nephropathy. This change is characteristic but probably not pathognomonic.

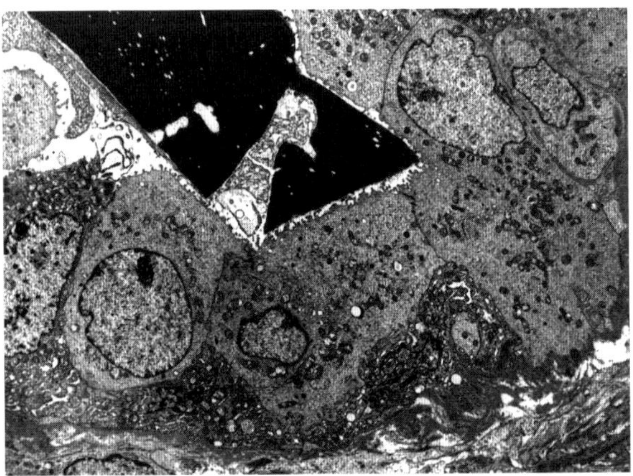

Figure 22-28

MYELOMA CAST NEPHROPATHY

Electron micrograph of a cast from a patient with myeloma cast nephropathy shows a large, "crackable," dense cast. This is characteristic but not pathognomonic.

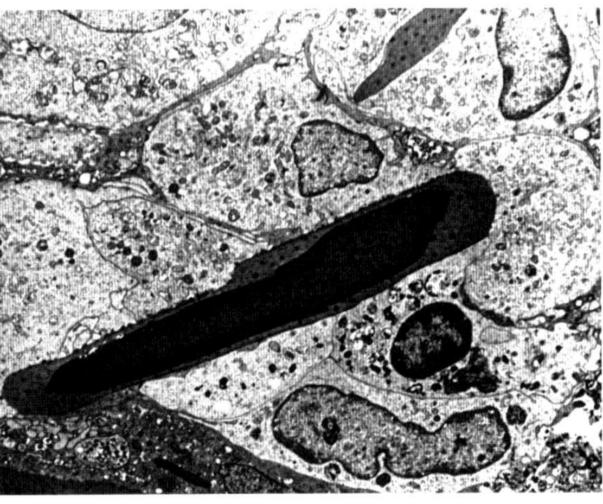

Figure 22-29

MYELOMA CAST NEPHROPATHY

Electron micrograph shows a cast surrounded by mononuclear cells, a probable stage in the giant cell formation.

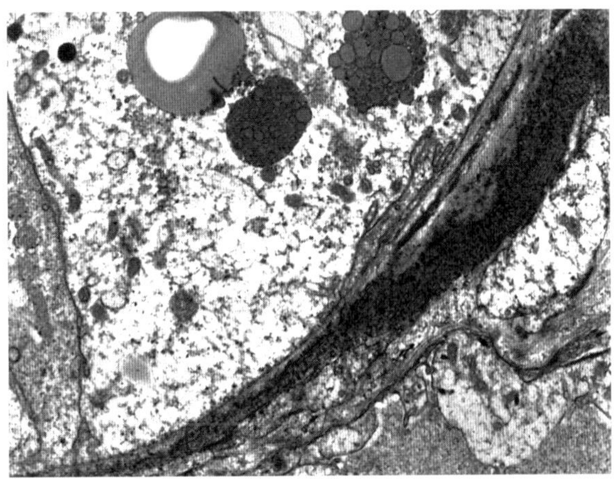

Figure 22-30

PLASMA CELL DYSCRASIA

Electron micrograph shows an electron-dense immune-type deposition in the tubular basement membrane. This patient had light chain deposition disease.

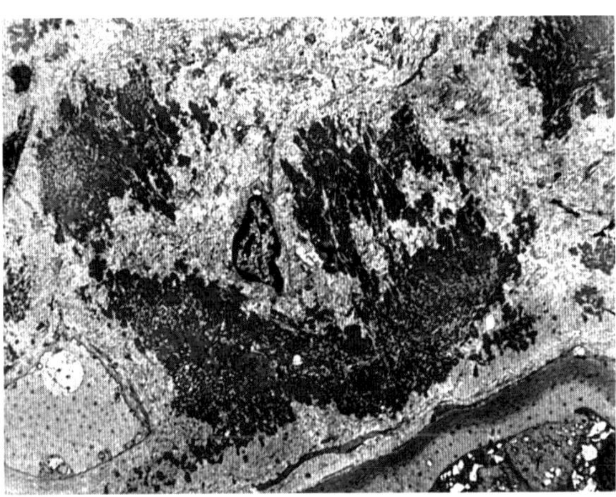

Figure 22-31

PLASMA CELL DYSCRASIA

Electron microscopy shows large electron-dense immune-type deposits in the renal interstitium. This patient had light chain deposition disease.

of light chain disease (usually associated with a monoclonal immunoglobulin deposition disease) (figs. 22-30, 22-31). In some patients with a plasma cell dyscrasia, the lysosomes of the tubular epithelium (especially the proximal tubular epithelium) contain large inclusions, probably representative of abnormal light chains that have been reabsorbed by the proximal tubular epithelium in their attempt to catabolize these filtered proteins (figs. 22-32, 22-33).

Special Studies. Immunocytochemistry for the detection of kappa and lambda light chains is usually not as sensitive as immunofluorescence on cryostat sections. If the renal sections (parenchyma or casts) are positive for one light chain but not the other (either kappa or lambda), then a diagnosis of plasma cell dyscrasia should be considered. There does not seem to be any specific heavy or light chain class or isotype that preferentially leads to myeloma cast nephropathy.

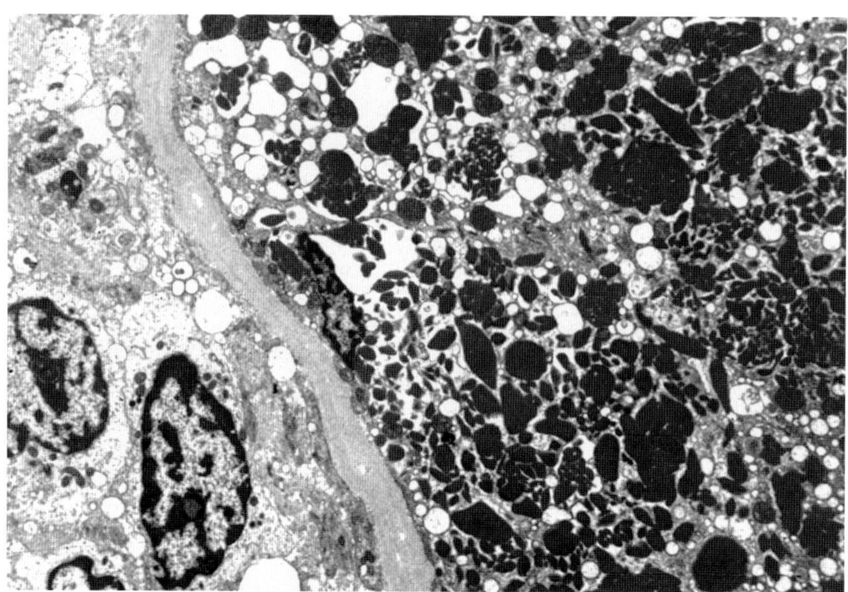

Figure 22-32

PLASMA CELL DYSCRASIA WITH TUBULAR EPITHELIAL CRYSTALS

These unusual inclusions are seen within the tubular epithelial lysosomes. This has been noted on many occasions with a plasma cell dyscrasia and probably represents reabsorption of the filtered light chain (electron micrograph).

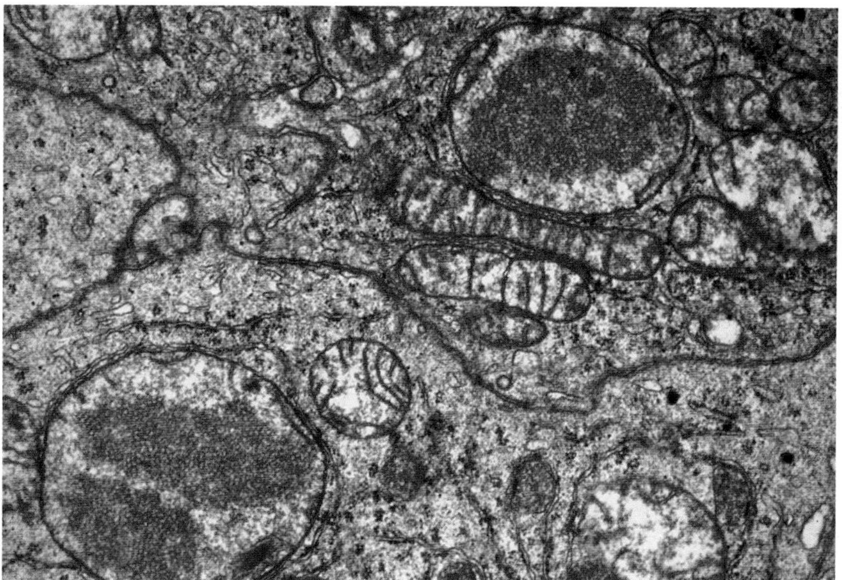

Figure 22-33

PLASMA CELL DYSCRASIA WITH TUBULAR EPITHELIAL CRYSTALS

Another patient with plasma cell dyscrasia and large inclusions within the lysosomes of the tubular epithelium (electron micrograph).

The most important special study is immunoelectrophoresis, with immunofixation of the serum and urine to confirm the presence of a monoclonal protein of the same light chain type. As noted before, immunocytochemical and lectin studies using a variety of antibodies and lectins with somewhat nephron-site specific abilities, have demonstrated that the giant cells are hematopoietic in origin, rather than tubular epithelial in origin (figs. 22-34, 22-35) (1,56). Other studies have shown intrarenal obstruction with "reflux" of Tamm-Horsfall protein throughout the nephron and into the renal interstitial spaces (fig. 22-36). In addition, immunocytochemical studies have demonstrated renal interstitial deposition of the light chains (figs. 22-37, 22-38).

Differential Diagnosis. There are a great many different clinical conditions that lead to renal insufficiency in a patient with a plasma cell dyscrasia, including amyloidosis, light chain deposition disease, dehydration, hypercalcemia, drug toxicity, acute tubular necrosis, interstitial inflammation, or radiocontrast toxicity. Renal biopsy is required for precise diagnosis.

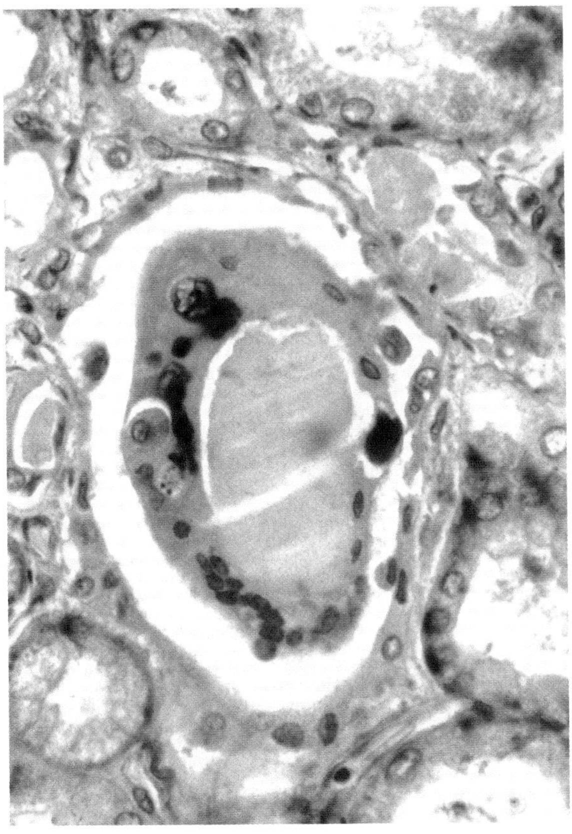

Figure 22-34

MYELOMA CAST NEPHROPATHY

This immunocytochemical stain shows the giant cells but not the tubular epithelial cells from this patient with characteristic myeloma cast nephropathy, suggesting that the giant cells are not of tubular origin (antivimentin stain).

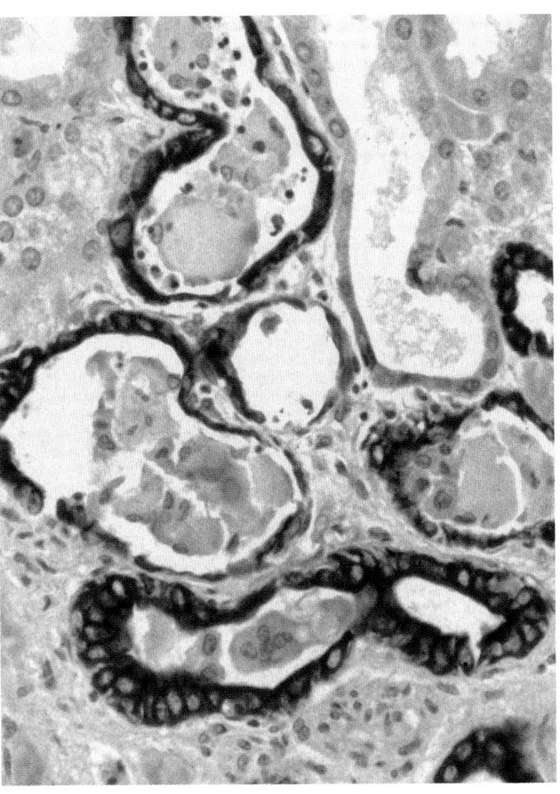

Figure 22-35

MYELOMA CAST NEPHROPATHY

The antisera to AE1/AE3 (cytokeratin) preferentially stains the distal collecting system. The giant cells stain with the vimentin stain (see figure 22-34) but not the immunocytochemical and lectin stains for epithelial (i.e., tubular) cells. Studies (56) suggest that the giant cells are indeed nontubular epithelial, and represent blood-borne hematopoietic cells (anti-AE1/AE3 cytokeratin antibody).

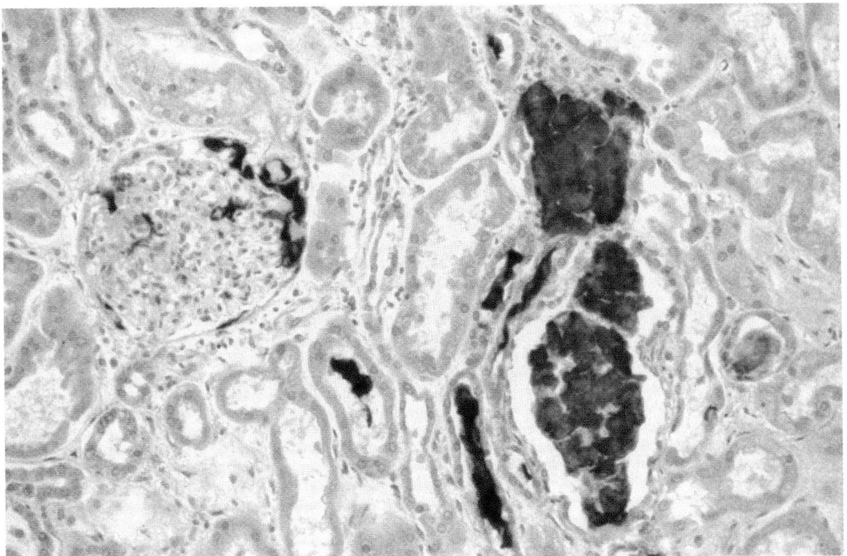

Figure 22-36

MYELOMA CAST NEPHROPATHY

These sections from a series of patients with myeloma cast nephropathy are stained with an antibody to Tamm-Horsfall protein (THP), which is normally produced in only the thick ascending limb of Henle's loop of the distal tubule. Note the large casts positive for THP throughout the tubular system. There is extravasation of THP from the tubular lumen into the nearby interstitium. This staining can be seen in a "retrograde flow" into Bowman's space (anti-Tamm-Horsfall protein).

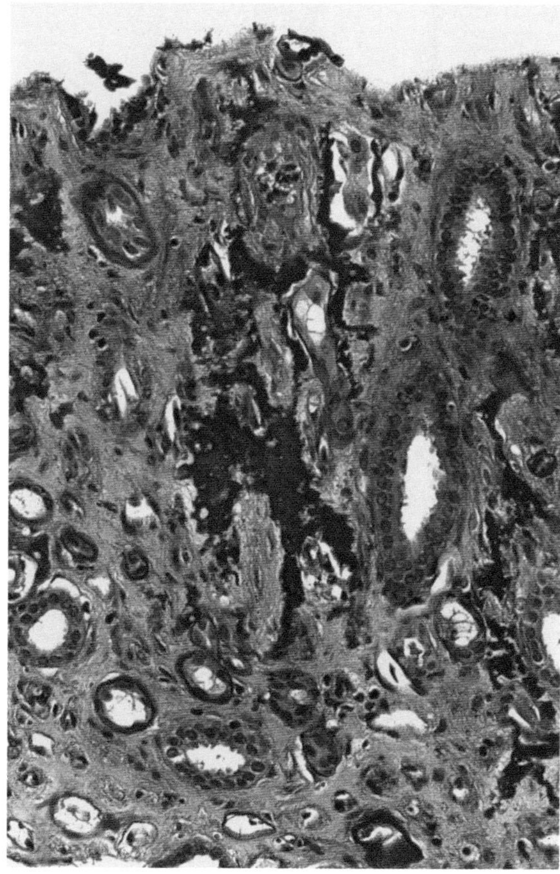

Figure 22-37

MYELOMA CAST NEPHROPATHY: KAPPA LIGHT CHAIN DEPOSITION IN THE RENAL INTERSTITIUM

Intensely PAS-positive material is deposited in the tissues between the tubules.

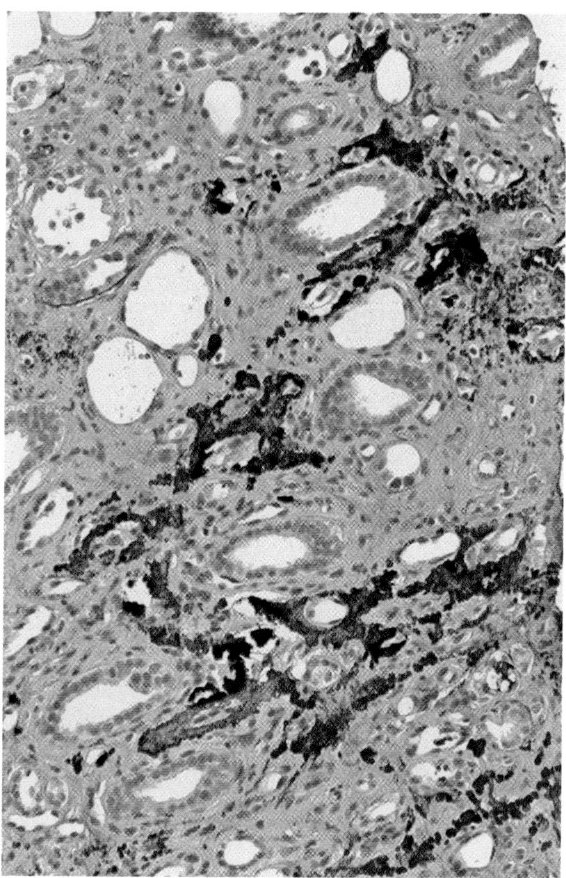

Figure 22-38

MYELOMA CAST NEPHROPATHY

Immunocytochemical stain for kappa light chains shows that the acellular interstitial material is kappa light chain (lambda light chain immunocytochemistry was negative) (antikappa light chain). (Courtesy of Dr. T. Nadasdy, Rochester, NY.)

The characteristic changes of the cast nephropathy noted above are not entirely pathognomonic for a plasma cell dyscrasia, although they are usually, in the proper setting, quite characteristic. Somewhat similar casts can be seen in many conditions leading to end-stage kidney disease. Casts with polymorphonuclear leukocytes are most commonly be seen in patients with acute infectious pyelonephritis, obstruction, and even in patients with severe and acute tubular necrosis. Casts with polymorphonuclear leukocytes and giant cells have been reported (45), although rarely, in patients with pancreatic or thyroid carcinoma and in a patient with tuberculosis treated with rifampin; however, these cases were reported in the older literature and lack immunologic studies to exclude a plasma cell dyscrasia (45). Recently a histologically similar pattern of casts has been seen in a transplant patient treated with a specific drug (rapamycin). The most difficult problem is differentiating Tamm-Horsfall casts, which may incite a mild cellular reaction resembling myeloma casts. Tamm-Horsfall casts are strongly PAS positive and fibrillar, whereas myeloma casts are at most only weakly PAS positive and harder in appearance.

Etiology and Pathogenesis. The pathogenesis is related to paraprotein deposits in the kidney (36). The nephrotoxic effects of monotypic light chain (kappa or lambda) immunoglobulins on the tubular epithelium lead to destruction of the tubular epithelium and obstruction of the tubular system by the large proteinaceous casts. These casts are composed of crystallized monoclonal light chains. The free immunoglobulin light chain (also termed Bence Jones protein) is believed to be directly toxic to the renal tubular epithelium and leads to obstruction downstream. Not all light chains are equally nephrotoxic (39,40,42,46,47,54).

A brief review of normal light chain synthesis and metabolism is in order. Normal plasma cells produce only entire immunoglobulin molecules and a slight excess of light chains. Each plasma cell produces either kappa or lambda light chains. The immunoglobulins are retained in the general circulation and excluded from the glomerular filtrate by virtue of their size; however, light chains, normally 20,000 to 40,000 molecular weight and existing as monomers or dimers, are freely filtered by the glomerulus and endocytosed by the proximal renal tubular epithelium, where they are normally metabolized/catabolized (28,62). Because of tubular reabsorption, only tiny amounts of light chains are normally excreted in the urine.

In 1847, Henry Bence Jones described urinary proteins in myeloma patients that precipitated on heating and then dissolved with cooling. These have been identified as light chains (or Bence Jones protein). In patients with multiple myeloma, the amount of light chain secreted into the blood and excreted into the urine is much greater than normal. The free light chains in these patients may be smaller or larger than normal with sizes generally ranging from 12,000 to 30,000 molecular weight; the heavier light chains are probably due to excess glycosylation. Certain physicochemical characteristics of the light chains (such as size, isoelectric point [pI], hydrophobicity, and state of aggregation) may affect glomerular clearance and tubular toxicity. Thus, in a plasma cell dyscrasia, a large unregulated amount of monotypic or monoclonal light chain is produced, which is filtered by the normal glomerulus. The filtered light chains apparently overwhelm the ability of the proximal tubular epithelium to catabolize them; certain specific light chains appear to be intrinsically nephrotoxic (or more precisely tubulotoxic) (33,41). Direct injury of the tubular epithelium by light chains is supported by the urinary excretion of other low molecular weight proteins in patients with myeloma (tubular proteinuria). The uncatabolized light chains continue to flow down the nephron, leading to large cast formation and even obstruction in the distal tubules and collecting ducts.

Not all Bence Jones proteins (light chains) are nephrotoxic (tubulotoxic). Some patients may have large amounts of light chain excretion for many years without evidence of alteration of renal tubular function. The physicochemical characteristics of the light chain that render it tubulotoxic are uncertain. Some investigators have suggested that the electrostatic interactions of the light chain (pI) with Tamm-Horsfall proteins predispose to precipitation (20,34,57). Bence Jones proteins can bind to specific sites of the Tamm-Horsfall protein, leading to coprecipitation and obstruction in the distal nephron (62a). It has been suggested that renal myeloma casts persist because of their resistance to urinary and macrophage proteases. Finally, the often-accompanying interstitial inflammation secondary to obstruction and rupture of the tubules, with release of tubular contents and inflammatory mediators, allows Tamm-Horsfall proteins to activate a variety of interstitial inflammatory cells, leading to cytokine release and production of proteases and reactive oxygen metabolites.

Renal disease in patients with plasma cell dyscrasias may be precipitated or potentiated by other nephrotoxins or insults that tend to reduce renal perfusion (11). These include dehydration, administration of radiopaque materials used in intravenous pyelograms (IVPs), hypercalcemia, and drugs (nonsteroidal anti-inflammatory drugs [NSAIDs] and antibiotics) (11). Other diseases or complications of multiple myeloma, such as hyperuricemia, chronic vascular disease, infectious pyelonephritis, and renal stones may further adversely affect renal function.

Treatment and Prognosis. Multiple myeloma is an inexorably progressive disease in which there is a steady increase in the number of neoplastic plasma cells, with the eventual development of renal failure, infection, or failure of the bone marrow with death. The median survival time is about 3 to 4 years. Most chemotherapeutic regimens include melphalan and prednisone, or combinations of adriamycin, vincristine, and decadron. Plasmapheresis has also been employed with limited success (64).

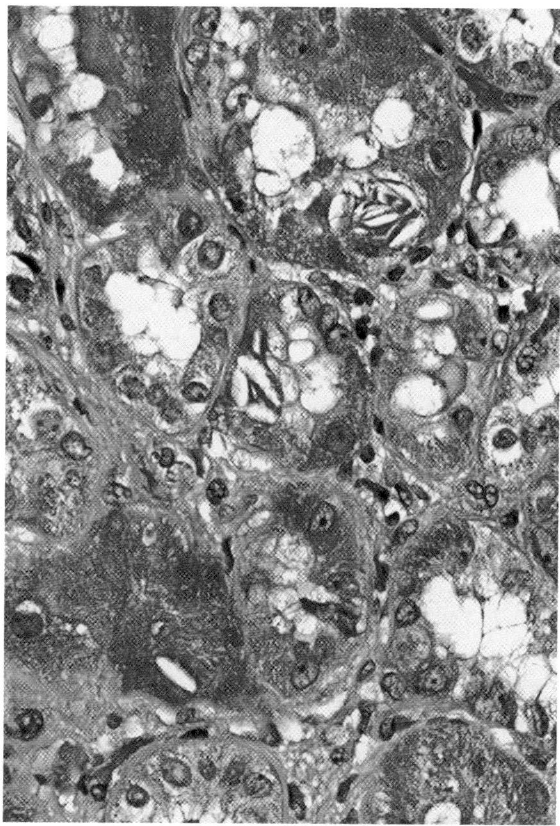

Figure 22-39

LIGHT CHAIN FANCONI'S SYNDROME

A number of elongated crystals are present within the renal tubular epithelium (Masson trichrome stain).

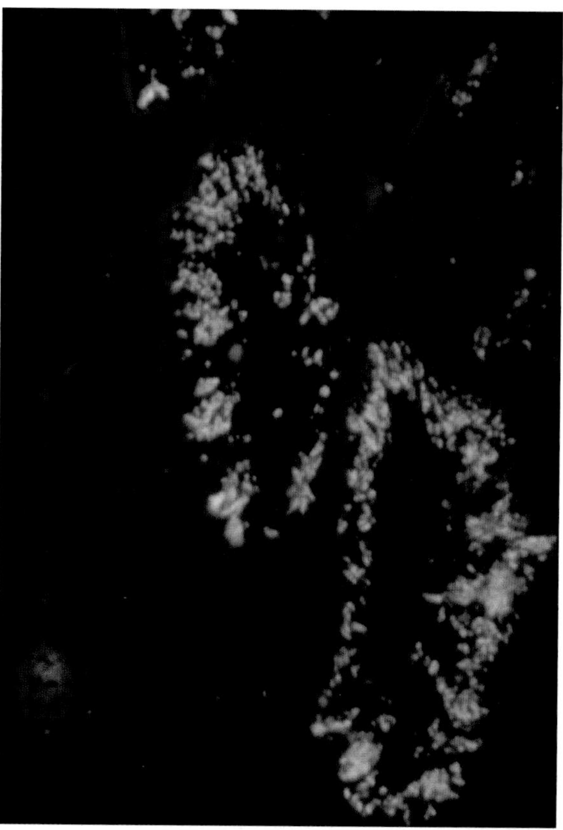

Figure 22-40

LIGHT CHAIN FANCONI'S SYNDROME

In the tubular epithelium there is intense staining of the crystals for kappa light chains (immunofluorescence with antikappa light chain).

Renal prognosis is poor (37). A minority of patients experience some improvement in renal function if treatment is instituted promptly (3,4, 13,16,19,36,37). Chemotherapy is aimed at decreasing the production of light chains whereas hydration and alkalinization of the urine reduce the likelihood of light chain precipitation in the tubules. Many patients require dialysis. Renal transplantation has been offered to those patients whose myeloma is in remission (55).

LIGHT CHAIN FANCONI'S SYNDROME

Light chain Fanconi's syndrome occurs in patients with Fanconi's syndrome who have aminoaciduria, renal glycosuria, phosphaturia, and renal tubular acidosis (7,30,31,43). These patients typically have a plasma cell dyscrasia with light chain deposition within the proximal tubular epithelium, usually involving a kappa light chain. This deposition, which may lead directly to tubular damage and precipitation of crystals, is found in the tubular cytoplasm.

Intracytoplasmic droplets and needle-like crystals can be seen in the altered renal tubular epithelium, even in regions away from tubular casts (fig. 22-39). Tubular crystals are often found in patients with partial or complete Fanconi's syndrome (figs. 22-40, 22-41). The crystals are often phosphotungstic acid-hematoxylin (PTAH) positive. By electron microscopy, rod- or needle-shaped crystals with substructure are identified within the proximal tubular cytoplasm (fig. 22-41).

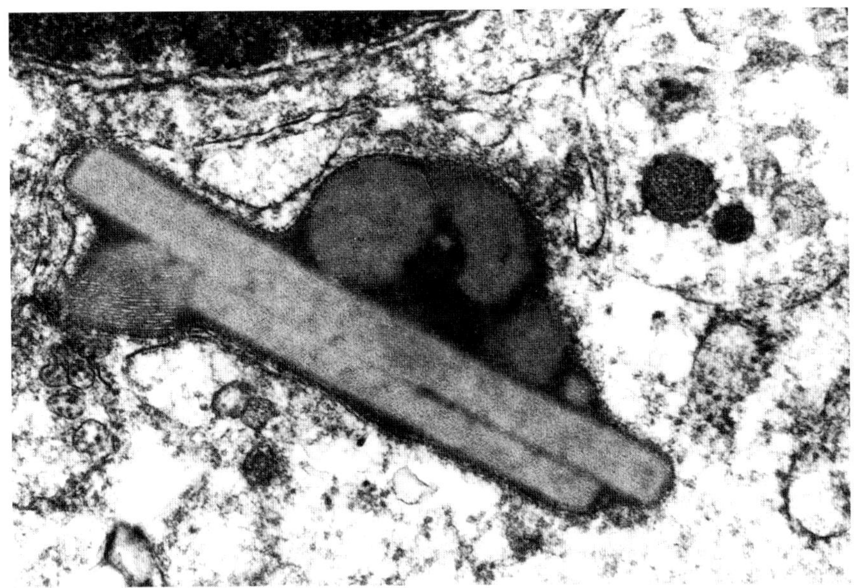

Figure 22-41

LIGHT CHAIN FANCONI'S SYNDROME

Large crystals are in the tubular epithelium (electron micrograph).

REFERENCES

1. Alpers CE, Magil AB, Gown AM. Macrophage origin of the multinucleated cells of myeloma cast nephropathy. Am J Clin Pathol 1989;92:662–5.
2. Barlogie B. Plasma cell myeloma. In: Beutler E, Lichtman MA, Coller BS, Kipps TJ, eds. Williams hematology, 5th ed. New York: McGraw-Hill; 1995:1109–26.
3. Bear RA, Cole EH, Lang A, Johnson M. Treatment of acute renal failure due to myeloma kidney. Can Med Assoc J 1980;123:750–3.
4. Bernstein SP, Humes HD. Reversible renal insufficiency in multiple myeloma. Arch Intern Med 1982;147:2083–6.
5. Burke JR Jr, Flis R, Lasker N, Simenhoff M. Malignant lymphoma with "myeloma kidney" acute renal failure. Am J Med 1976;60:1055–60.
6. Carson FL, Kingsley WB. Nonamyloid green birefringence following Congo red staining. Arch Pathol Lab Med 1980;104:333–5.
7. Chan KW, Ho FC, Chan MK. Adult Fanconi syndrome in kappa light chain myeloma. Arch Pathol Lab Med 1987;111:139–42.
8. Cohen AH, Border WA. Myeloma kidney. An immunomorphogenetic study of renal biopsies. Lab Invest 1980;42:248–56.
9. Cohen DJ, Sherman WH, Osserman EF, Appel GB. Acute renal failure in patients with multiple myeloma. Am J Med 1984;76:247–56.
10. DeFronzo RA, Cooke CR, Wright JR, Humphrey RL. Renal function in patients with multiple myeloma. Medicine 1978;57:151–66.
11. DeFronzo RA, Humphrey RL, Wright JR, Cooke CR. Acute renal failure in multiple myeloma. Medicine 1975;54:209–23.
12. Gallo G, Kumar A. Hematopoietic disorders. In: Silva FG, D'Agati VD, Nadasdy T, eds. Renal biopsy interpretation. New York: Churchill Livingstone; 1996:259–82.
13. Ganeval D, Rabian C, Guerin V, Pertuiset N, Landais P, Jungers P. Treatment of multiple myeloma with renal involvement. Adv Nephrol Necker Hosp 1992;21:347–70.
14. Ivanyi B. Frequency of light chain deposition nephropathy relative to renal amyloidosis and Bence Jones cast nephropathy in a necropsy study of patients with myeloma. Arch Pathol Lab Med 1990;114:986–7.
15. Ivanyi B. Renal complications in multiple myeloma. Acta Morph Hung 1989;37:235–43.
16. Johnson WJ, Kyle RA, Pineda AA, O'Brien PC, Holley KE. Treatment of renal failure associated with multiple myeloma. Arch Intern Med 1990;150:863–9.
17. Kapadia SB. Multiple myeloma: a clinicopathologic study of 62 consecutively autopsied cases. Medicine (Baltimore) 1980;59:380–92.

18. Kern WF, Laszik ZG, Nadasdy T, Silva FG, Bane BL, Pitha JV, eds. Plasma cell dyscrasias, monoclonal gammopathies, and the fibrillary glomerulopathies: multiple myeloma, light chain deposition disease, amyloidosis, fibrillary glomerulonephritis, and immunotactoid glomerulopathy. In: Atlas of renal pathology. Philadelphia: WB Saunders; 1999:212.
19. Korzets A, Tam F, Russell G, Feehally J, Walls J. The role of continuous ambulatory peritoneal dialysis in end-stage renal failure due to multiple myeloma. Am J Kidney Dis 1990;16:216–23.
20. Kumar S, Muchmore A. Tamm-Horsfall protein—uromodulin (1950-1990). Kidney Int 1990;37: 1395–401.
21. Kyle RA. "Benign" monoclonal gammopathy—after 20 to 35 years of follow-up. Mayo Clin Proc 1993;68:26–36.
22. Kyle RA. Monoclonal gammopathy of undetermined significance. Blood Rev 1994;8:135–41.
23. Kyle RA. Multiple myeloma and other plasma cell disorders. In: Hoffman R, Benz EJ Jr, Shattil SJ, Furie B, Cohen HJ, Silberstein LE, eds. Hematology: basic principles and practice. New York: Churchill Livingstone; 1995:1354–74.
24. Kyle RA. Multiple myeloma: review of 869 cases. Mayo Clin Proc 1975;50:29–40.
25. Kyle RA, Beard CM, O'Fallen WM, Kurland LT. Incidence of multiple myeloma in Olmsted County, Minnesota: 1978 through 1990, with a review of the trend since 1945. J Clin Oncol 1994;12:1577–83.
26. Levi DF, Williams RC Jr, Lindstrom FD. Immunofluorescent studies of the myeloma kidney with special reference to light chain disease. Am J Med 1968;44:922–33.
27. Lin J, Markowitz GS, Valeri AM, et al. Renal monoclonal immunoglobulin deposition disease: the disease spectrum. J Am Soc Nephrol 2001;12:1482–92.
28. Maack T. Renal handling of low molecular weight proteins. Am J Med 1975;58:57–64.
29. MacLennan IC, Drayson M, Dunn J. Multiple myeloma. BMJ 1994;308:1033–6.
30. Maldonado JE, Velosa JA, Kyle RA, Wagoner RD, Holley KE, Salassa RM. Fanconi syndrome in adults. A manifestation of a latent form of myeloma. Am J Med 1975;58:354–64.
31. Markowitz GS, Flis RS, Kambham N, D'Agati VD. Fanconi syndrome with free kappa light chains in the urine. Am J Kidney Dis 2000;35:777–81.
32. Matsuyama N, Joh K, Yamaguchi Y, et al. Crystalline inclusions in the glomerular podocytes in a patient with benign monoclonal gammopathy and focal segmental glomerulosclerosis. Am J Kidney Dis 1994;23:859–65.
33. McGeoch J, Falconer Smith J, Ledingham J, Ross B. Inhibition of active-transport sodium-potassium-A.T.P.ase by myeloma protein. Lancet 1978;2:17–8.
34. Melcion C, Mougenot B, Baudouin B, et al. Renal failure in myeloma: relationship with isoelectric point of immunoglobulin light chains. Clin Nephrol 1984;22:138–43.
35. Morel-Maroger L, Verroust P, Preud'Homme JL. Glomerular lesions in plasma cell dyscrasias. In: Rosen S, ed. Pathology of glomerular disease 1. New York: Churchill Livingstone; 1983:207–24.
36. Niesvizky R, Siegel D, Michaeli J. Biology and treatment of myeloma. Blood Rev 1993;7:24–33.
37. Port FK, Nissenson AR. Outcome of end-stage renal disease in patients with rare causes of renal failure. II. Renal or systemic neoplasms. Q J Med 1989;73:1161–5.
38. Preud'Homme JL, Aucouturier P, Touchard G, et al. Monoclonal immunoglobulin deposition disease: a review of immunoglobulin chain alterations. Int J Immunopharmacol 1994;16:425–31.
39. Preud'Homme JL, Morel-Maroger L, Brouet JC, et al. Synthesis of abnormal immunoglobulins in lymphoplasmacytic disorders with visceral light chain deposition. Am J Med 1980;69:703–10.
40. Preud'Homme JL, Morel-Maroger L, Brouet JC, Mihaesco E, Mery JP, Seligmann M. Synthesis of abnormal heavy and light chains in multiple myeloma with visceral deposition of monoclonal immunoglobulin. Clin Exp Immunol 1980;42:545–53.
41. Preuss HG, Hammack WJ, Murdaugh HV. The effect of Bence Jones protein on the in vitro function of rabbit renal cortex. Nephron 1968;5:210–6.
42. Pruzanski W. Clinical manifestation of multiple myeloma: relation to class and type M component. Can Med Assoc J 1976;114:896–7.
43. Raman SB, Van Slyck EJ. Nature of intracytoplasmic crystalline inclusions in myeloma cells (morphologic, cytochemical, ultrastructural and immunofluorescent studies). Am J Clin Pathol 1983;80:224–8.
44. Rayner HC, Haynes AP, Thompson JR, Russell N, Fletcher J. Perspectives in multiple myeloma: survival, prognostic factors and disease complications in a single center between 1975 and 1988. Q J Med 1991;79:517–25.
45. Reducka K, Gardiner GW, Sweet J, Vandenbroucke A, Bear R. Myeloma-like cast nephropathy associated with acinar cell carcinoma of the pancreas. Am J Nephrol 1988;8:421–4.
46. Sanders PW. Pathogenesis and treatment of myeloma kidney. J Lab Clin Med 1994;124:484–8.
47. Sanders PW, Booker BB. Pathobiology of cast nephropathy from human Bence Jones proteins. J Clin Invest 1992;89:630–9.
48. Sanders PW, Herrera GA, Kirk KA, Old CW, Galla JH. Spectrum of glomerular and tubulointerstitial renal lesions associated with monotypical immunoglobulin light chain deposition. Lab Invest 1991;64:527–37.
49. Schubert GE. [Myeloma kidney. I. Incidence of pathological-anatomical findings (author's transl).] Klin Wochenschr 1974;52:763–70.

50. Schwartz MM. The dysproteinemias and amyloidosis. In: Jennette JC, Olson JL, Schwartz MM, Silva FG, eds. Heptinstall's pathology of the kidney, 5th ed. Philadelphia: Lippincott-Raven; 1998:1321–69.
51. Sedmak DD, Tubbs RR. The macrophagic origin of multinucleated giant cells in myeloma kidney: an immunohistologic study. Hum Pathol 1987;18:304–6.
52. Sessa A, Torri Tarelli L, Meroni M, Ferrario G, Giordano F, Volpi A. Multinucleated giant cells in myeloma kidney: an ultrastructural study. Appl Pathol 1984;2:185–94.
53. Silva FG, Pirani CCL, Mesa-Tejada R, Williams GS. The kidney in plasma cell dyscrasias: a review and a clinicopathologic study of 50 patients. In: Fenoglio C, Wolff M, eds. Progress in surgical pathology. New York: Masson; 1983:131.
54. Solomon A, Weiss DT, Kattine AA. Nephrotoxic potential of Bence Jones proteins. N Engl J Med 1991;324:1845–51.
55. Spence RK, Hill GS, Goldwein MI, Grossman RA, Barker CF, Perloff LJ. Renal transplantation for end-stage myeloma kidney: report of a patient with long-term survival. Arch Surg 1979;114: 950–52.
56. Start DA, Silva FG, Davis LD, D'Agati V, Pirani CL. Myeloma cast nephropathy: immunohistochemical and lectin studies. Mod Pathol 1988;1:336–47.
57. Thomas DB, Davies M, Peters JR, Williams JD. Tamm Horsfall protein binds to a single class of carbohydrate specific receptors on human neutrophils. Kidney Int 1993;44:423–9.
58. Touchard G. Renal biopsy in multiple myeloma and in other monoclonal immunoglobulin-producing diseases. Ann Med Interne (Paris) 1992;143:80–3.
59. Vassar PS, Culling CF. Fluorescent amyloid staining of casts in myeloma nephrosis. Arch Pathol 1962;73:59–63.
60. Waugh DA, Ibels LS. Multiple myeloma presenting as recurrent obstructive uropathy. Aust N Z J Med 1980;10:555–8.
61. Winearls CG. Acute myeloma kidney. Kidney Int 1995;48:1347–61.
62. Wochner RD, Strober W, Waldmann TA. The role of the kidney in the catabolism of Bence Jones proteins and immunoglobulin fragments. J Exp Med 1967;126:207–21.
62a. Ying WZ, Sanders PW. Mapping the binding domain of immunoglobulin light chains for Tamm-Horsfall protein. Am J Pathol 2001:158:1859–66.
63. Zlotnick A, Rosenmann E. Renal pathologic findings associated with monoclonal gammopathies. Arch Intern Med 1975;135:40–5.
64. Zucchelli P, Pasquali S, Cagnoli L, Ferrari G. Controlled plasma exchange trial in acute renal failure due to multiple myeloma. Kidney Int 1988;33:1175–80.

23 RENAL STONES

Urinary stones, or calculi, are macroscopic concretions that form at any level of the urinary tract, from the kidney parenchyma to the urinary bladder. Most are renal stones arising in the kidney.

Renal stones may be silent, lying within the renal parenchyma for years without producing symptoms or significant renal damage, or they may obstruct the urinary flow causing ureteral colic. Characteristically, this excruciating pain, caused by contraction of the ureteral smooth muscle, passes down from the flank, curves anteriorly, and then descends toward the groin. The pain may vanish abruptly if the stone passes into the urinary bladder or is voided. In some cases, calculi cause obstruction without producing pain. The renal stones may produce ulceration of the urothelium and bleeding, leading to microscopic or more commonly macroscopic hematuria. Infection may be secondary to prolonged obstruction, compounded by the trauma/ulceration of the urothelium that is produced (1–3,10,14).

The larger stones lying within the renal pelvis (renal calyx or ureteropelvic junction) are often associated with urinary tract infection with pyonephrosis (pus in the renal pelvis) and hematuria. These large stones are often painless and may remain clinically silent for years. Small stones are more hazardous and painful because they may pass into the ureters and cause transient obstruction in one of the normal regions of ureteral narrowing: 1) renal pelvis-ureter junction; 2) where the ureter crosses the iliac vessels at the pelvic bone; 3) in the posterior pelvis where the ureter is crossed anteriorly by the pelvic vessels; and 4) especially where the ureter enters the urinary bladder.

Urolithiasis is a frequent clinical problem (34,35). It affects almost 10 percent of people in the United States sometime during their life and accounts for almost 1 percent of all hospital admissions. Males are much more often affected than females. Most stones in women are due to metabolic defects (e.g., cystinuria) or infection. The peak age of onset is between 20 and 30 years. Although most patients with renal stones do not have a known familial or hereditary predisposition to stone formation, some do. Certain inborn errors of metabolism, like gout, cystinuria, and primary hyperoxaluria, are examples of hereditary diseases manifested by excessive production and excretion of stone-forming substances (Table 23-1). Stones may lead to chronic partial obstruction and infection (14).

PATHOLOGIC CHANGES

Stones are unilateral in about four fifths of cases. Favored sites of formation are within the renal pyelocalyceal system, and to a lesser extent, the urinary bladder. The stones in the renal pelvis may be solitary or multiple, and quite large and even branching structures that create a cast of the renal pelvis and pyelocalyceal system as seen in the staghorn calculus (figs. 23-1–23-3). Alternately, renal stones may be small, about 2 to 3 mm in diameter. The stones may have a smooth exterior, or an irregular surface with a rough, jagged, or spicular appearance. Sometimes multiple stones are noted within the kidney.

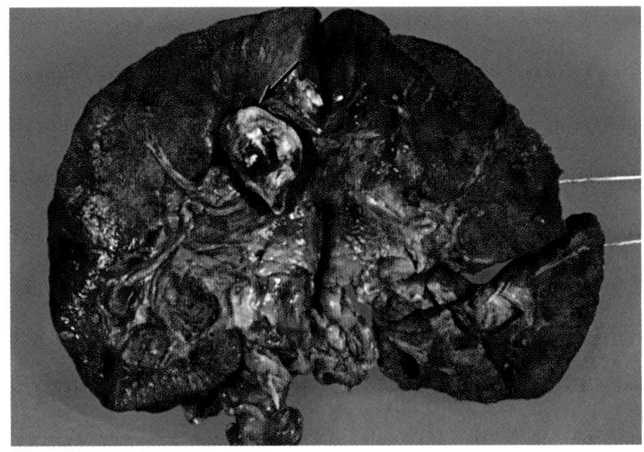

Figure 23-1

STONES IN THE RENAL PELVIS

The adjacent urothelium appears hemorrhagic and eroded.

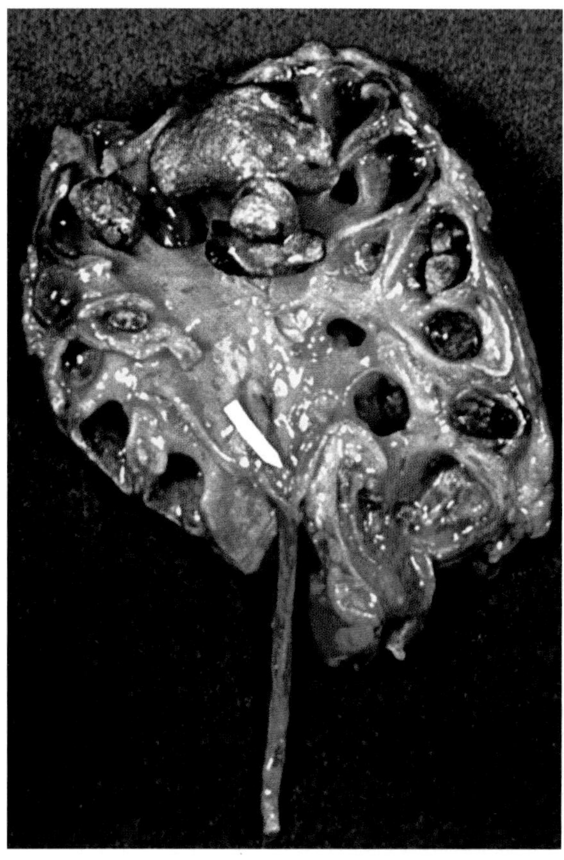

Figure 23-2
RENAL STONES WITH HYDRONEPHROSIS

The gross and radiologic appearances of renal stones depend on the chemical composition of the stone (Table 23-1). Thus, each type of renal stone is considered separately (fig. 23-4).

CALCIUM STONES

Calcium stones (calcium oxalate with or without calcium phosphate) comprise about three fourths of all renal stones. They are usually small (less than 1 to 2 cm in diameter), rounded to jagged, sharply circumscribed, and difficult to section with the scalpel (figs. 23-5–23-7). They are black, gray, or white. Calcium stones are radiopaque. Because calcium stones account for most cases of urolithiasis, the majority of renal stones (about 85 percent) are visible on noncontrast radiographs. On urinary analysis the crystals appear envelope shaped (1–3,6).

About 5 percent of patients with these stones have both hypercalcemia and hypercalciuria (secondary to hyperparathyroidism, sarcoidosis, or other causes of hypercalcemia) (19,22). Another 55 percent have hypercalciuria without hypercalcemia; this is caused by many factors, which include increased absorption of calcium from the intestine (so called absorptive hypercalciuria), intrinsic impairment of renal tubular reabsorption of calcium (renal hypercalciuria), or idiopathic fasting hypercalciuria with normal parathyroid function (11). About 20 percent have increased uric acid secretion (hyperuricosuric

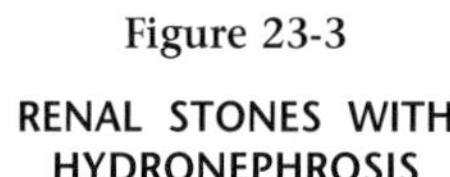

Figure 23-3
RENAL STONES WITH HYDRONEPHROSIS

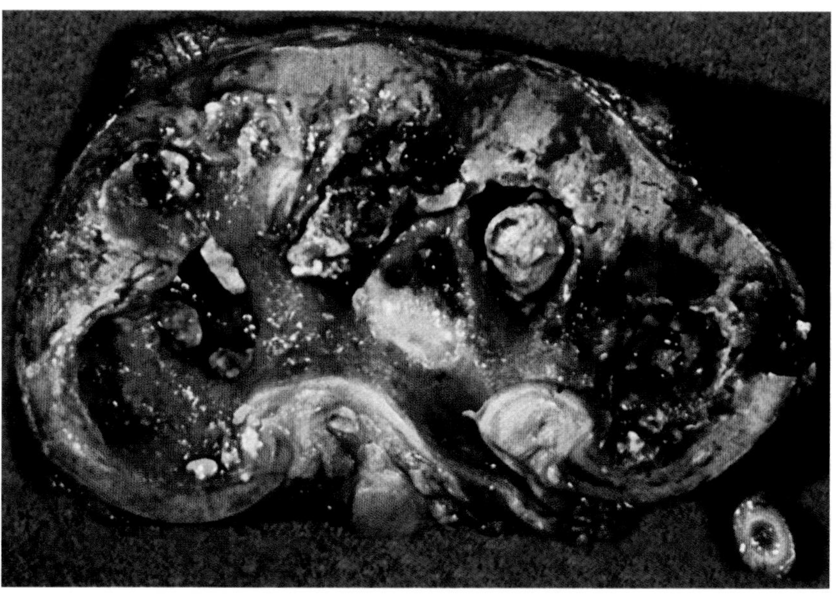

Table 23-1

PREVALENCE OF VARIOUS TYPES OF RENAL STONES[a]

	Percentage of All Stones
Calcium Oxalate (Phosphate)	75
Idiopathic hypercalciuria (without hypercalcemia: absorptive, renal, or idiopathic) (50%)	
Hypercalciuria and hypercalcemia (10%)	
Hyperoxaluria (5%)	
Enteric (4.5%)	
Primary (0.5%)	
Hyperuricosuria (enteric or primary) (20%)	
Hypocitraturia	
No known metabolic abnormality (15%-20%)	
Struvite (Magnesium Ammonium Phosphate) (Triple Stones)	10–15
(Associated with renal infections)	
Uric Acid	5–6
Associated with hyperuricemia	
Associated with hyperuricosurias	
Idiopathic (50% of uric stones)	
Cystine (Defective tubular reabsorption of cystine)	1–2
Brushite (Associated with renal tubular acidosis)	rare
Others or Unknown	±10

[a]Modified from table 21-13 from reference 5.

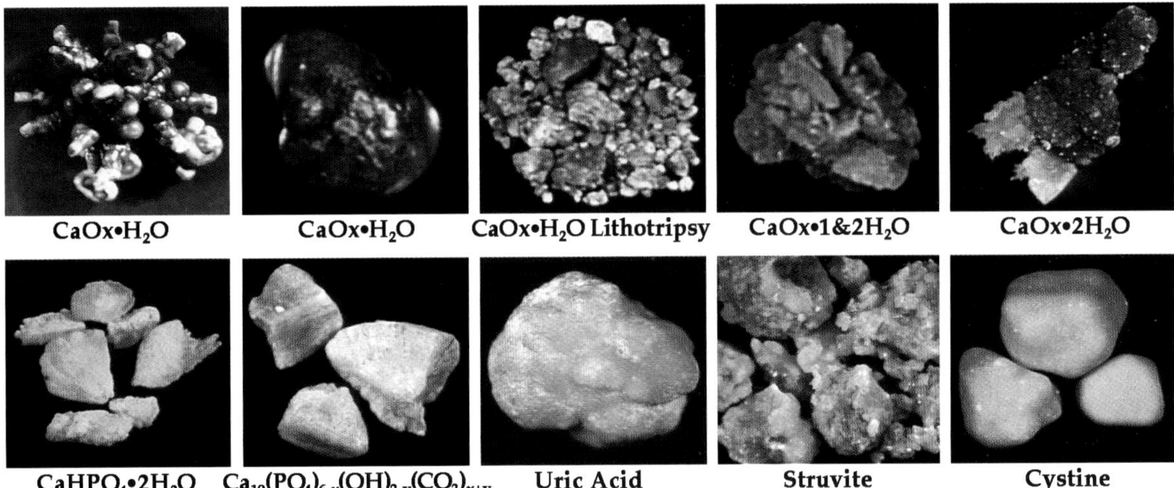

Figure 23-4

RENAL STONES (COMMON STONE TYPES)

The authors wish to acknowledge UroCor, Inc. for providing material used in this chapter (figs. 23-4–23-7, 23-10, 23-11, 23-13, and 23-14) that originates from their UroStone (SM) Metabolic Management System (Oklahoma City, Oklahoma). This system combines chemical analysis of stones, and 24-hour urine and serum analysis with a risk stratification for stone recurrence.

calcium stones), causing nucleation of calcium oxalate on uric acid crystals in the renal collecting tubules. There may or may not be associated hypercalciuria (36). Another 5 percent have hyperoxaluria (either acquired by overabsorption in the gut secondary to intestinal disease, or less commonly, as a hereditary condition [primary oxaluria]). The former (enteric hyperoxaluria)

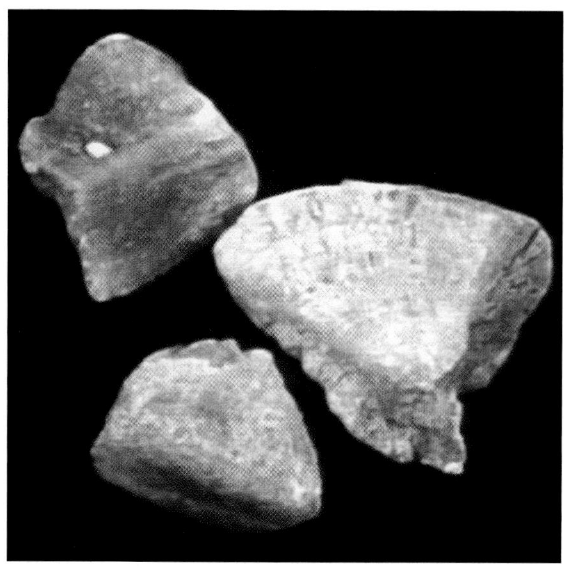

Figure 23-5

CALCIUM STONES

The stones are small, rounded to jagged, and rock hard.

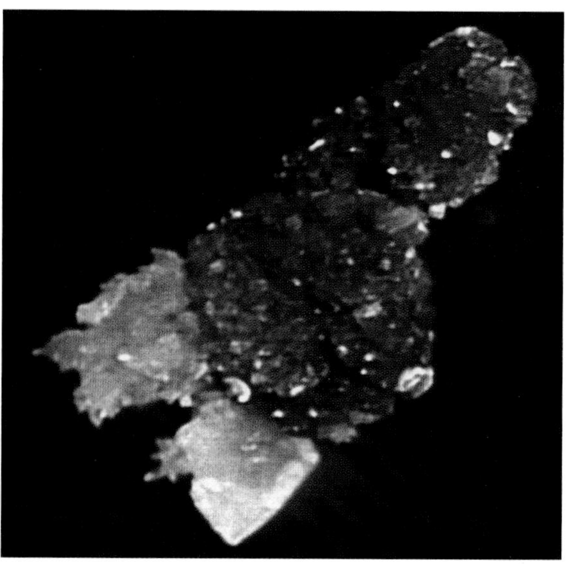

Figure 23-7

CALCIUM OXALATE DIHYDRATE STONES

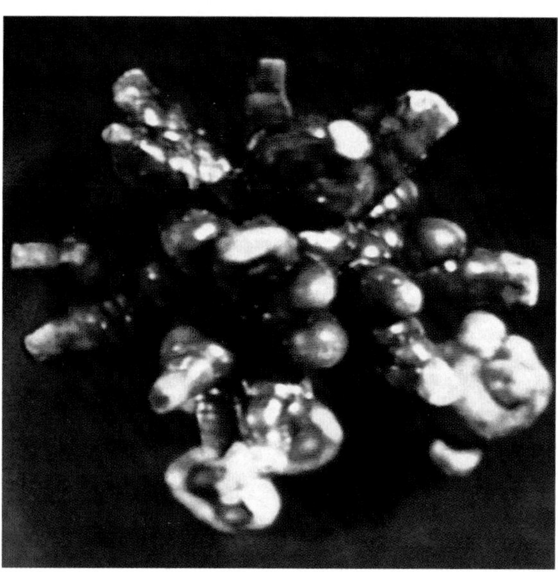

Figure 23-6

CALCIUM OXALATE MONOHYDRATE STONES

occurs in vegetarians whose diet is rich in oxalates. Decreased levels of citrate in the urine associated with chronic diarrhea and acidosis can produce calcium stones. In some patients with calcium stones, no direct cause is identified (idiopathic calcium stone disease).

NEPHROCALCINOSIS

Definition. The term nephrocalcinosis indicates the deposition of a marked number of calcium crystals within the renal parenchyma.

Clinical Features. Nephrocalcinosis occurs most frequently in patients with chronic hypercalcemia and hypercalciuria, which are secondary to the conditions shown in Table 23-2. Nephrocalcinosis is also seen in patients with human immunodeficiency virus (HIV), Bartter's syndrome, and cystic fibrosis, or following acute tubular necrosis or cortical necrosis. Renal transplant biopsies often show renal calcification. Renal calcifications also occur in many normal older individuals. Hypercalcemia itself can lead to significant impairment in renal function, even without evidence of deposition of calcium in the renal parenchyma.

The earliest manifestation of hypercalcemia is an inability to concentrate the urine, resulting in polyuria. Hypercalcemia may also lead to renal tubular acidosis (both proximal and distal). Patients may have nausea, vomiting, extracellular volume depletion, lethargy or other mental status changes, renal failure, and cardiac arrhythmias. There is little proteinuria and the urinary analysis shows little abnormality.

Table 23-2

CAUSES OF CHRONIC HYPERCALCEMIA AND HYPERCALCIURIA

Hyperparathyroidism (parathyroid adenomas or carcinomas)
Malignancies (parathyroid hormone [PTH])-related production by carcinomas or true PTH production by small cell carcinomas of the ovary or lung, or by osteolytic tumors/metastases by myeloma, lymphomas, or carcinomas)
Increased Intestinal Absorption of Calcium (such as vitamin D excess or sarcoidosis)
Increased Bone Turnover (such as with Paget's disease of the bone)

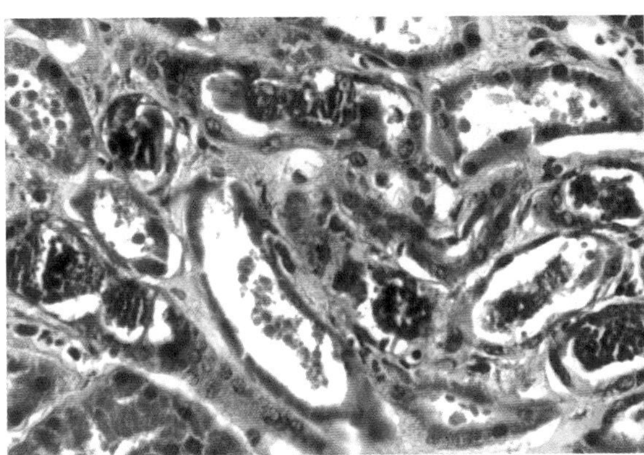

Figure 23-8

CALCIFICATION OF THE RENAL PARENCHYMA

This patient has nephrocalcinosis and renal calculi (hematoxylin and eosin [H&E] stain).

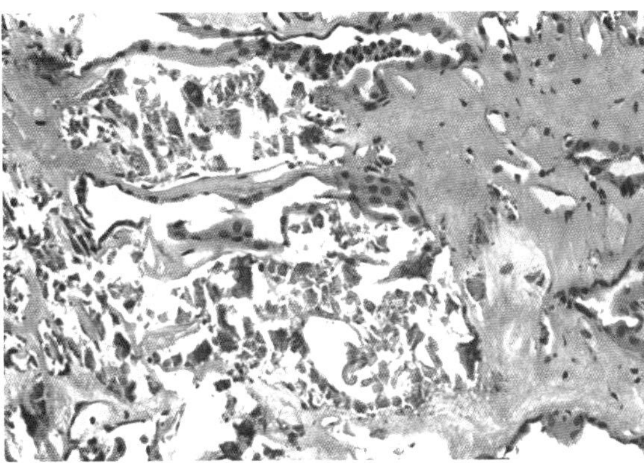

Figure 23-9

RANDALL'S PLAQUE

There is marked dystrophic calcification of the renal papillary tip (H&E stain).

Gross Findings. The kidneys are small to normal in size. The renal parenchyma may feel "gritty" on sectioning if there is significant renal deposition of calcium. The cut surfaces may show alternating areas of normal renal parenchyma and wedge-shaped scars (due to the accompanying vascular disease).

Light Microscopic Findings. There are basophilic calcifications in the tubular epithelium, tubular basement membrane regions, and nearby interstitial regions (fig. 23-8). Occasional calcifications within tubular epithelial cells or tubular lumens may be seen in normal older individuals or patients with proteinuria. The tubular epithelium is often atrophic. In severe or acute hypercalcemia there may be calcifications within the tubular lumens, appearing to obstruct the tubules.

Small foci or regions of calcification are noted in the renal papillae (if you have these to examine). These small linear or rounded deposits may cover the tips of the papillae and are termed Randall's plaques (fig. 23-9). They may serve as a nidus for further crystallization or organization of renal stones. They are otherwise not thought to be of any functional significance.

In chronic nephrocalcinosis there is calcification of the tubular basement membranes. This calcification appears most prominently in the proximal tubular regions; however, all segments of the nephron can be involved. The calcification can appear in both scarred regions and in regions of otherwise intact renal parenchyma. Calcifications may appear in sclerotic glomeruli or in Bowman's capsule. The calcification appears basophilic or as a purplish tinge when stained with hematoxylin and eosin (H&E). It can be accentuated with the use of the von Kossa stain for calcium.

Treatment and Prognosis. The treatment and prognosis of the patient depends primarily on the underlying disease process.

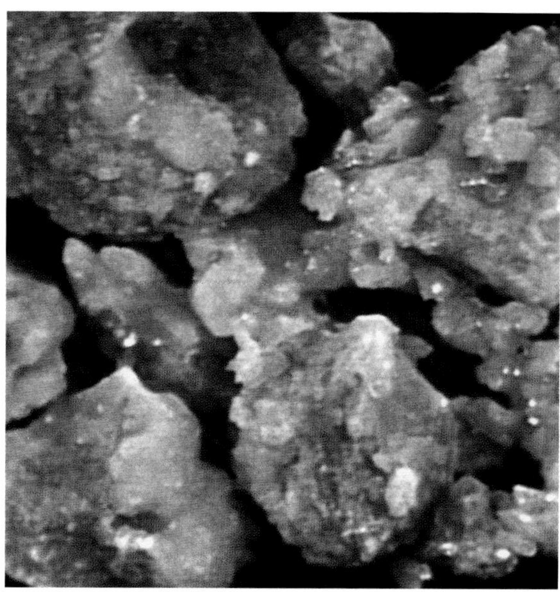

Figure 23-10

TRIPLE STONES (STRUVITE/UREASE STONES)

These tend to be large.

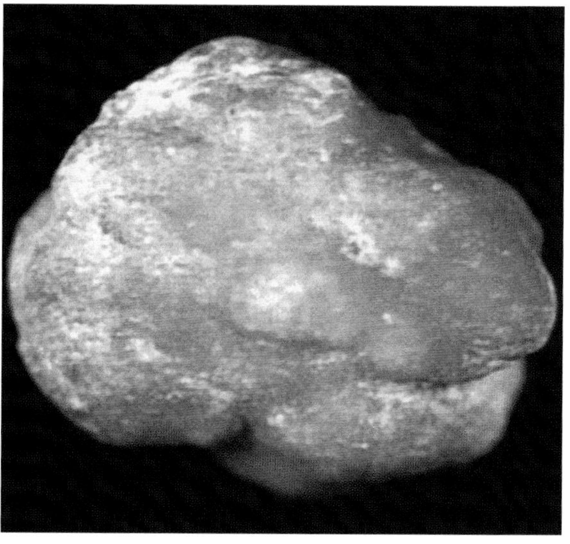

Figure 23-11

URIC ACID STONES

TRIPLE STONES

Struvite stones or urease stones are composed of magnesium ammonium phosphate and account for 10 to 15 percent of urinary calculi (fig. 23-10). They also contain some calcium apatite.

These are some of the largest renal stones. These stones may form huge branching structures that fill the renal pelvis and calyces (forming staghorn calculi). Staghorn calculi are almost always of this type and are associated with infections. They are yellow-tan.

Triple stones are formed in patients with urinary tract infections due to urea-splitting bacteria such as *Proteus* sp, some staphylococci, and other organisms but not *Escherichia coli* which does not make urease (23). Urea-splitting organisms convert urea to ammonia, which elevates the urine pH. The alkaline urine leads to precipitation of the magnesium ammonium phosphate salts. Once infection is well established, the renal stones grow and branch quite rapidly, forming staghorns with surprising speed. Bacterial infection is difficult to treat successfully because the organisms are inaccessible within the interstices of the stone. More than one third of patients with struvite stones have an underlying metabolic abnormality (such as primary hyperparathyroidism) which is the primary predisposing factor to nephrolithiasis. Secondary infection then leads to the formation of the struvite stones. On macroscopic examination of the urinary sediment, the typical struvite crystals are said to have a "coffin-lid" appearance. There may be widespread destruction of the renal parenchyma due to longstanding stones in the renal pelvis, with secondary infection (15).

URIC ACID STONES

Stones comprised primarily of uric acid account for about 5 percent of all kidney stones. They are white to orange, and may fill the renal pelvis (fig. 23-11). These stones are radiolucent. They occur in patients with hyperuricemia and hyperuricosuria, secondary to such conditions as gout (6). They are also seen in patients with leukemias and lymphomas (diseases with rapid cell turnover). In more than half of the patients with these calculi, however, there is no evidence of increased uric acid secretion in the urine (uricosuria), or hyperuricemia. In the latter group, an unexplained acid pH of the urine (less than 5.5) probably predisposes to uric acid stones because uric acid is relatively insoluble in acidic urine. Uric acid stones can dissolve during alkali therapy (if they are not already secondarily calcified). As noted above, hyperuricosuria is a risk factor for calcium

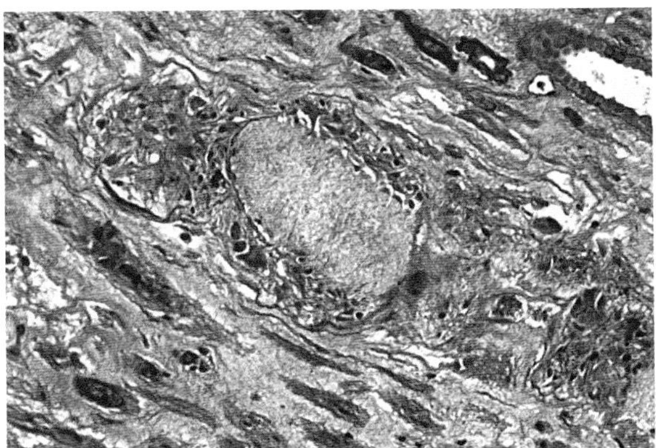

Figure 23-12

GOUTY TOPHUS IN THE RENAL MEDULLARY REGION

This patient has gout and renal calculi. The pale-staining crystals are usually surrounded by giant cells, as in this figure (H&E stain).

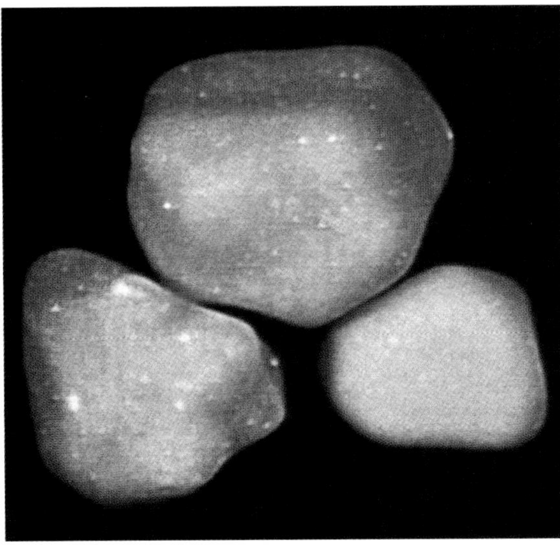

Figure 23-13

CYSTINE STONES

These stones are usually small and jagged.

stone formation probably because uric acid acts as a surface for nucleation. On examination of the urinary sediment, the uric acid crystals exhibit a diamond-shaped appearance.

Grossly, the kidneys are usually equally affected, unless there is unilateral obstruction by the stones. They are usually reduced in size and have a granularity or coarser scars on the surface. The renal medulla contains small white specks and occasionally radiating pale-yellow urate deposits. The pelvis may be dilated and contains the small uric acid stones.

Microscopically, the medullary collecting tubules contain crystals of monosodium urate (fig. 23-12). These crystals are elongated or rectangular and may be so fragmented as to appear amorphous. The crystals are best demonstrated in alcohol-fixed material, but may be preserved in material fixed in formol-saline solution. They are doubly refractile. In many deposits, the crystalline appearance and birefringence is lost, and a pale-staining, slightly amorphous substance is noted. The walls of the collecting tubules are often lost and the crystalline material appears to be in the medullary interstitium. There is often a rim of giant cells and other inflammatory mononuclear cells.

CYSTINE STONES

These stones are related to a genetic defect in the renal tubular transport of a number of amino acids, such as cystine, leading to decreased renal tubular reabsorption of cystine (6). Cystine stones are usually small and jagged in appearance. They are often sand-colored to yellow-brown, or greenish yellow, sometimes flecked with shiny crystallites (fig. 23-13). They are radiopaque, often showing a "sculpted wax" or "soap" appearance.

Cystinuria must be distinguished from cystinosis, which is a rare hereditary disorder with widespread intracellular accumulation of cystine and ensuing renal failure. In cystinuria, all renal deposits are extracellular (i.e., in the tubular lumens and pelvis). Cystine crystals identified by microscopic examination of the urinary sediment have a hexagonal appearance. High fluid intake is often effective in reducing stone formation; other patients require pharmacotherapy.

OTHER STONES

Rarely, other types of stones have been reported (fig. 23-14). Radiolucent xanthine stones occur in association with the rare hereditary disorder, xanthinuria, or as a complication of allopurinol therapy for hyperuricemia. A fascinating type of stone consisting entirely of matrix has been described in patients on maintenance dialysis. These stones have a laminated appearance (1–3).

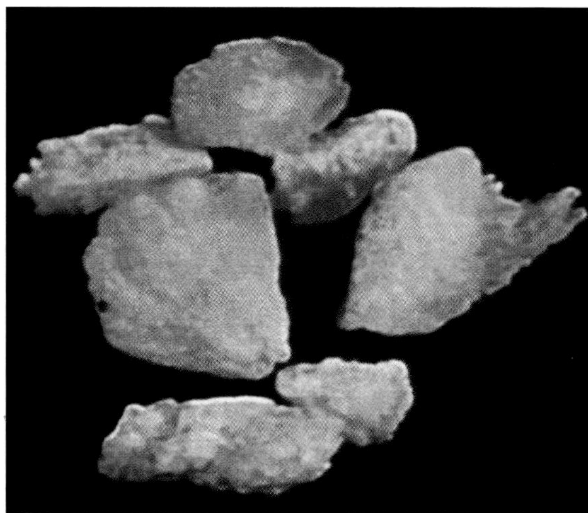

Figure 23-14

BRUSHITE STONES

STONES, LITHOTRIPSY, AND THE KIDNEY

Ordinarily, the kidneys remain intact and function well; however, small foci of calcification are common in the renal papillae and occur either as small round deposits, linear streaks, or plaques covering the tips of the papillae. These Randall plaques are calcifications in the distal portions of the renal medullary collecting ducts (of Bellini) and are seen in association with nephrolithiasis (28) (see above).

Although renal stones are an infrequent cause of severe renal injury and renal failure, some patients with nephrolithiasis develop progressive renal interstitial fibrosis and tubular atrophy. Longstanding renal disease, such as that seen in patients with hereditary stone diseases (cystinuria, primary hyperoxaluria), primary struvite stones, and infection-related stone disease associated with anatomic and functional urinary tract abnormalities and spinal cord injury, may increase the risk of renal failure (7,12,32).

During the last decade or so, extracorporeal shock wave therapy (ESWT) with the Dornier lithotriptor as well as percutaneous nephrostolithotomy have revolutionized the treatment of patients with urinary tract calculi. Up to four fifths of patients with stones that do not spontaneously pass in the urine receive these treatments. The success of ESWT begins to diminish with stones greater than 1 cm in diameter and is poor with stones larger than 2 cm. The fragmentation products of lower pole stones do not pass easily and stones in this location are probably better treated with percutaneous lithotripsy. Cystine stones are relatively refractory to ESWL. Thus, the two different therapies are utilized for different types and sizes of stones.

Most patients treated by ESWT have microscopic hematuria, which appears to be a result of renal parenchymal injury and not simply the result of stone fragmentation. The renal trauma ranges from focal renal parenchymal hemorrhages to large subcapsular or renal hematomas (which may require blood transfusions) (17,20,26, 37). Magnetic resonance imaging (MRI) scans have shown perirenal accumulation of fluid and loss of the corticomedullary junction. Experimental studies performed on canine kidneys suggest that the trauma is dose related and may include renal edema, hemorrhage, tubular dilatation, cast formation, and even some parenchymal fibrosis (9).

A small increase in the incidence of new cases of hypertension has been reported to occur within 2 years after treatment of patients with ESWT. Thus far, few clinical studies have shown loss of renal function after this therapy, although long-term effects remain to be determined.

DIFFERENTIAL DIAGNOSIS OF RENAL STONES

Any renal stone should be grossly described, photographed, and sent to a laboratory for chemical/metabolic analysis to determine the composition and guide future evaluation and therapy. A review of the clinical history may reveal a previous history of renal stones.

ETIOLOGY AND PATHOGENESIS OF RENAL STONES

There are many causes of stone formation (1–3). The most common and important factor is an increased urinary concentration of the constituent(s) of the renal stone that exceeds the solubility of that constituent in the urine, leading to supersaturation. Many compounds are supersaturated in the normal urine: the concentration of calcium oxalate in the normal urine is four times its solubility. Other factors also play a role, such as agent(s) that serve as a nidus for stone formation (i.e., nucleation), low urine volume which favors supersaturation, an altered pH, and possibly the presence of certain bacteria which influence the formation of a calculus. Possible nucleating factors in the urine include tubular epithelial cells and cellular debris, urinary casts, and crystals (such as uric acid crystals serving as nucleating factors for calcium oxalate stones) (18,21,24,28,31). Recent studies have suggested that certain tiny bacteria (so called nanobacteria) serve as a microscopic nidus for stone formation. Stone growth occurs by aggregation, with the orderly movement of ions out of solution onto the growing crystal. An organic matrix of various mucoproteins is present in all calculi and makes up 1 to 5 percent of the weight of the stone.

It is an enigma why many stones occur in the absence of these known factors. Conversely, many patients with hypercalciuria, hyperoxaluria, and hyperuricosuria do not have renal stones. This has led to a hypothesis that in certain cases stone formation is enhanced by a deficiency of inhibitors of crystal formation in the urine (such as nephrocalcin, uropontin, Tamm-Horsfall protein, citrate, glycosaminoglycans, diphosphonate, and pyrophosphate) (16,33). The pH of the urine is also important: a pH of less than 6.5 increases calcium phosphate saturation. Not all renal calculi are attributed to metabolic risk factors. Anatomic derangements, such as polycystic kidney disease, horseshoe kidney, and medullary sponge kidney, can predispose to stone formation. Current investigation is underway and the reader is referred to recent in-depth studies of the subject (21,31,33,35).

TREATMENT

Calculi can lead to a variety of complications including renal colic and urinary tract obstruction. Generally, smaller stones are more likely to cause abrupt complications because they are free to pass from the kidney into the ureter. Of course, calculi can also predispose to infection by causing destruction and trauma to the urothelium/transitional epithelium lining the pyelocalyceal/ureteral regions. Stones less than 3 to 5 mm in diameter are likely to pass spontaneously; stones larger than 7 mm are unlikely to do so. Stones less than 2 cm can often be treated with ESWL (25,29). Nephrolithotomy may be required for renal calculi greater than 2 cm in diameter or for stones in the renal lower pole that exceed 1 cm. Stones lodged in the distal ureter may be managed by ureteroscopic removal (8).

Without treatment, many patients who have had one stone experience at least one recurrence. After a first calcium stone, approximately 40 percent of untreated patients have another stone within 5 years, and another 40 percent within the next 25 years. Thus, determination of the chemical composition of the renal stone and investigation of possible predisposing factors provide necessary information to reduce the risk of recurrences (30,35). Multiple tiny stone fragments (gravel) may be filtered from the strained urine and analyzed to determine the composition of the stone. Prophylactic therapy, such as increased water ingestion, alterations of the urine pH, and citrate intake, and other drug therapies (e.g., thiazides) have been employed (1–3,4,13,27).

REFERENCES

1. Asplin JR, Favus MJ, Coe FL. Nephrolithiasis. In: Brenner BM, ed. Brenner and Rector's the kidney, 5th ed. Philadelphia: Saunders; 1996:1893–935.
2. Coe FL, Favus MJ. Nephrolithiasis. In: Brenner B, Rector F Jr, eds. The kidney, 4th ed. Philadelphia: WB Saunders; 1991:1728–67.
3. Coe FL, Parks JH. Nephrolithiasis: pathogenesis and treatment, 2nd ed. Chicago: Year Book Medical Publishers; 1988.
4. Consensus conference. Prevention and treatment of kidney stones. JAMA 1988;260:977–81.
5. Cotran RS, Kumar V, Collins T, eds. Robbins pathologic basis of disease (the kidney), 6th ed. Philadelphia: WB Saunders; 1999.
6. Cuppage FE, Chonko AM. Urate and uric acid nephropathy, cystinosis, and oxalosis. In: Tisher CC, Brenner BM, eds. Renal pathology: with clinical and functional correlations. Philadelphia: JB Lippincott; 1989:1335–62.
7. Daudon M, Lacour B, Jungers P, et al. Urolithiasis in patients with end stage renal failure. J Urol 1992;147:977–80.

8. Delaney CP, Creagh TA, Smith JM, Fitzpatrick JM. Do not treat staghorn calculi by extracorporeal shockwave lithotripsy alone! Eur Urol 1993;24:355–7.
9. Delius M, Jordan M, Eizenhoefer H, et al. Biological effects of shock waves: kidney hemorrhage by shock waves in dogs—administration rate dependence. Ultrasound Med Biol 1988;14:689–94.
10. Drach GW. Urinary lithiasis. In: Walsh P, Gittes R, Perlmutter A, Stamey T, eds. Campbell's urology. Philadelphia: WB Saunders; 1986:1094–190.
11. Favus MJ. Familial forms of hypercalciuria. J Urol 1989;141:719–22.
12. Gambaro G, Favaro S, D'Angelo A. Risk for renal failure in nephrolithiasis. Am J Kidney Dis 2001;37:233–43.
13. Hess B, Ackermann D, Essig M, Takkinen R, Jaeger P. Renal mass and serum calitriol in male idiopathic calcium renal stone formers: role of protein intake. J Clin Endocrinol Metab 1995;80:1916–21.
14. Hill GS. Urinary tract infections: general considerations. In: Hill GS, ed. Uropathology. New York: Churchill Livingstone; 1989:279–331.
15. Hoorens A, Van Der Niepen P, Keuppens F, Vanden Houte K, Kloppel G. Pseudotuberculous pyelonephritis associated with nephrolithiasis. Am J Surg Pathol 1992;16:522–5.
16. Kaiser ET, Bock SC. Protein inhibitors of crystal growth. J Urol 1989;141:750–2.
17. Kaude JV, Williams CM, Milner MR, Scott KN, Finlayson B. Renal morphology and function immediately after extracorporeal shock-wave lithotripsy. AJR Am J Roentgenol 1985;145:305–13.
18. Khan SR. Calcium oxalate crystal interaction with renal tubular epithelium, mechanism of crystal adhesion and its impact on stone development. Urol Res 1995;23:71–9.
19. Khan SR, Shevock PN, Hackett RL. Acute hyperoxaluria, renal injury and calcium oxalate urolithiasis. J Urol 1992;147:226–30.
20. Knapp PM, Kulb TB, Lingeman JE, et al. Extracorporeal shock wave lithotripsy-induced perirenal hematomas. J Urol 1988;139:700–3.
21. Kok DJ, Khan SR. Calcium oxalate nephrolithiasis, a free or fixed particle disease. Kidney Int 1994;46:847–54.
22. Lemann J Jr, Gray RW. Idiopathic hypercalciuria. J Urol 1989;141:715–8.
23. Lerner SP, Gleeson MJ, Griffith DP. Infection stones. J Urol 1989;141:753–8.
24. Lieske JC, Walsh-Reitz MM, Toback FG. Calcium oxalate monohydrate crystals are endocytosed by renal epithelial cells and induce proliferation. Am J Physiol 1992;262:F622–30.
25. Lingeman JE, Woods J, Toth PD, Evan AP, McAteer JA. The role of lithotripsy and its side effects. J Urol 1989;141:793–7.
26. Murray MJ, Chandhoke PS, Berman CJ, Sankey NE. Outcome of extracorporeal shockwave lithotripsy monotherapy for large renal calculi: effect of stone and collecting system surface areas and cost-effectiveness of treatment. J Endourol 1995;9:9–13.
27. Ohkawa M, Tokunaga S, Nakashima T, Orito M, Hisazumi H. Thiazide treatment for calcium urolithiasis in patients with idiopathic hypercalciuria. Br J Urol 1992;69:571–6.
28. Ohman S, Larsson L. Evidence for Randall's plaques to be the origin of primary renal stones. Med Hypotheses 1992;39:360–3.
29. Pak CY, Britton F, Peterson R, et al. Ambulatory evaluation of nephrolithiasis. Classification, clinical presentation and diagnostic criteria. Am J Med 1980;69:19–30.
30. Preminger GM. The metabolic evaluation of patients with recurrent nephrolithiasis: a review of comprehensive and simplified approaches. J Urol 1989;141:760–3.
31. Riese RJ, Riese JW, Kleinman JG, Weissner JH, Mandel GS, Mandel NS. Specificity in calcium oxalate adherence to papillary epithelial cells in cultures. Am J Physiol 1993;255:F1025–32.
32. Sarica K, Kupei S, Sarica N, Gogus O, Kilic S, Saribas S. Long-term follow-up of renal morphology and function in children after lithotripsy. Urol Int 1995;54:95–8.
33. Shiraga H, Min W, VanDusen WJ, et al. Inhibition of calcium oxalate crystal growth in vitro by uropontin: another member of the aspartic acid-rich protein superfamily. Proc Natl Acad Sci U S A 1992;89:426–30.
34. Smith LH. The medical aspects of urolithiasis: an overview. J Urol 1989;141:707–10.
35. Smith LH. The pathophysiology and medical treatment of urolithiasis. Semin Nephrol 1990;10:31– 52.
36. Tominaga Y, Grimelius L, Johansson H, et al. Histological and clinical features of non-familial primary parathyroid hyperplasia. Pathol Res Pract 1992;188:115–22.
37. Williams CM, Kaude JV, Newman RC, Peterson JC, Thomas WC. Extracorporeal shock-wave lithotripsy: long-term complications. AJR Am J Roentgenol 1988;150:311–5.
38. Wilson WT, Husmann DA, Morris JS, Miller GL, Alexander M, Preminger GM. A comparison of the bioeffects of four different modes of stone therapy on renal function and morphology. J Urol 1993;150:1267–70.

24 HYDRONEPHROSIS (OBSTRUCTIVE NEPHROPATHY)

Definition. Obstructive nephropathy is the term used for a myriad of pathologic/morphologic changes that occur in the kidney following obstruction of the urinary tract (hydronephrosis) (30–33,39,45). Obstruction to the flow of urine may occur at the level of the renal pelvis, ureter, urinary bladder, or portions of the urethra. The term hydronephrosis is usually used to denote dilatation of the renal pelvis and ureters. Obstructive nephropathy may result in irreversible renal damage.

Clinical Features. The signs and symptoms of patients with hydronephrosis depend on the rate of onset of the obstruction (i.e., either sudden or insidious), the location, the degree of obstruction (i.e., whether the obstruction is complete or partial), whether the obstruction is complicated by an infection or not, and the duration of the obstruction (i.e., short or prolonged) (13,31). The clinical manifestations also depend on whether the obstruction is unilateral or bilateral. Obstructive uropathy is a common entity that is treatable and often reversible (14,15,20,28,40).

The clinical presentation is quite variable and depends on the cause of the obstruction. Obstruction is secondary to functional or anatomic lesions that can be located anywhere in the urinary tract, from the renal tubules (e.g., crystals as in uric acid) to the urethral meatus. Complete sudden obstruction (as with a renal stone) may elicit an acute, severe, colic-like pain secondary to distention and contraction of the ureter. Partial obstruction may develop slowly and be clinically silent for a long time. Obviously, in unilateral ureteral obstruction the renal function as measured by blood urea nitrogen (BUN) and serum creatinine remains in the normal range, although the glomerular filtration rate (GFR) may be reduced. It is only with bilateral ureteral involvement and obstruction that renal function becomes severely impaired and an elevation in serum creatinine is detected (21,31).

In bilateral ureteral obstruction, the earliest findings may be polyuria, polydipsia, and nocturia, reflecting the loss of the renal concentrating ability (isosthenuria or hyposthenuria) (30–33). Renal tubular acidosis due to defects in urinary acidification may be identified. Renal tubular defects in the reabsorption of sodium, potassium, and glucose also occur. Whenever there is obstruction of the urinary tract, secondary infection may ensue and this may be the event that brings the patient to clinical attention. Surprisingly, unilateral severe obstruction with marked hydronephrosis may be clinically silent. In other cases, patients present with flank pain, enlarged tender kidney(s), or polycythemia.

Systemic hypertension has been associated frequently with hydronephrosis (1,37,42). Several possible mechanisms are proposed for this association, with a variable contribution for each in individual patients. In some cases, sodium retention with volume overload plays a major role, whereas in others there is activation of the renin-angiotensin system or even loss of medullary vasodepressor lipids (4,18,52). The extent to which these pathophysiologic processes are reversible is unclear, and only one third of patients who undergo surgery to correct the hydronephrosis return to normotensive levels.

The multiple causes of urinary tract obstruction (Table 24-1) and the subsequent hydronephrosis, are considered below. Obviously, the level of the obstruction dictates whether the obstruction is bilateral (e.g., at the level of the urinary bladder or urethra) or unilateral (involving only one ureter or pelvis). The obstruction can be intrinsic or extrinsic (external) to the urinary tract, and the lesions can be structural (organic) or functional (e.g., secondary to neurologic disorders) (2,13,16,22,30–34,41,43,53).

Approximately 0.5 percent of fetuses have been shown to have ureteral dilatation by ultrasound examination; most of these cases resolve by the end of the first year of life. Occasionally, the congenital urinary tract obstruction remains silent until adulthood (8,23,46).

Table 24-1

CAUSES OF OBSTRUCTION OF THE URINARY TRACT[a]

- **Intrinsic Causes**
  - Tumors
    - Benign tumors of renal pelvis, ureter, and bladder (e.g., fibrous polyp)
    - Malignant tumors of renal pelvis, ureter, bladder, and urethra
      - Transitional cell carcinoma
      - Squamous carcinoma
      - Sarcomas
        - Leiomyosarcoma
        - Hemangiosarcoma
        - Others
  - Infections
    - Renal pelvis and ureter
      - Malakoplakia
      - Xanthogranulomatous pyelitis and ureteritis
      - Pyeloureteritis cystica and glandularis
    - Urethra
      - Nongonococcal urethritis
      - Postgonococcal stricture
  - Renal and bladder calculi
  - Surgery-related lesions
    - Postoperative ureteral obstruction
    - Post-transplant obstruction
      - Surgical anastomosis
      - Rejection-mediated
      - Human polyoma virus (BK) infection
    - Post-traumatic urethral stricture
- **Extrinsic Causes**
  - Tumors
    - Direct extension lesions
      - Cervical carcinoma
      - Prostate carcinoma
      - Colorectal carcinoma
      - Ovarian and uterine carcinomas
    - Metastatic lesions
      - Breast carcinoma
      - Colon carcinoma
    - Tumor-related retroperitoneal fibrosis
      - Lymphomas
        - Hodgkin's disease
        - Non-Hodgkin's (principally histiocytic) lymphomas
      - Carcinomas: breast, stomach, prostate, cervix, colon, pancreas, ovary
    - Retroperitoneal neoplasms
  - Arterial obstruction
    - Aortic aneurysms
    - Aortic prostheses and bypasses
    - Iliac artery aneurysms
    - Arterial anomalies
      - Aberrant renal arteries
      - Others
  - Venous obstruction
    - Ovarian vein syndrome
    - Retrocaval ureter
    - Venous collaterals
  - Benign prostatic hyperplasia
  - Gynecologic conditions
    - Pregnancy
    - Ectopic pregnancy
    - Endometriosis
    - Pelvic inflammatory disease
    - Uterine prolapse
  - Surgery- and irradiation-related obstruction
    - Ureteral ligation
    - Postoperative retroperitoneal fibrosis
    - Radiation fibrosis
  - Gastrointestinal disease
    - Regional enteritis (Crohn's disease)
    - Ulcerative colitis
    - Lesions of the appendix
  - Retroperitoneal lesions
    - Idiopathic retroperitoneal fibrosis
    - Pelvic lipomatosis
    - Retroperitoneal hematomas
      - Traumatic
      - Anticoagulant related
      - Tumor related
        - Renal angiomyolipoma
        - Renal cell carcinoma
        - Wilms' tumor
        - Retroperitoneal hemangioma
  - Retroperitoneal cysts
    - Urogenital cysts
    - Mesocolic (enteric cysts)
    - Teratomas
    - Lymphatic cysts
  - Retroperitoneal abscesses
  - Miscellaneous
    - Renal pelvic cysts and diverticula
    - Ureteroceles
    - Ureteral cholesteatomas
    - Cerebrospinal fluid cysts, associated with ventriculoperitoneal shunts
    - Extrinsic fecal obstruction
    - Hydatid cysts
    - Foreign objects

[a]Modified from tables 20-4 and 20-5 from reference 33.

The most common cause of hydronephrosis in male children is the presence of posterior urethral valves, although other conditions may lead to infantile/pediatric obstruction, such as ureterocele and a variety of neurologic disorders (45). Congenital obstructive uropathy may be associated with other congenital abnormalities, such as unilateral renal agenesis, ectopia, dysplasia, or duplicated/fused kidneys (45).

Between childhood and the age of 60 years, urinary tract obstruction is much more common in women. The most common causes in

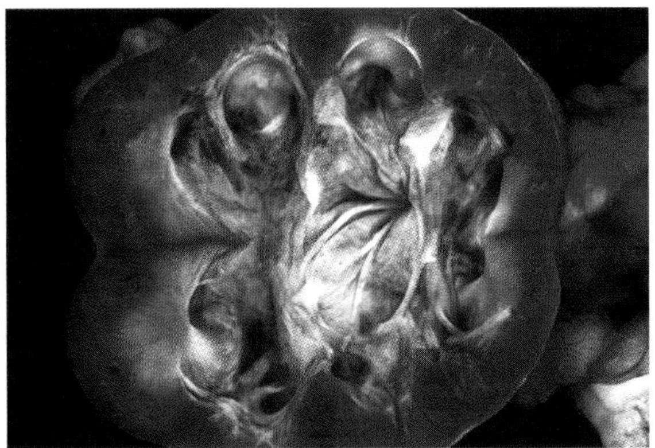

Figure 24-1

MILD TO MODERATE HYDRONEPHROSIS

There is mild to moderate dilatation of the renal pelvis but little ischemic atrophy of the overlying renal parenchyma.

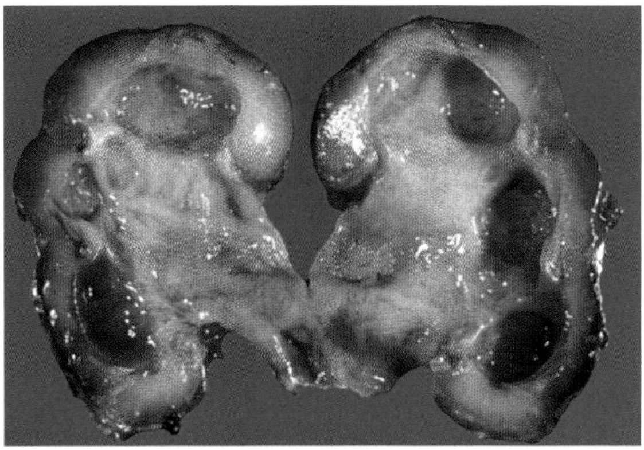

Figure 24-2

MARKED HYDRONEPHROSIS

In this infant with hydronephrosis, the renal pelvis is dilated with concomitant compression and blunting of the renal pelvic area (renal papillae are concave instead of their normal convex contour).

these patients are pregnancy (16,53) and gynecologic tumors (32,34), such as squamous cell carcinoma of the uterine cervix or endometrial adenocarcinoma. After the age of 60, the frequency of urinary tract obstruction increases in men, usually due to nodular hyperplasia of the prostate gland.

Gross Findings. The earliest renal change following complete urinary tract obstruction is a mild to moderate dilatation of the renal pelvis, with slight blunting of the renal calyces (fig. 24-1) (30,31). The weight of the kidney may be mildly increased owing to renal interstitial edema. After several days of continuing complete obstruction, the renal papillae become compressed, blunted, and flattened (assuming a concave instead of a normally convex shape). These morphologic changes are more apparent at the upper and lower poles than in the midregions of the kidney because the compound papillae at the poles permit the increased pressures (and the urinary fluid) to be transmitted into the overlying renal parenchyma more readily than do the simple papillae in the midregions. Simple papillae close under increased pressure, preventing reflux into the renal parenchyma, whereas the compound papillae remain open, allowing reflux into the kidney. There may be small regions of papillary necrosis due to further compromise of an already limited or tenuous vascular supply to that medullary region.

With continuing complete obstruction, or lengthy partial obstruction, there is progressive dilatation of the renal collecting systems and the renal pelvis, flattening of the papillae, and eventual thinning of the renal parenchyma (figs. 24-2, 24-3). This initial renal thinning occurs secondary to loss of the renal papillae and thinning of the renal medulla. As the disease progresses, the renal cortex begins to thin out as well. The renal parenchyma bulges outward between the fibromuscular septa that normally form the fibrous skeleton of the kidney. These septa radiate out like a fan from the renal hilum into the renal parenchyma and carry the segmental branches of renal arteries, veins, nerves, and lymphatics. The septa contain smooth muscle and adipose tissue as well. They are somewhat resistant to atrophy from pressure and offer some protection to the intervening renal cortex that forms the columns of Bertin.

The end stage of severe hydronephrosis is a pale kidney whose surface may appear bosselated, but is still reniform (figs. 24-4, 24-5) (31). There is often only a thin rim of renal parenchyma supported by fibrous septa radiating from the hilus. The renal parenchyma may be so thinned as to resemble parchment paper. When the markedly distended renal pelvis is drained of its fluid, the kidney collapses into a shapeless empty sac. The papillae disappear completely. As noted above, there is relative sparing of the

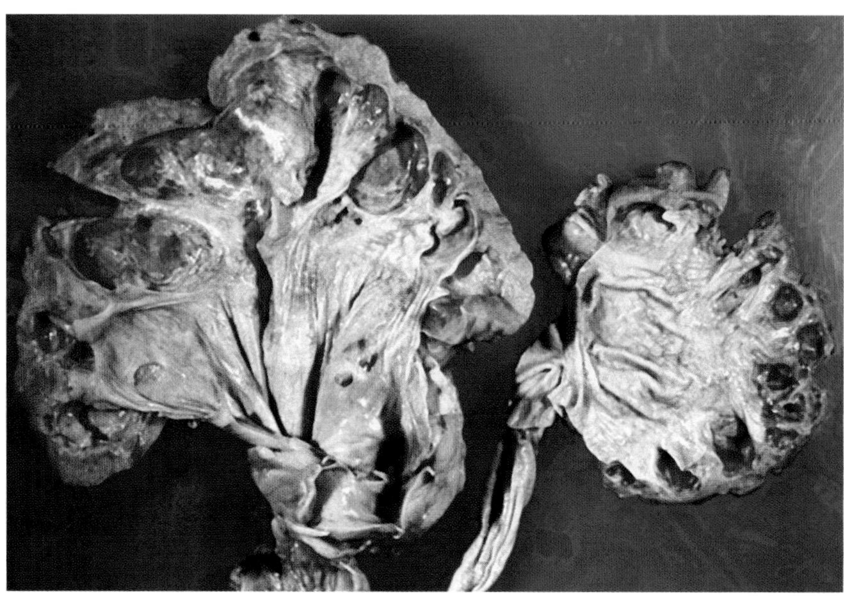

Figure 24-3

MARKED BILATERAL HYDRONEPHROSIS

There is progressive dilatation of the renal pelvis, with flattening of the papillae and thinning of the renal parenchyma. The renal cortex is extremely thinned.

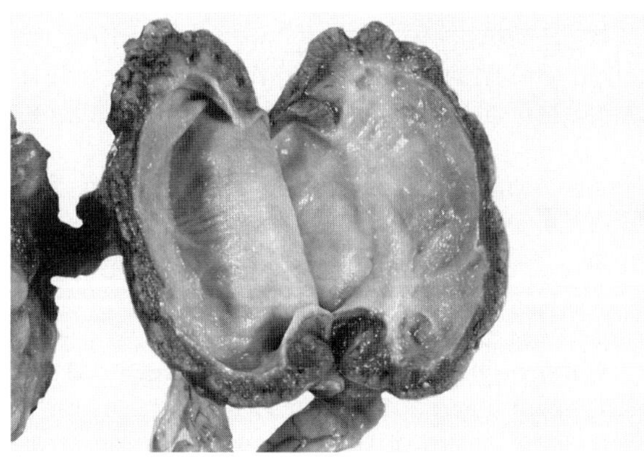

Figure 24-4

MARKED HYDRONEPHROSIS

There is marked dilatation of the renal pelvis with marked thinning of the overlying renal parenchyma. (Courtesy of Dr. J. Stejskal, Prague, Czech Republic and Dr. J. Pitha, Oklahoma City, OK.)

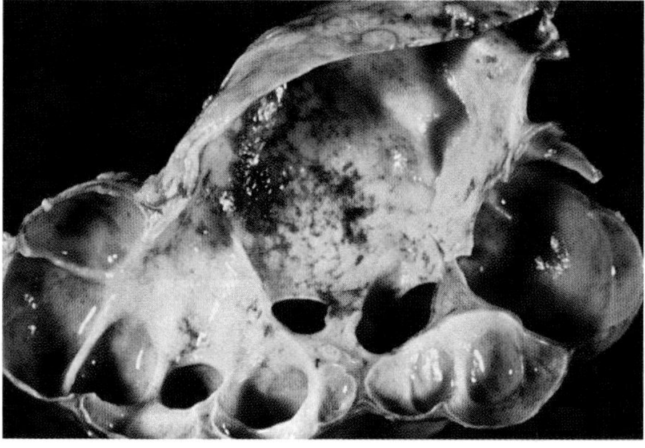

Figure 24-5

MARKED HYDRONEPHROSIS

There is marked dilatation of the renal collecting system with tremendous thinning of the renal parenchyma. All that remains of the renal parenchyma are the bridging fibromuscular septa that form the skeleton of the kidney.

columns of Bertin until very late in the hydronephrotic process when all portions (poles and midportions) are equally atrophic. The thin dilated sacs of atrophic kidney tissue often show splayed-out vessels of the atrophic parenchyma, resembling the veins in leaves.

Anatomic lesions of the upper urinary tract are less common causes of obstruction. The most common site of functional obstruction in the ureters is the ureteropelvic junction, which may have abnormally oriented muscle bundles, according to some investigators (9,10,24–26,41,49,50,51).

Light Microscopic Findings. The gross and microscopic appearances of hydronephrosis are similar, despite the multitude and disparity of the underlying causes (Table 24-1). The increased tension in the renal parenchyma leads to transformation of the renal interstitial cells into myofibroblasts, especially in the medulla and papillae. There is associated smooth muscle

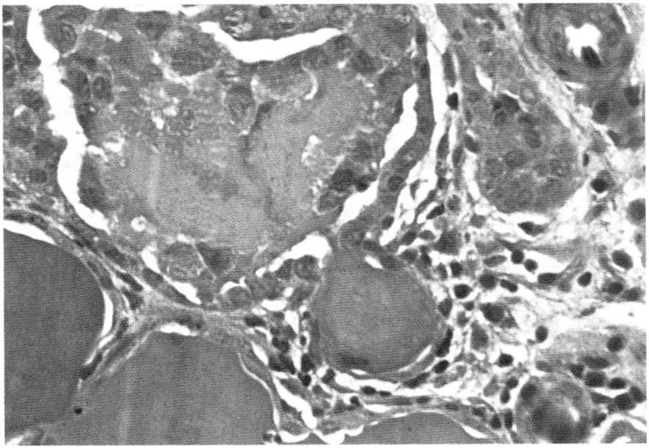

Figure 24-6

RUPTURED TUBULAR BASEMENT MEMBRANE

Periodic acid–Schiff (PAS)-positive cast-like material flows from the tubular lumen into the adjacent interstitium. This extravasation of tubular cast material is often noted in patients with renal obstruction (either intrarenal or extrarenal) (PAS stain).

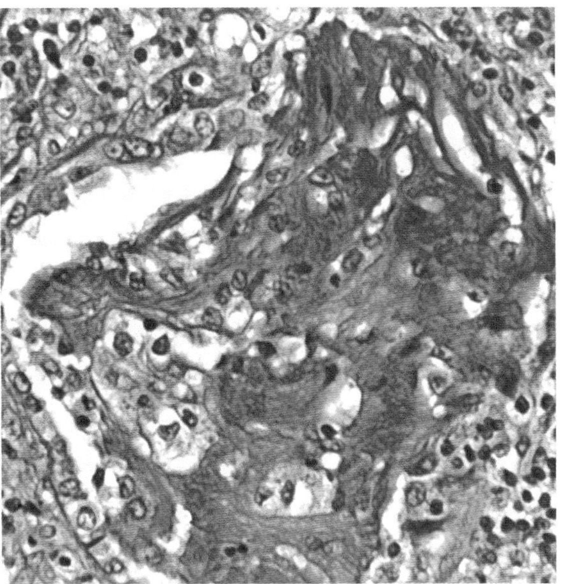

Figure 24-7

RUPTURED TUBULAR BASEMENT MEMBRANE

Microscopic examination of the renal parenchyma shows ischemic renal atrophy and PAS-positive acellular hyaline material in the renal interstitium. This represents Tamm-Horsfall protein (PAS stain).

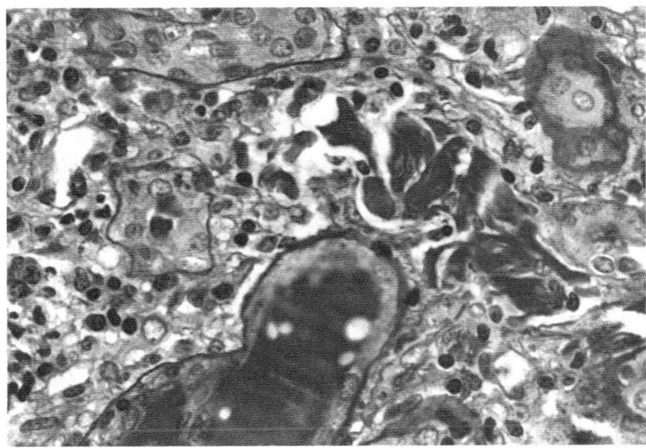

Figure 24-8

RUPTURED TUBULAR BASEMENT MEMBRANE

PAS-positive material is intratubular and interstitial. The latter represents extravasated fluid from the lumens of a patient with renal obstruction (PAS stain).

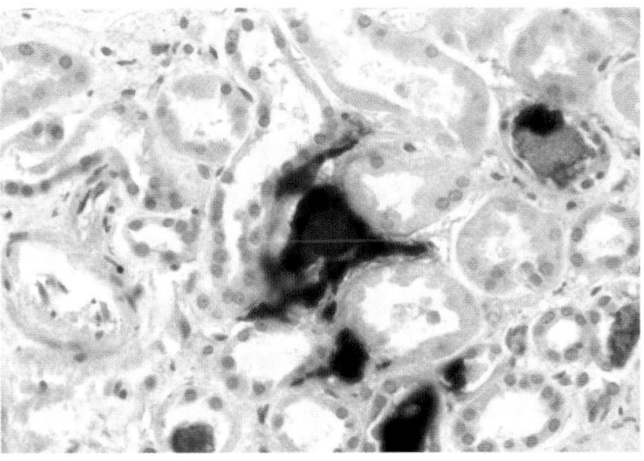

Figure 24-9

RUPTURED TUBULAR BASEMENT MEMBRANE

Immunocytochemical staining of an obstructed kidney with antibodies to Tamm-Horsfall protein. The intense staining is not only in the tubular lumens but also in the adjacent interstitium.

hyperplasia in the renal septa themselves. Studies have shown that in infants and small children these morphologic changes are even more pronounced, and a thick band of fibrous tissue and smooth muscle develops at the edge of the expanding renal pelvis (31).

The earliest microscopic renal parenchymal change is interstitial edema. There is also dilatation of the tubules and flattening of the tubular epithelium, particularly in the collecting ducts and the distal tubules. This dilatation of the collecting ducts is most prominent within the first day of obstruction, but may not be seen in pathologic specimens taken later. There is often loss of the periodic acid–Schiff (PAS)-positive

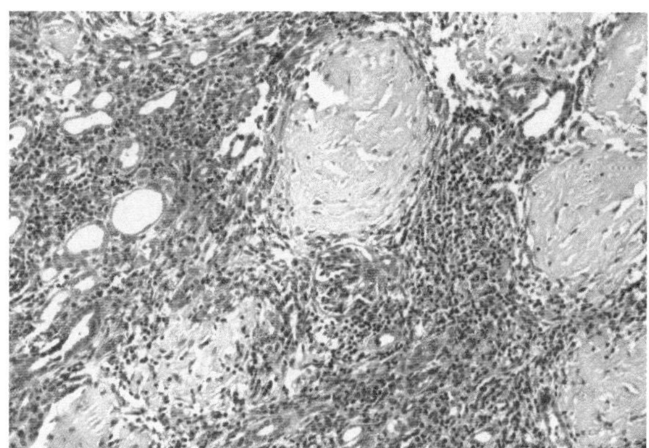

Figure 24-10

OBSTRUCTIVE NEPHROPATHY

Large lakes of slightly eosinophilic material are in the inflamed interstitium of the kidney. These represent chronic lesions of Tamm-Horsfall extravasation (hematoxylin and eosin [H&E] stain). (Courtesy of Dr. R. Mesa-Tejada, New York, NY.)

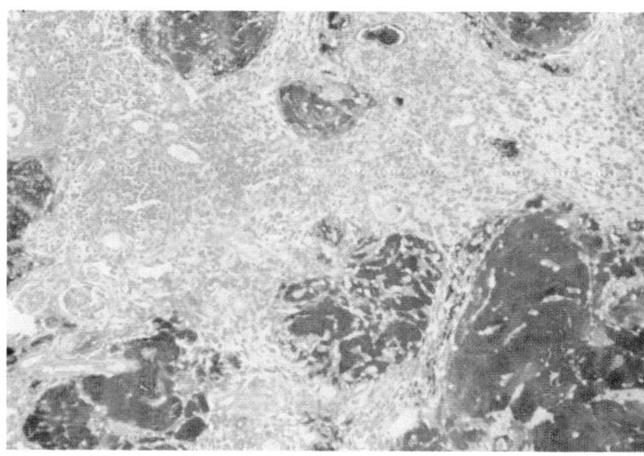

Figure 24-11

OBSTRUCTIVE NEPHROPATHY

The large interstitial lakes of acellular material stain markedly with the antibody to Tamm-Horsfall protein. (Courtesy of Dr. R. Mesa-Tejada, New York, NY.)

brush border of the proximal tubular epithelium. The interstitial peritubular capillaries are congested and may even develop microthrombi. Renal veins are dilated, although the arteries show few morphologic changes (31).

One very characteristic microscopic feature of urinary backflow (either in urinary tract obstruction or urinary reflux) is the presence of small to large, PAS-positive, acellular collections of Tamm-Horsfall protein in the peritubular spaces (due to rupture of the tubules), in the proximal tubular lumens, and in Bowman's space (figs. 24-6–24-11). Normally Tamm-Horsfall protein, which is produced in the medullary thick ascending limb of Henle, would only be identified in distal and collecting tubules. In hydronephrosis, the back-pressure from obstruction pushes the intratubular casts anterograde up the nephron. In the renal medulla and papillae there is ischemic atrophy. There may also be extensive hyaline degeneration of the interstitial collagen in the medulla. Although degeneration of medullary interstitial collagen is well recognized as an aging phenomenon, this process is much more accelerated in patients with hydronephrosis. This hyaline degeneration is often seen around the spiral arteries of the renal pelvis. There may be necrosis of the tubular epithelial cells lining the ducts of Bellini at the tips of the papillae, with exudation of neutrophils. Occasionally, there is cystic dilatation of the ducts of Bellini. Even the glomerular capillaries may be congested.

As the obstruction continues, the ischemic renal atrophy becomes more pronounced. The tubular atrophy and interstitial fibrosis appear to be more severe at the corticomedullary junction and in the superficial portions of the outer cortex. This is due to the pressure effects in the juxtamedullary nephrons (with their long loops of Henle) and Krogh's principle (that tissue farthest away from the incoming blood supply is most vulnerable to ischemia), respectively. As noted, the columns of Bertin are better preserved and the poles of the kidney tend to be more severely involved than the midportions (at least until the very late stages of hydronephrosis) (31).

There is only a mild chronic interstitial inflammation unless there is a secondary bacterial infection. Apoptotic tubular epithelial cells, as well as tubular mitotic figures, may be noted. Eventually, the tubular epithelial cells become quite thinned and simplified. There may be "thyroidization" of the tubules as well. The normal tubular profiles become distorted and irregular, with apparent out-pouchings or epithelial herniations. The tubular basement membranes are thickened. As noted above, the interstitium shows young fibroblast-like cells contributing to a cellular interstitial fibrosis. The tubules become increasingly separated from one another by the deposition of interstitial collagen (31).

The renal septa become more prominent because of atrophy of the surrounding parenchyma and because there is substantial hyperplasia and hypertrophy of the bundles of smooth muscle that extend radially into the cortex from the hilum. There is hyperplasia of the muscle layers of the renal veins in both the septa and within the renal parenchyma itself. These areas of smooth muscle hyperplasia are more prominent on the side of the veins toward the renal pelvis.

At the very end stages of the hydronephrotic process, the various components of the renal parenchyma, such as glomeruli and arteries/arterioles, leave almost no trace of their prior existence. The renal parenchyma has been reduced to a translucent, paper-thin wall between the thickened and prominent fibromuscular septal struts. All areas of the renal cortex are severely atrophic, including the poles, midportions, and even the columns of Bertin (31).

Immunofluorescence Findings. These are noncontributory.

Electron Microscopic Findings. The changes are nonspecific and reveal only the ultrastructural damage expected on the basis of the light microscopic findings. There may be widespread tubular epithelial cell changes, such as loss of brush border, vacuolated cytoplasm, increased number of lysosomes, and loss of basal interdigitations. There may be modest effacement of the visceral epithelial cell foot processes of glomeruli. With prolonged obstruction, the glomerular basement membranes become thickened, convoluted, and collapsed.

Etiology and Pathogenesis. The pathophysiologic mechanisms by which an obstruction in the urinary tract injures the kidney are incompletely understood. For many years, it was assumed that injury resulted entirely from increased pressure inside the renal pelvis, with secondary reflux of urine into the collecting ducts, and transmission of the increased pressure into the medulla. The pressure measured inside the renal pelvis in certain experimental models of hydronephrosis, however, is actually often only slightly increased and can be normal. It has now been shown that the renal damage is due to a combination of two important and related factors: markedly increased tension in the wall of the kidney due to the increased pressure and prominent renal vasoconstriction (3,6,19,27,29,35,36,44,47,48,54,55).

Many of the studies of obstructive nephropathy and hydronephrosis are from animal experimentation, usually involving manipulations leading to complete obstruction of the urinary tract (3,5–8,18,38,44,47). Clinically, partial obstruction is more common than complete obstruction and little is known about the changes that occur in the course of partial obstructive nephropathy (especially early) in man.

Acute experimental obstruction of the ureter leads to three responses related to the ureteral pressure and renal blood flow. Initially, the renal blood flow and ureteral pressure rise in parallel. The increased blood flow (vasodilatation) is confined to the renal cortex, with the tenuous medullary blood flow declining from the very onset. The second phase begins by about 2 hours and is manifested by vasoconstriction leading to reduction in renal blood flow as the renal pelvic pressures rise. Finally, the renal pelvic pressure drops (at about 5 hours) in concert with the reductions in glomerular filtration rate and renal blood flow. Subsequently, pressures in the renal pelvis and ureter, and the renal blood flow, continue to decline progressively. The blood flow decline continues to be much greater in the renal cortex, although perhaps the decreasing blood flow is more devastating in the tenuously supplied renal medulla (31,48).

It appears that the initial renal vasodilatation is secondary to intrarenal release of prostaglandin E2 (PGE2) and the vasoconstriction secondary to the release of thromboxane A2 (TXA2) and, importantly, activation of the renin-angiotensin system (7,35,52). The onset of the obstruction leads to an outpouring of lymphocytes and macrophages into the renal cortex, and this appears to be responsible for a marked release of cytokines, especially of tumor growth factor-beta and insulin-like growth factor type 1 (17). During this time, there is a period of major increase in interstitial cells and the transformation of these cells into myofibroblasts (11,12).

The increased tension on the renal parenchyma elongates and narrows the renal vasculature (especially the arcuate and segmental arteries). This is followed by narrowing and collapse of the postglomerular vasculature (54,55).

As noted above, virtually all of the pathogenetic data have been obtained from experimental models of acute and complete obstruction, whereas in the human most obstruction appears to be intermittent and incomplete, at least initially. In the few experimental studies of partial obstruction, it appears that the lesions progress slowly and may stabilize, typically at 2 to 4 weeks postobstruction. Renal blood flow may be increased, but the damage seems to occur during the period of increased intrapelvic pressure. These observations in experimental animals correlate with the clinical course of certain patients who remain stable over long periods of time, with little deterioration of renal function. There may be a balance between the emptying of the obstructed outlet and the reabsorption through pyelovenous and pyelotubular pathways sufficient enough to prevent further elevation of intrapelvic pressure.

Treatment and Prognosis. Treatment obviously depends on the underlying condition leading to the obstruction. The major question is how much of the renal function can be recovered after the obstruction is relieved. Prompt relief of obstruction (such as extraction of a renal stone) should lead to complete recovery. An end-stage, severely hydronephrotic kidney with a very thin cortex (several millimeters) will have no ability to recover. Between these two extremes, the situation with regards to renal recovery is far less clear (14,15,20,28,40).

The duration of the obstruction is clearly the most important factor in determining the ability to recover renal function. Experimental studies suggest that nearly complete renal recovery can occur if the acute obstruction is relieved within approximately 4 days (5,6,8). Some recovery of renal function can occur after obstruction of even 3 weeks' duration, although there may be some degree of irreversible renal damage and renal recovery can take up to several months (14). Of course, the exact relationship of these experimental conditions to the human condition is unclear, and the duration of obstruction in humans is not known with precision. In humans, recovery of renal function, as measured by function on an intravenous pyelogram (IVP) has been shown to occur even after 72 days of accidental ureteral obstruction (e.g., following a hysterectomy) (28). The renal recovery, however, may be partial and very little information exists on human unilateral function.

Some clinicians suggest that after the obstruction is relieved (e.g., by stent), the patient should be monitored for 2 weeks and the degree of renal function reevaluated with a renal isotopic scan. Diuresis may occur following relief of the obstruction; this is secondary to tubular injury and loss of function of apical transporters responsible for salt and water reabsorption. There may be a need for fluid and electrolyte support during the early interval following relief of the obstruction.

REFERENCES

1. Abramson M, Jackson B. Hypertension and unilateral hydronephrosis. J Urol 1984;132:746–8.
2. Antonakopoulos G, Fuggle W, Newman J, Considine J, O'Brien J. Idiopathic hydronephrosis. Light microscopic features and pathogenesis. Arch Pathol Lab Med 1985;109:1097–101.
3. Bander S, Buerkert J, Martin D, Klahr S. Long-term effects of 24-hr unilateral ureteral obstruction on renal function in the rat. Kidney Int 1985;28:614–20.
4. Berka JL, Alcorn D, Bertram JF, Ryan GB, Skinner SL. Effects of angiotensin converting enzyme inhibition on glomerular number, juxtaglomerular cell activity and renin content in experimental unilateral hydronephrosis. J Hypertens 1994;12:735–43.
5. Bogaert GA, Gluckman GR, Mevorach RA, Kogan BA. Renal preservation despite 35 days of partial bladder obstruction in the fetal lamb. J Urol 1995;154:694–9.
6. Buerkert J, Martin D, Head M, Prasad J, Klahr S. Deep nephron function after release of acute unilateral ureteral obstruction in the young rat. J Clin Invest 1978;62:1228–39.
7. Chen RN, Inman SR, Stowe NT, Novick AC. Role of endothelium-derived relaxing factor in the maintenance of renal blood flow in a rodent model of chronic hydronephrosis. Urology 1995;46:438–42.

8. Cheng EY, Maizels M, Chou P, Hartanto V, Shapiro E. Response of the newborn ureteropelvic junction complex to induced and later reversed partial ureteral obstruction in the rabbit model. J Urol 1993;150:782–9.
9. Costantinou C, Djurhuus J. Pyeloureteral dynamics in the intact and chronically obstructed multicaliceal kidney. Am J Physiol 1981;241: R398–411.
10. dell'Agnola CA, Carmassi L, Tadini B, Ghisoni L, Carmignani L. Predictability of duration and severity of congenital hydronephrosis as a cause of smooth muscle deterioration in pyelo-ureteral junction obstruction. Eur J Pediatr Surg 1992;2:274–6.
11. Diamond JR. Macrophages and progressive renal disease in experimental hydronephrosis. Am J Kidney Dis 1995;26:133–40.
12. Diamond JR, van Goor H, Ding G, Engelmyer E. Myofibroblasts in experimental hydronephrosis. Am J Pathol 1995;146:121–9.
13. Drake D, Stevens P, Eckstein H. Hydronephrosis secondary to ureteropelvic obstruction in children: a review of 14 years of experience. J Urol 1978;119:649–51.
14. Fallon B. Functional recovery in a kidney after prolonged, complete ureteric obstruction. Br J Urol 1977;49:72.
15. Fink R, Caridis D, Chmiel R, Ryan G. Renal impairment and its reversibility following variable periods of complete ureteric obstruction. Aust N Z J Surg 1980;50:77–83.
16. Fried AM. Hydronephrosis of pregnancy: ultrasonographic study and classification of asymptomatic women. Am J Obstet Gynecol 1979;135:1066–70.
17. Frokiaer J, Flyvbjerg A, Knudsen L. Obstructive nephropathy in the pig. Possible roles for insulin-like growth factor I. Urol Res 1992;20:335–9.
18. Frokiaer J, Pedersen EB, Knudsen L, Djurhuus JC. The impact of total unilateral ureteral obstruction on intrarenal angiotensin II production in the polycalyceal pig kidney. Scand J Urol Nephrol 1992;26:289–95.
19. Fung LC, Steckler RE, Khoury AE, McLorie GA, Chait PG, Churchill BM. Intrarenal resistive index correlates with renal pelvis pressure. J Urol 1994;152:607–11; discussion 612–3.
20. Gillenwater JY, Westervelt FB Jr, Vaughan ED Jr, Howards SS. Renal function after release of chronic unilateral hydronephrosis in man. Kidney Int 1975;7:1179–86.
21. Glassberg KI, Braren V, Duckett JW, et al. Suggested terminology for duplex systems, ectopic ureters and ureteroceles. J Urol 1984;132:1153–4.
22. Gleason PE, Kelalis PP, Husmann DA, Kramer SA. Hydronephrosis in renal ectopia: incidence, etiology and significance. J Urol 1994;151:1660–1.
23. Gloor JM. Management of prenatally detected fetal hydronephrosis. Mayo Clin Proc 1995;70:145–52.
24. Gosling JA, Dixon JS. The structure of the normal and hydronephrotic upper urinary tract. In: O'Reilly PH, Gosling JA, eds. Idiopathic hydronephrosis. New York: Springer Verlag; 1982:1–15.
25. Hanna MK, Jeffs RD, Sturgess JM, Barkin M. Ureteral structure and ultrastructure. Part IV. The dilated ureter, clinicopathological correlation. J Urol 1977;117:28–32.
26. Hanna MK, Jeffs RD, Sturgess JM, Barkin M. Ureteral structure and ultrastructure. Part II. Congenital ureteropelvic junction obstruction and primary obstructive megaureter. J Urol 1976;116:725–30.
27. Hanss BG, Lewy JE, Vari RC. Alterations in glomerular dynamics in congenital, unilateral hydronephrosis. Kidney Int 1994;46:48–57.
28. Hata M, Tachibana M, Deguchi N, Jitsukawa S. Recovery of renal function after 72 days of anuria caused by ureteral obstruction. J Urol 1983;130:537–8.
29. Hayashi K, Loutzenhiser R, Epstein M, Suzuki H, Saruta T. Multiple factors contribute to acetylcholine-induced renal afferent arteriolar vasodilation during myogenic and norepinephrine- and KCl-induced vasoconstriction. Studies in the isolated perfused hydronephrotic kidney. Circ Res 1994;75:821–8.
30. Hill GS. Basic physiology and morphology of hydronephrosis. In: Hill GS, ed. Uropathology. New York: Churchill Livingstone; 1989:467–515.
31. Hill GS. Calcium and the kidney, hydronephrosis. In: Jennette JC, Olson JL, Schwartz MM, Silva FG, eds. Heptinstall's pathology of the kidney, 5th ed. Philadelphia: Lippincott-Raven; 1998:891–936.
32. Hill GS. Intrinsic and extrinsic obstruction of the urinary tract. In: Hill GS, ed. Uropathology. New York: Churchill Livingstone; 1989:517–74.
33. Hill GS. Ureteropelvic junction obstruction. In: Hill GS, ed. Uropathology. New York: Churchill Livingstone; 1989:575–98.
34. Hubner WA, Plas EG, Porpaczy P. Hydronephrosis in malignant tumors: rationale and efficiency of endo-urological diversions. Eur J Surg Oncol 1993;19:27–32.
35. Huland H, Gonnermann D. Pathophysiology of hydronephrotic atrophy: the cause and role of active preglomerular vasoconstriction. Urol Int 1983;38:193–8.

36. Huland H, Leichtweiss HP, Augustin HJ. Effect of angiotensin II antagonist, alpha-receptor blockage, and denervation on blood flow reduction in experimental, chronic hydronephrosis. Invest Urol 1980;18:203–6.
37. Kawano S, Yano S, Takahashi S, Nomura Y, Ogata J. A case of hypertension due to unilateral hydronephrosis in a child. Eur Urol 1986;12:357–9.
38. Kennedy WA 2nd, Stenberg A, Lackgren G, Hensle TW, Sawczuk IS. Renal tubular apoptosis after partial ureteral obstruction. J Urol 1994;152:658–64.
39. Kern WF, Laszik ZG, Nadasdy T, Silva FG, Bane BL, Pitha JV, eds. Disorders of the interstitium: interstitial nephritis, pyelonephritis, papillary necrosis, analgesic nephropathy, and obstructive nephropathy (hydronephrosis). Atlas of renal pathology, Philadelphia: W.B. Saunders; 1999:136.
40. Lewis HY, Pierce JM. Return of function after relief of complete ureteral obstruction of 69 days duration. J Urol 1962;88:377–9.
41. Lowe FC, Marshall FF. Ureteropelvic junction obstruction in adults. Urology 1984;23:331–5.
42. Mizuiri S, Amagasaki Y, Hosaka H, et al. Hypertension in unilateral atrophic kidney secondary to ureteropelvic junction obstruction. Nephron 1992;61:217–9.
43. Monzen Y, Mori H, Wakisaka M, et al. Hydronephrosis caused by a left renal vein in a patient with horseshoe kidney: a case report. Radiat Med 1993;11:95–7.
44. Morrison AR, Benabe JE. Prostaglandins and vascular tone in experimental obstructive nephropathy. Kidney Int 1981;19:786–90.
45. Peters CA. Urinary tract obstruction in children. J Urol 1995;154:1874–83; discussion 1883–4.
46. Peters CA, Carr MC, Lais A, Retik AB, Mandell J. The response of the fetal kidney to obstruction. J Urol 1992;148:503–9.
47. Reif R, Kucera J, Obrucnik M, Kamarad V. Experimental hydronephrotic atrophy of the kidney in light microscopy. Acta Univ Palacki Olomuc Fac Med 1982;103:123–37.
48. Solez K, Ponchak S, Buono RA, et al. Inner medullary plasma flow in the kidney with ureteral obstruction. Am J Physiol 1976;231:1315–21.
49. Starr NT, Maizels M, Chou P, Branningan R, Shapiro E. Microanatomy and morphometry of the hydronephrotic "obstructed" renal pelvis in asymptomatic infants. J Urol 1992;148:519–24.
50. Stock JA, Krous HF, Hefferman J, Packer M, Kaplan GW. Correlation of renal biopsy and radionuclide renal scan differential function in patients with unilateral ureteropelvic junction obstruction. J Urol 1995;154:716–8.
51. Tokunaka S, Gotoh T, Koyanagi T, Miyabe N. Muscle dysplasia in megaureters. J Urol 1984;131:383–90.
52. Vari RC, Boineau FG, Lewy JE. Angiotensin or thromboxane receptor antagonism in rats with congenital hydronephrosis. J Am Soc Nephrol 1993;3:1522–9.
53. Weiss RE, Stone NN. Persistent maternal hydronephrosis after intra-abdominal pregnancy. J Urol 1994;152:1196–8.
54. Winterborn MH, France NE. Arterial changes associated with hydronephrosis in infants and children. Br J Urol 1972;44:96–104.
55. Wyker AT, Ritter RC, Marion D, Gillenwater JY. Mechanical factors and tissue stresses in chronic hydronephrosis. Invest Urol 1981;18:430–6.

25 THE END-STAGE KIDNEY

END-STAGE RENAL DISEASE

Definition. The deterioration of renal function in a patient with an acute rapidly progressive or chronic progressive renal disease may culminate in end-stage renal disease (ESRD) (5,54, 56). By this time, the glomerular filtration rate is less than one fifth the normal value and the patient requires renal replacement therapy in the form of dialysis or transplantation. ESRD is defined by the United States Renal Data System (USRDS) as renal failure continuing beyond a period of 90 days that requires extracorporeal renal dialysis to sustain life (5,47,54,56).

In the period of 1960 to 1980, bilateral nephrectomies were frequently performed on patients with ESRD for the treatment of intractable hypertension or in preparation for renal transplantation. A morphologic diagnosis of ESRD would be made on these nephrectomy or autopsy kidneys, often with no attempt to further classify and delineate the underlying disease. In the 1970s Schwartz and Cotran (50) studied 95 pretransplant nephrectomy specimens and were able to determine the primary renal disease in 90. By examination of glomeruli that were not in an advanced stage of sclerosis, they classified 34 of 47 specimens as chronic glomerulonephritis. This study showed that the original disease could be determined in many patients with advanced/end-stage kidneys with severe renal failure. This is important not only for clinical and demographic studies, but to determine the risk of recurrent disease in those undergoing renal transplantation (4).

Clinical Features. When the glomerular filtration rate reaches or falls below 9 mL/min, the patient usually becomes uremic. The signs and symptoms of uremia are listed in Table 25-1. Once the serum creatinine rises to over 8 to 9 mg/dL, the patient generally requires renal replacement therapy.

The clinical features of the patient approaching ESRD depend on: 1) the underlying renal disease which leads to the ESRD, and 2) any signs/symptoms of impending uremia (before renal replacement therapy can be administered). According to data from the USRDS (55,56), the major underlying diseases of new patients developing ESRD are diabetes (40 percent or more), hypertension (26 to 38 percent), and glomerulonephritis of some sort (usually unspecified; 12 to 16 percent); polycystic kidney disease accounts for 3 percent and urologic conditions another 3 percent. The remaining percentages are of unknown etiologies. Thus, in the United States, more than 60 percent of patients with ESRD have diabetes mellitus and hypertension. A number of investigators have discussed the effects of racial differences on the incidence and prognosis of renal diseases (53).

After beginning dialysis, the end-stage kidneys continue to undergo atrophic changes. The vascular tree continues to become narrow and obliterated, and the kidneys often develop cysts, renal tubular epithelial hyperplasia, and even epithelial neoplasms. Hemorrhage, pain, and even renal cell carcinoma can occur in this setting.

The frequency of ESRD in the 1990s, according to the USRDS, was approximately 1,000 patients/million population/year in the United States (5,56). Over the past 10 years, the rate of patients with ESRD requiring renal replacement therapy has increased about 8 percent/year. The incidence of ESRD is higher in the United States than in other industrialized countries such as Japan, France, the Netherlands, Canada, Poland, and Australia, probably because of greater acceptance of ESRD patients for renal replacement therapy in the United States. The cost of renal replacement therapy in the United States in 1996 was $14.5 billion (for approximately 300,000 patients), or about $50,000/year/patient (33,54).

The prevalence of ESRD is increasing at an alarming rate. In 2000, chronic kidney failure

Table 25-1

MANIFESTATIONS OF CHRONIC RENAL FAILURE[a]

General
- Nausea and vomiting
- Malnutrition
- Fluid overload/edema/occasional ascites
- Uriniferous breath
- Secondary oxalosis
- Painful myopathy

Heart
- Congestive heart failure
- Coronary artery disease/arteriosclerosis
- Uremic cardiomyopathy (dilated, hypertrophic)

Pericardium
- Uremic pericarditis ("bread and butter," fibrinous)
- Fluid accumulation with cardiac tamponade
- Constrictive pericarditis

Blood Vessels
- Oxalate deposition in media of arteries
- Atherosclerosis

Lung
- Pulmonary edema/congestion
- "Uremic pneumonitis" (acute respiratory distress syndrome with hyaline membranes)
- Metastatic calcification

Skin
- Sallow, yellow appearance (due to accumulations of carotene pigments)
- White frost (urea secreted through skin)

Beta-2-Microglobulin Amyloidosis/Deposition
- Articular surfaces of bone
- Periarticular connective tissue
- Nerve sheaths
- Carpal tunnel syndrome
- Destructive arthropathy (shoulders, knees)
- Bone cysts/fractures

Gastrointestinal Tract
- Inflammation/mucosal erosions and ulcerations
- Angiodysplasia
- Ischemia
- Amyloid deposition

Pancreas
- Acute pancreatitis/chronic pancreatitis

Hematopoietic System
- Hypoplastic anemia (multifactorial including relative deficiency of erythropoietin; normocytic, normochromic)
- Platelet dysfunction

Chronic Hepatitis
- Hepatitis C
- Hepatitis B

Central Nervous System
- Cerebrovascular disease/infarcts or hemorrhage
- Uremic encephalopathy
- Dialysis disequilibrium syndromes
- Dialysis dementia
- Delirium/coma/death

Secondary Parathyroid Hyperplasia

Renal Osteodystrophy
- Osteitis fibrosa
- Osteomalacia
- Adynamic bone disease

Hypertension (malignant, volume overload, associated with elevated plasma renin levels)

occurred in over 90,000 individuals in the United States. The current population of patients on dialysis is approximately 300,000 and 80,000 patients are living with transplanted kidneys. Both the prevalence and the incidence of ESRD are about twice what they were just 10 years ago (56). In fact, in the year 2000, the number of patients with newly diagnosed renal failure exceeded the number of patients who died of any single type of cancer except lung cancer. Caring for patients with ESRD consumes more than $18 billion/year in the United States alone. Six percent of the Medicare budget is used for this service (55).

Gross Findings. The macroscopic renal findings depend on the underlying renal disease leading to the ESRD (12,14,15). The length of time that the patient is on dialysis also affects the gross morphologic findings. Patients on dialysis have progressive renal atrophy, with some kidneys weighing as little as a few dozen grams (normal is 150 to 175 g/kidney) (figs. 25-1–25-3). When examined late in the course of ESRD, with or without dialysis, the kidneys are markedly reduced in size and may be so atrophic that the original disease cannot be determined. Thus, review of the clinical history and examination of the kidneys as early as possible in the course

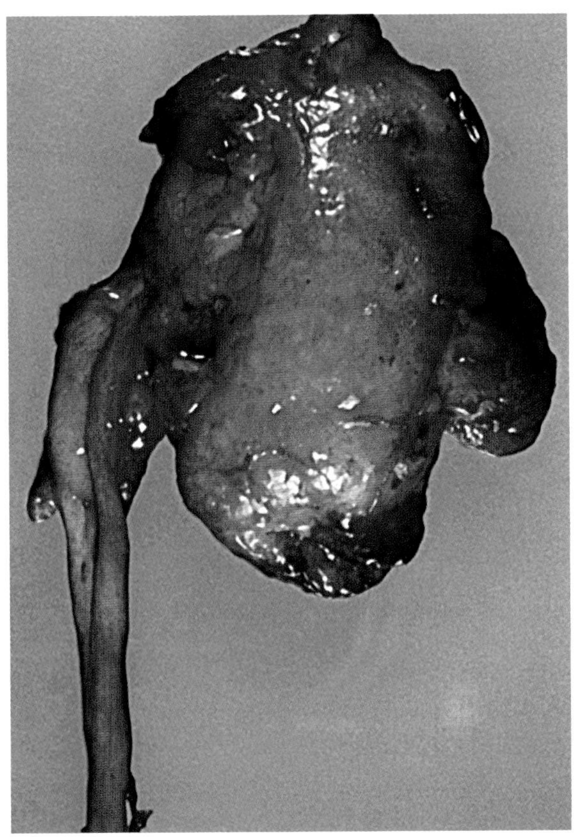

Figure 25-1

END-STAGE KIDNEY

The kidney is very small (less than 25 g). The cause of this unilaterally small kidney was uncertain.

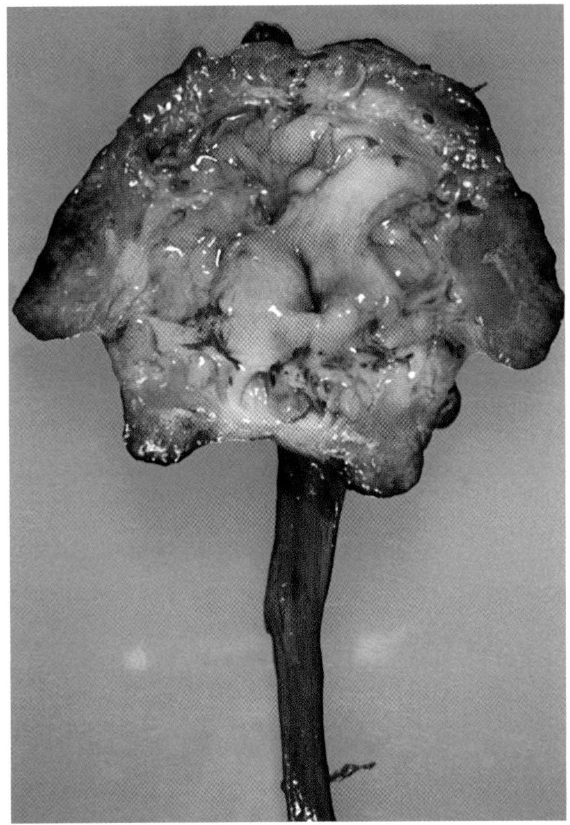

Figure 25-2

END-STAGE KIDNEY

Cross section of the kidney seen in figure 25-1. The "hyperplasia" of the peripelvic adipose tissue is apparent relative to atrophy of the renal parenchyma.

of the renal disease allows for a more specific and informed diagnosis than that of "end-stage kidney disease."

There may be some diagnostic gross and microscopic changes, even in advanced cases. According to Hughson (14,20), the end-stage kidney can be subdivided into at least four categories: 1) hypertensive vascular disease, 2) diabetic nephrosclerosis, 3) chronic pyelonephritis, and 4) glomerulonephritis of some sort.

Hypertensive Vascular Disease. Longstanding vascular disease (which may be primary or secondary to another renal disease) results in small kidneys. However, the kidneys are generally not as shrunken as those with severe chronic glomerulonephritis or chronic pyelonephritis. The cortical surface in hypertensive kidneys usually has a regular fine granularity (fig. 25-4), although large vascular scars may be present and confused

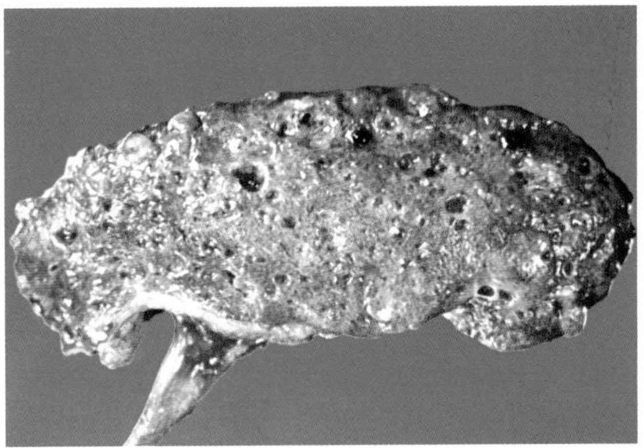

Figure 25-3

END-STAGE KIDNEY

The kidney is small and weighs less than 90 g. Note the granular surface and the numerous small cysts. The nature of the initial renal disease (i.e., the underlying disease) was not apparent in this patient.

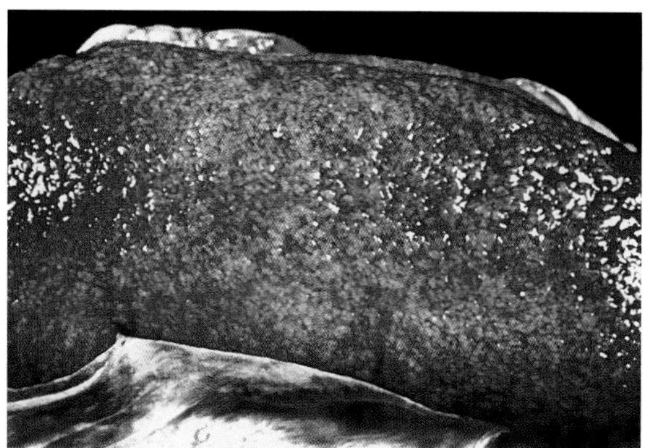

Figure 25-4

ADVANCED RENAL DISEASE SECONDARY TO VASCULAR DISEASE/HYPERTENSION

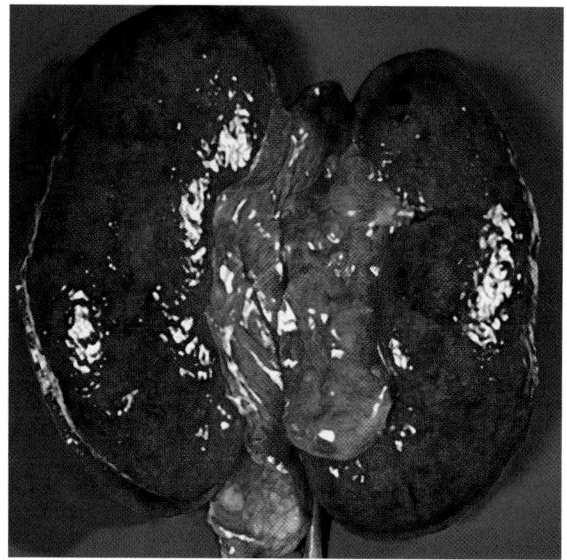

Figure 25-5

END-STAGE KIDNEY DISEASE SECONDARY TO MALIGNANT HYPERTENSION

Irregular blotching of the cortical surface is seen.

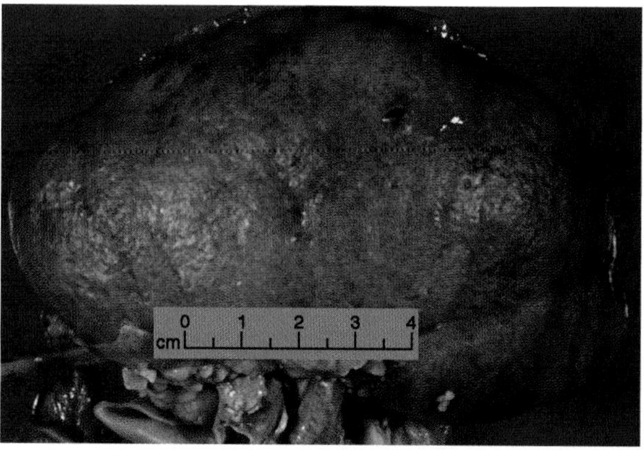

Figure 25-6

END-STAGE KIDNEY DISEASE SECONDARY TO ADVANCED DIABETIC NEPHROPATHY

This is a "large contracted kidney." Despite advanced tubular atrophy and interstitial fibrosis, the kidneys of diabetic patients are often enlarged.

with the broad-based scars of bonafide chronic pyelonephritis. The renal capsule usually strips fairly easily from the surrounding tissues. End-stage kidneys from patients with malignant hypertension are usually normal in size or only slightly smaller than normal (the latter if there was preexisting "benign" hypertension) (fig. 25-5).

Cross-section of the kidney shows a cortex that usually measures much less than the normal 6 to 7 mm in thickness. Petechial hemorrhages may be noted on the cut surface of the renal cortex if there is severe hypertension. Ideally, the larger blood vessels should be sectioned and studied macroscopically and microscopically. Unless there is true chronic pyelonephritis or papillary necrosis, the pyelocalyceal systems are intact, with convex papillae and no dilatation. The transitional mucosa appears normal and there is little chronic inflammation under the urothelium.

Diabetic Nephrosclerosis. The end-stage kidney secondary to diabetes mellitus is usually normal in size or may be even enlarged, the "large contracted kidney" of diabetes mellitus (fig. 25-6). The surface is usually granular, reflecting the underlying vascular disease.

Chronic Pyelonephritis. Typically, the broad-based, U-shaped cortical scars in patients with chronic pyelonephritis directly overlie the dilated, inflamed, damaged and distorted pyelocalyceal system (fig. 25-7). That is, the renal papillae, rather than normally convex and rounded, are distorted and concave. Because of this destruction of the terminal collecting tubules of the nephrons, the overlying nephrons that drain into these collecting ducts become obsolescent, thereby producing the U-shaped cortical scar. In these cortical areas, the renal parenchyma may be quite thin. In patients with

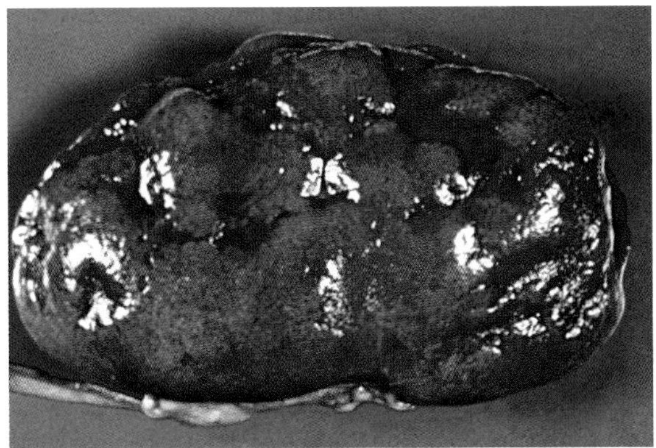

Figure 25-7

END-STAGE KIDNEY DISEASE SECONDARY TO CHRONIC PYELONEPHRITIS

Large scars are apparent on the cortical surface.

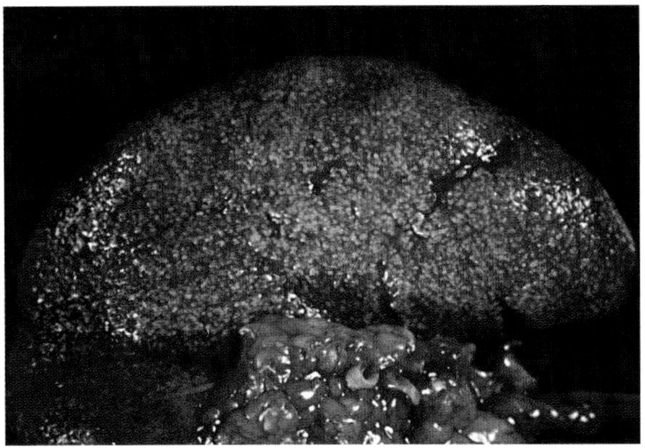

Figure 25-8

END-STAGE KIDNEY DISEASE SECONDARY TO CHRONIC GLOMERULONEPHRITIS (NOT OTHERWISE SPECIFIED)

There is a granular surface to this shrunken kidney.

bonafide chronic pyelonephritis, the pyelocalyceal system is lined by thickened, fibrotic, and chronically inflamed transitional mucosa.

Differentiating a scar of chronic pyelonephritis from a vascular (atherosclerotic) scar may be difficult. Both pyelonephritic and vascular cortical scars may be large and deep. Generally, the vascular scars are V-shaped, whereas scars in chronic pyelonephritis are U-shaped with irregular borders. Study of the vascular tree and especially the underlying pyelocalyceal system (as well as the clinical history) will often elucidate the underlying cause of the renal parenchymal scar. Sections must therefore include the renal papillae.

Glomerulonephritis. The kidneys of patients with progressive glomerulonephritis are usually much smaller than normal and the surface is granular (fig. 25-8). This granularity may be somewhat coarser than that seen with small vessel disease (arteriolar nephrosclerosis). On cross sectioning, the cortex is irregularly thinned and the corticomedullary junction is sometimes indistinct. These kidneys may be very small, weighing as little as 20 g. Sometimes, other underlying renal conditions that lead to ESRD may be elucidated or suspected by gross examination. Proper sectioning of the kidney allows study of the pyelocalyceal system for evidence of papillary disease (as in chronic pyelonephritis, analgesic nephropathy, or papillary necrosis).

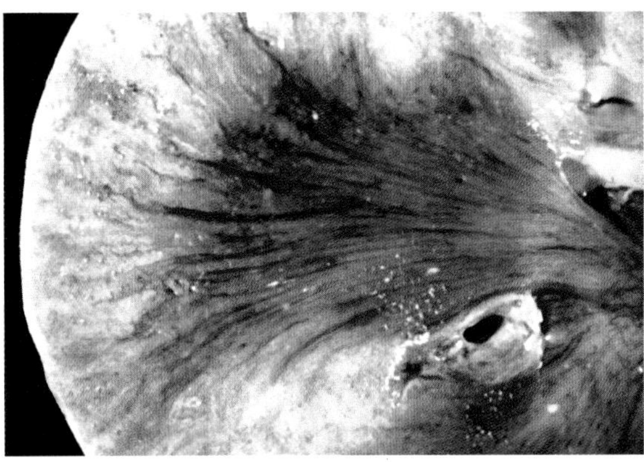

Figure 25-9

END-STAGE KIDNEY DISEASE SECONDARY TO AMYLOIDOSIS

Cross section of the kidney shows replacement of the renal parenchyma by "starchy" white material (amyloid).

Other glomerular diseases may lead to ESRD. In *amyloidosis*, the kidneys are firm, pale, and usually enlarged. The cortex is thick and has a waxy, gray, translucent appearance if the amyloidosis is widespread throughout the renal parenchyma (fig. 25-9). Even in the late stages of amyloidosis, the kidneys tend to be large and the surface slightly granular. The medulla is gray. Application of Lugol's iodine to the cut surface may disclose the presence of amyloidosis grossly, with its characteristic staining of the starchy

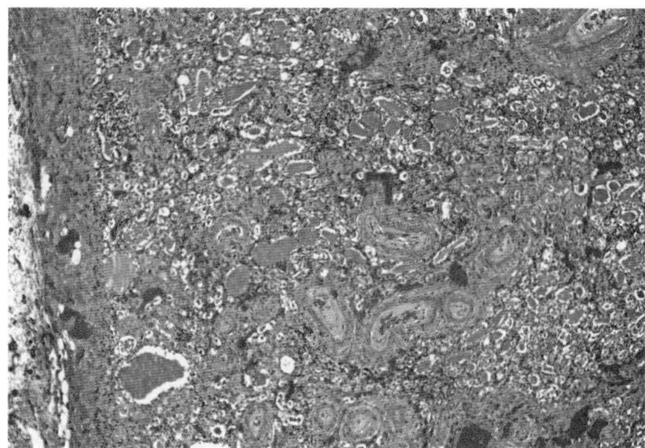

Figure 25-10

END-STAGE KIDNEY

Micrograph shows severe tubular atrophy, loss of tubular cells, and interstitial fibrosis (periodic acid–Schiff [PAS] stain).

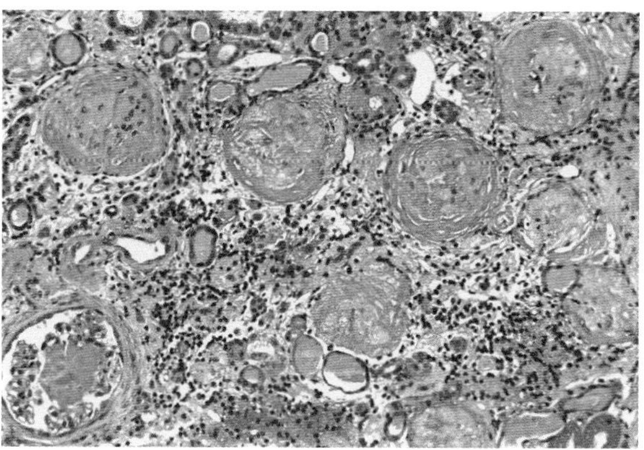

Figure 25-11

END-STAGE KIDNEY

Global glomerulosclerosis, tubular atrophy and dilatation, and interstitial fibrosis are seen. The globally sclerosed glomeruli are all very closely approximated, betraying the severe tubular atrophy that has taken place (hematoxylin and eosin [H&E] stain).

material. As the renal diseases progress, the renal cortical tissue undergoes continuing severe atrophy and the kidneys become smaller, with an irregular smooth or granular surface.

Diseases of the various renal compartments (glomerular, vascular, tubulointerstitial) eventually lead to progressive renal damage and the underlying initial cause of the renal disease may be impossible to determine in the late stages (38). As noted above, approximately one fourth to one third of kidneys of patients with ESRD receiving dialysis undergo cyst formation, resulting in the development of numerous cortical and medullary cysts.

Light Microscopic Findings. Irrespective of the initial cause of the renal injury leading to ESRD, eventually all four compartments of the kidney (glomeruli, vessels, tubules, and interstitium) become progressively damaged (figs. 25-10, 25-11) (14–20,25,35–38). The end-stage kidney shows advanced global glomerulosclerosis, tubular atrophy (of various forms), interstitial fibrosis, thickened blood vessels, and some degree of cystic change. Extensive oxalate deposition may be present. It has been said by Meadows (39) that the diagnosis of "end-stage renal disease" is a diagnosis of an "end-stage pathologist." Thus, one should attempt, with the use of a complete clinical history and careful examination of the kidney grossly and microscopically, to determine the underlying disease that led to the end-stage condition.

The best approach to the light microscopic examination of end-stage kidneys is to study microscopically each of the four renal components (glomeruli, tubules, interstitium, vessels) in a systematic fashion in order to identify morphologic features that may offer clues to the original disease (20). Whenever possible, the renal condition should be classified as one of the four major categories described above (vascular, diabetic, chronic pyelonephritic, or glomerular). Obviously, the task is more difficult when the kidney shows advanced damage and the renal parenchyma approaches total renal glomerular or tubulointerstitial atrophy (20,39).

Glomeruli. Even in advanced renal disease, usually at least some of the glomeruli are not globally sclerotic and may provide a clue to the underlying initial glomerular disease. These better preserved glomeruli may show proliferations or crescents that provide clues to a specific type of glomerular disease. Therefore, careful search for these less-affected and best-preserved glomeruli is recommended. For example, remnants of Kimmelstiel-Wilson nodules in damaged but most-preserved glomeruli point to an underlying diabetic nephropathy (fig. 25-12), whereas severe intracapillary or extracapillary (crescentic) proliferation may point to a form of glomerulonephritis. Glomerular synechiae (capsular adhesions) are produced in

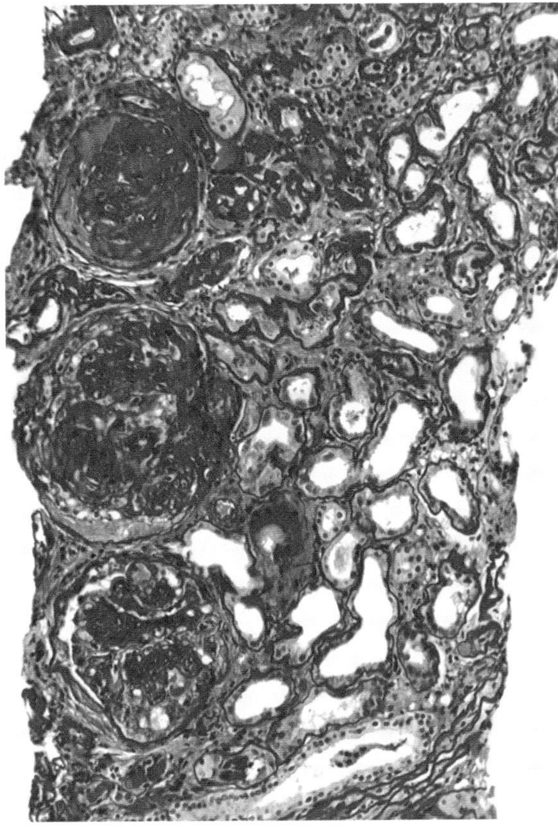

Figure 25-12

END-STAGE KIDNEY

The globally sclerosed glomeruli are enlarged, not retracted as most sclerotic glomeruli; this implies that something has been added to the sclerosed glomeruli. Remnants of Kimmelstiel-Wilson sclerotic mesangial nodules are seen in this patient with advanced diabetic nephropathy (PAS stain).

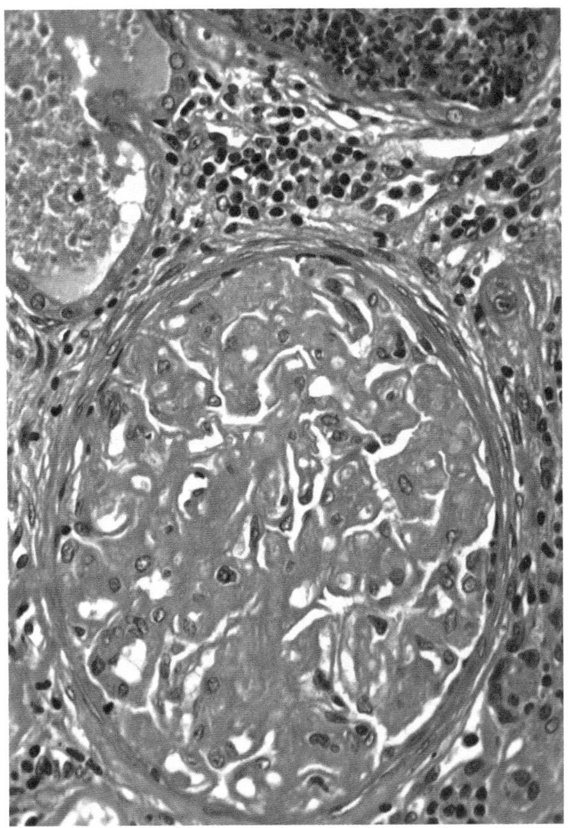

Figure 25-13

END-STAGE KIDNEY

The globally sclerotic glomerulus contains amorphous material; however, the glomerulus is not shrunken. Further examination revealed amyloid deposition throughout the glomeruli (H&E stain).

most forms of glomerulonephritis. During the collapse and solidification of the injured glomerular tuft, the basement membrane of Bowman's capsule is fragmented and focally lost; the hyalinized glomerulus becomes surrounded by small tubular structures (adenomatoid lesions or pseudotubules) (19). In end-stage diabetic glomerulosclerosis (fig. 25-12) or amyloidosis (fig. 25-13), the sclerotic glomeruli are large because something (sclerosis or amyloid fibrils) has been added to the glomerular tuft.

The obsolescent glomeruli in hypertensive patients often show total global sclerosis. In earlier stages, the less-affected glomeruli appear simplified, with wrinkling and thickening of the glomerular basement membranes (see figs. 25-19, 25-20). Collagen accumulates in Bowman's space, first near the vascular pole, and then extending throughout Bowman's space, with most of the poorly staining (by periodic acid–Schiff [PAS]) collagen noted at the vascular pole.

In ESRD due to membranoproliferative or membranous glomerulonephritis, the most preserved glomeruli may show diagnostic features of the underlying disease (fig. 25-14). In end-stage crescentic glomerulonephritis, there is often evidence of a previous crescentic process, denoted by large gaps or disruptions of the basal lamina of Bowman's capsules or more obvious recent crescent formation (figs. 25-15, 25-16).

As Meadows (39) has described, globally sclerotic glomeruli can, with time, merge imperceptibly with the adjacent inflamed interstitium. PAS,

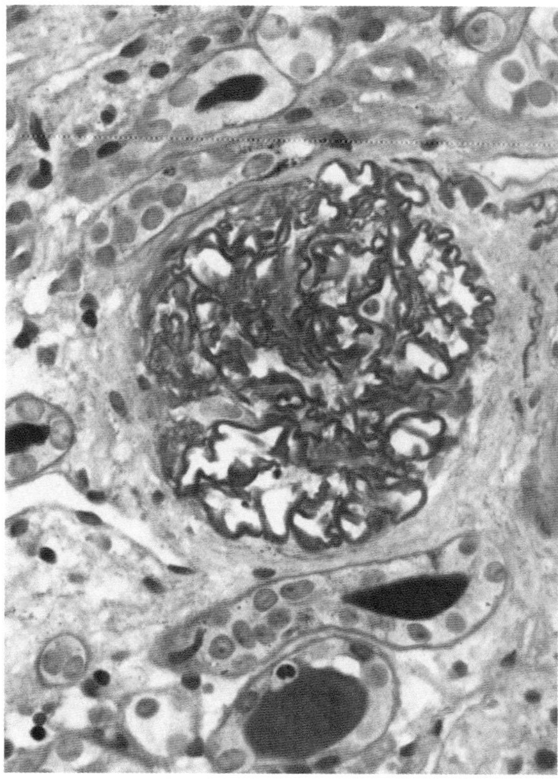

Figures 25-14

END-STAGE KIDNEY

This micrograph shows total global glomerulosclerosis in a renal transplant patient. The underlying nature of the end-stage renal disease (ESRD) is not apparent by light microscopy alone. Electron microscopy revealed recurrent dense deposit disease (PAS stain).

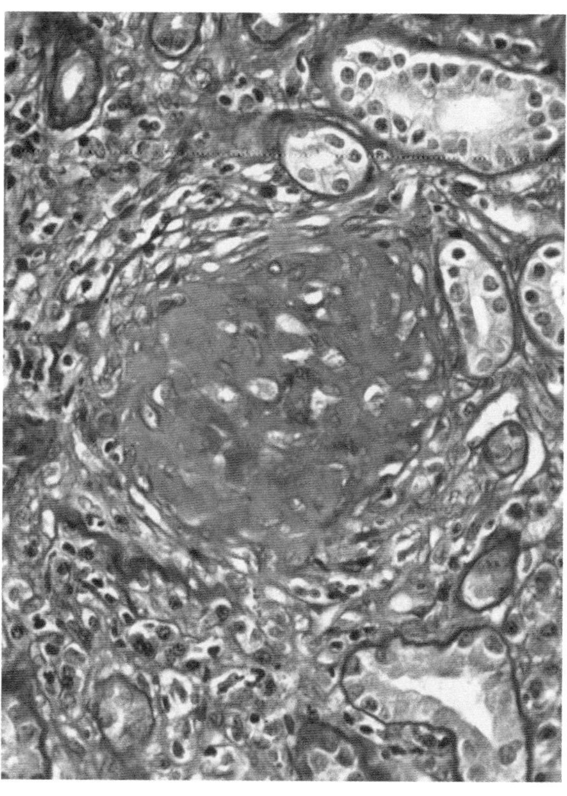

Figure 25-15

END-STAGE KIDNEY

This globally sclerotic glomerulus shows loss of or large breaks in Bowman's capsule, suggestive (though not pathognomonic) of a previous crescentic glomerulonephritis. The glomerulus is sometimes difficult to identify without PAS or other special stains (PAS stain).

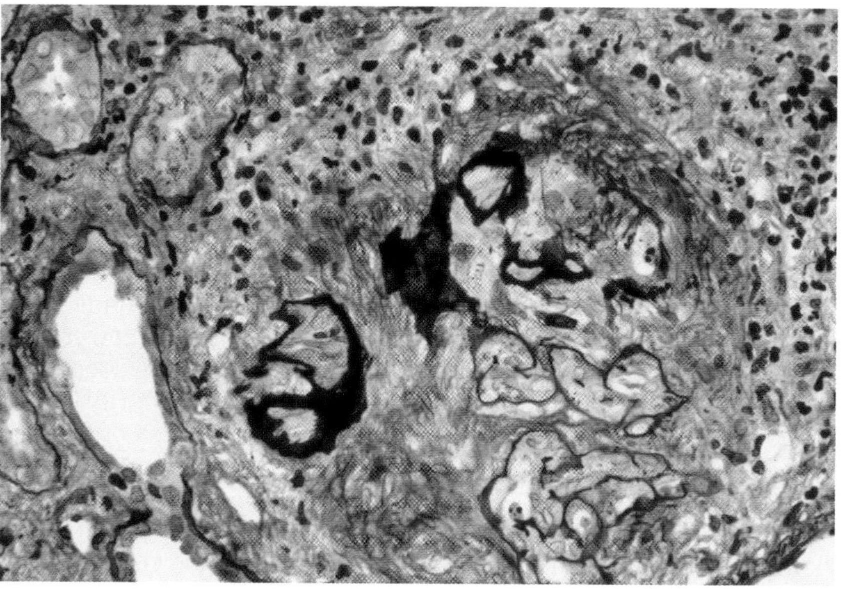

Figure 25-16

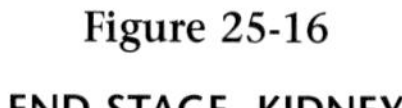

END-STAGE KIDNEY

The silver-positive Bowman's capsule is almost entirely destroyed in this patient with severe crescentic glomerulonephritis (Jones methenamine silver [JMS] stain).

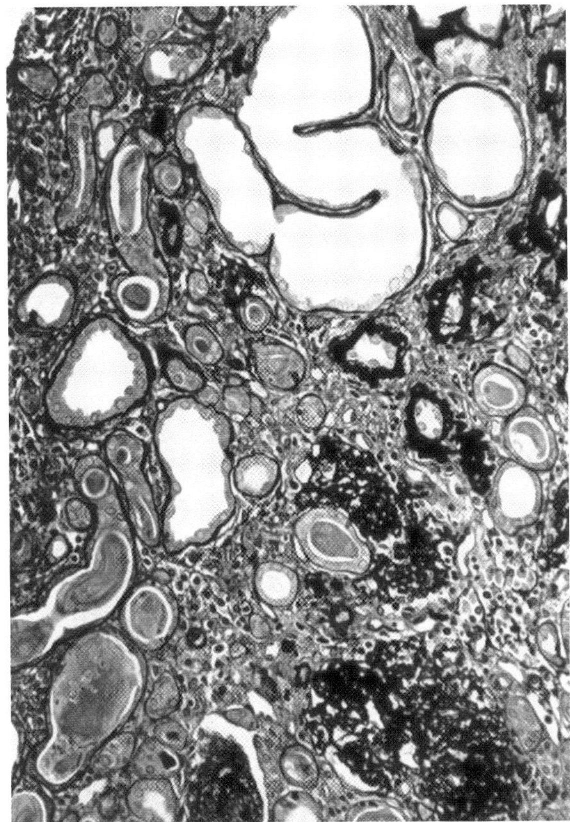

Figure 25-17

END-STAGE KIDNEY

The glomeruli merge imperceptibly in the adjacent inflamed and fibrotic interstitium. Sometimes only special stains, such as PAS or JMS, can accentuate very sclerotic glomeruli (JMS stain).

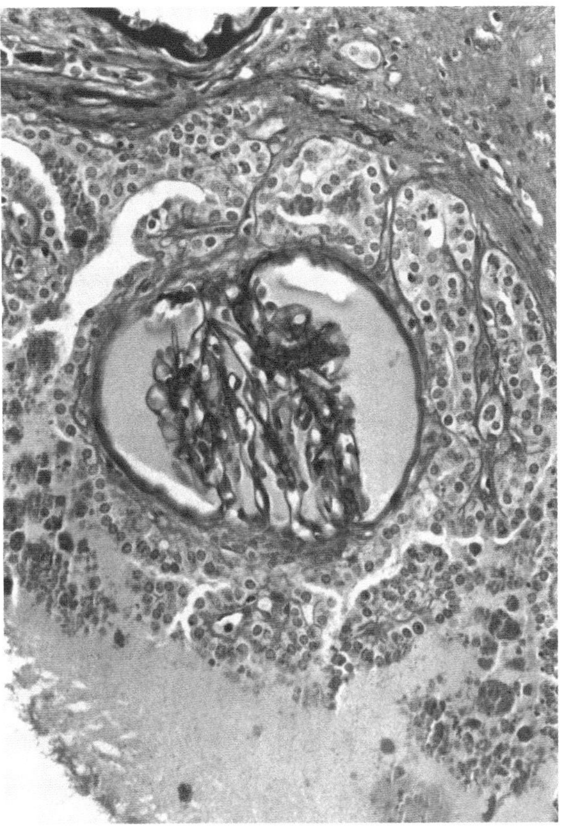

Figure 25-18

END-STAGE KIDNEY: EMBRYONAL HYPERPLASIA

There is marked proliferation adjacent to Bowman's capsule (PAS stain).

Jones methenamine silver (JMS), or trichrome stains can sometimes bring out these "disappearing" glomeruli (fig. 25-17).

In up to one third of patients of ESRD, there is embryonal hyperplasia of the epithelium of Bowman's capsule (fig. 25-18) (14,15,19,20). This is manifested by collections of small dark embryonal-appearing cells that have a delicate tubulopapillary structure surrounding hyalinized and obsolete glomerular tufts. The amount of embryonal hyperplasia varies and serial sections may be required to demonstrate its association with an underlying glomerulus. These proliferations can be twice the size of the glomerulus. In the early stage, the hyperplasia is derived from glomerular pseudotubules that are lined by single layers of embryonal cells. The embryonal cells are seen in about one third of children with ESRD. They tend to be found in the juxtamedullary cortex and similar dark cells have been found in tubules (occasionally with complex branching structures) that are not associated with obsolete glomeruli.

Tubules. Atrophic tubules have several appearances in ESRD. The "classic" atrophic tubule has a thick, occasionally lamellated and tortuous basement membrane, with a simplified tubular epithelium (figs. 25-21, 25-22). The "thyroidization" pattern is manifested by uniform, rounded tubules with a flattened, simplified renal tubular epithelium and abundant hyaline casts (figs. 25-23, 25-24). This pattern is reminiscent of the thyroid gland microscopically and is most commonly seen in patients with chronic pyelonephritis; however, it can be seen in virtually any advanced renal condition. "Endocrine"-type tubules are commonly seen in patients with

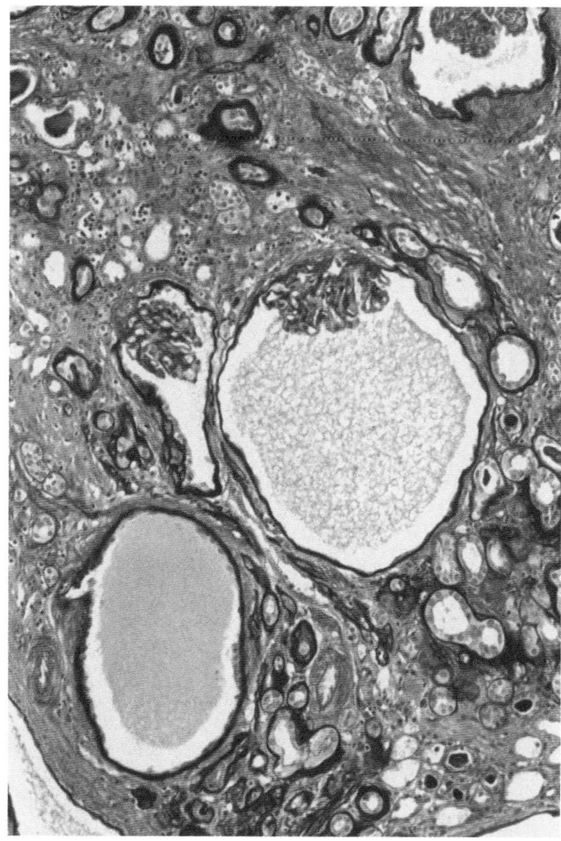

Figure 25-19

END-STAGE KIDNEY: GLOMERULAR ISCHEMIA

There is marked enlargement/expansion of Bowman's space. A small remnant of a glomerulus is without lobulation (PAS stain).

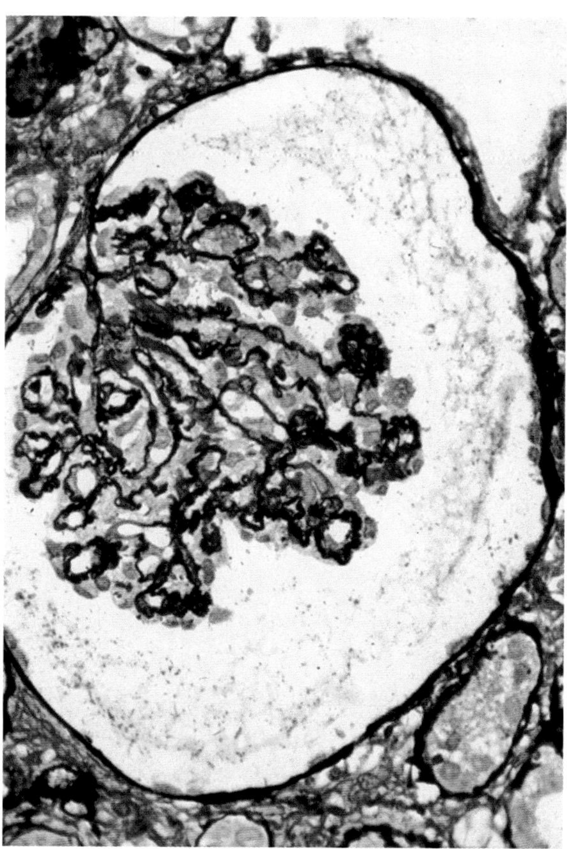

Figure 25-20

END-STAGE KIDNEY: GLOMERULAR ISCHEMIA

There is severe wrinkling and thickening of the glomerular capillaries secondary to severe ischemia (JMS stain).

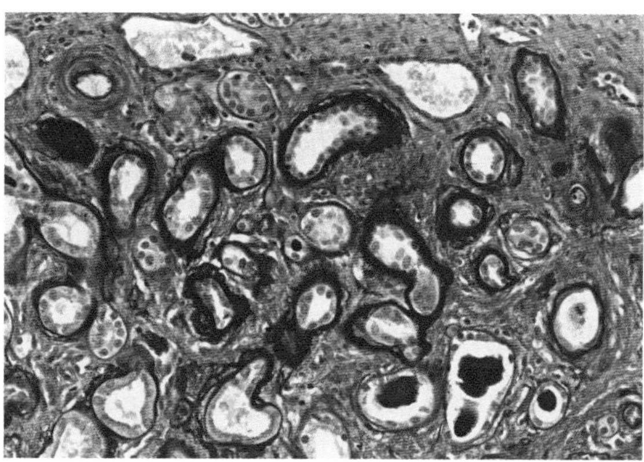

Figure 25-21

END-STAGE KIDNEY: CLASSIC TUBULAR ATROPHY

There is severe tubular atrophy with thickening and wrinkling of the tubular basement membranes. The tubular epithelial cells are uniform and appear undifferentiated (PAS stain).

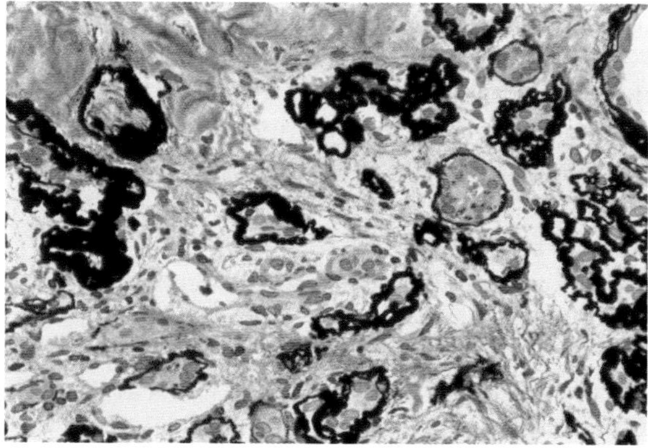

Figure 25-22

END-STAGE KIDNEY: CLASSIC TUBULAR ATROPHY

There is severe tubular atrophy with thickening and wrinkling of the tubular basement membranes (JMS stain).

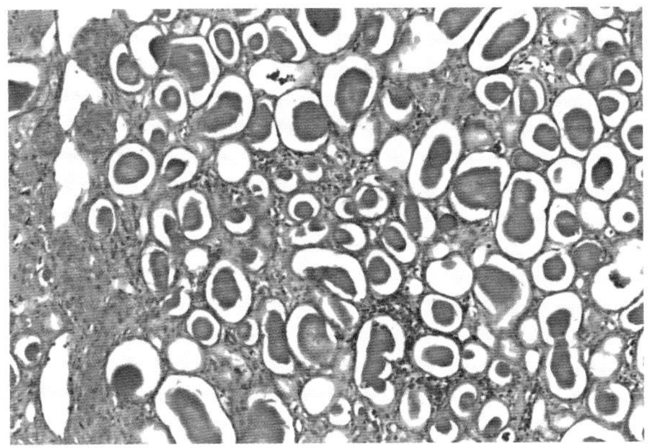

Figure 25-23

END-STAGE KIDNEY: TUBULAR ATROPHY OF THE "THYROIDIZATION" TYPE

The tubules are uniformly dilated and all contain similar-sized hyaline casts. The tubular epithelium is quite thin. Although this type of tubular atrophy is characteristic of chronic pyelonephritis, it is not pathognomonic, being seen in many different advanced renal conditions (PAS stain).

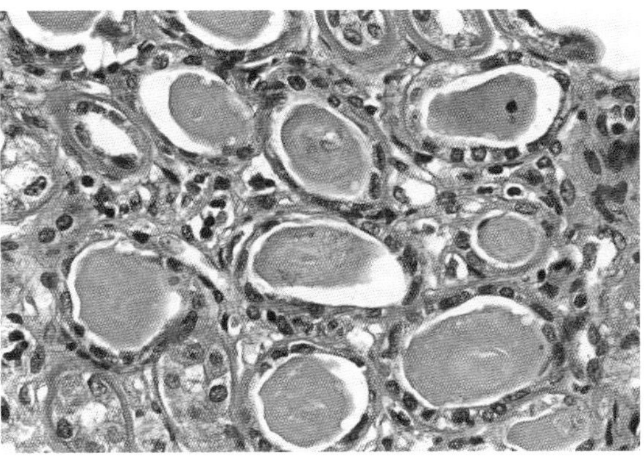

Figure 25-24

END-STAGE KIDNEY: TUBULAR ATROPHY OF THE "THYROIDIZATION" TYPE

This patient had bona fide chronic pyelonephritis (H&E stain).

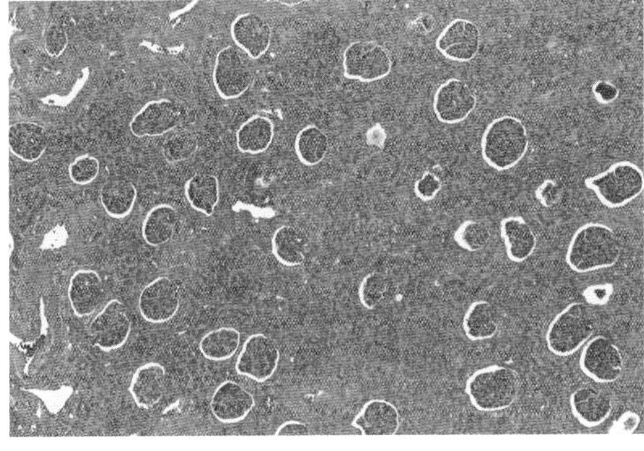

Figure 25-25

END STAGE KIDNEY SECONDARY TO RENAL ARTERY STENOSIS: "ENDOCRINE" TUBULES

These monotonous small tubules with cuboidal cells and virtually no lumen are often seen in patients with severe renal ischemia. There is glomerular sparing (H&E stain).

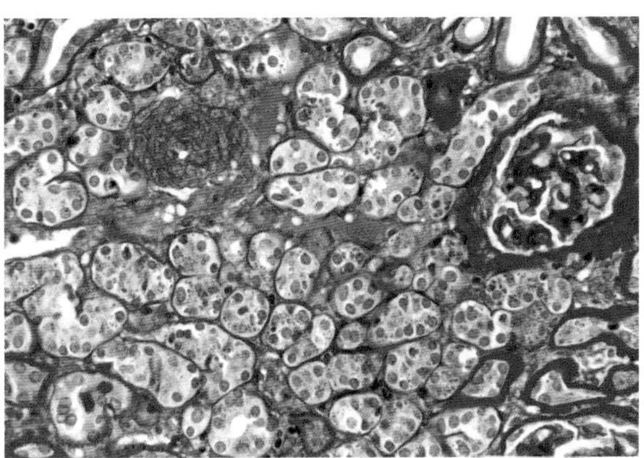

Figure 25-26

END-STAGE KIDNEY: ENDOCRINE TUBULES

PAS stain.

severe renal vascular disease and ischemia, and are comprised of small uniform tubules bunched closely together with very narrow or absent lumens, clear regular epithelial cells, and a relatively thin basement membrane (figs. 25-25, 25-26) (51). Ultrastructural studies show that these renal tubular epithelial cells are filled with mitochondria (fig. 25-27) (40). Tubular hypertrophy/hyperplasia may be seen in patients with severe proteinuria as well as those with severe renal parenchymal scarring and secondary tubular hypertrophy/hyperplasia (fig. 25-28). There may be dilatation of the tubules with what appear to be irregular tubular profiles (fig. 25-29).

In ESRD there is often marked separation of the renal tubules by interstitial fibrosis. This is best seen with the trichrome stain (fig. 25-30). Interstitial inflammation with lymphocytes and occasional plasma cells can be seen in any advanced renal disease. With special stains, mast cells can be identified within the interstitial inflammatory infiltrates. Interstitial inflammation

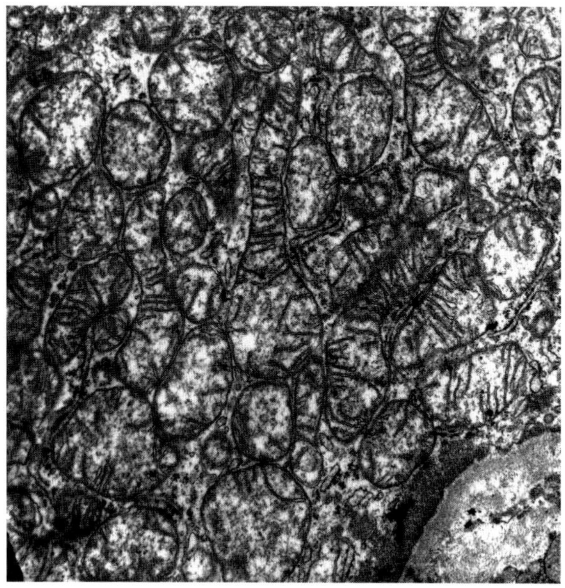

Figure 25-27

END-STAGE KIDNEY: ENDOCRINE TUBULES

Electron micrograph shows many mitochondria in the simplified tubular epithelial cells.

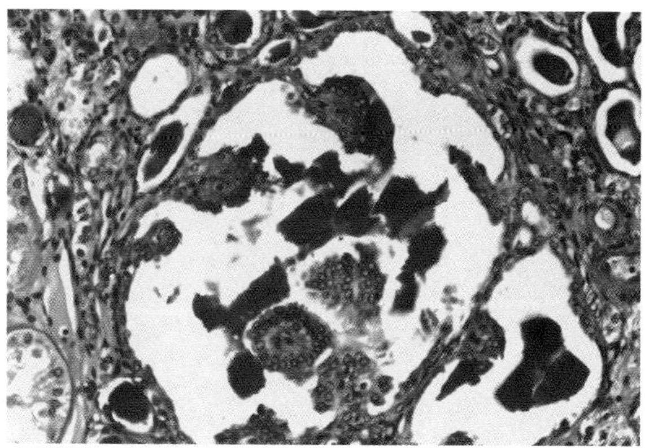

Figure 25-28

END-STAGE KIDNEY: TUBULAR HYPERPLASIA

With severe loss of the renal parenchyma, there is often hypertrophy of the residual nephrons as well as tubular hyperplasia, as noted here (Masson trichrome stain).

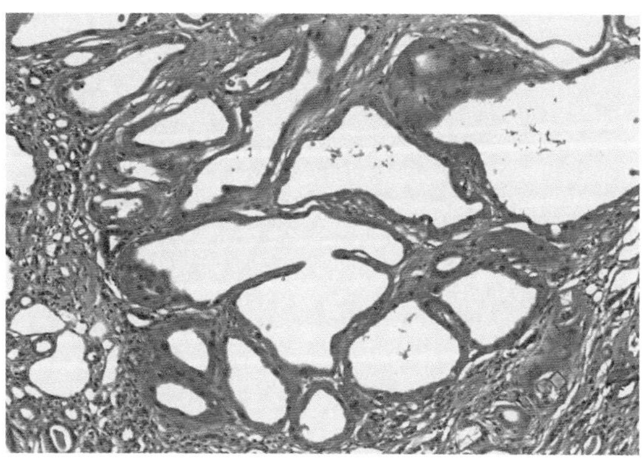

Figure 25-29

END-STAGE KIDNEY: TUBULAR DILATATION AND ABNORMALITIES OF THE TUBULAR CONTOUR

There is often patchy dilatation of the tubules, frequently with casts. In addition, the contour of the tubules is abnormal (H&E stain).

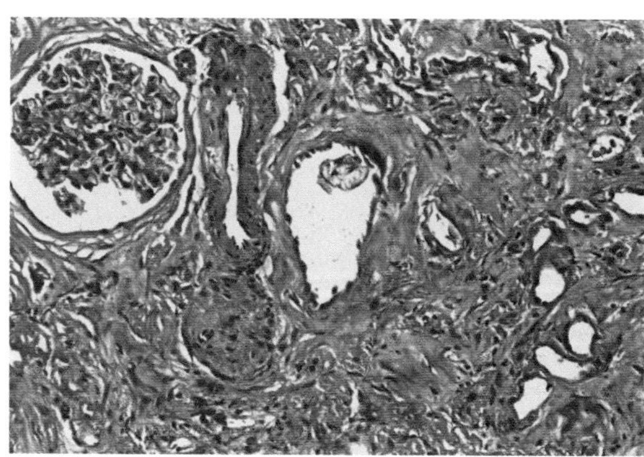

Figure 25-30

END-STAGE KIDNEY: INTERSTITIAL FIBROSIS

Interstitial fibrosis is best seen with the Masson trichrome stain.

may be even seen in advanced cases of diabetic nephropathy with severe vascular disease. In the proper clinical and morphologic setting, the finding of severe interstitial inflammation underlying the transitional urothelium at the pyelocalyceal system (renal papillae) is suggestive of true chronic pyelonephritis. Germinal centers may even be noted beneath the urothelium in chronic pyelonephritis. In some well-advanced cases of ESRD, the interstitial fibrotic regions have the staining characteristics of elastic tissue (i.e., positive with the Verhoeff-van Gieson stain). Myxoid connective tissue, metaplastic cartilage, and even woven bone have been noted occasionally in areas of severe interstitial fibrosis (11,14). Large acellular amorphous lakes of Tamm-Horsfall protein may be seen amid the inflamed interstitium (fig. 25-31).

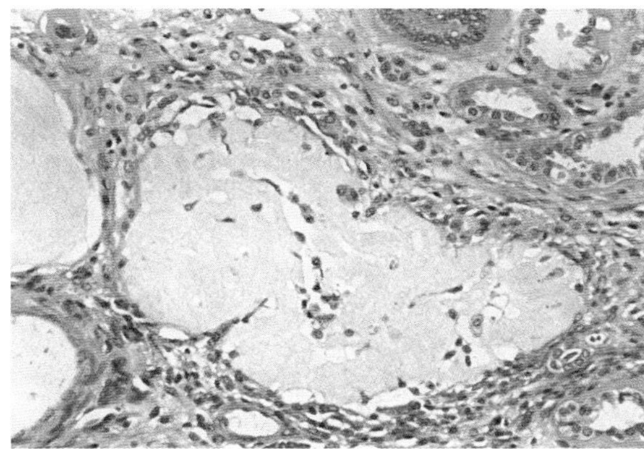

Figure 25-31

END STAGE KIDNEY: INTERSTITIAL COLLECTION OF TAMM-HORSFALL MATERIAL

This material, exuded into the interstitium from the disrupted tubule, is often lightly eosinophilic but intensely PAS positive (H&E stain).

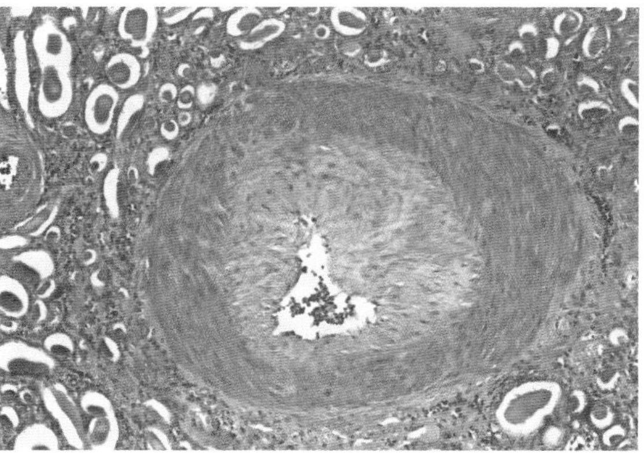

Figure 25-32

END-STAGE KIDNEY: VASCULAR LESION

The vessel walls are thickened and the vascular lumens are narrowed. The marked intimal hyperplasia (with ingrowth of the intima by modified medial smooth muscle cells) leads to narrowing of the arterial lumen (H&E stain).

Vessels. The renal arteries in patients with ESRD undergo severe fibrous intimal thickening and the lumens are extremely narrowed. The severity of this change is often related to the duration of dialysis. Renal arteries of all sizes are involved. The obliterative intimal fibrosis, with concentric thickening of the intima by collagenous connective tissue, contains a moderate number of spindle cells (figs. 25-32, 25-33). These spindle cells have been identified by electron microscopic and immunohistochemical stains as myointimal (smooth muscle) cells. This vascular lesion is thought to be an adaptive change to the increased vascular resistance caused by the loss of the peripheral microvascular tree (8,21,30,36,37,41,52). Musculomucoid intimal hyperplasia, identical to the lesions seen in patients with acute scleroderma, is often found, especially in patients with severe hypertension. There is a marked thickening of the intrarenal arteries by a mucoid ground substance containing many myointimal cells. There may be an apparent increase in vascularity secondary to atrophy of the intervening tubules, as well as an increase in the tortuosity of the arterioles (probably secondary to increased pressures within the vessels). (fig. 25-34). Within the end-stage kidney, small and medium-sized arteries may be occluded by concentric intimal fibroplasia with deep calcification (fig. 25-35) (28).

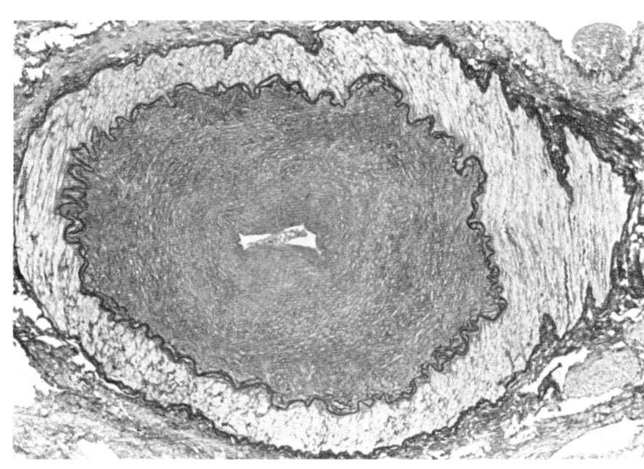

Figure 25-33

END-STAGE KIDNEY: VASCULAR LESION

Marked intimal fibroplasia internal to the internal elastic lamellae (Verhoeff-van Giesson elastic stain).

At times, the cells of the artery walls proliferate to form arteriolar nodules (14,16,37). These may be solid nodules of smooth muscle cells, resembling small leiomyomas, or they may resemble the plexiform vascular lesions seen in the small pulmonary arteries of patients with high-grade pulmonary hypertension. Fibrinoid necrosis of medium and small arteries can also be seen in patients with malignant hypertension. There is insudation of fibrin and dissection of red blood cells into the mucoid intima.

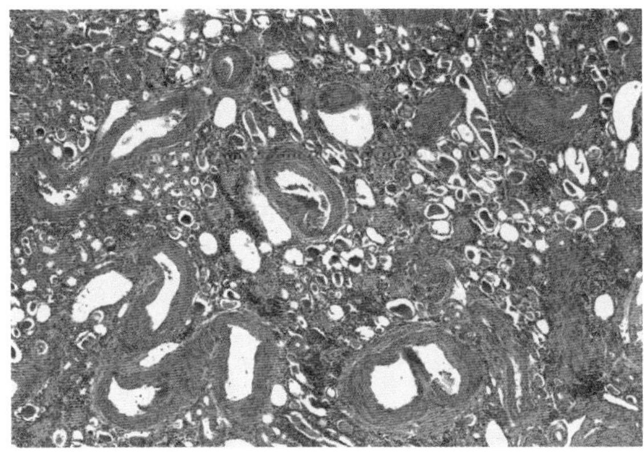

Figure 25-34

END-STAGE KIDNEY

There are multiple cross sections of the small perihilar arteries, suggestive of increased tortuosity of the blood vessels (H&E stain).

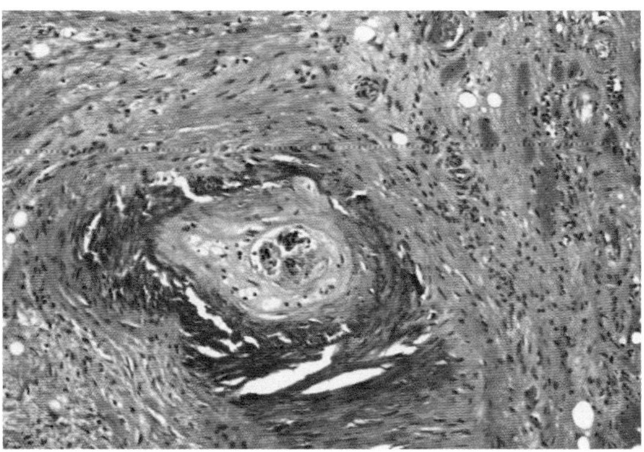

Figure 25-35

END-STAGE KIDNEY

There is marked intimal fibroplasia and severe dystrophic calcification of the vessel wall (H&E stain).

Renal veins are often thickened by the proliferation of hypertrophic smooth muscle (termed nodular phlebosclerosis). The walls of the thickened vein may enclose renal tubules composed of clear cuboidal cells.

Interstitium. Renal medullary fibrosis is difficult to identify and quantify (11). It is generally best to determine the degree of the interstitial fibrosis from sections of the renal cortex, especially with the use of the trichrome stain. In some cases of ESRD, there may be focal proliferation of smooth muscle around collecting ducts. Medullary interstitial cells may contain abundant glycogen, especially in kidneys removed for hypertension (18). Oxalosis has been found commonly in the kidneys of patients on dialysis (9). The oxalate crystals are found in the tubules, within the walls of the renal cysts, or embedded in the renal interstitium. In patients with ESRD due to analgesic nephropathy, there is typically evidence of prior papillary necrosis and calcification, with shedding or mummification of the necrotic papillae.

There may be juxtaglomerular granular cell hyperplasia in the kidneys of patients with ESRD (7,14). This is especially seen in patients with malignant hypertension and high plasma renin levels. Juxtaglomerular apparatuses (JGAs) may be identified even accompanying obsolete glomeruli. Granules can be seen in the hypertrophied medial smooth muscle cells of the afferent arterioles (called granular cell metaplasia) with the Bowie stain. Immunohistochemical stains utilizing antibodies to renin have shown intense staining in the glomeruli and afferent arterioles of patients with severe dialysis-resistant hypertension; in some of these cases the renin staining was noted in the arterioles even though most of the glomeruli had disappeared. There is less staining for renin in the kidneys of diabetic patients with advancing disease (7).

Immunofluorescence Findings. Immunofluorescent studies, even in advanced disease, may uncover an underlying immunologic glomerular disease. For example, patients with advanced global glomerulosclerosis due to immunoglobulin (Ig)A nephropathy often have intense glomerular staining for IgA. However, in globally sclerotic glomeruli (irrespective of cause) there is often nonspecific, nonimmunologic deposition of IgM and complement (C)3 in the scarred regions (fig. 25-36). Thus, evaluation of the least involved (least sclerotic) glomeruli or segments of preserved glomeruli is most useful.

Electron Microscopic Findings. Ultrastructural studies may be useful in diagnosing an immune complex glomerulonephritis (even in end-stage glomerular lesions) by the presence of discrete electron-dense immune-type deposits. However, distinguishing hyalinosis from true discrete immune deposits may be quite difficult, especially in areas of severe glomerular damage and sclerosis. Correlation with the immunofluorescence findings is particularly helpful because

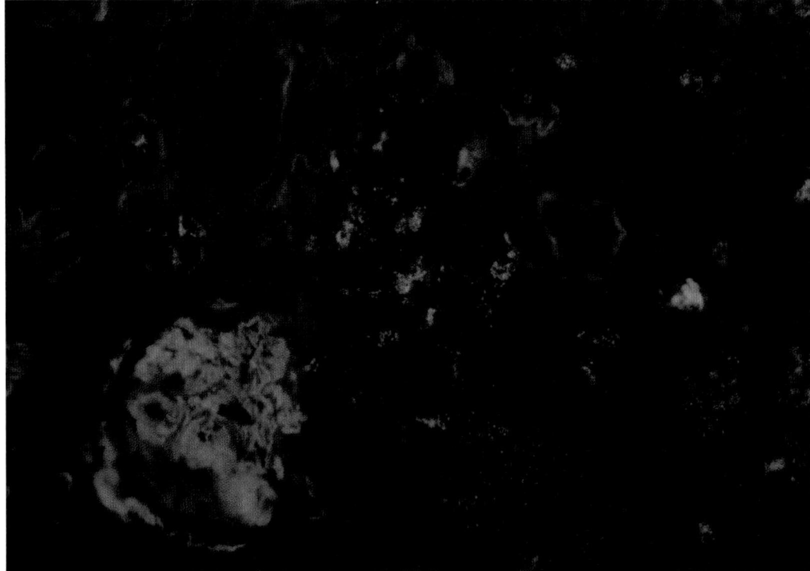

Figure 25-36

END-STAGE KIDNEY: GLOBAL GLOMERULOSCLEROSIS

Immunofluorescence for anti-albumin is positive in this sclerosed glomerulus. The original renal disease was not immune in nature. The nonspecific, nonimmunologic trapping of plasma proteins in damaged, sclerotic glomeruli is commonly seen.

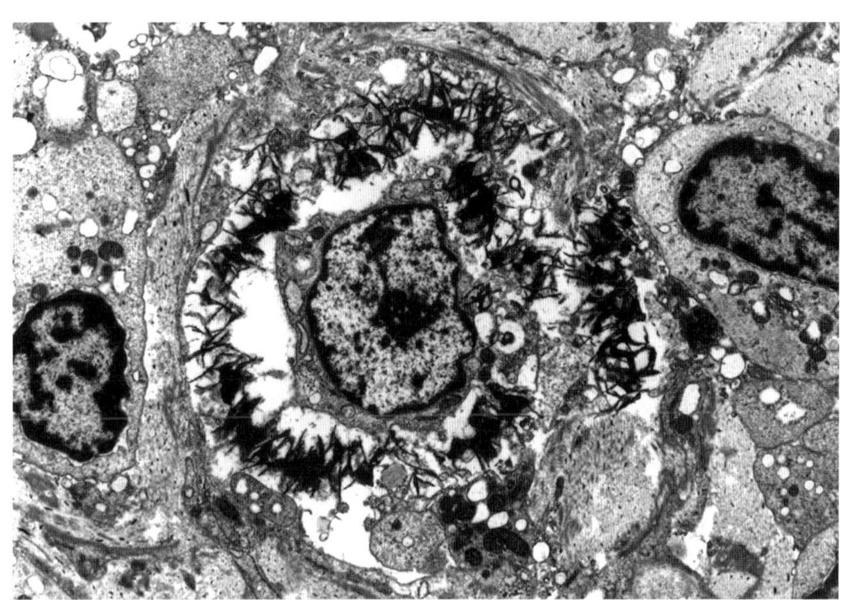

Figure 25-37

END-STAGE RENAL DISEASE

Ultrastructural examination of a renal tubule from a patient with severe ESRD. Large electron-dense spicules of calcium and calcified material are within the tubular basement membranes. The tubular epithelium is distorted. This patient had severe calciphylaxis.

hyaline usually stains only for IgM (with or without C3 and occasionally C1), whereas true immune deposits usually stain for other Ig classes (IgG, IgA), depending on the nature of the glomerulonephritis.

Electron microscopic studies of the tubules, interstitium, and vessels confirm the morphologic findings noted by light microscopy. Regions of plasmatic insudation (fibrin caps) in the sclerotic glomeruli of the diabetic patient need to be distinguished from the true, discrete, electron-dense immune-type deposits noted in immune complex glomerular disease (fig. 25-37).

Differential Diagnosis. The clinical history is quite important when trying to determine the initial cause of the patient's renal disease. If the patient has evidence of nephrotic-range proteinuria or severe hematuria (especially with dysmorphic red blood cells or red blood cell casts), then a presumptive diagnosis of a primary glomerular disease is appropriate. If the initial clinical findings are those only of severe hypertension, then a primary vascular disease should be considered.

Careful examination of the renal collecting systems (by intravenous pyelogram [IVP], retrograde pyelogram, gross examination) is important and can help secure the diagnosis of chronic pyelonephritis or analgesic nephropathy. Sections from the renal artery and vascular tree may be important if the entire kidney is available for study (from nephrectomy or autopsy).

Etiology and Pathogenesis. Irrespective of the initiating renal disease, progression to ESRD may occur and follows a complex course. In general, the reciprocal of the serum creatinine charted over time plots as a straight line for each individual patient. Indeed, this is how progression to renal replacement therapy is predicted by the nephrologist in the individual patient. The pathogenic mechanisms of progressive renal disease are complex and have been considered elsewhere (1,13,23,26,29,57). The etiology and pathogenic mechanisms involved in the acute injury of specific glomerular, tubular, interstitial, and vascular diseases are noted in those respective chapters. The morphologic findings in the diseased kidney are a result of the initial injury (e.g., immune complex, hypertension, drug toxicity, or ischemia) as is the subsequent tissue response to that injury. If the initial injury is severe enough or recurrent, and overwhelms the kidney's reparative mechanisms, then there may be progression of the renal damage. It appears that irrespective of the initial injury to the kidney, there may be a final common pathway to progressive renal injury (2,13,22,42–45,52).

With the loss of functional renal parenchyma, there is compensatory hypertrophy of the remaining nephrons. If a large number of glomeruli have been irreversibly damaged, then the remaining glomeruli are subjected to abnormally high plasma flow rates. There is loss of autoregulation (i.e., imbalance between the afferent and efferent arteriole). The resulting increase in the glomerular capillary pressure causes hyperperfusion injury that is associated with glomerulosclerosis and progressive glomerular injury. Increased glomerular filtration rates have been associated with glomerular hypertrophy and much experimental (and some clinical) work suggest a role for glomerular hypertrophy in the pathogenesis of progressive renal injury. Irrespective of the initial cause of the glomerular injury, at some point, even in the absence of the initiating injury, there may be progression of glomerulosclerosis and renal failure.

Recent experimental studies have suggested that prolonged severe proteinuria can directly cause tubular damage via several mechanisms. Macrophages recruited to the site of the injury release a number of injurious cytokines, leading to interstitial fibrosis. The intimate association between the tubules and the interstitial regions of the kidney are well recognized and agents leading to injury of one component not infrequently lead, through a variety of mechanisms, to injury of the other. Finally, in advanced and advancing renal injury, alteration and progressive destruction of one component of the kidney (i.e., glomerulus, tubules, interstitium, or vessels) will eventually lead to alteration and damage to the other renal components: thus, the final morphologic findings of the end-stage kidney.

Treatment and Prognosis. If the progression of the renal disease could be slowed, then there would be many savings, both financial and personal. Common strategies aimed at slowing the onset of ESRD often depends on the initial diagnosis of the clinical condition and the accepted therapy for that primary renal disease. Other general common strategies include: 1) avoidance of further renal insults if possible; 2) decreasing the systemic blood pressure; 3) controlling the diabetes, if present; 4) restricting oral protein intake; and 5) decreasing the proteinuria and glomerular hyperfiltration with a variety of medications including angiotensin-converting enzyme (ACE) inhibitors and/or angiotensin receptor blockaid (24,26,29,33,46,51).

About 60 percent of ESRD patients are treated by in-center hemodialysis; another 27 percent receive a functional renal transplant; and about 10 percent have peritoneal dialysis. The average life expectancy of a patient on hemodialysis is over 5 years (until the age of 55). A young patient with ESRD can expect to live more than 10 years. The two leading causes of death of patients on dialysis are cardiac (coronary artery disease, myocardial infarction; 21 percent) and infections (14 to 24 percent) (49,55). The death of patients following renal transplantation is considered elsewhere (4).

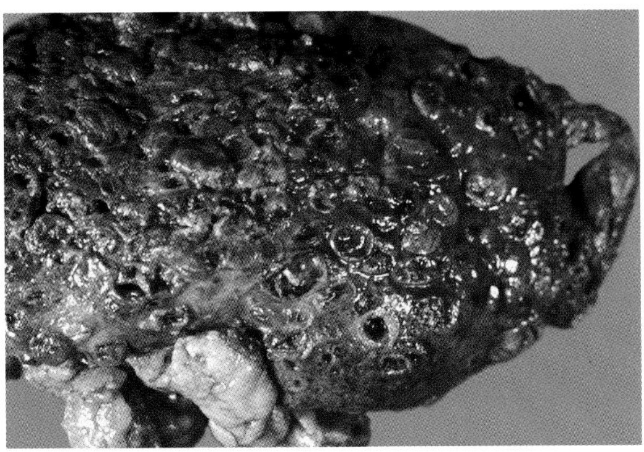

Figure 25-38

ACQUIRED CYSTIC DISEASE

The surface is irregular, and multiple small cysts encroach and replace the renal parenchyma. This is also termed "dialysis kidney."

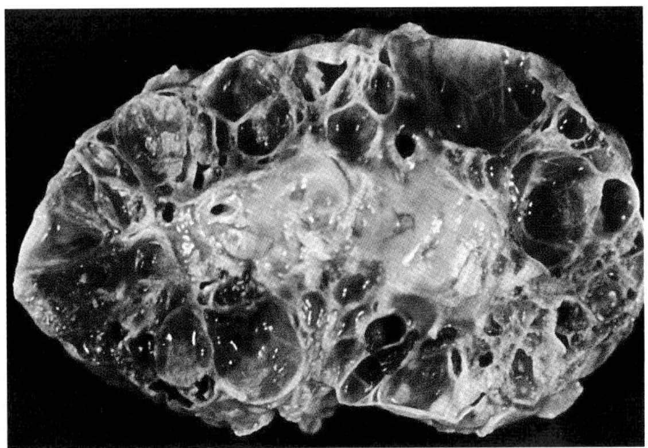

Figure 25-39

ACQUIRED CYSTIC DISEASE

Cross section of the kidney shows marked replacement of the renal parenchyma by numerous fluid-filled cysts. (Courtesy of Dr. M. Hughson, Jackson, MS.)

Other nonrenal complications include beta-2-microglobulin amyloidosis (often involving carpal tunnel or large joints) (27,32), aluminum bone disease, malignancy (48), and chronic hepatitis (B or C) (see Table 25-1).

Peritoneal clearance often becomes inadequate in up to a third of patients on continuous ambulatory peritoneal dialysis (CAPD) after 5 years or more. Sclerosing peritonitis is thought to be responsible for the loss of clearance in some patients. Fibrous peritoneal adhesions with the obliteration of the peritoneal cavity or bowel fibrosis with obstruction may occur.

ACQUIRED CYSTIC DISEASE ("DIALYSIS KIDNEY")

In 1977, two groups, Dunnill et al. (5) and McManus et al. (35), demonstrated that many end-stage kidneys obtained from patients on longstanding dialysis had a large number of renal cysts. This change appeared to be unique to patients on hemodialysis; the patients were not known to have a hereditary or preexisting cystic disease prior to the onset of renal failure. These authors coined the term acquired renal cystic disease (ACD). A few kidneys in these reports harbored renal cell carcinomas and adenomas. McManus et al. described the presence of hyperplastic, atypical cysts and related these hyperplastic changes to the development of the renal neoplasms (35,38). The marked cystic dilatation described by these authors is much different from the development of a few small cysts recognized for a century in chronically diseased kidneys. Radiologically, ACD has been defined as the presence of five or more cysts per kidney. Others have suggested that ACD should be defined as a cystic change involving at least 40 percent of the kidney volume. Thus, there is a discrepancy between the pathologic gross definition and the radiologic definition.

Subsequent radiologic studies of patients on hemodialysis have shown that diseased kidneys continue to atrophy up to 3 years after initiating dialysis, but at approximately 4 years, the kidney size increases as ACD begins to develop. ACD has now been reported in 10 to 80 percent of dialysis patients. Ninety percent of dialysis patients followed for longer periods of time (5 to 10 years) have ACD. Although there are some cases of ACD in patients with chronic renal failure who are not yet on dialysis, most patients with ACD have been on dialysis for at least several months. The cystic change is said to be more common in men and in patients with hypertension or glomerulonephritis (not diabetes). ACD has been described in patients on CAPD as well (42).

Intrarenal hemorrhage has been noted in about one sixth of the patients with ACD. The intrarenal hemorrhage can rupture into the retroperitoneum and be life-threatening.

Gross Findings. Kidneys with ACD range from quite small to large (figs. 25-38, 25-39), and weigh from 5 g to 800 g or more (average,

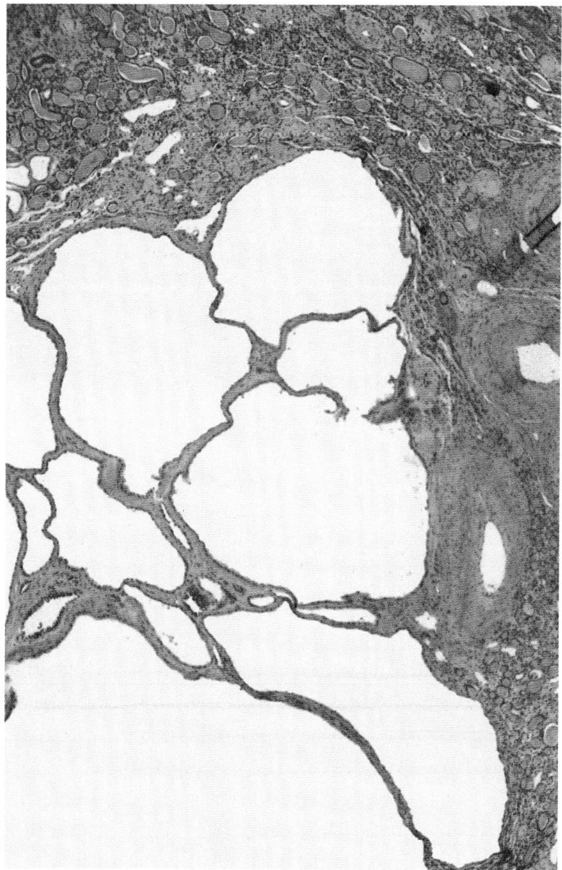

Figure 25-40

ACQUIRED CYSTIC DISEASE

The contour and outline of the renal tubule are markedly dilated and irregular (H&E stain).

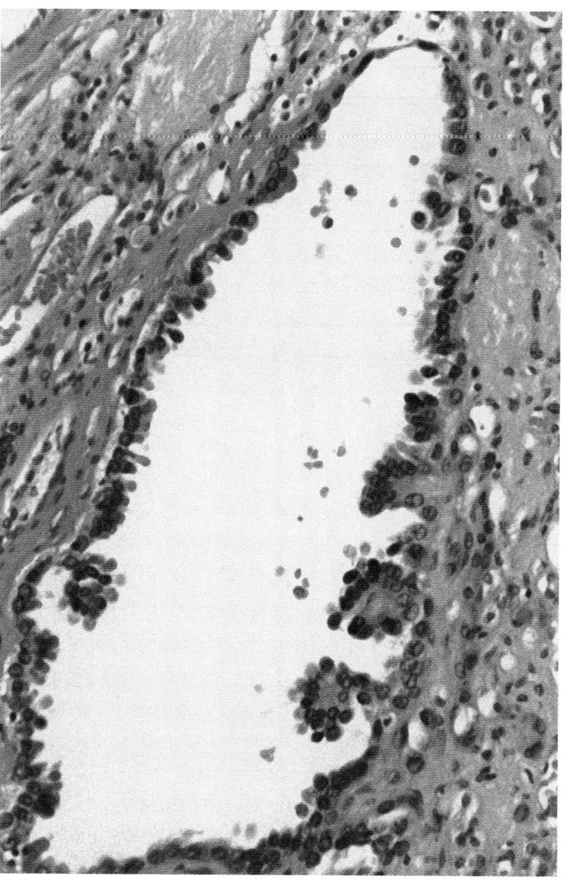

Figure 25-41

ACQUIRED CYSTIC DISEASE

There is proliferation of the tubular epithelium with small papillary projections into the dilated tubular lumen (H&E stain).

135 g). In some cases, the renal cysts are small, either clustered or evenly distributed throughout the spongy-appearing kidney, whereas in others the cysts are larger (2 to 3 cm in diameter). Cysts are mainly located in the renal cortex, but they can be found in the medulla. They are usually filled with clear to slightly cloudy, straw-colored fluid. Some cysts have a fluid that has a gelatinous consistency at room temperature (14,15,20,34,38).

The gross appearance of kidneys with ACD can resemble that of bona fide adult (autosomal dominant) polycystic kidney disease (ADPKD). However, the size of the kidney in these two conditions is quite different. In symptomatic patients with ADPKD, the kidney weighs from 1,000 to 2,000 g, whereas in patients with ACD, the majority of the kidneys studied have weighed less than 300 g. Obviously, clinical and family histories are important to differentiate between these two conditions.

Light Microscopic Findings. Most cysts in ACD, like cysts in hereditary forms of polycystic kidney disease, are lined by flattened, nondescript tubular epithelium (figs. 25-40, 25-41). Some cysts are lined by taller epithelium, which suggests histologically either proximal or distal tubular epithelium. Recent studies have suggested that the segment of the nephron undergoing the cystic dilatation can be determined with the use of immunohistochemical and lectin markers for different nephron segments (3). The cysts in ACD appear to arise from both proximal and distal tubular segments.

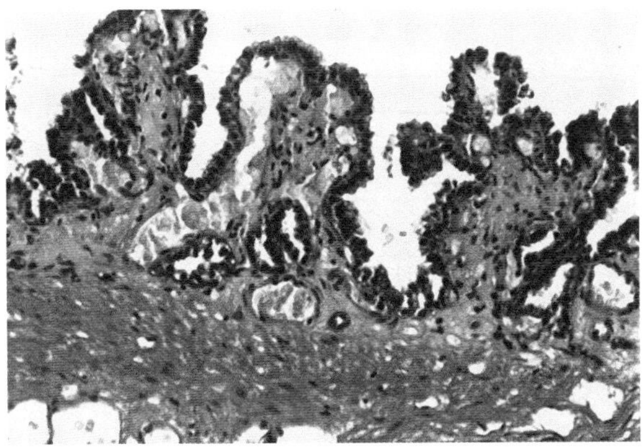

Figure 25-42

ACQUIRED CYSTIC DISEASE

There is papillary hyperplasia of the cystically dilated tubule (H&E stain).

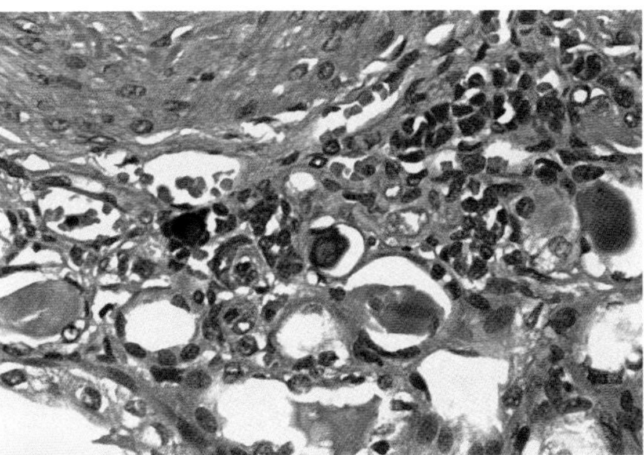

Figure 25-43

ACQUIRED CYSTIC DISEASE

There is calcium oxalate deposition in the atrophic tubules. The oxalate deposition is often seen within the tubular epithelium and in the adjacent interstitium in patients with acquired cystic disease (H&E stain).

In approximately one third of end-stage kidneys, cysts lined by tall columnar or small cuboidal epithelial cells show papillary epithelial hyperplasia (fig. 25-42). These have been called "atypical cysts" and may be found in end-stage kidneys with or without ACD (14,15,17, 34,35,38). Sometimes the renal epithelium of these atypical cysts shows dysplastic cytologic features and loss of nuclear polarity. These atypical cysts are more commonly seen in kidneys with renal cortical neoplasms and may represent preneoplastic lesions. Cystic dilatation of the glomeruli can also occur.

The renal parenchyma away from the cysts shows the constitutive background of globally sclerotic glomeruli, tubular atrophy, interstitial fibrosis, and obliterative intimal fibrosis of the arteries that characterizes ESRD. This is in contradistinction to ADPKD where the renal parenchyma between the cysts usually appears normal. However, after institution of dialysis in patients with ADPKD, the morphology merges. There may be marked calcium oxalate deposition in the dilated tubules, often noted within the tubular epithelium and in the adjacent interstitium. Calcium oxalate deposits can be seen with polarized microscopy (figs. 25-43, 25-44).

Special Studies. Nephron dissection techniques have shown that many of the renal cysts in patients with ACD begin as outpouchings or sacculations from the intact tubular segments. Nodules of collagen, elastic tissue, and duplicated tubular basement membranes are often

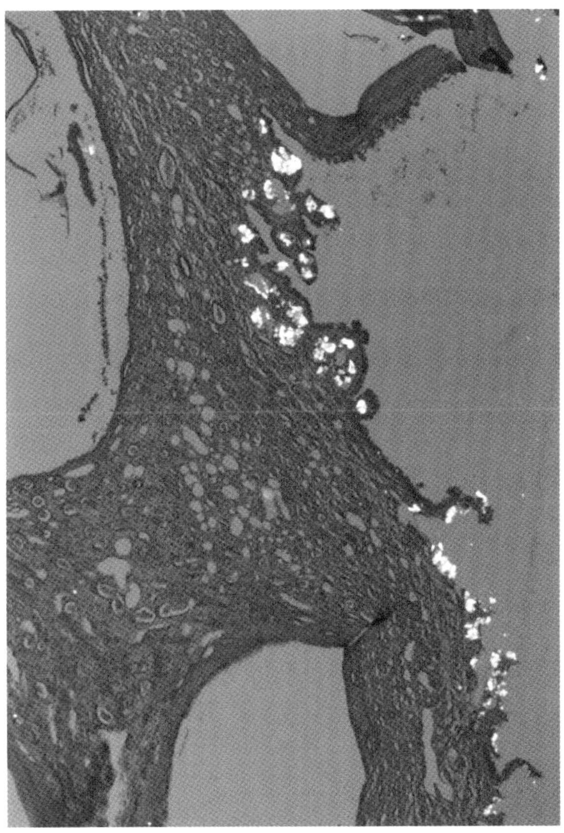

Figure 25-44

ACQUIRED CYSTIC DISEASE WITH CALCIUM OXALATE DEPOSITION

Polarization microscopy delineates the refractile oxalate crystals.

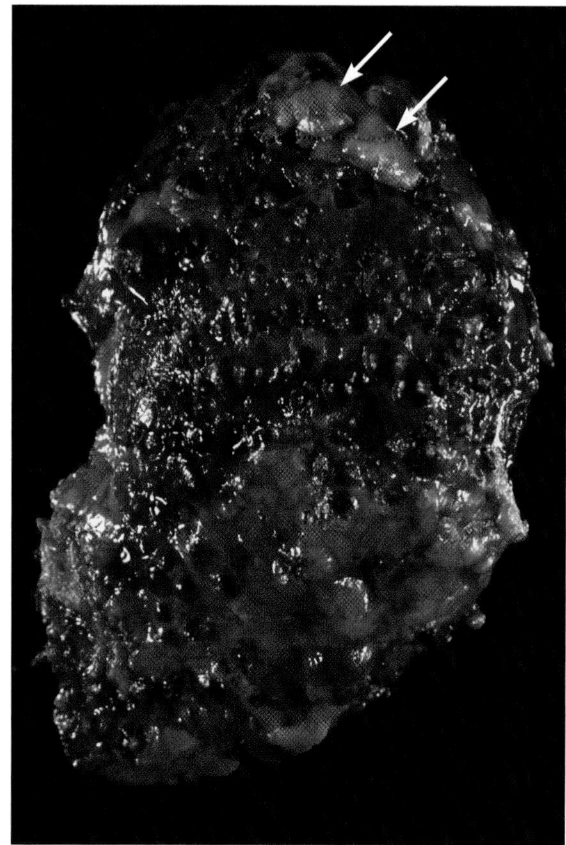

Figure 25-45

ACQUIRED CYSTIC DISEASE WITH MULTIPLE RENAL CELL CARCINOMAS

Tumors are seen in the kidney (arrows). This patient was on dialysis for an extended period of time. (Courtesy of Dr. M. Hughson, Jackson, MS.)

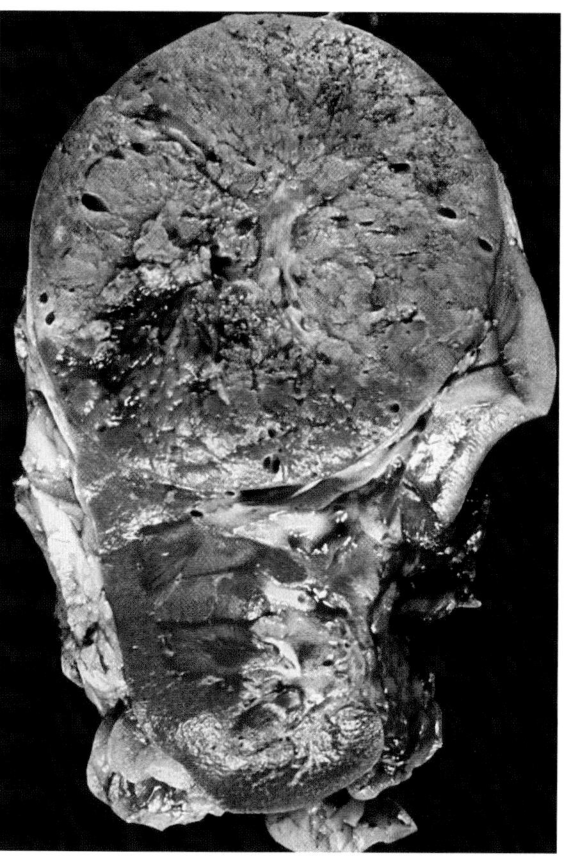

Figure 25-46

ACQUIRED CYSTIC DISEASE WITH LARGE RENAL CELL CARCINOMA

seen at the points of the cyst outpouching. Because of intracystic hemorrhage, some cysts contain hemosiderin in the epithelium and in the connective tissue of the cyst wall. The portion of the nephron involved has been studied with site-specific lectins and antibodies (3).

Etiology and Pathogenesis. The cause of ACD is not known. It has been suggested that following the loss of renal tissue, a renotropic growth factor is produced which promotes renal hypertrophy. Epidermal growth factor and transforming growth factor-alpha have been incriminated, but the growth substances are at present unknown. Tubular obstruction by oxalate crystals has also been suggested as a cause of ACD, but this is not widely accepted.

Renal Cell Tumors/Neoplasms in Acquired Cystic Disease

Renal cortical epithelial tumors (or neoplasms it appears) are found in about one sixth of end-stage kidneys (figs. 25-45, 25-46) (2,22,34,47). These tumors are of various sizes and are multiple in 9 to 10 percent of cases. Renal cell carcinoma has been described in about 6 percent of patients with ESRD (whether cystic or noncystic). Renal cell carcinoma is found 6 to 8 times more frequently in patients with ACD than in control groups without ACD, and at an average age that is about a decade younger than in the control group. Some have suggested that the severity of the change in cystic renal parenchyma (as determined by kidney weight) correlates with the risk of developing renal cell carcinoma.

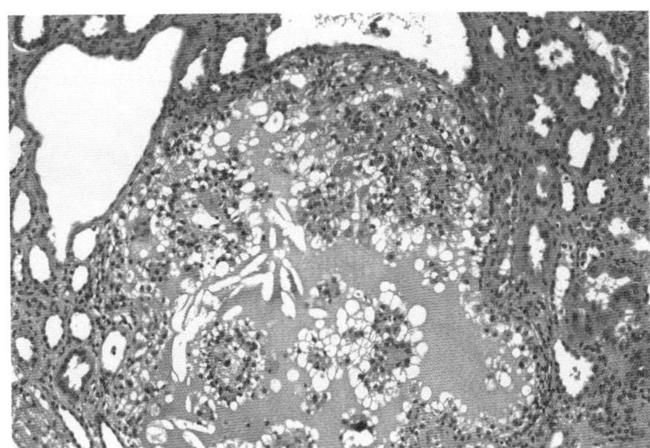

Figure 25-47

ACQUIRED CYSTIC DISEASE WITH RENAL CELL CARCINOMA

The histologic pattern is primarily one of a clear cell carcinoma.

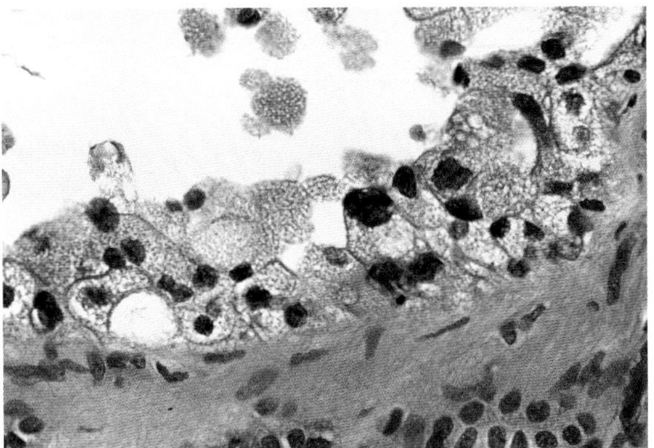

Figure 25-48

ACQUIRED CYSTIC DISEASE WITH RENAL CELL CARCINOMA

The cells lining this cyst are quite pleomorphic (a cystic clear cell carcinoma) (H&E stain).

The tumors may be small or large. Small tumors are well circumscribed and yellow to white. Most of the small tumors are situated in the superficial cortex just under the renal capsule, have a papillary architecture, and are thought to be adenomas with no clinical significance; however, these small subcapsular tumors may be clear cell carcinomas. Studies have shown that the risk of metastasis is low in clear cell neoplasms/carcinomas when their diameter is less than 3 cm (14).

Larger tumors often have a variegated appearance consisting of hemorrhage, cyst formation, or necrosis. Occasionally, these tumors are seen as mural nodules within renal cysts and may be papillary or clear cell in appearance. Clear cell carcinomas that invade the renal vein and perinephric tissue, and metastasize to regional lymph nodes and distant sites, such as the lung, have been well described.

Clear cell and papillary carcinomas occurring in patients with ACD are histologically identical to those that occur sporadically (figs. 25-47–25-49). It appears that papillary carcinoma is over-represented in the end-stage kidney compared with the clear cell variant (14,22). Most of the other subtypes or variants of renal cell carcinoma (e.g., chromophobe carcinoma, collecting duct carcinoma, oncocytoma) are not found with any frequency in patients with ACD or ESRD. Many of the renal carcinomas seen in patients with ESRD are incidental findings, of no clinical relevance. The major factors affecting the survival of these patients are age and the presence of cardiovascular disease.

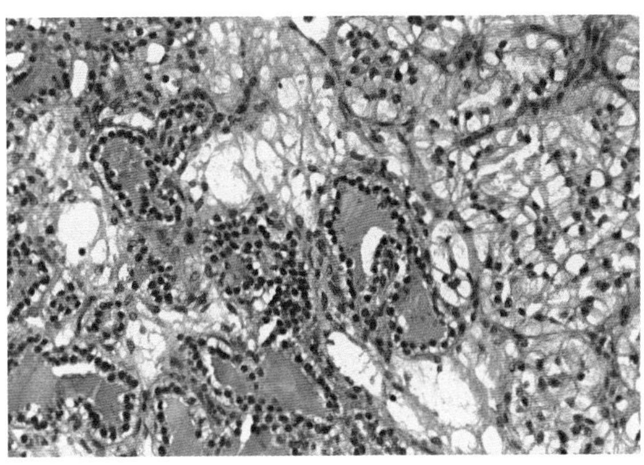

Figure 25-49

ACQUIRED CYSTIC DISEASE WITH RENAL CELL CARCINOMA

This is primarily a clear cell carcinoma (H&E stain).

The biologic behavior of tumors in patients with ESRD on hemodialysis seems to be more indolent than that of the sporadic renal carcinomas. Metastasis has only been observed in about 17 percent of patients with renal carcinoma on chronic hemodialysis. Cytogenetic studies of renal carcinomas in patients with ACD are underway, but few have been published.

REFERENCES

1. Bohle A, Biwer E, Christensen JA. Hyperperfusion injury of the human kidney in different glomerular diseases. Am J Nephrol 1988;8:179–86.
2. Budin RE, McDonnell PJ. Renal cell neoplasms. Their relationship to arteriolonephrosclerosis. Arch Pathol Lab Med 1984;108:138–40.
3. Deck MA, Verani R, Silva FG, et al. Histogenesis of renal cysts in end-stage renal disease (acquired cystic kidney disease): an immunohistochemical and lectin study. Am J Surg Pathol 1988;1:391.
4. Dlugosz BA, Bretan PN Jr, Novick AC, et al. Causes of death in kidney transplant recipients: 1970 to present. Transplant Proc 1989;21:2168–70.
5. Dunnill MS, Millard PR, Oliver D. Acquired cystic disease of the kidneys: a hazard of long-term intermittent maintenance dialysis. J Clin Pathol 1977;30:868–77.
6. Excerpts from the United States Renal Data System 1996 Annual Data Report. Am J Kidney Dis 1996;28(Suppl 2):S1–165.
7. Faraggiana T, Venkataseshan VS, Inagami T, Churg J. Immunohistochemical localization of renin in end-stage kidneys. Am J Kidney Dis 1988;12:194–9.
8. Fayemi AO, Ali M. Intrarenal vascular alterations in hemodialysis patients. A semiquantitative light microscopic study. Hum Pathol 1979;10:685–93.
9. Fayemi AO, Ali M, Braun EV. Oxalosis in hemodialysis patients: a pathologic study of 80 cases. Arch Pathol Lab Med 1979;103:58–62.
10. Gokal R. Quality of life in patients undergoing renal replacement therapy. Kidney Int 1993;40 (Suppl):S23–7.
11. Haggitt RC, Pitcock JA, Muirhead EE. Renal medullary fibrosis in hypertension. Hum Pathol 1971;2:587–97.
12. Heptinstall RH. Pathology of end-stage kidney disease. Am J Med 1968;44:656–63.
13. Hostetter TH, Olson JL, Rennke HG, Venkatachalam MA, Brenner BM. Hyperfiltration in remnant nephrons: a potentially adverse response to renal ablation. Am J Physiol 1981;241:F85–93.
14. Hughson MD. End-stage renal disease. In: Jennette JC, Olson JL, Schwartz MM, Silva FG, eds. Heptinstall's pathology of the kidney, 5th ed. Philadelphia: Lippincott-Raven; 1998:1371–408.
15. Hughson MD, Fox M, Garvin AJ. Pathology of the end-stage kidney after dialysis. Prog Reprod Genitourin Tract Pathol 1991;2:157.
16. Hughson MD, Harley RA, Hennigar GR. Cellular arteriolar nodules. Their presence in heart, pancreas, and kidney of patients with malignant nephrosclerosis. Arch Pathol Lab Med 1982;106:71–4.
17. Hughson MS, Hennigar GR, McManus JF. Atypical cysts, acquired renal cystic disease, and renal cell tumors in end-stage dialysis kidneys. Lab Invest 1980;42:475–80.
18. Hughson MD, McManus JF, Fitts CT, Williams AV. Studies of end-stage kidneys. III. Glycogen deposition in interstitial cells of the renal medulla. Am J Clin Pathol 1979;72:400–4.
19. Hughson MD, McManus JF, Hennigar GR. Studies on "end-stage" kidneys. II. Embryonal hyperplasia of Bowman's capsular epithelium. Am J Pathol 1978;91:71–84.
20. Hughson MD, Lajoie G. End-stage renal disease. In: Silva FG, D'Agati VD, Nadasdy T, eds. Renal biopsy interpretation. New York: Churchill Livingstone; 1996:357.
21. Hypertension in chronic renal disease. Kidney Int 1982;22:702–12.
22. Ishikawa I, Kovacs G. High incidence of papillary renal cell tumors in patients on chronic hemodialysis. Histopathology 1993;22:135–9.
23. Jacobson HR. Ischemic renal disease: an overlooked clinical entity? Kidney Int 1988;34:729–43.
24. Kasiske BL, Kalil RS, Ma JZ, Liao M, Keane WF. Effect of antihypertensive therapy on the kidney in patients with diabetes: a meta-regression analysis. Ann Intern Med 1993;118:129–38.
25. Kern WF, Laszik ZG, Nadasdy T, Silva FG, Bane BL, Pitha JV, eds. Atlas of renal pathology. Philadelphia: WB Saunders; 1999:113.
26. Klahr S, Levey AS, Beck G, et al. The effects of dietary protein restriction and blood-pressure control on the progression of chronic renal disease. Modification of Diet in Renal Disease Study Group. N Engl J Med 1994;330:877–84.
27. Kleinman KS, Coburn JW. Amyloid syndromes associated with hemodialysis. Kidney Int 1989;35:567–75.
28. Kunis CL, Markowitz GS, Liu-Jarin X, Fisher PE, Frei GL, D'Agati VD. Painful myopathy and end-stage renal disease. Am J Kidney Dis 2001;37:1098–104.
29. Levey AS, Greene T, Beck GJ, et al. Dietary protein restriction and the progression of chronic renal disease: what have all of the results of the MDRD study shown? Modification of Diet in Renal Disease Study Group. J Am Soc Neprol 1999;10:2426–39.

30. Lindner A, Charra B, Sherrard DJ, Scribner BH. Accelerated atherosclerosis in prolonged maintenance hemodialysis. N Engl J Med 1974;290: 697–701.
31. Llach F, Fernandez E. Overview of renal bone disease: causes of treatment failure, clinical observations, the changing pattern of bone lesions, and future therapeutic approach. Kidney Int 2003;87:S113–9.
32. Manske CL. Dialysis-related amyloidosis. J Lab Clin Med 1994;123:458–60.
33. Maschio G, Oldrizzi L. Introduction. Kidney Int 2000;57(Suppl 75):1.
34. Matson MA, Cohen EP. Acquired cystic disease: occurrence, prevalence, and renal cancers. Medicine (Baltimore) 1990;69:217–26.
35. McManus JF, Hughson MD. Focal atypical hyperplasia with cyst formation in end-stage/dialysis kidneys [Abstract]. Fed Proc 1978;37:676
36. McManus JF, Hughson MD. Histopathology of arteries and veins in the end-stage dialysis kidney. Pathol Ann 1979;14:23–59.
37. McManus JF, Hughson MD, Fitts CT, Williams AV. Studies on "end-stage" kidneys. Nodule formation in intrarenal arteries and arterioles. Lab Invest 1977;37:339–49.
38. McManus JF, Hughson MD, Hennigar GR, Fitts CT, Rajagopalan PR, Williams AV. Dialysis enhances renal epithelial proliferations. Arch Pathol Lab Med 1980;104:192–5.
39. Meadows R. Renal histopathology, 2nd ed. Oxford: Oxford University Press; 1978:154.
40. Nadasdy T, Laszik Z, Blick KE, Johnson DL, Silva FG. Tubular atrophy in the end-stage kidney: a lectin and immunohistochemical study. Hum Pathol 1994;25:22–8.
41. Nishi T, Bond C Jr, Brown G, Solez K, Heptinstall RH. A morphologic study of arterial intimal thickening in kidneys of dialyzed patients. Am J Pathol 1979;95:597–610.
42. Ogata K. Clinicopathologic study of kidneys from patients on chronic dialysis. Kidney Int 1990;37:1333–40.
43. Oldrizzi L, Rugiu C, De Biase V, Maschio G. The place of hypertension among risk factors for renal function in chronic renal failure. Am J Kidney Dis 1993;21:119–23.
44. Olson JL, de Urdaneta AG, Heptinstall RH. Glomerular hyalinosis and its relationship to hyperfiltration. Lab Invest 1985;52:387–98.
45. Olson JL, Heptinstall RH. Nonimmunological mechanisms of glomerular injury. Lab Invest 1988;59:564–78.
46. Pichette V, Querin S, Desmeules M, Ethier J, Copleston P. Renal functional recovery in end-stage renal disease. Am J Kidney Dis 1993;22:398–402.
47. Port FK, Fenton SS, Mazzuchi N. Introduction. ESRD Throughout the world: morbidity, mortality and quality of life. Kidney Int 1999;57(Suppl 74):S1–2.
48. Port FK, Ragheb NE, Schwartz AG, Hawthorne VM. Neoplasms in dialysis patients: a population-based study. Am J Kidney Dis 1989;14:119–23.
49. Rostand, SG, Drueke TB. Parathyroid hormone, vitamin D, and cardiovascular disease in chronic renal failure. Kidney Int 1999;56:383–92.
50. Schwartz MM, Cotran RS. Primary renal disease in transplant recipients. Hum Pathol 1976;7: 445–9.
51. Sekkarie MA, Port FK, Wolfe RA, et al. Recovery from end-stage renal disease. Am J Kidney Dis 1990;15:61–5.
52. Selye H, Stone H. Pathogenesis of the cardiovascular and renal changes which usually accompany malignant hypertension. J Urol 1946; 56:399–419.
53. Smith SR, Svetkey LP, Dennis VW. Racial differences in the incidence and prognosis of renal diseases. Kidney Int 1991;40:815–22.
54. Survival probabilities and causes of death. Am J Kidney Dis 1991;18(Suppl 2):S49–60.
55. Tokars JI, Alter MJ, Favero MS, Moyer LA, Bland LA. National surveillance of hemodialysis associated diseases in the United States, 1990. ASAIO J 1993;39:71–80.
56. United States Renal Data System. USRDS 2001 Annual Data System Report: atlas of end-stage renal disease in the United States. Bethesda, MD: National Institute of Diabetes and Digestive and Kidney Diseases; 2001.
57. Walser M. Progression of chronic renal failure in man. Kidney Int 1990;37:1195–210.

26 PATHOLOGY OF RENAL TRANSPLANTATION

INTRODUCTION

Although renal allotransplantation was introduced on a widespread scale nearly 40 years ago, the modern age of transplantation was ushered in around 1983 with the introduction of a new class of immunosuppressive agents, the calcineurin inhibitors. This has been followed by the more recent development of modern combination therapies. Even with improved immunosuppressive regimens, graft rejection remains the major cause of failure. Most patients with renal allografts have one or more episodes of graft dysfunction over their lifetime. Despite the recent introduction of diagnostic procedures such as fine needle aspiration and radionuclide scintigraphy, renal biopsy remains the most sensitive diagnostic tool for the diagnosis of rejection and other causes of graft dysfunction. Because of the relatively superficial location of the allograft in the iliac fossa (fig. 26-1), renal biopsies can be performed safely and repeatedly, with extremely low complication rates of less than 0.4 percent (21).

The causes of graft dysfunction are numerous, as outlined in Table 26-1. Because of the large number of conditions that can affect the allograft, sometimes in combination, renal transplantation pathology is one of the most challenging areas for the renal pathologist. The major entities that cause allograft dysfunction

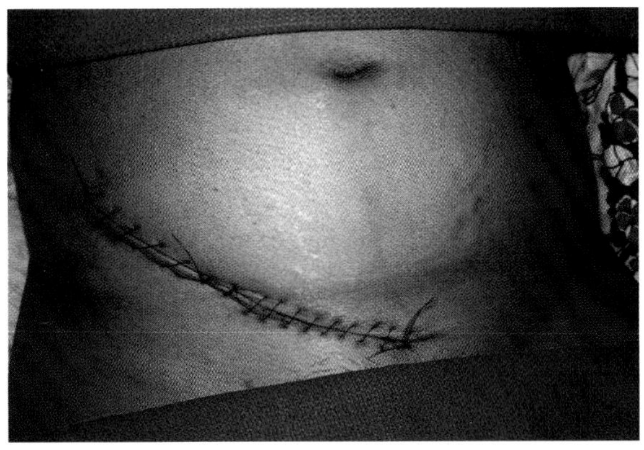

Figure 26-1

SITE OF SURGICAL IMPLANTATION

Location of the surgical scar over the right iliac fossa in a patient post renal transplantation.

Table 26-1

CAUSES OF RENAL ALLOGRAFT DYSFUNCTION

Rejection
- Primarily humoral (antibody mediated)
  - Hyperacute rejection
  - Acute antibody-mediated rejection
    - Acute tubular injury
    - Capillaritis (peritubular and glomerular)
    - Necrotizing arteritis (Banff/CCTT type III acute rejection)[a]
- Primarily cellular (T-cell mediated)
  - Acute cellular rejection
    - Tubulointerstitial (Banff/CCTT type I acute rejection)
    - Vascular (endarteritis) (Banff/CCTT type II acute rejection)
    - Glomerular (transplant glomerulitis/acute glomerulopathy)
- Chronic rejection (chronic allograft nephropathy) (mixed humoral and cellular pathogenesis/other factors)
  - Vascular (chronic transplant arteriopathy)
  - Tubulointerstitial
  - Glomerular (chronic transplant glomerulopathy)

Drug Toxicity
- Cyclosporine
- Tacrolimus (Prograf/FK506)
- OKT3

Acute Tubular Necrosis/Preservation Injury

Perfusion Injury

Major Artery/Vein Thrombosis or Stenosis

Obstruction

Infection

Drug-Induced Acute Interstitial Nephritis

De Novo Glomerular Disease

Recurrence of Original Renal Disease

Post-Transplant Lymphoproliferative Disease

[a]Banff = Conference of Banff, Canada; CCTT = Cooperative Clinical Trials in Transplantation.

include rejection, postoperative acute tubular necrosis, perfusion injury, drug toxicity (due to the calcineurin inhibitors—cyclosporine and tacrolimus), obstruction, major vascular occlusion, infection, allergic interstitial nephritis, recurrent or de novo glomerular disease, and posttransplant lymphoproliferative disease. In one prospective clinical trial, the clinical diagnosis after renal transplant biopsy differed from the prebiopsy diagnosis in 42 percent of episodes of graft dysfunction, often leading to a significant change in the clinical management (45).

HANDLING OF THE RENAL TRANSPLANT BIOPSY

Ideally, the clinician should provide two cores of tissue whenever possible (8), because rejection is notoriously focal in the early stages. The majority of the tissue is processed for light microscopic examination. A small portion of the biopsy is snap-frozen for immunofluorescence studies. Most investigators advocate the routine performance of immunofluorescence staining for complement (C)4d to exclude acute humoral rejection. Whether the full immunofluorescence panel of staining (for immunoglobulin [Ig]G, IgM, IgA, C3, C1q, fibrinogen, and kappa and lambda light chains) also needs to be performed in the early transplant period has been debated. Some pathologists would reserve doing the complete panel for those cases in which there is clinical evidence of glomerular dysfunction or light microscopic evidence of glomerular abnormalities. Generally, no tissue is sampled for electron microscopy unless the possibility of de novo or recurrent glomerular disease is suspected clinically, such as when there is new onset of nephrotic-range proteinuria or full nephrotic syndrome. Same day (rapid) processing of formalin-fixed transplant biopsy specimens is available in most centers. Rapid diagnosis from a frozen section preparation is much less reliable and may lead to diagnostic errors.

By the Banff 97 classification criteria (so named for the meeting place of the conference in Banff, Canada), an adequate biopsy contains 10 or more glomeruli and at least two arteries (48). In practice, however, the adequacy of the sample depends on the nature of the lesions identified. For example, a single artery with endothelialitis may be adequate to diagnose acute rejection, even if no glomeruli are sampled. A biopsy that contains medulla is inadequate to rule out acute rejection. Subcapsular cortex often shows inflammation and fibrosis, in the absence of acute rejection. This is because the capsular collateral circulation of the transplant kidney is interrupted following transplantation, producing a narrow subcapsular band of tubular atrophy, interstitial fibrosis, and inflammation (with or without tubulitis) that is not representative of the changes in the deeper cortex (fig. 26-2). Thus, a biopsy that contains exclusively subcapsular cortex may be inadequate.

ALLOGRAFT REJECTION

Allograft rejection is an immunologic response mounted by the recipient to foreign donor antigens displayed in the allograft, primarily human leukocyte antigen (HLA) class I and class II antigens. The role of minor transplantation antigens and endothelial antigens is less well defined. Rejection can be classified into hyperacute, acute, and chronic forms depending on the timing of the rejection and the pathologic features. Acute rejection can be subclassified morphologically and pathogenetically into two major subtypes: 1) primarily antibody mediated (humoral) and 2) primarily T-cell mediated (cellular).

Hyperacute Rejection

Definition. Hyperacute rejection is an immediate form of graft rejection that is entirely humoral (antibody mediated) and is generally irreversible. It occurs within minutes to hours of placement of the surgical anastomosis. In some cases, clinical evidence of rejection may be delayed for 24 to 48 hours *(delayed hyperacute rejection)*.

Clinical Features. At implantation, the allograft kidney becomes cyanotic, dusky blue, and flaccid within minutes of establishing the renal artery anastomosis. If tissue is taken at surgery for frozen section there is usually little if any bleeding because of widespread thrombotic occlusion of the renal microvasculature, even though the hilar pulse is preserved. Presentation is with primary graft failure (failure to develop any urine output following transplantation). Those with delayed hyperacute rejection may develop oligoanuria after a brief period of initial graft function.

Other features include fever, thrombocytopenia, elevated levels of fibrin split products, and intravascular hemolysis. A renal scan is helpful to demonstrate marked reduction or abolition of renal blood flow. The diagnosis is supported by the demonstration in the pretransplant serum of donor-specific antibodies to T cells, B cells, monocytes, or endothelium.

Gross Findings. The kidney parenchyma appears purple-blue, with a soft, flaccid consistency. If several days have passed before the kidney is explanted, there may be complete hemorrhagic infarction and swelling of the kidney (fig. 26-3). Occlusive thrombi may be detected macroscopically in the medium-sized and large arteries (fig. 26-3).

Light Microscopic Findings. The earliest features are vascular endothelial swelling and necrosis accompanied by neutrophil margination within peritubular and glomerular capillaries and small arteries (fig. 26-4). The endothelium lifts off the vascular basement membranes. Microthrombosis of glomerular capillaries, arterioles, and small arteries by fibrin-platelet thrombi rapidly ensues, leading to ischemic injury to all renal compartments (figs. 26-5, 26-6). Patchy tubular necrosis evolves rapidly into total renal infarction.

In the later stages there is, frequently, interstitial hemorrhage associated with mild neutrophil infiltration of the interstitium (fig. 26-5). Mononuclear inflammatory infiltrates and

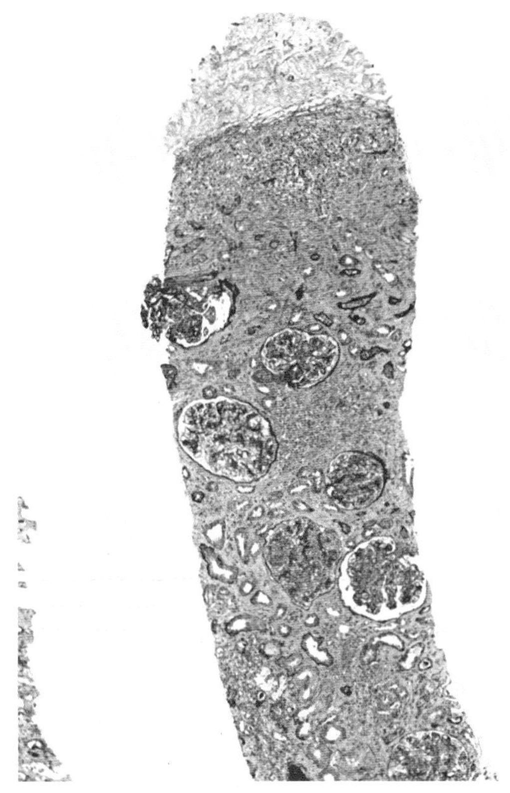

Figure 26-2

SUBCAPSULAR SCAR

Needle core biopsy specimen from an allograft 5 months post-transplantation shows a zone of subcapsular fibrosis and tubular atrophy, with relative preservation of the deeper cortex. Subcapsular scars are commonly seen in the allograft due to interruption of capsular collateral vessels (hematoxylin and eosin [H&E] stain).

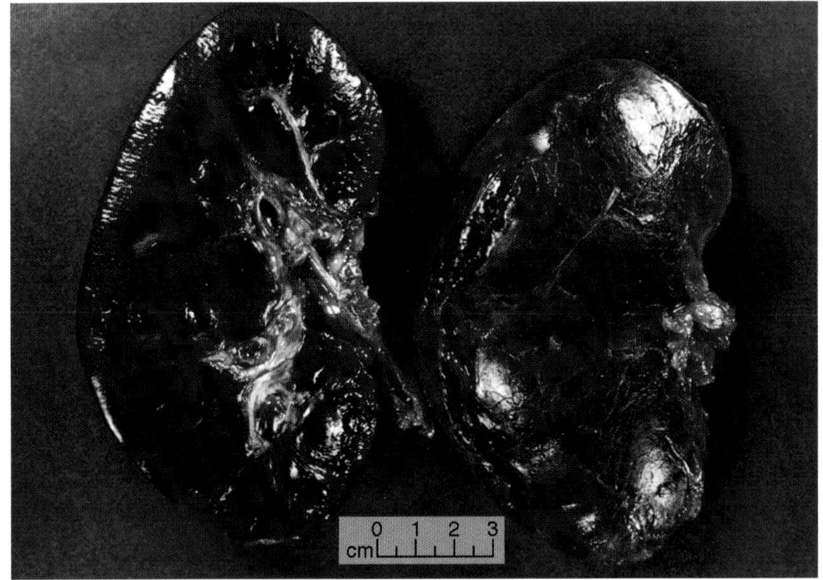

Figure 26-3

HYPERACUTE REJECTION

The explanted kidney is swollen, hemorrhagic, and diffusely infarcted. The interlobar arteries contain grossly identifiable thrombi.

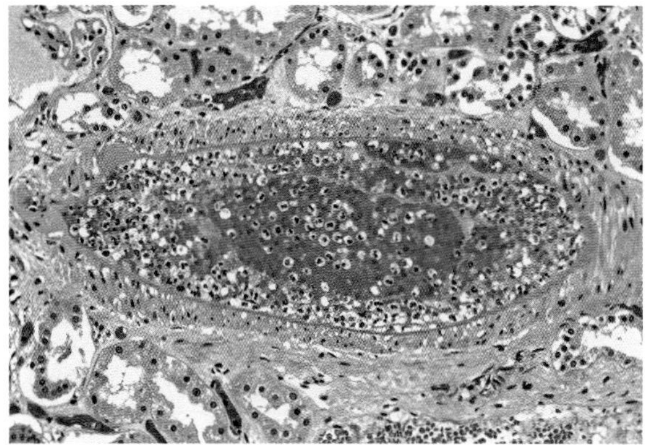

Figure 26-4

HYPERACUTE REJECTION

The earliest light microscopic findings are vascular congestion and neutrophil margination. This medium-sized artery is congested with erythrocytes and contains abundant marginating neutrophils that adhere to the swollen and denuded vascular endothelium. There is not yet evidence of intravascular fibrin thrombosis (H&E stain).

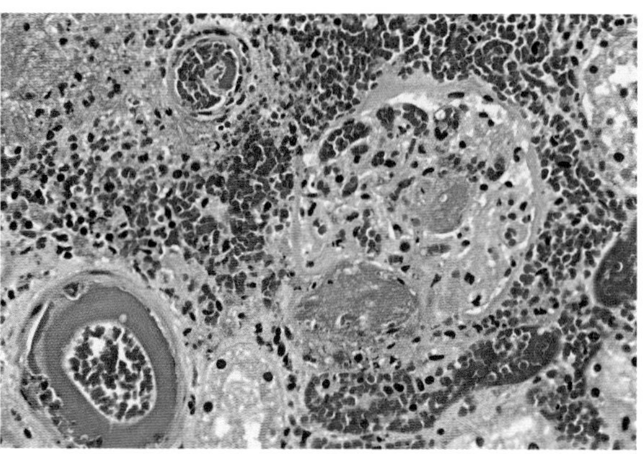

Figure 26-5

HYPERACUTE REJECTION

Several hours after the onset of hyperacute rejection, there is fibrin thrombosis of the arterioles and glomerular capillaries associated with interstitial hemorrhage (H&E stain).

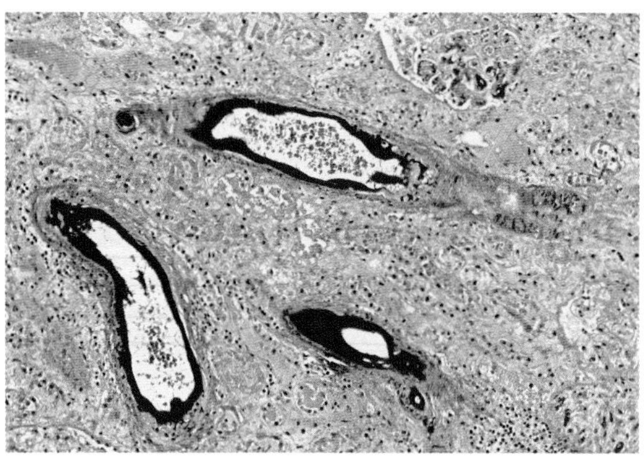

Figure 26-6

HYPERACUTE REJECTION

The Masson trichrome stain highlights the residual fuchsinophilic intravascular thrombosis despite complete cortical infarction.

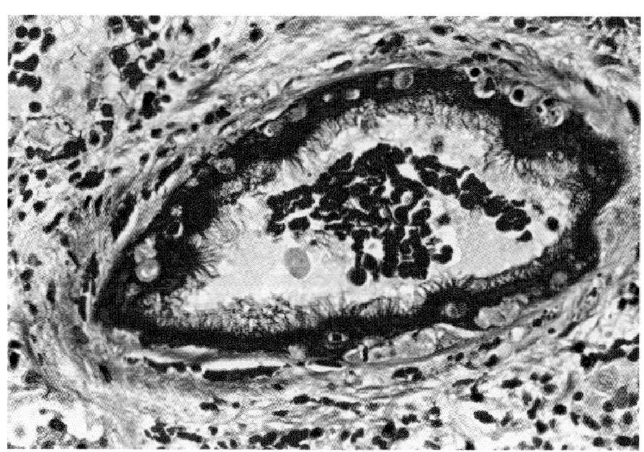

Figure 26-7

HYPERACUTE REJECTION

Fibrillar strands of fibrin adhere to the denuded arterial surface, and relatively spare the central lumen containing erythrocytes (Masson trichrome stain).

tubulitis are not features of this condition. Despite the infarcted state of the kidney, it is usually possible to discern intravascular microthrombi throughout the microvasculature, especially with the help of special stains such as trichrome, which stains fibrin red; Fraser-Lendrum, which stains fibrin orange; and phosphotungstic acid-hematoxylin (PTAH) which stains fibrin purple (figs. 26-7–26-9).

Immunofluorescence Findings. Because hyperacute rejection is antibody mediated, the diagnosis is aided by the detection of linear to semilinear staining for IgM or IgG, as well as C3 and C4d, along the surfaces of interstitial and glomerular capillaries, arterioles, and small arteries (fig. 26-10). IgM is usually more readily identifiable than IgG. In many cases, especially in specimens taken later in the course of hyperacute rejection, immunoglobulin may not be detectable. This is probably due to rapid shedding and clearing of endothelial-bound immunoglobulins from damaged vessels. C4d

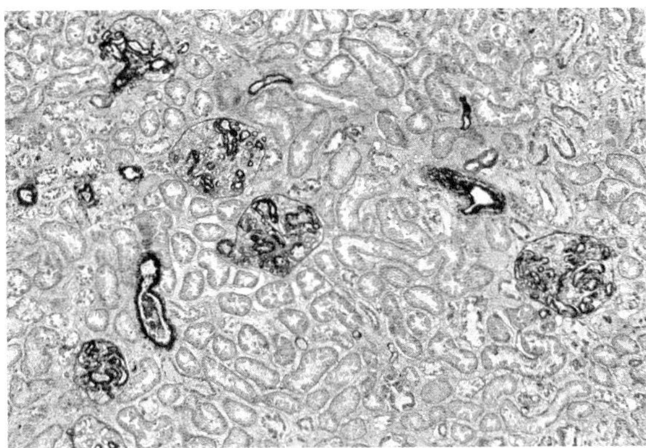

Figure 26-8

HYPERACUTE REJECTION

Phosphotungstic acid-hematoxylin (PTAH) stain for fibrin highlights the microthrombosis in small arteries and glomerular capillaries.

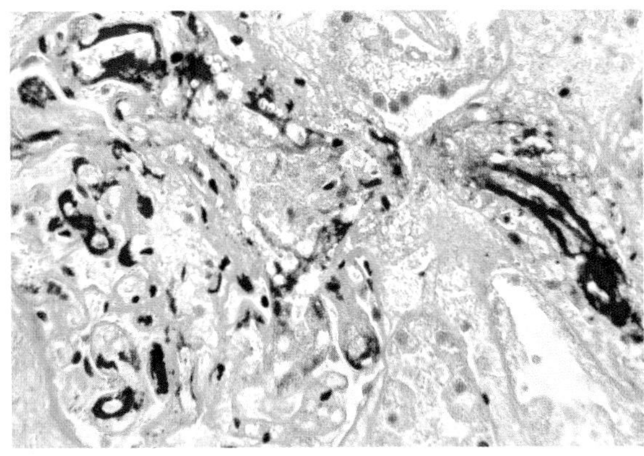

Figure 26-9

HYPERACUTE REJECTION

The Fraser-Lendrum stain shows red-pink stained fibrin in the afferent arteriole and glomerular capillaries.

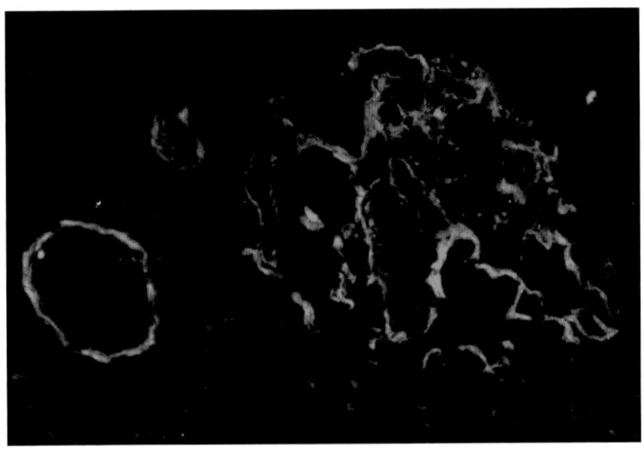

Figure 26-10

HYPERACUTE REJECTION

There is delicate (1+) semilinear staining for IgM along the endothelial surfaces of a preglomerular arteriole and the glomerular capillaries (immunofluorescence micrograph).

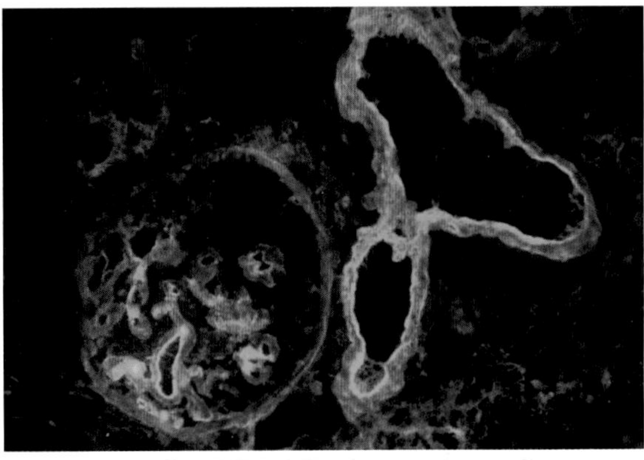

Figure 26-11

HYPERACUTE REJECTION

Strong (3+) staining for fibrin outlines the glomerular capillaries and small arteries (immunofluorescence micrograph).

may not be detectable in some specimens, perhaps because of the degree of tissue necrosis or insufficient time for it to bind covalently to the microvasculature. There is strong staining for fibrin-related antigen throughout the microvasculature and often focally in the interstitium, corresponding to areas of interstitial hemorrhage (fig. 26-11). In the event of renal infarction, the necrotic parenchyma may emit a diffuse yellowish autofluorescence.

Electron Microscopic Findings. The glomerular capillaries and small arteries are narrowed or occluded by fibrin-platelet thrombi and marginated neutrophils, with stasis of red blood cells. There is swelling, necrosis, and shedding of endothelial cells. In many instances, the endothelium is completely desquamated, with fibrin forming on the denuded glomerular or vascular basement membranes. No electron-dense deposits are identified. The tubules are in varying stages of coagulation necrosis.

Differential Diagnosis. The differential diagnosis includes other conditions that can cause primary graft failure (i.e., graft nonfunction ab initio). Diagnostic considerations include acute tubular necrosis, perfusion injury, and major vascular occlusion. Acute tubular necrosis is easily identified by renal biopsy. Perfusion injury may mimic hyperacute rejection by light microscopy, because it can cause vascular thrombosis, neutrophil margination, endothelial injury, and acute tubular necrosis. However, perfusion injury usually has less severe and less extensive neutrophil margination, thrombosis, and hemorrhage than hyperacute rejection. Moreover, immunofluorescence reveals no immunoglobulin deposits along the endothelial surfaces, although fibrin may be intensely positive. Major arterial occlusion leads to bland renal necrosis with little if any neutrophil margination or microthrombosis.

Etiology and Pathogenesis. Hyperacute rejection is mediated by preformed circulating antibodies to donor endothelial cells, such as ABO blood group antigens, HLA class I antigens, or less commonly, HLA class II antigens (8,17). Fortunately, this form of rejection is extremely rare (affecting less than 0.2 percent of transplants) due to standard cross-match tests that screen for donor-specific antibody prior to transplantation. Nevertheless, some cases fail to be averted because antibody titers are below the level of sensitivity of currently available cross-match tests or because the antibodies are directed to vascular-endothelial antigens that are not routinely screened for. Cold agglutinin IgM antibodies have also been incriminated in some cases of hyperacute rejection where the graft has not been adequately warmed prior to reperfusion. Preformed antibodies may have been acquired in the course of previous transplantations, pregnancy, or blood transfusions.

Graft injury occurs within minutes to hours of the establishment of the renal arterial flow. It is mediated by the binding of an antibody (usually of the IgM class) to the surface of graft endothelial cells at all levels of the vascular tree, with particularly severe involvement of glomerular capillaries, interstitial capillaries, and small arteries. Activation of complement causes the release of chemotactic complement fractions C3a and C5a, which attract neutrophils. Endothelial lysis is mediated by the generation of membrane attack complex C5b-9, leading to denudation of endothelium, activation of the coagulation cascade, production of occlusive fibrin-platelet thrombi, and subsequent renal infarction.

Treatment and Prognosis. There is no currently effective treatment for hyperacute rejection. The graft must be removed promptly to prevent dangerous systemic serum sickness–like reactions. Experimental approaches, such as plasmapheresis, adsorption of immunoglobulin on protein A columns, and complement antagonists, have not gained widespread use in man.

Acute Antibody-Mediated Rejection

Definition. Acute antibody-mediated rejection can arise any time following transplantation. Clinically and morphologically, it resembles a slow form of hyperacute rejection with predominant injury to the vascular compartment. Synonyms are *acute humoral rejection* and *accelerated vascular rejection*.

Clinical Features. The incidence of this form of rejection fell with the introduction of cyclosporine in the 1980s (8). However, its true incidence in the modern era may be under-recognized. Immunofluorescence staining for C4d and search for donor-specific antibodies reveal a higher incidence of acute antibody-mediated rejection than previously recognized (27). Presentation is with rapid development of graft failure after an initial period of good graft function, usually within the first 3 months of transplantation. Clinical features include sudden elevation of serum creatinine, sometimes accompanied by reduced urine output and graft tenderness.

Gross Findings. The kidney is enlarged and swollen, with focal hemorrhage and infarcts.

Light Microscopic Findings. The earliest finding is neutrophil margination in peritubular interstitial capillaries (fig. 26-12). Later there is endothelial injury, neutrophil margination, and thrombosis of glomerular capillaries, interstitial capillaries, and small arteries, producing lesions that resemble those of hyperacute rejection (figs. 26-13, 26-14). Glomerular endothelial necrosis is often accompanied by mesangiolysis, a dissolution of the mesangial matrix similar to that seen in other forms of thrombotic microangiopathy.

Larger arteries may display transmural arteritis or medial necrosis of the fibrinoid type, with permeation of fibrin and plasma proteins into the vessel wall, accompanied by necrosis of myocytes. Transmural arteritis, with or without fibrinoid and smooth muscle necrosis, is classified as *type/grade III acute rejection* by both the

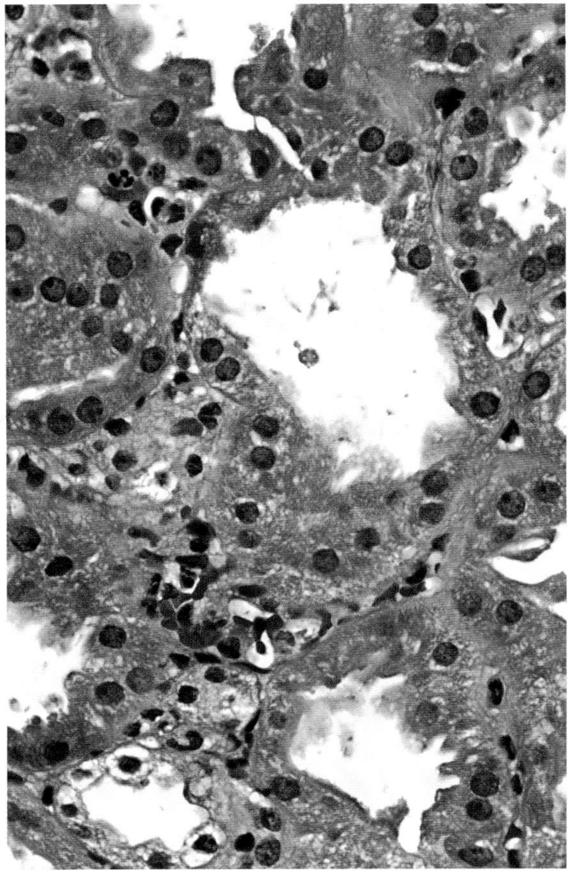

Figure 26-12

ACUTE ANTIBODY-MEDIATED (HUMORAL) REJECTION

The earliest finding is margination of neutrophils in the peritubular interstitial capillaries (H&E stain).

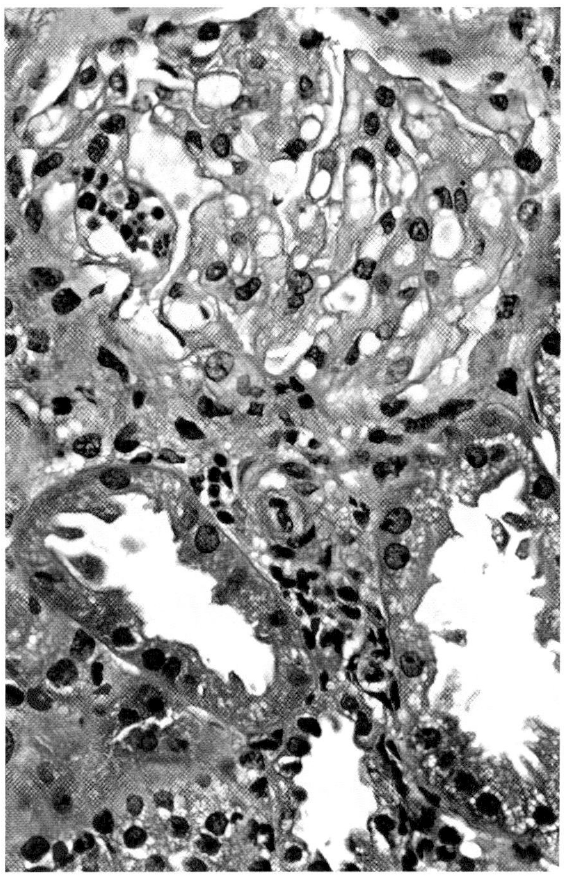

Figure 26-13

ACUTE ANTIBODY-MEDIATED (HUMORAL) REJECTION

In the same specimen as in figure 26-12, there is focal neutrophil margination in glomerular capillaries (H&E stain).

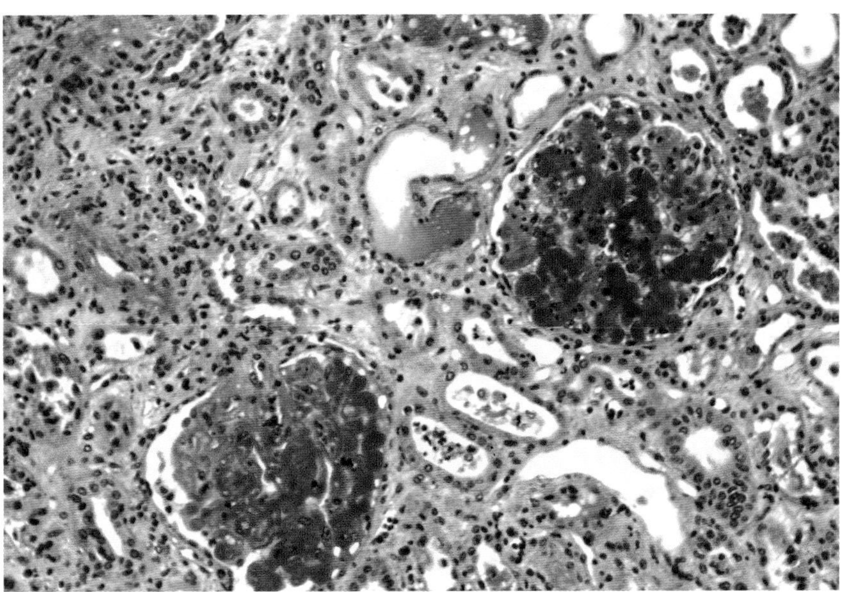

Figure 26-14

ACUTE ANTIBODY-MEDIATED (HUMORAL) REJECTION

A severe example shows massive glomerular capillary thrombosis and neutrophil margination. A component of cellular tubulointerstitial rejection is also present (H&E stain).

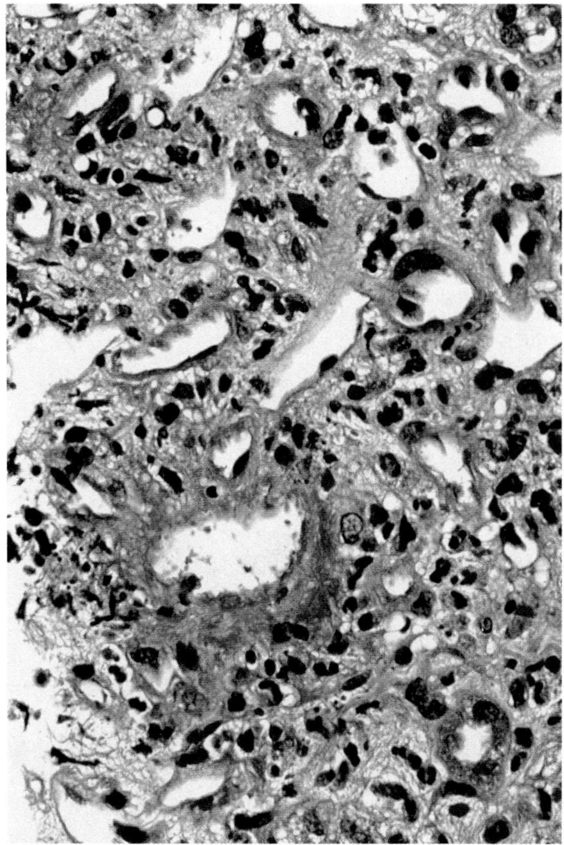

Figure 26-15

ACUTE ANTIBODY-MEDIATED (HUMORAL) REJECTION

There is fibrinoid necrosis of individual interstitial capillaries. Note the associated neutrophilic interstitial infiltrate (H&E stain).

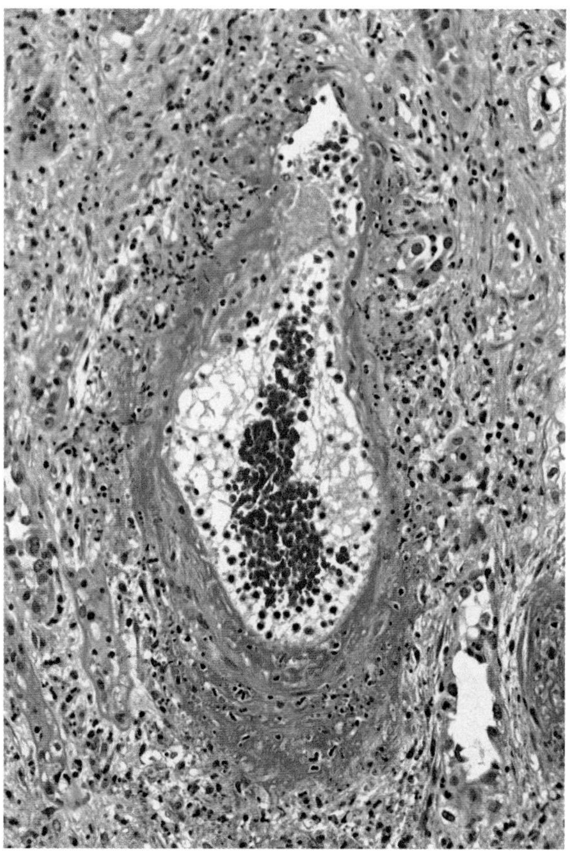

Figure 26-16

ACUTE ANTIBODY-MEDIATED (HUMORAL) REJECTION

An interlobar artery shows circumferential transmural fibrinoid necrosis and medial inflammation by neutrophils and lymphocytes. These findings resemble those of the necrotizing arteritis seen in microscopic polyangiitis (H&E stain).

Cooperative Clinical Trials in Transplantation (CCTT) and the Banff 97 criteria (9,48). Lesions with transmural neutrophil or lymphocytic infiltration and medial fibrinoid necrosis closely resemble the lesions of microscopic polyangiitis seen in native kidneys (figs. 26-15–26-17). There is little, if any, mononuclear inflammatory infiltration of the interstitium or tubulitis. Associated acute tubular necrosis or degenerative changes are common. In some cases, patchy cortical infarction occurs. There may be focal interstitial microhemorrhage involving the cortex or medulla.

In a minority of cases, a component of cellular rejection accompanies the acute humoral rejection. In this circumstance, interstitial mononuclear infiltrates and tubulitis may be present.

In 2003, the Banff criteria for the grading of acute antibody-mediated rejection were promulgated (Table 26-2) (47). Type (grade) I is a biopsy with features of acute tubular necrosis, minimal inflammation, and C4d positivity in peritubular capillaries. Type (grade) II is capillary margination and/or thrombosis, accompanied by C4d positivity in peritubular capillaries. The capillary margination may be in the form of glomerulitis or polymorphonuclear and/or mononuclear leukocytes in peritubular capillaries. Type (grade) III refers to arterial transmural arteritis or fibrinoid necrosis, accompanied by C4d positivity in peritubular capillaries. Although serologic demonstration of donor-specific antibody is still required for definitive diagnosis of acute antibody-mediated rejection, the presence of these histologic findings and C4d positivity allows a presumptive diagnosis.

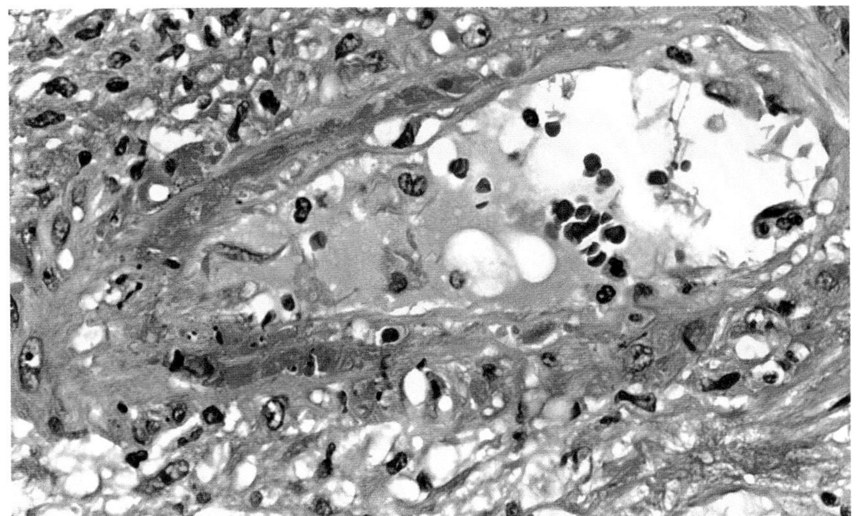

Figure 26-17

ACUTE ANTIBODY-MEDIATED (HUMORAL) REJECTION

There is transmural eccentric fibrinoid necrosis with leukocytoclasia of a small artery. The necrotic myocytes have a smudgy, hypereosinophilic appearance. The arterial endothelium appears swollen and focally denuded (H&E stain).

Table 26-2

BANFF 97 CRITERIA FOR ACUTE RENAL (CELLULAR) ALLOGRAFT REJECTION[a]

Borderline Changes ("Suspicious" for Acute Rejection)[b]	Interstitial inflammation involving 10-25% of the cortex and tubulitis with 1-4 mononuclear cells/tubular cross section or group of 10 tubular cells, in the absence of intimal arteritis
Type (Grade) IA	Interstitial inflammation involving >25% of the cortex and tubulitis with >4 mononuclear cells per tubular cross section or per group of 10 tubular cells
Type (Grade) IB	Significant interstitial inflammation involving >25% of the cortex and foci of severe tubulitis (>10 mononuclear cells per tubular cross section or per group of 10 tubular cells)
Type (Grade) IIA	Mild to moderate intimal arteritis (v1)
Type (Grade) IIB	Severe intimal arteritis (comprising >25% of the luminal area) (v2)
Type (Grade) III	Transmural arteritis and/or arterial fibrinoid change and necrosis of medial smooth muscle cells (v3)
UPDATED BANFF 97 CRITERIA FOR ACUTE ANTIBODY-MEDIATED REJECTION[c,d]	
Type (Grade) I	ATN-like[e], minimal inflammation, C4d+
Type (Grade) II	Capillary-leukocyte margination and/or thromboses, C4d+
Type (Grade) III	Arterial-v3 (transmural arteritis and/or arterial fibrinoid change and necrosis of medial smooth muscle cells), C4d+

[a]Modified from reference 48.
[b]For the assessment of tubulitis, atrophic tubules and scarred areas of cortex should not be graded.
[c]Modified from reference 47.
[d]Rejection due, at least in part, to documented antidonor antibody ("suspicious for" if antibody not demonstrated).
[e]ATN = acute tubular necrosis.

Immunofluorescence Findings. In some cases it is possible to demonstrate IgG or IgM and C3, in addition to fibrin, along the endothelial aspect of glomerular and interstitial capillaries (figs. 26-18, 26-19). However, more often, routine immunofluorescence is disappointingly negative. Recently, Colvin and colleagues (7) introduced a more sensitive diagnostic test, staining for C4d in peritubular capillaries (fig. 26-20) (11,27). The staining of peritubular capillaries for C4d should be bright and diffuse to be considered positive. After antibody binds to antigen on the endothelium, C4 is proteolytically cleaved by activated C1 into C4a and C4b. Bound C4b is converted to C4d, a proteolytically inactive 44-kDa peptide that binds covalently to the endothelium and

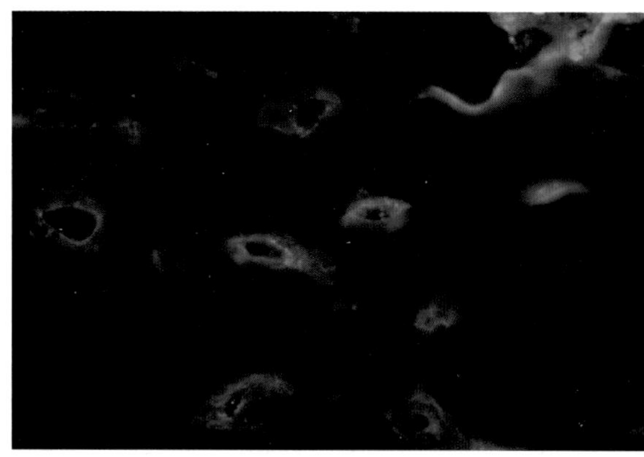

Figure 26-18

ACUTE ANTIBODY-MEDIATED (HUMORAL) REJECTION

Staining for complement component C3 outlines the endothelial aspect of the peritubular interstitial capillaries (immunofluorescence micrograph).

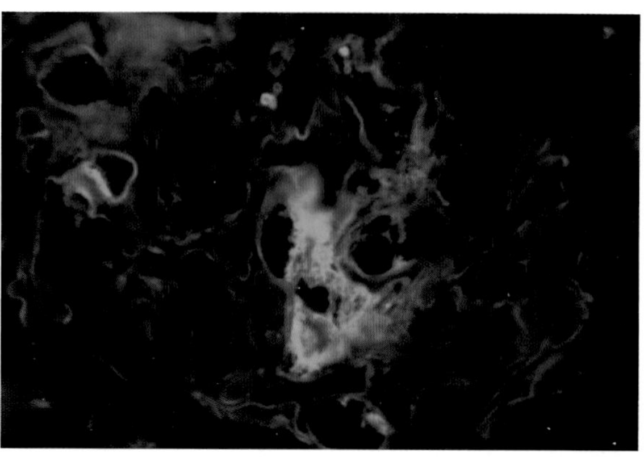

Figure 26-19

ACUTE ANTIBODY-MEDIATED (HUMORAL) REJECTION

There is strong (3+) staining for fibrin in the thrombosed glomerular capillaries (immunofluorescence micrograph).

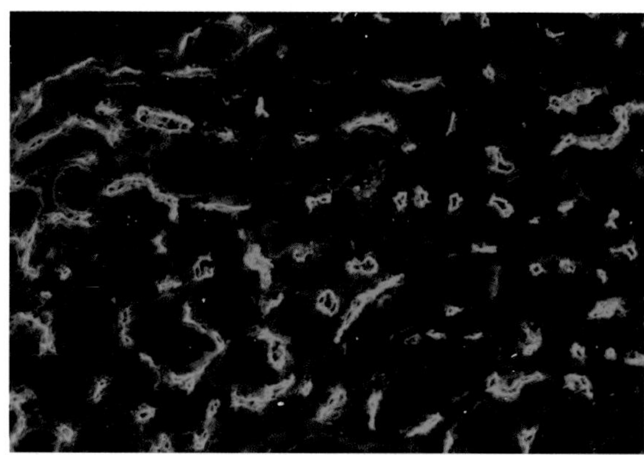

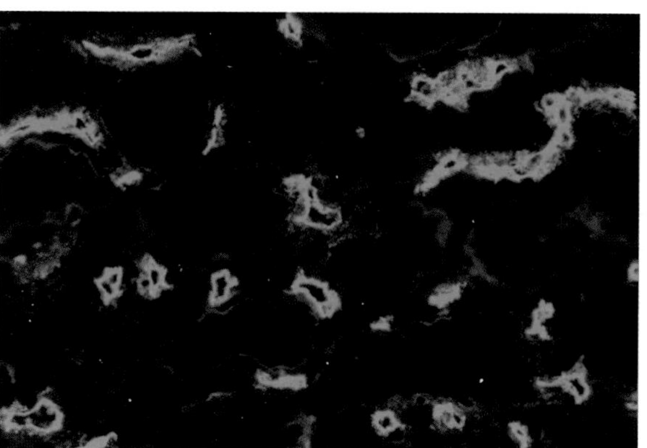

Figure 26-20

ACUTE ANTIBODY-MEDIATED (HUMORAL) REJECTION

Left: Low-power view shows strong and diffuse staining for complement component C4d in the distribution of the peritubular interstitial capillaries.

Right: High-power view illustrates the distribution of C4d. Staining outlines the walls of the peritubular capillaries that are located between the cortical tubules. The intervening tubules, which can be recognized as larger epithelial-lined structures, appear negative (left and right, immunofluorescence micrograph).

resists degradation, serving as a durable marker of complement activation by the classic pathway that can persist in the graft for up to 60 days (27). C4d may be the earliest identifiable abnormality, preceding the development of neutrophil margination or microvascular fibrin thrombi (11,27). Staining for C4d in peritubular capillaries is 95 percent sensitive and 96 percent specific for donor-specific antibodies (27).

Electron Microscopic Findings. Glomerular capillary lumens are narrowed by swelling and hypercellularity of the endothelial cells, obliterating the fenestrations. There is focal detachment of endothelium from the glomerular basement membrane, with deposition of fibrillar fibrin in the subendothelial space and the capillary lumen. The lamina interna rara may be widened by subendothelial, electron-lucent, flocculent material ("fluff") consistent with the degraded products of coagulation. Neutrophil margination and erythrocyte stasis are common, even in capillaries lacking overt intravascular coagulation. Arterioles and arteries are focally narrowed by endothelial swelling and denudation, and the intraluminal and intimal accumulation of fibrin and insuded electron-dense plasma proteins, accompanied by myocyte necrosis. No electron-dense immune-type deposits are seen.

Differential Diagnosis. The differential diagnosis of acute humoral rejection includes thrombotic microangiopathy secondary to calcineurin inhibitor toxicity (cyclosporine or tacrolimus), anticardiolipin syndrome (sometimes associated with hepatitis C infection), viral infection (due to parvovirus B19 or cytomegalovirus), and recurrent hemolytic uremic syndrome (2,3, 10,38,46). The presence of neutrophils in peritubular capillaries is the most helpful histologic feature for distinguishing acute humoral rejection from these other entities. If demonstrable, peritubular capillary positivity for IgG, IgM, C3, and/or C4d supports a diagnosis of acute antibody-mediated rejection, which should be confirmed by serologic demonstration of donor-specific antibodies.

Etiology and Pathogenesis. This form of rejection is antibody mediated, usually through donor-specific HLA class I antibodies (17). A minority of cases are mediated by antibodies to class II major histocompatability complex (MHC) antigens or by antibodies to non-MHC endothelial antigens. Risk factors include historically positive cross match, positive panel reactive analysis (PRA), and sensitization through prior transplantation.

Treatment and Prognosis. Plasmapheresis combined with the administration of mycophenolate mofetil and tacrolimus may be successful in eliminating donor-specific antibodies and reversing the acute humoral rejection (44). Prior to the introduction of this therapeutic regimen, prognosis was poor, with a graft recovery rate of only 50 to 60 percent compared to over 95 percent for acute cellular rejection (53). Intravenous immunoglobulin (IVIG) and anti-CD20 have also been used to prevent or treat antibody-mediated rejection.

ACUTE CELLULAR REJECTION

Acute cellular rejection (sometimes referred to merely as *acute rejection*) is the most common form of renal allograft rejection and is primarily T-cell mediated. Although most cases of acute cellular rejection occur 1 to 6 weeks post-transplantation, they may develop even years later, especially in situations where the level of immunosuppression has been reduced. Acute cellular rejection may target all four renal compartments: glomeruli, tubules, interstitium, and blood vessels, in varying combinations and degrees of involvement. The most common pattern of injury is tubulointerstitial, accounting for half to three quarters of cases of acute rejection. Involvement of blood vessels in the form of endarteritis affects less than half of patients and glomerular involvement in the form of transplant glomerulitis is found in fewer than 10 percent (8).

Approximately 30 percent of patients who receive kidney transplants from cadavers develop an episode of acute rejection in the first post-transplant year. Most of these occur within the first 3 months. Acute cellular rejection is usually heralded by an abrupt asymptomatic elevation in serum creatinine over a period of several days to weeks. If severe, it may be accompanied by reduction in urine output. Fever and graft tenderness, previously considered manifestations of rejection, are rare in the modern era of calcineurin inhibitors.

In patients with mild acute cellular rejection, the kidney is enlarged, pale, and swollen. In patients with severe forms, the kidney is enlarged and mottled, with focal hemorrhagic discoloration and patchy infarction (fig. 26-21). The corticomedullary junction may be accentuated due to medullary congestion. In rare instances, the kidney may rupture (fig. 26-22). The donor ureter may also demonstrate hemorrhagic infarction.

Tubulointerstitial (Type I) Acute Rejection

Light Microscopic Findings. The hallmark of type I acute cellular rejection is interstitial infiltration by mononuclear leukocytes, accompanied by interstitial edema, tubulitis, and acute tubular injury (fig. 26-23). Tubulitis is defined as leukocyte migration across the tubular basement membrane to infiltrate the tubular epithelium (fig. 26-24). Tubulitis involving nonatrophic tubules is considered more significant than tubulitis involving atrophic tubules. Tubulitis is best diagnosed using the periodic acid–Schiff (PAS) stain to outline the tubular basement membranes (fig.

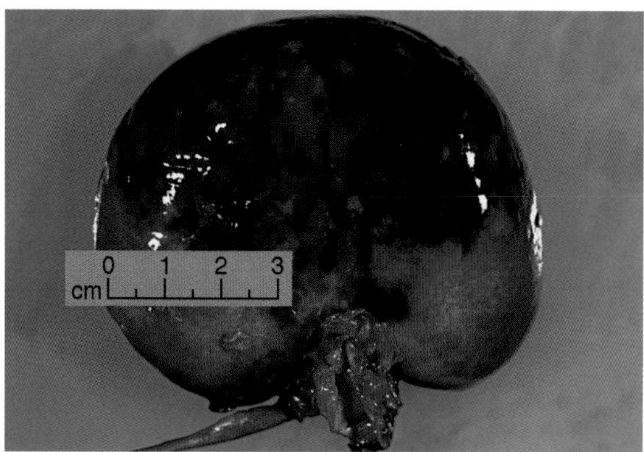

Figure 26-21

ACUTE CELLULAR REJECTION

Renal allograft explanted from a pediatric patient shows focal discrete infarcts at the poles and hemorrhagic discoloration of the parenchyma.

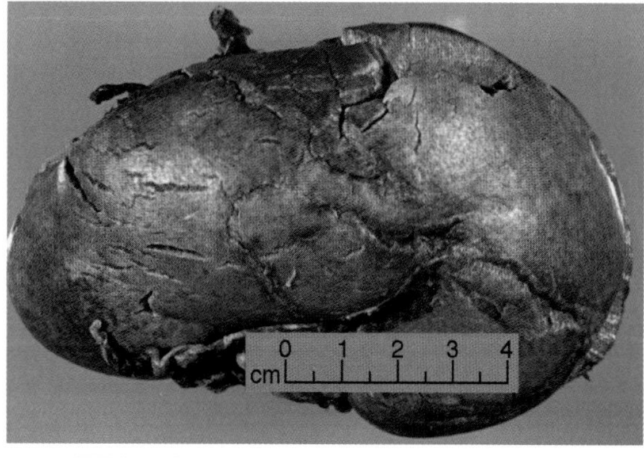

Figure 26-22

ACUTE ALLOGRAFT RUPTURE

The ruptured (formalin-fixed) kidney in a case of acute cellular rejection with massive interstitial edema. The tears over the cortical surfaces are due to rapid expansion of the renal parenchyma.

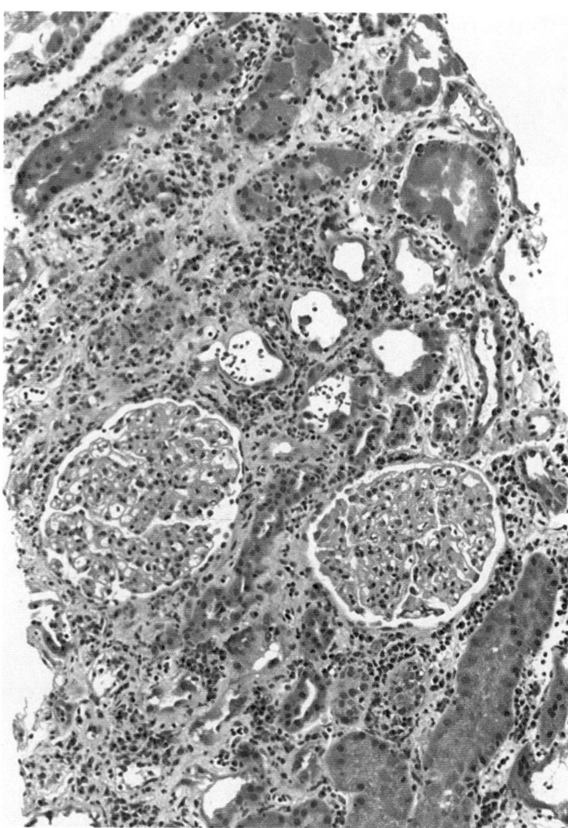

Figure 26-23

ACUTE CELLULAR REJECTION (TYPE I)

The major histologic hallmarks of acute rejection, namely, interstitial inflammation, edema, tubulitis, and tubular injury, are illustrated in this low-power view (H&E stain).

26-25). Infiltrating leukocytes have smaller and darker nuclei than those of tubular epithelial cells. In formalin-fixed specimens, there is sometimes a clear halo surrounding the leukocytes and separating them from the adjacent tubular epithelial cells. Tubulitis is usually accompanied by evidence of acute tubular injury in the form of degenerative and regenerative tubular changes, including individual cell necrosis or apoptosis, enlarged regenerative nuclei with nucleoli, epithelial thinning or detachment, cytoplasmic basophilia, and mitotic figures (fig. 26-26). Rupture of the tubular basement membrane (tubulorrhexis) may be seen (fig. 26-27). Interstitial edema is defined as expansion of the interstitium by pale-staining interstitial fluid, causing separation of the tubules. The interstitial infiltrate is predominantly perivascular early in the rejection process but becomes more peritubular and diffusely distributed in full-blown rejection.

It is important to recognize that interstitial inflammation alone is inadequate to diagnose type I acute rejection. Biopsies performed in clinically stable grafts in the course of research protocols have demonstrated that significant interstitial infiltrates may be present in nonrejecting allografts, especially in the first month post-transplant, where they may play a role in the acquisition of immunologic tolerance. To diagnose acute cellular rejection of the tubulointerstitial type the additional histologic features of tubulitis

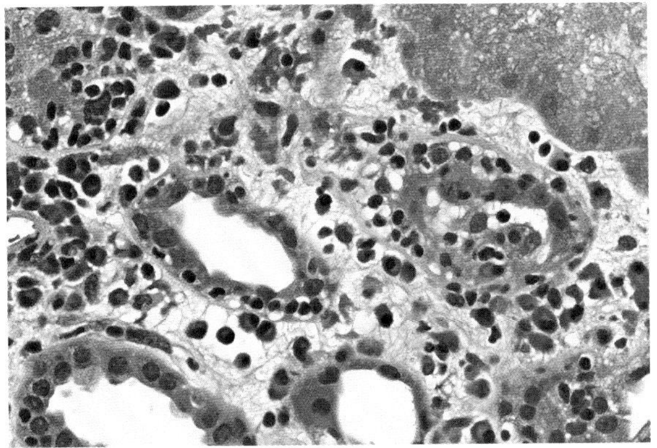

Figure 26-24

ACUTE CELLULAR REJECTION (TYPE I)

High-power view shows separation of the tubules by edema and inflammatory infiltrates of lymphocytes and plasma cells. There is extensive leukocytic infiltration of the tubular epithelium (tubulitis) accompanied by tubular degenerative changes (H&E stain).

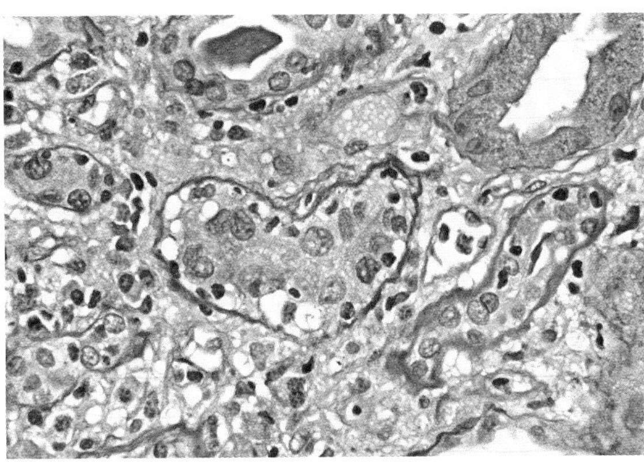

Figure 26-25

ACUTE CELLULAR REJECTION (TYPE I)

Tubulitis is best appreciated with the periodic acid–Schiff (PAS) stain, which outlines the tubular basement membranes. Lymphocytes that invade the tubular epithelium are often surrounded by a pericellular clear zone or halo.

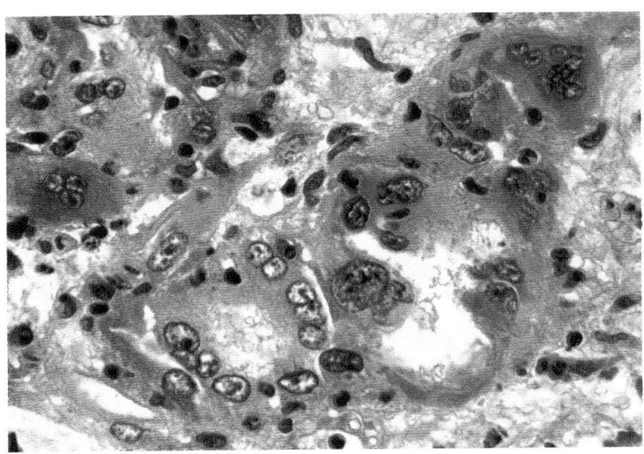

Figure 26-26

ACUTE CELLULAR REJECTION (TYPE I)

The marked regenerative nuclear atypia of the proximal tubules mimics viral inclusions (H&E stain).

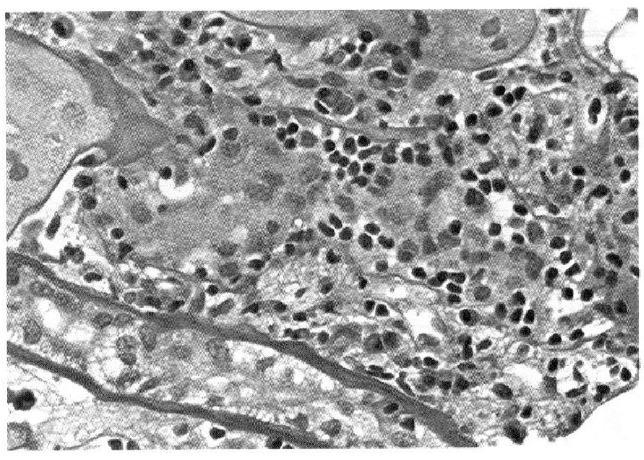

Figure 26-27

ACUTE CELLULAR REJECTION (TYPE I)

The tubule at the center displays severe tubulitis and almost complete destruction (tubulorrhexis) of the tubular basement membrane (PAS stain).

involving nonatrophic tubules and acute tubular injury are necessary.

The composition of the interstitial inflammatory infiltrate is mixed, consisting predominantly of T lymphocytes, lymphoblasts, and macrophages, with a smaller contribution by plasma cells, granulocytes (neutrophils, eosinophils, and basophils), and natural killer (NK) cells. In some cases, the infiltrate may be particularly rich in plasma cells or eosinophils (fig. 26-28). Immunophenotypic studies have revealed that while CD4-positive T cells are common in early rejection, particularly in the perivascular areas, CD8 cells usually predominate in fully developed acute rejection (4). Both CD4 and CD8 cells may infiltrate the tubular epithelium in areas of tubulitis (fig. 26-29). Some forms of acute rejection are unusually rich in plasma cells (plasma cell–rich acute rejection), without evidence of ongoing viral infection or post-transplant lymphoproliferative disease (fig. 26-28).

Several groups have attempted to define the threshold of injury needed to definitively

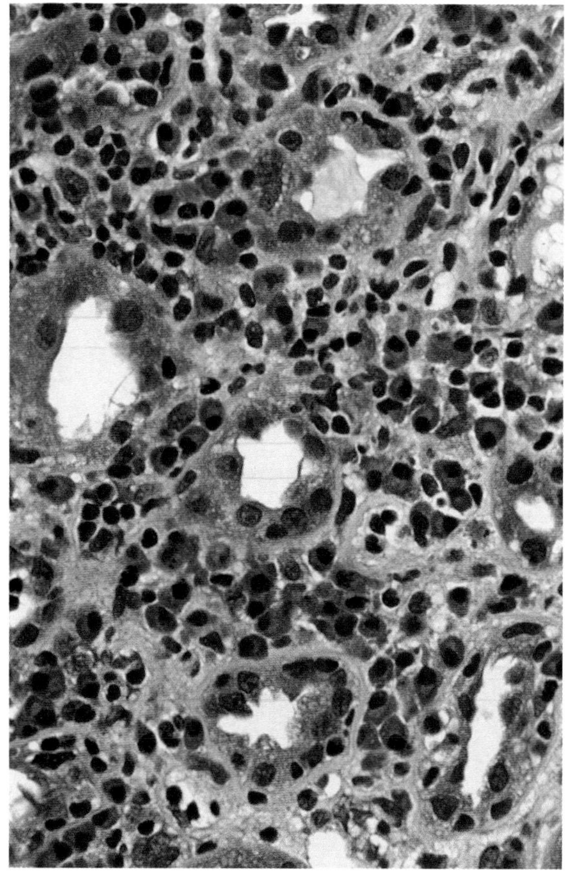

Figure 26-28

ACUTE CELLULAR REJECTION (TYPE I)

An example with a plasma cell–rich interstitial inflammatory infiltrate. Plasma cell–rich acute rejection is more likely to occur more than 6 months post-transplant and is associated with a poorer prognosis than typical acute cellular rejection (H&E stain).

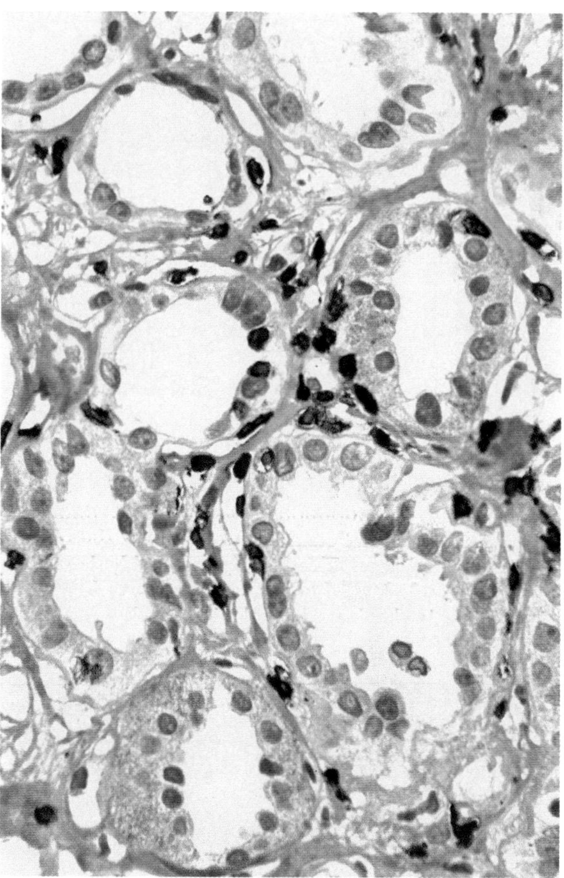

Figure 26-29

ACUTE CELLULAR REJECTION (TYPE I)

The majority of the intersitial lymphocytes are CD8-positive T cells (immunostain for CD8).

diagnose acute cellular rejection (9,48). By the Banff 97 criteria, mild acute rejection (type/grade IA) requires interstitial inflammation involving greater than 25 percent of the cortical surface area together with tubulitis of more than four cells per tubular cross section (or per group of 10 tubular cells) in one or more tubules (48). Interstitial inflammation involving 10 to 25 percent of the cortex, with tubulitis numbering less than four cells per tubular cross section qualifies as borderline (suspicious) rejection. Banff type/grade IB rejection is defined as tubulitis numbering more than 10 infiltrating leukocytes per tubular cross section (or per group of 10 tubular cells) and involvement of at least 25 percent of the cortex by interstitial mononuclear infiltrates (48).

The CCTT criteria simplify this schema by requiring at least 5 percent of the cortex to have interstitial inflammation for type I (mild acute) rejection if there are at least two of three additional features: edema, tubular degeneration/injury, or reactive lymphoblasts (9). Tubulitis must be identified, involving at least three tubules in 10 serial high-power fields (40X) from the areas with the most infiltrate. The CCTT criteria do not place a limit on the number of infiltrating lymphocytes required to define significant tubulitis. Thus, acute rejection type I by the CCTT criteria lumps together the Banff 97 categories of borderline, grade IA, and grade IB rejection (although not all borderline lesions will meet all criteria for CCTT type I acute rejection).

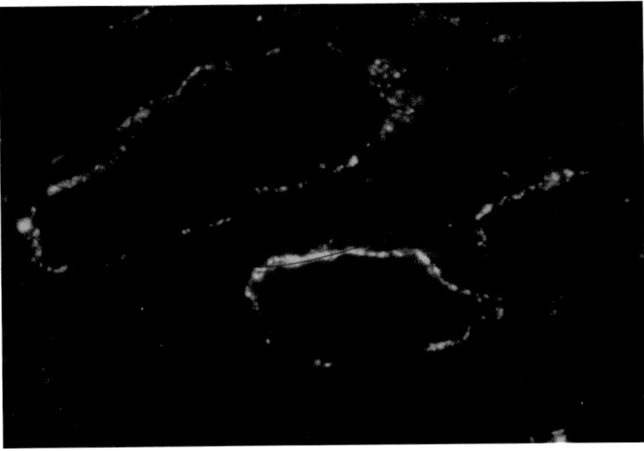

Figure 26-30

ACUTE CELLULAR REJECTION (TYPE I)

By routine immunofluorescence, the only finding is semilinear to granular staining for C3 along the tubular basement membranes. This finding is probably due to immunoglobulin-independent activation of complement in areas of tubulorrhexis associated with tubulitis.

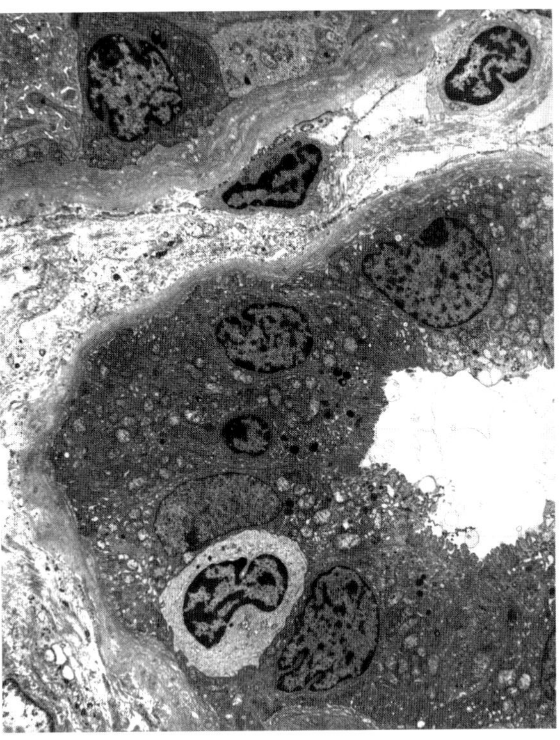

Figure 26-31

ACUTE CELLULAR REJECTION (TYPE I)

In areas of tubulitis, the lymphocytes that infiltrate the tubular epithelium are easily recognized by their clear cytoplasm (electron micrograph).

Immunofluorescence Findings. Fluorescence microscopy is not particularly helpful in the diagnosis of type I acute cellular rejection. The only finding may be focal staining of tubular basement membranes for C3 in a semilinear to granular pattern (fig. 26-30). No co-deposits of immunoglobulin are found. It is likely that tubulitis-induced damage to tubular basement membranes causes Ig-independent activation of C3, similar to what may be seen in other forms of acute interstitial nephritis. There may be focal staining for fibrinogen in the edematous interstitium.

Electron Microscopic Findings. In areas of tubulitis, activated lymphocytes with prominent cytoplasm insinuate between tubular epithelial cells, and are associated with tubular degenerative and regenerative changes. These infiltrating lymphocytes can often be identified by their pale cytoplasm and rounded cell contours (fig. 26-31).

Differential Diagnosis. Acute tubulointerstitial rejection must be differentiated from various forms of viral infection (such as with BK polyoma virus or adenovirus), acute bacterial or fungal pyelonephritis, drug-induced acute interstitial nephritis, and post-transplant lymphoproliferative disease (10). The diagnostic features of these conditions are described below.

Etiology and Pathogenesis. Acute cellular rejection involves T-cell–mediated cytotoxicity to tubular cells. Tubular expression of D-related (DR) antigen, interleukin (IL)-8, V cell adhesion molecule (VCAM)-1 and ICAM-1 have all been shown to be upregulated in acute cellular rejection and may be important in the mediation of the T-cell infiltration (fig. 26-32). T-cell recruitment and cellular cytotoxicity to the tubular epithelium is effectuated by the release of a panoply of cytokines, including interferon gamma, tumor necrosis factor-alpha and -beta, interleukins such as IL-2 and IL-6, perforin, and granzyme B. Although some investigators have attempted to grade the rejection by quantifying the levels of mRNA for these cytokines in biopsy material or urine, these techniques are too specialized and difficult to apply to the routine work-up of renal biopsies (25,55).

Treatment and Prognosis. Episodes of rejection are treated with antirejection therapy, which differs from the maintenance therapy used for the long-term prevention of renal allograft

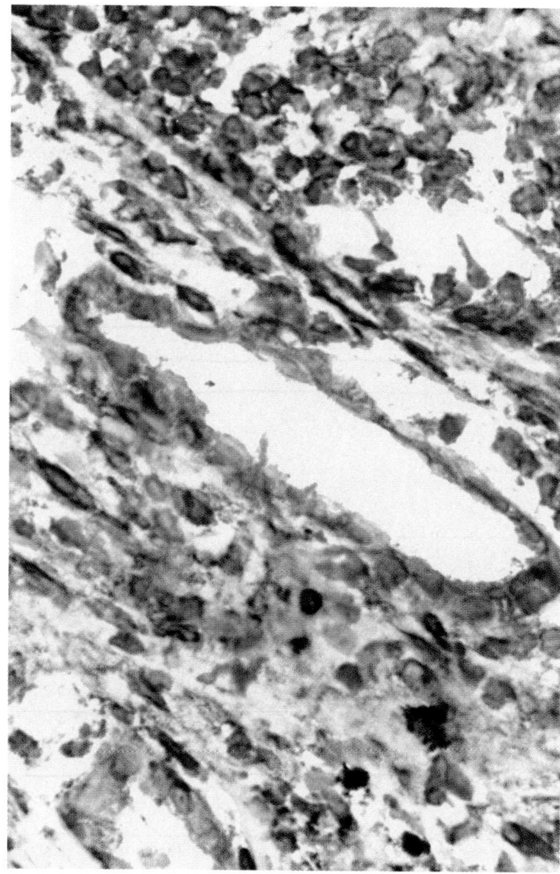

Figure 26-32

ACUTE CELLULAR REJECTION (TYPE I)

There is upregulation of class II D-related (DR) antigen on tubular epithelial cells and interstitial leukocytes (immunostain for HLA-DR).

rejection. Maintenance therapy consists of a triple drug regimen that includes a corticosteroid plus an immunophilin-binding agent (cyclosporine or tacrolimus) plus a lymphocyte proliferation inhibitor (azathioprine or mycophenolate mofetil). Antirejection therapies usually consist of high-dose intravenous corticosteroids, polyclonal antilymphocyte sera raised in horses (ATG) or rabbits (thymoglobulin), or OKT3, a noncomplement-fixing monoclonal antibody directed at the CD3 molecular complex. In randomized prospective multicenter trials, OKT3 reversed 94 percent of first acute rejection episodes, compared to 75 percent for high-dose corticosteroids (8). Plasma cell–rich rejection is more likely to occur late in the course of transplantation (more than 6 months post-transplant) and patients appear to have a worse prognosis than with the usual form of acute cellular rejection (39).

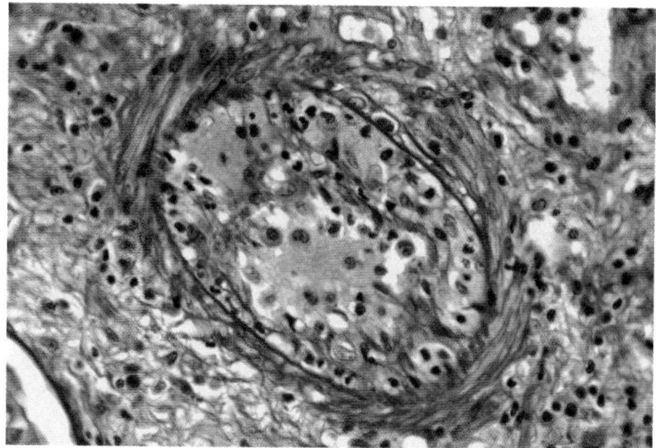

Figure 26-33

ACUTE CELLULAR REJECTION (TYPE II)

Endarteritis characterized by intimal edema and lymphocytic inflammation expands the intima of a small artery. The media is not involved (H&E stain).

Vascular (Type II) Acute Rejection

Definition. Cellular rejection of blood vessels is defined by the presence of endarteritis. Synonyms include *endothelialitis, endovasculitis,* and *intimal arteritis.* This lesion is the most specific lesion of acute rejection.

Light Microscopic Findings. Endarteritis occurs when mononuclear cells infiltrate beneath the vascular endothelium (fig. 26-33). The adherence of lymphocytes to the luminal surface of the endothelium is suspicious for, but inadequate evidence to define, this lesion (figs. 26-34, 26-35). The presence of lymphocytes in the perivascular adventitia is also insufficient to diagnose endarteritis. In severe examples, the undermining of the endothelium by lymphocytes may be accompanied by intimal expansion due to edema and fibrin deposition (fig. 26-36). There may be endothelial swelling, proliferation, and degeneration, however, the media is uninvolved. Endarteritis is more common in large arteries (interlobar, arcuate, subarcuate) than interlobular arteries or arterioles. Thus, it may not be sampled in a smaller, relatively superficial biopsy. The infiltrating lymphocytes include both CD4 and CD8 T cells as well as monocytes. Endarteritis is often present in association with features of tubulointerstitial rejection.

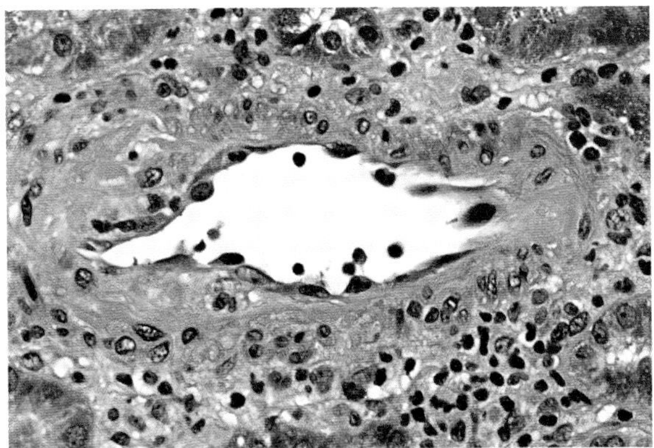

Figure 26-34

ACUTE CELLULAR REJECTION

An artery shows leukocyte margination and adhesion to the swollen vascular endothelium. This finding is suspicious for, but insufficient to diagnose, endarteritis (H&E stain).

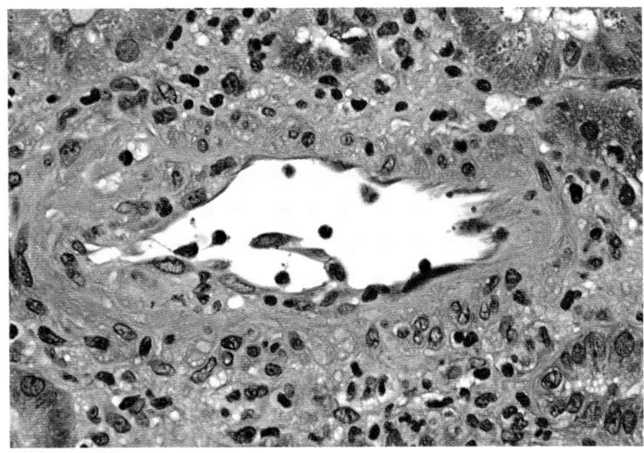

Figure 26-35

ACUTE CELLULAR REJECTION (TYPE II)

A serial section of the artery shown in figure 26-34 now displays the diagnostic feature of endarteritis, namely, focal undermining of the endothelium by infiltrating lymphocytes that have burrowed into the intima beneath the endothelium. The presence of a single vessel with this finding qualifies as type II rejection (H&E stain).

Endarteritis is the defining feature of type/grade II (moderate) acute rejection by both the CCTT and the Banff 97 classification criteria (9,48). The presence of even a single vessel with endarteritis upgrades the rejection to grade II. The Banff 97 classification distinguishes between mild to moderate (IIA) and severe (IIB) intimal arteritis (severe defined as comprising more than 25 percent of the luminal area). No distinction is made between the severity of the endarteritis in the CCTT criteria.

Immunofluorescence Findings. Immunofluorescence is typically negative for immunoglobulins. This is not surprising because endovasculitis is primarily a form of cellular, not humoral, rejection. Coarse intimal deposits of IgM, C3, and C1 may occur due to nonspecific trapping in areas of insuded plasma proteins within the swollen intima. The vascular lesions may exhibit positivity for fibrinogen in the expanded intima.

Electron Microscopic Findings. The arterial endothelium is undermined by infiltrating lymphocytes, accompanied by endothelial swelling and denudation, and by intimal edema and fibrin deposition. The media is typically intact.

Differential Diagnosis. Endarteritis (grade II rejection) must be distinguished from lesions of thrombotic microangiopathy and the necrotizing and/or transmural arteritis of grade III rejection.

Etiology and Pathogenesis. The pathogenesis of type/grade II rejection primarily involves cell-mediated immunity to vascular endothelium. Upregulation of the important mediators HLA-DR, ICAM-1, and VCAM-1 on vascular endothelium occurs. In some instances, a humoral component may contribute to the vascular injury, but its role is less well defined. By contrast, most type/grade III rejections are primarily humorally mediated. Some type/grade III rejections, however, especially those with transmural as well as intimal mononuclear cell

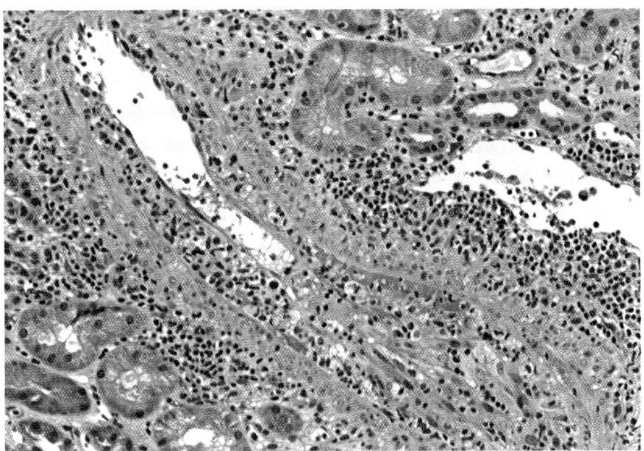

Figure 26-36

ACUTE CELLULAR REJECTION (TYPE II)

A large artery shows severe endarteritis with intimal fibrin deposition. Despite the severe involvement of the intima, the media appears intact (H&E stain).

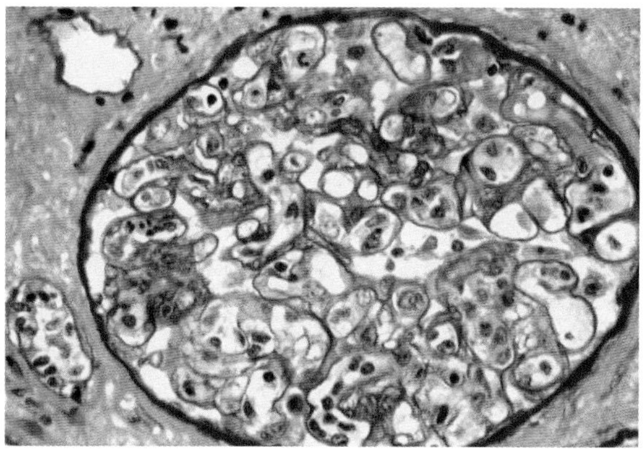

Figure 26-37

TRANSPLANT GLOMERULITIS

The glomerulus is hypercellular due to endothelial cell swelling and many intracapillary marginated leukocytes. There are no double contours of the glomerular basement membrane, distinguishing this glomerular lesion from transplant glomerulopathy (PAS stain).

inflammation, have a major cell-mediated component, are C4d negative, and are not associated with demonstrable donor-specific antibody.

Treatment and Prognosis. In general, antirejection therapy is less effective for treating the vascular lesions of acute cellular rejection than the tubulointerstitial lesions (41). Patients with endarteritis have a 61 percent 1-year graft survival rate when given antirejection therapy (compared to 29 percent for those with necrotizing arteritis) (26). OKT3 is the preferred antirejection regimen for grade II rejection. The response of patients with Banff 97 grade IIB rejection is worse than those with grade IIA, thereby justifying the distinction between these grades (15).

Glomerular Lesions (Transplant Glomerulitis)

Definition. In most cases of acute cellular rejection, glomeruli are unaffected. In approximately 10 percent of cases, however, there is prominent and diffuse infiltration of the glomerular tuft by mononuclear leukocytes, analogous to the endothelialitis seen in the arteries. This process has been termed *transplant glomerulitis* or *allograft glomerulitis*.

Glomerulitis is graded in the Banff 97 classification scheme by the percentage of glomeruli affected (g1, less than 25 percent; g2, 25 to 75 percent; and g3 more than 75 percent). However, it is not used as a criterion for acute cellular rejection in either the Banff or the CCTT classification because its significance remains controversial (9,48).

Light Microscopic Findings. Glomerular capillary lumens are narrowed or occluded by infiltrating T cells (both CD4 and CD8) and monocytes (CD68), together with swelling and mild proliferation of glomerular endothelial cells (fig. 26-37). Intracapillary fibrin is usually not a feature. Mild mesangial proliferation may be present, however, most of the hypercellularity is intraluminal. In fact, many of the infiltrating mononuclear leukocytes have the appearance of marginated intracapillary cells (61). In severe cases, the transplant glomerulitis is diffuse and global; in others, the process may be relatively focal and segmental. Transplant glomerulitis is usually accompanied by tubulointerstitial and/or vascular features of acute rejection. In about 5 percent of cases, however, it is the predominant histologic manifestation of the acute rejection.

Immunofluorescence Findings. Variable glomerular reactivity for fibrin, immunoglobulins (IgM and/or IgG), C3, and C1 is seen in a semilinear subendothelial distribution. This immune staining is generally of low intensity and scant.

Electron Microscopic Findings. Glomerular capillary lumens are severely narrowed or occluded by endothelial swelling and hypercellularity, with loss of endothelial fenestrations. Mononuclear leukocytes are closely apposed to the endothelial cells but generally do not infiltrate the mesangium (fig. 26-38). Subendothelial accumulation of electron-lucent fluffy material or fibrin strands is sometimes observed. No immune-type electron-dense deposits are identified.

Differential Diagnosis. Transplant glomerulitis must be differentiated from recurrent or de novo forms of proliferative glomerulonephritis (such as IgA nephropathy, lupus nephritis, acute postinfectious glomerulonephritis) as well as forms of glomerular thrombotic microangiopathy (such as recurrent or de novo hemolytic uremic syndrome, cyclosporine toxicity). Immunofluorescence and electron microscopy demonstrate the absence of glomerular immune deposits. Transplant glomerulitis must also be distinguished from transplant glomerulopathy, a more chronic glomerular lesion of the allograft

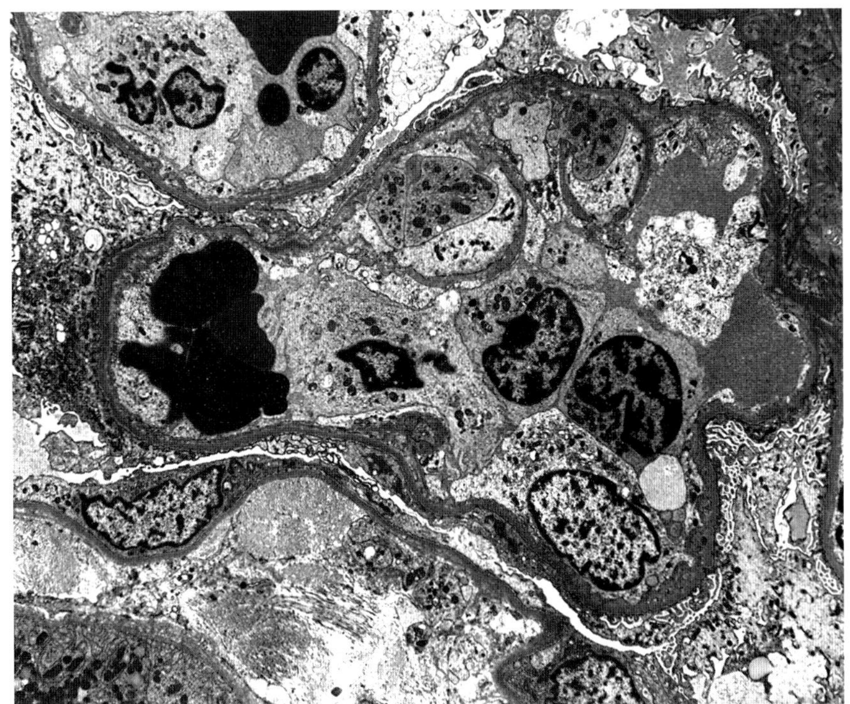

Figure 26-38

TRANSPLANT GLOMERULITIS

The glomerular capillary lumens are engorged with marginated mononuclear leukocytes. The endothelial cells appear swollen, and the fenestrae are obliterated. No electron-dense deposits are identified. The foot processes are focally effaced (electron micrograph).

in which there are membranoproliferative features, including double contours of glomerular basement membranes (see below).

Etiology and Pathogenesis. Transplant glomerulitis is considered a form of cellular rejection to the glomerulus, presumably directed primarily to the glomerular endothelium. Although early reports suggested that this lesion might represent a manifestation of cytomegalovirus (CMV) infection in the allograft, this association has not been substantiated. Nevertheless, it is possible that intercurrent CMV infection or other viral infections may promote acute rejection through upregulation of class II antigens and adhesion molecules on graft endothelial cells.

Treatment and Prognosis. Patients with transplant glomerulitis usually respond to the same antirejection therapy used for those with tubulointerstitial acute rejection or endovasculitis. OKT3 appears to be the most effective agent.

CHRONIC REJECTION (CHRONIC ALLOGRAFT NEPHROPATHY)

Definition. Chronic rejection refers to the gradual diminution in graft function that develops inexorably over months to years in association with irreversible immunologic injury to the allograft. In addition to a chronic immunologic attack on the renal parenchyma, other factors, such as a maladaptive response to loss of functioning nephrons with hyperfiltration in remnant nephrons, ischemia, hypertension, and chronic calcineurin inhibitor toxicity, may contribute to the development of chronic renal allograft injury (16). These insults lead to progressive tubular atrophy, interstitial fibrosis, glomerular sclerosis, and arteriosclerosis. To emphasize the multifactorial nature of the chronic renal injury, the Banff classification has introduced the term chronic allograft nephropathy.

Clinical Features. Chronic rejection/chronic allograft nephropathy is characterized by a slowly progressive decline in the glomerular filtration rate, often accompanied by proteinuria that may reach nephrotic levels. In some individuals, chronic rejection supervenes after one or more clinical episodes of acute rejection, whereas in others it develops insidiously without overt bouts of acute rejection. Donor (perioperative) transplant biopsies are useful to quantify the degree of baseline chronic donor-transmitted disease in the allograft and assess its contribution to the findings of chronic allograft nephropathy (24).

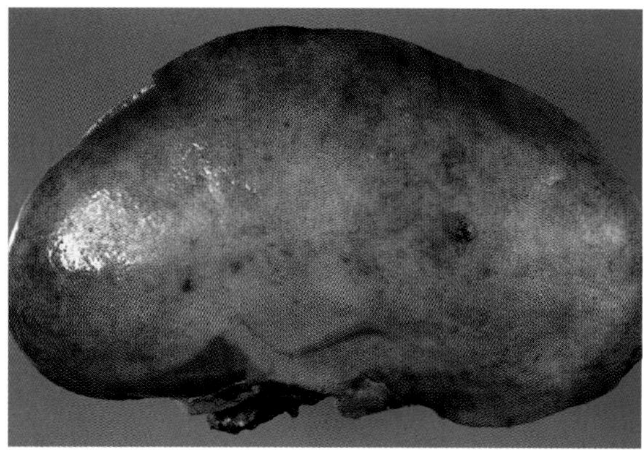

Figure 26-39

CHRONIC REJECTION

This renal allograft removed for irreversible graft failure appears pale tan with a smooth, fibrotic cortical surface. Despite the end-stage allograft failure, the kidney is not markedly shrunken; it is only slightly small because of the extensive expansion of the interstitium by fibrosis.

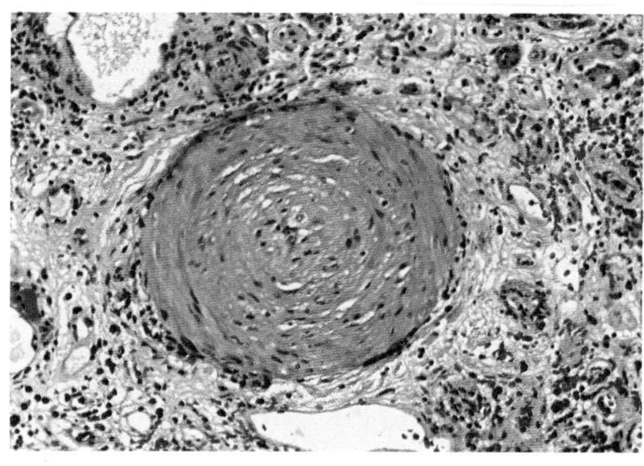

Figure 26-40

CHRONIC REJECTION

Chronic transplant arteriopathy has caused complete arterial occlusion by concentric, onion-skin, intimal fibroplasia, without evidence of residual endarteritis (H&E stain).

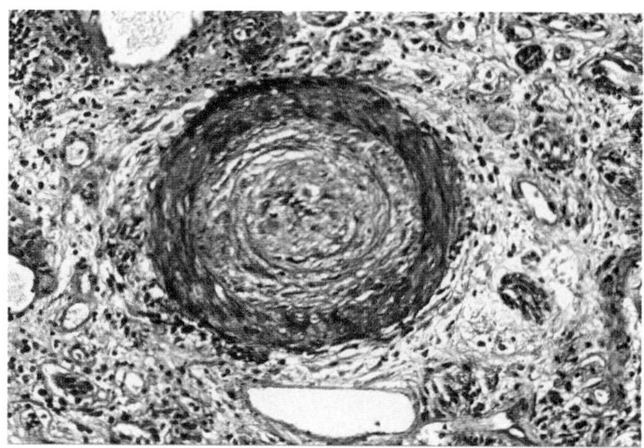

Figure 26-41

CHRONIC REJECTION

The same artery seen in figure 26-40 shows an intima thickened by trichrome blue–stained collagenous matrix. There is marked fibrosis of the adjacent cortical interstitium (Masson trichrome stain).

Chronic rejection remains the major cause of graft failure, accounting for a 10-year graft survival rate of 40 percent for cadaveric grafts, 50 percent for parental (one haplotype mismatch) grafts, and 70 percent for HLA identical grafts (6). Although antirejection therapy is extremely effective in reversing acute rejection episodes and improving one-year graft survival rates, modern immunosuppressive regimens have not appreciably altered the long-term graft survival rates.

Gross Findings. The kidney is firm, pale tan, and shrunken (fig. 26-39).

Light Microscopic, Immunofluorescence, and Electron Microscopic Findings. *Vascular Lesions.* Chronic vascular rejection, known as *chronic transplant arteriopathy,* is the most specific morphologic lesion of chronic rejection (20,31). It is characterized by progressive narrowing and occlusion of medium-sized and large caliber arteries by dense onion skin–type intimal fibroplasia (fig. 26-40). Small arteries and arterioles may also be involved, but usually to a lesser degree. The trichrome stain demonstrates concentric layers of abundant blue-staining collagen within the intima (fig. 26-41). The vascular elastic membranes are often duplicated and frayed, but without discrete ruptures. Intimal foam cells may be observed (fig. 26-42). At this stage the vascular endothelium is intact and the media is typically uninvolved. There is often residual sparse leukocyte infiltration of the thickened arterial intima and adventitia, inflammatory features which distinguish this lesion from the ordinary arteriosclerosis of hypertension or aging.

Tubulointerstitial Lesions. The tubulointerstitial features of chronic rejection are relatively nonspecific, consisting of extensive interstitial fibrosis and tubular atrophy (fig. 26-43). In areas, the tubular architecture may be effaced, with loss of recognizable tubular basement membranes. In some patients, there is smouldering, ongoing

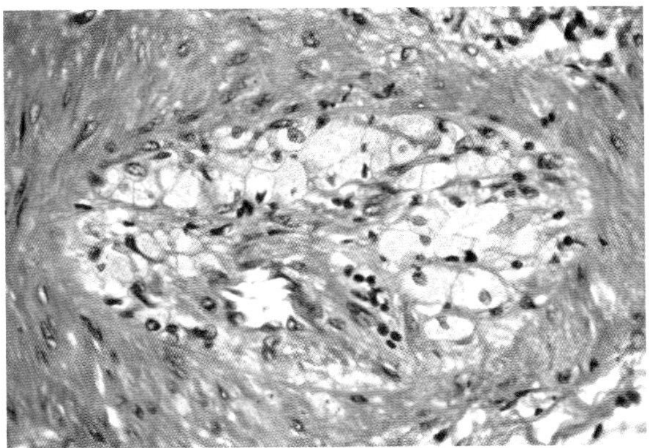

Figure 26-42

CHRONIC REJECTION

A narrowed artery contains many intimal foam cells. There is residual mild lymphocytic inflammation of the sclerotic intima (H&E stain).

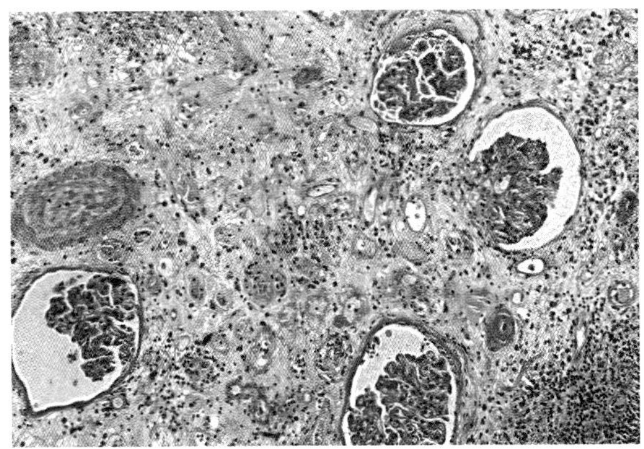

Figure 26-43

CHRONIC REJECTION

There is severe and diffuse tubular atrophy, interstitial fibrosis, and ischemic glomerulosclerosis. An interlobular artery is severely narrowed by intimal sclerosis (Masson trichrome stain).

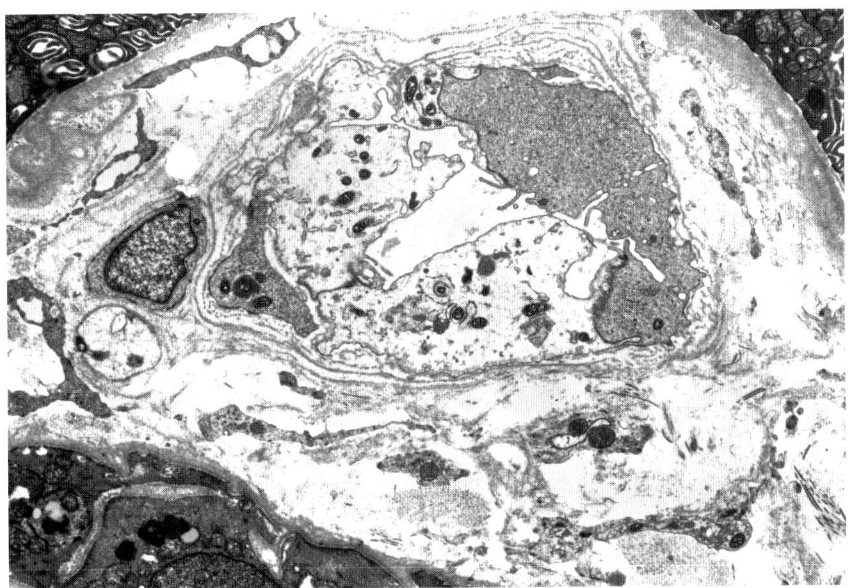

Figure 26-44

CHRONIC REJECTION

By electron microscopy, lamellation of the interstitial capillary basement membranes is seen. The interstitial capillary endothelium appears swollen. (Courtesy of Dr. K. Solez, Alberta, Canada.)

rejection in the form of interstitial inflammation and tubulitis involving atrophic or remaining nonatrophic tubules. In some end-stage allografts, particularly those with obliterative transplant arteriopathy, the renal parenchyma becomes mummified with interstitial and vascular calcifications as well as osteoid formation. In circumstances where immunosuppression has been withdrawn for some weeks or months prior to nephrectomy for end-stage graft failure, lesions of acute vascular and tubulointerstitial rejection may develop superimposed on a background of chronic vascular and tubulointerstitial disease. By electron microscopy, there may be thickening and lamellation of the basement membranes of interstitial capillaries (fig. 26-44) (19,29,37,42). By immunofluorescence, many cases of chronic rejection exhibit staining for C4d in the thickened walls of peritubular interstitial capillaries (28).

Glomerular Lesions. The glomerular lesions of chronic rejection assume several forms. In some cases, the lesions are relatively nonspecific in character, with ischemic-type global wrinkling, thickening, and retraction of the glomerular

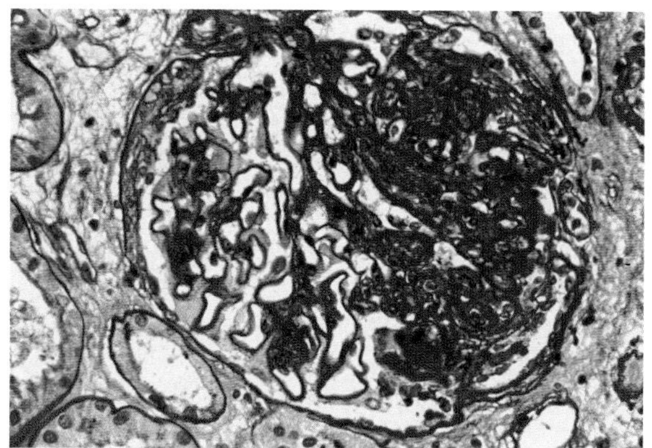

Figure 26-45

CHRONIC TRANSPLANT GLOMERULOPATHY

There are lesions of focal segmental glomerulosclerosis in the setting of chronic allograft nephropathy. This glomerular lesion is commonly encountered in chronic allografts and probably results, in part, from hyperfiltration in remnant nephrons following loss of renal mass due to chronic allograft nephropathy (PAS stain).

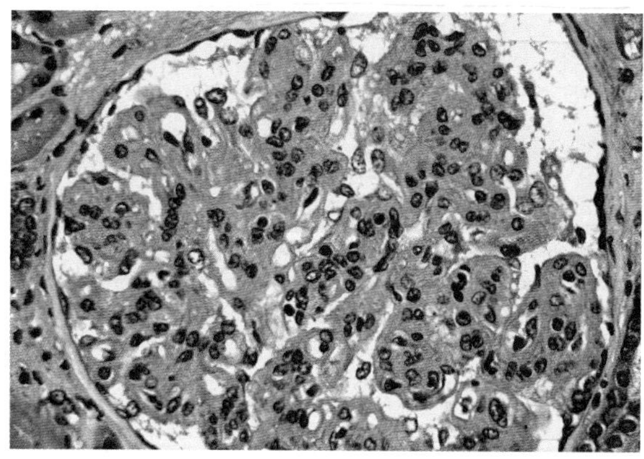

Figure 26-46

CHRONIC TRANSPLANT GLOMERULOPATHY

The glomerulus displays membranoproliferative features, with global mesangial hypercellularity, narrowing of capillary lumens, and lobular accentuation of the tuft (H&E stain).

basement membrane together with contraction of the glomerular tuft. In the Banff 93 classification, this lesion was termed *ischemic glomerulopathy* (56). In some individuals, nonsclerotic glomeruli are hypertrophied and develop a pattern of focal segmental glomerular sclerosis similar to that seen in other secondary forms of focal segmental sclerosis mediated by reduced renal mass and hyperfiltration injury (fig. 26-45).

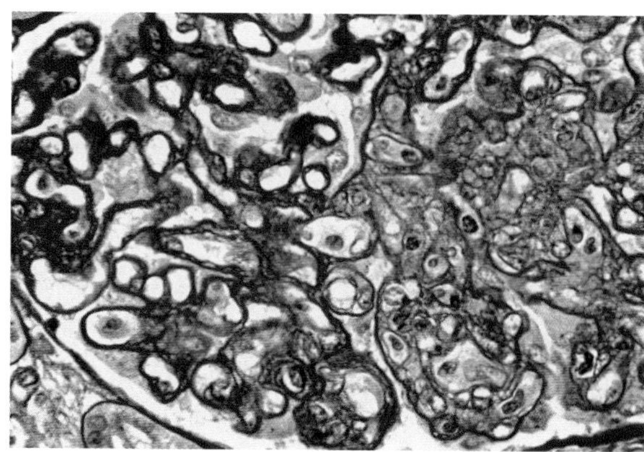

Figure 26-47

CHRONIC TRANSPLANT GLOMERULOPATHY

There is irregular replication of the glomerular basement membrane, producing double contours, accompanied by segmental mesangial interposition and segmental reticulation of the mesangial matrix (mesangiolysis) (PAS stain).

In some patients, particularly those with nephrotic proteinuria and full nephrotic syndrome, the glomeruli develop membranoproliferative features consistent with transplant glomerulopathy. This lesion is superficially similar to membranoproliferative glomerulonephritis type 1 (fig. 26-46). On close inspection, however, the lesion actually more closely resembles the membranoproliferative pattern seen with the chronic thrombotic microangiopathies. Histologic features include mesangial proliferation and sclerosis, mesangial interposition, thickening and double contours of the glomerular basement membranes, mesangiolysis, and rarely, crescents (fig. 26-47). There are often marginated mononuclear leukocytes within the glomerular capillaries, a finding also seen in transplant glomerulitis (fig. 26-48).

By immunofluorescence, there is mild to moderate semilinear to granular staining of the glomerular capillary walls and mesangium with antisera to IgM, C3, and C1, with variable staining for fibrin. Unlike idiopathic membranoproliferative glomerulonephritis type 1, transplant glomerulopathy usually does not stain for IgG.

Electron microscopy shows a widening of the subendothelial zone by flocculent, relatively electron-lucent material similar to that seen in chronic thrombotic microangiopathies (fig. 26-49). This subendothelial material is often incorporated into the glomerular capillary wall by a thin layer of newly formed basement membrane beneath the endothelium, producing a double contour (18). Mesangial interposition may be seen between the layers of basement membrane. Endothelial cells are often swollen, and fenestrae are lost. The glomerular basement membrane itself is frequently thickened and may have a complex lamellated texture. There is variable effacement of foot processes. Electron-dense deposits are not identified, a feature which helps to distinguish this lesion from recurrent or de novo membranoproliferative glomerulonephritis type 1.

Etiology and Pathogenesis. The pathogenesis of chronic rejection involves complex mechanisms of humoral and cellular immunity, upregulation of adhesion molecules on the vascular endothelium, and release of growth factors and inflammatory and fibrogenic cytokines such as platelet-derived growth factor (PDGF), tumor necrosis factor (TNF), IL-1, and transforming growth factor (TGF)-beta. These cellular factors promote progressive vascular myointimal proliferation and sclerosis, glomerular sclerosis, and interstitial fibrosis. Nonimmunologic mechanisms of hyperfiltration, hypertension, and hyperlipidemia are important contributing factors.

Transplant glomerulopathy is thought to represent a manifestation of chronic immunologic rejection to the glomerular endothelium, analogous to the intimal proliferative and sclerosing lesions seen in arteries. Some cases have been shown on repeat biopsies to develop from the more acute lesion of transplant glomerulitis.

Differential Diagnosis. Transplant arteriopathy must be differentiated from arteriosclerosis related to aging or hypertension. The presence of intimal mononuclear inflammatory cells and foam cells are distinguishing features of transplant arteriopathy. Transplant glomerulopathy

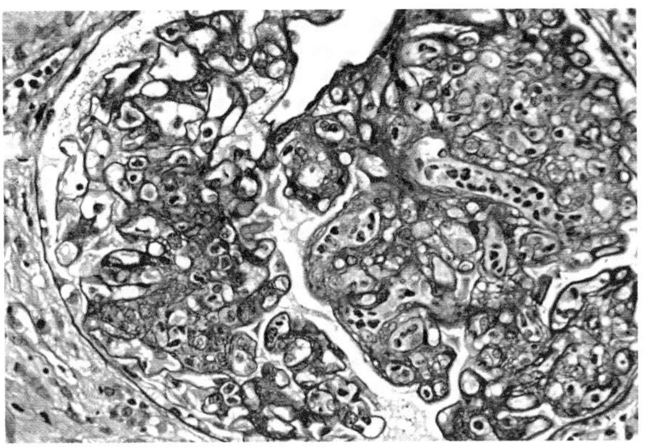

Figure 26-48

CHRONIC TRANSPLANT GLOMERULOPATHY AND TRANSPLANT GLOMERULITIS

In addition to double contours of the glomerular basement membrane, there are many marginated intracapillary mononuclear leukocytes (PAS stain).

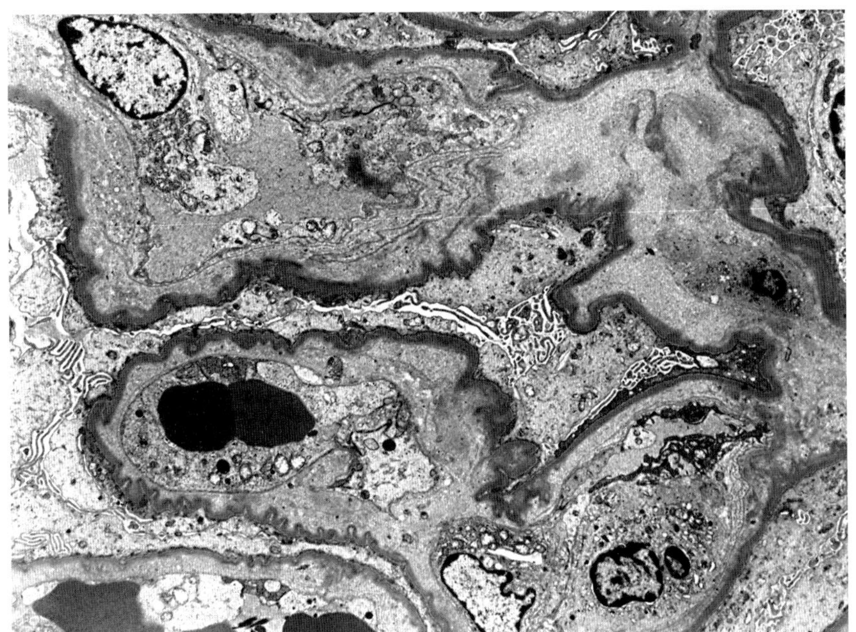

Figure 26-49

CHRONIC TRANSPLANT GLOMERULOPATHY

Electron-lucent material replaces the mesangium and expands the subendothelial zones. A new layer of subendothelial membrane produces double contours. The endothelium is swollen, with loss of fenestrations. These findings resemble those seen in other forms of chronic thrombotic microangiopathy (electron micrograph).

Table 26-3

CCTT CRITERIA FOR ACUTE RENAL ALLOGRAFT REJECTION[a,b]

Type I	At least 5 percent of the cortex must have interstitial mononuclear infiltration with at least two of the following three features present: edema, tubular degeneration/injury, or activated lymphocytes. In addition, tubulitis must be present, with at least a total of three tubules affected in 10 serial high-power (40X) fields from the areas with the most infiltrate.
Type II	Arterial or arteriolar mononuclear cell endothelial inflammation (endothelialitis or endarteritis) is present (with or without features of type I). A threshold of at least one cell *under* the endothelium is required. A lymphocyte adherent to the luminal surface of an endothelial cell is not sufficient for this diagnosis.
Type III	Arterial or arteriolar fibrinoid necrosis or transmural inflammation is present and may or may not be accompanied by thrombosis, parenchymal necrosis/recent infarction, or hemorrhage.

[a]For the assessment of tubulitis, atrophic tubules and scarred areas of cortex should not be graded.
[b]CCTT = Cooperative Clinical Trials in Transplantation; data from reference 9.

must be distinguished from membranoproliferative glomerulonephritis (recurrent or de novo). The absence of electron-dense deposits by electron microscopy and the presence of subendothelial flocculent material typical of chronic thrombotic microangiopathy support a diagnosis of transplant glomerulopathy. Moreover, transplant glomerulopathy usually lacks the prominent endocapillary proliferation and uniform marked hyperlobulation characteristic of membranoproliferative glomerulonephritis type I. Finally, transplant glomerulopathy must be distinguished from glomerular lesions of chronic thrombotic microangiopathy related to recurrent hemolytic uremic syndrome or calcineurin inhibitor toxicity. In this differential, a prior history of hemolytic uremic syndrome in the native kidney and the presence of other features of calcineurin inhibitor toxicity, such as nodular hyaline arteriolopathy, may be helpful.

CLASSIFICATION OF REJECTION

There are two major classification systems for the standardized grading of acute rejection, the Banff and the CCTT. The Banff classification was originally published in 1993 by Solez et al. (56) and was significantly modified in 1997 (48). In 2003, an update to the Banff 97 classification was made to accommodate newer understanding of acute antibody-mediated rejection (47). The modifications made in 1997 bring the Banff 97 schema close to the classification devised by the National Institutes of Health (NIH)-sponsored CCTT (9). The criteria for grading rejection by these two systems are outlined in Tables 26-2–26-4. The Banff 93 schema was hampered by the reliance on grading the severity of the tubulitis and endothelialitis, which is necessarily subjective. The mixing of tubulitis and endothelialitis in grade II rejection and the inclusion of endothelialitis, arterial fibrinoid necrosis, or parenchymal hemorrhage or infarction in grade III rejection created heterogeneous groupings (56). Kappa scores showed poor interobserver reproducibility using the Banff 93 schema.

The CCTT criteria have the advantage of simplicity and improved reproducibility. The rationale for the separation of grade I and grade II on the basis of endothelialitis is supported by studies showing that it is the presence or absence of endothelialitis that carries the greatest prognostic import. The severity of tubulitis per se does not appear to influence the responsiveness to antirejection therapy (9). Nevertheless, the distinction between Banff 97 grade IA and IB rejection appears justified based on a study showing a higher incidence of graft loss in grade IB than IA rejection (36).

There is no universal consensus on how individual centers should grade acute rejection. Because of the widely recognized value of both the Banff 97 and the CCTT classification systems, it is wise to use either one or both systems when reporting allograft biopsy diagnoses. The Banff 93 classification is now considered outmoded and should not be used.

The grading of chronic rejection has not been addressed by the CCTT criteria. In the Banff system, the chronic rejection (or chronic allograft nephropathy) is graded as mild, moderate, or severe depending on the severity of the

Table 26-4

DEFINITIONS APPLIED TO CCTT CRITERIA[a]

Interstitial Edema: Tubular separation (tubular basement membranes showing no points of direct contact) by interstitial fluid accumulation, resulting in clear or pale areas. Trichrome stain, when used, shows slender connective tissue fibers separated by irregular nonstaining areas.

Tubular Injury: Tubules lined by epithelial cells that may show one or more alterations, such as thinning, detachment, vacuolization, individual cell necrosis, nuclear enlargement, cytoplasmic basophilia, or mitotic activity. In rejection, the injury is seen primarily in association with the infiltrate.

Tubulitis: Tubular inflammation in which one or more mononuclear cells have penetrated into tubules and are located between tubular epithelial cells or between tubular cells and their basement membranes.

Activated Lymphocytes: Lymphocytes that are larger than normal (small or resting lymphocytes), which have basophilic cytoplasm, a large vesicular nucleus with an open chromatin pattern, and one or more nucleoli.

Endothelialitis (also known as Endarteritis or Endovasculitis): Intimal inflammation resulting from infiltration of one or more mononuclear cells into the subendothelial space of arteries or, less commonly, arterioles, usually associated with endothelial cell cytoplasmic and nuclear enlargement.

Fibrinoid Necrosis: Necrosis of arterial or arteriolar medial and intimal layers and replacement by homogeneous eosinophilic fibrin-like material. Nuclear debris is also usually present, and sometimes thrombi are present.

Glomerulitis: Segmental or global glomerular hypercellularity due to mononuclear cell infiltration and in severe form termed acute allograft glomerulopathy, with endothelial cell enlargement resulting in occlusion of capillary loops.

[a]Modified from reference 9.

tubular atrophy and interstitial fibrosis (48). It is reasonable to grade tubular atrophy and interstitial fibrosis involving more than 10 percent but less than 25 percent of the cortex as mild, 25 to 50 percent as moderate, and more than 50 percent as severe. This system does not factor in the chronic lesions that may be present in the glomeruli and vessels. In some cases, there may be disproportionately severe injury to one compartment, such as arteries, which may not be reflected in the assessment of chronicity by this method. The Banff 97 system actually addresses this issue by the use of chronic indices (graded on a scale of 0 to 3) for glomeruli (cg), interstitium (ci), tubules (ct), and vessels (cv). Some pathologists prefer to describe the degree (mild, moderate, or severe) of chronic injury in each of the four renal compartments within the body of the microscopic description.

CALCINEURIN INHIBITOR NEPHROTOXICITY

In 1983, the introduction of a new class of immunosuppressive agents, the calcineurin inhibitors, revolutionized the field of organ transplantation. The two major agents in this class, cyclosporine and tacrolimus (Prograf/FK506), act by inhibiting calcineurin, a cytoplasmic phosphatase required for the production of the activated form of the IL-2 gene promoter factor, NF-AT. The superior efficacy of these agents in inhibiting CD4 lymphocyte activity has been counterbalanced by potential nephrotoxicity (12,33–35). The renal toxicity may be difficult to diagnose in renal allograft recipients because of the confounding features of intercurrent rejection (32). However, similar nephrotoxicity has also been documented in heart, liver, and bone marrow transplant recipients as well as in nontransplant patients receiving cyclosporine for various autoimmune and inflammatory disorders. Virtually all the potential nephrotoxicities outlined below for cyclosporine also hold true for tacrolimus, a related fungal metabolite, although a patient's susceptibility to nephrotoxicity may vary for each agent (52).

Cyclosporine and tacrolimus nephrotoxicities occur in acute and chronic forms that can affect all four compartments of the kidney, including tubules, interstitium, blood vessels, and glomeruli. These subgroups of toxicity are outlined in Table 26-5. The presence of rejection does not exclude a diagnosis of cyclosporine toxicity. Therefore, careful clinical-pathologic correlation is often required to make a correct diagnosis.

Table 26-5

CYCLOSPORINE AND TACROLIMUS TOXICITY

Type	Renal Biopsy Findings
Acute	
Functional (Vasoconstriction)	No morphologic abnormalities
Toxic Tubulopathy	Isometric tubular vacuolization, microcalcification, tubular giant mitochondria
Acute Arteriolopathy	Microthrombosis (HUS-like syndrome), endothelial and myocyte necrosis[a]
Chronic	
Vascular	Hyaline arteriolopathy
Tubulointerstitial	Striped fibrosis, diffuse interstitial fibrosis and tubular atrophy
Glomerulopathy	Secondary focal and segmental glomerulosclerosis

[a]HUS= hemolytic uremic syndrome.

Functional Toxicity

Definition. Cyclosporine or tacrolimus administered in pharmacologic doses may cause reductions in renal plasma flow and glomerular filtration rate, without producing structural renal lesions.

Clinical Features. Functional toxicity is most common in the early post-transplant period, but may occur at any time. It is often, but not invariably, correlated with elevated serum levels of cyclosporine.

Light Microscopic Findings. The renal biopsy typically displays no morphologic abnormalities. Some observers have described margination of mononuclear leukocytes in peritubular capillaries as the only morphologic finding. Thus, the diagnosis of functional toxicity should be entertained in any patient with an acute elevation in the serum creatinine level in the absence of morphologic findings that can account for the level of renal functional impairment.

Pathogenesis. Functional toxicity is mediated by an imbalance between vasoconstrictive and vasodilatory forces, favoring vasoconstriction. Abnormal levels of eicosanoids such as prostaglandin (PG)E2, PGI2, and thromboxanes as well as increased activity of endothelin have all been implicated.

Treatment and Prognosis. Functional toxicity is fully reversible on lowering of the cyclosporine/tacrolimus dose.

Prolonged Post-Transplant Oligoanuria

Allografts with any degree of post-transplant acute tubular necrosis are particularly sensitive to calcineurin inhibitors as induction therapy, which may delay recovery from the acute tubular necrosis. The findings on biopsy are essentially those of postoperative acute tubular necrosis described below. Because of this potential toxicity, cyclosporine is usually withheld until good allograft function has been fully established. Prolongation of recovery from acute tubular necrosis may also occur in patients treated with the new macrolide immunosuppressant, sirolimus (Rapamycin, Rapamune), which binds to the same intracellular immunophilin as tacrolimus.

Acute Tubular Toxicity (Toxic Tubulopathy)

Definition. Toxic tubulopathy is defined as a clear vacuolization of the cytoplasm of proximal tubular cells. It most commonly involves the S2 and S3 (straight) segments (fig. 26-50).

Clinical Features. Presentation is with acute allograft dysfunction. This reversible form of cyclosporine toxicity correlates with elevated cyclosporine serum levels in some, but not all, cases. Its incidence has fallen over the past decade with the lowering of cyclosporine maintenance doses.

Light Microscopic Findings. The cytoplasmic vacuolization is often termed "isometric" because it produces vacuoles of similar size (fig. 26-50). It may appear extremely focal, affecting only a few tubular cross sections in a given biopsy (fig. 26-51). The involved tubules may exhibit dysmorphic, crenelated nuclei (fig. 26-52). Toxic tubulopathy is best depicted in formalin-fixed tissue using the hematoxylin and eosin (H&E) or trichrome stains. With the trichrome stain, the clear vacuoles contrast with the red-staining cytoplasm of adjacent uninvolved tubules (fig. 26-53). Other light microscopic features include

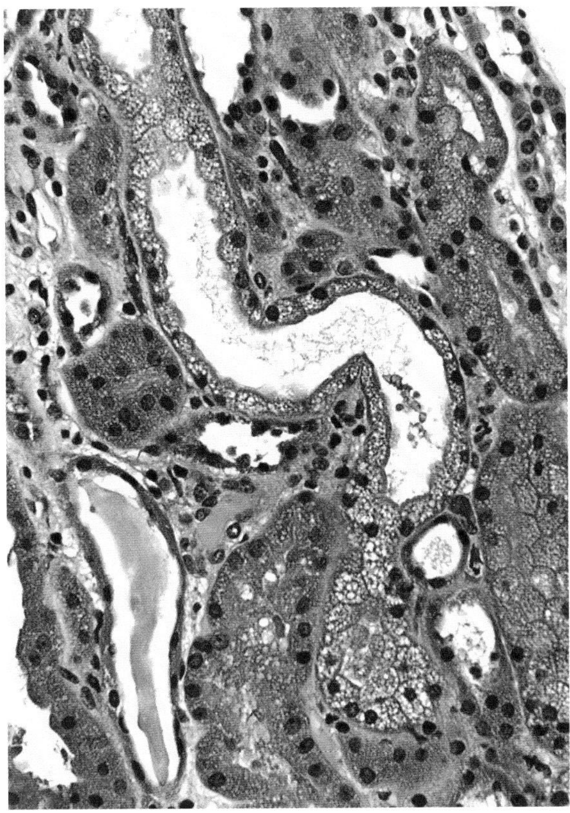

Figure 26-50

CYCLOSPORINE TOXIC TUBULOPATHY

The cytoplasm of the straight segment of the proximal tubule has clear vacuolization. More subtle, ill-defined vacuolization is also seen in some of the adjacent proximal tubules (H&E stain).

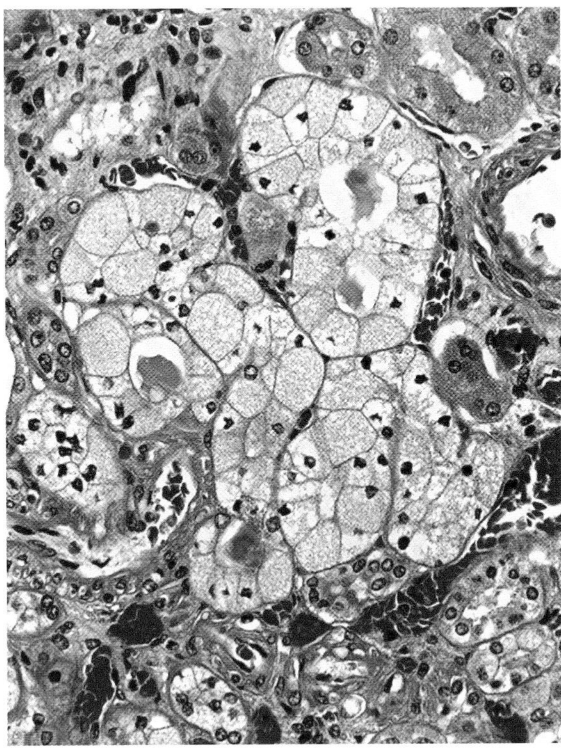

Figure 26-51

CYCLOSPORINE TOXIC TUBULOPATHY

A well-developed example with isometric tubular vacuolization and some dysmorphic nuclei. The involved tubules stand out at low power because of their cytoplasmic pallor. These changes were found at autopsy in the kidney of a cardiac transplant recipient who was treated with high-dose cyclosporine (H&E stain).

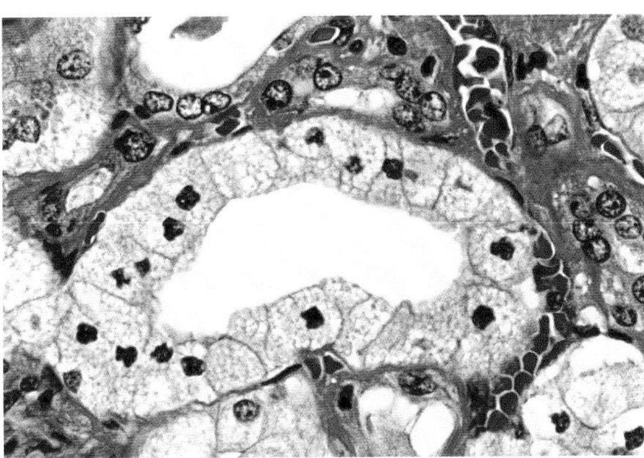

Figure 26-52

CYCLOSPORINE TOXIC TUBULOPATHY

On high-power magnification, the vacuoles appear isometric and the tubular nuclei appear condensed and crenelated (H&E stain).

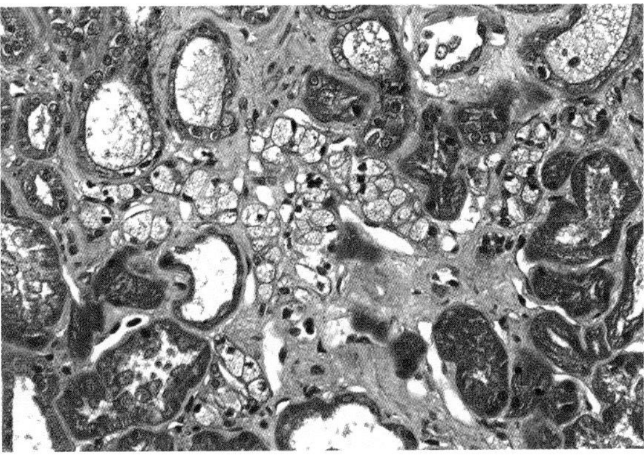

Figure 26-53

CYCLOSPORINE TOXIC TUBULOPATHY

Tubules with cyclosporine toxicity are readily identified at low power with the Masson trichrome stain because their cytoplasm appears clear, contrasting with the red staining cytoplasm of adjacent uninvolved proximal tubules.

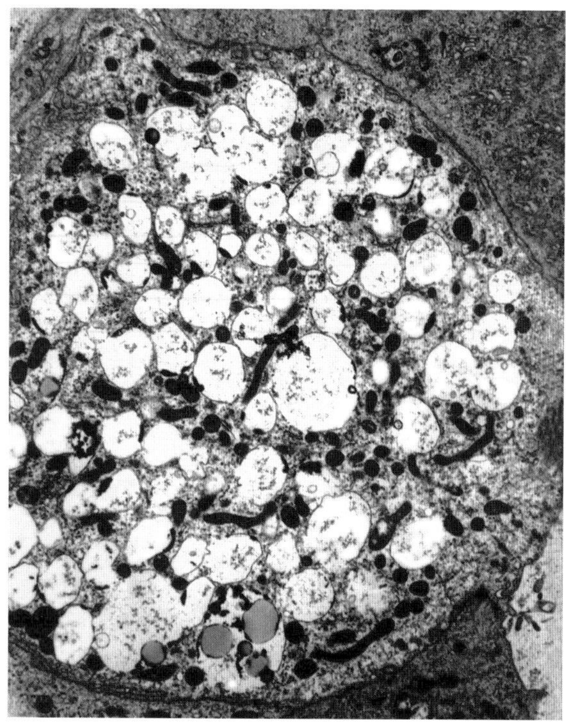

Figure 26-54

CYCLOSPORINE TOXIC TUBULOPATHY

Ultrastructurally, the clear intracytoplasmic vacuoles within proximal tubules correspond to dilated endoplasmic reticulum containing aqueous electron-lucent fluid (electron micrograph).

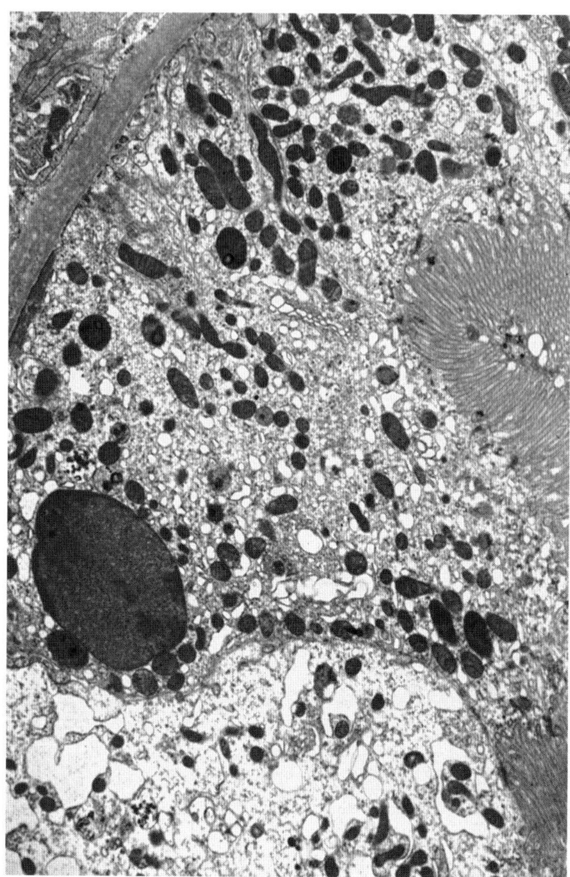

Figure 26-55

CYCLOSPORINE TOXIC TUBULOPATHY

A proximal tubular cell contains a giant mitochondrion which is many times larger than the adjacent normal mitochondria. It has only a few identifiable cristae internal to the outer mitochondrion membrane (electron micrograph).

increased numbers of tubular phagolysosomes, producing eosinophilic cytoplasmic inclusions, and tubular calcifications. Interstitial inflammation and tubulitis are not features of this condition.

Electron Microscopic Findings. Ultrastructurally, the tubular cytoplasmic vacuoles correspond to regular rounded dilatations of the smooth endoplasmic reticulum by aqueous fluid (not lipid) (fig. 26-54). There may be focal giant mitochondria (fig. 26-55).

Differential Diagnosis. The entities in the differential diagnosis include radiocontrast nephropathy, tubular vacuolization due to ischemia, osmotic nephrosis due to intravenous immunoglobulin (IVIG) preparations (now used to treat some cases of antibody-mediated rejection), and tubular reabsorption of lipid (usually in the setting of nephrotic-range proteinuria and lipiduria). The morphologic changes of cyclosporine toxic tubulopathy are indistinguishable by light and electron microscopy from those of radiocontrast nephrotoxicity. In ischemic acute tubular necrosis, the tubular vacuoles tend to be coarser and more irregular in size and distribution, with associated tubular simplification and loss of the brush border. By contrast, in cyclosporine toxic tubulopathy, the tubular vacuoles are extremely fine and regular, and the brush border is preserved. The vacuoles in osmotic nephrosis due to IVIG administration tend to be larger, often causing massive ballooning of the tubular cytoplasm.

Treatment and Prognosis. Acute toxic tubulopathy is fully reversible following lowering of the dose of the offending agent.

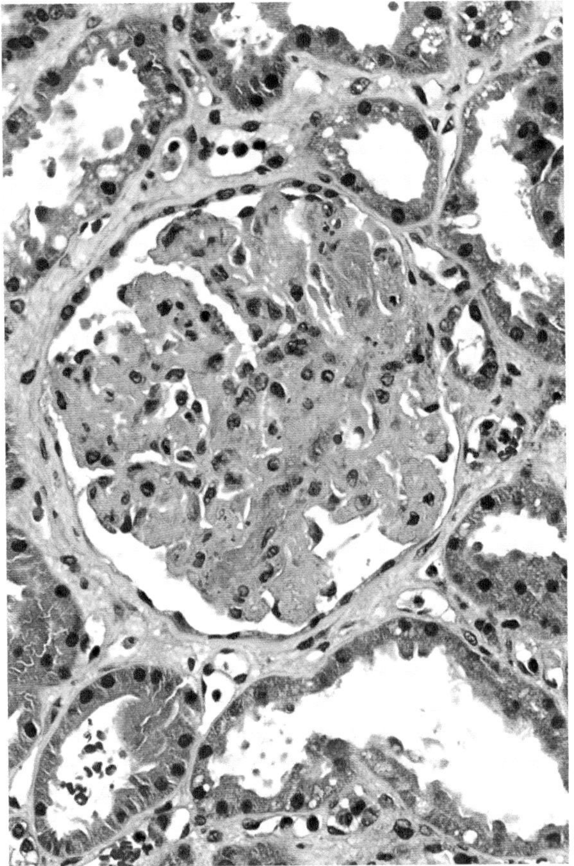

Figure 26-56

CYCLOSPORINE-INDUCED HEMOLYTIC UREMIC SYNDROME

Glomerular capillaries are occluded by endothelial necrosis and intracapillary fibrin thrombosis. The histologic findings resemble those seen in other forms of hemolytic uremic syndrome (H&E stain).

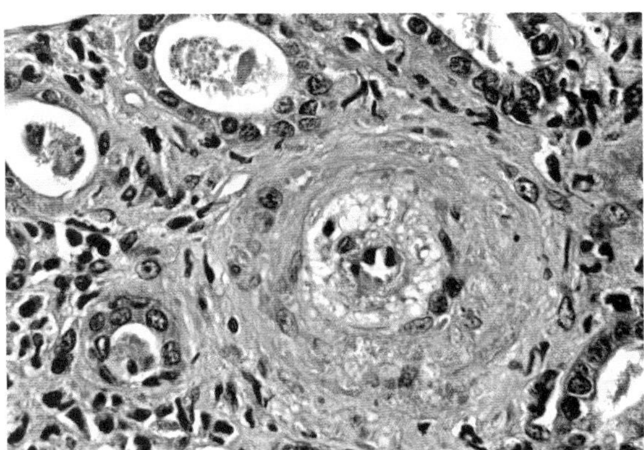

Figure 26-57

CYCLOSPORINE-INDUCED HEMOLYTIC UREMIC SYNDROME

An artery shows mucoid intimal edema in the setting of thrombotic microangiopathy (H&E stain).

Acute Vascular Toxicity (Hemolytic Uremic Syndrome)

Definition. Acute vascular toxicity is a form of calcineurin inhibitor toxicity with features of acute thrombotic microangiopathy that predominantly affects the distal portions of the renal arterial tree, namely, interlobular arteries, arterioles, and glomerular capillaries.

Clinical Features. Presentation is with acute allograft dysfunction manifested by a sudden rise in serum creatinine. In severe cases, there may be full-blown systemic findings of hemolytic uremic syndrome (including thrombocytopenia, microangiopathic hemolytic anemia, and acute oligoanuric renal failure).

Light Microscopic Findings. There is focal fibrin thrombosis of small arteries, arterioles, and glomerular capillaries, sometimes associated with myocyte necrosis. When glomeruli are involved, there may be associated mesangiolysis, endothelial swelling and necrosis, and entrapment of distorted erythrocytes (schistocytes) in the glomerular tuft (fig. 26-56). Mucoid intimal edema may affect the interlobular arteries (fig. 26-57).

Immunofluorescence Findings. There is glomerular and vascular positivity for fibrin/fibrinogen, with less intense positivity for IgM and C3. The staining for IgM probably reflects nonspecific trapping of this large immunoglobulin in areas of thrombosis (fig. 26-58).

Electron Microscopic Findings. There is fibrin thrombosis of glomerular capillaries with endothelial necrosis, mesangiolysis, and subendothelial accumulation of electron-lucent flocculent material, consistent with degraded products of coagulation. No immune-type electron-dense deposits are seen.

Differential Diagnosis. The differential diagnosis includes acute humoral rejection, endarteritis, perfusion injury, and recurrent hemolytic uremic syndrome in the allograft (23). The absence of neutrophil margination in glomerular capillaries and peritubular capillaries, and the absence of linear endothelial staining for immunoglobulin or complement (most notably C4d in peritubular capillaries) are findings

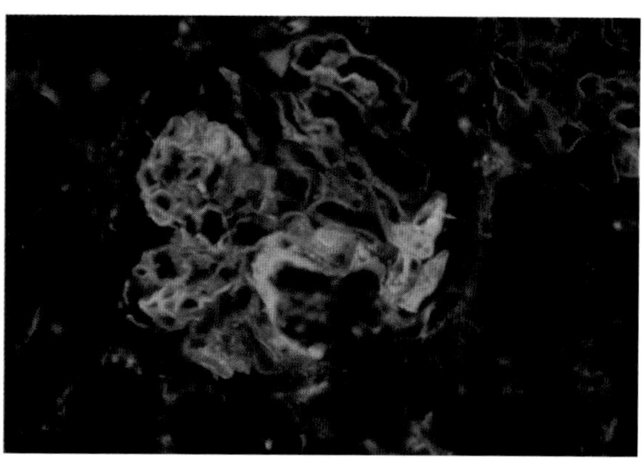

Figure 26-58

CYCLOSPORINE-INDUCED HEMOLYTIC UREMIC SYNDROME

There is strong staining of the glomerular capillaries for fibrin (immunofluorescence micrograph).

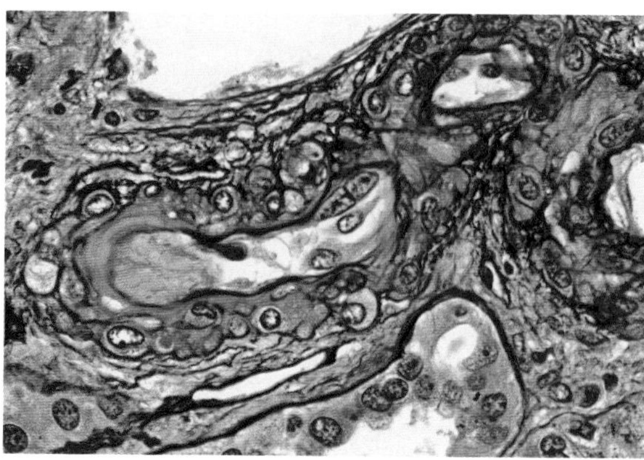

Figure 26-59

CYCLOSPORINE ACUTE VASCULAR TOXICITY

There is swelling and focal necrosis, with "drop-out" of individual medial myocytes. The necrotic myocytes leave an acellular defect in the medial wall where they used to reside (Jones methenamine silver [JMS] stain).

that favor cyclosporine-induced hemolytic uremic syndrome over acute humoral (antibody-mediated) rejection. The absence of a mononuclear inflammatory infiltration of the intima of small arteries militates against endarteritis. The clinical history and time course are usually helpful to exclude perfusion injury, which is limited to the immediate post-transplant period. Patients with a prior history of hemolytic uremic syndrome (especially the nonepidemic form) involving their native kidneys appear to be particularly susceptible to the development of acute vascular toxicity secondary to calcineurin inhibitors in the allograft.

Etiology and Pathogenesis. Acute vascular toxicity is mediated by direct endothelial toxicity, as well as platelet-aggregating effects.

Treatment and Prognosis. The clinical outcome varies. Some patients recover renal function following the lowering of the dose of cyclosporine or tacrolimus, while others develop irreversible renal damage. A response to plasma infusion or exchange has been reported in anecdotal cases.

Chronic Toxicity

Definition. Chronic calcineurin inhibitor toxicity is a form of chronic nephrotoxicity that may target the vascular, tubulointerstitial, and glomerular compartments (33,34).

Clinical Features. There is a gradual diminution in graft function that is indistinguishable clinically from chronic rejection/chronic allograft nephropathy. Some, but not all, patients have a history of elevated serum levels of cyclosporine or tacrolimus.

Pathologic Findings. *Vascular Lesions.* The most distinctive lesions are the vascular lesions, which are referred to as *cyclosporine arteriolopathy* or *hyaline arteriolopathy* (33,34). The preglomerular arterioles and most distal portions of the interlobular arteries are preferentially affected. An acute process of swelling, vacuolization, and necrosis of individual medial myocytes gives way to myocyte drop-out and replacement by hyaline (figs. 26-59–26-62). The lacunae left by the necrotic myocytes are filled by proteinaceous hyaline material. This medial hyalinosis extends into the outermost boundaries of the media, and produces a beaded circular pattern that is referred to as "pearl-necklace" appearance.

By immunofluorescence, the vascular lesions stain for IgM, C3, and C1 in the areas of hyalinosis, with more variable positivity for fibrin (fig. 26-63). In severe examples, the arteriolar lumen may be severely compromised or occluded by intimal hyalinosis, producing the features of obliterative arteriolopathy (figs. 26-64, 26-65).

Tubulointerstitial Lesions. Chronic tubulointerstitial lesions usually accompany the arteriolopathy. These take the form of linear zones of tubular atrophy and interstitial fibrosis often referred to as "striped fibrosis" (fig. 26-66).

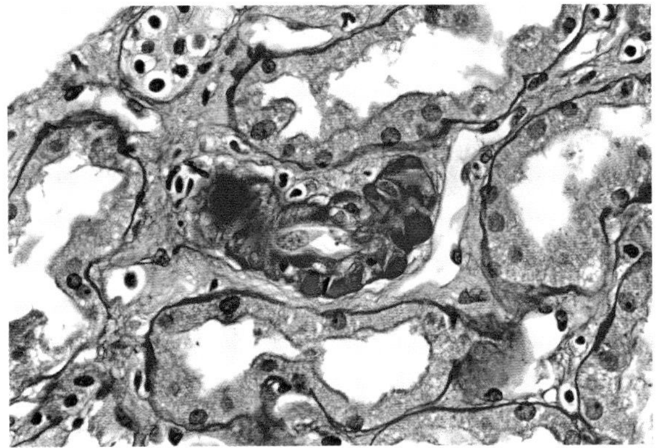

Figure 26-60

CYCLOSPORINE HYALINE ARTERIOLOPATHY

Beaded medial hyalinosis extends into the outermost media of this small arteriole (PAS stain).

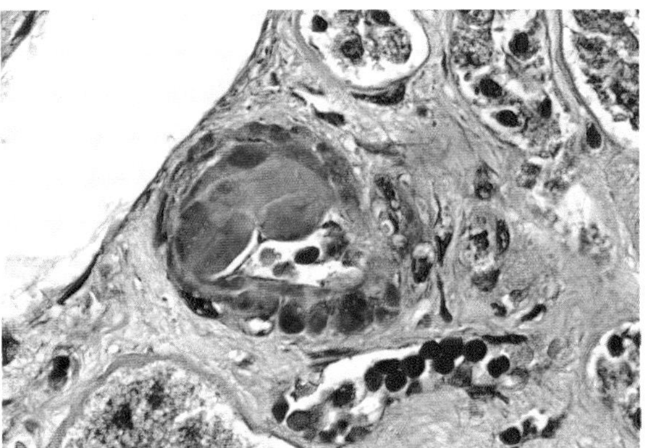

Figure 26-61

CYCLOSPORINE HYALINE ARTERIOLOPATHY

There is intimal and medial hyalinosis forming beaded deposits that replace the spaces previously occupied by individual myocytes (Masson trichrome stain).

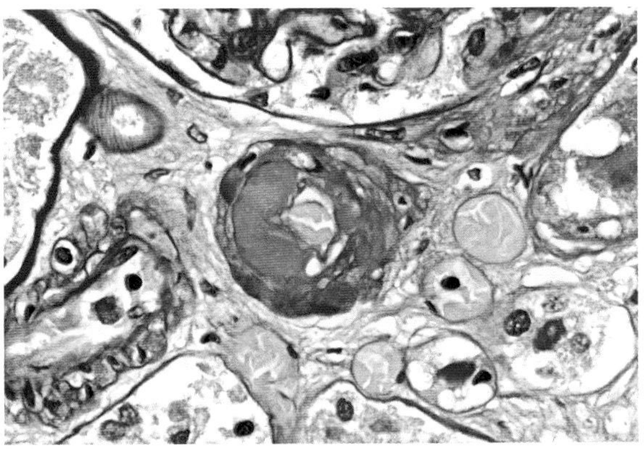

Figure 26-62

CYCLOSPORINE HYALINE ARTERIOLOPATHY

The vessel wall is paucicellular and almost entirely replaced by hyaline, which occupies both the intima and media. An uninvolved normal arteriole is seen to the left (PAS stain).

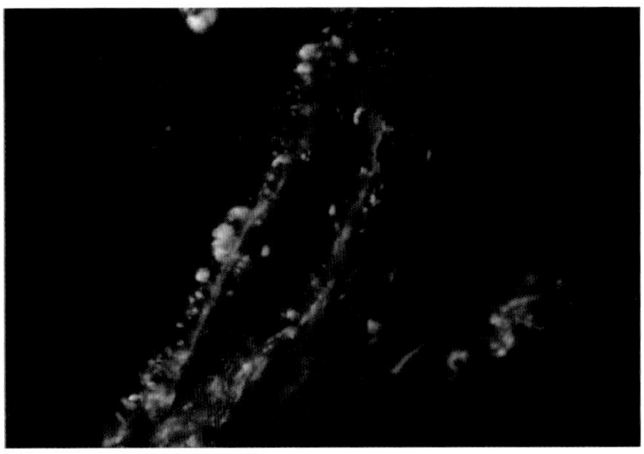

Figure 26-63

CYCLOSPORINE HYALINE ARTERIOLOPATHY

There is staining for C3 in the distribution of the intimal and medial hyaline deposits, producing a "pearl necklace" beaded appearance (immunofluorescence micrograph).

Experimental evidence in rats suggests that these striped areas correspond to the medullary rays, an area of the nephron particularly vulnerable to ischemic injury. As chronic cyclosporine toxicity progresses, the interstitial fibrosis and tubular atrophy assume a more diffuse distribution (fig. 26-67). Although a mild to moderate interstitial mononuclear infiltrate may be present, tubulitis is not a feature (32).

Glomerular Lesions. In some patients with chronic cyclosporine toxicity, nephrotic-range proteinuria develops. These patients often have a secondary pattern of focal and segmental glomerulosclerosis, with hypertrophy of remnant nephrons (fig. 26-68). This pattern of glomerular injury is likely a maladaptive response to loss of functioning nephrons rather than a direct form of toxicity to the glomerular constituents.

Differential Diagnosis. Chronic cyclosporine toxicity may be difficult to differentiate from chronic rejection because interstitial fibrosis, interstitial inflammation, and tubular atrophy may occur in both conditions. A stripe-like distribution of tubulointerstitial scarring, the presence

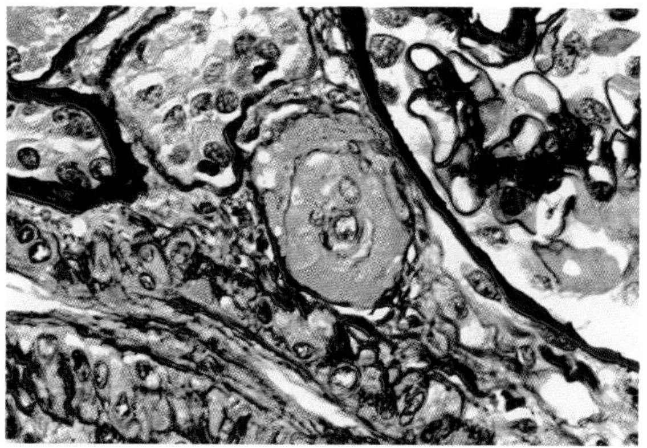

Figure 26-64

CYCLOSPORINE HYALINE ARTERIOLOPATHY

A severe example with obliterative hyalinosis. The entire wall is replaced by nonargyrophilic hyaline material, with loss of any recognizable medial myocytes (JMS stain).

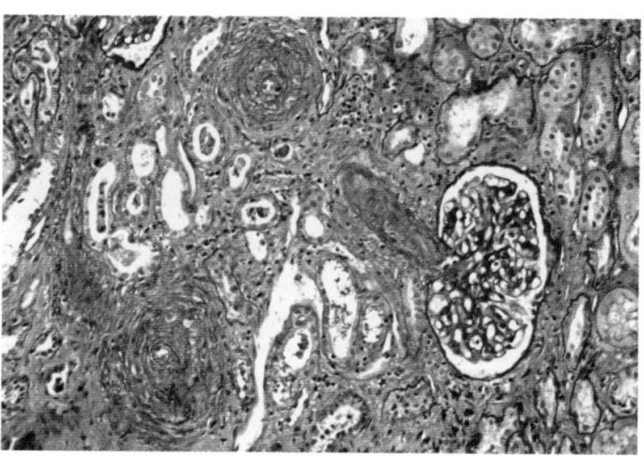

Figure 26-65

CYCLOSPORINE CHRONIC ARTERIOLOPATHY

There is occlusion of many interlobular arteries and preglomerular arterioles by expansile intimal sclerosis of the type seen in chronic thrombotic microangiopathies. The lesions are in the interlobular arteries and preglomerular arterioles, and extend to the glomerular hilus (PAS stain).

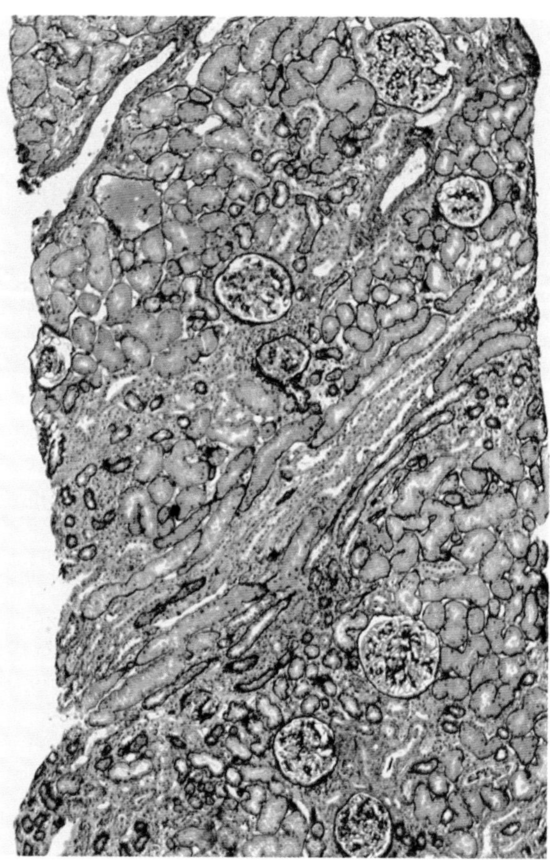

Figure 26-66

CYCLOSPORINE STRIPED FIBROSIS

There are linear bands of tubular atrophy and interstitial fibrosis that parallel the medullary rays (JMS stain).

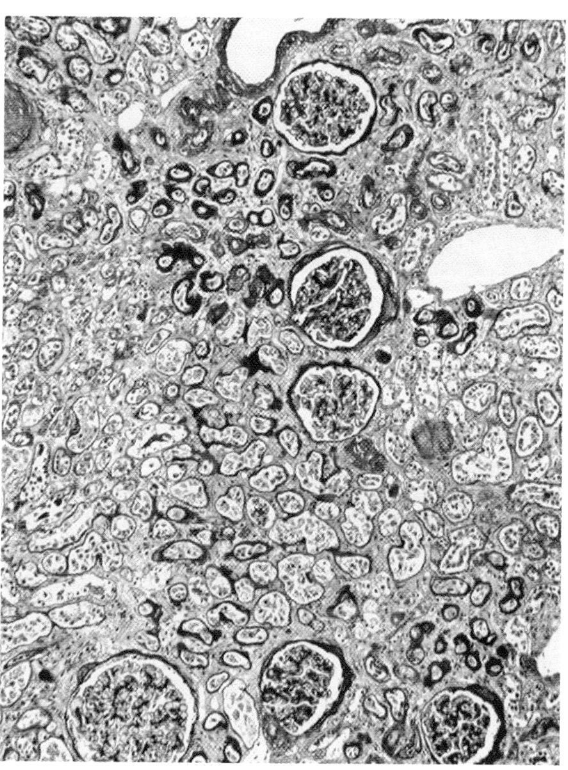

Figure 26-67

CYCLOSPORINE TOXICITY

Diffuse interstitial fibrosis and tubular atrophy are seen in a specimen from a cardiac transplant recipient who developed chronic renal insufficiency and eventual end-stage renal failure. The fibrotic interstitium contains a sparse lymphocytic infiltrate, without evidence of tubulitis (PAS stain).

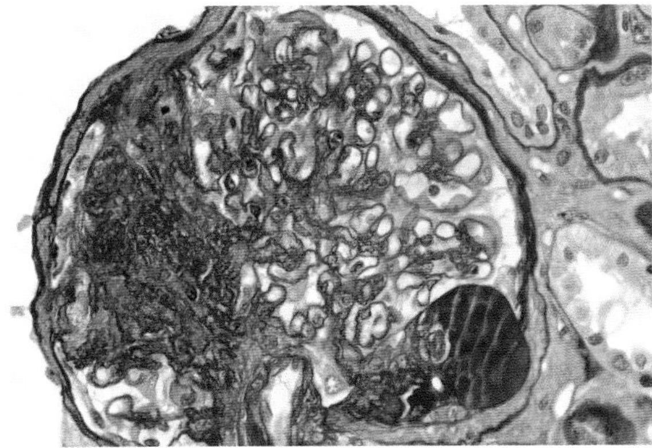

Figure 26-68

CYCLOSPORINE TOXICITY

In chronic cyclosporine toxicity, lesions of focal and segmental glomerulosclerosis and hyalinosis may be accompanied by the development of nephrotic-range proteinuria. These segmental lesions probably arise from loss of renal mass due to chronic cyclosporine toxicity, leading to hyperfiltration injury in remnant nephrons (PAS stain).

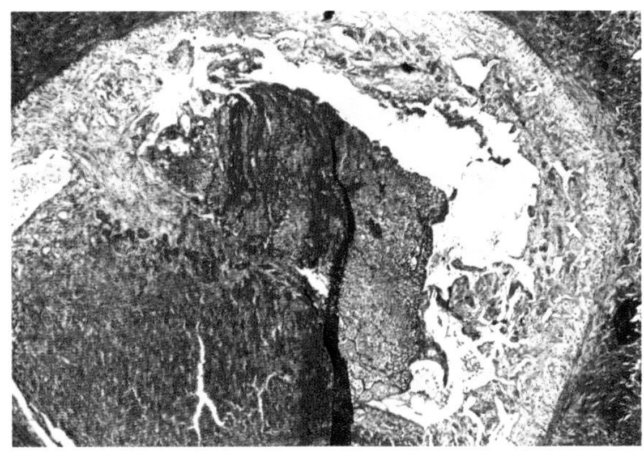

Figure 26-69

RENAL VEIN THROMBOSIS

Acute thrombosis following treatment with OKT3 has nearly occluded the renal vein. There was secondary hemorrhagic infarction of the kidney, necessitating nephrectomy (Masson trichrome stain).

of tubular vacuolization, and the presence of hyaline arteriolopathy help identify chronic cyclosporine nephrotoxicity (32,58,62). On the other hand, the absence of tubulitis, the absence of endarteritis, and the absence of arterial fibrointimal hyperplasia involving arcuate and interlobar arteries help to exclude chronic rejection.

Cyclosporine arteriolopathy must be differentiated from the vascular lesions seen in aging, hypertension, or diabetes. In the latter three conditions, the arteriolar hyaline predominantly affects the intima, hyalinosis rarely extends into the outermost media, and individual myocyte necrosis is not observed.

The secondary glomerular pattern of focal segmental glomerulosclerosis must be differentiated from idiopathic focal sclerosis (either recurrent or de novo). The presence of other obvious features of chronic calcineurin inhibitor toxicity and the absence of full nephrotic syndrome (despite nephrotic-range proteinuria) argue against idiopathic focal segmental glomerulosclerosis.

Treatment and Prognosis. Chronic toxicity due to the calcineurin inhibitors tends to be irreversible. In cardiac transplant patients who are often maintained on higher doses of cyclosporine than renal transplant recipients, nephrotoxicity may lead to end-stage renal failure requiring renal transplantation.

OKT3 TOXICITY

There are rare reports that high doses of OKT3 may induce allograft thrombosis at the level of the glomerular capillaries or large vessels, such as the main renal artery or vein (fig. 26-69). These prothrombotic effects have been linked to the cytokine storm that follows OKT3-induced release of TNF, IL-2, and interferon-gamma, which in turn trigger endothelial activation, with associated increased endothelial expression of leukocyte adhesion factors and tissue factor procoagulant. In some cases, acute renal vein thrombosis has led to graft rupture in the early post-transplant period.

ACUTE TUBULAR NECROSIS/PRESERVATION INJURY

Definition. Acute tubular necrosis in the allograft is a common form of acute tubular injury that usually results from prolonged warm or cold ischemia time; it typically manifests in the immediate postoperative period (43). It is a common initial complication of cadaveric renal transplantation. It may also affect living donor allografts if the surgery has been technically difficult, causing prolonged operative time and warm ischemia.

Clinical Findings. Patients present with primary graft failure and absence of urine output that may last from days to weeks, depending

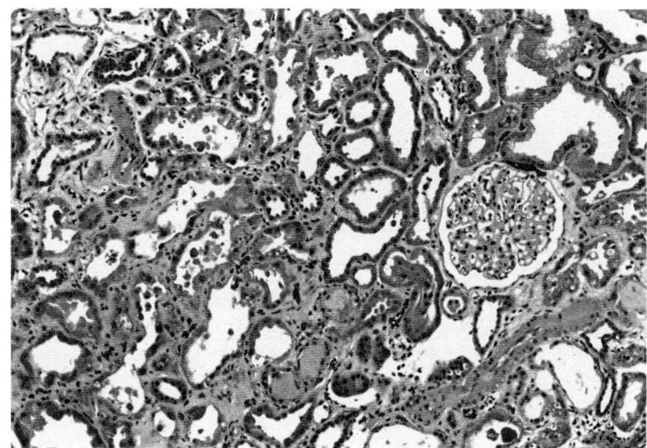

Figure 26-70

ACUTE TUBULAR NECROSIS

Post-transplant acute tubular necrosis occurred secondary to prolonged warm ischemia time in this patient with primary cadaveric graft failure. There is ectasia of proximal tubules with flattening and focal coagulation necrosis of tubular epithelial cells. Mild interstitial edema and sparse inflammation are seen, without tubulitis (H&E stain).

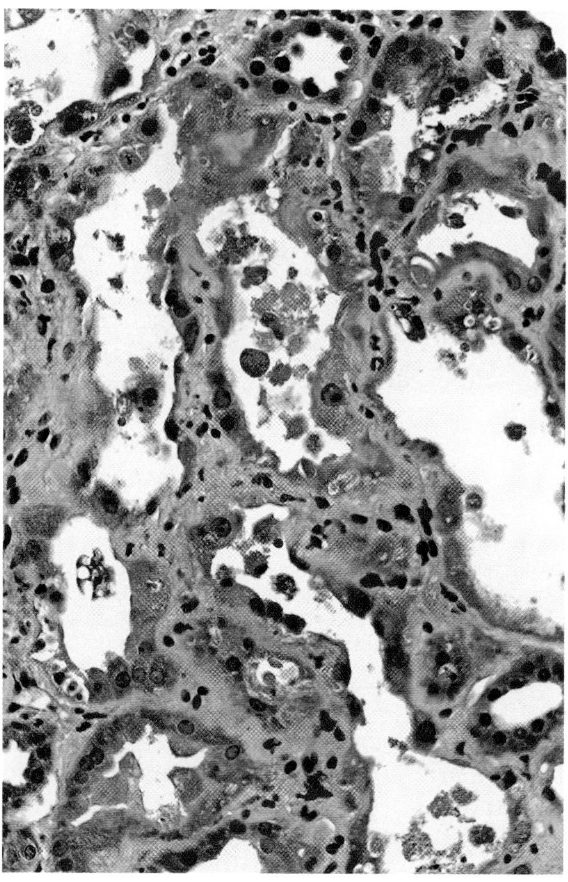

Figure 26-71

ACUTE TUBULAR NECROSIS

High-power view of figure 26-70 shows individual necrotic tubular epithelial cells with focal apoptotic bodies and desquamation of cells into the tubular lumen (H&E stain).

on the severity of the ischemic insult. Acute tubular necrosis may also affect the allograft after a period of initial graft function, following the same types of ischemic or toxic tubular insults that can cause acute tubular necrosis in the native kidney.

Light Microscopic Findings. There is diffuse tubular damage in the form of loss of brush border, focal epithelial coagulation necrosis and apoptosis, cytoplasmic basophilia, and enlarged regenerative nuclei with nucleoli (figs. 26-70, 26-71). In severe examples, clusters of desquamated necrotic tubular epithelial cells are identified in the tubular lumen. The interstitium is expanded by mild edema. Although there may be a sparse interstitial mononuclear infiltrate, tubulitis is not seen.

After prolonged ischemia, some grafts have a more severe form of preservation injury that includes vascular endothelial damage with thrombosis of small arteries, arterioles, and glomerular capillaries, and focal infarction (fig. 26-72).

Differential Diagnosis. A renal biopsy is often necessary to differentiate prolonged acute tubular necrosis from acute rejection (13). In acute tubular necrosis, there is extensive tubular damage without significant interstitial inflammation, and without evidence of tubulitis or endovasculitis. Severe preservation injury accompanied by intravascular coagulation may be difficult to distinguish from hyperacute or accelerated vascular rejection. The absence of neutrophil margination in interstitial peritubular capillaries and the negativity for immunoglobulin and C4d by immunofluorescence are features of severe perfusion injury.

Treatment and Prognosis. The patient is maintained on dialysis until there is restoration of urine output and recovery of renal function. Because the allograft is sensitive to the toxic effects of calcineurin inhibitors or sirolimus during this period, these agents should be withheld until renal function has been restored.

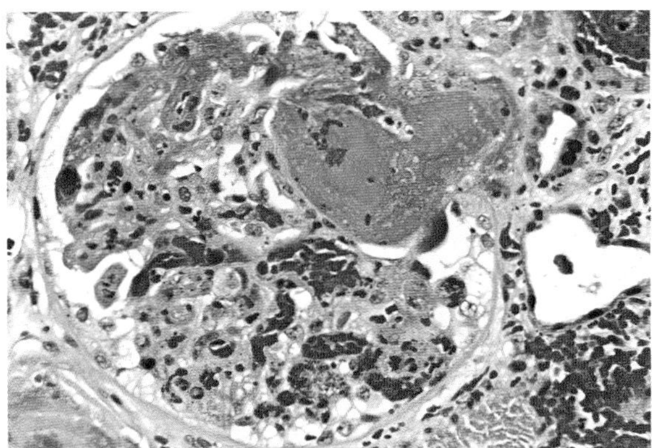

Figure 26-72

PRESERVATION INJURY

This allograft kidney, which had been subjected to prolonged warm ischemia time prior to transplantation, developed intraglomerular thrombi and neutrophil margination that mimicked hyperacute rejection at biopsy. The graft eventually recovered function after 3 weeks of hemodialysis (H&E stain).

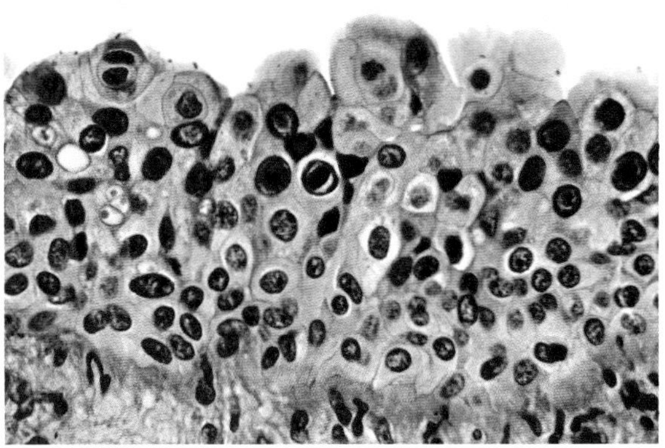

Figure 26-73

CYTOMEGALOVIRUS PYELITIS

The characteristic intranuclear viral inclusions are present in the pelvic urothelium of a renal allograft (H&E stain).

PERFUSION INJURY

Grafts that have been perfused with cold storage solutions, either by machine or manually prior to transplantation, may have delayed function. The injury is primarily to the endothelium, with microvascular thrombosis in glomerular capillaries and small arteries. Perfusion injury can be differentiated from hyperacute rejection by the absence of neutrophil margination and C4d deposition in peritubular capillaries. Graft perfusion continues to be used in many centers, particularly for the preservation of cadaveric kidneys from marginal donors.

INFECTIONS

A variety of viral, bacterial, fungal, and protozoal infections may occur in the renal allograft. Bacterial pyelonephritis and fungal pyelonephritis are covered in the chapter on renal infections. Discussion here is limited to viral agents: CMV, BK polyomavirus, and adenovirus.

Cytomegalovirus Infection

CMV can cause acute allograft infection as well as promoting graft rejection by indirect effects. Viral intranuclear and cytoplasmic inclusions are identified in tubular cells, glomerular endothelial cells, and interstitial capillary endothelial cells, as well as in urothelial cells of the renal pelvis (fig. 26-73). In some patients, occasional viral intranuclear and cytoplasmic inclusions are identified without a significant inflammatory reaction. In unusual cases, an acute tubulointerstitial nephritis is present, with more widespread cytopathic viral changes. There have also been rare examples of acute glomerulonephritis with glomerular viral inclusions.

BK Polyomavirus Infection

BK virus, named for the initials of the first patient in whom it was described, is a member of the papova virus family and is related to both the JC and simian virus (SV)40 viruses. It is a common cause of acute tubulointerstitial nephritis in the allograft due to reactivation of latent infection in an immunocompromised host (40,49,50). This form of tubulointerstitial nephritis closely mimics acute rejection because it is associated with a prominent mononuclear inflammatory infiltrate (including lymphocytes and plasma cells) with active tubulitis. The intranuclear viral inclusions can easily be mistaken for the enlarged regenerative nuclear atypia seen in acute rejection. The main feature of the polyomavirus inclusions is the presence of enlarged nuclei with smudgy, ground-glass, basophilic inclusions that completely replace the nuclear chromatin (fig. 26-74). Some infected cells may contain a more amphophilic discrete inclusion surrounded by a halo. There is focal viral cytolysis with shedding of infected cells into the tubular lumen (fig. 26-75).

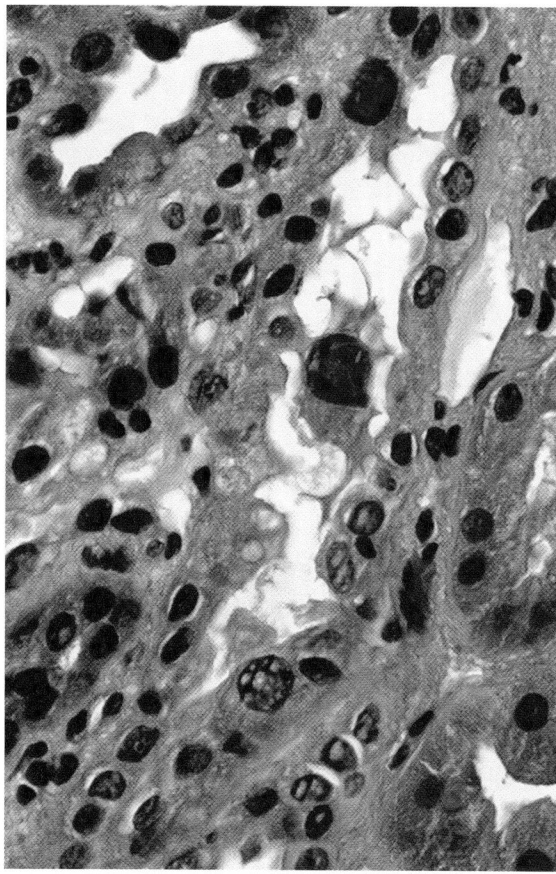

Figure 26-74

BK POLYOMA VIRUS

Large basophilic inclusions with a ground-glass appearance are present in individual tubular epithelial cells of the cortical collecting ducts (H&E stain).

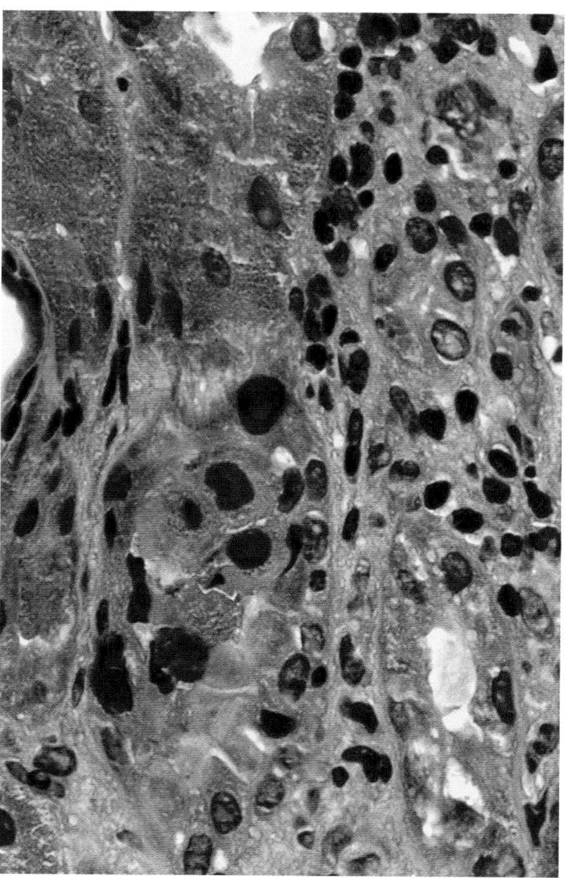

Figure 26-75

BK POLYOMA VIRUS

The viral cytolysis leads to shedding of tubular cells containing large amphophilic inclusions into the tubular lumen. Mild tubulitis is also present, mimicking acute rejection (H&E stain).

In mild cases, the infection is relatively focal, predominantly involving the collecting tubules. In severe forms, the virus involves the cortical tubules more diffusely. Infection may even extend to parietal epithelial cells, with focal crescent formation.

Confirmation of BK polyomavirus infection is possible using immunostains for SV40 directed to the large T antigen (fig. 26-76). Electron microscopic analysis reveals clusters of intranuclear, rounded, electron-dense virions measuring 40 to 45 nm in diameter and arranged in parallel linear arrays (figs. 26-77, 26-78) (40). The viral inclusions are readily demonstrated in the urine sediment.

It is essential to differentiate this condition from acute rejection because treatment strategies are diametrically opposed. Patients with BK polyomavirus infection respond to lowering of immunosuppression but no specific antiviral agents have proven effective. Severe infections often lead to irreversible graft failure.

Adenovirus Infection

In the renal allograft, adenovirus infection can produce a necrotizing and hemorrhagic acute tubulointerstitial nephritis. The intranuclear viral inclusions tend to involve many epithelial cells in a given tubule. Infected cells have enlarged basophilic nuclei with a smudged appearance, as well as more discrete intranuclear inclusions with a surrounding halo. Immunostains for adenovirus antigens are helpful to confirm the

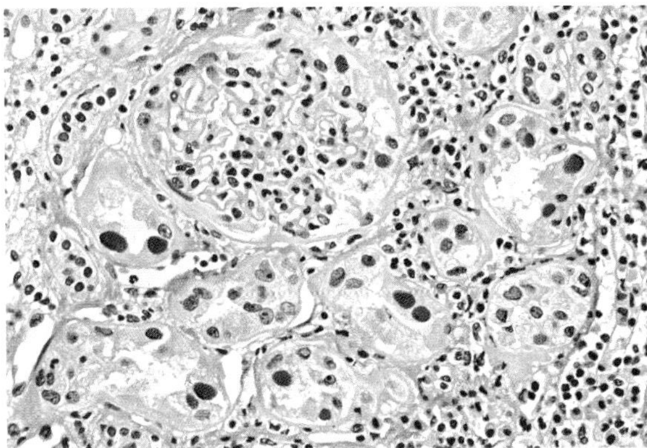

Figure 26-76

BK POLYOMA VIRUS

The SV40 immunostain gives strong nuclear positivity to the infected proximal tubular cells, which have enlarged nuclei corresponding to intranuclear inclusions. Some nuclear positivity is also seen in the distribution of parietal epithelial cells (immunoperoxidase stain).

diagnosis. Electron microscopy reveals intranuclear arrays of virions that range from 75 to 80 nm in diameter. Features that distinguish adenovirus infection from acute rejection include more extensive interstitial hemorrhage and a less prominent interstitial inflammatory infiltrate.

ACUTE (ALLERGIC) INTERSTITIAL NEPHRITIS

Patients with a renal allograft may develop drug-induced acute interstitial nephritis, similar to that in the native kidney. Common inciting drugs include antibiotics such as the beta-lactams and sulfonamides. Patients usually present with an acute rise in serum creatinine, with or without eosinophiluria. The presence of rash, fever, and eosinophilia are helpful diagnostic clues. The light microscopic findings are identical to those of allergic interstitial nephritis in the native kidney and include patchy or diffuse interstitial inflammation by lymphocytes, monocytes, and eosinophils, associated with interstitial edema, tubulitis, and tubular degenerative changes. All of these findings can also be seen in acute rejection. In addition to the clinical context, helpful morphologic findings favoring allergic interstitial nephritis include eosinophil infiltration of the tubules (eosinophilic tubulitis) and focal interstitial granulomas, features not generally seen in acute rejection. In addition, extensive involvement of the outer medulla, as much or more than the involvement of the cortex, suggests drug-induced interstitial nephritis. Nonetheless, in some cases it is extremely difficult and may be impossible to make a clinical-pathologic diagnosis of drug-induced interstitial nephritis in the presence of inflammation meeting Banff 97 criteria for acute rejection.

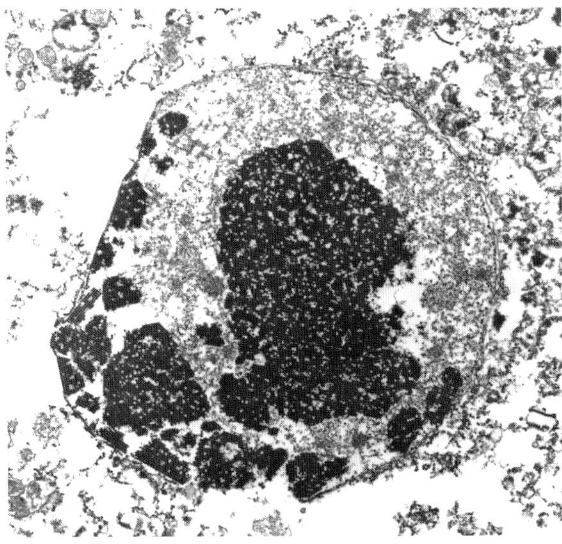

Figure 26-77

BK POLYOMA VIRUS

Ultrastructural appearance of an infected degenerating tubular epithelial cell containing many intranuclear virions in parallel formation (electron micrograph).

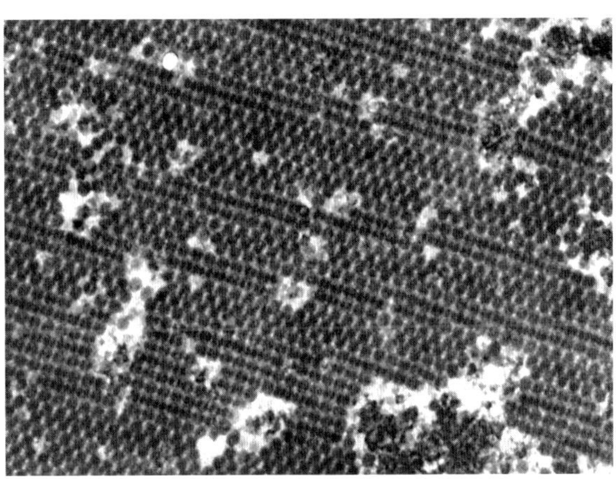

Figure 26-78

BK POLYOMA VIRUS

High-power view of the intranuclear virions from a desquamated, lysed tubular epithelial cell shows regular linear arrays of rounded, 45-nm virions (electron micrograph).

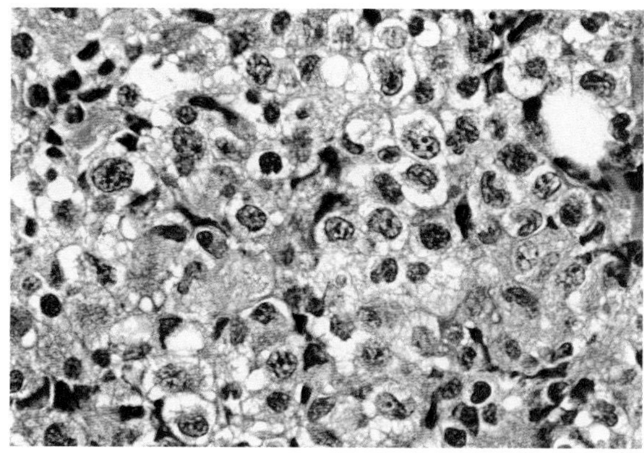

Figure 26-79

POST-TRANSPLANT LYMPHOPROLIFERATIVE DISEASE

The specimen shows a dense infiltrate of atypical lymphoid cells with enlarged hyperchromatic nuclei (H&E stain).

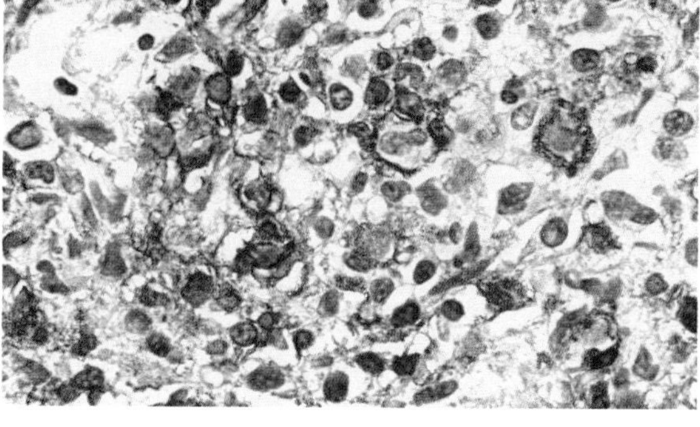

Figure 26-80

POST- TRANSPLANT LYMPHOPROLIFERATIVE DISEASE

Many of the atypical lymphoid cells are positive for CD20, indicating B lymphocytes (immunoperoxidase stain).

POST-TRANSPLANT LYMPHOPROLIFERATIVE DISEASE

Definition. Post-transplant lymphoproliferative disease (PTLD) is a predominantly extranodal, usually Epstein-Barr virus (EBV)-associated lymphoproliferative disorder that develops in the immunocompromised transplant recipient. It encompasses a spectrum of lesions from polymorphic to monomorphic, and ranging from plasmacytic hyperplasia to polymorphic B-cell hyperplasia to frank immunoblastic lymphoma or multiple myeloma (22,51).

Clinical Features. Patients often have an acute mononucleosis-like syndrome, with fever, lymphadenopathy, and splenomegaly. Common extranodal sites of involvement include the central nervous system, gastrointestinal tract, and lung, with the transplant kidney a relatively infrequent site. PTLD complicates approximately 1 percent of adult renal transplants, with a 10-fold higher incidence in pediatric transplant recipients due to the higher rate of primary EBV infections in this group.

The kidney is involved in about 15 percent of kidney transplant recipients with PTLD, but less than 1 percent of heart transplant recipients. In some patients, the kidney may be the exclusive site of involvement. Renal involvement by PTLD usually manifests with acute allograft dysfunction. In some cases, there may be ureteric obstruction due to the tumor mass.

Gross Findings. The kidney may contain irregular serpiginous zones of necrosis and discrete tumor nodules.

Light Microscopic Findings. There is a dense, often nodular, interstitial infiltration by atypical lymphoid cells. In the polymorphic forms, the lymphoid cells exhibit a range of B-cell differentiation that includes immunoblasts, plasma cells, large cleaved or noncleaved cells, and small round lymphocytes. Some cells have marked nuclear atypia (fig. 26-79). In the monomorphic forms, the infiltrate is more monotonous in appearance, resembling lymphoma. PTLD may produce tubulitis and venulitis that mimics acute rejection.

Special Studies. PTLD can easily be mistaken for acute rejection, and a proper diagnosis requires a high index of suspicion. The easiest and most helpful ancillary test is immunostaining of formalin-fixed, paraffin-embedded tissue for L26, an antibody to CD20 expressed on B lymphocytes (fig. 26-80). A CD20 immunostain typically stains the majority of lymphocytes in PTLD, whereas there is a preponderance of T lymphocytes (CD3 positive) in acute rejection. Demonstration of clonality with kappa or lambda immunostains or immunoglobulin gene rearrangement studies is helpful in the monomorphic forms, however, the infiltrate is usually polyclonal in polymorphic PTLD. Special stains for EBV virus, such as immunostains for EBNA-2 and LMP-1 as well as in situ hybridization for EBER, provide confirmatory evidence of PTLD.

Differential Diagnosis. The major entity in the differential diagnosis is acute rejection. Differentiation is especially difficult in cases of plasma cell–rich acute rejection (39). In PTLD, the tubulitis is usually less severe than expected for the intensity of the interstitial infiltrate. Although veins are frequently infiltrated in PTLD, endovasculitis involving arteries is not a feature.

Etiology and Pathogenesis. PTLD is linked to latent or primary infection with EBV, which can infect and immortalize B cells. In the transplant setting, excessive immunosuppression leads to uncontrolled proliferation of EBV-transformed B cells. Thus, PTLD often arises in the setting of refractory acute rejection.

Treatment and Prognosis. The mainstay of treatment is reduction or total discontinuation of immunosuppression. Antiviral agents, such as acyclovir or ganciclovir, are commonly administered. Interferon-alpha or anti-CD20 antibodies may also be effective. Cases of frank lymphoma may require the addition of chemotherapy or radiation. Mortality is over 60 percent for monomorphic, but less than 10 percent for polymorphic, forms.

RECURRENT GLOMERULAR DISEASE

Definition. When the same glomerular disease that was documented in the native kidney develops in the allograft kidney, it is designated a recurrent glomerular disease.

Clinical Features. Numerous glomerular diseases have been reported to recur with varying frequency in the allograft (5,8,54). Since 20 to 40 percent of renal transplants are performed in patients with end-stage glomerular disease, the potential for disease recurrence in this population should not be underestimated. Only some of these recurrences cause graft failure. In many cases, recurrent disease is an incidental finding in a patient with acute rejection.

The glomerular disease that recurs at the highest rate (95 to 100 percent) is dense deposit disease (membranoproliferative glomerulonephritis type II), although less than 15 percent of affected patients lose their graft to recurrent disease. Other conditions that commonly recur in the allograft include membranoproliferative glomerulonephritis type I (recurrence rate 40 to 70 percent), IgA nephropathy and Henoch-Schönlein purpura nephritis (30 to 50 percent), focal segmental glomerulosclerosis (30 to 40 percent), and hemolytic uremic syndrome (nonepidemic form; 30 percent). Lower rates of recurrence are reported for membranous glomerulopathy (10 percent), antiglomerular basement membrane (anti-GBM) disease (5 to 10 percent), and lupus nephritis (less than 5 percent). Most recurrences occur within the first 6 months post-transplantation. In some cases, as in recurrent focal segmental glomerulosclerosis, nephrotic syndrome may develop as early as several days post-transplantation.

Systemic diseases that commonly recur in the allograft include diabetic nephropathy, amyloidosis, oxalosis, and Fabry's disease.

Pathologic Findings. Recurrent disease in the allograft has the same light microscopic, immunofluorescence, and electron microscopic features as the disease occurring in the native kidney. Because of the transplant setting, however, there may be background changes of acute or chronic rejection.

Differential Diagnosis. Routine histology should be supplemented by immunofluorescence and electron microscopy in cases where recurrent glomerular disease is suspected on the basis of the clinical presentation or light microscopic findings. Recurrent glomerulonephritis in the allograft must be differentiated from transplant glomerulitis and transplant glomerulopathy. The absence of immune deposits by immunofluorescence and electron microscopy helps to differentiate transplant glomerulopathy from recurrent primary membranoproliferative glomerulonephritis.

DE NOVO GLOMERULAR DISEASE

When the allograft develops a primary glomerular disease that is different from the native kidney disease, this is defined as a de novo glomerular disease (5). Knowledge of the original disease that led to end-stage renal failure is essential to exclude a recurrent process.

The onset of de novo glomerular disease is often heralded by the new appearance of proteinuria, nephrotic syndrome, active urinary sediment, or reduced renal function, depending on

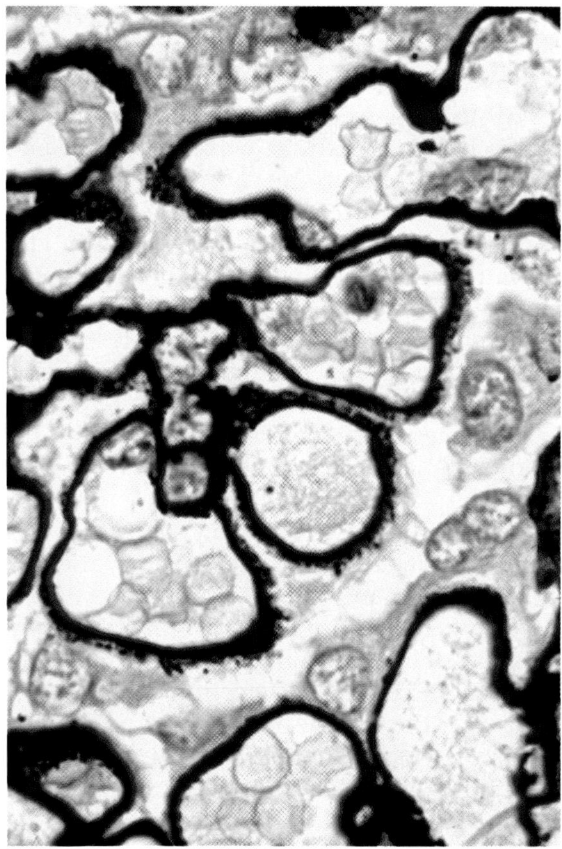

Figure 26-81

DE NOVO MEMBRANOUS GLOMERULOPATHY

There are glomerular basement membrane spikes identical to those seen in membranous glomerulopathy of the native kidney (JMS stain).

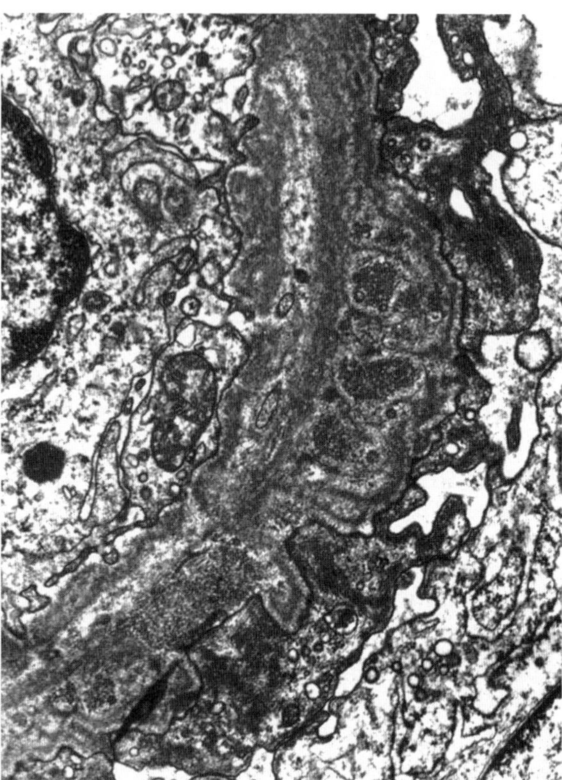

Figure 26-82

DE NOVO MEMBRANOUS GLOMERULOPATHY

There are subepithelial electron-dense deposits separated by basement membrane spikes. In addition, there is widening of the subendothelial zone by electron-lucent flocculent matrix with double contours, indicating combined features of membranous glomerulopathy and transplant glomerulopathy (electron micrograph).

the nature of the glomerular disease. As in the case of recurrent disease, it is unusual for de novo glomerular disease to cause graft loss, and many cases are diagnosed as an incidental finding in a patient with intercurrent rejection.

De Novo Membranous Glomerulopathy

The most common glomerular disease to occur de novo in the transplant is membranous glomerulopathy (1,60). The incidence of de novo membranous glomerulopathy in large biopsy series ranges from 2 to 5 percent and would likely be higher if immunofluorescence and electron microscopy were performed routinely on all allograft biopsies. Most cases are diagnosed with stage 1 to 2 membranous alterations, and subepithelial deposits tend to be small (fig. 26-81) (60). Some cases have mixed features of transplant glomerulopathy, with subendothelial electron lucent "fluff," causing widening of the lamina rara interna (fig. 26-82). The demonstration that de novo membranous glomerulopathy occurs in the allograft, but not in the remnant glomeruli of the patient's native kidney, suggests that it develops as a sequela of allograft rejection, possibly mediated by in situ formation of immune deposits through antibodies directed to minor transplantation antigens (59,60).

De Novo Antiglomerular Basement Membrane Disease

Anti-GBM disease occurs de novo in up to 15 percent of kidneys transplanted for end-stage hereditary nephritis (14). Most cases of hereditary nephritis are caused by a mutation in the gene that encodes the alpha 5 subunit of collagen IV. Goodpasture's antibody is directed to the alpha 3 subunit of collagen IV. It has been proposed that mutations in alpha 5 cause failure of incorporation of alpha 3 into the glomerular basement membrane, such that alpha 3 presented in the allograft is viewed as foreign antigen to which an immune response is then mounted. In some patients, linear IgG is detected in the glomerular capillary walls, without overt nephritis. In others, there may be severe crescentic glomerulonephritis leading to graft failure.

De Novo Focal Segmental Glomerulosclerosis

A common pattern of glomerular injury to occur de novo in the transplant is focal segmental glomerulosclerosis, which develops in 10 to 20 percent of allografts. This is a nonspecific pattern that may occur as a complication of ischemia, hypertension, chronic rejection, cyclosporine toxicity, and hyperfiltration injury. It is likely that only a small fraction of patients, particularly those presenting with full nephrotic syndrome, have true idiopathic focal segmental glomerulosclerosis occurring de novo in the transplant kidney. Collapsing glomerulopathy, a variant of focal sclerosis, also may occur as a de novo glomerular disease in the allograft (30,57). Some of these patients have a zonal distribution of the glomerular lesions that follows the distribution of chronic transplant arteriopathy. The geographic distribution of the collapsing lesions and the absence of nephrotic syndrome are features that suggest an ischemic etiology in some cases of de novo collapsing glomerulopathy.

REFERENCES

1. Antignac C, Hinglais N, Gubler MC, Gagnadoux MF, Broyer M, Habib R. De novo membranous glomerulonephritis in renal allografts in children. Clin Nephrol 1988;30:1–7.
2. Baid S, Pascual M, Cosimi AB, et al. Viruses and thrombotic microangiopathy. Transplantation 1999;6:710–1.
3. Baid S, Pascual M, Williams WW Jr, et al. Renal thrombotic microangiopathy associated with anticardiolipin antibodies in hepatitis C-positive renal allograft recipients. J Am Soc Nephrol 1999;10:146–53.
4. Bishop GA, Hall BM, Duggin GG, Horvath JS, Sheil AG, Tiller DJ. Immunopathology of renal allograft rejection analyzed with monoclonal antibodies to mononuclear cell markers. Kidney Int 1986;29:708–17.
5. Cameron JS. Recurrent primary disease and de novo nephritis following renal transplantation. Pediatr Nephrol 1991;5:412–21.
6. Cecka JM. The UNOS scientific renal transplant registry—ten years of kidney transplants. In: Terasaki PI, ed. Clinical transplants 1997. Los Angeles: UCLA Tissue Typing Laboratory; 1998.
7. Collins AB, Schneeberger EE, Pascual M, et al. Complement activation in acute humoral renal allograft rejection: diagnostic significance of C4d deposits in peritubular capillaries. J Am Soc Nephrol 1999;10:2208–14.
8. Colvin RB. Renal transplant pathology. In: Jennette JC, Olson JL, Schwartz ML, Silva FG, eds. Heptinstall's pathology of the kidney. Philadelphia: Lippincott-Raven; 1998:1409–540.
9. Colvin RB, Cohen AH, Saiontz C, et al. Evaluation of pathologic criteria for acute renal allograft rejection: reproducibility, sensitivity, and clinical correlation. J Am Soc Nephrol 1997;8:1930–4.
10. Colvin RB, Mauiyyedi S. Differential diagnosis between infection and rejection in renal allografts. Transplant Proc 2001;33:1778–9.
11. Crespo M, Pascual M, Tolkoff-Rubin N, et al. Acute humoral rejection in renal allograft recipients. I. Incidence, serology and clinical characteristics. Transplantation 2001;71:652–8.
12. D'Agati VD. Morphologic features of cyclosporine nephrotoxicity. Contrib Nephrol 1995;114:84–110.
13. Gaber LW, Gaber AO, Tolley EA, Hathaway DK. Prediction by postrevascularization biopsies of cadaveric kidney allografts of rejection, graft loss, and preservation nephropathy. Transplantation 1992;53:1219–25.

14. Gobel J, Olbricht CJ, Offner G, et al. Kidney transplantation in Alport's syndrome: long term outcome and allograft anti-GBM nephritis. Clin Nephrol 1992;38:299–304.
15. Haas M, Kraus ES, Samaniego-Picota M, Racusen LC, Ni W, Eustace JA. Acute renal allograft rejection with intimal arteritis: histologic predictors of response to therapy and graft survival. Kidney Int 2002:61:1516–26.
16. Halloran PF, Melk A Barth C. Rethinking chronic allograft nephropathy: the concept of accelerated senescence. J Am Soc Nephrol 1999;19:167–81.
17. Halloran PF, Schlaut J, Solez K, Srinivasa NS. The significance of the anti-class I response. II. Clinical and pathologic features of renal transplants with anti-class I-like antibody. Transplantation 1992;53:550–5.
18. Hsu HC, Suzuki Y, Churg J, Grishman E. Ultrastructure of transplant glomerulopathy. Histopathology 1980;4:351–67.
19. Ivanyi B, Fahmy H, Brown H, Szenohradszky P, Halloran PF, Solez K. Peritubular capillaries in chronic renal allograft rejection: a quantitative ultrastructural study. Hum Pathol 2000;31: 1129–38.
20. Kasiske BL, Kalil RS, Lee HS, Rao KV. Histopathologic findings associated with a chronic, progressive decline in renal allograft function. Kidney Int 1991;40:514–24.
21. Kiss D, Landmann J, Mihatsch M, Huser B, Brunner FP, Thiel G. Risks and benefits of graft biopsy in renal transplantation under cyclosporin-A. Clin Nephrol 1992;38:132–4.
22. Knowles DM, Cesarman E, Chadburn A, et al. Correlative morphologic and molecular genetic analysis demonstrates three distinct categories of posttransplantation lymphoproliferative disorders. Blood 1995;85:552–65.
23. Lahlou A, Lang P, Charpentier B, et al. Hemolytic uremic syndrome. Recurrence after renal transplantation. Groupe Cooperatif de l'Ile-de-France (GCIF). Medicine 2000:79:90–102.
24. Legendre C, Thervet E, Skhiri H, et al. Histologic features of chronic allograft nephropathy revealed by protocol biopsies in kidney transplant recipients. Transplantation 1998:65:1506–9.
25. Li B, Hartono C, Ding R, et al. Noninvasive diagnosis of renal-allograft rejection by measurement of messenger RNA for perforin and granzyme B in urine. N Engl J Med 2001;344: 947–54.
26. Matas AJ, Sibley R, Mauer M, Sutherland DE, Simmons RL, Najarian JS. The value of needle renal allograft biopsy. I. A retrospective study of biopsies performed during putative rejection episodes. Ann Surg 1983;197:226–37.
27. Mauiyyedi S, Crespo M, Collins AB, et al. Acute humoral rejection in kidney transplantation. II. Morphology, immunopathology, and pathologic classification. J Am Soc Nephrol 2002;13:779–87.
28. Mauiyyedi S, Pelle PD, Saidman S, et al. Chronic humoral rejection: identification of antibody mediated chronic renal allograft rejection by C4d deposits in peritubular capillaries. J Am Soc Nephrol 2001;12:574–82.
29. Mazzucco G, Motta M, Segoloni G, Monga G. Intertubular capillary changes in the cortex and medulla of transplanted kidneys and their relationship with transplant glomerulopathy: an ultrastructural study of 12 transplantectomies. Ultrastruct Pathol 1994;18:533–7.
30. Meehan SM, Pascual M, Williams WW, et al. De novo collapsing glomerulopathy in renal allografts. Transplantation 1998;65:1192–97.
31. Mihatsch MJ, Nickeleit V, Gudat F. Morphologic criteria of chronic renal allograft rejection. Transplant Proc 1999:31:1295–7.
32. Mihatsch MJ, Ryffel B, Gudat F. The differential diagnosis between rejection and cyclosporine toxicity. Kidney Int 1995;52(Suppl)S63–9.
33. Mihatsch MJ, Theil G, Ryffel B. Cyclosporine nephrotoxicity. Adv Nephrol Necker Hosp 1988;17:303–20.
34. Mihatsch MJ, Thiel G, Ryffel B. Morphologic diagnosis of cyclosporine nephrotoxicity. Sem Diagn Pathol 1988;5:104–21.
35. Mihatsch MJ, Theil G, Spichtin HP, et al. Morphological findings in kidney transplants after treatment with cyclosporine. Transplant Proc 1983;15(Suppl 1):2821–35.
36. Minervini MI, Torbenson M, Scantlebury V, et al. Acute renal allograft rejection with severe tubulitis (Banff 1997 grade IB). Am J Surg Pathol 2000;24:553–8.
37. Monga G, Mazzucco G, Novara R, Reale L. Intertubular capillary changes in kidney allografts: an ultrastructural study in patients with transplant glomerulopathy. Ultrastruct Pathol 1990; 14:201–9.
38. Murer L, Zacchello G, Bianchi D, et al. Thrombotic microangiopathy associated with parvovirus B19 infection after renal transplantation. J Am Soc Nephrol 2000;11:1132–7.
39. Nadasdy T, Krenacs T, Kalmar KN, Csajbok E, Boda K, Ormos J. Importance of plasma cells in the infiltrate of renal allografts. An immunohistochemical study. Pathol Res Pract 1991;187:178–83.
40. Nickeleit V, Hirsch HH, Binet IF, et al. Polyomavirus infection of renal allograft recipients: from latent infection to manifest disease. J Am Soc Nephrol 1999;10:1080–9.

41. Nickeleit V, Vamvakas EC, Pascual M, Poletti BJ, Colvin RB. The prognostic significance of specific arterial lesions in acute renal allograft rejection. J Am Soc Nephrol 1998;9:1301–8.
42. Oikawa T, Morozumi K, Koyama K, et al. Electron microscopic peritubular capillary lesions: a new criterion for chronic rejection. Clin Transplant 1999;13(Suppl 1);24–32.
43. Olsen S, Burdick JF, Keown PA, Wallace AC, Rasusen LC, Solez K. Primary acute renal failure ("acute tubular necrosis") in the transplanted kidney: morphology and pathogenesis. Medicine 1989;68:173–87.
44. Pascual M, Saidman S, Tolkoff-Rubin N, et al. Plasma exchange and tacrolimus-mycophenolate rescue for acute humoral rejection in kidney transplantation. Transplantation 1998;66: 1460–4.
45. Pascual M, Vallhonrat H, Cosimi AB, et al. The clinical usefulness of the renal allograft biopsy in the cyclosporine era: a prospective study. Transplantation 1999;67:737–41.
46. Pham PT, Peng A, Wilkinson AH, et al. Cyclosporine and tacrolimus-associated thrombotic microangiopathy. Am J Kidney Dis 2000;36:844–50.
47. Racusen LC, Colvin RB, Solez K, et al. Antibody-mediated rejection criteria—an addition to the Banff 97 classification of renal allograft rejection. Am J Transplant 2003;3:708–14.
48. Racusen LC, Solez K, Colvin RB, et al. The Banff 97 working classification of renal allograft pathology. Kidney Int 1999;55:713–23.
49. Randhawa PS, Demetris AJ. Nephropathy due to polyomavirus type BK. N Engl J Med 2000;342: 1361–3.
50. Randhawa PS, Finkelstein S, Scantlebury V, et al. Human polyoma virus-associated interstitial nephritis in the allograft kidney. Transplantation 1999;67:103–9.
51. Randhawa PS, Magnone M, Jordan M, Shapiro R, Demetris AJ, Nalesnik M. Renal allograft involvement by Epstein-Barr virus associated post-transplant lymphoproliferative disease. Am J Surg Pathol 1996;20:563–71.
52. Randhawa PS, Shapiro R, Jordan ML, Starzl TE, Demetris AJ. The histopathological changes associated with allograft rejection and drug toxicity in renal transplant recipients maintained on FK506. Clinical significance and comparison with cyclosporine. Am J Surg Pathol 1993;17:60–8.
53. Salmela KT, von Willebrand EO, Kyllonen LE, et al. Acute vascular rejection in renal transplantation—diagnosis and outcome. Transplantation 1992;54:858–62.
54. Schwarz A, Krause PH, Offermann G, Keller F. Recurrent and de novo renal disease after kidney transplantation with or without cyclosporine A. Am J Kidney Dis 1991;17:524–31.
55. Sharma VK, Bologa RM, Li B, et al. Molecular executors of cell death—differential intrarenal expression of Fas ligand, Fas, granzyme B and perforin during acute and/or chronic rejection of human renal allografts. Transplantation 1996;62:1860–6.
56. Solez K, Axelsen RA, Benediktsson H, et al. International standardization of criteria for the histologic diagnosis of renal allograft rejection: the Banff working classification of kidney transplant pathology. Kidney Int 1993;44:411–22.
57. Stokes MB, Davis CL, Alpers CE. Collapsing glomerulopathy in renal allografts: a morphological pattern with diverse clinicopathologic associations. Am J Kidney Dis 1999;33:658–66.
58. Taube DH, Neild GH, Williams DG, et al. Differentiation between allograft rejection and cyclosporin nephrotoxicity in renal transplant recipients. Lancet 1985;2:171–4.
59. Thoenes GH, Pielsticker K, Schubert G. Transplantation-induced immune complex kidney disease in rats with unilateral manifestations in the allografted kidney. Lab Invest 1979;41:321–33.
60. Truong L, Gelfand J, D'Agati V, et al. De novo membranous glomerulonephropathy in renal allografts: a report of ten cases and review of the literature. Am J Kidney Dis 1989;14:131–44.
61. Tuazon TV, Schneeberger EE, Bhan AK, et al. Mononuclear cells in acute allograft glomerulopathy. Am J Pathol 1987;129:119–32.
62. Verani RR, Flechner SM, Van Buren CT, Kahan BD. Acute cellular rejection or cyclosporine A nephrotoxicity? A review of transplant renal biopsies. Am J Kidney Dis 1984;4:185–91.

Index*

*Numbers in boldface indicate table and figure pages.

B

C

D

I

K

L

M

N

O

R

S

T

U

V

W

X

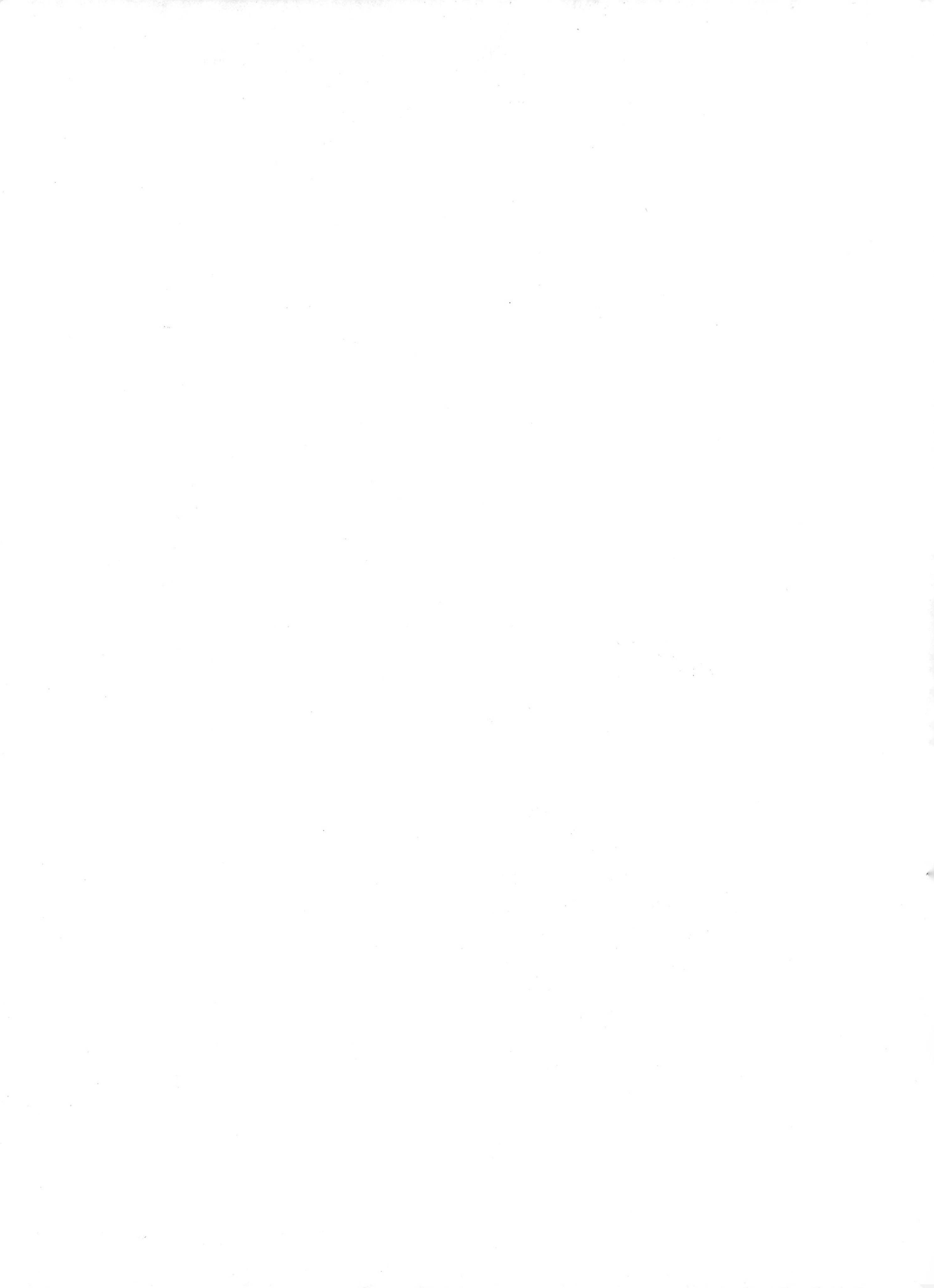